The Haemolytic Anaemias

VOLUME 3

The Auto-Immune Haemolytic Anaemias

For Churchill Livingstone
Publisher : Michael Parkinson
Project Editor : Dilys Jones
Copy Editor: Robin Watson
Production Controller: Lesley W. Small
Sales Promotion Executive: Marion Pollock

The Haemolytic Anaemias

VOLUME 3

The Auto-Immune Haemolytic Anaemias

Sir John Dacie
MD (Lond) FRCP (Lond) FRCPath FRS
Emeritus Professor of Haematology,
University of London, Royal Postgraduate
Medical School, London, UK

THIRD EDITION

CHURCHILL LIVINGSTONE
EDINBURGH LONDON MADRID MELBOURNE NEW YORK AND TOKYO 1992

CHURCHILL LIVINGSTONE
Medical Division of Longman Group UK Limited

Distributed in the United States of America by Churchill
Livingstone Inc., 650 Avenue of the Americas, New York,
N.Y. 10011, and by associated companies, branches and
representatives throughout the world.

First published 1992

ISBN 0-443-03502-4

British Library of Cataloguing in Publication Data
A catalogue record for this book is available from the British
Library.

Library of Congress Cataloging in Publication Data
A catalog record for this book is available from the Library of
Congress.

The
publisher's
policy is to use
**paper manufactured
from sustainable forests**

Printed in Great Britain by The Bath Press, Avon

Preface

In this volume on the auto-immune haemolytic anaemias I have attempted to continue the story of their understanding and treatment from the point I had reached when Part II of the second edition of *The Haemolytic Anaemias* was published in 1962. The result has been a volume greatly increased in size. This increase in size reflects the substantial advances that have taken place in the last 30 years in our understanding of the structure of antibodies and of the mechanism and regulation of their formation and of the genesis of auto-immune diseases; and it also reflects the burgeoning understanding of the complexity of the human blood-group antigens and of the complement system and also of the way in which the body deals with antibody-affected erythrocytes.

As in the science and practice of other branches of medicine, these advances have closely followed advances in understanding and technical progress in the more fundamental biological and physical sciences. This has been as true in relation to the haemolytic anaemias of auto-immune origin as it has been in the hereditary haemolytic anaemias that I attempted to describe in the first two volumes of this book. However, despite the many important and seminal advances in understanding that have been made, a great deal is still not fully understood: in particular, the reason why certain people, even infants, suffer from auto-immune haemolytic anaemia — in reality a rather rare group of disorders — while the great majority of us fail to do so. This individual proneness to suffer from a particular illness is one of the great mysteries of clinical medicine and is of course not confined to auto-immune blood diseases. The solution to the mystery seems to lie in the patient's individuality, i.e. his or her genetic make-up, coupled with the effect of his or her environment. But exactly how the interaction between nature and nurture can lead in certain individuals to severe and perhaps fatal disease is the key question for which a complete answer is not yet forthcoming.

In this present volume I have attempted to describe in chronological order what has been discovered and by whom, as I tried to do when writing the relevant chapters in the book's earlier editions. I debated whether I should start in the early 1960s and omit detailed descriptions of what had been discovered earlier and had been described in the second (1962) edition of this book. I decided, however, not to do this. In fact, the foundations of our present knowledge were securely laid in the late 1940s and 1950s, if not earlier, and are in my view an integral part of the story. This book thus attempts to cover the whole history of our understanding of the auto-immune haemolytic anaemias from the beginning of the century until the early 1990s. I had planned also to include a description of haemolytic disease of the newborn and the drug immune haemolytic anaemias. I abandoned this idea when it became clear to me that including these important topics would make the book too large and delay unnecessarily its publication. I plan to deal with them, as well as the secondary auto-immune haemolytic anaemias and paroxysmal nocturnal haemoglobinuria, in Volume 4 of this book.

I am very grateful to friends who have encouraged me to undertake the present volume, and I have to thank particularly Professor Lucio Luzzatto and Professor Alan Waters for their support and advice and those who have generously allowed me to reproduce illustrations from their own work which I have felt to be particularly revealing. A list of these illustrations and my acknowledgement to the authors and publishers follow in a separate section. The photomicrographs new to this edition were kindly taken for me by Mr W. F. Hinks of the Department of Medical Illustration at the Royal Postgraduate Medical School (RPMS). I am indebted, too, to the Department of Medical Illustration for preparing excellent prints of certain of the figures.

The exacting task of typing the whole of the text, and the tables and index, too, has been undertaken by my wife, without whose encouragement, patience and skill creating this book would have been almost impossible.

I wish to thank warmly, too, Miss Eleanor Lloyd and Mrs Sylvia Barnes of the Department of Haematology at the RPMS for valued help with photocopying, and Miss Joan Ferguson, Librarian of the Royal College of Physicians, Edinburgh, and the library staff of the RPMS, the Royal Society of Medicine and the Royal Society, for their much appreciated assistance. Messrs Churchill Livingstone have been unfailingly helpful.

London 1992   John Dacie

Acknowledgements

I am greatly indebted to the following authors and publishers for copyright permission to reproduce the figures referred to below.

Chapter 22. Fig. 22.2: The Lancet (*Lancet*, **i**, 652, 1932). Fig. 22.3: Dr S. N. Swisher and Postgraduate Medicine (*Postgrad. med.*, **40**, 378, 1966). Fig. 22.4: Professor C. Salmon and The American Journal of Medicine (*Amer. J. Med.*, **56**, 61, 1974). Fig. 22.5: Springer-Verlag, France (*Rev. Hémat.*, **6**, 316, 1951). Fig. 22.6 and 22.7: Professor A. Waters and Blackwell Scientific Publications. (*Clin. lab. Haemat.*, **6**, 219, 1984).

Chapter 23. Fig. 23.3: Dr G. B. Weiss and Wiley-Liss, a division of John Wiley and Sons, Inc. (*Amer. J. Hemat.*, **17**, 433, 1984), (© Wiley-Liss, 1984). Fig. 23.7: Dr W. H. Zinkham. Fig. 23.10: Professor G. Sansone and Edizioni Minerva Medica (*Minerva pediat.* (*Torino*), **9**, 270, 1957). Fig. 23.18: Dr J. L. Liesveld and Grune and Stratton Inc. (*Blood*, **69**, 820, 1987). Figs. 23.19 and 23.20: Dr U. M. Hegde and Professor E. C. Gordon-Smith and The British Medical Association (*Brit. med. J.*, **ii**, 1444, 1977). Fig. 23.21: Professor C. L. Conley and The American Medical Association (*J. Amer. med. Ass.*, **244**, 1688, 1980). Fig. 23.22: Professor C. L. Conley and The New England Journal of Medicine (*New Engl. J. Med.*, **306**, 281, 1982). Fig. 23.28: Professor G. Sirchia and Blackwell Scientific Publications (*Brit. J. Haemat.*, **19**, 411, 1970). Fig. 23.29: Dr G. L. Scott and Munksgaard International Publishers Ltd. (*Scand. J. Haemat.*, **8**, 53, 1971). Fig. 23.30: Dr E. Kaplan and Elsevier Publishing Company. (*Clin. chim. Acta*, **38**, 301, 1972).

Chapter 24. Fig. 24.3: Dr S. Suzuki and Academic Press Inc. (*Clin. Immunol. Immunopath.*, **21**, 247, 1981). Fig. 24.4: Dr N. Costea and Grune and Stratton Inc. (*Blood*, **69**, 820, 1987).

Chapter 25. Fig. 25.1: The Athlone Press (*Lectures on the Scientific Basis of Medicine* (1957–58, 7, 59, 1959). Fig. 25.4 and 25.5: Dr A. E. G. Kr. von dem Borne and Blackwell Scientific Publications (*Clin. exp. Immunol.*, **4**, 333, 1969). Fig. 25.6: Dr P. Lalezari and Blackwell Scientific Publications (*Brit. J. Haemat.*, **21**, 131, 1971). Fig. 25.7. and 25.8: Professor F. Stratton and The Lancet (*Lancet*, **i**, 1388, 1960).

Chapter 27. Fig. 27.1: Professor F. Stratton and Blackwell Scientific Publications (*Clin. lab. Haemat.*, **5**, 387, 1983). Fig. 27.2. and 27.3: Dr J. Freedman and The American Association of Blood Banks (*Transfusion*, **22**, 511 and 515, 1982). Fig. 27.4. and 27.5: Dr T. O. Sýmanski and Grune and Stratton Inc. (*Blood*, **55**, 48, 1980). Figs. 27.6: Drs M. Ali and J. G. Kelton and The American Association of Blood Banks (*Transfusion*, **28**, 29, 1988). Fig. 27.7: Dr K. Rickard and The British Medical Association (*Arch. Dis. Childh.*, **46**, 102, 1969).

Chapter 28. Figs. 28.2 and 28.3: The Royal Society of Medicine (*Proc. roy. Soc. Med.*, **50**, 647, 1957).

Chapter 29. Figs. 29.1 and 29.2: Blackwell Scientific Publications (*Brit. J. Haemat.*, **3**, 153, 1957). Fig. 29.3: Blackwell Scientific Publications (*Brit. J. Haemat.*, **2**, 321, 1956). Fig. 29.4: Dr L. Marsh and Blackwell Scientific Publications (*Brit. J. Haemat.*, **7**, 200, 1961). Fig. 29.5: Professor V. Hoffbrand and Blackwell Scientific Publications (*Brit. J. Haemat.*, **15**, 381, 1968). Fig. 29.6: The Royal Society of Medicine (*Proc. roy. Soc. Med.*, **48**, 211, 1955).

Chapter 30. Fig. 30.1: Dr T. Feizi and The Royal Society of Medicine (*Proc. roy. Soc. Med.*, **59**, 1109, 1966).

Chapter 32. Fig. 32.1: Georg Thieme Verlag. Fig. 32.2: Professor G. Garratty and Grune and

Stratton Inc. (*Blood*, **38**, 491, 1971). Fig. 32.5: Dr J. A. Hernandez and J. B. Lippincott Co. (*Amer. J. clin. Path.*, **81**, 787, 1984). Fig. 32.6: Professor D. G. Nathan and The Massachusetts Medical Society, (*New Engl. J. Med.*, **284**, 1250, 1971).

Chapter 34. Fig. 34.1: Professor W. F. Rosse and The Rockefeller University Press (*J. exp. Med.*, **123**, 969, 1966). Fig. 34.2: Blackwell Scientific Publications (*Clin. exp. Immunol.*, 7, 401, 1970). Fig. 34.3: Dr D. L. Brown. Fig. 34.4: Dr D. L. Brown and Professor D. Nelson. Figs. 34.5 and 34.6: Blackwell Scientific Publications (*Brit. J. Haemat.*, **6**, 154, 1960). Fig. 34.7: Blackwell Scientific Publications (*Brit. J. Haemat.*, **6**, 222, 1960). Fig. 34.8: Dr D. L. Brown and Blackwell Scientific Publications (*Brit. J. Haemat.*, **19**, 499, 1970). Fig. 34.10: Dr S. O. Schwartz and Charles B. Slack Inc. (*Amer. J. med. Sci.*, **196**, 769, 1938).

Chapter 35. Figs. 35.1 and 35.2: The British Council (*Brit. med. Bull.*, **15**, 67, 1959). Fig. 35.4: The Rockefeller University Press (*J. clin. Invest.*, **50**, 734, 1971). Fig. 35.6: Dr R. S. Schwartz and Grune and Stratton Inc. (*Blood*, **19**, 483, 1962). Figs. 35.7a and b: Professor J. Richmond and The Lancet (*Lancet*, **ii**, 127, 1963).

Fig. 35.8: Grune and Stratton Inc. (*Progr. Hemat.*, **6**, 82, 1969). Figs. 35.9, 35.12, 35.13 and 35.14: Blackwell Scientific Publications (*Brit J. Haemat.*, **2**, 237, 1956). Fig. 35.15: Blackwell Scientific Publications (*Brit. J. Haemat.*, **6**, 122, 1960). Fig. 35.16: Dr Ten Pas and Charles B. Slack Inc. (*Amer. J. med. Sci.*, **251**, 63, 1966). Fig. 35.17: Dr M. J. Wilmers and The Lancet (*Lancet*, **ii**, 915, 1963). Fig. 35.18: Grune and Stratton Inc. (*Progr. Hemat.*, **6**, 82, 1969). Fig. 35.19: The British Medical Association (*Brit. med. J.*, **ii**, 381, 1970). Fig. 35.20: Dr C. F. Abilgaard and Acta Paediatrica Scandinavica (*Acta paediat. scand.*, **65**, 375, 1976). Fig. 30.21: Dr Y. S. Ahn and The American Medical Association (*J. Amer. med. Ass.*, **249**, 2189, 1983). Fig. 35.22: Dr O. Andersen and Acta Paediatrica Scandinavica (*Acta paediat. scand.*, **73**, 145, 1984). Fig. 35.23: Dr H. Oda and C. V. Mosby Co. (*J. Pediat.*, **107**, 744, 1985). Fig. 35.25: Grune and Stratton Inc. (*Progr. Hemat.*, **6**, 82, 1969). Fig. 35.27: Professor W. F. Rosse and The Rockefeller University Press (*J. clin. Invest.*, **52**, 493, 1976). Fig. 35.28: The New York Academy of Sciences (*Ann. N.Y. Acad. Sci.*, **124**, 422, 1965).

Contents of Volume 3

21. The auto-immune haemolytic anaemias: introduction   1

22. Auto-immune haemolytic anaemia (AIHA): warm-antibody syndromes I: 'idiopathic' types: history and clinical features   6

23. Auto-immune haemolytic anaemia (AIHA): warm-antibody syndromes II: 'idiopathic' types: haematological and biochemical findings   54

24. Auto-immune haemolytic anaemia (AIHA): warm-antibody syndromes III: serological findings 1: introduction; the direct antiglobulin test and other ways of demonstrating erythrocyte sensitization   94

25. Auto-immune haemolytic anaemia (AIHA): warm-antibody syndromes IV: serological findings 2: auto-antibodies in serum   127

26. Auto-immune haemolytic anaemia (AIHA): warm-antibody syndromes V: serological findings 3: specificity of the auto-antibodies   158

27. Auto-immune haemolytic anaemia (AIHA): warm-antibody syndromes VI: Coombs-negative (DAT-negative) haemolytic anaemia; positive direct antiglobulin tests in normal subjects and in hospital patients; polyagglutinability and haemolytic anaemia   183

28. Auto-immune haemolytic anaemia (AIHA): cold-antibody syndromes I: 'idiopathic' types: clinical presentation and haematological and serological findings   210

29. Auto-immune haemolytic anaemia (AIHA): cold-antibody syndromes II: immunochemistry and specificity of the antibodies; serum complement in auto-immune haemolytic anaemia   240

30. Auto-immune haemolytic anaemia (AIHA): cold-antibody syndromes III: haemolytic anaemia following mycoplasma pneumonia   296

31. Auto-immune haemolytic anaemia (AIHA): cold-antibody syndromes IV: haemolytic anaemia following infectious mononucleosis and other virus infections   313

32. Auto-immune haemolytic anaemia (AIHA): cold-antibody syndromes V: paroxysmal cold haemoglobinuria (PCH)   329

33. Auto-immune haemolytic anaemia (AIHA): aetiology   363

34. Auto-immune haemolytic anaemia (AIHA): pathogenesis   392

35. Auto-immune haemolytic anaemia (AIHA): treatment   452

Index   521

Contents of Volume 1

1. Introduction and classification of the haemolytic anaemias

2. The erythrocyte: structure and metabolism; life-span and fate in health, and mechanisms and consequences of a shortened life-span. Haemoglobin catabolism

3. Haemolytic anaemia in man: clinical findings, blood picture and other pathological changes, methods of investigation, diagnosis and treatment

4. Hereditary spherocytosis (HS)

5. Hereditary elliptocytosis (HE)

6. Hereditary stomatocytosis and allied disorders (hereditary haemolytic anaemias with altered cation permeability of the erythrocyte membrane); Rh$_{null}$ disease; hereditary acanthocytosis; McLeod syndrome etc.

7. Hereditary enzyme-deficiency haemolytic anaemias I: introduction and pyruvate-kinase deficiency

8. Hereditary enzyme-deficiency haemolytic anaemias II: deficiencies of enzymes of the Embden-Meyerhof (EM) pathway other than pyruvate kinase and of enzymes involved in purine and pyrimidine metabolism

9. Hereditary enzyme-deficiency haemolytic anaemias III: deficiency of glucose-6-phosphate dehydrogenase

10. Hereditary enzyme-deficiency haemolytic anaemias IV: glutathione synthetase deficiency; glutamylcysteine synthetase deficiency; glutathione reductase deficiency; glutathione peroxidase deficiency, and 6-phosphogluconate dehydrogenase deficiency

Index

Contents of Volume 2

11. Sickle-cell disease I: history, genetics and geographical distribution of haemoglobin S; clinical aspects of sickle-cell trait and homozygous sickle-cell disease

12. Sickle-cell disease II: haematological findings and laboratory diagnosis of homozygous sickle-cell disease and sickle-cell trait; screening programmes for haemoglobinopathies

13. Sickle-cell disease III: compound heterozygosity for haemoglobin S and β-thalassaemia or other abnormal β-chain variant haemoglobin or hereditary persistence of fetal haemoglobin; effect of α-thalassaemia or α-chain variant haemoglobins on homozygous sickle-cell anaemia

14. Sickle-cell disease IV: pathology, the sickling phenomenon and pathogenesis

15. Sickle-cell disease V: treatment and antenatal diagnosis

16. Haemoglobin C, haemoglobin C Harlem, haemoglobin D, haemoglobin E and haemoglobin O: effect of the combination of these haemoglobins with another abnormal haemoglobin or thalassaemia

17. The unstable haemoglobin haemolytic anaemias

18. The thalassaemias I: history, heterogeneity, and clinical and haematological features

19. The thalassaemias II: pathology, pathogenesis and molecular genetics

20. The thalassaemias III: differential diagnosis, antenatal diagnosis and treatment

Index

The auto-immune haemolytic anaemias: introduction

The term acquired haemolytic anaemia is used to describe a situation in which the life-span of the erythrocytes is significantly reduced for reasons other than genetic defects of the cells themselves. An accelerated rate of erythrocyte destruction *in vivo* (increased haemolysis) is quite common in disease and can be produced by a variety of different mechanisms. The degree to which haemolysis is increased varies greatly from patient to patient—from slight acceleration which has no clinical effect to a marked shortening of the erythrocytes' life-span leading to serious illness.

Three clinical types of acquired haemolytic anaemia can be distinguished: (1) the increased haemolysis dominates the clinical picture and is apparently unaccompanied by any other co-existing disease—these cases are often referred to as primary or idiopathic acquired haemolytic anaemias; (2) the increased haemolysis, which may or may not dominate the clinical picture, is associated with some well-defined underlying disease or abnormality—these cases are often referred to as secondary or symptomatic acquired haemolytic anaemias, and (3) the increased haemolysis follows the taking of a drug or exposure to a toxin or chemical.

From the point of view of the mechanism of the increased haemolysis, there are two main types of acquired haemolytic anaemia: those brought about by antibodies acting against antigens on the surface of the patients' erythrocytes (immune haemolytic anaemias) and those in which mechanisms other than antibody–antigen interaction are responsible (non-immune haemolytic anaemias).

The immune types of acquired haemolytic anaemia can be grouped into two broad categories:

1. The responsible antibodies are auto-antibodies, i.e. they are formed by the patient himself or herself—these are the auto-immune haemolytic anaemias (AIHAs)
2. The antibodies are allo-antibodies, i.e. they were formed by some person other than the patient, as in haemolytic disease of the newborn.

THE AUTO-IMMUNE HAEMOLYTIC ANAEMIAS (AIHAs): CLASSIFICATION

The AIHAs, although uncommon clinically, have probably been studied in greater detail than any other type of auto-immune disorder. As mentioned, they may be grouped into two broad categories: primary cases—so-called idiopathic AIHA—and secondary AIHAs accompanying and complicating a well-defined associated disease. Most frequently, the associated disease is a malignant lymphoma or another auto-immune disorder, such as systemic lupus erythematosus (SLE). Other cases have followed exposure to certain drugs or a virus or *Mycoplasma pneumoniae* infection. The precise causation (aetiology) of both groups of AIHA remains obscure (see Chapter 33).

This volume of *The Haemolytic Anaemias* (Volume 3) will deal with idiopathic AIHA and the secondary AIHAs which are clearly associated with overt infections, i.e. those following mycoplasma pneumonia or infectious mononucleosis or other virus infections. The secondary AIHAs, i.e. those that are drug-dependent or associated with malignant lymphomas and some other tumours, and those associated with other auto-immune disorders, will be dealt with in

Volume 4, as will haemolytic disease of the newborn and other allo-immune haemolytic anaemias.

Cases of AIHA can be classified, too, according to the nature of the anti-erythrocyte auto-antibodies the patient is forming: i.e., whether they are 'warm' antibodies, which react well (perhaps maximally) at body temperature (37°C), or 'cold' antibodies, which react strongly at low temperatures, e.g. 4°C, and react less well as the temperature rises and usually fail to react at all at 37°C. The clinical syndrome the patients suffer from depends not only on the amount of auto-antibody he or she is forming but also on the nature of the antibody, of which its thermal range is an important component.

The proportion of secondary to primary cases has varied considerably in different authors' series. To some extent this has depended on the particular interests of the physician, haematologist or serologist reporting the data: in particular, on whether he or she is known to be interested in auto-immune diseases other than AIHA or specializes in haematological malignancies as well as haemolytic anaemia. Another factor has been the thoroughness with which the existence of an underlying disease has been sought. It has become clear, too, that the longer the patients are followed-up the higher the proportion of secondary cases becomes.

Early published data were quoted by Dacie (1962, p. 342). For instance, Lal and Speiser (1957) listed 48 out of 97 cases of warm-antibody AIHA as being secondary in type. Other early data included cold-antibody as well as warm-antibody cases: van Loghem, van der Hart and Dorfmeier (1958) reported that 67 out of 122 cases were secondary, Revol et al. (1958), seven out of 27 cases and Dausset and Colombani (1959) 35 out of 128 cases. Dacie's (1962) data comprised 167 cases of which 108 were judged to be idiopathic (primary) and 59 secondary. In the larger series reported by Dacie and Worlledge (1969) a higher proportion was judged to be secondary, i.e. 111 idiopathic to 99 secondary warm-antibody cases (including 11 cases attributed to drug therapy, mostly α-methyldopa); and 46 idiopathic to 39 secondary cold-antibody cases (Table 21.1).

Table 21.1 Relative incidence of different types of auto-immune haemolytic anaemia. RPMS series 1947–68.

Type of disorder	No. of patients	Sex	
		Males	Females
Warm AIHA			
Idiopathic	111	46	65
Assoc. with drugs*	11	1	10
Secondary			
Assoc. with lymphomas, etc.	37	14	23
SLE	16	1	15
Other possible or probable auto-immune disorders	21	8	13
Infections and miscellaneous	13	9	4
Ovarian teratoma	1	0	1
Totals	210	79	131
Cold AIHA			
Idiopathic (cold haemagglutinin disease)	38	16	22
Secondary			
Assoc. with atypical or mycoplasma pneumonia	23	5	18
Infectious mononucleosis	2	1	1
Lymphomas	7	3	4
PCH			
Idiopathic	8	7	1
Secondary	7	4	3
Totals	85	36	49

*α-Methyldopa 7, chlordiazepoxide (Librium) 2, mefenamic acid (Ponstan) 1, flufenamic acid and indomethazine 1. [Reproduced by permission from Dacie and Worlledge (1969).]

The data of Videbaek (1962) and Pirofsky (1969, 1975) contrast markedly with the above-quoted figures. Videbaek reported that he had studied 41 patients between 1951 and 1961. Only five were classified as apparently primary, the remaining 36 were secondary cases (approximately 90%). Videbaek stressed how careful investigation and even several years' observation were necessary to rule out an underlying disease, especially SLE or a malignant systemic disease. Pirofsky, too, stressed the paramount importance of searching for evidence of underlying disease and of prolonged follow-up: thus only 44 out of 234 of his cases were judged by him to be idiopathic, i.e. 18.8%. He contrasted this low percentage to a mean percentage of 57.2 in the seven series he quoted (Pirofsky, 1969, his Table 11). Pirofsky remarked, however, that his 'patient population is characterized by many leukemia and lymphoma patients undergoing constant followup'. 114 of his 234 warm-antibody patients belonged in fact to this group — all had been deliberately investigated for evidence of AIHA.

Pirofsky (1969) devoted six chapters (comprising 165 pages) of his monograph to the secondary AIHs, under the headings Leukemias, Lymphomas, Infectious Disease, Collagen Disease and Diseases of Hypersensitivity, The Gastrointestinal Tract, and Miscellaneous Diseases. As already implied, these secondary cases represented 81.2% of the 234 patients of his personal series.

Data reported earlier by Homberg et al. (1967) from France also indicated a predominance of secondary cases: thus the disorder was considered to be idiopathic in only 35 out of 95 patients suffering from AIHA (of various serological types). A more recent analysis from France has, too, given a similar result (Salmon, Homberg and Habibi, 1975b): of 514 cases, 174 (34%) were classified as idiopathic (including 33 cases of chronic cold-haemagglutinin disease) and 340 as secondary. In Thailand, too, the proportion of idiopathic to secondary cases seems to be similar, 31 out of the 100 cases reported by Kruatrachue and Sirisinha (1977) being idiopathic.

Petz and Garratty (1980) summarized the data reported from six centres on the relative incidence of idiopathic and secondary cases: of 656 cases 45% had been idiopathic, 55% secondary. They mentioned two factors that had possibly contributed to the large differences in incidence at the different centres: one was the nature of the centre, the other was a different interpretation as to what constituted a related underlying disease. They listed 15 disorders as being frequently associated with warm-antibody AIHA, i.e., chronic lymphocytic leukaemia, Hodgkin's disease, non-Hodgkin's lymphomas, thymomas, multiple myeloma, Waldenström's macroglobulinaemia, systemic lupus erythematosus, scleroderma, rheumatoid arthritis, infectious disease — especially childhood viral syndromes, hypogammaglobulinaemia, dysglobulinaemias, other immune deficiency syndromes, ulcerative colitis, and ovarian dermoid cyst.

The importance of prolonged follow-up and of a careful enquiry into a patient's past history is also illustrated by Conley's (1981) review of warm-antibody AIHA patients who had been attending the Johns Hopkins Hospital. In a retrospective study of 33 patients whose illness would 'in the past have been designated "idiopathic"', he found evidence of an associated immunologically-mediated disorder in 19 of them. The disorders listed included thrombocytopenic purpura, hypo- and hyper-thyroidism, Hashimoto's thyroiditis, polyarthritis, rheumatic fever, rheumatoid arthritis, immune complex nephritis, agranulocytosis attributed to propylthiouracil, eczema, urticaria and chronic asthma. An additional three patients developed a lymphoma, 2–10 years after AIHA had been diagnosed. The medium follow-up of the whole series had been 4 years.

All authors who have reported on large series of patients agree that cases attributed to warm antibodies far outnumber those brought about by cold antibodies.

Early personal data reported by Dacie (1962, p. 342) comprised 129 warm-antibody cases to 46 cold-antibody cases, a ratio of approximately 2.8:1. Later, Dacie and Worlledge (1969) reported on a total of 295 cases of which 210 were of the warm type and 85 of the cold type, a ratio of approximately 2.5:1. Their data are reproduced in Table 21.1, which includes a breakdown of the secondary cases into several main categories. The more recent data of Petz and Garratty (1980), based on a total of 347 cases (of which 43 were drug-induced), revealed a higher ratio still, namely, approximately 6.7:1.

More recently, Engelfriet and his co-workers (1987) reported on a serological analysis of 2400 cases that had been investigated since 1961 at the Central Laboratory of the Netherlands Red Cross Transfusion Service in Amsterdam. Of these patients, 1999 had formed warm auto-antibodies, 391 cold auto-antibodies and 10 both warm and cold auto-antibodies. The warm to cold antibody ratio was approximately 5.1:1.

Early reports and reviews on the clinical and laboratory aspects of AIHA include those of Dameshek and Schwartz (1940), Dameshek (1951), Dreyfus, Dausset and Vidal (1951), Young, Miller and Christian (1951), Dacie (1954,

1959, 1962), Lejeune (1954), Dausset (1956), Crosby and Rappaport (1957), Hennemann (1957), Letman (1957), Schubothe (1957, 1958, 1959), Oettgen and Kindler (1959) and Braaker (1960). These reviews taken together provide a revealing and comprehensive picture of the state of knowledge at the time they were written. Dameshek and Schwartz's (1940) review and the monographs of Hennemann (1957) and Schubothe (1958, 1959) are particularly valuable because of their extensive bibliographies.

Reviews that have been published more recently include those of Videbaek (1962), Pirofsky (1965, 1969, 1975, 1976), Schwartz and Costea (1966), Allgood and Chaplin (1967), Homberg et al. (1967), Dacie and Worlledge (1969, 1975), Worlledge and Blajchman (1972), Pirofsky and Bardana (1974), Dacie (1975, 1979), Degos, Clauvel and Seligmann (1975), Salmon, Homberg and Habibi (1975a, b), Issitt (1977), Leddy and Swisher (1978), Sokol, Hewitt and Stamps (1981), Worlledge (1982), Lalezari (1983), Sokol and Hewitt (1985), Engelfriet et al. (1987) and Gibson (1988).

Pirofsky's (1969) monograph *Autoimmunization and the Autoimmune Hemolytic Anemias*, Petz and Garratty's (1980) *Acquired Immune Hemolytic Anemias*, Issitt's *Applied Blood Group Serology* (1985, 3rd edn) and Rosse's (1990) *Clinical Immunopathology: Basic Concepts and Clinical Applications* were particularly important additions to the literature.

REFERENCES

ALLGOOD, J. W. & CHAPLIN, H. JNR (1967). Idiopathic acquired autoimmune hemolytic anemia. A review of forty-seven cases treated from 1955 through 1965. *Amer. J. Med.*, **43**, 254–273.

BRAAKER, J. (1960). Zur Klinik der durch Autoantikörper bedingten erworbenen hämolytischen Anämien. *Praxis*, **49**, 209–214.

CONLEY, C. L. (1981). Immunologic precursors of autoimmune hematologic disorders. Autoimmune hemolytic anemia and thrombocytopenic purpura. *Johns Hopkins med. J.*, **149**, 101–109.

CROSBY, W. H. & RAPPAPORT, H. (1957). Autoimmune hemolytic anemia. I. Analysis of hematologic observations with particular reference to their prognostic value. A survey of 57 cases. *Blood*, **12**, 42–55.

DACIE, J. V. (1954). *The Haemolytic Anaemias: Congenital and Acquired*, pp. 164–216. Churchill, London.

DACIE, J. V. (1959). Acquired haemolytic anaemias. *Brit. med. Bull.*, **15**, 67–73.

DACIE, J. V. (1962). *The Haemolytic Anaemias: Congenital and Acquired. Part II—The Auto-immune Haemolytic Anaemias*, 2nd edn, 377pp. Churchill, London.

DACIE, J. V. (1975). Autoimmune hemolytic anemia. *Arch. intern. Med.*, **135**, 1293–1300.

DACIE, J. (1979). Forty years' experience with autoimmune haemolytic anaemia (Emily Cooley Lecture). In: *A Seminar on Laboratory Management of Hemolysis*, pp. 71–86. American Association of Blood Banks.

DACIE, J. V. & WORLLEDGE, S. M. (1969). Auto-immune hemolytic anemias. In *Progr. Hemat.*, **6**, (ed. by E. B. Brown), pp. 82–120. Grune & Stratton, New York.

DACIE, J. V. & WORLLEDGE, S. (1975). Auto-allergic blood diseases. In *Clinical Aspects of Immunology* (ed. by P. G. H. Gell, R. R. A. Coombs and P. J. Lachmann), pp. 1149–1182. Blackwell Scientific Publications, Oxford.

DAMESHEK, W. (1951). Anémie hémolytique acquise. Physiopathologie. Considérations sur l'auto-immunisation et le traitement. *Rev. Hémat.*, **6**, 255–266.

DAMESHEK, W. & SCHWARTZ, S. O. (1940). Acute hemolytic anemia (acquired hemolytic icterus, acute type). *Medicine (Baltimore)*, **19**, 231–327.

DAUSSET, J. (1956). *Immuno-Hématologie, Biologique et Clinique*. Éditions Médicales, Flammarion, Paris.

DAUSSET, J. & COLOMBANI, J. (1959). The serology and the prognosis of 128 cases of autoimmune hemolytic anemia. *Blood*, **14**, 1280–1301.

DEGOS, L., CLAUVEL, J. P. & SELIGMANN, M. (1975). Anémies hémolytiques auto-immunes idiopathiques: étude du pronostic des formes chroniques. *Actualites Hématologiques*, 9th Series. Masson, Paris.

DREYFUS, B., DAUSSET, J. & VIDAL, G. (1951). 1. Étude clinique et hématologique de douze cas d'anémie hémolytique acquise avec auto-anticorps. *Rev. Hémat.*, **6**, 349–368.

ENGELFRIET C. P., OUWEHAND, W. H., VAN'T VEER, M. B., BECKERS, D., MAAS, N. & VON DEM BOURNE, A. E. G. KR. (1987). Autoimmune hemolytic anaemias. *Bailliere's clin. Immunol. Allergy*, **1**, 251–267.

GIBSON, J. (1988). Autoimmune hemolytic anemia: current concepts. *Aust. N. Z. J. Med.*, **18**, 625–637.

HENNEMANN, H. H. (1957). *Erworbene hämolytische*

Anämian: Klinik und Serologie, 198 pp. VEB Georg Thieme, Leipzig.

HOMBERG, H. C., GERBAL, A., ROCHANT, H., NAJMAN, A., COMBRISSON, A., SALMON, CH., DUHAMEL, G. & ANDRÉ, R. (1967). Implications cliniques de la nouvelle classification immunologique des anémies hémolytiques avec auto-anticorps. *Nouv. Rev. Hémat.*, 7, 407–414.

ISSITT, P. D. (1977). Autoimmune hemolytic anemia and cold hemagglutinin disease: clinical disease and laboratory findings. In: *Progress in Clinical Pathology*, Vol. VII (ed. by M. Stefanini et al.), pp. 137–163. Grune and Stratton, New York.

ISSITT, P. D. (1985). *Applied Blood Group Serology*, 3rd edn, 683 pp. Montgomery Scientific Publications, Miami.

KRUATRACHUE, M. & SIRISINHA, S. (1977). Autoimmune haemolytic anaemias in Thailand. *Scand. J. Haemat.*, 19, 61–67.

LAL, V. B. & SPEISER, P. (1957). Untersuchungen über Zusammenhänge zwischen erworbenen hämolytischen Anämien, klassischen Blutgruppen, Rhesusfactor, Geschlecht und Alter. *Blut*, 3, 15–19.

LALEZARI, P. (1983). Autoimmune hemolytic disease. In: *Recent Advances in Clinical Immunology* (ed. by R. A. Thompson and N. R. Rose), pp. 69–90. Churchill Livingstone, Edinburgh.

LEDDY, J. P. & SWISHER, S. N. (1978). Acquired immune hemolytic disorders (including drug-induced hemolytic anemia). In: *Immunological Diseases*, Vol. 2, 3rd edn (ed. by M. Samter), pp. 1187–1227. Little, Brown and Co., Boston.

LEJEUNE, E. (1954). Les syndromes hémolytiques acquis: étude clinique et immunologique à propos de 28 observations. Imprimerie des Beaux-Arts, Camille Annequin, Lyon.

LETMAN, H. (1957). Auto-immune haemolytic anaemia. *Dan. med. Bull.*, 4, 143–147.

OETTGEN, H. F. & KINDLER, M. (1959). Die chronische erworbene hämolytische Anämie: klinische und immunologische Untersuchungen an 47 Fällen. *Folia haemat.* (Frankfurt), 4, 22–76.

PETZ, L. D. & GARRATTY, G. (1980). *Acquired Immune Hemolytic Anemias*, 456 pp. Churchill Livingstone, New York.

PIROFSKY, B. (1965). Serologic and clinical findings in autoimmune hemolytic anemia. *Ser. haemat.*, 9, 47–60.

PIROFSKY, B. (1969). *Autoimmunization and the Autoimmune Hemolytic Anemias*, 537 pp. Williams and Wilkins, Baltimore.

PIROFSKY, B. (1975). Immune haemolytic disease: the autoimmune haemolytic anaemias. *Clinics Haemat.*, 4, 167–180.

PIROFSKY, B. (1976). Clinical aspects of autoimmune hemolytic anemia. *Seminars Hemat.*, 8, 251–265.

PIROFSKY, B. & BARDANA, E. J. JNR (1974). Autoimmune hemolytic anemia: I. Clinical aspects. *Ser. haemat.*, 7, 367–375.

REVOL, L., LEJEUNE, E., BRIZARD, C.P., JOUVENCEAUX, A. & PERRIN, N. (1958). Contribution à l'étude systématique des tests globulaires et sériques dans les syndromes hémolytiques (à propos d'une statistique de 2,400 examens). *Sang*, 29, 416–425.

ROSSE, W. R. (1990), *Clinical Immunohematology: Basic Concepts and Clinical Applications*. 677 pp. Blackwell Scientific Publications, Boston.

SALMON, C., HOMBERG, J. C. & HABIBI, B. (1975a). Immunologie des anémies hémolytiques auto-immunes (Première partie). *Rev. franç. Transf. Immuno-hémat.*, 18, 301–320.

SALMON, C., HOMBERG, J. -C. & HABIBI, B. (1975b). Immunologie des anémies hémolytiques auto-immunes (Deuxième partie). *Rev. franç. Transf. Immuno-hémat.*, 18, 497–513.

SCHUBOTHE, H. (1957). Der erworbenen hämolytischen Anämien. B. Die Klinik der autoimmunhämolytischen Erkrankungen. In: *Immunopathologie in Klinik und Forschung und das Problem der Autoantikörper* (ed. by P. Miescher, and K. O. Vorlaender), p. 196. Georg Thieme, Stuttgart.

SCHUBOTHE, H. (1958). *Serologie und klinische Bedeutung der Autohämantikörper*, 284 pp. Karger, Basel.

SCHUBOTHE, H. (1959). Serologie und Klinik der Autoimmunhämolytischen Erkrankungen. *Ergebn. inn. Med. Kinderheilk.*, 11, 466–624.

SCHWARTZ, R. S. & COSTEA, N. (1966). Autoimmune hemolytic anemia: clinical correlations and biological implications. *Seminars Hemat.*, 3, 2–26.

SOKOL, R. J. & HEWITT, S. (1985). Autoimmune hemolysis: a critical review. CRC *crit. Rev. Oncol/Hemat.*, 4, 125–154.

SOKOL, R. J., HEWITT, S. & STAMPS, B. (1981). Autoimmune haemolysis: an 18-year study of 865 cases referred to a regional transfusion centre. *Brit. med. J.*, 282, 2023–2027.

VAN LOGHEM, J. J. JNR, VAN DER HART, M. & DORFMEIER, H. (1958). Serologic studies in acquired hemolytic anemia. *Proc. 6th int. Congr. int. Soc. Hemat.*, Boston, 1956, pp. 858–868. Grune and Stratton, New York.

VIDEBAEK, A. (1962). Primary (idiopathic) auto-immune haemolytic anaemia. *Acta med. scand.*, 171, 449–462.

WORLLEDGE, S. (revised by Hughes Jones, N. C. and Bain, B.) (1982). Immune haemolytic anaemia. In *Blood and its Disorders*, 2nd edn. (ed. by R. M. Hardisty and D. J. Weatherall), pp. 479–513. Blackwell Scientific Publications, Oxford.

WORLLEDGE, S. M. & BLAJCHMAN, M. A. (1972). The autoimmune haemolytic anaemias. *Brit. J. Haemat.*, 23, Suppl., 61–69.

YOUNG, L. E., MILLER, G & CHRISTIAN, R. M. (1951). Clinical and laboratory observations on autoimmune hemolytic disease. *Ann. intern. Med.*, 35, 507–517.

Auto-immune haemolytic anaemia (AIHA): warm-antibody syndromes I: 'idiopathic' types: history and clinical features

Early history 6

Later history: a summary 11

Synonyms and eponyms 11

Race and genetic factors 12
    ABO blood groups 14
    HLA types 14

Clinical features of warm-antibody auto-immune haemolytic anaemia 15
    Sex 15
    Age 15
    Incidence in the population 16

Symptoms and course of the disease 16

Physical signs 17
    Jaundice 18
    Liver 18
    Spleen 18

Unusual complications and associations 19

Auto-immune haemolytic anaemia in pregnancy 19
    Case reports 21
    'Coombs-negative' AIHA in pregnancy 22
    Prognosis for the patient and for her infant 24
    Transient AIHA in infants born to mothers suffering from warm-antibody AIHA 24

Auto-immune haemolytic anaemia in infancy and childhood 25
    Age 30
    Sex 31
    Course 31

Auto-immune haemolytic anaemia in association with ITP (Evans syndrome) 34

Immunopancytopenia 36

Auto-immune haemolytic anaemia in immune deficiency syndromes 39

EARLY HISTORY

Hayem (1898) is generally credited with giving the first recognizable description of acquired haemolytic anaemia under the title 'Ictère infectieux chronique splénomégalique' and of differentiating anaemia with jaundice from disease of the liver. It was in France, too, that the first observations were made that suggested that haemolytic anaemia might be caused by the development of auto-antibodies. From 1908 onwards, Widal, Abrami and Brulé (1908a,b;1909) in a series of papers gave the first accurate descriptions of 'l'ictère hémolytique acquis.' Significantly, they stressed that autohaemagglutination was characteristic of the cases they studied and Le Gendre and Brulé (1909), in emphasizing the differences between the congenital and acquired forms of haemolytic jaundice, stated that in the acquired form 'auto-agglutination des hématies restait constamment,

intense et rapide, prenait une veritable valeur diagnostique.'

Other important observations were made in France at about the same time. Chauffard and Troisier (1908) and Chauffard and Vincent (1909) described as suffering from 'ictère hémolysinique' and 'hémoglobinurie hémolysini-que' patients in whom intense haemolysis was taking place in vivo and whose sera appeared to contain abnormal haemolysins.

Eason (1918) described a boy of 17 (who had earlier shown signs of purpura) who was anaemic and who had increased osmotic fragility and was diagnosed as suffering from acholuric jaundice (haemolytic icterus) of a chronic acquired form.

These pioneer studies were to some extent forgotten in the succeeding decades, and 30 years or so passed without much progress being made. Several publications, however, certainly deserve mention. In 1925, Lederer described three patients who had suffered from acute haemolytic episodes of sudden onset and of short duration. In each case recovery seemed to take place following blood transfusion. Brill (1926), too, reported what appeared to be a similar type of case and subsequently Lederer (1930) described three further patients.

These reports were followed by a description by Parsons (1931) of five children who became acutely anaemic in consequence it was thought of a preceding infection. Three of the children recovered rapidly: in two the disorder was less acute and ran a more chronic course. Parsons described their illness in the following terms: it was preceded 'by abdominal pain and diarrhea and vomiting, leading to an acute and grave anemia which was characterized by a spontaneous and rapid recovery'. The blood picture was interpreted as being typical of a severe destruction of red blood cells, with an intense marrow reaction resulting in 20 000–40 000 per c.mm white cells and many reticulated cells. Soon, descriptions of patients giving similar histories started to appear in the medical press of countries other than the United States, e.g. by Parkes Weber (1931) in England and by Kühl (1931) and Altmann (1932) in Germany. While the identity of these cases with auto-immune haemolytic anaemia is in doubt, some, at least, probably were examples of the syndrome. In none, however, were serological studies carried out.

Lederer's and Brill's reports of hyperacute and short-lived haemolytic anaemia were soon followed by descriptions of other cases of apparently acquired origin and of uncertain cause and outlook, the severity of which was variable but generally initially less than that of Lederer's cases but greater than that of typical congenital acholuric jaundice [hereditary spherocytosis (HS)]. Davidson (1932), O'Donoghue and Witts (1932), Lovibond (1935), Dyke and Young (1938), Lescher, Osborn and Bates (1939), McGavack (1939) and Mason (1943) described cases of this type.

The merit of Dyke and Young's (1938) paper, in which they described six cases of chronic macrocytic haemolytic anaemia, is that they clearly distinguished them from hereditary spherocytosis, on the basis of the macrocytic blood picture and the often poor and uncertain

response to splenectomy. Once more, however, serological findings were not mentioned.

There was confusion, too, at this time between acquired haemolytic anaemia and a latent hereditary haemolytic anaemia first appearing in adult life, and in England (at least throughout the 1930s), although not, for example, in Germany (Heilmeyer and Albus, 1936), the current teaching was that many, perhaps most, cases of apparently 'acquired' haemolytic anaemia (icterus) were in fact really examples of congenital acholuric jaundice that had previously been latent and had presented no symptoms (Dawson, 1931; Murray-Lyon, 1935; Vaughan, 1936; Duthie, 1937; Israëls and Wilkinson, 1938). The usual, although not invariable, presence of spherocytosis and increased osmotic fragility in both types of case and the lack of a reliable and distinguishing serological test go a long way to explain this confusion.

There are reports, too, published well before Lederer's first paper, of patients who seem very likely in retrospect to have suffered from the same syndrome. Teeter's (1907) description of a 6-year-old girl who recovered from 'leukanemia', read before the Society of Alumni of Bellevue Hospital, New York, is a notable example. The following is an abbreviated version of his description.

The child had been perfectly well previously except for an attack of measles 2–3 years previously. On the 4th May 1905 she developed general malaise, and that night she began to vomit. The next day vomiting was incessant and her temperature reached 103°F. By the 6th May she had ceased vomiting but was very restless, and during the day passed 'about one pint of bloody urine'. It was noticed that she was becoming very pale 'with a slight icteric tint'. On the 7th May the liver was found to be enlarged and the spleen palpable two fingers' breadth below the ribs. She was restless and delirious but had ceased vomiting and the urine no longer contained blood. Her blood picture was as follows: erythrocytes 1 530 000/c.mm; haemoglobin 20%; leucocytes 132 800/c.mm; neutrophils 59%, myelocytes 11%, unclassified cells 6%; nucleated red cells 20 000/c.mm, 10% megaloblasts, 68% normoblasts. By the 10th May her condition had improved; and on the 11th May the erythrocyte count had risen and the leucocyte count had fallen to 36 000/c.mm, of which 56% were neutrophils, 5% myelocytes and 4% unclassified cells, and the nucleated erythrocyte count had fallen to 10 800/c.mm.

Thereafter, improvement was rapid and progressive: 3 months after the onset of her illness her haemoglobin was 100% and the child 'seemed normal in every respect'.

Teeter concluded that his patient had suffered from a 'toxemia of unknown origin, but producing a rapid destruction of red cells with marked stimulation of the bone marrow and spleen, so that all the cells character-istic of leukemia appeared in large numbers in the circulation. The destruction of the red cells is so pronounced that the blood findings also resembled those of a pernicious anemia.' Two (rather poor) photomicrographs are reproduced in Teeter's paper. The first is of a blood film made at the time of the first blood examination: this shows, in addition to many leucocytes, autoagglutination (probably) and micro-spherocytosis (possibly). The second (a better photo-graph) is of a blood film made 8 days later: although recognized by Teeter as looking practically normal, some microspherocytes are clearly visible.

O'Donoghue and Witts's (1932) review entitled 'The acute haemolytic anaemia of Lederer' deserves special mention. Three cases already published in Guy's Hospital Reports were redescribed and a description of a fourth patient was added. O'Donoghue and Witts also referred to 32 additional cases described in other journals. They recognized that the rate of haemolysis varied from patient to patient and that in the most acute cases haemoglobinuria was often a striking symptom. Untreated, the disease was considered to have a high mortality; transfusion was, however, usually dramatically curative. O'Donoghue and Witts stressed that when haemolysis was most acute the leucocyte count might reach extraordinary high levels (see p. **79**), and that there might be real difficulty (and impor-tance) in distinguishing between acute haemolytic anaemia and acute leukaemia; they cited several reports of patients that had been described as suffering from 'acute leukaemia with recovery'. Finally, they concluded that Lederer's anaemia appeared to be a specific illness due to an infec-tion of unknown nature which affected both sexes apparently equally and that although it might occur at any age it was most frequent in the first two decades.

Parsons and Hawksley (1933) in their extensive review of the anaemias of infancy and childhood devoted a major section to acute haemolytic anaemia (Lederer type). They mentioned four patients referred to earlier (Parsons, 1931) and reported that they had seen five more patients; eight of these children had recovered, five having responded 'remarkably' to transfusion. They referred also to four more children who had suffered from a less severe form of the disease (subacute haemolytic anaemia), all of whom had recovered without transfusion. They emphasized that the same disease might 'affect not only the erythron but also the myeloid and platelet systems', with the result that 'the marrow may be completely paralysed during the period of haemolysis'.

In 1938 Dameshek and Schwartz (1938a) once again reported the presence of abnormal haemolysins in patients suffering from acute (acquired) haemolytic anaemia. They also showed clearly, both in man and in guinea-pigs injected experimentally with anti-erythrocyte sera, that spherocytosis and increased osmotic fragility might develop during the course of acquired haemolytic anaemia (Dameshek and Schwartz, 1938b).

It is most interesting to re-read Dameshek and Schwartz's first paper (1938a) in an attempt to discover the type of lysin they had encountered. They had studied three patients who had become severely anaemic within a few days or weeks. In their Case 3 spherocytes were reported as being conspicuous and osmotic fragility was increased. There was, however, no mention of auto-agglutination. Sera from Cases 2 and 3 lysed approximately one-third to one-half of quite a large number of erythrocyte samples, irrespective of their ABO groups: with the serum from Case 2 (who was group O) six out of 19 tests were positive with O cells; and with the serum of Case 3 (who was group B), 32 out of 55 tests were positive with O or B cells. The serum from Case 1, which had been obtained during the patient's convalescence, lysed one out of three samples of O cells. These results suggest that the lysis was being brought about by a complement-fixing warm or high-thermal-amplitude cold auto-antibody which was reacting with an antigen outside the ABO system.

The fact that Dameshek and Schwartz could not determine the exact nature of their haemolysin (or haemolysins) does not detract from the importance of their observations. Their concept that 'haemolysins' of one type or another were the cause of many cases of apparently acquired haemolytic anaemia was further developed by Dameshek and Schwartz (1940) in a lengthy review. The importance of this review at the time it was published can hardly be exaggerated. It extended to 195 pages, included 380 references, and embodied an exhaustive discussion of all aspects of acute acquired haemolytic anaemia, including its possible treatment, extending back to the beginning of the century.

Dameshek and Schwartz's main conclusions were as follows: that 'acute non-congenital (acquired) hemolytic icterus (anemia)' had been first described by Widal, Abrami and Brulé and by Chauffard and his collaborators in 1901–1908; that at least four, possibly five, different types of 'iso-hemolysins' had been described in various haemolytic syndromes; that similar syndromes could be produced experimentally in animals by the use of haemolytic immune sera comparable to those that had been found in human cases and that it was 'not improbable' that haemolysins of various types and 'dosages' were responsible for the various types of human haemolytic disease; that spherocytosis and increased osmotic fragility are the end-results of the activity of haemolysins on mature erythrocytes and not due to faulty production by an abnormal marrow; that spherocytes are almost always present in acutely ill patients, their number depending upon the rapidity of haemolysis; that the macrocytic picture sometimes seen may be due to the presence of large numbers of reticulocytes in the peripheral blood, and that the bone marrow in such cases is normoblastic and shows none of the features of a megaloblastic anaemia.

Dameshek and Schwartz further concluded that acute haemolytic anaemia is not a benign disease as had usually been depicted and that blood transfusion was not always curative; splenectomy, on the other hand, might have an almost immediate beneficial effect in many cases. Their final paragraph is produced below:

'The various hemolytic syndromes, both congenital and acquired, may be classified as fulminating (with hemoglobinuria), acute, subacute and chronic. Spherocytosis and increased fragility may occur in both the congenital and acquired varieties. "Acute hemolytic anemia" is the acute variety of acquired hemolytic icterus (anemia). This type is at times associated with the presence of hemolysins in the serum ("hemolysinic icterus"). The terms "hemolytic icterus" and "hemolytic anemia" are interchangeable. Because of the many prior descriptions, the eponym "Lederer's" anemia appears to be unwarranted.'

Dameshek and Schwartz's general thesis that haemolysins were responsible for the development of many cases of acquired haemolytic anaemia was, however, viewed with some scepticism by their contemporaries, a major difficulty being that the postulated 'haemolysins' could not be demonstrated by the techniques then available in the great majority of cases—the three patients that Dameshek and Schwartz had themselves described were clearly exceptional. Several more years were to pass before this difficulty was resolved and Dameshek and Schwartz's views were vindicated, at least in relation to *acquired* haemolytic anaemia. [They were incorrect in extrapolating their concept of the role of haemolysins to *congenital* haemolytic jaundice (hereditary spherocytosis): while correct in questioning that spherocytosis was pathognomonic of the disorder, they were wrong in suggesting that it might be caused by the 'more or less continued action of an hemolysin'.]

In 1946, Boorman, Dodd and Loutit published their classic paper in which they described how they had applied the antiglobulin test of Coombs, Mourant and Race (1945) to 39 patients suffering from haemolytic anaemia. Twenty-eight of these patients were considered to be suffering from congenital acholuric jaundice (hereditary spherocytosis): in none of them were washed erythrocytes agglutinated by a diluted anti-human globulin serum. In striking contrast the erythrocytes of all of the five patients thought to have acquired acholuric jaundice were agglutinated, while in a further six patients, who had been diagnosed as suffering from miscellaneous types of haemolytic anaemia, the test was negative. Boorman, Dodd and Loutit concluded that the agglutination test 'will discriminate the congenital from the acquired form of acholuric jaundice, and that it indicated that the acquired form is due to a process of immunization, whereas the congenital form is not.' [Recently, Dodd (1984) has given a delightful account of the excitement that these results created.]

Boorman, Dodd and Loutit's results with their anti-human globulin serum were concordant with the data on erythrocyte survival that had been obtained a few years earlier using the Ashby method of differential agglutination (see Vol.1, pp. 22 and 108). Brown and his co-workers (1944) had not only showed that compatible erythrocytes transfused to patients with acquired haemolytic anaemia might survive far less well than in normal recipients, but they also showed that the data when plotted against time on arithmetic graph paper formed a markedly curved line instead of the almost straight line found normally. They concluded that the curve indicated that the erythrocytes were being eliminated by exponential mechanisms that were different from the mechanisms giving rise to the almost straight line found in health and also that the exponential mechanisms were 'probably of the nature of a process of destruction acting at random on the erythrocytes irrespective of their age or other characteristic. Loutit and Mollison's similar but more extensive data were not published until 1946 (Loutit) and 1947 (Loutit and Mollison).

In Loutit and Mollison's paper eight examples of idiopathic AIHA were referred to: in seven of them the elimination of transfused erythrocytes was very rapid; it was relatively slow, but still abnormal in one patient. In some of the patients the graph of elimination was curved and roughly exponential in form. In one patient the rate of elimination was much slower after splenectomy than before splenectomy.

Mollison (1947) described observations made on five cases of idiopathic AIHA. Once again, normal erythrocytes were shown to be rapidly destroyed after transfusion to the patients. In each case elimination of half the tranfused cells took place in 6 days or less; in one patient 45% of the transfused blood was eliminated within the first 9 hours of transfusion. Other similar observations were reported by Mollison (1951, p. 124). In a personally studied patient who died of a hyperacute haemolytic anaemia (Dacie, 1954, p. 202, Case 12) Mollison found that normal erythrocytes were destroyed almost as fast as they were transfused to the patient. Lüdin (1948) also demonstrated the rapid elimination of normal erythrocytes from the circulation of a patient suffering from macrocytic haemolytic anaemia of the 'Dyke–Young' type.

Selwyn and Hackett (1949) showed that not only was there a markedly increased rate of elimination of normal erythrocytes transfused to three patients suffering from idiopathic AIHA, but that the normal cells become sensitized (as shown by their reaction with antiglobulin serum) in the recipients' circulation before they were eliminated. They also carried out the reverse procedure of transfusing the blood of patients into normal recipients. In two experiments they found that the patients' blood was eliminated at an increased rate for the first 10–15 days after transfusion; thereafter, elimination took place at the normal rate. The transfused cells remained sensitized until they were eliminated. It appeared, however, that antibody was also transferred from the patients' to the recipients' erythrocytes as the majority of the recipients' erythrocytes became sensitized after the transfusion as judged by their agglutination by antiglobulin serum.

It seemed likely that the relatively good or even normal survival of a patient's erythrocytes in a normal recipient was due to elution of the antibody from the patient's cells in vivo and transference to the recipient's cells, as well as to the fact that the patient's cells were no longer exposed to further sensitization when circulating in a normal environment.

Owren (1949) similarly studied the survival of the sensitized erythrocytes of an AIHA patient when transfused to a normal recipient, as well as that of normal erythrocytes transfused to the patient. The normal erythrocytes were quickly destroyed, half being eliminated in 6–7 days. As in Selwyn and Hackett's experiments, the elimination of the patient's cells took place in two phases; first, a rapid fall within 3 days to about 35% of the immediate post-transfusion count, and then a much slower elimination, which was still incomplete 80 days after the transfusion. Owren found that the transfused (patient's) cells gave positive antiglobulin tests during the first 3 days after transfusion at the time when the cells were being rapidly eliminated.

The early studies referred to above clearly demonstrated that normal erythrocytes are destroyed unusually rapidly after transfusion to patients suffering from AIHA. Unfortunately, however, the Ashby method was incapable of determining how fast the patient's own erythrocytes were being destroyed in his or her own circulation. The ^{51}Cr technique, which was introduced into clinical practice in 1950 (see Vol. 1, p. 30), proved, on the other hand, capable of answering this question. Because of this, and also because only small volumes of blood (e.g. 10–20 ml) need to be labelled, the ^{51}Cr technique largely superseded the Ashby technique in studying erythrocyte survival after transfusion. In AIHA it has been mainly used in establishing the presence of minor degrees of increased haemolysis, in demonstrating the specificity of an auto-antibody and, by virtue of its penetrating radiation, in combining erythrocyte survival studies with surface counting over the liver and spleen to assess the site(s) of erythrocyte destruction (p. **477**).

A further important advance, of a technical nature, was the discovery of Morton and Pickles (1947) that the agglutination of erythrocytes by antibodies could often be enhanced if the cells under test were first exposed to the action of the proteolytic enzyme trypsin, and, moreover, that 'incomplete' antibodies that failed to cause the agglutination of cells when suspended in saline would do so if the cells had first been exposed to trypsin. Trypsinized cells and, subsequently, cells pre-treated by other enzymes (papain, ficin, bromelin, etc.), as well as the complement-sensitive paroxysmal nocturnal haemoglobinuria (PNH) cells, were to prove to be most valuable tools in the demonstration and characterization of the antibodies in acquired haemolytic anaemia. The use of antiglobulin sera and of enzyme-treated erythrocytes contributed greatly to the understanding of the pathogenesis of acquired haemolytic anaemia by making it possible to demonstrate the presence of incomplete auto-antibodies in many cases in which other techniques had failed to do so.

LATER HISTORY: A SUMMARY

The seminal reports of Boorman, Dodd and Loutit (1946) and of Morton and Pickles (1947) led to the antibodies of AIHA being extensively studied in the next decade and subsequently. As mentioned earlier, two main types of auto-antibody — warm and cold — were soon recognized and the clinical syndromes associated with their presence clearly defined. Advances in biochemical and biophysical technique — for instance, the development of electrophoresis and immunoelectrophoresis and the availability of ultracentrifuges — allowed the chemical and physical nature of the auto-antibodies to be more precisely established, and the rapidly expanding knowledge of the human blood-group antigens was soon applied to the exacting task of defining

the antibodies' specificity. Antiglobulin sera, monospecific for globulin class and for complement and its components proved to be most useful laboratory reagents.

Another major event was the advent of the synthetic corticosteroid drugs and immunosuppressive agents and the demonstration of their value in treatment. Finally, in this short summary of some of the main events in the development of knowledge of the AIHAs subsequent to the introduction of the antiglobulin test, mention should be made of the recognition of auto-immune haemolytic anaemias in mammalian species other than man. All the above-mentioned discoveries and advances in knowledge are discussed in detail in later sections of this book.

SYNONYMS AND EPONYMS

L'ictère hémolytique acquis (Widal, Abrami and Brulé, 1909); erworbener hämolytischer splenomegalischer Ikterus, Typus Hayem–Widal (Micheli, 1911); acquired acholuric jaundice (haemolytic icterus) (Eason, 1918); acute hemolytic anemia (Lederer, 1925; Dameshek and Schwartz, 1940); immunohemolytic anemia (Evans et al., 1951); autoimmune hemolytic disease (Young, Miller and Christian, 1951); antiglobulin-positive hemolytic anemia (Osgood, 1961).

Some Continental workers (e.g. Marcolongo, 1953) have referred to different forms of idiopathic acquired haemolytic anaemia by the eponyms 'Hayem–Widal', 'Dyke–Young', 'Loutit' and 'Lederer–Brill', whilst the term 'Lederer's anaemia (anemia)' was at one time quite widely used in British and American literature, e.g. by Joules and Masterman (1935) and McGavack (1939). It seems, however, in retrospect to have been unwise to have attempted to separate on the basis mainly of clinical differences cases of acquired haemolytic anaemia of unknown origin into subgroups labelled by eponyms, e.g. into the 'Lederer type' (acute transient) or 'Dyke–Young type' (chronic macrocytic), unless the distinction could have been backed by real differences in aetiology or pathogenesis.

The eponyms 'Hayem–Widal' (Micheli, 1911,

etc.), recalling pioneer clinical and serological observations or 'Loutit' (Maier, 1948; Schulthess, 1949; Heilmeyer, 1950; Fleischhacker, 1952; Heni and Blessing, 1954; Stephinger, 1954), recalling the first demonstration of positive antiglobulin tests in acquired haemolytic anaemia, are more worthy of perpetuation, and an amalgam of the three names to 'Hayem–Widal–Loutit anaemia' would not be inappropriate; but it suffers from being uninformative compared with 'auto-immune haemolytic anaemia' (AIHA) and can hardly be recommended.

RACE AND GENETIC FACTORS

As far as is known, warm-antibody AIHA is not confined to any particular race or races. However, most of the published case reports have dealt with patients of Caucasian origin. Vietnamese (Le-Xuan-Chat, 1958) and Japanese (Fukuoka and Ando, 1965) are, however, known to have been affected. Amongst Allgood and Chaplin's (1967) 47 patients there were four blacks, an incidence of 9%. This was contrasted with a 14% incidence of black patients admitted to the hospital's medical service during an 8-month period. There is, however, considerable evidence for the role of genetic factors other than that of race. Thus more than one case of AIHA has been recorded in the same family and in other families AIHA in one member of the family has been associated with another type of auto-immune disease in another member. Such occurrences have received considerable attention in the literature. More than one case of AIHA in the same family is, however, most unusual, although probably less rare than at one time it seemed to be. The author (Dacie, 1969), for instance, recorded that he had up to the time of writing seen only one example of a family incidence — a sister and a brother both affected with AIHA — out of more than 100 such patients he had personally studied. Details of these two patients are summarized in Table 22.1, and other recorded cases are listed in Table 22.2.

Amongst the relationships listed in Table 22.2 are four sets of twins (Schmid, 1969; Zuelzer et al., 1970; Habibi et al., 1974; Pérez-Mateo and

Table 22.1 Clinical and serological data of two patients, a sister and brother, who suffered from warm-antibody AIHA.*

	Sister	Brother
Clinical features	Thrombocytopenia when aged 29	AIHA when aged 62
	Splenectomy when aged 32	
	AIHA when aged 40	
	Died from acute AIHA when aged 42	
Blood group	B CDe/cde	B CDe/cde
Direct antiglobulin test	IgG	IgG
Specificity of eluted antibodies	Anti-C Anti-e	Anti-e
Specificity of auto-antibodies in serum	Anti-C (high titre) Anti-e (high titre)	Anti-C (low titre) Anti-e (moderate titre)
Spherocytosis	Marked	Marked
Intravascular haemolysis	Present	Absent

*Modified from Dacie and Worlledge (1975).

Tascón, 1982) of which three sets were reported as being identical. It seems, however, that if a patient suffering from warm-antibody AIHA has an identical twin it is not inevitable that the twin will develop the same condition. Dacie (1954, p. 197) reported such an occurrence: the patient (Case 9) was followed up for 20 years after the initial diagnosis had been made and during this time her twin remained apparently free from the disease.

Patients who suffer from warm-antibody AIHA in whose family one or more other members suffer from an immunologically mediated disorder other than AIHA are more frequently encountered. Dreyfus (1964), in a valuable review which included 116 references, mentioned the occurrence of chronic thrombocytopenia, polyarteritis nodosa, rheumatoid arthritis, pernicious anaemia and hypogammaglobulinaemia; he added that he had demonstrated one or more abnormalities in the serum immune globulins of eight out of 15 relatives of two of his patients with chronic AIHA. Pirofsky (1968, 1969) reported that one or more relatives of eight out of 43 of his patients (approximately 20%) had suffered from a wide range of

Table 22.2 Occurrences of AIHA in more than one member of a family.*

Reference	Relationship and age at onset (years, except where stated)
Kissmeyer-Nielson, Bent-Hansen and Kieler (1952)	Mother (61) and daughter (23)
Fialkow, Fudenberg and Epstein (1964); Olanoff and Fudenberg (1983)	Mother (72) and son (33)
Hennemann and Krause (1964)	Two sisters (18 and 14)
Dobbs (1965)	Sister (55) and brother (38); a further sister (35) possibly affected
van Loghem (1965)	Two children had 'symptoms of acquired hemolytic anemia' 'Two brothers developed autoimmune hemolytic anemia'
Cordova et al. (1966)	Mother (40) and daughter (8)
Schwartz and Costea (1966)	Sister (57) and brother (who had died earlier of AIHA and lymphosarcoma)
Shapiro (1967)	Sister (3 months) and two brothers (3 and 4 months)
Pirofsky (1968, 1969)	Two sisters (66 and 49) and brother (48)
Seip, Harboe and Cyvin (1969)	Two sisters (4 and 12)
Pollock, Fenton and Barrett (1970)	Brother (14) and sister (19); also paternal aunt
Zuelzer et al. (1970)	Identical twin girls (1 and $2\frac{1}{2}$)
Blajchman et al. (1971)	Mother and daughter (12)
Dacie and Worlledge (1975)	Sister (40) and brother (62) (See also Table 22.1)
Roth et al. (1975)	Brother (20) and two sisters (17 and 15)
Toolis et al. (1977)	Two sisters (66 and 62)
Conley (1981)	Two sisters (68 and 60)
Reynolds, Vengelen-Tyler and More (1981)	Mother and son (14)
Pérez-Mateo and Tascón (1982)	Twin brothers (21 and 23)
Boling et al. (1983)	Two sisters (71 and 73)
Horowitz, Borcherding and Hong (1984)	Two families with two affected sisters (7 months and 6, and 12 months and 9 months)

*Conley and Savarese (1989) gave in a Table interesting details of other disorders accompanying the AIHA in most of the patients referred to above, and in other members of their families.

probable or possible auto-immune disorders, including glomerulonephritis, pernicious anaemia, Stevens–Johnson syndrome, rheumatoid arthritis, systemic lupus erythematosus (SLE) and thrombocytopenic purpura. Hodgkin's disease and chronic granulocytic leukaemia had also been included in the list.

The incidence in Conley's (1981) more recent series of warm-antibody AIHA patients was considerably higher: 14 out of 33 patients had family members known to have suffered from an immunologically mediated disorder similar to those listed by Pirofsky or from a lymphoma or leukaemia.

Lippman and his co-workers (1982) reported a detailed study of a large family, one of whose members, a female aged 22, had experienced a severe but short-lived (< 3 months) episode of warm-antibody AIHA (appearing during the course of asymptomatic infectious mononucleosis). She also suffered from hypothyroidism and her serum contained anti-thyroid and anti-gastric antibodies. Thirty-three living relatives in three generations and 11 spouses were studied. None had AIHA; but five relatives in three generations had hyperthyroidism, and single relatives had, respectively, asthma, ulcerative colitis or acute leukaemia. Six relatives had raised titres of anti-nuclear antibody and the serum of six others bound abnormal amounts of single-stranded DNA. The serum of one relative gave a false-positive reaction for syphilis. Two relatives had hypergammaglobulinaemia and three relatives (and one spouse) had raised levels of IgA and three relatives raised levels of IgM. The direct antiglobulin reaction was positive in two relatives (and one spouse). Statistical analysis showed highly significant differences for immune-mediated diseases and serological abnormalities between the relatives and the spouses. The HLA genotypes (A, B, Cw, DR, DRw) were ascertained for the patient and all except three of her relatives, but no evidence of linkage of any abnormality with HLA type was established—the odds were 100:1 against.

Lippman and his co-workers (1982) studied in a similar way a large kindred in which the proband had idiopathic thrombocytopenic purpura (ITP) and also eight families in which 21 members suffered from SLE. The data from these families were similar to those obtained from the family the proband of which had had AIHA. Lippman et al. concluded that their study suggested that in each of the 10 families an autosomal dominant genetic factor, not linked to the HLA genes, had led to an enhanced predisposition to auto-immune diseases and serological abnormalities. They pointed out that several varieties of immune deficiency with different patterns of inheritance are known to predispose to auto-immune disorders including AIHA, chronic ITP and SLE (see Ch. 33, p. 371).

Mousa et al. (1985) recorded the occurrence of severe chronic anaemia and erythroblastopenia, which responded to treatment with prednisone, in a 21-year-old female whose mother suffered from DAT-positive AIHA and thrombocytopenia.

In their most recent review from the Johns Hopkins Hospital, Conley and Savarese (1989) recorded in considerable detail the occurrence in patients with AIHA of other auto-immune and lymphoproliferative disorders, and emphasized, too, the frequent association of abnormal serological reactions and abnormalities in the concentrations of the serum immunoglobulins. In a table listing reported cases of familial incidences of AIHA such associations are particularly striking— both in the patients affected with AIHA (the propositi) and in their siblings and more remote family members. The inescapable conclusion is that genetic influences play a significant role in the genesis of AIHA and in auto-immune disorders in general. In Conley and Savarese's concluding but nevertheless cautious words: 'Our observations support the view that an abnormality of cells of the immune system, often genetically determined, may predispose to serologic changes, immune deficiency, autoimmune diseases and neoplasia' (see also p. 371).

ABO blood groups

Hunt and Lucia (1953) claimed to have demonstrated a statistically significant increase of group O in cases of acquired haemolytic anaemia: 78% of 27 patients were group O compared with 48% of their controls. These observations were supported by further figures from Australia, Clemens and Walsh (1955) reporting that 64% of 66 patients with acquired haemolytic anaemia (giving positive direct antiglobulin tests) were group O. However, this apparent association between group O and AIHA was not confirmed by subsequent reports based on larger series. Lal and Speiser (1957) found that 39% of 97 cases of the idiopathic warm-antibody

type were group O, a figure not significantly different from that of the general population. Dunsford and Owen (1960) came to the same conclusion: out of 127 patients with acquired haemolytic anaemia (giving positive antiglobulin tests) 47.2% were group O compared with 45.4% of their controls. Dacie's (1962, p. 348) data also did not support any strong association with group O. The ABO group of 120 patients (warm and cold antibodies) were: 40% group O, 44% group A, 13.5% group B and 2.5% group AB.

More recently, Sokol, Hewitt and Stamps (1981) reported that the ABO and Rh genotypes of 865 patients with idiopathic or secondary warm- or cold-antibody AIHA investigated at a blood transfusion centre over an 18-year period did not differ from those of a control population.

HLA types

The possibility that proneness to develop AIHA might be associated with the presence of a particular HLA antigen or haplotype has prompted several detailed studies. No very clear pattern has, however, emerged.

Da Costa and co-workers (1974) compared the incidence of 14 HLA-A antigens and three HLA-W antigens in 56 patients with IgG or complement on their erythrocytes with that in 613 normal controls. Twelve of the patients were suffering from idiopathic AIHA; 10 were receiving α-methyldopa and gave positive antiglobulin tests; 29 patients were suffering from lymphomas or conditions in which immune complexes circulate; five had positive antiglobulin tests for no discernible cause. Compared with the controls, there was a significant increase in the incidence of HLA-A1 and HLA-A8 antigens. The results reported by Clauvel et al. (1974) were, however, substantially different. They had studied 31 patients with idiopathic AIHA and found a higher than normal incidence of HLA-A3 but normal incidences of HLA-A1, HLA-A7 and HLA-A8. Dausset and Hors (1975), too, reported an increase in HLA-A3 but no deviation in other HLA antigens, especially HLA-A7. They considered, however, that their series of idiopathic AIHA patients —11 males and 25 females, all unrelated—was too small for any conclusions to be drawn. Different again were the data obtained by Abdel-Khalik et al. (1980), who studied 20 patients with warm-antibody AIHA and 40 normal controls. The incidence of HLA-B8 and of homozygosity for HLA-BW6 was found to be increased. Antigens that were not significantly prevalent in the patient group included HLA-A1, HLA-A3 and HLA-DRW3.

It is interesting to note that Toolis et al. (1977) had reported that both the two sisters (out of five siblings) who developed AIHA possessed the HLA antigens A1, B7 and B8.

CLINICAL FEATURES OF WARM-ANTIBODY AUTO-IMMUNE HAEMOLYTIC ANAEMIA

Sex

Both sexes are affected, but as in other auto-immune disorders, e.g. SLE, the majority of patients are female. The reason for the sex difference remains obscure.

Sacks, Workman and Jahn (1952) reviewed 147 cases of acquired haemolytic anaemia that had been reported in the literature as well as 19 patients of their own and stated that two-thirds of the patients were female.

Dausset and Malinvaud (1954) and Dausset and Colombani (1958, 1959) similarly reported an excess of females, 61% of 93 patients with idiopathic AIHA being female. They recorded, however, that 60% of 35 patients suffering from secondary AIHA were male.

Lal and Speiser (1957) reported that 55% of 49 patients with idiopathic AIHA and 62% of patients with secondary AIHA were female.

Dacie's (1962, p. 342) findings were: 58% of 108 patients with idiopathic AIHA and 66% of 59 patients with secondary AIHA were female. Dacie and Worlledge (1969) reported almost exactly the same percentages, 59% of 111 idiopathic patients and 64% of 88 secondary cases being female (Table 21.1, p. 2). Allgood and Chaplin (1967) had had a similar experience: 60% of their 47 patients with the idiopathic disease were female.

Pirofsky's (1969, p. 25) data are particularly interesting. While 64% of 44 patients with idiopathic AIHA were female, when idiopathic and secondary cases were considered together the incidence in males and females was found to be exactly the same. This seems to have been brought about by the relatively high proportion of patients in his secondary AIHA series who had either chronic lymphocytic leukaemia or a lymphoma.

Silverstein and co-workers (1972), who reviewed the survival of 117 patients who had been treated at the Mayo Clinic between 1955 and 1965, reported that 61 were female and 56 male. [Six patients (three with SLE and three with a lymphoma), whose sex was not recorded, were subsequently excluded from the series.]

A more recent report from South-East Asia also reveals a marked female preponderance, 25 of Kruatrachue and Sirisinha's (1977) 31 patients with idiopathic AIHA being female.

Age

The age distribution of 125 patients suffering from warm-antibody AIHA investigated by the

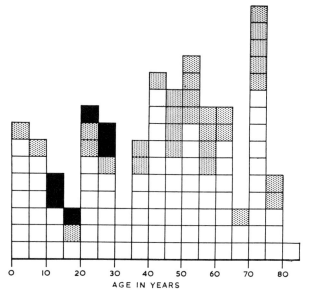

Fig. 22.1 Age distribution of 125 patients suffering from auto-immune haemolytic anaemia of the warm-antibody type.
Open squares = idiopathic cases; dotted squares = secondary cases (excluding SLE); filled-in squares = cases associated with systemic lupus erythematosus (SLE).

author in the late 1940s and 1950s is shown in Fig. 22.1. As the figure illustrates, subjects of all ages are affected, from infants in the first few months of life to elderly people. The age incidence of secondary warm-antibody AIHA reflects the age incidences of the associated diseases, e.g., patients suffering from SLE and AIHA are characteristically young (female) adults.

Data published subsequently on age incidence closely conform to the pattern outlined above and illustrated in Fig. 22.1.

Allgood and Chaplin's (1967) 47 idiopathic warm-antibody patients were aged between 10 and 80 years. Most were aged between 30 and 70, with a peak at 50–60; their mean age was 48.6.

Pirofsky (1969, p. 23) recorded an age range of 1 month to 87 years: 73% of his patients were over 40 years of age, with a peak incidence between 60 and 70. Most of his large series of warm-antibody patients were, however, suffering from secondary AIHA, and a relatively high proportion had chronic lymphocytic leukaemia and were over 40 years of age.

Kruatrachue and Sirisinha (1977), reporting on 100 Thai patients, also found a wide age range—from early childhood to 80 years. Idiopathic AIHA appeared, however, to be occurring at a relatively early age, most of the patients being between 15 and 30 (an age-range similar to that of patients whose AIHA was associated with SLE).

Incidence in the population

Letman (1957) calculated that the incidence of warm-antibody AIHA in a Danish population was 1 in 75 000 per annum. Pirofsky's (1969, p. 22) much larger experience led him to much the same conclusion: he calculated that an average of 29 cases seen annually over a 9-year period indicated that the incidence in Oregon, where he stated that the population is largely of Scandinavian extraction, was approximately 1 in 80 000 per annum.

Böttiger and Westerholm (1973) reported that 161 cases of AIHA (of all types) had been recorded within a 5-year period in the Uppsala region of Sweden—an incidence of approximately 2.6 per 100 000 per annum. Women predominated (63%), particularly in the 15–34 years age-group. In both sexes the incidence increased markedly after the age of 50.

In the United Kingdom, in the Sheffield area, Sokol, Hewitt and Stamps (1981) calculated that the incidence of auto-immune haemolytic anaemia (all types) was less than 2 per 100 000 until the age of 40; it then rose steeply to a maximum of approximately 2 per 100 000 at the age of 70.

SYMPTOMS AND COURSE OF THE DISEASE

AIHA is a most variable disorder and almost every grade of severity may be met with. In some patients the illness is a chronic one extending over years and the only symptoms complained of may be those common to chronic mild anaemia of any cause, e.g., undue tiredness and mild dyspnoea on exertion. In more severely affected patients the intensity of the anaemia often leads to serious dyspnoea and incapacity. At the other end of the scale the patient may be free from symptoms and not be significantly anaemic, despite serological signs of auto-immunization, e.g. a positive direct antiglobulin test. Hennemann (1963) emphasized the existence of occult (latent) cases of this type. Sometimes, chronic jaundice may be the patient's chief complaint, but this is a very variable symptom. In the most severely affected patients— often infants or young children, although not exclusively so—the onset may be sudden instead of being insidious, the chief features of the disease being rapidly increasing anaemia and increasing jaundice, often accompanied by pyrexia, and in the worst cases by a state of shock-like prostration.

Haemoglobinuria may be present as in the patients described by Lederer (1930), and 'acute haemolytic anaemia' is then an apt descriptive label. Fortunately, such cases are rare. Massive haemoglobinuria does not as a rule last more than a few days. If it persists despite all attempts at treatment, the outlook is grave; but Miller, Shumway and Young (1957) nevertheless reported the gradual recovery of a 14-year-old negress after 14 days' haemoglobinuria. Acute renal insufficiency seldom seems to follow haemoglobinuria. It was, however, reported by Payne, Spaet and Aggeler (1955) in an unusual ('Coombs-negative') case.

Occasionally, a patient suffers from repeated attacks of haemolysis separated by spontaneous remissions. Young and Miller (1953) described for instance a patient who had suffered from six episodes of acute haemolysis within 4 years of the initial attack for which splenectomy had been performed (see also Fig. 35.13, p. 475). According to Crosby (1955) and Crosby and Rappaport (1957), haemolytic crises are more frequent in the (cold) winter months. In children, as has been emphasized, the disease not infrequently appears as an acute (sometimes fulminating) disorder, fortunately often of relatively short duration (a matter of weeks or even days), but chronic and relapsing cases also occur (see p. 32).

Dreyfus, Dausset and Vidal (1951) referred to the occurrence of superficial thrombophlebitis and the frequent presence of gallstones (usually causing no symptoms) in long-standing cases.

Young, Miller and Christian (1951) and Young and Miller (1953) also mentioned thrombophlebitis as a troublesome symptom and as occurring repeatedly in association with haemolytic episodes.

The course of auto-immune haemolytic anaemia is thus unpredictable. Nevertheless, Dausset and Malinvaud (1954), while stressing that the course of the disease is very variable, thought that they found evidence in some patients of a fairly constant pattern: first, an acute or 'sensitization' phase; then a long-continued phase of 'compensated desensitization'. Eight patients out of their series recovered completely but it took on the average 3 years for this to happen.

Occasionally, the signs and symptoms of thrombocytopenic purpura are associated with or have preceded those of haemolytic anaemia [Evans's (Evans) syndrome (see p. 34)].

Amongst rarely recorded symptoms are precordial pain (with ECG evidence pointing to infarction) and headache (associated with an abnormal EEG), both attributed by Christen, Jaccottet and Wuilleret (1958) to microthrombi formed by agglutinated erythrocytes. Dreyfus, Dausset and Vidal (1951) recorded the presence in one of their patients of a complex neurological syndrome which cleared up almost completely when the haemolytic process was alleviated following splenectomy.

Idiopathic warm-antibody AIHA often starts without apparent cause, but sometimes there is a history of a recent infection of some sort: certainly clinical relapse may be precipitated in this way. Christen, Jaccottet and Wuilleret (1958) reported that a bee sting precipitated a relapse in one of their patients.

It is uncertain whether drug-taking is ever a precipitating factor. Where this has seemed possible [e.g. in de Gruchy's (1954) Case 6 who had received butazolidine] the patient's underlying disease may have been the more (or perhaps the only) important factor.

The relatively early reports summarized above give a detailed picture of the clinical syndromes of warm-antibody AIHA as witnessed by clinicians in the 1950s. They are particularly valuable because they illustrate the course of the disease at a time when corticosteroid therapy was only just being introduced and when for many patients blood transfusion and splenectomy had been the only treatments available. More recent reports often describe the symptoms and course of AIHA as modified by relatively effective treatment.

Valuable reviews published in the 1960s include those of Videbaek (1962), Schwartz and Costea (1966), Allgood and Chaplin (1967) and Pirofsky's (1969) monograph.

Schwartz and Costea (1966) commented that although the onset of idiopathic warm-antibody AIHA was generally insidious an abrupt onset with flu-like or abdominal symptoms was not rare. Symptoms were tolerated usually for 1–2 months before medical advice was sought; occasionally, weakness and fatigue had lasted for as much as 1 year. Allgood and Chaplin (1967) stated that in their series of 47 patients the mean duration of symptoms before diagnosis had been 6–9 months; the range was 10 days to 36 months. Pyrexia had been present at the onset in 27%. Pirofsky (1969, p. 33) recorded a lower incidence of pyrexia—18% (compared with 41% in his much larger series of secondary cases); he also made the point that the clinical pattern of the disease (in idiopathic cases) largely depended on the rate of erythrocyte destruction, the ability of the patient's bone marrow to compensate for this, the consequent rapidity with which the erythrocyte mass was reduced and the ability of the patient to 'acclimatize' to this reduction.

Prognosis and mortality. These important aspects are discussed in Chapter 35, pp. 497–502.

PHYSICAL SIGNS

The following descriptions generally refer to patients at the start of their illness or before it has been modified by treatment.

Pallor. This varies from mild to extremely severe. On the whole, patients with idiopathic AIHA tend to be more anaemic and are generally more seriously ill than are patients suffering from a hereditary haemolytic anaemia such as hereditary spherocytosis, and it is not uncommon for the erythrocyte count to be as low as $1.0-1.3 \times 10^{12}/l$ and the haemoglobin to be 3–5 g/dl in the most severely affected patients.

[In exceptionally severely affected patients, in addition to extreme pallor combined with jaundice there may be noticeable cyanosis, affecting particularly the lips, nose, cheeks and ears. This cyanosis is presumably secondary to peripheral vascular stasis brought about by intravascular auto-agglutination. Cyanosis occurs in a more marked and regular form in less anaemic and less seriously ill patients suffering from the cold-haemagglutinin disease (see p. 217). In a patient described by Sézary, Kipfer and Gharib (1938) cyanosis of the skin took the form of a network of violet bands ('livedo annularis'*). A similar appearance was observed by the writer in a patient, seen through the courtesy of Dr. J. Sakula (Dacie, 1962, Case 7), who had formed a most unusual and potent auto-antibody causing auto-agglutination at 37°C.]

Owren (1949) noted the phenomenon of 'sludged blood' in the conjunctival vessels of a severely anaemic male aged 74. (The patient's erythrocytes underwent agglutination *in vitro* in his own serum and in normal sera of the same blood-group.)

Jaundice. Usually the patient is visibly jaundiced to a moderate degree. The hyperbilirubinaemia is due as a rule in large measure to an excess of unconjugated bilirubin; the jaundice is thus typically acholuric in nature. In seriously ill patients, however, significant amounts of conjugated bilirubin may circulate in the plasma, the direct Hijmans van der Bergh reaction may be positive, and bile pigment may also appear in the urine. The presence of large amounts suggests actual liver damage, focal areas of necrosis being not uncommonly found in fatal cases (see p. 431). The data of Tisdale, Klatskin and Kinsella (1959) indicate that some conjugated bilirubin often finds its way into the blood stream when the rate of excretion of pigment is greatly accelerated.

Purpura. This is not commonly found (but see p. 34, under Evans syndrome).

Liver. The liver is often slightly enlarged, particularly in the most anaemic patients. According to Schwartz and Costea (1966), it is palpable in two-thirds of patients and is occasionally very tender. Pirofsky (1969, p. 34), however, recorded it as being palpable in only 32% of his 44 patients.

Liver function may be seriously affected in very seriously ill patients. Shirey and co-workers (1987), for instance, described how a female patient aged 22 had suffered from recurrent episodes of intravascular haemolysis. Her liver progressively enlarged and its function deteriorated. Eventually she died in hepatic coma. The liver failure was attributed to auto-agglutination within the liver sinuses (see also p. 431). The antibody responsible was most unusual; it was a warm-reacting IgM (see p. 113).

Spleen. The spleen is probably always considerably enlarged, varying, according to Dameshek and Schwartz (1940), from one-and-a-half to five times its normal size. Usually it is readily palpable; however, it may not be felt at the onset of an acute attack. It is unusual for an enlarged spleen to reach the umbilicus and on the whole the degree of splenomegaly is less than that found in hereditary spherocytosis (Rappaport and Crosby, 1957). Sometimes the spleen is tender on palpation; especially is this true in acute haemolytic episodes.

Schwartz and Costea (1966) stated that the spleen is palpable in approximately one-half of the patients at the time of diagnosis; they added that it might be expected to enlarge by approximately 0.5 cm as every month passes in an untreated case and also that the presence of a spleen greater than 8 cm in size should generate suspicion of an underlying malignancy. Pirofsky (1969, p. 34) recorded that the spleen was palpable in approximately 50% of his 44 idiopathic cases.

Lymph nodes. They are not usually significantly enlarged but the writer has seen one case where enlargement of the inguinal nodes due to myeloid metaplasia led to the clinical diagnosis of reticulosarcoma. Pirofsky (1969, p. 34) recorded enlarged lymph nodes in 23% of his 44 patients thought to suffer from the idiopathic disease.

Other physical signs. The other organs of the body usually appear to be essentially normal on physical examination except for the effects that anaemia may have on them.

---

*'Livedo annularis' was illustrated by Schubothe (1957); 'livedo reticularis' is an alternative term (see p. 267).

Unusual complications and associations

One most unusual complication is gangrene of the skin of the fingers and elsewhere. This was reported by Kölbl (1955) in an infant during an acute haemolytic episode which developed soon after vaccination; it was attributed to the effects of intravascular auto-agglutination. In another unusual case signs of cutaneous porphyria developed in an adult suffering from auto-immune haemolytic anaemia (Bousser et al., 1963).

The occurrence of warm-antibody AIHA in patients already suffering from a genetic defect affecting haemoglobin formation, i.e. sickle-cell disease, β°-thalassaemia, the Swiss type of HPFH, Hb-H disease and Hb-E, has already been referred to in Volume 2 of this book (pp. 56, 435, 441, 463).

Moskowitz (1970) described AIHA in a patient with erythrocyte G6PD deficiency.

Gasser (1954, p. 170) described a 3-year-old boy who responded satisfactorily to splenectomy for what appeared to be classical hereditary spherocytosis (HS). However, 3 weeks after the operation he became jaundiced again and was then found to have developed a DAT-positive AIHA. He recovered from this, and when re-examined 2 years later the DAT was found to be negative. Erythrocyte osmotic resistance had, however, persisted, as in typical HS after splenectomy.

Siddoo (1954) described a 47-year-old male, suffering from a subacute DAT-positive AIHA, who died as the result of loss of blood from oesophageal varices. At necropsy he was found to have had haemochromatosis complicated by a hepatoma.

Leonardi and Gregoris (1956) described a 17-year-old female who apparently developed PNH after she had recovered from an acute severe DAT-positive AIHA. Four years later all the tests for auto-immunization and for PNH had by then become negative.

AUTO-IMMUNE HAEMOLYTIC ANAEMIA IN PREGNANCY

Incidence. Haemolytic anaemia apparently appearing for the first time during the course of a pregnancy has been recognized for many years. Osler (1919), for instance, gave details of a case he referred to 'as a typical example of the so called toxic or haemolytic anaemia of pregnancy'. The patient, who had become severely anaemic in the last trimester of pregnancy, was delivered of a stillborn infant at the 7th month. After delivery her recovery was rapid and uninterrupted. It certainly seems possible that this patient had suffered from an auto-immune haemolytic anaemia. Witts (1932), too, in his third Goulstonian Lecture on the Pathology and Treatment of Anaemia, devoted half of it to the 'haemolytic anaemia of pregnancy'. This he regarded as a rare disease—one, however, with a copious but hardly critical literature. His definition was, however, precise. In his own words: 'for over a century it has been realised that there is a severe anaemia of pregnancy which affects women who were in perfect health before conception, which occurs in the absence of any signs of infection, and which disappears completely if the patient survives her pregnancy and puerperium'. Witts's knowledge of the disease was remarkably complete and accords—except in respect of a realization of its auto-immune origin —with present-day descriptions. He described how the disease usually began in the third trimester, reached a crisis at the time of delivery or in the puerperium and then typically subsided, usually completely, quickly thereafter. Delivery was often premature and the maternal death rate high, between 1917 and the time of his report (1932) approximately 30%. Witts made the significant point that there was a risk of relapse in subsequent pregnancies and that there were more records of relapse than of normal subsequent pregnancies. Recovery, he said, never took place until the fetus was expelled: it was (in the untransfused patient) associated 'with an outpouring of immature red cells and rapid regeneration of the blood'. He illustrated this in a figure based on data published by Jungmann (1914) (Fig. 22.2). The clinical and haematological findings in 'haemolytic anaemia of pregnancy' did not differ, Witts concluded, from those of 'acute haemolytic anaemia' affecting a non-pregnant person except for the fact of pregnancy.

Despite the many case reports in the literature, haemolytic anaemia of pregnancy was, and still is,

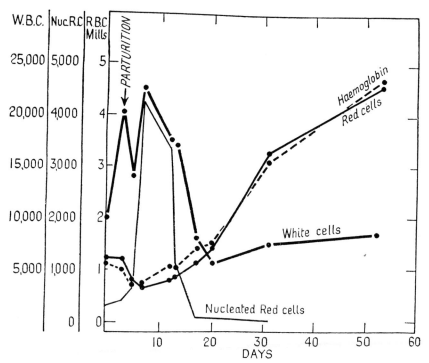

Fig. 22.2   Spontaneous recovery after parturition in a case of haemolytic anaemia of pregnancy.
[From Witts (1932).]

a rare disorder. Witts (1932), for instance, quoted Beckman (1921–1922) as describing six cases of severe pernicious or pernicious-like anaemia in 60 000 pregnancies in Vienna, between 1902 and 1920. Three of these patients may well have suffered from acquired haemolytic anaemia. Figures published more recently confirm its rarity.

Lillie, Gatenby and Moore (1954) described one such occurrence in 4,314 pregnancies. Borglin and Hackl (1964) referred to 10 similar cases out of a total of 34 cases of various types of haemolytic anaemias in pregnancy recorded in the literature between 1925 and 1960 and also to 10 patients of their own seen in a 10-year period. Borglin and Hackl stressed the frequency of crises of haemolysis and the high rate of abortion (22%) and that the perinatal mortality, including death from prematurity, was also high (9%).

The early reports mentioned above suffer inevitably from incomplete investigation and lack of a precise diagnosis. Lescher's (1942) series of eight patients thought to have suffered from acute haemolytic anaemia (Lederer type) come into this category. Haemolytic crises had developed *post partum* in the majority of the patients and in at least two instances sepsis appears to have been a major causal factor.

The history of the patient described by Bromberg, Toaff and Ehrenfeld (1948) is interesting. A woman aged 27 became severely anaemic in her eighth pregnancy (Hb 6.1 g/dl) and had a high reticulocyte count (24%). There was no previous history of anaemia. After delivery, improvement was spontaneous, but she remained anaemic (Hb 7.5–9 g/dl). After 4 years she became pregnant again; her haemoglobin fell to 4.5 g/dl and the reticulocyte count rose to 26%.

The subsequent descriptions in this chapter of 'haemolytic anaemia of pregnancy' refer solely to cases of proved auto-antibody causation or to cases in which an auto-immune causation appeared to be highly likely. [Pregnant women may suffer, of course, from many other types of haemolytic anaemia—from HS to PNH. It does, however, seem likely that 'haemolytic anaemia of pregnancy', as described by Witts (1932), is probably always of auto-immune causation.]

Case reports of AIHA in pregnancy

Amongst the early descriptions in the literature of apparent idiopathic warm-antibody AIHA are those of Evans and Duane [1949, Case 6 (F.R.), who was also severely thrombocytopenic], Frumin et al. (1953), Wagner and Maresch (1955) and Wirtheimer (1957).

More recent reports include those of Silverstein, Aaro and Kempers (1966), Swisher (1966) (Fig. 22.3), Letts and Kredenster (1968), de Groot (1969), Zara and Bolis (1972), Chaplin et al. (1973), Baumann and Rubin (1973), Vanhaeverbeck et al. (1974), Kageyama et al. (1975), Jain et al. (1977), Yam et al. (1980), Sacks, Platt and Johnson (1981), Sokol, Hewitt and Stamps (1982) and Issaragrisil and Kruatrachue (1983).

Sokol, Hewitt and Stamps (1982), who had written from a Blood Transfusion Centre, reviewed the clinical and serological records of 20 pregnant women in whom erythrocyte auto-

antibodies had been detected. Seven had suffered from overt haemolysis, while the direct antiglobulin test was positive in 17. It was concluded that auto-antibodies against erythrocytes were to be found in 1 in 50 000 pregnancies compared with an estimated incidence in a control population (non-pregnant females aged between 16 and 40) of 0.2 per 50 000.

The above accounts deal with patients in whom AIHA appeared apparently for the first time in pregnancy as well as with patients with established AIHA whose illness underwent an exacerbation during pregnancy.

Chaplin and co-workers (1973) were able to collect from the literature reports of haemolytic anaemia occurring in 19 pregnancies (16 patients) for which they considered that the evidence for an acquired origin was unequivocal and for which an auto-immune mechanism was certain or at least likely. The direct antiglobulin test on maternal erythrocytes was positive in seven pregnancies, negative in five and not carried out in seven. (In

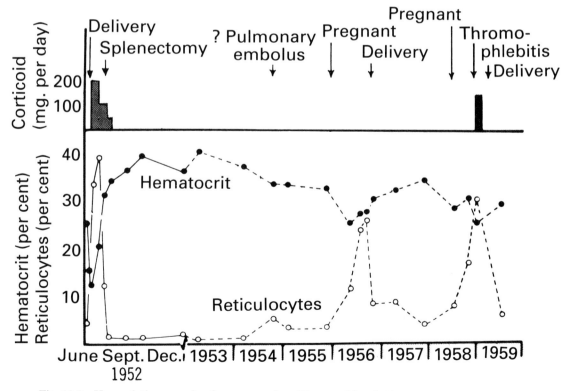

Fig. 22.3   Haemolytic anaemia of pregnancy in a 25-year-old patient.
Occurrence of AIHA in three successive pregnancies. [Reproduced by permission from Swisher (1966).]

the seven patients in whom the test was negative or had not been carried out and to whom corticosteroids had *not* been given, the diagnosis, Chaplin et al. admitted, remained in doubt.)

Chaplin and co-workers also described in considerable detail how their own patient, known to have suffered from relapsing haemolytic anaemia and thrombocytopenia, fared during pregnancy. Haemolysis accelerated in the 34–40th week and this was associated with a fall in the platelet count to $120 \times 10^9/l$. The patient responded well to carefully adjusted doses of prednisone and a live infant was delivered. Chaplin et al. pointed out that in the 19 cases they reviewed increased haemolysis had been present at conception in four; it was first documented during the pregnancy in the remainder, in four, however, not until the last trimester. The rate of haemolysis accelerated in 18 of the 19 patients as pregnancy proceeded: in nine pregnancies the haemoglobin fell to below 5 g/dl; in eight to within 5–8 g/dl. Following delivery, eight of the patients experienced complete remissions, eight partial remissions. Of particular interest is the acceptance by Chaplin et al. of five patients as probably suffering from auto-immune haemolysis despite the fact that the results of the direct antiglobulin test had been negative ('Coombs-negative AIHA'). A number of such cases have in fact been described (see below), and it is particularly interesting that quite often haemolytic anaemia has developed in more than one pregnancy, with apparent complete remission between pregnancies ('recurrent Coombs-negative AIHA in pregnancy').

'COOMBS-NEGATIVE' AIHA IN PREGNANCY

In 1941 the present author, in collaboration with the late Dr. E. ff. Creed and Professor P. L. Mollison, studied a patient who suddenly developed a severe haemolytic anaemia when 30 weeks pregnant. There was no spherocytosis but erythrocyte survival studies (published by Mollison, 1947) showed that transfused normal cells were completely eliminated (on two occasions) within 20 days. Caesarean section was

eventually carried out and the blood picture was found to be normal 4 months later. Of particular interest is the fact that this patient developed what appeared to be a similar episode in a subsequent pregnancy (in the late 1940s). On this occasion the direct antiglobulin test (DAT) carried out on a blood sample kindly provided by Professor W. M. Davidson was found to be negative. The status of this patient in the intervening years is not known.

The history of the patient described by Craig and Turner (1955) closely resembles that of Creed's patient (see above). She developed a severe haemolytic anaemia during the latter half of two successive pregnancies but in each instance recovered from the anaemia after delivery. Spherocytes were absent from the blood film, osmotic fragility was normal and all tests for auto-antibodies were negative. Transfusion produced only transient rises in haemoglobin and this was taken to indicate that the haemolytic mechanism was not an intrinsic one.

Burt and Prichard (1957), Bateman, Hutt and Norris (1959), Jankelowitz, Eckerling and Joshua (1960) and Mallarmé et al. (1965) described patients who developed severe haemolytic anaemia in pregnancy which appeared to respond to treatment with corticosteroids although the DAT was negative.

Ess and Friederici (1958) described a patient with a chronic, apparently acquired, haemolytic anaemia who had developed severe crises after infections and after pregnancy. The DAT was negative throughout. However, she appeared to respond to cortisone and prednisone.

The history of the patient described by Söderhjelm (1959) is especially interesting. At the age of 20 she developed thyrotoxicosis; when aged 21, and again when 23, she suffered from episodes of severe haemolytic anaemia complicated by megaloblastic change: when aged 30 and 35 she had further similar episodes of haemolytic anaemia when pregnant. The DAT was repeatedly found to be negative. Her first infant appeared to be normal; her second, although at first not anaemic, became progressively anaemic and jaundiced within 2 weeks of birth, and its spleen became palpable. Reticulocyte responses followed the administration in sequence of folic acid, liver and cortisone, and it eventually recovered completely.

Letts and Kredenster's (1968, 1969) reports are also particularly interesting. Their patient had a long history of Evans syndrome, starting with severe thrombocytopenia when 6 years old. She was splenectomized when aged 12. When aged 18, she developed severe AIHA with a positive DAT. One year later, when she was pregnant, haemolytic anaemia recurred and at 32 weeks she gave birth to a stillborn infant. Eluates from its erythrocytes showed that it had suffered from haemolytic anaemia serologically identical with that of its mother. Six months later the patient was pregnant again. This time, however, the blood picture at 38 weeks was apparently normal, the DAT was negative, and she gave birth to a healthy infant. Finally, as described by Letts and Kredenster (1969), during a third pregnancy she developed severe thrombo-cytopenia (platelet count 2 x 10^9/l), moderate anaemia (haemoglobin 8–10 g/dl) and a slightly raised serum bilirubin (1–2 mg/dl). The DAT was negative on this occasion and no free antibodies could be detected using enzyme-treated erythrocytes. She was delivered of an infant who recovered eventually after suffering from severe neonatal purpura. The patient herself remained severely thrombocytopenic after delivery and died of a cerebral haemorrhage 5 weeks later.

A further remarkable case was described by Eldor, Yatzin and Hershko (1975). Their patient, aged 25 at the time of a second pregnancy, had suffered from an undiagnosed anaemia during her first pregnancy. During her second pregnancy she again became anaemic and by the 8th month the haemoglobin was 7.0 g/dl with 9% reticulocytes. The DAT and indirect antiglobulin test were negative. A healthy girl was deliv-ered at term: at birth the infant was not anaemic, but when 4 weeks old its haemoglobin was found to have fallen to 7.8 g/dl; at 12 weeks it was 5.3 g/dl, with 15.2% reticulocytes, at which time it was transfused. It then appeared to recover spontaneously. Three days after delivery the ^{51}Cr T$_{50}$ of the erythrocytes of its mother (the patient) was only 9 days; 2 years later when her haemoglobin was 13.2 g/dl the ^{51}Cr T$_{50}$ was 20 days.

Four similar patients were described by Hershko et al. (1976). All were thought to have developed unequivocal signs of acquired haemolytic anaemia in seven pregnancies. An auto-immune mechanism was considered to be responsible, despite the fact that the DAT was persistently negative: transfused blood was destroyed rapidly and the patients responded favourably to corticosteroid therapy. Two of the infants developed transient haemolytic anaemia, and this was attributed to passage of auto-antibodies across the placenta.

Goodall and his co-workers (1979) described some interesting studies carried out on the blood of a 29-year-old woman who was 36 weeks pregnant and had developed a moderately severe haemolytic anaemia. She had previously been in good health and there was no evidence of haemolytic disease in other members of her family. The increased haemolysis gradually subsided after delivery. The DAT was negative and no unusual antibodies could be detected in her serum. There was slight spherocytosis.

Autohaemolysis was slightly increased and this was increased, not decreased, by the addition of glucose: it was, however, decreased by glucose and insulin. Goodall et al. suggested that the patient's erythrocytes had been altered by placental lactogen and/or prolactin in such a way as to make them abnormally dependent on insulin for the uptake of glucose. On the other hand, they were unable to exclude an immune origin for the haemolysis.

Yam and co-workers (1980) described three patients suffering from haemolytic anaemia during pregnancy. In two of them the DAT was positive; in the third it was, however, negative. 'I .... (third) patient was in the second trimester of her 8th pregnancy, and her haemoglobin was then 9.6 g/dl and there were 10.3% reticulocytes. (She had had a haematocrit of 29%, with 7% reticulocytes during her 7th pregnancy.) Spherocytes were obvious in blood films. Despite the DAT being negative when carried out by conventional means using standard antiglobulin sera, the comple-ment-fixation antibody consumption (CFAC) test of Gilliland, Leddy and Vaughan (1970) was positive: this test indicated an average of 212 antibody (IgG) molecules on each erythrocyte, the normal upper limit being 25 molecules per cell. The patient's anaemia was controlled satisfactorily by prednisone therapy. After delivery her reticulocyte count fell to normal and the CFAC test revealed less erythrocyte sensitization (52 molecules per cell, 2 weeks *post partum*). The infant was anaemic at birth and had an average of 250 molecules IgG on each erythrocyte, a value which fell to less than 25 (a normal result) 14 days later.

Whether positive CFAC tests would be obtainable in the majority of pregnant patients who suffer from 'Coombs-negative AIHA' is a matter for speculation. It seems probable that the test would be positive in those patients, at least, whose haemolysis can be readily controlled by corticosteroid therapy.

More recent reports of Coombs-negative AIHA in pregnancy include those of Starksen, Bell and Kickler (1983) and Lumley et al. (1991).

Starksen, Bell and Kickler (1983) described two patients of their own and reviewed the course of events in 10 other women (19 pregnancies in all). In 14 out of 18 pregnancies haemolysis was first noticed in the 1st or 2nd trimesters; it resolved within 5 months of delivery in each case. Haemolysis recurred in a second pregnancy in six out of 12 women and for the third time in two out of six women. All seven patients who were treated with corticosteroids responded favourably. Four out of the 19 infants born to the affected mothers suffered from transient haemolysis.

Lumley and co-workers (1991) described in an abstract how they had treated a 25-year-old pregnant woman with a transfusion-dependent DAT-negative acquired haemolytic anaemia by means of intravenous IgG at a high dosage (5g/kg within 8 days). She responded partially and her transfusion requirement was reduced to one-third. She was subsequently maintained on a reduced dose of IgG (2 g/kg within 10 days) and was eventually delivered at 37 weeks of an unaffected infant. This was the patient's third pregnancy. Remarkably, she had similarly suffered from transfusion-dependent haemolytic anaemia in two previous pregnancies. Between pregnancies, haemolysis had persisted but at a reduced rate which she had been able to compensate for.

AIHA IN PREGNANCY: PROGNOSIS FOR THE PATIENT AND FOR HER INFANT

The reports outlined above indicate that AIHA occurring in pregnancy may have serious consequences, both for the patient and for her infant. Fortunately, the occurrence is relatively rare. In patients suffering from a pre-existing AIHA who become pregnant, anaemia typically becomes more severe, especially in the last trimester, and blood transfusion may then be necessary. Corticosteroids are, however, usually of benefit, and they do not seem to harm the developing fetus if given in only moderate dosage. The perinatal mortality and the incidence of stillbirth are, however, both increased; and an infant born to a severely affected mother may be expected to show signs of haemolytic disease of the newborn, i.e., transient auto-immune haemolytic anaemia (see below).

The role of pregnancy in causing exacerbations of auto-immune diseases in general was discussed in an interesting review by Gleicher (1986). Both improvement and exacerbation have been reported in SLE for instance. In some cases, when there is exacerbation, this is particularly severe in the immediate post-partum period, reflecting perhaps 'rebound' after a period of enhanced suppressor cell activity.

TRANSIENT AIHA IN INFANTS BORN TO MOTHERS SUFFERING FROM WARM-ANTIBODY AIHA

As referred to above, women affected with warm-antibody AIHA have given birth to infants showing signs of overt increased haemolysis. Jaundice often increases rapidly after birth and exchange transfusion may be required. The DAT is likely to be positive and auto-antibody probably demonstrable in the infant's serum. Increased haemolysis eventually, however, subsides; and the infants may be expected to become perfectly normal in a matter of weeks or a few months. Some infants, however, have appeared normal at birth and have shown no obvious signs of increased haemolysis.

Burt and Prichard (1957) reported that the haemoglobin of the infant born to their patient, who had suffered from 'Coombs-negative' AIHA, fell to 11.1 g/dl and that the infant's serum bilirubin rose to 27 mg/dl. Recovery followed two exchange transfusions. The first infant born to Letts and Kredenster's (1968) patient, who had suffered from long-continued severe Evans syndrome, was stillborn and showed signs of erythroblastosis. Elution of antibody from its erythrocytes showed that it was similar to that coating its mother's erythrocytes. Her third infant was born with severe thrombocytopenia but the DAT was negative—as was the test carried out on her own erythrocytes at this period in her illness.

Chaplin and his co-workers (1973) reported that the infant of the patient they had followed in detail throughout her pregnancy suffered from hyperbilirubinaemia within 48 hours of birth. Its haemoglobin, at birth 18.4 g/dl, with 6.5% reticulocytes, fell to half the cord-blood level at the 8th week. The DAT was weakly positive at birth; it was barely positive at 70 days and clearly negative at 110 days. Chaplin et al. recorded in their review of 19 cases of AIHA in pregnancy that seven of the infants were reported to have given positive antiglobulin tests.

Yam and co-workers (1980), who described three patients in detail—one with a negative DAT, reported that one of their infants gave a weakly positive test, although it was not anaemic, the second a negative test, despite the fact that the test was positive with the mother's erythrocytes, and the third a negative test—this was the infant born to the mother whose erythrocytes also failed to react with the standard reagents. It was particularly interesting to note that this infant's cells, nevertheless, were shown to carry on an average 250 molecules of IgG at birth—10 times the normal amount. The baby was then anaemic; within 14 days, however, the average IgG load had fallen to 25 molecules.

As already mentioned, Starksen, Bell and Kickler (1983), who reviewed the outcome of 19 pregnancies in women suffering from Coombs-negative AIHA in pregnancy, reported that four of the infants born to the affected mothers had suffered from transient haemolysis.

AUTO-IMMUNE HAEMOLYTIC ANAEMIA IN INFANCY AND CHILDHOOD

It has been realized for many years that children, even young infants, might suffer from acquired haemolytic anaemia of obscure origin and that the disorder, although rare, might be of great severity, with a sudden onset and signs of massive haemolysis. Indeed, three of Lederer's (1925, 1930) six patients described as suffering from 'acute hemolytic anemia (probably of infectious origin)' were children aged 16 months, 6 months and 3 years, respectively. The disease in these children was of short duration and they all recovered after being transfused. In retrospect, it is not, of course, possible to be certain that they had suffered from auto-immune haemolytic anaemia but this may well have been so. The same comment applies to other early descriptions of acute haemolysis of short duration affecting children published subsequent to Lederer's reports and before the introduction of the antiglobulin test, e.g. by Lazarus (1930), Parsons (1931), Parsons and Hawksley (1933), Dunlop and Sanders (1934), Patterson and Stewart Smith (1936), Giordano and Blum (1937, Case 1), Baxter and Everhart (1938), Hamilton (1939), Atkinson (1940), Hoyer (1941), David and Minot (1944), Meier (1944), Murano (1946), Fisher (1947, Cases 13 and 14), Lamy et al. (1950) and Berrey and Watson (1951).

As already referred to (p. 8), Parsons (1931), in his account of the anaemias of infancy and early childhood, mentioned under the heading of anaemia due to infection the occurrence in small children of an acute and grave anaemia which was characterized by a spontaneous and rapid recovery. Their blood picture was reported to be 'typical of a severe destruction of red blood cells with an intense marrow reaction', with the 'circulation flooded with reticulated red cells'. Three children were mentioned in which the disease had run an acute short course and two in which it was more chronic. Parsons and Hawksley's (1933) review has also been referred to earlier (p. 8). Atkinson's (1940) account of Lederer's anaemia is also valuable. Thirty children (21 were male, 9

female) and 29 adults were referred to, all described in the literature between 1925 and 1938. The children were aged between 5 months and 13 years; haemoglobinuria had occurred in eleven of them; seven died, 23 had recovered. Details of their blood counts were also given: the minimum erythrocyte count recorded was $0.52 \times 10^{12}/l$; the maximum leucocyte count was $97 \times 10^9/l$.

Following the introduction of the antiglobulin test, it did not take long for it to be realized that young patients did indeed suffer from AIHA and that the disorder in childhood often differed substantially with respect to clinical manifestations and course, and in haematological and serological findings, from that seen most frequently in adults. Perhaps because of these differences, and because of its often dramatic nature, the literature on AIHA in childhood is, despite the rarity of the disease, quite extensive. To summarize its main characteristics: its onset is often sudden — over perhaps a few days at the most; often, although by no means always, the attack has been preceded by an overt infection, often presumed to be viral; haemolysis is often massive, the erythrocyte count falling perhaps to less than $1.0 \times 10^{12}/l$ if the patient is not transfused; there may be haemoglobinuria; slightly more male than female children are affected; the prognosis is relatively good, with most of the children recovering completely, well within 3 months; most of the children respond to high-dose corticosteroid therapy, and splenectomy need seldom be contemplated; severe haemolysis may be accompanied by hyperleucocytosis; thrombocytopenia is uncommon but does occur; the serological findings are variable — in the majority of cases the antibodies are of the warm type, with or without complement components (e.g. C3d) adsorbed to erythrocytes; cold antibodies, except for the Donath–Landsteiner antibody, are rarely responsible for the haemolysis.

Recent reviews dealing with the course and

Table 22.3 Selected case reports in chronological order of auto-immune haemolytic anaemia in infants and children.

Reference	Sex and age of patient	Summary of clinical features and haematological findings	Serological findings
Denys and van den Broucke (1947)	M. 7½ months	Sudden onset of severe haemolysis; transfused, eventually splenectomized. Marked erythroblastaemia	DAT and IAT pos
Meyer (1951)	M. 13 months	Sudden onset of severe haemolysis. Transfused; eventually recovered after ACTH therapy	DAT pos
Gasser and Holländer (1951, 1952)	7 weeks	Sudden onset of severe haemolysis and thrombocytopenia; 'pseudoleukaemic lymphocytosis'; erythrophagocytosis. Died	DAT and IAT pos; complete and incomplete auto-antibodies; erythrocytes 'polyagglutinable'
Gasser (1952)	F. 5½ years	Acute onset of haemolysis 1 week after otitis media. Haemoglobinuria and purpura. Died	DAT strongly pos
Gasser (1952)	M. 3 years	Appeared at first to have classic HS. Splenectomy. 3 weeks later haemolytic crisis; erythrophagocytosis	DAT at first neg; strongly pos at time of haemolytic crisis
Betke et al. (1953)	3 years	Sudden onset of severe haemolysis 10 days after Coxsackie A-virus infection; erythrophagocytosis, reticulocytopenia	DAT pos; cold-agglutinin titre 128
Rose and Nabarro (1953) (All four patients became ill within a 16-day period)	(1) F. 6 months	Sudden onset of severe haemolysis. Treated with ACTH; eventually recovered	DAT pos
	(2) F. 3 years	Sudden onset of severe haemolysis. Treated with ACTH; eventually recovered	DAT not undertaken at onset; neg when recovering
	(3) F. 8 years	Sudden onset of severe haemolysis. Recovered after a single blood transfusion	DAT not undertaken at onset: pos at 18th week when recovered; eventually neg
	(4) M. 8 years	Sudden onset of severe haemolysis. Transfused. Responded to ACTH but relapsed several times. Splenectomy ineffective; eventually recovered	DAT pos; still pos 30 weeks after onset
Chaptal et al. (1954)	M. 18 months	Sudden onset of acute haemolysis after atypical pneumonia. Eventually died after three crises	DAT pos
Bowman (1955)	F. 22 months	Pallor for 1 year; eventually severe haemolysis. Recurrent purulent otitis media; reticulocytopenia; exchange transfusion; relapse responded to cortisone	DAT pos
Niemann et al. (1956)	M. 1 year	Sudden onset of severe haemolysis (?) following influenza A-virus infection. Treated with corticosteroids and splenectomy. Recovered in 2 months	DAT pos
O'Connor, Vakiener and Watson (1956)	(1) F. 4 years	Subacute onset of severe haemolysis; mumps preceded onset. Treated with ACTH and splenectomy; recovered after c. 1 year	DAT pos
	(2) F. 8 months	Sudden onset of acute haemolysis. Remissions with corticosteroids; relapses following infections. Splenectomy little influence	DAT pos
Dausset et al. (1957)	M. 2½ years	Sudden onset of acute haemolysis; haemoglobinuria for 4 days. Recovered after transfusions and steroids	DAT pos; warm haemolysin present

Table 22.3 (*contd*)

Reference	Age/Sex	Clinical course	Serology
Larson (1957)	(1) 13 months	10 weeks' history of haemolysis. Many transfusions; little response to ACTH. Died	DAT pos
	(2) F. 12 years	1 month's history of haemolysis. Responded to ACTH and cortisone; eventually recovered	DAT pos
Miller, Shumway and Young (1957)	(1) 13 months	Sudden onset of haemolysis. Gradual response to cortisone	DAT pos
	(2) M. 8 years	Chronic haemolysis. Splenectomy ineffective; gradual response to steroids	DAT pos
	(3) F. 14 years	Acute onset; 14 days' haemoglobinuria. Gradual recovery	DAT pos
Saxena and Saraswat (1957)	5 months	Responded to prednisone	DAT pos; neg after treatment with prednisone
Horveno et al. (1958)	F. 5 months	Splenectomy followed by rapid recovery	DAT pos; neg on recovery
Colletta, Schettini and di Francesco (1959)	M. 11 months	Recovered after corticosteroid therapy	
Di Piero (1959)	M. 4 years, 7 months	Responded to cortisone	DAT pos
Gelli and Vignale (1959)	M. 4 years	Acute onset; then relapsing course with haemolysis persisting for 18 months	DAT pos; neg after treatment with cortisone
Roget, Beaudoing and Jobert (1959)	14 months	Died despite many transfusions, ACTH and corticosteroid therapy and splenectomy	
Laski et al. (1960, 1961)	(1) M. $5\frac{1}{2}$ months	Sudden onset of severe haemolysis. Given numerous transfusions and prednisone. Spontaneous remission after 5 weeks	DAT pos. Anti-e and anti-f in serum
	(2) M. $2\frac{1}{2}$ months	Sudden onset of severe haemolysis. Given many transfusions and prednisone. Remitted after 3 months	DAT neg at first, then pos. Anti-D in serum
Negri, Pototschnig and Mailo (1960)	9 months	Severe haemolysis. Died after 3 months despite many transfusions, including four exchange transfusions	DAT and IAT pos
Cortesi (1961)	F. 16 months	Sudden onset of severe haemolysis. Treated with corticosteroids, ACTH and transfusion. Recovered	DAT and IAT pos
Coutel, Bretagne and Morel (1962)	M. 9 years	Sudden onset of severe haemolysis; moderate thrombocytopenia. Transfusions and exchange transfusion resulted in only transient benefit. Remitted when given ACTH and corticosteroid	DAT and IAT pos
Günther and Bube (1962)	M. $3\frac{1}{2}$ years	Sudden onset of severe haemolysis; also severe thrombocytopenia and reticulocytopenia. Recovered completely after 10 weeks	DAT and IAT pos

Table 22.3 (*contd*)

Ritz and Haber (1962)	M. 6 weeks	Sudden onset of severe haemolysis; reticulocytopenia. Received transfusions, ACTH and prednisone. Relapsing course; at 17 months slightly anaemic, with 3.5% reticulocytes	DAT and IAT pos; DAT still pos at 17 months
Wilmers and Russell (1963)	F. $2\frac{1}{2}$ months	Sudden onset of severe haemolysis 24 hours after injection of triple antigen. Given many transfusions; failed to respond to steroids and splenectomy. Remitted about 2 weeks after thymectomy (see p. 483)	DAT and IAT pos
de Veber (1964)	M. 6 years	Sudden onset of severe haemolysis; haemoglobinuria. Transfused twice; recovered quickly	DAT not possible because erythrocytes lysed. IAT weak pos
Gross and Newman (1964)	M. $9\frac{1}{2}$ months	Insidious onset of haemolysis. Severe anaemia. Received transfusions and prednisone. Recovered after c. 200 days	DAT and IAT pos. Anti-D and non-specific auto-antibody
Scholer and Germano (1964)	M. 13 years	Subacute onset of severe haemolysis. Received ACTH and recovered within 3 months; relapsed after 2 years, then remitted and no further relapses for 6 years	DAT pos. Anti-e auto-antibody
Oski and Abelson (1965)	F. 8 weeks	Sudden onset of severe haemolysis, associated with reticulocytopenia and thrombocytopenia. Died after an illness lasting c. $4\frac{1}{2}$ months. Had failed to respond to corticosteroids, 6MP, thymectomy and splenectomy	DAT pos. Anti-M, anti-c and anti-E auto-antibodies.
Seip, Harboe and Cyvin (1969, Case 2)	F. 12 years	Thrombocytopenia, haemolysis and neutropenia starting 1 week after a respiratory illness. Received blood transfusions and prednisone. Remitted after 2–3 months	DAT pos (anti-IgG pos, anti-C trace)
Hirooka et al. (1970)	M. $3\frac{1}{2}$ years	Subacute onset of haemolysis. Treated by blood transfusions, corticosteroids and splenectomy for over 2 years without sustained benefit. Eventually thymectomized, with gradual improvement over next 2 years	DAT pos, mixed γ and non-γ type
Bossi and Wagner (1972)	M. 5 months	Onset 3 weeks after triple vaccine inoculation. Severe haemolysis. Cytomegalovirus isolated from urine. Received blood transfusions and prednisone without sustained benefit; after 2 months given azathioprine and remitted	DAT pos (anti-IgG pos, anti-IgM weak, anti-C neg). Anti-f (ce) and anti-c auto-antibodies
Lamagnère et al. (1972)	F. 32 months M. 15 months	Sudden onset of haemolysis 4–8 days after acute throat infection	{ DAT pos (anti-IgG neg, anti-IgM, anti-C pos)
Peters et al. (1974)	M. 6 weeks	Sudden onset of severe haemolysis. Treated by blood transfusions and exchange transfusions without sustained benefit; responded to corticosteroids and recovered within 2 months. Developed rise in antibody titre to cytomegalovirus	DAT pos (anti-IgG pos, anti-C pos)

Table 22.3 *(contd)*

Reference	Sex, age	Clinical notes	DAT
Johnson and Abildgard (1976)	F. 4 months	Acute onset of haemolysis. Failed to respond to ACTH, heparin, cyclophosphamide and splenectomy. Died	DAT strongly pos
	M. 4 months	Acute onset of haemolysis. Failed to respond to corticosteroids, azathioprine, splenectomy and thymectomy. Died after an illness lasting 7 months	DAT strongly pos. 7S warm agglutinin; no specificity demonstrated
Hegde, Gordon-Smith and Worlledge (1977)	F. 9 years	Acute onset of severe haemolysis; reticulocytopenia lasting 3 months. Received blood transfusions and prednisone without sustained benefit; remitted following splenectomy	DAT persistently neg
Haneberg et al. (1978)	M. 4 months	Acute onset of haemolysis 4 days after 2nd injection of DPT vaccine	DAT pos
	F. 7 months	Acute onset of haemolysis 2 days after 2nd injection of DPT vaccine	DAT pos
	M. $10\frac{1}{2}$ months	Acute onset of haemolysis; had had polio vaccine at $3\frac{1}{2}$, $4\frac{1}{2}$ and $5\frac{1}{2}$ months and DTP vaccine at 9 months	DAT pos
Miyazaki et al. (1980)	M. 10 years	Severe haemolysis, developing 6 years after onset of Duchenne's muscular dystrophy	DAT pos (anti-IgG pos, anti-C pos)
Carapella de Luca et al. (1984)	F. 8 months	Severe haemolysis; reticulocytopenia and marrow erythroid hypoplasia. Relapsing course; eventually remitted after *c.* 18 months from onset. Received transfusions, prednisone and azathioprine without sustained benefit.	DAT pos (anti-IgG pos, anti-IgM weak pos, anti-C3d pos)

pos = positive, neg = negative.
DAT = direct antiglobulin test.

prognosis, and the clinical and serological findings, in quite large series of patients include those of Zuelzer et al. (1970), Habibi *et al.* (1974), Buchanan, Boxer and Nathan (1976), Zupánska et al. (1976), Carapella de Luca et al. (1979), Heisel and Ortega (1983), Miyazaki et al. (1983) and Sokol et al. (1984).

Early case reports, incorporating the results of serological investigations, include those of Denys and van den Brouke (1947), Debré et al. (1950), Gasser and Holländer (1951, 1952), Gasser (1952, 1954), Millichap (1952), Betke et al. (1953), Chaptal et al. (1954), Bowman (1955), Fontan et al. (1955), Neimann et al. (1956), O'Connor, Vakiener and Watson (1956), Dausset et al. (1957), Miller, Shumway and Young (1957), Larson (1957), Saxena and Saraswat (1957), Verger and Moulinier (1957), Sansone (1957), Christen, Wuilleret and Jaccottet (1958), Coletta and Schettini (1958), Horveno et al. (1958), Roget, Beaudoing and Jobert (1959), Di Piero (1959) and Coletta, Schettini and di Francesco (1959) (see also Table 22.3).

The majority of the infants referred to in the above reports were aged between 2 and 18 months. Debré and co-workers (1950), however, mentioned that two of their five patients had been infants as young as 15 and 19 days old, respectively. Negri, Pototschnig and Maiolo (1960) reviewed the literature and reported a further case of their own—a 9-month-old infant. The 29 case reports they reviewed dealt with infants aged between 2 and 13 months of which eight had died. In the 1950s the outlook for an affected child was thus serious, despite the fact that the majority recovered apparently completely and often quite rapidly.

Significant case reports published in the 1960s and 1970s, and subsequently, include those of Laski et al. (1960, 1961), Cortesi (1961), Coutel et al. (1962), Günther and Bube (1962), Ritz and Haber (1962), Bartolozzi et al. (1963), Wilmers and Russell (1963), de Veber (1964), Gross and Newman (1964), Scholer and Germano (1964), Oski and Abelson (1965), Seip, Harboe and Cyvin (1969), Hirooka et al. (1970), Paolucci et al. (1970), Bossi and Wagner (1972), Lamagnère et al. (1972), Peters et al. (1974), Carapella-de-Luca et al. (1976), Johnson and Abildgard (1976), Hegde, Gordon-Smith and Worlledge (1977), Haneberg et al. (1978) and Becton and Kinney (1986) (see also Table 22.3). Homberg, Bonnet-Gajdos and Salmon (1970), in a review, referred to 12 patients with AIHA, out of a total of 420 studied at a Blood Transfusion Centre between 1936 and 1968, who were infants or small children aged between 1 month and 4 years in age.

More recent case reports of outstanding interest include those of Greenberg et al. (1980), Issitt et al. (1982), Carapella De Luca et al. (1984), Becton and Kinney (1986), Sander, Hardy and van Meter (1987) and Hadnagy (1989).

Age

As already mentioned, young children, often less than 1 year old, are most frequently affected. Data reported by recent reviewers are summarized below. It is particularly interesting to note that when the cases are stratified into acute or subacute and chronic categories, it is the younger children in particular who have suffered from the more acute (and more transient) illnesses.

Homberg, Bonnet-Gajdos and Salmon (1970) recorded that of 59 patients aged 20 or less, thirty were less than 4 years of age. Zuelzer et al. (1970) reported similarly: of 28 patients aged 14 years or less, 18 were less than 4 years old; eight were aged less than 1 year.

Habibi and co-workers' (1974) series comprised 80 children. The peak incidence was during the first 4 years of life (Fig. 22.4). Of 34 children categorized as acute transient cases, 28 (82%) were less than 4 years of age. Compared to this high percentage, only 21 (46%) of 46 children who suffered from chronic AIHA were in this age-group.

Zupańska et al. (1976) reported similarly: seven out of 13 children with acute illnesses had been less than 5 years of age, compared to six out of 12 children with subacute illnesses and none of the six children who had had a chronic illness.

Data reported more recently from Italy, Japan, England and West Germany have provided support for the same two points: namely, that AIHA in children predominately affects young children and infants and that this is particularly true of acute cases of short duration.

Carapella de Luca and co-workers (1979), who reviewed the clinical, haematological and serological data in 29 cases, found that 19 of the children were less

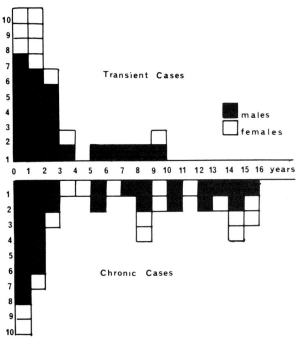

Fig. 22.4   Age distribution in 80 children with AIHA.
[Reproduced by permission from Habibi et al. (1974).]

Sex

In contrast to AIHA in adults, male rather than female infants and children seem to be predominately affected. Thus, out of a total of 216 infants and children referred to in eight review papers summarized in the previous section 126 were male and 90 female. There are indications, too, that the male predominance is greater in younger children, and in those who are acutely ill, than in older children and in those with a more chronic illness.

Homberg, Bonnet-Gajdos and Salmon (1970) stated that of 12 children aged less than 4 years, seven had been males; and Zuelzer et al. (1970) reported that ten out of 18 children aged 4 years or less were males, compared with three males to seven females in the group who were more than 5 years of age.

Habibi et al. (1974) recorded a male to female ratio of 27 : 10 in acutely ill children less than 10 years of age, compared to 29 : 17 in chronically ill children aged less than 16 years (Fig. 22.4).

Zupańska et al. (1976) reported that 17 out of 31 children aged between 3 months and 14 years had been males; and Carapella de Luca et al. (1979) stated that 18 out of 29 children under 12 years of age had been males. Miyazaki and co-workers' (1983) figures were 9 males to 7 females in a group of acutely ill children, compared with 7 males to 11 females in those who had had a chronic illness. Sokol and co-workers (1984) reported that the male to female ratio had been 2.5 : 1 in children less than 5 years of age; in older children, however, both sexes had been equally affected. Seven out of the 12 children aged less than 6 years, referred to by Salama and Mueller-Eckhardt (1987), had been females.

than 4 years of age. Miyazaki and co-workers (1983) reported on 34 children: 16 of them had suffered from acute AIHA; 14 were less than 4 years of age. Sokol and co-workers (1984) reported that 65% of 42 children they had investigated for AIHA had been seen before their 5th birthday. Salama and Mueller-Eckhart (1987), who described a series of 12 children who had presented with warm-antibody AIHA associated with unusual serological findings [the presence of non-complement-fixing IgM auto-antibodies (see p. 128)], reported that eight were infants under 1 year of age.

Hadnagy (1989) described what is possibly a unique occurrence. His patient was an infant girl who was deeply jaundiced at birth in July 1976. The DAT was positive although there was no evidence of feto/maternal incompatibility. In 1977 and 1978 the child was found to be moderately severely anaemic and to have 14%–23% reticulocytes. The DAT was still positive; it became transitorily negative after prednisone therapy only to become positive again when the dose of prednisone was reduced. Splenectomy was carried out when the child was $3\frac{1}{2}$ years old. Haemolysis persisted after the operation although it was less intense; it was still continuing in June 1989 when the child was last examined. Her serum immunoglobulins were apparently normal except that before splenectomy the IgA had been as low as 60 mg/dl. There was no family history of anaemia.

COURSE: PRODROMAL FEATURES, INTENSITY AND DURATION OF HAEMOLYSIS, COMPLICATIONS, PROGNOSIS AND MORTALITY

The often-reported frequency of an antecedent, acute infection, suspected of being, or established as, of viral origin has already been referred to. In Homberg, Bonnet-Gajdos and Salmon's (1970) 12 patients, there was a rapid onset of haemolysis, with overt haemoglobinuria in at least some of them, which had developed, associated with pyrexia, 3–10 days after an attack of rhinopharyngitis and laryngotracheitis. The children's spleen was not as a rule palpable at the onset of their illness, but the liver was usually enlarged. Within 2 months they had recovered completely. [The serological findings in this series of patients were characteristic and almost uniform. The direct antiglobulin test was positive with an anti-complement serum and often positive, too, with an anti-yM (IgM) serum; it was negative with an anti-yG (IgG) serum.] Homberg, Bonnet-Gajdos and Salmon emphasized the similarity between the clinical picture they had observed and the earlier descriptions of Lederer (1925) and Brill (1926).

Zuelzer and his co-workers (1970) reported on three categories of patients, 28 in all:

1. In seven children, aged between 10 weeks and $3\frac{1}{2}$ years, haemolysis had begun acutely, accompanied by pyrexia; it was preceded or accompanied in two children by diarrhoea, in two by a respiratory tract infection. Enlargement of the spleen and a slight generalized enlargement of lymph nodes were present. Atypical lymphocytes were noted in their blood. Six of these children recovered, with or without corticosteroid therapy, in 1–4 months. One child died in the acute phase, and at necropsy there was evidence of widespread infection with cytomegalovirus (CMV). Their serum immunoglobulins were generally normal.

2. In eight children, aged between 4 months and 13 years, the onset of haemolysis was acute in six, indeterminate in two. Their illness was prolonged, lasting from 1 to 6 years, but all eventually recovered. One child had a transient butterfly rash; a minor degree of lymph-node enlargement was a frequent feature. Two children had recurrent thrombocytopenia, two had repeated respiratory tract infections.

3. This group comprised 13 children aged 4 months to 13 years and a premature newborn infant in whose blood CMV had been detected. The onset of haemolysis was indeterminate or acute, and its duration was prolonged, up to 11 years. Seven of the children suffered from growth failure, and intercurrent infections or other complications were frequent; eight of the children died. The serum immunoglobulins were frequently abnormal; IgA was absent in two of the children and its concentration subnormal in three.

Of the 80 patients referred to by Habibi et al.

(1974), 34 had illnesses categorized as acute and transient. In 23 of the children haemolysis appeared to have been precipitated by well-defined infections: most had had rhinopharyngitis, but there were single instances of pneumonia, measles, varicella and viral hepatitis. In 21 of the children the onset was sudden: 15 had had haemoglobinuria and some had suffered from a shock-like state. In contrast, 13 children became anaemic within 2–3 days without particular abruptness. The spleen became moderately enlarged in 10 children and the liver became 'mildly' enlarged in eight (all infants). Underlying disorders were uncommon, as opposed to their frequency in chronic cases (see below). None of the children died: all recovered within 3 months of the onset of their illness. The remaining 46 patients referred to by Habibi et al. had chronic illnesses, and an underlying or associated disorder was present in 24 of them, ITP, SLE or a complex immune deficiency syndrome being the most frequent. The onset was acute in only one-third of the cases. Once established, the increased haemolysis was intermittent or continuous, and the childrens' illness lasted for months or years. Seventeen of them, however, eventually recovered; but nine died, mostly of complications of an underlying disorder.

Zupańska and co-workers (1976) referred to 44 children of whom 31 had warm-antibody acute, subacute or chronic AIHA and 13 cold-antibody acute or chronic AIHA. In over 50% the onset had been preceded by an acute infection or immunization; in 16% there was evidence of a chronic underlying disorder. In the latter group haemolysis was prolonged. Eleven of the 13 acutely-ill children recovered completely; two, however, died of complications, e.g. haemorrhage, pneumonia, renal failure. Zupańska et al. stressed that the prognosis was in general good and that death was unlikely to be caused by anaemia *per se*; severe thrombocytopenia was, however, an adverse factor.

Of the 29 children referred to by Carapella de Luca et al. (1979), 15 had transient AIHA (lasting less than 3 months) and 14 chronic AIHA (persisting for more than 3 months). Eight children in each series had had a prodromal acute infection and the onset of haemolysis had been acute in approximately half of those in each series. In three children there was evidence of CMV infection. Four of the children in the transient AIHA group and six in the chronic AIHA group had autoimmune-related underlying disorders. Fourteen

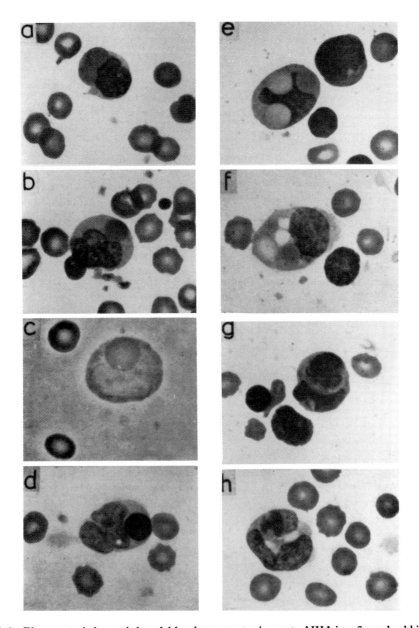

Fig. 22.5   Phagocytosis by peripheral-blood monocytes in acute AIHA in a 7-week-old infant.
[Reproduced by permission from Gasser and Holländer (1951).]

patients recovered fully; eight died, three of a lymphoma, one of immunodeficiency and renal failure, two of hyperacute haemolysis (associated in one with renal failure) and two of unknown causes.

Miyazaki and co-workers (1983) described the course of illness in 34 Japanese children. Sixteen had an acute transient illness preceded by an acute infection in 14 of them; four had haemoglobinuria. Eighteen children had suffered from chronic haemolysis, and this had been preceded by an acute infection in only two of

them. Four children in this group had an underlying disorder, compared with none of the children in the acute group. Twenty-six patients eventually recovered fully; in four haemolysis persisted. Four died (11.8%): all of them had an underlying illness — lymphoma, muscular dystrophy, SLE or severe combined immunodeficiency.

Sokol and co-workers' (1984) series of AIHA patients comprised 42 children and adolescents; it included 16 children with warm-antibody AIHA and

17 who had developed paroxysmal cold haemoglobin-uria (PCH) associated with the Donath–Landsteiner antibody. In 28 patients haemolysis had appeared to follow an acute infection, and in most cases the onset had been acute. Recovery had usually been rapid and 83% of the patients recovered fully in less than 6 months. Two patients only had an underlying auto-immune-related disorder, i.e. SLE or polyarthropathy. Two patients died: one was a girl aged 3 years and 9 months who died of hyperacute haemolysis within 12 hours of admission to hospital; the other was a boy aged 14 years who died of a haemolytic crisis and miliary tuberculosis 4 years after the onset of haemolysis and subsequent apparent complete recovery—he had developed, too, thrombocytopenia for which he had undergone splenectomy 1 year before his death.

Many of the case reports that have been already referred to are of very great interest and, while there is often a close general similarity between the clinical and laboratory findings, each case has, too, as might be expected, its own unique features.

Gasser and Holländers' (1951, 1952) patient was a male infant who, after a normal birth, developed hyperacute haemolysis and severe thrombocytopenia when 7 weeks old. There was, too, initially a remarkable 'pseudoleukaemic' leucocytosis of 60×10^9 cells per litre of which 50×10^9/l were small lymphocytes. This leucocytosis subsided to 8.5×10^9 cells per litre 6 days after admission to hospital and blood transfusion. In an attempt to correct increasing thrombocytopenia, splenectomy was carried out but the child died of haemorrhage shortly afterwards. An unusual feature was the presence of many monocytes acting as erythrophages in the peripheral blood (Fig. 22.5), and particularly in venous blood from the spleen. Monocytes in blood from the spleen could, too, be seen phagocytosing neutrophils and platelets, and it was concluded that the child had formed auto-antibodies against neutrophils and platelets as well as against erythrocytes.

AUTO-IMMUNE HAEMOLYTIC ANAEMIA IN ASSOCIATION WITH IDIOPATHIC THROMBOCYTOPENIC PURPURA (ITP) (EVANS SYNDROME)

Ever since the publications of Fisher (1947), Evans and Duane (1949) and Evans et al. (1951) especial interest has been taken in the occurrence of thrombocytopenia and apparent ITP in association with AIHA of the warm-antibody type.

Fisher (1947) had reviewed under the title 'The Cryptogenic Acquired Haemolytic Anaemias' 18 cases of haemolytic anaemia taken from the records of the Radcliffe Infirmary, Oxford. Case 15 was a female aged 69 who developed transient purpura and polyarthritis, followed by a haemolytic crisis. Her haemoglobin had been recorded to have been as low as 30%, reticulocyte count as high as 52%, and neutrophil and platelet counts as low as 900 and 20 000 per μl, respectively. There was marked spherocytosis. Splenectomy had been followed by a further haemolytic crisis and later by a recurrence of thrombocytopenia and purpura. The Coombs (DAT) test was found to be positive after splenectomy. Fisher thought that her syndrome corresponded with those described by Frank (1925) as 'splenopathic leucopenia', and by Wiseman and Doan (1942) as 'primary splenic leucopenia'. In discussing her illness, Fisher wrote: 'The red-cell component was deficient because of excessive destruction due to sensitization by a globulin of immune antibody type. It seems reasonable to postulate a similar rather than a dissimilar pathological process to account for the deficiency in the other two components, the platelets and the neutrophils.'

Evans and Duane (1949) reported that five out of 11 patients with acquired haemolytic anaemia had had persistently low platelet counts and that one of them had suffered from purpura. In two of them there was, too, symptomless leucopenia, and it was suggested that the patients had been forming auto-antibodies against platelets and leucocytes in addition to those acting against erythrocytes.

The idea that the haemolytic anaemia, thrombocytopenia and leucopenia might have a similar pathogenesis was further developed by Evans and his co-workers (1951). Out of 18 patients with AIHA, 10 had normal platelet (and leucocyte) counts, four patients had thrombocytopenia and no purpura, and four had thrombocytopenia and the clinical signs of purpura (one patient had tuberculosis of the spleen). In addition, it was reported that in six out of 11 patients with thrombocytopenia but without haemolytic anaemia the direct antiglobulin test was, nevertheless, positive. Two of Evans's patients suffering from haemolytic anaemia and purpura were women, both of whom were pregnant; in these patients, and in a male patient, haemolytic anaemia and thrombocytopenia and purpura appear to have developed simultaneously.

It is now realized that low platelet counts are found quite commonly in AIHA and that clinically obvious purpura is not infrequent. Moreover, in some of the cases it has been possible to demonstrate that the thrombocytopenia is associated with the presence of antibodies active against platelets, i.e. that the patient is suffering from idiopathic thrombocytopenic purpura (ITP) as well as AIHA. The combination is now widely referred to as the Evans syndrome. In Evans and his co-workers' own words, there exists a 'spectrum-like relationship between acquired hemolytic anemia and thrombocytopenic purpura'; 'on the one hand, acquired hemolytic anemia with sensitization of the red cells is often accompanied with thrombocytopenia, while, on the other hand, primary thrombocytopenic purpura is frequently accompanied with red cell sensitization with or without hemolytic anemia'. They suggested that the terms 'immunohemolytic anemia', 'immune thrombocytopenia' and 'immunopancytopenia' were appropriate descriptions for the disorders and pointed out that whereas only two of 466 miscellaneous patients had given positive direct antiglobulin tests (DATs) and none out of 75 normal subjects, as many as 14 out of 24 patients suffering from disseminated lupus, periarteritis nodosa, nephrosis or rheumatic fever, all disorders also thought to have an immunological basis, had given positive DATs.

Subsequent to the reports of Fisher and of Evans and his co-workers referred to above, many other patients suffering from both AIHA and severe thrombocytopenia were soon described or mentioned, e.g. by Gasser and Holländer (1951), Kissmeyer-Nielson, Bent-Hansen and Kieler (1952), Loeb, Seaman and Moore (1952),

Wiener et al. (1952), Flückiger, Hässig and Koller (1953), Young and Miller (1953), Bernard et al. (1954), Crosby (1955), Baumgartner (1956), Müller and Weinreich (1956), Niemann et al. (1956), Weiner, Whitehead and Walkden (1956, Case 2), Crosby and Rappaport (1957) and Harris-Jones, McLellan and Owen (1958).

Crosby and Rappaport (1957) reported that five out of 16 surviving patients with idiopathic AIHA had had severe thrombocytopenia (10–86 $\times$ 10^9/l platelets), and that of 18 patients who had died, 12 had been thrombocytopenic (14–90 $\times$ 10^9/l platelets).

Dausset and Colombani (1959) reviewed the clinical histories of 83 patients with warm-antibody AIHA. Eleven (13.2%) had suffered from thrombocytopenic purpura; in three patients purpura had preceded haemolytic anaemia; in five they developed simultaneously, and in three purpura followed haemolytic anaemia.

AIHA has even supervened in patients who had previously undergone splenectomy for thrombocytopenic purpura. Waugh (1932) described a probable example of this occurrence, the patient being a woman aged 39 who died of fulminating haemolytic anaemia: 4 years previously she had undergone splenectomy for chronic thrombocytopenic purpura. The patients described by Dacie (1954, p. 202) as Case 12 and by Dacie (1962, p. 439) as Case 7 both similarly developed severe AIHA after having been splenectomized. Case 12 was a female who had had her spleen removed for chronic thrombocytopenic purpura 11 years before she died, when aged 43, of very severe AIHA*. Case 7 was a boy who died of very severe AIHA when 11 years of age: he had first developed acute thrombocytopenic purpura when aged 3, and had been splenectomized when aged 6.

Case reports of additional patients described in the 1960s who had AIHA and severe thrombocytopenia, often in association with haemorrhagic symptoms, and reviews of the literature, include those of Kintzel and Schmidt (1960), Lees, Fisher and Shanks (1960), Brunner and Frick (1962), Günther and Bube (1962), Silverstein and Heck (1962), Brunet, Najean and Bernard (1964), Ando (1965), Matthews (1965),

---

*This patient's brother subsequently developed severe AIHA (see Table 22.1).

Hörder, Manrique and Weinreich (1966), Silverstein, Aaro and Kempers (1966), Tattersall (1967), Sievers, Lehtinen and Aho (1968) and Letts and Kredenster (1969). More recent descriptions include those of Heck and Gehrmann (1973), Mönch, Breithaupt and Mueller-Eckhardt (1981), Hansen, Sørensen and Astrup (1982), Pegels et al. (1982) and Cuesta et al. (1986).

In 1977 Zucker-Franklin and Karpatkin reported the result of a most interesting study which strongly supported the concept of a close association between AIHA and ITP. They used an electron microscope to study buffy-coat preparations and platelet-rich plasma obtained from 17 patients with chronic ITP. The plasma was submitted to three successive centrifugations at 2500 g, 25 000 g and 27 000 g, respectively. (Two of the patients were in remission and five had undergone splenectomy.) Electron microscopy revealed many small platelet fragments in the plasma samples, and in 15 of the patients small fragments of erythrocytes were also present, identified by their electron density and osmophilia. Similar small fragments were not found in the plasma of normal or asplenic (but otherwise normal) individuals. There was little evidence of erythrophagocytosis by monocytes in the buffy-coat preparations, although a very few of the cells had engulfed erythrocyte fragments similar in size to those free in the plasma. Zucker-Franklin and Karpartkin concluded that their patients were suffering from subclinical increased haemolysis as well as destroying platelets. None, however, gave positive DATs when their erythrocytes were tested with routine (commercial) antisera; seven out of 10, however, reacted weakly when tested with anti-C3d and anti-C3b sera.

Crosby (1955) and Crosby and Rappaport (1957) had stressed in their retrospective reviews that when thrombocytopenia is present in patients who have AIHA the outlook was grave: twelve out of 17 patients with thrombocytopenia had died compared with five out of 16 patients without thrombocytopenia. Chertkow and Dacie (1956), too, in their review of the response of patients with AIHA to splenectomy concluded that the chances of recovery were probably less good in patients who were thrombocytopenic than in those with normal platelet counts. The histories of the patients described by Dacie [1954, p. 202 (Case 12)] and Dacie [1962, p. 389 and p. 439 (Cases 4 and 7)] certainly support the contention that the development of major degrees of thrombocytopenia is a serious event. It has to be added, however, that the high death-rates referred to above were derived from the histories of patients for most of whom the only available treatment was blood transfusion or splenectomy. At the present time the outlook for patients with Evans syndrome is probably much better.

IMMUNOPANCYTOPENIA

Some patients are known to have developed granulocytopenia as well as haemolytic anaemia and thrombocytopenia. Fisher's (1947) report and prescient conclusion has already been referred to. Evans and his co-workers (1951) mentioned four patients who were leucopenic and gave details of one of them, a woman aged 47, whose total leucocyte count was $1.7 \times 10^9/l$, of which 70% were neutrophils. Davis and his co-workers (1952, Case 4) described a 46-year-old man whose reticulocyte count was zero at the time of a severe anaemic crisis; the leucocyte count was $0.5 \times 10^9/l$ and platelet count $78 \times 10^9/l$. Splenectomy was eventually carried out and a 1700 g spleen removed. The patient eventually recovered. Young and Miller (1953) described a patient with a 22-year history of anaemia, leucopenia, thrombocytopenia and splenomegaly who was eventually splenectomized with benefit. Wasastjerna (1954) referred to a patient who had a long-standing mild haemolytic anaemia with a positive DAT, chronic neutropenia and a slightly low platelet count, whose serum contained a leucocyte-agglutinating factor.

Baumgartner (1956) described a boy aged 11 who developed severe warm-antibody AIHA and after experiencing a remission suffered from acute thrombocytopenic purpura and subsequently granulocytopenia. Antibodies active against his platelets and leucocyte agglutinins were demonstrated in his serum. Müller and Weinreich (1956), in a paper entitled 'Immunpancytopenien' reported the presence of leucocyte and platelet antibodies in a 70-year-old woman who had moderately severe thrombocytopenia, granulocytopenia and haemolytic anaemia associated with a positive antiglobulin test. Crosby and Rappaport (1957) mentioned in their survey of 57 AIHA patients that leucocyte counts were normal or increased in all but six of them at the time of haemolytic crises. One of their patients whose AIHA was associated with ITP was leucopenic. The patient described by Harris-Jones, McLellan and Owen (1958), too, had at one time a leucocyte count as low as $2 \times 10^9/l$ (42% neutrophils).

Evers, Kretschmer and Mueller-Eckhardt (1973) described a female patient aged 41 who gave a long history of recurrent leucopenia and AIHA. 'Auto-lymphocytotoxins' were demonstrated in her serum.

Fagiolo (1974) described a 35-year-old man who for 5 months had suffered from neuropsychiatric symptoms. He was found to be severely anaemic (Hb 5.4 g/dl, with 15% reticulocytes) and to be moderately neutropenic (total leucocytes 3.9×10^9/l, of which 65% were neutrophils). Fragments of erythrocytes could be seen in blood films. The DAT was positive with anti-IgA and anti-C sera. Cytotoxic antibodies against neutrophils and lymphocytes were demonstrated in his serum and also agglutinins active against platelets. The patient died and histological sections showed diffuse deposition of fibrin in arterioles and capillaries, especially in vessels in the kidney, heart and spleen. A

diagnosis of thrombotic thrombocytopenic purpura and auto-immune pancytopenia was suggested.

Fagiolo (1976) reviewed the occurrence of leucopenia and thrombocytopenia in 32 patients with AIHA, all but two being adults. Twenty-seven had suffered from idiopathic AIHA; in five the AIHA was associated with an underlying (non-malignant) disease. Leucopenia was present in 59%, thrombocytopenia similarly in 59%; both conditions were present in 41%. Specific antibodies active against granulocytes were identified in 81%, anti-platelet antibodies in 91%. The haemolytic anaemia, leucopenia and thrombocytopenia developed independently and responded differently to immunosuppressive treatment. Thrombocytopenic purpura was present in six patients. Fagiolo concluded that AIHA was often a manifestation of a complex auto-immune syndrome that

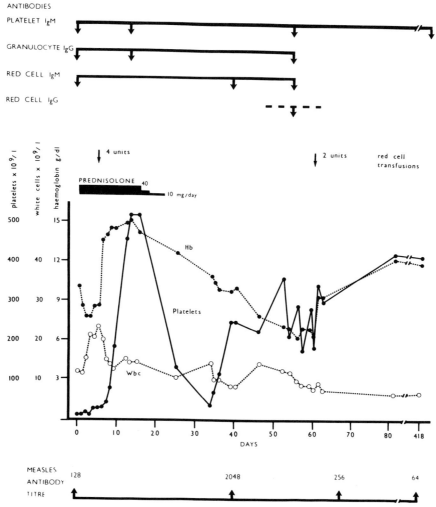

Fig. 22.6   Peripheral blood picture and serological findings in a 39-year-old woman who developed acute ITP and AIHA following measles.
[Reproduced by permission from Chapman et al. (1984).]

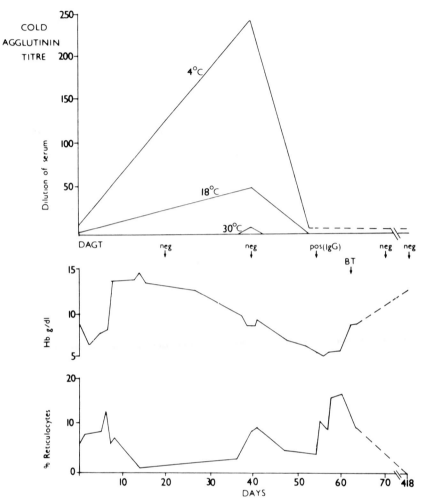

Fig. 22.7   Changes in haemoglobin and reticulocyte count in relation to the titre and thermal amplitude of an IgM anti-I antibody and to the appearance of an IgG warm auto-antibody.
Same patient whose treatment and course are illustrated in Fig. 22.6. [Reproduced by permission from Chapman et al. (1984).]

commonly involved the development of antibodies specific for leucocytes and platelets as well as against erythrocytes.

Pui, Willimas and Wang (1980) reviewed 164 cases of ITP and 15 of AIHA in children: eleven had had both conditions; seven had neutropenia also (0.15–0.8 × 10⁹/l neutrophils). Their illness was usually chronic and relapsing and treatment was generally not satisfactory. The direct antiglobulin test was positive in all of them, the indirect test positive in five; tests for platelet antibodies were positive in two and negative in four: tests for granulocyte antibodies were positive in three and negative in two, and for lymphocytotoxic antibodies positive in two and negative in three. The seven patients as a group had suffered from 28 platelet

relapses, 18 neutrophil relapses and nine erythrocyte relapses.

Mönch, Breithaupt and Mueller-Eckhardt (1981) described the presence of membrane-bound and free platelet auto-antibodies in a 65-year-old woman with AIHA and moderately severe thrombocytopenia.

Pegels and co-workers (1982), using an immunofluorescent test for auto-antibodies, studied 24 patients with AIHA and ITP or INP (immuno-neutropenia): 16 had AIHA plus ITP; one AIHA plus INP; seven AIHA plus ITP plus INP. Antibodies active against erythrocytes, platelets and granulocytes were demonstrated. Moreover, it appeared that the antibodies were separate entities, i.e. target-cell specific. They were most readily demonstrated attached to the membrane of the cells, and in only a few of the cases was it possible to show that antibodies (usually reacting weakly) were free in the serum. Granulocyte antibodies were eluted from granulocytes obtained from some of the patients who presented with clinical evidence of Evans syndrome only. Pegels et al. were more successful in finding antibodies against erythrocytes free in serum than in demonstrating antibodies against platelets or granulocytes; they suggested, however, that this might well be due to the test they had used being less successful in detecting platelet and granulocyte antibodies than erythrocyte antibodies.

Miller and Beardsley (1983) described three unrelated children suffering, concurrently or successively, from neutropenia, thrombocytopenia and haemolytic anaemia. One of them developed reticulocytopenia. They were 7, 12 and 14 years of age and suffered, too, from other probable auto-immune disorders: e.g. asthma and gastritis, an enlarged thymus, and pulmonary infiltrates, lymph-node enlargement and a cerebellar mass which underwent involution after steroids had been given. The DAT was positive, and anti-platelet and anti-leucocyte antibodies were present. In two of the children it was possible to show that the anti-erythrocyte and anti-platelet antibodies were separate entities which did not cross-react. Miller and Beardsley considered that a generalized disorder of immune regulation was basically responsible for the childrens' illness.

Chapman and co-workers (1984) described the interesting history of a 39-year-old black woman who developed acute thrombocytopenic purpura and autoimmune haemolysis apparently as a sequel to measles. A platelet IgM antibody and an IgM anti-I antibody of moderate titre and thermal amplitude, as well as a warm IgG auto-antibody, appeared to be responsible for the thrombocytopenia and haemolysis (Figs. 22.6 and 22.7). The DAT was originally negative using anti-IgG, -IgM, -IgA and -C3d sera, but had become positive with an anti-IgG serum at the time of a second haemolytic crisis (Fig. 22.7). An IgG anti-granulocyte antibody was also demonstrable, but the patient did not become neutropenic. She eventually fully recovered clinically; the platelet auto-antibody was, however, still detectable 1 year later. The platelet, granulocyte and erythrocyte antibodies appeared to be separate entities and not a single cross-reacting antibody.

Details of two further patients with 'idiopathic combined immunocytopenia' were given by Wiesneth et al. (1985). Auto-antibodies active against erythrocytes, platelets and granulocytes were demonstrated in each case.

AUTO-IMMUNE HAEMOLYTIC ANAEMIA IN IMMUNE DEFICIENCY SYNDROMES

Ever since the early 1960s it has been realized that not infrequently in AIHA there is substantial evidence of deficiency of the patient's immune mechanisms. Thus substantial reductions in the concentrations of the serum immunoglobulins have been reported in patients of all ages. AIHA has developed, too, as a complication in children afflicted with a variety of congenital or familial immune deficiency syndromes and also in adults suffering from hypogammaglobulinaemia of apparently acquired origin. As is to be expected, many of these patients suffered from repeated infections in consequence of their immune deficiency. The combination of warm-antibody AIHA and immune deficiency syndromes has attracted a good deal of attention and many reports of the occurrence are now available. In Table 22.4 are listed a selection: the table illustrates the remarkable diversity of immune defects with which AIHA has been associated.

Earlier descriptions of adults suffering from apparently acquired 'idiopathic' hypogammaglobulinaemia associated with splenomegaly and hypersplenism were reviewed by Citron (1957) and Prasad, Reiner and Watson (1957).

Citron (1957) referred to 45 cases of agammaglobulinaemia described in the literature. The spleen had been enlarged in six of the patients; three had undergone splenectomy and in two of them anaemia had been relieved. No evidence was found suggestive of an abnormal immunological mechanism and Citron concluded that the increased haemolysis (and neutropenia) in these patients was a direct consequence of the splenic enlargement.

Prasad, Reiner and Watson (1957) reported similarly. They referred to 17 patients, two of whom were under their care. Nine of the patients were anaemic, and in at least six of them this appeared to be haemolytic in origin (Collins and Dudley, 1955; Rohn, Behnke and Bond, 1955; Standaert and De Moor, 1955; Martin, Gordon and McCullough, 1956; Prasad, Reiner and Watson, 1957). In none of these patients was there

Table 22.4 Interesting case reports in chronological order of auto-immune haemolytic anaemia associated with immune defects (excluding patients with an overt lymphoma or thymoma).

Reference	Sex and age of patient	Summary of clinical features and haematological findings	Serological findings	Nature of immune defects; serum immunoglobulins
Fudenberg and Solomon (1961, Case 2)	M. 65 years	Good health until severe haemolysis	DAT pos	Hypogammaglobulinaemia; γG markedly diminished; α_2G low
Fritz (1962)		ITP; little haemolysis. Died of septicaemia	DAT pos	Hypogammaglobulinaemia
Breton et al. (1963)	9 months	Many infections. Fluctuating severe haemolysis	DAT pos	Hypogammaglobulinaemia; β_2A absent, β_2 macroglobulin $\uparrow$; lymphopenia
van Loghem–Langereis et al. (1965)	F. 59 years	Glomerulonephritis; urinary tract infection; haemolysis. Died of septicaemia	DAT neg. Immune adherence test pos	Hypogammaglobulinaemia. Circulating $\beta_2M/7S\gamma G$ complexes
Schaller et al. (1966)	F. 20 weeks	Nephritis and haemolysis. Died of pneumocystis pneumonia	DAT pos	Familial hypogammaglobulinaemia; severe lymphoid hypoplasia; lymphopenia. IgG and IgA $\uparrow$, IgM $\downarrow$
Hobbs, Russell and Worlledge (1967)	(1) F. 44 years	Severe haemolysis, then severe ITP. Splenectomy; infections subsequently	DAT pos (anti-IgG). Auto-antibody: some anti-c specificity	Dysgammaglobulinaemia Type IV C; IgG $\downarrow$, IgA $\downarrow$, IgM $\uparrow$
	(2) F. $2\frac{1}{2}$ years	Chronic haemolysis. Died of lung infection (CMV)	DAT pos (anti-IgG)	Dysgammaglobulinaemia, Type IV C; IgG N, IgA almost absent, IgM$\uparrow$
Straub and Sachtleben (1967)	M. 6 years	Undersized; total alopecia; chronic bronchitis, severe haemolysis	DAT and IAT pos	Severe deficiency of Ig A and IgM; partial deficiency of IgG
Hennemann and Rentsch (1968)	F. 65 years	Chronic haemolysis of $2\frac{1}{2}$ year duration	DAT pos	Hypogammaglobulinaemia; IgG, IgA and IgM $\downarrow$
Robbins, Skinner and Pearson (1969) [also Pearson, Robbins and Skinner (1967)]	M. 6 years	Recurrent infections. Severe haemolysis	DAT pos. Anti-LW auto-antibody	X-linked hypogammaglobulinaemia; IgG and IgM $\downarrow$, IgA always absent
Stoelinga, van Munster and Slooff (1969)	M. 12 years	Infections since infancy. Severe haemolysis	DAT pos	Severe IgM defect, probably familial (parents consanguineous) IgG N, IgA $\uparrow$, IgM $\downarrow$
Zuelzer et al. (1970, Cases 7 and 11)	(1) F. $2\frac{1}{2}$ years	Acute haemolysis	DAT pos	IgG N, IgA $\downarrow$, IgM $\downarrow$
	(2) F. $2\frac{1}{2}$ years (identical twins)	Acute haemolysis	DAT pos	IgG $\downarrow$, IgA $\downarrow$, IgM absent
Bergström et al. (1973)	F. 70 years	Recurrent infections; malabsorption syndrome. Chronic haemolysis	DAT pos (anti-IgG, anti-IgM, anti-C)	IgA absent, IgG $\uparrow$, IgM N
Ghosh and Harris-Jones (1974)	(1) F. 18 years	Severe haemolysis ('Coombs-negative')	DAT neg. Auto-antibody (IgG) eluted	IgG N, IgA $\downarrow$, IgM N
	(2) F. 12 years	Severe haemolysis ('Coombs-negative')	DAT neg. Auto-antibody (IgG) eluted	IgG $\downarrow$, IgA $\downarrow$, IgM N
Ballow, Dupont and Good (1976)	M. 3 years	Wiscott–Aldrich syndrome. Severe (ultimately fatal) haemolysis developed during treatment with transfer factor	DAT pos	IgG and IgA N, IgM $\downarrow$

Table 22.4 (contd)

Reference	Patient	Clinical features	DAT	Laboratory findings
Sandler and Zlotnick (1976)	F. 56 years	Chronic haemolysis	DAT pos (intermittently)	Familial IgA deficiency (mother and son). IgA virtually absent in both (son, aged 25, in good health)
Blanchette et al. (1978)	(1) M. 17 years	Relapsing haemolysis; severe thrombocytopenia; otitis media	DAT pos (anti-IgG)	Severe IgA deficiency, IgG ↓, IgM ↓ or N
	(2) M. 13 years	Relapsing haemolysis; severe thrombocytopenia; otitis media	DAT pos (anti-IgG)	IgA ↓, IgG and IgM N
Rich et al. (1979)	M. 5 years	Purine nucleoside phosphorylase deficiency. Minor infections. Severe haemolysis	DAT pos (anti-IgG and anti-C)	Severe lymphopenia; T cell dysfunction. IgG and IgM ↑, IgA N
Webster et al. (1981)	(3) M. 21 years	Previous thrombocytopenia; chronic haemolysis, with acute episodes; splenomegaly; eczema	DAT pos (anti-IgG)	IgG ↓, IgM ↓, IgA ↓
	(4) M. 22 years	Chronic haemolysis, neutropenia and thrombocytopenia; hepatosplenomegaly, liver granuloma; eczema and recurrent infections	DAT pos (anti-IgG)	IgG ↓, IgM ↓, IgA ↓
	(5) F. 50 years	Chronic haemolysis. Earlier thrombocytopenia and neutropenia; eczema; severe varicella; splenomegaly and splenectomy	DAT pos (anti-IgG and anti-C3d)	IgG ↓, IgM ↓, IgA absent
Bloomfield, Stockdill and Bernetson (1982)	F. 8 months	Moderate haemolysis; eosinophilia. Juvenile pemphigoid	DAT pos (anti-IgG and anti-C)	Thymic hypoplasia and T lymphocyte deficiency. IgG, IgA and IgM N; IgE markedly raised
Hansen, Sørensen and Astrup (1982)	M. 26 years	Recurrent haemolysis and severe ITP over a 10-year period (Evans syndrome)	DAT pos (anti-IgG and anti-C3d)	Sporadic IgA deficiency: IgG and IgM N, IgA virtually absent
Schreiber et al. (1983)	(1) F. 26 and 32	AIDS. Two patients had brisk haemolysis	DAT pos [anti-IgG + anti-C (1) and anti-IgG (3)]	Lymphopenia
	(2) M. 31 and 44			
Horowitz, Borcherding and Hong (1984)	(1) F. 7 months	Recurrent infections and reurrent haemolysis	DAT pos (anti-IgG)	T-suppressor cell deficiency; normal immunoglobulins
	(2) F. 12 months	Acute haemolysis	DAT pos (anti-IgG)	
Cuesta et al. (1986)	F. 10 years	Moderately severe haemolysis, severe thrombocytopenia; also chronic active hepatitis and focal glomerulonephritis	DAT pos (anti-IgG and anti-C3)	IgA absent, IgG ↑, IgM N
Rapoport, Rowe and McMican (1988)	M. 29 years	AIDS Severe haemolysis	DAT pos (anti-IgG and anti-C)	

Other patients giving similar histories and with similar laboratory findings in whom a lymphoma or thymoma was shown to be present will be referred to in Vol. 4 of this book.

pos = positive; neg = negative; N = normal.
DAT = direct antiglobulin test.

Table 22.5 Serum immunoglobulin levels in 84 patients with warm–antibody AIHA.

IgG	N	N	N	N	N	N	N	N	N	N	N	N	N	N	
IgA	↓	N	↓	↓	↓	N	N	↓	N	↓	N	↓	N	N	
IgM	↓	N	↑	↓	↑	↓	N	↓	→	↑	↑	N	↑	N	Number of patients
Idiopathic	**8**	5	4	3	3	1	**2**	1	2	1	**2**	1	0	14	48
α-Methyldopa	0	0	0	0	1	2	0	1	0	0	0	0	0	11	15
Secondary															
Lymphoma	1	2	1	0	1	0	0	1	0	0	1	0	0	3	9
Other auto-immune diseases	0	1	2	1	2	1	1	0	0	0	0	0	0	6	12
Total															84

N = within normal range; ↓ below −2 S.D. of normal mean; ↑ above + 2 S.D. of normal mean. Deficiency of IgA is indicated in bold type.
[Data abstracted from Blajchman et al. (1969).]

positive evidence that their increased haemolysis was auto-immune; in particular the DAT (when carried out) was negative.

A further case of acquired hypogammaglobulinaemia associated with splenomegaly was described by Thompson and Johnson (1962). Their patient, a woman aged 51, gave a 4-year history of recurrent infections. She was moderately anaemic (haemoglobin 67%) and there were 4%–6% of reticulocytes. The DAT was negative. Treatment with intramuscular gammaglobulin resulted in clinical improvement but haemolysis persisted.

Still earlier descriptions of patients who appear likely to have suffered from the same syndrome, but in whom no information as to their serum globulins is available, include the five patients described by Wiseman and Doan (1942) under the title 'primary splenic neutropenia' and Cases 5 and 7 of Kracke and Riser (1949), referred to as suffering from 'acquired hemolytic anemia of unknown cause' and 'primary splenic panhematopenia', respectively.

The discovery that AIHA might develop in association with major, and clinically important, immunoglobulin deficiency naturally led to the systematic search for possible immunoglobulin deficiencies in patients who had AIHA but presented no clinical evidence of any abnormality of their immune system other than the development of auto-antibodies against erythrocytes (and perhaps platelets and leucocytes, too). The data

of Blajchman and co-workers (1969), which had been obtained by a modification of the Mancini immuno-precipitation method using antisera specific for IgG, IgA and IgM, provided some answers. In only 34 out of 84 patients who had developed warm-type AIHA were the results of the quantitative estimation of the three immunoglobulins normal. IgA was the immunoglobulin most commonly present in abnormal (usually reduced) concentration, but as many as 13 different combinations of immunoglobulin deficiency or excess were demonstrated. Forty-eight of the 84 patients were considered to be suffering from idiopathic AIHA: in only 14 were the results normal (Table 22.5). It is interesting to note, in contrast, that the results were normal in as many as 11 out of 15 patients whose disease had apparently been precipitated by treating their hypertension with α-methyldopa.

The finding of the association between deficiency, or less commonly excess, of serum immunoglobulins and the development of auto-antibodies is clearly of great significance in relation to the problem as to why and how auto-immunization against an individual's own blood cells can take place. This important and difficult question is considered in Chapter 33 (pp. 363–391).

REFERENCES

ABDEL-KHALIK, A., PATON, L., WHITE, A. G. & URBANIAK, S. J. (1980). Human leucocyte antigens A, B, C and DRW in idiopathic 'warm' autoimmune haemolytic anaemia. *Brit. med. J.*, **280**, 760–761.

ALLGOOD, J. W. & CHAPLIN, H. JNR (1967). Idiopathic acquired autoimmune hemolytic anemia. A review of forty-seven cases treated from 1955 through 1965. *Amer. J. Med.*, **43**, 254–273.

ALTMANN, F. (1932). Akute (hämolytische, febrile oder infektiöse) Anämie (Lederer). *Z. Kinderheilk.*, **53**, 112–117.

ANDO, S. (1965). Clinical studies on autoimmune hemolytic anemia. II. Observations on the clinical features of autoimmune hemolytic anemia of the warm-antibody type with the mixed type. *Acta haemat. jap.*, **28**, 631–634.

ATKINSON, F. R. B. (1940). Lederer's Anaemia. *Brit. J. child. Dis.*, **37**, 35–40.

BALLOW, M., DUPONT, B. & GOOD, R. A. (1976). Autoimmune hemolytic anemia in Wiskott–Aldrich

syndrome during treatment with transfer factor. *J. Pediat.*, **83**, 772–780.

BARTOLOZZI, G., PAVARI, E., GUAZZELLI, C. & MARIANELLI, L. (1963). Anemia emolitica autoimmune in un lattante. *Riv. Clin. pediat.*, **72**, 249–267.

BATEMAN, D. R. E., HUTT, M. S. R. & NORRIS, P. R. (1959). A case of acquired haemolytic anaemia in pregnancy. *J. Obstet. Gynaec. Brit. Emp.*, **66**, 130–132.

BAUMANN, R. & RUBIN, G. (1973). Autoimmune hemolytic anemia during pregnancy with hemolytic disease in the newborn. *Blood*, **41**, 293–297.

BAUMGARTNER, W. (1956). Maladie par autoaggression. Akute hämolytische Anämie, thrombocytopeniche Purpura und Granulocytopenie. *Helv. med. Acta*, **23**, 324–330.

BAXTER, E. W. & EVERHART, M. W. (1938). Acute hemolytic anemia (Lederer type). *J. Pediat.*, **12**, 357–362.

BECKMAN, M. (1921–1922). Zur perniziosen und perniziosaartigen Graviditätsanämie. *Monat. Geburtsh. Gynäk.*, **56**, 119–128.

BECTON, D. L. & KINNEY, T. R. (1986). An infant girl with severe autoimmune hemolytic anemia: apparent anti-Vel specificity. *Vox Sang.*, **51**, 108–111.

BERGSTRÖM, K., BRITTON, M., HANSON, L. Å., HOLM, G., KARDOS, M. & WESTER, P. O. (1973). IgA deficiency and autoimmune haemolytic anaemia. *Scand. J. Haemat.*, **11**, 87–91.

BERNARD, J., DAUSSET, J., MALINVAUD, G. & LESUEUR, G. (1954). Anémies, leucopénies, thrombopénies immunologiques. Association d'anticorps dirigés contre les trois lignes cellulaires du sang. *Bull. Soc. méd. Hôp. Paris*, **70**, 651–666.

BERREY, B. H. & WATSON, J. D. (1951). Acquired hemolytic anemia. Report of a case in an infant with discussion of several etiological factors which may have been operative. *Arch. Pediat.*, **68**, 10–27.

BETKE, K., RICHARZ, H., SCHUBOTHE, H. & VIVELL, O. (1953). Beobactungen zu Krankheitsbild, Pathogenese und Ätiologie der akuten erworbenen hämolytischen Anämie (Lederer-Anämie). *Klin. Wschr.*, **31**, 373–380.

BLAJCHMAN, M. A., DACIE, J. V., HOBBS, J. R., PETTIT, J. E. & WORLLEDGE, S. M. (1969). Immunoglobulins in warm-type autoimmune haemolytic anaemia. *Lancet*, **ii**, 340–344.

BLAJCHMAN, M. A., HUI, Y. T., JONES, T. E. & LUKE, K. H. (1971). Familial autoimmune hemolytic anemia with an autoantibody demonstrating U specificity. *Program of the 24th Annual Meeting of the American Association of Blood Banks, Chicago*, 1971, p. 82.

BLANCHETTE, V. S., HALLET, J. J., EHMPHILL, J. M., WINKETSTEIN, J. A. & ZINKHAM, W. H. (1978). Abnormalities of the peripheral blood as a presenting feature of immunodeficiency. *Amer. J. Hemat.*, **4**, 87–92.

BLOOMFIELD, S., STOCKDILL, G. & BARNETSON, R. ST. C. (1982). Thymic hypoplasia, auto-immune haemolytic anaemia and juvenile pemphigoid in an infant. *Brit. J. Dermat.*, **106**, 353–355.

BOLING, E. P., WEN, J., REVEILLE, J. D., BIAS, W. B., CHUSED, T. M. & ARNETT, F. C. (1983). Primary Sjogren's syndrome and autoimmune hemolytic anemia in sisters. A family study. *Amer. J. Med.*, **74**, 1066–1071.

BOORMAN, K. E., DODD, B. E. & LOUTIT, J. F. (1946). Haemolytic icterus (acholuric jaundice) congenital and acquired. *Lancet*, **i**, 812–814.

BORGLIN, N. E. & HACKL, H. (1964). Hämolytische Anämie und Gravidität. *Wien. klin. Wschr.*, **76**, 844–847.

BOSSI, E. & WAGNER, H. P. (1972). Autoimmune hemolytic anemia and cytomegalovirus infection in a six months old child, treated with azathioprine. *Helv. paediat. Acta*, **27**, 155–162.

BÖTTIGER, L. E. & WESTERHOLM, B. (1973). Acquired haemolytic anaemia. I. Incidence and aetiology. *Acta med. scand.*, **193**, 223–226.

BOUSSER, J., CHRISTOL, D., GAJDOS, A., GAJDOS-TOROK, M., LUMBROSO, P. & NETTER, A. (1963). Porphyrie cutanée de l'adulte apparue après une anémie hémolytique à auto-anticorps. *Bull. Soc. méd. Hôp. Paris*, **114**, 665–671.

BOWMAN, J. M. (1955). Acquired hemolytic anemia. Use of replacement transfusion in a crisis. *Amer. J. Dis. Child.*, **89**, 226–232.

BRETON, A., WALBAUM, R., BONIFACE, L., GOUDEMAND, M. & DUPONT, A. (1963). Lymphocytophtisie avec dysgammaglobulinémie chez un nourrisson. *Arch. franç. Pédiat.*, **20**, 131–146.

BRILL, I. C. (1926). Acute febrile anemia. A new disease? *Arch. intern. Med.*, **37**, 244–247.

BROMBERG, Y. M., TOAFF, R. & EHRENFELD, E. (1948). Acute crises in chronic haemolytic anaemia induced by pregnancy. *J. Obstet. Gynaec. Brit. Emp.*, **55**, 325–329.

BROWN, G. M., HAYWARD, O. C., POWELL, E. O. & WITTS, L. J. (1944). The destruction of transfused erythrocytes in anaemia. *J. Path. Bact.*, **56**, 81–94.

BRUNET, P., NAJEAN, Y. & BERNARD, J. (1964). Étude de dix cas d'association d'anémie hémolytique idiopatique immunologique et de purpura thrombopénique. *Sem. Hôp. Paris*, **40**, 294–302.

BRUNNER, H. E. & FRICK, P. G. (1962). Simultaneous thrombocytopenic purpura and autoimmune haemolytic anaemia. *Germ. med. Mthly*, **7**, 289–291.

BUCHANAN, G. R., BOXER, L. A. & NATHAN, D. G. (1976). The acute and transient nature of idiopathic immune hemolytic anemia in childhood. *J. Pediat.*, **88**, 780–783.

BURT, R. L. & PRICHARD, R. W. (1957). Acquired hemolytic anaemia in pregnancy: report of a case. *Obstet. and Gynec.*, **10**, 444–450.

CARAPELLA DE LUCA, E., CASADEI, A. M., DI PIERO, G., MIDULLA, M., BISDOMINI, C. & PURPURA, M. (1979). Auto-immune haemolytic anaemia in childhood. Follow-up in 29 cases. *Vox Sang.*, **36**, 13–20.

CARAPELLA-DE-LUCA, E., DI PIERO, G., MALAGUZZI, VALERI, O. & PURPURA, M. (1976). Presentazione di 14 casi di anemia emolitica autoimmune in èta pediatrica. *Minerva pediat. (Torino)*, **19**, 611–613.

CARAPELLA DE LUCA, E., STEGAGNO, M., MORINO, G., BALLATI, G. & LORENZINI, F. (1984). Prolonged reticulocytopenia and transient erythroid hypoplasia in a child with autoimmune haemolytic anaemia. *Haematologica*, **69**, 315–320.

CHAPLIN, H. JNR, COHEN, R., BLOOMBERG, G., KAPLAN, H. J., MOORE, J. A. & DORNER, I. (1973). Pregnancy and idiopathic autoimmune haemolytic anaemia: a prospective study during 6 months gestation and 3 months *post-partum. Brit. J. Haemat.*, **24**, 219–229.

CHAPMAN, J. F., METCALFE, B., MURPHY, M. F.,

BURMAN, J. F. & WATERS, A. H. (1984). Sequential development of platelet, neutrophil and red cell autoantibodies associated with measles infection. *Clin. lab. Haemat.*, **6**, 219–228.

CHAPTAL, J., CAZAL. P., JEAN, R., LOUBATIERES, R., CAMPO, C. & RIBSTEIN, M. (1954). Anémie hémolytique mortelle par auto-anticorps au cours de l'évolution de une syndrome de réticulite, d'origine virale probable, chez un nourrison. Action temporaire du traitement hormonal sur l'hémolyse: étude histologique. *Pédiatrie*, **9**, 445–449.

CHAUFFARD, M. A. & TROISIER, J. (1908). Anémie grave avec hémolysine dans la sérum; ictère hémolysinique. *Sem. méd.*, **28**, 345.

CHAUFFARD A. & VINCENT, C. (1909). Hémoglobinurique hémolysinique avec ictère polycholique aigu. *Sem. méd.*, **29**, 601–604.

CHERTKOW, G. & DACIE, J. V. (1956). Results of splenectomy in auto-immune haemolytic anaemia. *Brit. J. Haemat.*, **2**, 237–249.

CHRISTEN, J. -P., JACCOTTET, M. & WUILLERET, B. (1958). Anémie hémolytique immunologique par auto-anticorps, 1e partie: clinique. *Helv. paediat. Acta*, **13**, 131–139.

CITRON, K. M. (1957). Agammaglobulinaemia with splenomegaly. *Brit. med. J.*, **i**, 1148–1151.

CLAUVEL, J. P., MARCELLI-BARGE, A., GAUTIER COGGIA, I., POIRIER, J. C., BANAJAM, A. & DAUSSET, J. (1974) HL-A antigens and idiopathic autoimmune hemolytic anemias. *Transplant Proc.*, **6**, 447–448.

CLEMENS, K. & WALSH, R. J. (1955). Blood groups and acquired haemolytic anaemia. *Aust. J. Sci.*, **17**, 136–137.

COLETTA, A. & SCHETTINI, F. (1958). Contributo allo studio dell'anemia emolitica acquisata autoimmune nel lattante. *Pediatria*, **66**, 60–70.

COLETTA, A., SCHETTINI, F. & DI FRANCESCO, L. (1959). Sull' anemia emolitica acquisita autoimmune nel lattante. *Pediatria*, **67**, 203–215.

COLLINS, H. D. & DUDLEY, H. R. (1955). Agammaglobulinemia and bronchiectasis. *New Engl. J. Med.*, **252**, 255–259.

CONLEY, C. L. (1981). Immunologic precursors of autoimmune hematologic disorders. Autoimmune hemolytic anemia and thrombocytopenic purpura. *Johns Hopk. med. J.*, **149**, 101–109.

CONLEY, C. L. & SAVARESE, D. M. F. (1989). Biologic false-positive serologic tests for syphilis and other serologic abnormalities in autoimmune hemolytic anemia and thrombocytopenic purpura. *Medicine (Baltimore)*, **68**, 67–84.

COOMBS, R. R. A., MOURANT, A. E. & RACE, R. R. (1945). A new test for the detection of weak and 'incomplete' Rh agglutinins. *Brit. J. exp. Path.*, **26**, 255–266.

CORDOVA, M. S., BAEZ-VILLASENOR, J., MENDEZ, J. J. & CAMPOS, E. (1966). Acquired hemolytic anemia with positive antiglobulin (Coombs' test) in mother and daughter. *Arch. intern. Med.*, **117**, 692–695.

CORTESI, M. (1961). Un caso di anemia emolitica acuta da autoanticorpi in una bambina della prima infanzia. *Minerva pediat. (Torino)*, **13**, 1375–1379.

COUTEL, Y., BRETAGNE, J. & MOREL, H. (1962). Anémie hémolytique aiguë idiopathique avec auto-anticorps chauds chez un enfant de 9 ans. Guérison. *Arch. franç. Pédiat.*, **19**, 253–261.

CRAIG, G. A. & TURNER, R. L. (1955). A case of symptomatic haemolytic anaemia in pregnancy. *Brit. med. J.*, **i**, 1003–1005.

CROSBY, W. H. (1955). The clinical aspects of immunologic hemolytic anemia. *Sang*, **26**, 3–6.

CROSBY, W. H. & RAPPAPORT, H. (1957). Autoimmune hemolytic anaemia. I. Analysis of hematologic observations with particular reference to their prognostic value. A survey of 57 cases. *Blood*, **12**, 42–55.

CUESTA, B., FERNÁNDEZ, J., PARDO, J., PÁRAMO, J. A., GOMEZ, C. & ROCHA, E. (1986). Evan's [sic] syndrome, chronic active hepatitis and focal glomerulonephritis in IgA deficiency. *Acta haemat. (Basel)*, **75**, 1–5.

DA COSTA, J. A. G., WHITE, A. G, PARKER, A. C. & GRIGOR, G. B. (1974). Increased incidence of HL-A1 and 8 in patients showing IgG or complement coating on their red cells. *J. clin. Path.*, **27**, 353–355.

DACIE, J. V. (1954). *The Haemolytic Anaemias: Congenital and Acquired*, 525 pp. Churchill, London.

DACIE, J. V. (1962). *The Haemolytic Anaemias: Congenital and Acquired. Part II—The Auto-immune Haemolytic Anaemias*, 377 pp. Churchill, London.

DACIE, J. V. (1969). Modern concepts on autoimmune haemolytic anaemia. *Folia allergol.*, **16**, 370–379.

DACIE, J. V. & WORLEDGE, S. M. (1969). Auto-immune hemolytic anemias. In *Progress in Hematology VI* (ed. by E. B. Brown and C. V. Moore), pp. 82–120. Grune and Stratton, New York.

DACIE, J. V. & WORLEDGE, S. (1975). Auto-allergic blood diseases. In *Clinical Aspects of Immunology* (ed. by P. G. H. Gell, R. R. A. Coombs and P. J. Lachmann), pp. 1149–1182. Blackwell Scientific Publications, Oxford.

DAMESHEK, W. & SCHWARTZ, S. O. (1938a). The presence of hemolysins in acute hemolytic anemia; preliminary note. *New Eng. J. Med.*, **218**, 75–80.

DAMESHEK, W. & SCHWARTZ, S. O. (1938b). Hemolysins as the cause of clinical and experimental hemolytic anemias. With particular reference to the nature of spherocytosis and increased fragility. *Amer. J. med. Sci.*, **196**, 769–792.

DAMESHEK, W. & SCHWARTZ, S. O. (1940). Acute hemolytic anemia (acquired hemolytic icterus, acute type). *Medicine (Baltimore)*, **19**, 231–327.

DAUSSET, J. & COLOMBANI, R. (1958). Étude statistique et pronostique de 100 cas d'anémie hémolytique immunologique. *Acta haemat. (Basel)*, **20**, 137–146.

DAUSSET, J. & COLOMBANI, J. (1959). The serology and the prognosis of 128 cases of autoimmune hemolytic anemia. *Blood*, **14**, 1280–1301.

DAUSSET, J., COLOMBANI, R., JEAN, R. G., CANLORBE, P. & LELONG, M. (1957). Sur un cas d'anémie hémolytique aiguë de l'enfant avec présence d'une hémolysine immunologique et d'un pouvoir anticomplémentaire du sérum. *Sang*, **28**, 351–363.

DAUSSET, J. & HORS, J. (1975). Some contributions of the HL-A complex to the genetics of human diseases. *Transplant. Rev.*, **22**, 44–74.

DAUSSET, J. & MALINVAUD, G. (1954). Les anémies hémolytiques acquises avec auto-anticorps: évolution, pronostic et traitement d'après l'étude de 54 cas. *Sem. Hôp. Paris*, **30**, 3130–3137.

DAVID, J. K. JNR & MINOT, A. S. (1944). Acute hemolytic anemia in infancy. Report of a case with demonstration of hemolytic activity of serum. *Amer. J. Dis. Child.*, **68**, 327–329.

DAVIDSON, L. S. P. (1932). Macrocytic haemolytic anaemia. *Quart. J. Med.*, **25**, (N.S.1), 543–578.

DAVIS, L. J., KENNEDY, A. C., BAIKIE, A. G. & BROWN, A. (1952). Haemolytic anaemias of various types treated with ACTH and cortisone. Report of ten cases, including one of acquired type in which erythropoietic arrest occurred during a crisis. *Glasgow med. J.*, **33**, 263–285.

DAWSON OF PENN, LORD (1931). Haemolytic icterus (Hume Lectures). *Brit. med. J.*, **i**, 963–966 (Lecture II).

DE GROOT, A. W. (1969). Een Zwangere met hemolytische anemie. *Ned. Tijdschr. Verloskunde Gynaecol.*, **69**, 283–286.

DE GRUCHY, G. C. (1954). The diagnosis and management of acquired haemolytic anaemia. *Aust. Ann. Med.*, **3**, 106–115.

DE VEBER, L. L. (1964). A case of Lederer's anemia (acute acquired hemolytic anemia). *Canad. med. Ass. J.*, **90**, 370–373.

DEBRÉ, R., MOZZICONACCI, P., BUHOT, S., GUINAND-DONIOL, J. & HERRAULT, A. (1950). Anémies hémolytiques aiguës curables de l'enfance. *Arch. franç. Pédiat.*, **7**, 168–171.

DENYS, P. & VAN DEN BROUCKE, J. (1947). Anémie hémolytique acquise et réaction de Coombs. *Arch. franç. Pédiat.*, **4**, 205–217.

DI PIERO, G. (1959). Su una nuova osservazione di anemia emolitica acquisata in età pediatrica. *Haematologica*, **44**, 489–500.

DOBBS, C. E. (1965). Familial auto-immune hemolytic anemia. *Arch. Intern. Med.*, **116**, 273–276.

DODD, B. E. (1984). First tests with anti-human globulin on the red cells of patients suffering from haemolytic anaemia. *Vox Sang.*, **46**, 183–184.

DREYFUS, B. (1964). Rôle probable d'un facteur héréditaire dans le déterminisme de certaines anémies hémolytiques par auto-anticorps. *Nouv. Rev. franç. Hémat.*, **4**, 669–690.

DREYFUS, B., DAUSSET, J. & VIDAL, G. (1951). I. Étude clinique et hématologique de douze cas d'anémie hémolytique acquise avec auto-anticorps. *Rev. Hémat.*, **6**, 349–368.

DUNLOP, H. A. & SANDERS, A. G. (1974). Acute haemolytic anaemia. *Lancet*, **i**, 1169–1170.

DUNSFORD, I. & OWEN, G. (1960). Distribution of the ABO blood groups in cases of acquired haemolytic anaemia. *Brit. med. J.*, **i**, 1172–1173.

DUTHIE, E. S. (1937). Acquired haemolytic jaundice with unusual features. *Lancet*, **i**, 1167–1169.

DYKE, S. C. & YOUNG, F. (1938). Macrocytic haemolytic anaemia associated with increased red cell fragility. *Lancet*, **ii**, 817–821.

EASON, J. (1918). Remarks on acquired acholuric jaundice (haemolytic icterus). *Edinb. med. J.*, **20**, 158–171.

ELDOR, A., YATZIN, S. & HERSHKO, C. (1975). Relapsing Coombs-negative haemolytic disease in pregnancy with haemolytic disease in the newborn. *Brit. med. J.*, **4**, 625.

ESS, H. & FRIEDERICI, L. (1958). Klinische und serologische Relationen bei erworbenen hämolytischen Anämien. *Ärztl. Wschr.*, **13**, 457–468.

EVANS, R. S., & DUANE, R. T. (1949). Acquired hemolytic anemia. I. The relation of antibody activity to activity of the disease. II. The significance of thrombocytopenia and leukopenia. *Blood*, **4**, 1196–1213.

EVANS, R. S., TAKAHASHI, K., DUANE, R. T., PAYNE, R. & LIU, C. -K. (1951). Primary thrombocytopenic purpura and acquired hemolytic anemia. Evidence for a common etiology. *Arch. Intern. Med.*, **87**, 48–65.

EVERS, K. G., KRETSCHMER, V. & MUELLER-ECKHARDT, CH. (1973). Immunohämolytische Anämie und chronische Leukozytopenie mit Autozytotoxinen. *Dtsch. med. Wschr.*, **98**, 532–534.

FAGIOLO, E. (1974). Thrombotic thrombocytopenic purpura with autoimmune pancytopenia. A case report. *Acta haemat. (Basel)*, **52**, 356–361.

FAGIOLO, E. (1976). Platelet and leukocyte antibodies in auto-immune hemolytic anemia. *Acta haemat. (Basel)*, **56**, 97–106.

FIALKOW, P. J., FUDENBERG, H. & EPSTEIN, W. V. (1964). 'Acquired' antibody hemolytic anemia and familial aberrations in gamma globulins. *Amer. J. Med.*, **36**, 188–199.

FISHER, J. A. (1947). The cryptogenic acquired haemolytic anaemias. *Quart. J. Med.*, **16**, 245–262.

FLEISCHHACKER, H. (1952). Hämolytische Anämie vom Typ Loutit. *Wien. Z. inn. Med.*, **33**, 438–444.

FLÜCKIGER, P., HÄSSIG, A. & KOLLER, F. (1953). Über den Thrombocytens-Coombs-Test. *Schweiz. med. Wschr.*, **83**, 1035–1036.

FONTAN, VERGER, MARCHAND, MOULINIER, & LAGARDE (1985). Anémie hémolytique acquise du nourrisson avec présence d'anticorps chauds agglutinants. *Arch. franç. Pédiat.*, **12**, 323–326.

FRITZ, E. (1962). Gleichzeitiges Vorkommen von Autoaggressions Krankheiten des Blutes und Antikörpermangelsyndrom. *Münch. med. Wschr.*, **104**, 1269–1272.

FRUMIN, A. M., SMITH, E. M., TAYLOR, A. G. & DRATMAN, M. B. (1953). Acquired hemolytic anemia in pregnancy treated with ACTH and cortisone. *Amer. J. Obstet. Gynec.*, **65**, 421–423.

FUDENBERG, H. & SOLOMON, A. (1961). 'Acquired agammaglobulinaemia' with auto-immune hemolytic disease: graft-versus-host reaction? *Vox Sang*, **6**, 68–79.

FUKUOKA, Y. & ANDO, S. (1965). Clinical studies on autoimmune hemolytic anemia. II. Observations on the clinical features of autoimmune hemolytic anemia of the warm-antibody type with the mixed type. *Acta haemat. jap.*, **28**, 631–634.

GASSER, C. (1952). Akute erworbene hämolytische Anämien mit Immunkörpernachweis und Erythrocytenphagocytose im peripherien Blut. *Schweiz. med. Wschr.*, **82**, 42–43.

GASSER, C. (1954). Hämolyse und erworbene hämolytische Erkrankungen. *Helv. paediat. Acta*, **9**, 135–175.

GASSER, C. & HOLLÄNDER, L. (1951). Anémie hémolytique acquise aiguë. Provoquée par des auto-anticorps, accompagnée de purpura thrombocytopénique, chez un nourrisson de 7 semaines. *Rev. Hémat.*, **6**, 316–333.

GASSER, C. & HOLLÄNDER, L. (1952). Akute durch autoantikörper bedingte hämolytische Anämie, einhergehend mit thrombocytopenischer Purpura bei einem Säugling. *Ann. Paediat.*, **178**, 340–342.

GELLI, G. & VIGNALE, A. M. (1959). Anemia emolitica acquisita immunologica a decorso cronico. *Minerva pediat.*, **11**, 82–86.

GHOSH, M. L. & HARRIS-JONES, J. N. (1974). Coombs-negative autoimmune hemolytic anemia and immunoglobulin deficiency. *Amer. J. clin. Path.*, **62**, 40–46.

GILLILAND, B. C., LEDDY, J. P. & VAUGHAN, J. H. (1970). The detection of cell-bound antibody on complement-coated human red cells. *J. clin. Invest.*, **49**, 898–906.

GIORDANO, A. S. & BLUM, L. L. (1937). Acute hemolytic anemia (Lederer type). *Amer. J. med. Sci.*, **194**, 311–320.

GLEICHER, N. (1986). Pregnancy and autoimmunity. *Acta haemat. (Basel)*, **76**, 68–77.

GOODALL, H. B., HO-YEN, D. O., CLARK, D. M., THOMSON, M. A. R., BROWNING, M. C. K. & CROWDER, A. M. (1979). Haemolytic anaemia of pregnancy. *Scand. J. Haemat.*, **22**, 185–191.

GREENBERG, J., CURTIN-COHEN, M., GILL, E. M. & COHEN, A. (1980). Prolonged reticulocytopenia in autoimmune hemolytic anemia of childhood. *J. Pediat.*, **97**, 784–786.

GROSS, S. & NEWMAN, A. J. (1964). Auto-immune anti-D specificity in infancy. *Amer. J. Dis. Child.*, **108**, 181–183.

GÜNTHER, F. W. & BUBE, F. W. (1962). Zur Diagnostik und Therapie der parakuten hämolytischen Anämie in Verbindung mit Thrombozytopenie durch AutoimmunKörper (Evans-Syndrom). *Arch. Kinderheilk.*, **167**, 155–159.

HABIBI, B., HOMBERG, J. -C., SCHAISON, G. & SALMON, C. (1974). Autoimmune hemolytic anemia in children. A review of 80 cases. *Amer. J. Med.*, **56**, 61–69.

HADNAGY, C. S. (1989). Severe chronic autoimmune haemolytic anaemia presenting [as] haemolytic disease of the newborn. *Lancet*, **ii**, 749 (letter).

HAMILTON, D. G. (1939). A case of acute haemocytolytic anaemia with haemoglobinuria. *Med. J. Aust.*, **i**, 305–307.

HANEBERG, B., MATRE, R., WINSNES, R., DALEN, A., VOGT, H. & FINNE, P. H. (1978). Acute hemolytic anemia related to diphtheria–pertusis–tetanus vaccination. *Acta pediat. Scand.*, **67**, 345–350.

HANSEN, O. P., SØRENSEN, C. H. & ASTRUP, L. (1982). Evans' syndrome in IgA deficiency. Episodic autoimmune haemolytic anaemia and thrombocytopenia during a 10 years observation period. *Scand. J. Haemat.*, **29**, 265–270.

HARRIS-JONES, J. N., McLELLAN, D. M. & OWEN, G. (1958). Haemolytic anaemia following thrombocytopenic purpura. *Brit. med. J.*, **i**, 624–625.

HAYEM, G. (1898). Sur une variété particulière d'ictère chronique. Ictère infectieux chonique splénomégalique. *Presse médicale*, **6**, 121–125.

HECK, J. & GEHRMANN, C. (1973). Probleme des Evans Syndroms. Klinischer und nuklearmedizinischer Beitrag. *Dtsch. med. Wschr.*, **98**, 1163–1168.

HEGDE, U. M., GORDON-SMITH, E. C. & WORLLEDGE, S. M. (1977). Reticulocytopenia and 'absence' of red cell autoantibodies in immune haemolytic anaemia. *Brit. med. J.*, **ii**, 1444–1447.

HEILMEYER, L. (1950). Die hämolytischen Anämien. *Sang*, **21**, 105–141.

HEILMEYER, L. & ALBUS, L. (1936). Die hämolytische Hypersplenie. Beitrag zur Frage des erworbenen hämolytischen Ikterus. *Dtsch. Arch. klin. Med.*, **178**, 89–102.

HEISEL, M. A. & ORTEGA, J. A. (1983). Factors influencing prognosis in childhood autoimmune hemolytic anemia. *Amer. J. ped. Hemat./Oncol.*, **5**, 147–152.

HENI, F. & BLESSING, K. (1954). Beschreibung zweier schwerer erworbener idiopathischer hämolytischer Anämien. *Klin. Wschr.*, **32**, 481–485.

HENNEMANN, H. H. (1963). Okkulte (latente) erworbene hämolytische syndrome. *Dtsch. med. Wschr.*, **88**, 2288–2293.

HENNEMANN, H. H. & KRAUSE, H. (1964).

Chronische Thrombozytopenie (Morbus Werlhof) und erworbene hämolytische Anämie bei zwei Schwestern. *Dtsch. med. Wschr.*, **89**, 1161-1166.

HENNEMANN, H. H. & RENTSCH, I. (1968). Idiopathische autoimmunhämolytische Anämie mit Hypogammaglobulinämie. *Klin. Wschr.*, **46**, 156-157.

HERSHKO, C., BERREBI, A., RESNITZKY, P. & ELDER, A. (1976). Relapsing haemolytic anaemia of pregnancy with negative antiglobulin reaction. *Scand. J. Haemat.*, **16**, 135-140.

HIROOKA, M., YOSHIOKA, K., OHNO, T., KUBOTA, N. & IKEDA, S. (1970). Autoimmune hemolytic anemia in a child treated with thymectomy. *Tohoku J. exp. Med.*, **101**, 227-235.

HOBBS, J. R., RUSSELL, A. & WORLLEDGE, S. M. (1967). Dysgammaglobulinaemia type IVC. *Clin. exp. Immun.*, **2**, 589-599.

HOMBERG, J. -C., BONNET-GAJDOS, M. & SALMON, C. (1970). L'anémie hémolytique aiguë transitoire CγM chez l'enfant après rhino-pharyingite. *Nouv. Rev. Hémat.*, **10**, 9-18.

HOMBERG, H. C., GERBAL, A., ROCHANT, H., NAJMAN, A., COMBRISSON, A., SALMON, CH., DUHAMEL, G. & ANDRÉ, R. (1967). Implications cliniques de la nouvelle classification immunologiques des anémies hémolytiques avec auto-anticorps. *Nouv. Rev. Hémat.*, **7**, 407-414.

HÖRDER, M., MANRIQUE, R. & WEINREICH, J. (1966). Über gleichzeitig auftretende Thrombozytopenie und erworbene hämolytische Anämie. *Med. Welt. (Stuttg.)*, **17**, (N.F.), 1502-1507.

HOROWITZ, S.D., BORCHERDING, W. & HONG, R. (1984). Autoimmune hemolytic anemia as a manifestation of T-suppressor-cell deficiency. *Clin. Immunol. Immunopath.*, **33**, 313-323.

HORVENO, HERVOUET, HARROUSSEAU & GUYOT-TRICHET (1958). L'anémie hémolytique par auto-anticorps due nourrisson (à propos d'un cas personnel). *Nourrisson*, **46**, 6-30.

HOYER, K. (1941). Et tilfaelde af febril haemolytisk anaemi af Lederer-typen. *Nord. Med.*, **12**, 3387-3390.

HUNT, M. L. & LUCIA, S. P. (1953). The occurrence of acquired hemolytic anemia in subjects of blood group O. *Science*, **118**, 183-184.

ISRAËLS, M. C. G. & WILKINSON, J. F. (1938). Haemolytic (spherocytic) jaundice in the adult. *Quart. J. Med.*, **7**, 137-150.

ISSARAGRISIL, S. & KRUATRACHUE, M. (1983). An association of pregnancy and autoimmune haemolytic anaemia. *Scand. J. Haemat.*, **31**, 63-68.

ISSITT, P. D., GRUPPO, R. A., WILKINSON, S. L. & ISSITT, C. H. (1982). Atypical presentation of acute phase, antibody-induced haemolytic anaemia in an infant. *Brit. J. Haemat.*, **52**, 537-543.

JAIN, G., AGARWAL, S., DASH, S. C. & GREWAL, K. S. (1977). Autoimmune hemolytic anemia and fetal loss. *J. Ass. Phycns India*, **25**, 765-776.

JANKELOWITZ, T., ECKERLING, B. & JOSHUA, H. (1960). A case of acquired haemolytic anaemia associated with pregnancy. *S. Afr. med. J.*, **34**, 911-913.

JOHNSON, C. A. & ABILDGARD, C. F. (1976). Treatment of idiopathic autoimmune hemolytic anemia in children. Review and report of two fatal cases in infancy. *Acta pediat. scand.*, **65**, 375-379.

JOULES, H. & MASTERMAN, L. M. (1935). The acute haemolytic anaemia of Lederer. *Brit. med. J.*, **ii**, 150-154.

JUNGMANN, P. (1914). Beitrage zur Kenntnis der Schwangershaftsanämie. *Münch. med. Wschr.*, **61**, 414-417.

KAGEYAMA, T., IWAKOSHI, K., TSUMOTO, S., TODA, H. & KIMOTO, S. (1975). A case of autoimmune hemolytic anemia in pregnancy and delivery. *Bull. Osaka med. Sch.*, **21**, 140-145.

KINTZEL, H. -W. & SCHMIDT, G. (1960). Perakute hämolytische Anämie (typ Lederer) nach thrombocytopenischer Purpura beim Kinde. *Z. Kinderheilk*, **83**, 362-368.

KISSMEYER-NIELSEN, F., BENT-HANSEN, K. & KIELER, J. (1952). Immuno-hemolytic anemia with familial occurrence. *Acta med. scand.*, **144**, 35-39.

KÖLBL, H. (1955). Klinik und Therapie der akuten erworbenen hämolytischen Anämien im Kindesalter. *Öst.Z. Kinderheilk.*, **11**, 27-51.

KRACKE, R. R. & RISER, W. H. JNR (1949). The problem of hypersplenism. *J. Amer. med. Ass.*, **141**, 1132-1139.

KRUATRACHUE, M. & SIRISINHA, S. (1977). Autoimmune haemolytic anaemias in Thailand. *Scand. J. Haemat.*, **19**, 61-67.

KÜHL, (1931). Ein Fall von akuter Anämie. *Klin. Wschr.*, **10**, 1053 (Abstract).

LAL, V. B. & SPEISER, P. (1957). Untersuchungen über Zusammenhänge zwischen erworbenen hämolytischen Anämien, klassischen Blutgruppen, Rhesusfactor, Geschlecht und Alter. *Blut*, **3**, 15-19.

LAMAGNÈRE, J. P., LEROY, J., AVRIL, J., LAUGIER, J. & DESBUQUOIS, G. (1972). Anémie hémolytique aiguë transitoire à auto-anticorps (gamma M)-C' de l'enfant. *Pédiatrie*, **27**, 749-756.

LAMY, M., JAMMET, M. -L., AUSSANNAIRE, M. & BOURNIQUE, R. (1950). Trois cas d'anémie hémolytique acquise observés dans le premier âge. *Arch. franç. Pédiat.*, **7**, 171-174.

LARSON, A. (1957). Chronic idiopathic autoimmune hemolytic disease in childhood. *Acta paediat. (Uppsala)*, **46**, 144-151.

LASKI, B., WAKE, E. J., BAIN, H. W. & GUNSON, H. H. (1961). Autohemolytic anemia in young infants. *J. Pediat.*, **59**, 42-46.

LASKI, B., WAKE, B., GUNSON, H. & BAIN, H. W. (1960). Idiopathic acquired hemolytic anemia in two young infants. *Amer. J. Dis. Child.*, **100**, 524-525 (Abstract).

LAZARUS, S. D. (1930). Acute hemolytic anemia in childhood. *Amer. J. Dis. Child.*, **40**, 1063–1068.

LE GENDRE & BRULÉ (1909). Ictère hémolytique congenital et ictère hémolytique acquis. *Presse méd.*, **17**, 70 (Abstract).

LE-XUAN-CHAT (1958). Les anémies hémolytiques par auto-anticorps au Vietnam (Étude préliminaire). *Sang*, **29**, 620–629.

LEDERER, M. (1925). A form of acute hemolytic anemia probably of infectious origin. *Amer. J. med. Sci.*, **170**, 500–510.

LEDERER, M. (1930). Three additional cases of acute hemolytic (infectious) anemia. *Amer. J. med. Sci.*, **179**, 228–236.

LEES, M. H., FISHER, O. D. & SHANKS, J. M. (1960). Case of immune aplastic haemolytic anaemia with thrombocytopenia. *Brit. med. J.*, **i**, 110–111.

LEONARDI, P. & GREGORIS, L. (1956). Anemia emolitica acuta idiopatica auto-immunoanticorpale con singulare comportamento globulare simulante la malattia di Marchiafava-Micheli. *Acta med. patav.*, **16**, 392–404.

LESCHER, F. G. (1942). The grave anaemias in pregnancy and the puerperium. Report of 17 cases. *Lancet*, **ii**, 148–151.

LESCHER, F. G., OSBORN, G. R. & BATES, J. J. G. (1939). Atypical haemolytic anaemias. *Quart. J. Med.*, **8**, 335–351.

LETMAN, H. (1957). Auto-immune haemolytic anaemia. *Dan. med. Bull.*, **4**, 143–147.

LETTS, H. W. & KREDENSTER, B. (1968). Thrombocytopenia, hemolytic anemia and two pregnancies. Report of a case. *Amer. J. clin. Path.*, **49**, 481–486.

LETTS, H. W. & KREDENSTER, B. K. (1969). Thrombocytopenia, hemolytic anemia, three pregnancies, and death. A supplementary case report. *Amer. J. clin. Path.*, **51**, 780–783.

LILLIE, E. W., GATENBY, P. B. B. & MOORE, H. C. (1954). A survey of anaemia in 4,314 cases of pregnancy. *Irish. J. med. Sci.*, 6th series, 304–310.

LIPPMAN, S. M., ARNETT, F. C., CONLEY, C. L., NESS, P. M., MEYERS, D. A. & BIAS, W. B. (1982). Genetic factors predisposing to autoimmune diseases. Autoimmune hemolytic anemia, chronic thrombocytopenic purpura, and systemic lupus erythematosus. *Amer. J. Med.*, **73**, 827–840.

LOEB, V. JNR, SEAMAN, W. B. & MOORE, C. V. (1952). The use of thorium dioxide sol (Thorotrast) in the roentgenologic demonstration of accessory spleens. *Blood*, **7**, 904–914.

LOUTIT, J. F. (1946). In discussion on the life and death of the red blood corpuscle. *Proc. roy. Soc. Med.*, **39**, 757–760.

LOUTIT, J. F. & MOLLISON, P. L. (1946). Haemolytic icterus (acholuric jaundice), congenital and acquired. *J. Path. Bact.*, **58**, 711–728.

LOVIBOND, J. L. (1935). Macrocytic haemolytic anaemia. *Lancet*, **ii**, 1395–1399.

LÜDIN, H. (1948). Zur Differentialdiagnose hämolytischer Anämien. *Acta haemat. (Basel)*, **1**, 28–33.

LUMLEY, S. P., MANSON, L., MURPHY, W. G. & LUDLAM, C. A. (1991). Unexplained haemolytic anaemia of pregnancy with negative direct antiglobulin test: response to high dose IV IgG. *Brit. J. Haemat.*, **77** (Suppl), 18.

MCGAVACK, T. H. (1939). Acute hemolytic (Lederer's?) anemia. *New Eng. J. Med.*, **220**, 140–142.

MAIER, C. (1948). Der Typus Loutit, eine neue Form von erworbenen hämolytischer Anämie. *Schweiz. med. Wschr.*, **78**, 983–984.

MARCOLONGO, F. (1953). Anemie emolitiche acquisate da auto-immunizzazione. *Rec. Progr. Med.*, **15**, 1, 137–239.

MALLARMÉ, J., AUZÉPY, P., BERCOVICI, J. P. & LÉVY, J. (1965). Un cas d'anémie hémolytique acquise, avec leucopenie et thrombopenie, de la grossesse. *Nouv. Rev. franç. Hémat.*, **5**, 765–768.

MARTIN, C. M., GORDON, R. S. & MCCULLOUGH, N. B. (1956). Acquired hypogammaglobulinemia in an adult. Report of a case, with clinical and experimental studies. *New Engl. J. Med.*, **254**, 449–456.

MASON, V. R. (1943). Acquired hemolytic anemia. *Arch. intern. Med.*, **72**, 471–493.

MATTHEWS, R. J. (1965). Idiopathic autoimmune hemolytic anemia and idiopathic thrombocytopenic purpura associated with diffuse hypergammaglobulinemia, amyloidosis, hypoalbuminemia, and plasmacytosis. *Amer. J. Med.*, **39**, 972–983.

MEIER, K. (1944). Die akute hämolytische Anämie vom Typ Lederer–Brill. *Ann. Paed.*, **162**, 140–161.

MEYER, J. F. (1951). Idiopathic acquired hemolytic anemia in an infant. Successful treatment with corticotropin (ACTH). *Amer. J. Dis. Child.*, **82**, 721–725.

MICHELI, F. (1911). Unmittelbare Effekte der Splenektomie bei einem Fall von erworbenen hämolytischen splenomegalischen Ikterus, Typus Hayem–Widal. *Wien. klin. Wschr.*, **24**, 1269–1274.

MILLER, B. A. & BEARDSLEY, D. S. (1983). Autoimmune pancytopenia of childhood associated with multisystem disease manifestations. *J. Pediat.*, **103**, 877–881.

MILLER, G., SHUMWAY, C. N. JNR & YOUNG, L. E. (1957). Auto-immune hemolytic anemias. *Pediat. Clin. N. Amer.*, **4**, 429–444.

MILLICHAP, J. G. (1952). Acute idiopathic haemolytic anaemia. *Arch. Dis. Childh.*, **27**, 222–229.

MIYAZAKI, S., FUKUDA, S., SHIBATA, R., KUROKAWA, T., GOYA, N., KOBAYASHI, T. & FUKUDA, T. (1980). A case of autoimmune hemolytic anemia associated with Duchenne's muscular dystrophy. *Acta haemat. jap.*, **43**, 685–688.

MIYAZAKI, S., NAKAYAMA, K., AKABANE, T., TAGUCHI, N., AKATSUKA, J., NAGAO, T., TSUJINO, G. & NAKAGAWA, T. (1983). Follow-up study of 34 children with autoimmune hemolytic anemia. *Acta haemat. jap.*, **46**, 6–10.

MOLLISON, P. L. (1947). The survival of transfused erythrocytes, with special reference to cases of acquired haemolytic anaemia. *Clin. Sci.*, **6**, 137–172.

MOLLISON, P. L. (1951). *Blood Transfusion in Clinical Medicine*, 456 pp. Blackwell Scientific Publications, Oxford.

MÖNCH, H., BREITHAUPT, H. & MUELLER-ECKHARDT, C. (1981). Immunological studies in a case of Evans' syndrome. *Blut*, **42**, 27–32.

MORTON, J. A. & PICKLES, M. M. (1947). Use of trypsin in the detection of incomplete anti-*Rh* antibodies. *Nature (Lond.)*, **159**, 779–780.

MOSKOWITZ, R. M. (1970). Autoimmune hemolytic anemia in a patient with a deficiency of red cell glucose-6-phosphate dehydrogenase activity. *Johns Hopk. med. J.*, **126**, 139–145.

MOUSA, M. E., NIMKHEDKAR, K., KUMAR, V. & JAIN, S. C. (1985). Coexistence of red cell aplasia and autoimmune haemolytic anaemia in a family. *Haematologia*, **18**, 201–203.

MÜLLER, W. A. & WEINREICH, J. (1956). Immun-pancytopenien. *Klin. Wschr.*, **34**, 505–509.

MURANO, G. (1946). Contributo alla conoscenza dell' anemia di Lederer. *Haematologica*, **28**, 183–255.

MURRAY-LYON, R. M. (1935). Familial acholuric jaundice simulating Lederer's anaemia. *Brit. med. J.*, **i**, 50–52.

NEGRI, M., POTOTSCHNIG, C. & MAIOLO, A. T. (1960). L'anemia emolitica da autoanticorpi nella prima infanzia. Presentazione di un caso. *Minerva pediat. (Torino)*, **12**, 656–666.

NEIMANN, P., MICHON, P., PIERSON, M. & LASCOMBES, G. (1956). L'anémie hémolytique acquise par auto-anticorps, chez le nourrisson. *Arch. franç. Pédiat.*, **13**, 247–256.

O'CONNOR, W. J., VAKIENER, J. M. & WATSON, R. J. (1956). Idiopathic acquired hemolytic anemia in young children. *Pediatrics*, **17**, 732–738.

O'DONOGHUE, R. J. L. & WITTS, L. J. (1932). The acute haemolytic anaemia of Lederer. *Guy's Hosp. Rep.*, **82**, 440–456.

OLANOFF, L. S. & FUDENBERG, H. H. (1983). Familial autoimmunity: twenty years later. *J. clin. lab. Immunol.*, **11**, 105–111.

OSGOOD, E. E. (1961). Antiglobulin-positive hemolytic anemias. *Arch. intern. Med.*, **107**, 313–323.

OSKI, F. A. & ABELSON, N. M. (1965). Autoimmune hemolytic anemia in an infant. Report of a case treated unsuccessfully with thymectomy. *J. Pediat.*, **67**, 752–758.

OSLER, W. (1919). Observations of the severe anaemias of pregnancy and the post-partum state. *Brit. med. J.*, **i**, 1–3.

OWREN, P. A. (1949). Acquired hemolytic jaundice. *Scand. J. clin. Lab. Invest.*, **1**, 41–48.

PAOLUCCI, G., ROSITO, P., MANCINI, A., VIVARELLI, F., MASI, M. & GIOVANARDI, E. (1970). Considerazioni clinico-terapeutiche su quattro casi di anemia emolitica autoimmune dell' infanzia. *Haematologica*, **55**, 509–521.

PARKES WEBER, F. (1931). Severe acute haemoglobinuria in a boy. *Proc. roy. Soc. Med.*, **25**, 715–716.

PARSONS, L. G. (1931). The anemias of infancy and early childhood. Some observations. *J. Amer. med. Ass.*, **97**, 973–979.

PARSONS, L. G. & HAWKSLEY, J. C. (1933). Studies in the anaemias of infancy and early childhood. Part V. The haemolytic (erythronoclastic) anaemias of later infancy and childhood: with special reference to the acute haemolytic anaemia of Lederer and the anaemia of von Jaksch. *Arch. Dis. Childh.*, **8**, 184–210.

PATTERSON, H. W. & STEWART SMITH, G. (1936). Acute haemolytic anaemia of Lederer in a child. *Lancet*, **ii**, 1096–1097.

PAYNE, R., SPAET, T. H. & AGGELER, P. M. (1955). An unusual antibody pattern in a case of idiopathic acquired hemolytic anemia. *J. Lab. clin. Med.*, **46**, 245–254.

PEARSON, H. A., ROBBINS, J. B. & SKINNER, R. G. (1967). Autoimmune hemolytic anemia in a patient with congenital hypogammaglobulinemia. *Ped. Res.*, **1**, 215 (Abstract).

PEGELS, J. G., HELMERHORST, F. M., VAN LEEUWEN, E. F., VAN DER PLAS-VAN DALEN, C., ENGELFRIET, C. P. & VON DEM BORNE, A. E. G. KR. (1982). The Evans syndrome: characterization of the responsible autoantibodies. *Brit. J. Haemat.*, **51**, 445–450.

PÉREZ-MATEO, M. & TASCÓN, A. (1982). Anemia hemolítica autoinmune idiopática en unos hermanos gamelos. *Med. clin. (Barcelona)*, **79**, 476 (Letter).

PETERS, R. W., JACOBS, R. A., FINKELSTEIN, J. Z. & MYHRE, B. A. (1974). Autoimmune hemolytic anemia in a 6-week-old infant. *Amer. J. Dis. Child.*, **127**, 268–270.

PIROFSKY, B. (1968). Hereditary aspects of autoimmune hemolytic anemia; a retrospective analysis. *Vox Sang.*, **14**, 334–347.

PIROFSKY, B. (1969). *Autoimmunization and the Autoimmune Hemolytic Anemias*, 537 pp. Williams and Wilkins, Baltimore.

POLLOCK, J. G., FENTON, E. & BARRETT, K. E. (1970). Familial autoimmune haemolytic anaemia associated with rheumatoid arthritis and pernicious anaemia. *Brit. J. Haemat.*, **18**, 171–182.

PRASAD, A. S., REINER, E. & WATSON, C. J. (1957). Syndrome of hypogammaglobulinemia, splenomegaly and hypersplenism. *Blood*, **12**, 926–932.

PUI, C. -H., WILLIMAS, J. & WANG, W. (1980). Evans syndrome in childhood. *J. Pediat.*, **97**, 754–758.

RAPOPORT, A. P., ROWE, J. M. & MCMICAN, A. (1988). Life-threatening autoimmune hemolytic anemia in a patient with the acquired immune deficiency syndrome. *Transfusion*, **28**, 190–191.

RAPPAPORT, H. & CROSBY, W. H. (1957). Auto-immune hemolytic anemia. II. Morphologic observations and clinicopathologic correlations. *Amer. J. Path.*, **33**, 429–449.

REYNOLDS, M. V., VENGELEN-TYLER, V. & MORE, P. A. (1981). Autoimmune hemolytic anemia associated with autoanti-Ge. *Vox Sang.*, **41**, 61–67.

RICH, K. C., ARNOLD, W. J., PALELLA, T. & FOX, I. H. (1979). Cellular immune deficiency with autoimmune hemolytic anemia in purine nucleoside phosphorylase deficiency. *Amer. J. Med.*, **67**, 172–176.

RITZ, N. D. & HABER, A. (1962). Autoimmune hemolytic anemia in a 6-week-old child. *J. Pediat.*, **61**, 904–910.

ROBBINS, J. B., SKINNER, R. G. & PEARSON, H. A. (1969). Autoimmune hemolytic anemia in a child with congenital X-linked hypogammaglobulinemia. *New Engl. J. Med.*, **280**, 75–79.

ROGET, J., BEAUDOING, A. & JOBERT (1959). Un cas d'anémie hémolytique par auto-anticorps chez un nourrisson de 14 mois. Echec de toutes les thérapeutiques. *Pédiatrie*, **14**, 530–536.

ROHN, R. J., BEHNKE, R. H. & BOND, W. H. (1955). Acquired agammaglobulinemia with hypersplenism. A case report. *Amer. J. med. Sci.*, **229**, 406–412.

ROSE, B. S. & NABARRO, S. N. (1953). Four cases of acute acquired haemolytic anaemia in childhood treated with A.C.T.H. *Arch. Dis. Childh.*, **28**, 87–90.

ROTH, P., MORELL, A., HUNZIKER, H. R., GEHRI, P. & BUCHER, U. (1975). Familiäre autoimmunhämolytische Anämie (AIHA) mit negativem Coombs-Test, Lymphozytopenie und Hypogammaglobulinämie. *Schweiz. med. Wschr.*, **105**, 1584–1585.

SACKS, D. A., PLATT, L. D. & JOHNSON, C. S. (1981). Autoimmune hemolytic disease during pregnancy. *Amer. J. Obstet. Gynec.*, **140**, 942–946.

SACKS, M. S., WORKMAN, J. B. & JAHN, E. F. (1952). Diagnosis and treatment of acquired hemolytic anemia. *J. Amer. med. Ass.*, **150**, 1556–1559.

SALAMA, A. & MUELLER-ECKHARDT, C. (1987). Autoimmune haemolytic anaemia in childhood associated with non-complement binding IgM autoantibodies. *Brit. J. Haemat.*, **65**, 67–71.

SANDER, R. P., HARDY, N. M. & VAN METER, S. A. (1987). Anti-Jk^a autoimmune hemolytic anemia in an infant. *Transfusion*, **27**, 58–60.

SANDLER, S. G. & ZLOTNICK, A. (1976). IgA deficiency and autoimmune hemolytic disease. Report of familial occurrence and discussion of the implications of transfusion therapy. *Arch. intern. Med.*, **136**, 93–94.

SANSONE, G. (1957). Anemie emolitiche acute idiopatiche a genesi autoimmunitaria nell'infanzia. *Minerva pediat. (Torino)*, **9**, 270–273.

SAXENA, K. M. & SARASWAT, K. D. (1957). Acquired haemolytic anaemia. *J. Ind. med. Ass.*, **29**, 403–405.

SCHALLER, J., DAVIS, S. D., CHING, Y.-C., LAGUNOFF, D., WILLIAMS, C. P. S. & WEDGWOOD, R. J. (1966). Hypergammaglobulinaemia, antibody deficiency, auto-immune haemolytic anaemia and nephritis in an infant with a familial lymphopenic immune defect. *Lancet*, **ii**, 825–829.

SCHMID, F. R. Unpublished observations quoted by Pirofsky (1969).

SCHOLER, H. & GERMANO, G. (1964). Perakute Hämolyse bei jugendlichen Personon. *Schweiz. med. Wschr.*, **94**, 1391–1395.

SCHREIBER, Z. A., LOH, S. H., CHARLES, M. & ABEEDE, L. S. (1983). Autoimmune hemolytic anemia in patients with acquired immune deficiency syndrome. *Blood*, **62**, 117a (Abstract 370).

SCHUBOTHE, H. (1957). Der erworbenen hämolytischen Anämien. B. Die Klinik der autoimmunhämolytischen Erkrankungen. In *Immunopathologie in Klinik und Forschung und das Problem der Autoantikörper* (ed. by P. Miescher and K. O. Vorlaender), p. 196. Georg Thieme, Stuttgart.

SCHULTHESS, G. VON (1949). Der Typus Loutit, eine neue Form von erworbener hämolytischer Anämie. *Acta haemat. (Basel)*, **2**, 1–13.

SCHWARTZ, R. S. & COSTEA, N. (1966). Autoimmune hemolytic anemia: clinical correlations and biological implications. *Seminars Hemat.*, **3**, 2–26.

SEIP, M., HARBOE, M. & CYVIN, K. (1969). Chronic autoimmune hemolytic anemia in childhood with cold antibodies, aplastic crisis and familial occurrence. *Acta paediat. scand.*, **58**, 275–280.

SELWYN, J. G. & HACKETT, W. E. R. (1949). Acquired haemolytic anaemia: survival of transfused erythrocytes in patients and normal recipients. *J. clin. Path.*, **2**, 114–120.

SÉZARY, A., KIPFER, H. & GHARIB, M. (1938). 'Livedo annularis' et crises de cyanose chez un sujet atteint de maladie hémolytique avec grande auto-agglutination des hématies. *Bull. Soc. méd. Hôp. Paris*, **54**, 1710–1716.

SHAPIRO, M. (1967). Familial autohemolytic anemia and runting syndrome with **Rh$_o$**-specific autoantibody. *Transfusion*, **7**, 281–296.

SHIREY, R. S., KICKLER, T. S., BELL, W., LITTLE, B., SMITH, B. & NESS, P. M. (1987). Fatal immune hemolytic anemia and hepatic failure associated with a warm-reacting IgM autoantibody. *Vox Sang.*, **52**, 219–222.

SIDDOO, J. K. (1954). Acquired hemolytic anemia associated with hemochomatosis. *Arch. intern. Med.*, **93**, 977–981.

SIEVERS, K., LEHTINEN, M. & AHO, K. (1968). Development of immune haemolytic anaemia and thrombocytopenia in a chronic biologic false-positive reactor for syphilis. *Scand. J. Haemat.*, **5**, 264–270.

SILVERSTEIN, M. N., AARO, L. A. & KEMPERS, R. D. (1966). Evans' syndrome and pregnancy. *Amer. J. med. Sci.*, **252**, 206–211.

SILVERSTEIN, M. N., GOMES, M. R., ELVEBACK, L. R., REMINE, W. H. & LINMAN, J. W. (1972). Idiopathic acquired hemolytic anemia. Survival in 117 cases. *Arch. intern. Med.*, **129**, 85–87.

SILVERSTEIN, M. N. & HECK, F. J. (1962). Acquired hemolytic anemia and associated thrombocytopenic purpura: with special reference to Evans' syndrome. *Proc. Staff Meetings Mayo Clin.*, **37**, 122–128.

SÖDERHJELM, L. (1959). Non-spherocytic haemolytic anaemia in mother and new-born infant. *Acta paediat. scand.*, **48**, Suppl. 117, 34–39.

SOKOL, R. J., HEWITT, S. & STAMPS, B. (1981). Autoimmune haemolysis: an 18-year study of 865 cases referred to a regional transfusion centre. *Brit. med. J.*, **282**, 2023–2027.

SOKOL, R. J., HEWITT, S. & STAMPS, B. K. (1982). Erythrocyte autoantibodies, autoimmune haemolysis and pregnancy. *Vox Sang.*, **43**, 169–176.

SOKOL, R. J., HEWITT, S., STAMPS, B. K. & HITCHEN, P. A. (1984). Autoimmune haemolysis in childhood and adolescence. *Acta haemat. (Basel)*, **72**, 245–257.

STANDAERT, L. & DE MOOR, P. (1955). L'agammaglobulinémie chez l'adulte. *Acta clin. belg.*, **10**, 477–492.

STARKSEN, N. F., BELL, W. R. & KICKLER, T. S. (1983). Unexplained hemolytic anemia associated with pregnancy. *Amer. J. Obstet. Gynec.*, **146**, 617–622.

STEPHINGER, J. (1954). Klinische Beobachtungen, Verlauf und Behandlung hämolytischer Anämien vom Typ Loutit. *Klin. Wschr.*, **32**, 1046–1049.

STOELINGA, G. B. A., VAN MUNSTER, P. J. J. & SLOOFF, J. P. (1969). Antibody deficiency syndrome and autoimmune haemolytic anaemia in a boy with isolated IgM deficiency. Dysimmunoglobulinaemia type 5. *Acta paediat. scand.*, **58**, 352–362.

STRAUB, E. & SACHTLEBEN, P. (1967). Autoaggresive Antikörper bei antikörpermangel syndrom. *Mschr. Kinderheilk.*, **115**, 527–531.

SWISHER, S. N. (1966). Acquired hemolytic disease. *Postgrad. Med. Minn.*, *U.S.A.*, **40**, 378–386.

TATTERSALL, M. H. N. (1967). Thrombocytopenic purpura in patient with autoimmune haemolytic anaemia, successfully treated with mercaptopurine. *Brit. med. J.*, **iii**, 93–94.

TEETER, C. E. (1907). Recovery from leukanemia. *J. Amer. med. Ass.*, **48**, 608–609.

THOMPSON, E. N. & JOHNSON, R. J. (1962). A case of primary idiopathic hypogammaglobulinaemia associated with haemolytic anaemia. *Postgrad. med. J.*, **38**, 292–295.

TISDALE, W. A., KLATSKIN, G. & KINSELLA, E. D.

(1959). The significance of the direct-reacting fraction of serum bilirubin in hemolytic jaundice. *Amer. J. Med.*, **26**, 214–227.

TOOLIS, F., PARKER, A. C., WHITE, A. & URBANIAK, S. (1977). Familial autoimmune haemolytic anaemia. *Brit. med. J.*, **i**, 1392.

VANHAEVERBEEK, M., DELVOYE, P., GAUSSET, P. & MASSART-GUIOT, TH. (1974). Anémie hémolytique auto-immune au cours de la grossesse. *J. Gynéc. Obstét. Biol. reprod. (Paris)*, **4**, 227–234.

VAN LOGHEM, J. J. (1965). Some comments on autoantibody induced red cell destruction. *Ann. N. Y. Acad. Sci.*, **124**, 465–476.

VAN LOGHEM-LANGEREIS, E., PEETOOM, F., VAN DER HART, M., VAN LOGHEM, J. J., BOSCH, E. & GOUDSMIT, R. (1965). The occurrence of gammaglobulin/anti-gammaglobulin complexes in a patient suffering from hypogammaglobulinaemia and haemolytic anaemia. *Proc. 10th Congr. int. Soc. Blood Transf., Stockholm 1964. Bibliotheca haemat.*, **23**, 55–61.

VAUGHAN, J. M. (1936). *The Anaemias*, 2nd edn., pp. 230 and 250. Oxford University Press.

VERGER & MOULINIER (1957). Anémie hémolytique avec auto-anticorps du nourrisson. *J. Méd. Bordeaux*, **134**, 531–533.

VIDEBAEK, A. (1962). Primary (idiopathic) auto-immune haemolytic anaemia. *Acta med. scand.*, **171**, 449–462.

WAGNER, K. & MARESCH, W. (1955). Hämolytische Anämie und inkomplette Rhesus-Antikörper (anti-c̄) bei eines Schwangeren. *Wien. klin. Wschr.*, **67**, 856–858.

WASASTJERNA, C. (1954). Leukocyte-agglutinins in a case of chronic granulocytopenia and hemolytic anemia. *Acta med. scand.*, **144**, 355–360.

WAUGH, T. R. (1932). Acquired haemolytic jaundice in a woman previously splenectomized for essential thrombocytopenia. *Folia haemat. (Lpz.)*, **48**, 248–260.

WEBSTER, A. D. B., PLATT-MILLS, T. A. E., JANNOSSY, G., MORGAN, M. & ASHERSON, G. L. (1981). Autoimmune blood dyscrasias in five patients with hypogammaglobulinemia: response of neutropenia to vincristine. *J. clin. Immunol.*, **1**, 113–118.

WEINER, W., WHITEHEAD, J. P. & WALKDEN, W. J. (1956). Acquired haemolytic anaemia. Clinical and serological observations of two cases. *Brit. med. J.*, **i**, 73–77.

WIDAL, F., ABRAMI, P. & BRULÉ, M. (1908a). Les ictères d'origine hémolytique. *Arch. Mal. Coeur*, **1**, 193–231.

WIDAL, F., ABRAMI, P. & BRULÉ, M. (1908b). Auto-agglutinations des hématies dans l'ictère hémolytique acquis. *C. R. Soc. Biol. (Paris)*, **64**, 655–657.

WIDAL, F., ABRAMI, P. & BRULÉ, M. (1909). Rétrocession des symptômes cliniques et des troubles hématiques au cours des ictères hémolytiques acquis. *Bull. Soc. méd. Hôp. Paris*, **28**, 73–85.

WIENER, A. S., SAMWICK, A. A., MORRISON, M. & LOEWE, L. (1952). Acquired hemolytic anemia. *Amer. J. clin. Path.*, **22**, 301–312.

WIESNETH, M., PFLIEGER, H., FRICKHOFEN, N. & HEIMPEL, H. (1985). Idiopathic combined immunocytopenia. *Brit. J. Haemat.*, **61**, 339–348.

WILMERS, M. J. & RUSSELL, P. A. (1963). Autoimmune haemolytic anaemia in an infant treated by thymectomy. *Lancet*, **ii**, 915–917.

WIRTHEIMER, C. (1957). Grossesse et anémie hémolytique, *Brux.-méd.*, **37**, 539–547.

WISEMAN, B. K. & DOAN, C. A. (1942). Primary splenic neutropenia; a newly recognized syndrome closely related to congenital hemolytic icterus and essential thrombocytopenic purpura. *Ann. intern. Med.*, **16**, 1097–1117.

WITTS, L. J. (1932). The pathology and treatment of anaemia. Lecture III. The haemolytic anaemia of pregnancy (Part 2 of third Goulstonian lecture). *Lancet*, **i**, 652–657.

YAM, P., WILKINSON, L., PETZ, L. D. & GARRATTY, G. (1980). Studies on hemolytic anemia in pregnancy with evidence for autoimmunization in a patient with a negative direct antiglobulin (Coombs') test. *Amer. J. Hemat.*, **8**, 23–29.

YOUNG, L. E. & MILLER, G. (1953). The long-term picture in autoimmune hemolytic disease. *Trans. Ass. Amer. Phycns*, **66**, 190–199.

YOUNG, L. E., MILLER, G. & CHRISTIAN, R. M. (1951). Clinical and laboratory observations on autoimmune hemolytic disease. *Ann. intern. Med.*, **35**, 507–517.

ZARA, C. & BOLIS, P. F. (1972). Anemia emolitica da autoanticorpi in gravidanza (descrizione di due casi). *Ann. Ostet. Ginec.*, **93**, 468–472.

ZUCKER-FRANKLIN, D. & KARPATKIN, S. (1977). Red-cell and platelet fragmentation in idiopathic autoimmune thrombocytopenic purpura. *New Engl. J. Med.*, **297**, 517–523.

ZUELZER, W. W., MASTRANGELO, R., STULBERG, C. S., POULIK, M. D., PAGE, R. H. & THOMPSON, R. I. (1970). Autoimmune hemolytic anemia. Natural history and viral–immunologic interactions in childhood. *Amer. J. Med.*, **49**, 80–93.

ZUPAŃSKA, B., LAWKOWICZ, W., GÓRSKA, B., KOZLONSKA, J., OCHOCKA, M., ROKICKA-MILEWSKA, R., DERULSKA, D. & CIEPIELEWSKA, D. (1976). Autoimmune haemolytic anaemia in children. *Brit. J. haemat.*, **34**, 511–520.

Auto-immune haemolytic anaemia (AIHA): warm-antibody syndromes II: 'idiopathic' types: haematological and biochemical findings

Blood picture   *54*
  Blood films   *54*
  Absolute values   *57*
  Auto-agglutination   *57*
  Erythrophagocytosis   *59*
  Erythroblastaemia   *60*
  Spherocytosis   *62*
Osmotic fragility (OF)   *63*
Autohaemolysis   *66*
  Mechanical fragility (MF)   *66*
Reticulocytes   *67*
Siderocytes   *67*
Bone marrow   *67*
  Megaloblastic erythropoiesis   *68*
Reticulocytopenia   *69*
'Aplastic' crises   *69*
  Role of parvovirus   *76*

Leucocytes   *77*
  Erythrocyte neutrophil rosetting   *78*
Platelets   *78*
Effect of splenectomy on the blood picture   *80*
Biochemical findings   *80*
  Serum proteins   *80*
  Abnormal serological reactions   *81*
  Biological false-positive tests for syphilis   *81*
Haemoglobinaemia   *84*
  Haptoglobins   *84*
Serum bilirubin   *85*
Urine   *85*
Faeces   *85*
Erythrocyte metabolism   *86*
  Acetylcholinesterase   *86*
  Erythrocyte membrane proteins   *88*
  Erythrocyte lipids   *88*

BLOOD PICTURE

There are two features that indicate strongly that a patient is suffering from a haemolytic anaemia of auto-immune origin: one is the presence of auto-agglutination of the erythrocytes and the other is evidence of erythrophagocytosis. Other features, such as spherocytosis and polychromasia, although often present to a marked degree in AIHA are, of course, to be seen in other types of haemolytic anaemia.

Anaemia

The degree to which a patient is anaemic varies considerably, but in an untreated patient the erythrocyte count may fall as low as $1–2 \times 10^{12}/l$ or even lower (Table 23.1). Characteristically, the anaemia is macrocytic rather than normocytic. The macrocytosis is 'regenerative' in nature and is associated with a raised reticulocyte count, the macrocytes being derived from macronormoblasts rather than from megaloblasts.

Blood films

Anisocytosis is usually a marked feature; this is brought about by the presence of microsphero-cytes with reduced erythrocyte diameter and macrocytes usually staining diffusely basophilic—these are the reticulocytes. If there is marked spherocytosis and a high reticulocyte count, the degree of anisocytosis may be striking, the microspherocytes being as small as 5 µm in diameter and the disc-like macrocytes as large as 10 µm (Fig. 23.1). The spherocytes typically have a rounded contour. Poikilocytes are generally not conspicuous in AIHA. However, in some patients small numbers of pear-shaped cells may be present. Rather rarely, small thin projections from the surface of some of the erythrocytes may be seen (Dacie, 1962, p. 354) (Fig. 23.2).

Table 23.1 Representative haematological data in cases of auto-immune haemolytic anaemia of the idiopathic warm-antibody type.

Patient	Erythrocytes (minimum) $\times 10^{12}/l$	Haemoglobin (minimum) g/dl	MCV (mean) fl	MCHC (mean) (%)	Reticulocytes (maximum) (%)	Leucocytes (range) per µl	Platelets (range) per µl	Bilirubin (maximum) per dl	Comment
Mild cases									
L. M. (Case 8 of Dacie, 1954)	1.9	8.4	110	35	11.5	8000	110 000–120 000	1.2	Spontaneous recovery
S. H. (Case 9 of Dacie, 1954)	2.7	10.0	100	37	14.5	7000–8000	190 000	1.9	Clinical cure followed splenectomy (Fig. 172)
Serious cases									
A. A. (Case 8)		5.6		32	57	6000–14 000	130 000–430 000	4.1	Auto-antibody of anti-e specificity. Died of broncho-pneumonia
E. B. (Case 12)	2.0	3.7	123	30	69	10 000–20 000	160 000–320 000	8.0	Moderate improvement followed splenectomy (Fig. 174)
R. D.* (Case 13)	2.1	7.1	147	27	68	15 000–40 000	60 000–580 000	3.5	Splenectomy failed to benefit the patient. Haemolysis controlled by high doses of steroids (Fig. 178)
Fatal cases									
J. L. (Case 11 of Dacie, 1954)	1.2	5.0	111	33	30	15 000–28 000	100 000–110 000	5.0	Never fit for splenectomy
R. E. (Case 12 of Dacie, 1954)	1.4	4.5	106	43	32	21 000	220 000–270 000		Died in an acute crisis. Splenectomy 11 years previously for thrombocytopenic purpura
J. H. (Case 4)		3.9		29	51	12 000–20 000	2000–4000		Died with severe thrombocytopenia. Not fit for splenectomy
D. P.* (Case 7)	2.2	5.2	107	32	7.9	3300–8700	10 000–26 000		Alternating haemolytic anaemia and thrombocytopenia. Splenectomy carried out 5 years before. 'Warm' haemolysin. Died in acute crisis

Table 23.1 (*contd*)

Cases with complications

C. J. (Case 5) (folic-acid deficiency)	6.2			29	20	1600–7000	90 000–350 000	2.6	Responded well to steroids and folic acid (Chanarin, Dacie and Mollin, 1959) (Fig. 143)
E. M. (Case 6) (massive splenomegaly with leuco-penia)	2.1	6.1	102	32	9.5	1000–2100	100 000–160 000	4.9	Responded well to splenectomy ('simple' hyperplasia of spleen) (Fig. 144)

*After splenectomy.
Unless specified otherwise, the Case and Figure numbers refer to patients described by Dacie (1962).

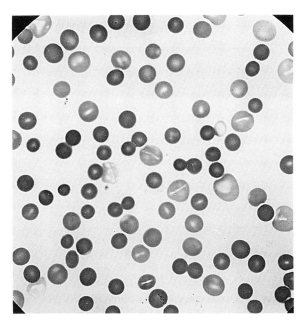

Fig. 23.1   Photomicrograph of a blood film from a patient with warm-antibody AIHA.
Spherocytosis and anisochromasia are conspicuous. Some of the spherocytes are adhering together in pairs. The large pale staining macrocytes are reticulocytes. x 700.

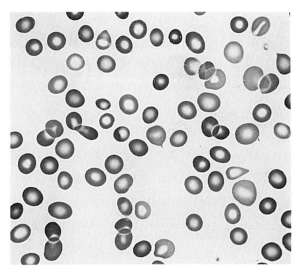

Fig. 23.2   Photomicrograph of a blood film from a patient with idiopathic warm-antibody AIHA.
There is a minor degree of spherocytosis and anisochromasia. A few poikilocytes are present and the cell in the centre of the field has a small thin projection from its surface. x 700.

Farolino and co-workers (1986) have more recently raised the question of the role of the spleen in the causation of tear-drop poikilocytes (dacryocytes) in the peripheral blood of patients with AIHA. They described two patients in whom tear-drop cells were conspicuous: in the first patient they disappeared from the peripheral blood within 2 weeks of splenectomy: in the second (who had Hodgkin's disease and AIHA) the number of tear-drop cells markedly diminished following prednisone and standard anti-Hodgkin's disease therapy which had caused the spleen to shrink. Farolino et al. concluded that the tear-drop deformity might be the consequence of extramedullary erythropoiesis or perhaps result from the passage of erythrocytes through an abnormal spleen.

Polychromasia is often obvious, reflecting the height of the reticulocyte count. Punctate basophilia is not a marked feature. Pappenheimer bodies can, however, usually be seen in films made from patients who have undergone splenectomy; they are rarely seen if the spleen is *in situ* (see later, under Siderocytes, p. 67).

Absolute values

The MCV is usually substantially raised, reflecting the increased percentage of reticulocytes usually present. The MCH is usually normal and the MCHC within the normal range, too, but it is likely to be above normal in patients in whom there is marked spherocytosis. Representative data are given in Table 23.1.

Spurious high values for MCV (and low values for erythrocyte count) may result from the use of automated cell counters if auto-agglutinated cells fail to separate and are counted as doublets or triplets (Brittin et al., 1969). Weiss and Bessman (1984) recorded how in two patients the automated MCV value varied erratically from 89 to 162 fl, and from 113 to 128 fl, respectively. In both patients volume distribution curves showed abnormal triplet and/or doublet cell peaks (Fig. 23.3).

Auto-agglutination

Massive auto-agglutination, easily visible to the naked eye, is a characteristic feature in patients with cold-antibody AIHA, if their blood has been allowed to cool to room temperature (15–25°C). Less intense auto-agglutination, which is not so obvious to the naked-eye and persisting in blood

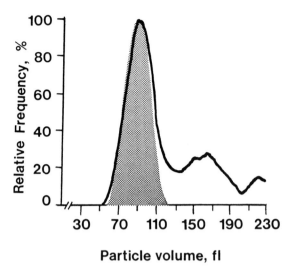

Fig. 23.3   Distribution of MCV (particle volume) in a patient with AIHA, as recorded by an automated cell counter.
There are two, and possibly three, volume peaks.
[Reproduced by permission from Weiss and Bessman (1984).]

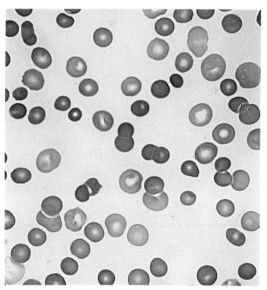

Fig. 23.4   Photomicrograph of a blood film from a patient with idiopathic warm-antibody AIHA.
There is moderately marked spherocytosis and some auto-agglutination. x 700.

kept at 37°C, is a quite common feature of the blood of patients suffering from warm-antibody AIHA if they are severely affected. In Figs 23.4 and 23.5 are illustrated various degrees of auto-agglutination. The spherocytes, in particular, tend to stick together in pairs or larger clumps. The agglutination appears to be brought about by the mutual adhesion of cells coated by incomplete antibodies when the cells are suspended in a medium of high protein content such as plasma. Exceptionally, the agglutination results from the action of an auto-agglutinin, active at 37°C, in which case the consequent agglutination may be massive.

As already mentioned (p. 6), auto-agglutination was referred to in the first decade of this century by French physicians in their early descriptions of 'l'ictère hémolytique acquis'. Moreover, it was thought to be a feature which distinguished acquired from congenital cases of haemolytic jaundice. Its presence has often been referred to in subsequent descriptions of acquired haemolytic anaemia, both before and after the recognition that many of the cases are caused by the formation of anti-erythrocyte auto-antibodies.

Early case reports in which auto-agglutination was noted to be a striking feature include those of Troisier

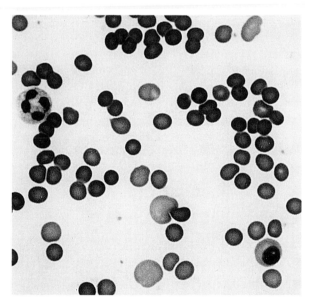

Fig. 23.5   Photomicrograph of a blood film from a patient with warm-antibody AIHA.
There is marked spherocytosis and definite auto-agglutination. x 700.

and Cattan (1932), Greenwald (1938), Ravault, Girard and Joud (1939), Hargraves, Herrell and Pearman (1941), Reisner and Kalkstein (1942), Evans (1943), Mason (1943), Young and Lawrence (1946) and Renner and McShane (1947). It seems likely that most, if not all, of the patients described in the case reports cited above were suffering from warm-antibody AIHA. Hahn and Lüttgens (1949), in a lengthy review of the occurrence of auto-agglutination in haemolytic icterus, recognized three categories: that due to cold auto-agglutinins, cold auto-agglutinins with extended thermal range, and warm auto-agglutinins, respectively.

Erythrophagocytosis

As already referred to, the presence in the peripheral blood of monocytes (or rarely neutrophils) that have phagocytosed erythrocytes is a pointer to an auto-immune haemolytic anaemia. Phagocytosis by circulating monocytes and fixed macrophages is in fact an important mechanism for the elimination from the circulation of erythrocytes that have been damaged by auto-antibodies and/or complement (see Chap. 34). In practice, erythrophagocytosis is most easily seen in films made from the buffy coat of peripheral blood (Zinkham and Diamond, 1952; de Gruchy, 1954) (Figs 23.6 and 23.7). Sometimes, however, so many erythrophages are present that they can be found without too much difficulty in films of whole uncentrifuged blood (Fig. 23.8). Another way that has been suggested to increase their number is to make films from blood withdrawn from the finger after its circulation has been obstructed for a short while (Ehrlich's test) (Schubothe and Müller, 1955; Wolf, 1956).

Case reports in which the presence of erythrophagocytosis was described include those of Hargraves, Herrell and Pearman (1941), Landolt (1946), Berrey and Watson (1951), Gasser and Holländer (1951) (Fig. 22.5, p. 33), Gasser (1952, 1954), Zinkham and Diamond (1952), Betke et al. (1953), de Gruchy (1954), Kölbl (1955), Schubothe and Müller (1955), Wolf (1956), Sansone (1957), Pisciotta, Downer and Hinz (1959) and Greenberg et al. (1980). Most of the erythrophages noted in the case reports cited above were monocytes; phagocytosis by neutrophils was, however, recorded by Hargraves, Herrell and Pearman (1941).

Hargraves, Herrell and Pearman's (1941) patient was a 54-year-old male who eventually recovered after an acute haemolytic episode: in this exceptional case not only were erythrocytes being phagocytosed by monocytes and neutrophils but the phagocytic cells were themselves surrounded by agglutinated

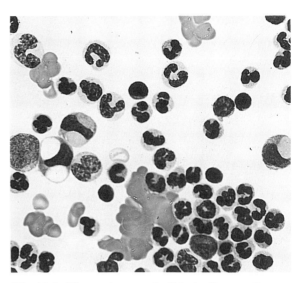

Fig. 23.6   Photomicrograph of the buffy coat of a patient with severe idiopathic AIHA (Case 7, Dacie, 1962, p. 439).
There is gross auto-agglutination and many of the monocytes are acting as erythrophages. x 700.

spheroidally shaped erythrocytes [Fig. 23.9 and Sansone (1957) below].

Landolt (1946), who described how a 6-year-old girl had died of acute haemolytic anaemia after an illness lasting only 7 days, reported that 14% and 28% (two counts) of her circulating monocytes were acting as erythrophages.

Gasser and Holländer's (1951) 7-week-old male infant has already been referred to (Fig. 22.5). Monocytes phagocytosing erythrocytes (up to six per cell) were particularly frequent in blood obtained from the spleen.

Zinkham and Diamond (1952) described erythrophagocytosis in the peripheral blood of two infants, one with acute and the other with more chronic AIHA. The erythrophages were noted to be much more numerous in films made from the buffy coat of centrifuged blood after it had been incubated for $\frac{1}{2} - 2$ hours at $37°C$ than in peripheral blood films made in the ordinary way.

de Gruchy (1954) looked for erythrophagocytosis in the buffy-coat films of eight patients with AIHA: erythrophages were seen in five of them, all actively haemolysing; none was seen in one other actively haemolysing patient and in two remitting cases.

Schubothe and Müller (1955) described erythrophagocytosis in the finger blood of three patients with warm-antibody AIHA after the circulation in a finger had been obstructed by a ligature and the finger then submerged in water at $40°C$ for 30 minutes.

Sansone (1957), who described three children with acute AIHA, stressed the value of looking at wet prepa-

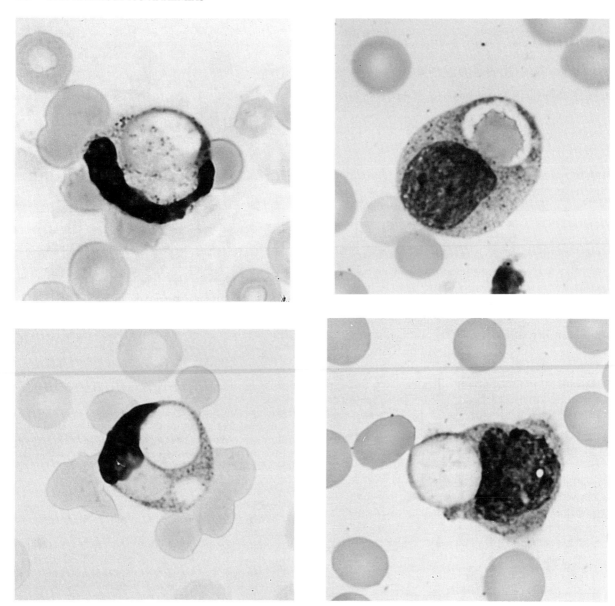

Fig. 23.7   Four photomicrographs of monocytes acting as erythrophages in the buffy coat of a 8-month-old infant suffering from acute AIHA.
x 2000. (Reproduced by the courtesy of Dr. W. H. Zinkham.)

rations of blood by phase-contrast microscopy. He illustrated the occurrence of erythrophagocytosis and the adhesion of erythrocytes to monocytes, a phenomenon he described as 'aspetti a margherita' (Fig. 23.10).

Erythroblastaemia

Erythroblasts, mainly polychromatic normoblasts,

are often present in the peripheral blood of patients suffering from warm-antibody AIHA; they are, however, only present in large numbers when haemolysis is rapid and the reticulocyte count is markedly raised. The largest numbers are likely to be seen in patients in whom increased haemolysis and anaemia have persisted after splenectomy: then the erythroblast count may

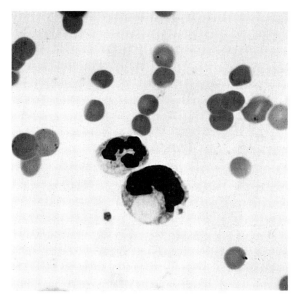

Fig. 23.8   Photomicrograph of a peripheral blood film of a patient with very severe warm-antibody AIHA (Case 12 of Dacie, 1954, p. 202).
There is marked spherocytosis and auto-agglutination. The monocyte towards the centre of the field is acting as an erythrophage. x 1000.

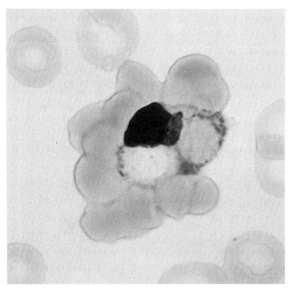

Fig. 23.9a

dyserythropoietic changes, e.g. nuclear budding, as illustrated by Troisier and Cattan (1932). (See also Fig. 23.11.)

Early case reports of patients (described as suffering from acquired haemolytic jaundice or acute haemolytic anaemia), in whose blood erythroblastaemia was a notable feature, include those of Kaznelson (1924),

even exceed the total leucocyte count. In seriously anaemic patients the normoblasts may show

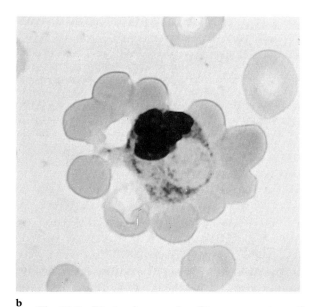

b

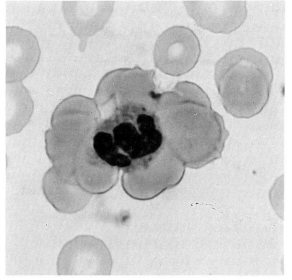

c

Fig. 23.9   Photomicrographs of two monocytes acting as erythrophages and one neutrophil surrounded by a cluster of spherocytes in the buffy coat of an 8-month-old infant suffering from acute AIHA.
x 2000. (Reproduced by the courtesy of Dr. W. H. Zinkham.)

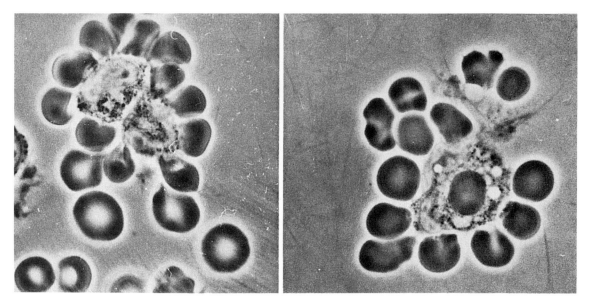

Fig. 23.10   Photomicrographs of the peripheral blood of a child with acute AIHA showing adhesion of spherocytes to monocytes.
A wet preparation, as viewed by phase-contrast microscopy. [Reproduced by permission from Sansone (1957).]

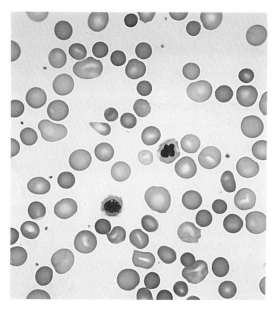

Fig. 23.11   Photomicrograph of a blood film from a patient with warm-antibody AIHA.
There is marked spherocytosis and anisocytosis, and the normoblast in the centre of the field has a fragmented nucleus. x 700.

Lederer (1925), Reynolds (1930), Castex, Steingart and Poletti (1932), Troisier and Cattan (1932), Waugh (1932), Dameshek and Schwartz (1938a, 1940), Ravault, Girard and Joud (1939), Sterner (1940–1941), Hanssen (1943) and David and Minot (1944). The patients described in the above reports were all severely anaemic and none had had, of course, the benefit of treatment with corticosteroids. Their erythroblast counts had been as high as 20 000 per μl.

Later reports of acutely anaemic patients (in whom auto-antibodies had been demonstrated), and in whom there was marked erythroblastaemia, include those of Pisciotta, Downer and Hinz (1959) and Martin and Kilian (1960). Martin and Kilian's patient had relapsed three times after splenectomy, and on each occasion increasing the dosage of corticosteroid led to high reticulocyte and nucleated cell counts, the latter reaching the exceptionally high total of $190 \times 10^9/l$ of which $160 \times 10^9/l$ were erythroblasts. The report of Coutel, Bretagne and Morel (1962) is much more typical. Their patient, a boy aged 9 years, had 30% erythroblasts out of a total of $18 \times 10^9/l$ nucleated cells at a time his erythrocyte count had fallen to $1.0 \times 10^{12}/l$. Splenectomy had, however, not been carried out.

Spherocytosis

As described in Volume 1 of this book (p. 67), it was not until the publications of Dameshek and Schwartz (1938a, b; 1940) that it came to be realized and was generally accepted that spherocytosis was a common and important accompaniment of haemolytic anaemias that were of acquired origin, in addition to being a characteristic finding in the disorder now generally referred to as hereditary spherocytosis (HS). Dameshek and Schwartz (1938a,b) not only demonstrated spherocytosis in human cases of acute acquired haemolytic anaemia, they also showed that spherocytosis (microspherocytosis) was a characteristic finding in acute antibody-induced haemolytic anaemia that had been produced experimentally in guinea-pigs (Fig. 3.4, Vol. 1, p. 68). [The same change had, in fact, been described and illustrated many years previously by Muir and McNee (1912) in rabbits to which haemolytic immune sera had been administered (Fig. 3.3, Vol. 1, p. 67), although the microspherocytes so produced had not been specifically named.]

The mechanism by which spherocytes are produced in antibody-produced haemolytic anaemias is now fairly well understood. It is not a direct effect of antibody on the erythrocyte surface (as is the case, for instance, with the spherocytosis caused by the toxin of *Cl. welchi*), it results from injurious contact between antibody- and/or complement-coated erythrocytes and phagocytic cells which possess receptors which are specific for the FC fragment of antibodies or the third component of complement (C3) (see Ch. 34).

In practice, although spherocytosis is often easily recognized in the blood films of patients with warm-antibody AIHA, the phenomenon is not always present, at any rate to a marked degree, even if the patient under study is actively haemolysing. The reason for the case-to-case differences in spherocytosis is not wholly understood: presumably it depends on the nature of the antibodies, as well as the number of antibody molecules being produced, and on subtle antibody-to-antibody differences in the degree to which the erythrocyte surface is damaged by antibody or antibody/complement action. In Figs 23.1, 23.2, 23.4 and 23.5 are illustrated blood films from patients suffering from warm-antibody AIHA. The photographs illustrate patient-to-patient differences in spherocytosis and also how spherocytosis may or may not be combined with auto-agglutination. As with the visual appreciation of spherocytosis, large patient-to-patient differences in osmotic fragility (OF) are apparent if OF is measured quantitatively (see below).

OSMOTIC FRAGILITY (OF)

Increased OF has been known for many years to be a striking finding in some cases of acquired haemolytic anaemia. This was so, for instance, in one of the three patients reported by Dameshek and Schwartz (1938a) as suffering from acute haemolytic anaemia. She was 44 years old and became rapidly anaemic over a 5-day period: her haemoglobin fell to 22%; there were 21% reticulocytes and osmotic lysis commenced in 0.72 g/dl NaCl. Haemoglobinuria followed a blood transfusion. However, she eventually recovered completely after splenectomy, and 7 weeks later OF was normal. Dameshek and Schwartz realized that the increase in OF was a reflection of a marked but transient microspherocytosis.

It is now realized that OF is, in fact, usually moderately or markedly increased in most cases of warm-antibody AIHA and that the increase runs parallel with the degree of spherocytosis present. In patients in remission, on the other hand, the OF is likely to be normal or at the most only very slightly increased even if the DAT is still positive. Greatly increased OF, on the other hand, is always associated with clinically serious haemolysis. Observations on a series of patients investigated by the author are summarized in Fig. 23.12: OF was strictly normal in five out of the 22 cases and only just increased in a further four patients. Two of the patients in whom the OF was normal or only minimally increased were acutely ill and died of their disease, and the others were in an active haemolytic phase; one had undergone splenectomy. Splenectomy is not necessarily associated with a diminution in OF—unless the patient goes into remission following the operation. The patient with the greatest increase in OF recorded in Fig. 23.12 [Case 12 of Dacie (1954, p. 202)] had in fact undergone splenectomy previously. Young, Miller and Christian (1951), too, referred to a patient who suffered repeated relapses after splenectomy: on each occasion relapse was marked by an increase in osmotic (and mechanical) fragility.

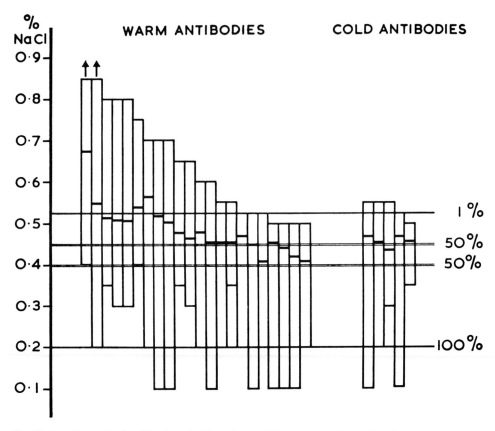

Fig. 23.12   Osmotic-fragility data in 22 patients with warm-antibody AIHA in an active phase of their disease, and in five patients with cold-antibody AIHA, also in an active phase of their disease.

The saline concentration producing 1% lysis (top thin horizontal bar), 50% lysis (thick horizontal bar) and 100% lysis (bottom thin horizontal bar are recorded. ↑ denotes > 1% lysis. The upper and lower thin horizontal lines represent the normal upper limit for initial (1%) lysis and the normal lower limit for complete (100%) lysis, respectively. The two double horizontal lines represent the upper and lower normal limits for 50% lysis (MCF).

Young and Miller (1953) summarized their experience and compared their data on spherocytosis and osmotic and mechanical fragility (MF) with those of a larger series of HS patients. They concluded that spherocytes were usually found in AIHA, and that OF and MF were usually increased; the changes were, however, less regular than in HS. Thirteen AIHA patients had been studied at a time of maximal increase in OF and 12 patients at a time when their haemolysis was quiescent and their OF was normal or minimally increased. The mean increase in OF of the fresh blood of the patients not in remission was similar to that of the HS patients but the increase in OF resulting from incubation for 24 hours at 37°C was less striking. In contrast, the mean OF of the fresh blood of the patients in remission (half of whom had been splenectomized) was normal and after incubation was less than normal (presumably a post-splenectomy effect).

More recently, in an interesting study, von dem Borne and co-workers (1971) were able to show that a close relationship exists between increase in osmotic fragility (recorded as the NaCl concentration producing 50% lysis) and the in-vivo survival of the patient's erythrocytes (recorded as the ^{51}Cr $T_{\frac{1}{2}}$) (Fig. 23.13). They were able to show that normal erythrocytes, known to react *in vitro* with the warm auto-antibodies of an AIHA patient, became, after as little as 48 hours in the patient's circulation, as fragile as the patient's own erythrocytes (Fig. 23.14). In complete contrast, the fragility of erythrocytes shown *in vitro* not to be affected by the auto-antibodies of a similar patient remained unaltered for at least 4 days after injection into the patient's circulation.

As already referred to, the marked case-to-case

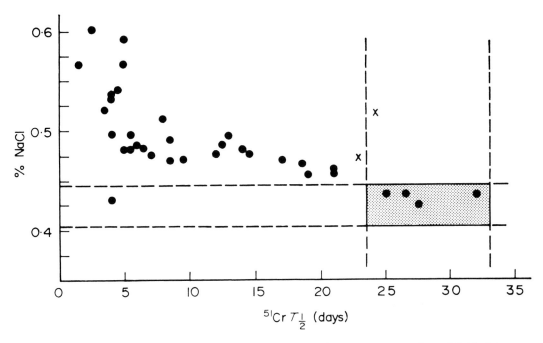

Fig. 23.13   Relationship between osmotic fragility, expressed as the concentration of NaCl giving 50% lysis, in patients with IgG warm-antibody AIHA.
The stippled area indicates the normal range. [Reproduced by permission from von dem Borne et al. (1971).]

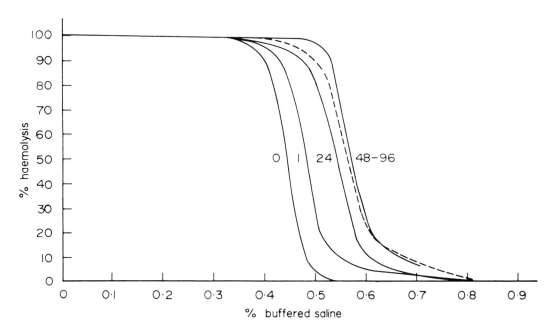

Fig. 23.14   Change in osmotic fragility of transfused normal erythrocytes, shown to react *in vitro* with the auto-antibodies of a patient with warm-antibody AIHA, after transfusion to the patient.
The figures represent hours after the transfusion. [Reproduced by permission from von dem Borne et al. (1971).]

differences in spherocytosis and OF which characterize human AIHA (and its experimental counterpart as demonstrated by Dameshek and Schwartz in their guinea-pigs to which haemolytic immune sera had been administered) are not easily explainable. But amongst the factors which seem likely to contribute to the differences are: the potency of the patient's antibodies as spherocyte producers; the ability of the patient's phagocytic system to remove antibody-damaged erythrocytes from the blood stream; the ability of the patient's marrow to produce reticulocytes — which are more osmotically resistant than adult erythrocytes; and the extent to which the reticulocytes are being damaged by the antibodies. Bearing in mind the individuality of the patient with respect to each of the variables mentioned above, marked patient-to-patient differences in spherocytosis and OF, and indeed in the blood picture as a whole, are perhaps only to be expected.

Osmotic fragility after 24 hours' incubation at 37°C

Increases in OF, often but not invariably greater than normal, are produced by incubating the blood of patients with warm-antibody AIHA for 24 hours at 37°C. It seems unlikely, however, that study of the changes in OF produced by incubation has any practical application in diagnosis as is the case with hereditary spherocytosis (HS). Data on seven patients were recorded by Dacie, (1962, Fig. 131, p. 363). The data of Young and Miller (1953) have been referred to in the previous section.

AUTOHAEMOLYSIS

The rate at which the blood of patients suffering from warm-antibody AIHA undergoes spontaneous lysis during incubation under sterile conditions for 24–48 hours is usually significantly increased, but it may be normal, even in the presence of active haemolysis [Dacie (1962, Table 16, p. 365)]. Occasionally, however, lysis is obvious even within an hour or so of collection, and in one of the author's patients [Case 12 of Dacie (1954, p. 204)] it was impossible to obtain unhaemolysed serum or plasma. It is significant that in these patients spherocytosis was intense, and it seems probable that the very rapid lysis was

due more to be disintegration of markedly spherocytic cells than to immune-body lysis involving complement. Young and co-workers (1956) also referred to the very rapid lysis of the erythrocytes of two patients in haemolytic crisis; they contrasted this with a rate of lysis only just above the normal in the same patients during quiescent phases of their disease.

Selwyn (1953) studied the effect on lysis of maintaining a high concentration of glucose throughout the incubation period. In four out of five patients with warm auto-antibodies glucose had less than its normal effect in diminishing lysis, and in one severely ill patient with marked spherocytosis and a rapid rate of autohaemolysis glucose had absolutely no effect in diminishing lysis.

Young and co-workers (1956) extended this work, They also observed, in a study of six patients, that the addition of glucose caused in most instances a slight increase in autohaemolysis rather than a decrease. Adenosine, on the other hand, generally caused a greater reduction in autohaemolysis than in hereditary spherocytosis (HS).

Verloop and Bakker-v. Aardenne (1958) and Verloop, Bakker-v. Aardenne and Ricci (1959) reported further observations. Three patients with idiopathic AIHA were studied; two showed markedly increased autohaemolysis rates (18% and 23.5% lysis at 48 hours). Haemolysis was substantially reduced by the presence of glucose. One of these patients was studied before and after splenectomy. After splenectomy the rate of autohaemolysis was markedly diminished although OF after incubation remained increased.

Two factors acting in opposite directions probably determine the rate of autohaemolysis on incubation: one is the degree of spherocytosis; the other is the proportion of reticulocytes present — spherocytes being sensitive to incubation while reticulocytes are resistant.

Mechanical fragility (MF)

The MF of the erythrocytes has seldom been studied in warm-antibody AIHA. However, Young, Miller and Christian (1951) referred to two patients both of whom developed increased erythrocyte MF in haemolytic crises. The change was noticed to run more or less parallel with increases in OF (see also Young and Miller, 1953). Shaub and Maier (1956) referred briefly to six patients, in five of whom the MF was increased. Two of the patients had a normal OF and in another patient who went into remission the MF remained abnormal longer than did the OF. Shaub and Maier concluded that the estimation of mechanical fragility was a delicate method of assessing the intensity of a haemolytic process. Bakker-v. Aardenne, Verloop and van Boetzelaer (1958) summarized the results of carrying out the test on five patients with idiopathic AIHA: MF was abnormal in three of these patients using fresh blood and abnormal in two when incubated blood was tested. They, too, concluded that the result of MF and OF tests do not always run parallel and that the former was less dependent on 'sphering' of the erythrocytes.

RETICULOCYTES

A persistently raised reticulocyte count in the peripheral blood is the typical finding in warm-antibody AIHA, and in actively haemolysing patients the count may exceed 50% (Table 23.1, p. 55). Reynolds (1930) reported a count as high as 95% in a severely anaemic 21-year-old male considered to be suffering from acquired hemolytic jaundice and Neimann and co-workers (1956) recorded a count of 90% in a 13-month-old male child, as part of an exceptional blood picture in which erythroblasts outnumbered leucocytes by a ratio of 2:1. A reticulocytosis is, however, not always present, and a low percentage of reticulocytes (1–3%), or even their virtual absence, is a not uncommon finding (see p. 69).

Siderocytes

As in other haemolytic anaemias after splenectomy, siderocytes are often present in the peripheral blood in large numbers (see Vol. 1, p. 88). McFadzean and Davis (1947), in an early account of iron-staining inclusions in erythrocytes, recorded their findings in seven patients with acquired haemolytic anaemia before and after splenectomy. Before splenectomy the maximum percentages ranged from less than 1 to 11; after splenectomy in the same patients the figures were 16–88%. The rise in count reflects the circulation of erythrocytes, particularly reticulocytes, from which the spleen when *in situ* had extracted siderotic granules, probably while the cells were in passage between the pulp and the splenic sinuses.

BONE MARROW

As in other haemolytic anaemias, the bone marrow normally undergoes hypertrophy. This is roughly proportional to the intensity of the haemolysis. Thus red marrow spreads into the shafts of the long bones where in adults little haemopoiesis normally takes place. The fat spaces normally present may almost if not entirely disappear. The hypertrophy is primarily due to hyperplasia of erythropoietic cells with the result that the erythroid:myeloid ratio may even exceed unity. Bone-marrow aspiration biopsy shows that erythropoiesis is typically normoblastic in type. Mitotic figures are frequent.

As haemolysis becomes intense, erythropoiesis tends to become abnormal: in some cases there is a tendency for the nuclei of mature normoblasts to break up into two or more lobes of varying size, and for Howell–Jolly bodies to be present in the cytoplasm of some of the normoblasts; many 'macronormoblasts' with bulky cytoplasm may be present and the nuclei of partly ripened cells may appear megaloblast-like (Remy, 1952) (Figs. 23.15 and 23.16). Bare normoblast nuclei are usually conspicuous in the cytoplasm of phagocytic reticulum cells.

The amount of iron demonstrable by Perls's reaction is usually small, no doubt due to a rapid reutilization of iron in the marrow for the synthesis of haemoglobin. However, in some marrows the developing normoblasts and marrow

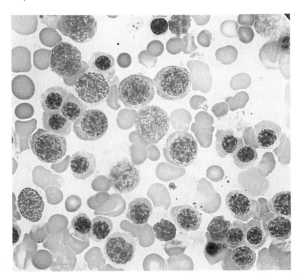

Fig. 23.15   Photomicrograph of a bone-marrow film of a patient with severe warm-antibody AIHA.
Erythropoiesis predominates and is 'macronormoblastic' or even possibly megaloblastic. x 700.

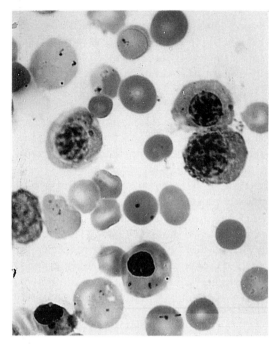

Fig. 23.16   Photomicrograph of a bone-marrow film of a patient with severe warm-antibody AIHA (Case 12 of Dacie, 1962, p. 684).
Stained by Perls's reaction to show siderotic granules. Erythropoiesis is macronormoblastic or even possibly megaloblastic. x 1260.

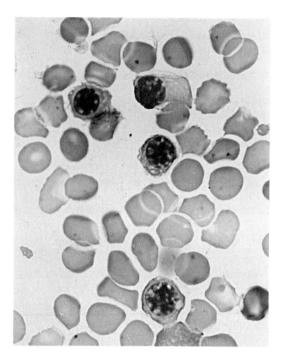

Fig. 23.17   Photomicrograph of a bone-marrow film of a patient with severe warm-antibody AIHA.
Stained by Perls's reaction to show siderotic granules. The same patient whose marrow is shown in Fig. 23.16, after a favourable response to corticosteroids and splenectomy. Erythropoiesis is now normoblastic. x 1260.

reticulocytes contain excessive numbers of unusually large siderotic granules (Fig. 23.16). In one patient (Dacie, 1962, p. 686, Case 12) these were observed to revert to normal following remission induced by steroids and splenectomy (Fig. 23.17).

Occasionally, erythrophagocytosis may be seen in sections of bone marrow. It is less frequently seen in films of marrow made from aspirated material. This is probably because most of the fixed phagocytic cells, if aspirated at all, remain embedded in fragments of marrow tissue. Herrador and De Castro (1960), however, reported seeing phagocytosis of both leucocytes and erythrocytes in the marrow film of one patient.

Megaloblastic erythropoiesis

The abnormal marrow findings described above have some features in common with megaloblastic erythropoiesis, e.g., the 'open' appearance of some of the cell nuclei, the Howell–Jolly bodies and the fragmenting nuclei. It is in fact possible, but unproved, that they *are* signs of early megaloblastic change, due perhaps to local deficiency of haemopoietic factors resulting from the very great demands of a hyperactive marrow. Overt megaloblastic erythropoiesis certainly occurs, as in other types of haemolytic anaemia, but it has not often been reported.

Tosatti (1947) described a 23-year-old male who developed an acute haemolytic anaemia associated with haemoglobinuria, considered to be of Lederer type. Megaloblasts were present in bone-marrow films at the height of the haemolysis. The patient made a spontaneous recovery.

Gruelund (1950) described an example of severe acquired haemolytic anaemia (probably of the autoimmune type) in an elderly woman whose marrow was partially megaloblastic, and referred to several earlier cases in the literature of haemolytic anaemia plus 'pernicious anaemia' or of 'pernicious anaemia' accompanied by increased osmotic fragility. Probably in most instances of this kind there is some additional cause of a conditioned deficiency of haemopoietic factors, such as latent malabsorption syndrome or pregnancy, which leads to folate deficiency. Subsequently reported cases include those of Baikie and Pirrie (1956), Rubio and Burgin (1957), Chanarin, Dacie and Mollin (1959) (Fig. 3.47, Vol. 1), Söderhjelm (1959), Willoughby et al. (1961) and Ryder (1965). The auto-immune status of Baikie and Pirrie's patient's illness was doubtful — she responded to vitamin B_{12}, and no cause for the folate deficiency other than the haemolytic anaemia could be demonstrated in Chanarin, Dacie and Mollin's patient. Rubio and Burgin's patient was thought to be suffering from coincidental genuine pernicious anaemia. Ryder's patient, who had AIHA complicating Hodgkin's disease, was folate-deficient.

Issitt and co-workers' (1982) patient was a black male aged 22 months whose haemoglobin stabilized at 11.9–12.2 g/dl with 2.3–6.1% reticulocytes after treatment with folic acid.

Reticulocytopenia

The literature is quite extensive and reflects the interest in the atypical in preference to the typical, but it also reflects the clinical importance of reticulocytopenia. Its occurrence has been recognized for many years. Parsons (1938), for instance, in a general review of haemolytic anaemia in childhood, wrote 'severe cases [of Lederer's anaemia] may show at first an aregenerative phase', but he gave no details. In Table 23.2 are listed a selection of case reports in which reticulocytopenia was highlighted.

Several reviews are available which illustrate the frequency of marked reticulocytopenia. Crosby and Rappaport (1956) reported that 15 out of 34 patients with idiopathic AIHA were reticulocytopenic at the time of crisis—and only three out of the 15 patients survived. Allgood and Chaplin (1967) recorded the reticulocyte percentage in 47 idiopathic cases as ranging from 0.1 to 72.9: five patients (10%) had less than 5%; 23 (49%) had between 5 and 20%; 19 (41%) had more than 20%. Pirofsky (1969, p. 48) tabulated the reticulocyte percentage in 35 untreated idiopathic cases: nine patients (26%) had less than 2% (in five there were between 0.0 and 0.3%); eight patients (23%) had between 2.0 and 4.9%; eight patients (23%) had between 5.0 and 9.9%, and ten patients (29%) had more than 10%.

More recently, Liesveld, Rowe and Lichtman (1987) reported from Rochester, New York, on a retrospective study of the erythropoietic responses of 109 consecutive patients who had suffered from

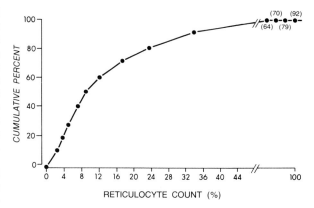

Fig. 23.18 Cumulative percentage of percent reticulocyte counts at first diagnosis in 108 cases of AIHA of varied type.
Reproduced by permission from Liesveld, Rowe and Lichtman (1987).

various types of auto-immune haemolysis. Fifty-one of these patients were judged to have had primary warm-antibody AIHA. Their reticulocyte counts ranged from 0.4 to 92% (Fig. 23.18): the mean was 18% and the median 9%, and 20% of the patients had an initial count of less than 4%. Reticulocytopenia was about equally frequent in the warm- and cold-antibody cases and in the primary and secondary cases. The bone marrow had been examined in just over one-half of the reticulocytopenic patients: erythropoiesis was hyperplastic in three-quarters, and in only one patient was there erythroid hypoplasia.

'APLASTIC' CRISES

As can be seen in Table 23.2, peripheral-blood reticulocytopenia in patients with warm-antibody AIHA may be associated with either erythroblastopenia—an 'aplastic' marrow—or erythroid hyperplasia. Hyperplasia seems to be the more common finding, as least as judged from published case reports (Table 23.2). The reticulocytopenia may be short-lived or long-continued (and life-threatening), and is frequently, but not invariably, accompanied by thrombocytopenia and/or leucopenia.

There seem to be several possible mechanisms for the reticulocytopenia: destruction of erythroblasts by the action of an auto-antibody which

Table 23.2 Reticulocytopenia in warm antibody auto-immune haemolytic anaemia

Reference	Sex and age of patient	Minimum haemoglobin	Reticulocytes in peripheral blood	Other findings; outcome
Evans (1943)	F. 32 years	20%	At first 26%, later absent	Severe thrombocytopenia. Splenectomy:improvement in platelet count; no change in erythrocyte count
Stats, Wasserman and Rosenthal (1948)	M. 5 years	Erythrocytes $1.16 \times 10^{12}/l$	1%	Acute haemolysis with haemoglobinuria. Marked erythroid hyperplasia. Transfused; eventual complete recovery
Dacie and de Gruchy (1951, Case 5)	F. 56 years	4.1 g/dl	0.5%	Severely ill; haemoglobinuria. Splenectomy. Ultimately recovered
Davis et al. (1952)	M. 46 years	14%	0.0%	Severely ill. Leucopenia and thrombocytopenia as well as reticulocytopenia during crisis; marrow erythroblastopenia. Splenectomized; eventually recovered
Millichap (1952, Case 4)	F. 10 months	20%	<1%	Marked marrow erythroid hyperplasia. DAT pos. Splenectomy; died 1 month later
Bonham Carter, Cathie and Gasser (1954)	M. 4 years, 6 months	17%	0.0%	Severely ill; relapsing course. Reticulocytopenia and marrow erythroblastopenia lasted 17 months. Transfused repeatedly; received cortisone and ACTH. Splenectomized: eventually recovered
Eisemann and Dameshek (1954)	F. 58 years	5.6g	0.0%	Chronic course. DAT pos. Sustained by repeated transfusions. Marrow erythroid hypoplasia (almost complete absence of erythroblasts). Eventually recovered after splenectomy
Bousser et al. (1955)	F. 38 years		Prolonged reticulocytopenia	Severe relapsing course. Prolonged marrow erythroblastopenia; thrombocytopenia. DAT pos
Bowman (1955)	F. 22 months	2.1 g/dl	0.1%	Marrow erythroblastopenia. DAT pos. Replacement transfusion; eventually responded to cortisone
Seip (1955)	14 years		Absent for almost 4 months	Marrow erythroblastopenia; leucopenia and thrombocytopenia. DAT pos. Splenectomy
Wagner (1955)	F. 13 years		Absent	DAT pos. Died after an acute illness of 8 days' duration
Beickert (1956)	M. 69 years		<1%	Marrow erythroid hyperplasia. DAT pos. Failed to respond to splenectomy. Died
Martoni and Musiani (1956)	M. 6 months	40%	<1%	Two prolonged crises of marrow erythroblastopenia. DAT pos. Splenectomy. Eventually recovered
Müller and Weinreich (1956, Case 3)	F. 18 months	5 g/dl	0.6%	Leucopenia. DAT pos. Splenectomy: 1680 g spleen. Marrow fibrosis and extramedullary haemopoiesis
Veras and Manios (1956)	F. 18 months		At first 40–60%, then absent	Marrow erythroblastopenia, with almost complete absence of erythroblasts. DAT pos. Died

Table 23.2 (contd)

Reference	Patient	Hb	Reticulocytes	Comments
Hennemann and Falck (1957)	(1) M. 56 years		< 0.5%	(1) Marrow erythroid hyperplasia. Died.
	(2) M. 61 years		5%, usually less	(2) 3-year history of 'aplastic' anaemia. Marrow erythroid hyperplasia. DAT pos. Died of haemolytic crisis and reticulocytopenia
Burston et al. (1959)	(1) M. 76 years		0.3%	Marrow erythroblastopenia, leucopenia and thrombocytopenia. DAT pos.
	(2) M. 68 years	3.7 g/dl	< 0.1%	Marrow erythroblastopenia, leucopenia. DAT pos. Died: Tb found at necropsy
Harley and Dods (1959, Case B)	15 months		0.5%	Haemolysis persisted for 2 years. Reticulocytopenia persisted for 16 weeks after splenectomy. Eventually recovered
Lees, Fisher and Shanks (1960)	F. 2 months	3.9 g/dl	Absent	Marrow erythroblastopenia, thrombocytopenia. DAT neg at first, then pos. Splenectomy: recovered.
Meyer and Bertcher (1960)	M. 51 years	5.7 g/dl	Absent	Transient complete marrow erythroblastopenia. DAT pos. Responded to corticosteroids and ACTH.
Laski et al. (1961)	M. 2½ months	3.0 g/dl	'Low'	DAT at first neg, then pos
Ritz and Haber (1962)	M. 6 weeks	5.0 g/dl	0.2%	Long relapsing course. Marrow erythroblastopenia. DAT pos. Remitted on ACTH
Mallarmé et al. (1965)	F.		0.5%	'Haemolytic anaemia of pregnancy'. Leucopenia and thrombocytopenia. DAT neg. Responded to corticosteroids; recovered after delivery
Letts and Kredenster (1968)	F.	6.0 g/dl	0–1%	Long-continued Evans syndrome dating from childhood and persisting through two pregnancies. Reticulocytopenia after splenectomy. Marrow erythroid hyperplasia. DAT pos.
Celada, Farquet and Muller (1977)	F. 75 years	4.0 g/dl	0.2%	Terminal phase of chronic illness. Six episodes of haemolysis responded to prednisone and azathioprine. Marrow erythroid hyperplasia (98% of cells sideroblasts); dyserythropoietic changes
Hegde, Gordon-Smith and Worlledge (1977)	(1) F. 9 years	3.8 g/dl	0.6%	Marrow erythroid hyperplasia. DAT neg. Recovered after splenectomy
	(2) M. 41 years	5.7 g/dl	0.5%	Chronic relapsing course. Marrow erythroid hyperplasia, leucopenia, thrombocytopenia. DAT neg. Responded to corticosteroids.
	(3) M. 13 years	2.9 g/dl	3.0%	Chronic course. DAT neg, then weakly pos. Eventually responded to azathioprine
Seewan (1979)	F. 66 years	4.5 g/dl	0–03%	Marrow erythroid hyperplasia. Reticulocytopenia lasted for at least 6 weeks. DAT pos. Eventually recovered.

Table 23.2 (*contd*)

Reference	Patient	PCV / Hb	Duration of reticulocytopenia	
Conley, Lippman and Ness (1980); Conley et al. (1982)	(1) F. 52 years	PCV 10%	10 days	All five patients had intensely cellular erythroid marrow
	(2) F. 78 years	PCV 9%	4 days	
	(3) F. 53 years	PCV 10%	90 days	
	(4) M. 39 years	PCV 9%	8 days	
	(5) F. 49 years	PCV 8%	160 days	
Greenberg et al. (1980)	(1) F. 4 months	4.5 g/dl	0.2%	Prolonged reticulocytopenia; marrow erythroid hyperplasia. DAT neg, then pos. Eventually recovered
	(2) M. 13 years	7.2 g/dl	0.2%	Prolonged reticulocytopenia; marrow erythroid hyperplasia. DAT pos. Eventually recovered
Hansen, Sørensen and Astrup (1982)	M. 26 years	3.5 g/dl	0.9%	IgA deficiency. Recurrent haemolysis and thrombocytopenia over a 10-year period. Marrow erythroblastopenia. DAT pos
Hauke et al. (1983)	F. 43 years	3.5 g/dl	Absent	Past history of rheumatoid arthritis. Marrow erythroid hyperplasia; some dyserythropoietic features. Received 38 units of blood in 24 days. Responded to prednisone, splenectomy and azathioprine. Eventually recovered
Miller and Beardsley (1983, Case 4)	M. 12 years	4.4 g/dl	0.1%	Chronic relapsing course. Leucopenia and thrombocytopenia. DAT pos
Carapella De Luca et al. (1984)	F. 8 months	5.2 g/dl	0.7%	Relapsing course. Prolonged reticulocytopenia. Marrow erythroid maturation arrest. DAT pos. Eventual recovery
Celada (1984, Case 2)				Marrow erythroid hyperplasia, with ring sideroblasts. Died 5 weeks after start of reticulocytopenia. Had been treated with immunosuppressive drugs
Mangan et al. (1984)	M. 67 years	6.1 g/dl		Patient had chronic lymphocytic leukaemia. At first high reticulocytosis; later reticulocytopenia and marrow erythroid hypoplasia (< 1% erythroblasts). Eventually recovered
Bertrand et al. (1985); Lefrère et al. (1986)	M. 12 years	6.0 g/dl	Absent	Marrow erythroid hypoplasia (3% erythroblasts); leucopenia and thrombocytopenia. IgM anti-parvovirus antibodies demonstrated. Recovered within a few days
Rapoport, Rowe and McMican (1988)	M. 29 years		1–2%	AIDS. Severe AIHA, indistinguishable from idiopathic disease. DAT pos

may or may not be distinct from that acting on reticulocytes and mature erythrocytes; destruction of reticulocytes (and mature erythrocytes) in the marrow and peripheral blood by an antibody that spares erythroblasts; inhibition by some means of erythroblast maturation, and 'hypersplenism'. The fact that some patients (with either hypoplastic or hyperplastic erythroid marrows) respond favourably to high doses of cortico-steroids or immunosuppressive drugs implicates an immune process. The role of the spleen, other than as a site of haemolysis, is uncertain. Splenectomy is probably no more a specific remedy in reticulocytopenic patients than it is in patients who have responded to auto-immune haemolysis with a sustained reticulocytosis.

Another mechanism resulting in erythroid hypoplasia that is quite distinct from the auto-immune mechanisms discussed in the previous paragraph is infection by parvovirus. This seems, however, to be a rare cause of erythroblastopenia in AIHA and, judging from the aplastic crises reported in hereditary spherocytosis and sickle-cell anaemia, only likely to be responsible for short-lived crises.

In relation to reticulocytopenia being produced by auto-antibody action, the experimental study of Linke (1952) is significant. An anti-rat-erythrocyte haemolytic serum administered to 45 rats caused severe reticulocytopenia in 18 of them. This developed within a few hours, and it seemed likely that the haemolytic serum was acting on bone-marrow erythroblasts.

A similar explanation was advanced by Eisemann and Dameshek (1954) and Gasser (1955). Eisemann and Dameshek, however, suggested, as an alternative, that 'hypersplenism' might be responsible. Their patient recovered after splenectomy, although reticulocytes did not appear in the peripheral blood until 18 days after the operation. The infants reported by Martoni and Musiani (1956) and by Lees, Fisher and Shanks (1960) also may have been benefited by splenectomy. In the patient of Bonham Carter, Cathie and Gasser (1954), however, splenectomy had no apparent beneficial effect and in Linke's experimental haemolytic anaemias three rats previously splenectomized developed reticulo-cytopenia.

It is noteworthy that Steffen (1955) and Pisciotta and Hinz (1956) demonstrated by means of the antiglobulin test that bone-marrow erythroblasts of several patients with AIHA were 'coated' by auto-antibodies. Rossi, Diena and Sacchetti (1957), too, showed that erythroblasts, even immature basophilic ones, were agglutinable by auto-antibodies of both the warm and cold types, and Sacchetti, Diena and Rossi (1957) reported visible evidence of damage to erythro-blasts when these were cultured *in vitro* in serum from AIHA patients.

Some recent reports

Hegde, Gordon-Smith and Worlledge (1977) described three patients (two children and one adult) who had low reticulocyte counts (0.5–3%) despite being severely anaemic and whose bone marrow showed erythroid hyperplasia. Erythrophagocytosis was conspicuous in bone-marrow aspirates in Cases 1 and 3. The patients were unusual, too, in that the DAT was negative in Case 1 and initially negative and then positive later (complement components only) in Cases 2 and 3. All three eventually recovered after prolonged relapsing courses (Figs 23.19 and 23.20). Hegde, Gordon-Smith and Worlledge demonstrated in Case 1 that ^{59}Fe accumulated in the spleen within 24–48 hours of administration, associated with a fall-off in radioactivity over the sacrum. This was interpreted as indicating trapping and subsequent destruction of labelled patients' erythrocytes in the spleen. They suggested in relation to the cause of the reticulo-cytopenia that 'If the antigenic sites [with which the auto-antibody interacted] were strongly expressed on a large proportion of young red cells or reticulocytes, these cells would be destroyed, giving rise to an accumulation of cells on which these antigenic sites were poorly expressed. The concentration of antibody on these surviving cells could therefore be too low to be detected by the DAGT'.

Conley, Lippman and Ness (1980) and Conley and his co-workers (1982) stressed the life-threatening nature of reticulocytopenia. In their 1980 paper they referred to four patients under the title 'Autoimmune hemolytic anemia with

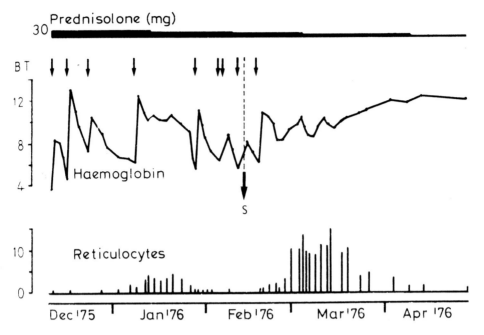

Fig. 23.19   Failure of haemolysis and reticulocytopenia to respond to modest dosage of prednisolone, with remission following splenectomy (S). BT = blood transfusion.
Case 1 of Hegde, Gordon-Smith and Worlledge (1977). Reproduced by permission.

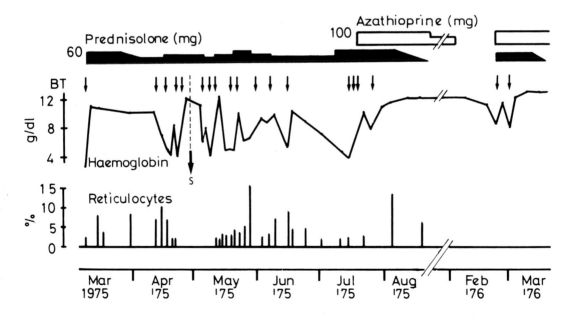

Fig. 23.20   Severe haemolysis and reticulocytopenia following reduction in prednisolone dosage, with remission following treatment with azathioprine.
Splenectomy (S) had been ineffective. BT = blood transfusion. Case 3 of Hegde, Gordon-Smith and Worlledge (1977). Reproduced by permission.

reticulocytopenia. A medical emergency', and described their condition on admission to the Johns Hopkins Hospital as 'stuporous', 'comatose', 'extremely pale, jaundiced with air hunger and tachycardia', and 'moribund', respectively. All were rescued by immediate blood transfusion (Figs 23.21 and 23.22). All four patients, and a fifth patient described in addition in their 1982 paper, had bone marrow in which erythroid cells, mainly late and polychromatic erythroblasts, predominated. In one patient they demonstrated that ^{59}Fe was retained in the bone marrow and did not appear in the peripheral blood until spontaneous recovery from the reticulocytopenia took place; they also showed that the auto-antibody reacted more strongly with a suspension of normal erythrocytes that was reticulocyte-poor than with a suspension that was reticulocyte-enriched. They concluded that the auto-antibody

in the patient they had studied appeared to have some effect on maturing erythroblasts that retarded their proliferation and prevented their extrusion into the circulation and that the presence of polychromatic cells in the marrow indicated that maturation was continuing but probably at a reduced rate. They also pointed out that their in-vitro experiments indicated that reticulocytes were not likely to have been preferentially destroyed.

Hauke and co-workers (1983) described some in-vitro studies which indicated that their patient was forming an auto-antibody which inhibited the growth of early erythroid cells. Their patient, a male aged 43, was severely anaemic; he had a hyperplastic erythroid marrow and initially no reticulocytes in the peripheral blood. He received 38 units of blood within 24 days and eventually made a good recovery, after high-dose prednisone, splenectomy and azathioprine therapy.

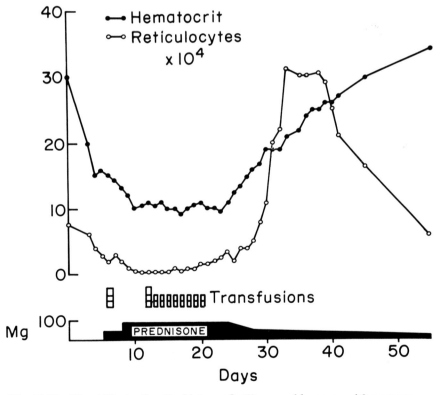

Fig. 23.21   Chart illustrating the history of a 52-year-old woman with a severe uncompensated idiopathic warm-antibody AIHA, accompanied by severe reticulocytopenia.
   She was treated with prednisone and by blood transfusion and eventually made a complete recovery. [Reproduced by permission from Conley, Lippman and Ness (1980).]

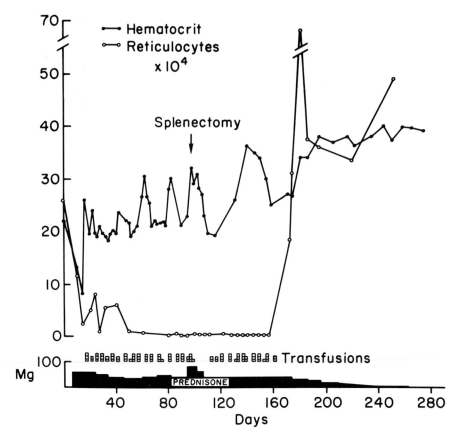

Fig. 23.22   Chart illustrating the history of a 49-year-old woman with a severe uncompensated idiopathic warm-antibody AIHA who failed to respond to prednisone therapy or to splenectomy.
Recovery was spontaneous after a prolonged period of reticulocytopenia. [Reproduced by permission from Conley et al. (1982).]

Bone-marrow culture showed that his plasma inhibited the growth of erythroid progenitor cells (BFU-E) derived from his own marrow, or normal marrow, but had no effect on granulocyte or mixed colony formation. Hauke et al. suggested that the patient's splenomegaly was responsible for concurrent leucopenia and thrombocytopenia and they pointed out that the inhibitory activity of the patient's plasma disappeared simultaneously with the warm auto-antibody in his plasma active against peripheral blood erythrocytes.

Mangan and co-workers (1984) provided evidence for the simultaneous presence of two auto-antibodies in a male patient, aged 67, who had warm-antibody AIHA and an underlying chronic lymphocytic leukaemia. At one time he had an active erythropoietic marrow and up to 60% reticulocytes. Later, the reticulocyte count fell to 0.4–0.6%. The DAT was strongly positive and his marrow was markedly erythroblastopenic (<1% erythroid cells). His serum was found to contain two distinct IgG auto-antibodies — a complement-independent anti-e and a complement-dependent inhibitor of the growth in marrow cultures of erythroid colony- and burst-forming units. Following cortico-steroid therapy and extracorporeal immune adsorption, the serum IgG level was reduced to 27%, at which point it was no longer possible to demonstrate inhibition of the growth of erythroid progenitor cells *in vitro*. Simultaneously, reticulocytes reappeared in the peripheral blood.

Role of parvovirus. Bertrand and co-workers (1985) and Lefrère and co-workers (1986) described a 12-year-old boy in whom a crisis of pancytopenia was accompanied by evidence of infection with parvovirus. He was admitted to hospital with a haemoglobin of 6 g/dl, $1.8 \times 10^9/l$ leucocytes and $77 \times 10^9/l$ platelets. Reticulocytes were absent from the peripheral blood and there was marked marrow erythroblastopenia (3% erythroblasts). Immunological and virological studies revealed anti-HPV IgM antibodies; the DAT was positive and antinuclear antibodies (titre 20) were present. He was transfused and recovered quickly, leucocytes and platelets reaching peaks 10 days or so after admission and reticulocytes a little later. The DAT remained positive and spherocytes were seen in blood films. In this case the erythroblastopenic crisis, which was apparently virus-induced, was the initial manifestation of a severe and persistent AIHA.

LEUCOCYTES

The total leucocyte count varies within wide limits in warm-antibody AIHA. The count is usually well above 10 x 10⁹/l when haemolysis is active (Table 23.1), mainly due to an increase in neutrophils. However, as already referred to (p. 36), some patients are chronically neutropenic, in which case the platelet count is usually low, too (and possibly the reticulocyte count as well (immunopancytopenia)). In such patients leucocyte auto-antibodies, plus possibly hypersplenism, are probably responsible for the neutropenia.

In hyperacute haemolytic episodes the leucocyte count is usually markedly raised and counts well in excess of 20 x 10⁹/l are commonly found. In such cases myelocytes and promyelocytes, and even an occasional myeloblast, may circulate in the peripheral blood, so much so that their presence may lead to leukaemia being considered as a possible diagnosis (O'Donoghue and Witts, 1932).

Data on leucocyte counts in several large series of patients who had had warm-antibody AIHA are summarized below.

Crosby and Rappaport (1957) reviewed the leucocyte picture in 34 patients: the total count was normal or increased in all but six during crises of haemolysis. Marked leucocytosis, in which neutrophils predominated, characteristically followed splenectomy and counts exceeding 30 × 10⁹/l were found as an agonal phenomenon in several patients.

Allgood and Chaplin (1967) reported data from 47 patients. Their total leucocyte counts ranged from 2.25 to 23.7 × 10⁹/l: six (13%) were leucopenic at diagnosis (counts < 5 × 10⁹/l); 25 (53%) had counts within the normal range (5–10 × 10⁹/l); 16 (34%) had leucocytoses (counts > 10 × 10⁹/l).

Pirofsky (1969, p. 46) reviewed the counts of 39 patients. They ranged from 1.4 to 37 × 10⁹/l: more than half the patients had counts within the normal range; six were leucopenic (counts < 2 × 10⁹/l): seven had high counts (13.1– 37 × 10⁹/l). (One patient had a count of 108 × 10⁹/l, but this was thought to be an allergic response to penicillin — there were 88% eosinophils.)

Habibi and co-workers (1974) reported on 80 children. Twenty-five of 34 children who had had acute AIHA had leucocytoses of 10–50 × 10⁹/l, sometimes with promyelocytes and myelocytes amounting to up to 20% of the cells. Leucocytoses were present, too, in 22 of the 46 patients who developed a chronic illness, particularly if haemolysis had been acute at its onset. Eight children were leucopenic, but all of them were non-idiopathic cases.

Liesveld, Rowe and Lichtman (1987) reviewed the initial leucocyte counts of 108 patients suffering from various types of auto-immune haemolysis (Figs 23.23 and 23.24). The counts ranged from 1.5 to 137 × 10⁹/l: the mean was 10.6 × 10⁹/l and median 9.0 × 10⁹/l. (Three of the patients had chronic lymphocytic leukaemia and their counts were excluded from the data when the mean was calculated.) Fourteen of the patients had counts of less than 4.5 × 10⁹/l—all were

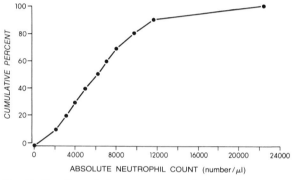

Fig. 23.23   Cumulative percentage of absolute neutrophil counts at first diagnosis in 102 patients with AIHA of varied type.

[Reproduced by permission from Liesveld, Rowe and Lichtman (1987).]

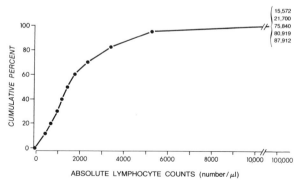

Fig. 23.24   Cumulative percentage of absolute lymphocyte counts at first diagnosis in 102 patients with AIHA of varied type.

[Reproduced by permission from Liesveld, Rowe and Lichtman (1987).]

forming warm antibodies and half of them were judged to have had primary AIHA. Forty per cent of the patients had initial counts exceeding 11×10^9/l.

Data for leucocyte counts (probably total nucleated-cell counts in most instances), extracted from some of the early case reports of hyperacute acquired haemolytic anaemia are recorded in Table 23.3. They illustrate how high the counts may be in such cases. A reaction to 'stress' plus stimulation by products of intravascular haemolysis are probably important factors in producing the leucocytoses, and it is interesting to note that similar rises in leucocyte count have been reported in crises of haemolysis (e.g. in favism) in which immunological action and infection play no part in causation (Vol. 1, p. 383).

Erythrocyte neutrophil rosetting

In the 2nd edition of this book (Part III), Dacie (1967, p. 937) described under the title 'Hypersplenic haemolytic anaemia' a 37-year-old male who had a chronic haemolytic anaemia associated with moderate splenomegaly. The DAT was persistently negative and no abnormal antibodies could be demonstrated in his serum. Splenectomy was carried out, and 4 months later there were no signs of continuing haemolysis. An unusual feature was the presence in blood films of neutrophils surrounded by a rosette of erythrocytes (Fig. 23.25). The same phenomenon was subsequently described by Pettit, Scott and Hussain (1976). Their patient was a 28-year-old male who also suffered from a chronic acquired haemolytic anaemia. In this case, however, the DAT was positive using anti-complement sera. Pettit, Scott and Hussain noted that the neutrophil rosetting, which affected more than 75% of the neutrophils, was visible only in films made from blood anticoagulated with EDTA; it was not present when heparin or sodium citrate had been used as anticoagulant or in films made from uncoagulated blood. They pointed out that the better known adhesion of platelets to neutrophils likewise appeared to be EDTA-dependent.

The mechanism and significance of erythrocyte neutrophil rosetting is obscure.

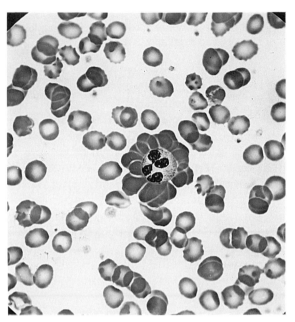

Fig. 23.25 **Photomicrograph of the blood film of a 37-year-old man with a DAT-negative 'hypersplenic haemolytic anaemia'.**
A neutrophil is surrounded by a rosette of erythrocytes. x 700.

PLATELETS

The quite frequent association of thrombocytopenia with idiopathic warm-antibody AIHA has been discussed in some detail on pp. 34–39. Thrombocytosis, on the other hand, is a much rarer event, and marked increases, comparable to the leucocytoses accompanying acute crises of haemolysis seem seldom, if ever, to occur.

Crosby and Rappaport (1957), who tabulated the platelet counts of 29 patients, recorded only two counts above 400×10^9/l, i.e. 430 and 440×10^9/l, respectively. Allgood and Chaplin (1967), on the other hand, reported that as many as 11 out of 45 patients (24%) had counts on presentation that exceeded 400×10^9/l. Pirofsky's (1969, p. 47) figures were, however, comparable with those of Crosby and Rappaport: only one out of 31 patients had a count exceeding 300×10^9/l, i.e. 1000×10^9/l. Habibi and co-workers (1974), in their review of 80 children with AIHA, did not mention the occurrence of thrombocytosis. Heisel and Ortega (1983), however, recorded a mean platelet count at diagnosis of 421×10^9/l (range 191–583 $\times 10^9$/l) in nine children suffering from acute (transient) AIHA and a mean count of 195×10^9/l (range 15–795 $\times$

Table 23.3 Hyperleucocytosis in acute acquired haemolytic anaemia

Reference	Age and sex of patient	Minimum erythrocyte count ($\times 10^{12}$/l)	Maximum leucocyte count (μl)	History and outcome
Teeter (1907)	F. 6 years	1.0	132 800 (59% neutrophils, 11% myelocytes, 6% unclassified)	Acute haemolysis, 'leukanemic' blood picture. Recovered
Lederer (1925)	(1) M. 19 years	1.87	33 000	3-day history. Recovered after blood transfusion
	(2) M. 16 months		52 000	3-day history. Recovered after blood transfusion
	(3) F. 35 years	0.78	37 000	6-day history. Gradually recovered after three blood transfusions
Lederer (1930)	(1) M. 24 years	0.99	44 000	3-day history. Recovered after blood transfusion
	(2) M. 2 years	1.07	39 600	2-day history. Recovered after blood transfusion
	(3) M. 6 months	0.95	81 000	6-day history. Recovered after blood transfusion
Baxter and Everhart (1938)	F. 7 years	0.95	33 500	Acute onset 2 weeks after a respiratory infection
Landolt (1946)	F. 6 years, 7 months	1.10	46 500	Died after an acute 7-day illness
Gasser and Holländer (1951)	M. 7 weeks	0.87	60 000 (77% lymphocytes)	Hyperacute haemolysis and severe thrombocytopenia. Splenectomy. Died 17 days after admission
Gasser (1952, 1954)	F. 5½ years		87 000	Pseudoleukaemic blood picture; total nucleated cell count 103 000/μl. Died of a hyperacute illness lasting 3 days
Lillie, Gatenby and Moore (1954)	F.	1.0	45 000	Acute haemolytic anaemia of pregnancy. Recovered after delivery of macerated fetus
Braaker (1960)	M. 4 years		99 700 (30% lymphocytes)	Acute haemolysis associated with otitis media

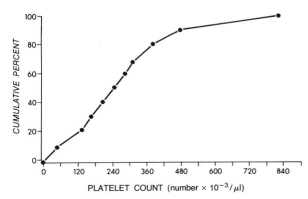

Fig. 23.26 Cumulative percentage of platelet counts at first diagnosis in 95 patients with AIHA of varied type.
[Reproduced by permission from Liesveld, Rowe and Lichtman (1987).]

10^9/l) in 16 children suffering from chronic AIHA (ten had counts of $< 150 \times 10^9$/l at diagnosis).

Liesveld, Rowe and Lichtman (1987) recorded the initial platelet counts of 85 patients (Fig. 23.26). Thirteen patients were judged to be thrombocytopenic: (platelet count $< 120 \times 10^9$/l): all were forming warm antibodies and six of them had been diagnosed as suffering from ITP. Sixteen patients had thrombocytosis (platelet count $> 400 \times 10^9$/l; 13 were forming warm antibodies, two had secondary cold-antibody AIHA and one patient (a child) appeared to be forming both warm and cold antibodies.

Impairment of platelet aggregation in AIHA.

Russell, Keenan and Frais (1978) described a 30-year-old woman who developed during the course of a DAT-positive haemolytic anaemia an obscure platelet defect. This had become apparent during plasmapheresis carried out as treatment for restricted circulation in her left hand which had led to gangrene of the finger tips. Tests showed an impaired platelet aggregation response to collagen and ADP. She was treated with azathioprine, and 1 month later the haemoglobin had risen to 13.1 g/dl and the platelets aggregated normally in the presence of collagen and ADP.

EFFECT OF SPLENECTOMY ON THE BLOOD PICTURE

The changes vary from patient to patient, depending essentially on the response to splenectomy. If haemolysis persists, then a marked rise in the numbers of circulating erythroblasts may be expected (e.g., as reported by Pisciotta, Downer and Hinz, 1959), so much so that the erythroblast count may exceed the total leucocyte count. The platelet count may be expected to rise after splenectomy, as in patients with other types of haemolytic anaemia, that is if there is no concomitant immune platelet-destroying mechanism. The same applies to the total leucocyte count: in the absence of an immune leucocyte-destroying mechanism the count will rise.

The extent to which the morphology of the erythrocytes will change once the spleen is removed depends, too, on the effect its removal has had on the rate of haemolysis: spherocytosis if persistent and marked will mask any tendency to target-cell formation.

Siderocytes may be present in small numbers before splenectomy, occasionally in quite large numbers (Remy, 1952). Douglas and Dacie (1953) reported on 19 patients before splenectomy: the average count was 2.3%, with a range of 0–21%; the largest numbers were found in patients in whom haemolysis was most active. After splenectomy (13 patients), the average count was 20%, with a range of 1–67%.

BIOCHEMICAL FINDINGS

Serum proteins

The relatively frequent association of abnormal serum immunoglobulin (Ig) levels, particularly deficiency of IgA, in idiopathic warm-antibody AIHA has already been described (p. 39).

Earlier studies carried out before specific anti-IgG, IgA and IgM sera became available had not revealed any consistent pattern. Charbonnier and Dausset (1953), however, using a microelectrophoresis technique, had found decreased percentages of α and β globulins in relation to total serum proteins in seven out of nine patients with idiopathic warm-antibody AIHA; γ globulins, on the other hand, were moderately elevated in six of the nine patients.

Christenson and Dacie (1957), too, who submitted the sera of 38 similar patients to paper electrophoresis, found that the concentrations of albumin and total globulins were generally normal except for occasional decreases in α_2 and β globulins and increases in γ globulin. An abnormal peak in the β–γ region was, however, produced by the serum of one patient.

As described on p. 43, Blajchman and his co-workers (1969) found that the serum (Ig) concentrations were within the normal range in only 37 out of 88 patients with warm-antibody AIHA. IgA was the Ig most commonly present in abnormal (usually reduced) concentration, but as many as 13 different combinations of Ig deficiency or excess were demonstrated.

Further data were reported by Kretschmer and Mueller-Eckhardt (1972). IgG, IgA, IgM and β1A globulins were determined in serum at the time of maximum haemolysis in 21 AIHA patients. Dysgammaglobulinaemia (increases or decreases in Ig concentration) was demonstrable in 57% of the patients, the commonest abnormality being decreases in IgG (eight patients) or IgM (nine patients). There appeared to be no correlation between the type of serum IgG abnormality and the auto-antibody class or type of disease. Clinical improvement was associated with a tendency for the Ig concentrations to become more normal, and it appeared, too, that complement fixation to the erythrocytes was correlated with a decrease in serum β1A globulin (complement) concentration.

Mueller-Eckhardt and co-workers (1977) reported on the serum immunoglobulin (Ig) levels in 56 warm-antibody AIHA patients, 43 of whom had been repeatedly studied; 33 had idiopathic AIHA. Serum Ig abnormalities were demonstrated in 44 of the patients (79%)—in 91% of the symptomatic cases and in 70% of the idiopathic cases. The concentration of IgM was abnormal in 28 patients—usually it was raised; that of IgA and IgG was abnormal in 15 patients each—either raised or lowered concentrations. No significant differences were demonstrated between the degree or type of dysgammaglobulinaemia and serological and clinical findings, e.g., the degree of positivity of the DAT and severity of anaemia were not correlated with serum Ig levels.

The findings quoted above confirmed the earlier report of Blajchman et al. (1969) which emphasized the frequency and diversity of serum IgG abnormalities in warm-antibody AIHA; the German data differed, however, in as much as they did not confirm the special frequency of reduced levels of serum IgA that Blajchman et al. had observed.

Abnormal serological reactions

It has been realized since the middle 1960s that not only might the concentration of the serum immunoglobulins be quantitatively abnormal but that the patients' sera might react abnormally with a variety of organ-specific or non-organ-specific antigens.

van Loghem (1965) mentioned that in 'idiopathic hemolytic anemia' auto-antibodies against tissue antibodies 'frequently occur', but gave no details. Tan and Chaplin (1968) referred to 26 patients with warm-antibody AIHA, none of whom showed any evidence of a collagen disease or a benign or malignant lymphoproliferative disorder: antinuclear (ANF) antibodies were detected at low titres (20 or less) in 10 of them—an incidence of 39% compared with 3% in controls. None of the patients forming the antinuclear antibodies gave a positive LE-cell test, and precipitating antibodies, as found in SLE, were not demonstrable.

Blajchman's (1971) observations were based on a larger series of patients. Thirty-eight females and 22 males had warm-antibody AIHA: 16% of their sera contained low-titre (20 or less) antibodies against ANF (compared with 4.2% in controls) and 5% contained antibodies against mitochondria (compared with 0% in controls). Interestingly, the increases were only significant in the female patients. Blajchman also looked for antibodies active against gastric parietal cells, thyroid cytoplasmic antigens and smooth muscle, but did not detect any significant differences in their (low) incidence between the patients and controls. He concluded that, as in other auto-immune diseases, the incidence of non-organ-specific antibodies in the sera of warm-antibody AIHA patients was higher than normal.

Salmon and Homberg (1971) also gave details of the occurrence of anti-cardiolipids, anti-nuclear and anti-organ-specific antibodies in 109 patients with idiopathic or secondary AIHA. Anti-nuclear antibodies were most frequently present (32%); next frequent were anti-thyroid antibodies (14%), anti-cardiolipid antibodies (12%) and rheumatoid factors (10%).

Biological false-positive tests for syphilis

The fact that the serum of certain patients with acquired haemolytic anaemia reacted positively with the cardiolipin antigen used in the

Table 23.4 Biological false positive (BFP) reactions in auto-immune haemolytic anaemia

Reference	Sex and age of patients (years)	Serological reactions	Type of AIHA and outcome
Davidson (1932, Case 8)	F. 45	WR weak, then neg	Relapsing severe haemolysis. Eventually recovered
Rosenthal and Corten (1937)	F. 62	WR strongly pos	Severe haemolysis; auto-agglutination. Died
Kracke and Hoffman (1943)	F. 32	WR and Kahn tests pos; became neg after splenectomy	Chronic haemolysis. Auto-agglutination at room temperature; hyperglobulinaemia. Died
Lubinski and Goldbloom (1946)	M. 11½	WR and Kline test pos	Acute haemolysis. High-thermal-amplitude auto-agglutination. Died
Rubinstein (1948)	M. 50	WR transitorily strongly pos; Kahn and Kline tests neg	Subacute haemolysis. Transfused. Eventually recovered
Gatman and Hamilton (1949)	M. 69	Kahn test pos with eluate from erythrocytes (WR neg); Kahn test and WR neg with serum	Chronic severe haemolysis. Transfused. Gradual recovery
Kracke and Riser (1949, Case 5)	F. 22	Kahn test pos; neg after splenectomy	Subacute haemolysis; hypersplenism
Rosenthal, Komninos and Dameshek (1953)	F. 33	Kahn and Hinton tests pos; Hinton test neg when in remission	Severe haemolysis. DAT pos. Remitted after corticosteroid treatment
Dacie (1954, p. 205, Case 13)	F. 54	WR and Kahn tests pos; both tests neg 3 years after splenectomy	Chronic haemolysis. DAT pos. High-thermal-amplitude cold antibody; also possibly separate warm haemolysin
Hennemann (1955)	F. 22	Kahn and Meinicke tests pos; became neg after splenectomy. WR neg throughout	Relapsing severe haemolysis; also leucopenia and thrombocytopenia. Recovered after splenectomy
Christen and Jaccottet (1958)	M. 13	WR pos	Chronic AIHA. DAT pos
Jenkins and Marsh (1961)	Three females aged 43–58	WR and Price's reaction pos; TPI test neg (one patient)	Severe AIHA. DAT pos. Antibodies in serum specifically active against stored erythrocytes
Dacie (1962, p. 374, Case M.J.)	F. 73	WR pos	Subacute haemolysis. DAT pos. High-thermal-amplitude cold antibody, plus incomplete warm antibody
Videbaek (1962, Case 3)	F. 35	WR pos, noted first when aged 17	Severe relapsing haemolysis. DAT pos. Eventually recovered
Shulman and Harvey (1964)	F. 65	'Serologic test', TPI test neg	Chronic haemolysis. DAT pos. Thrombocytopenia. Also long-standing rheumatoid arthritis, Hashimoto's thyroiditis and Sjögren's syndrome

Table 23.4 (*contd*)

Schwartz and Costea (1966)	F. 50	BFP reaction consistently pos	Chronic haemolysis. Lymphosarcoma (Mickulicz's syndrome)
Sievers, Lehtinen and Aho (1968)	M. 49	WR, Kahn, Kolmer, VDRL tests pos; TPI test neg	Chronic haemolysis. DAT pos. Unusual cold antibody plus IgG antibody
Oken et al. (1973)	M. 42	VDRL test pos; Treponema test neg	Chronic haemolysis. DAT pos. Hypergammaglobulinaemia. ? NZB syndrome in man
Conley and Savarese (1989)	(1) M. 63	Standard tests pos when aged 19 and 40. TPI test pos when aged 40	Severe haemolysis. DAT pos (anti-IgG and anti-C). Well 12 years after onset
	(2) F. 45	Standard tests pos when aged 22; TPI test neg	Severe haemolysis. DAT pos (anti-IgG). Well when aged 59
	(3) F. 26	Flocculation tests pos when aged 20; TPI test neg	Severe haemolysis during pregnancy. DAT pos later (aged 47). Relapsed and died aged 56. DAT pos (anti-IgG and anti-C)
	(4) M. 46	BFP reaction pos when aged 22 and subsequently; VDRL pos when aged 44	Severe relapsing haemolysis; also thrombocytopenia. DAT pos (anti-IgG and anti-C)
	(7) F. 53	VDRL test pos; TPI test neg	Severe persistent haemolysis. DAT pos (anti-IgG and anti-C)
	(10) F. 67	VDRL test pos; Reiter test neg	Severe haemolysis. DAT pos. 10 years later, acute relapse (? Waldenström's disease). Died aged 84
	(11) F. 42	VDRL test pos; TPI test neg	Relapsing haemolysis. DAT pos (anti-IgG and anti-C). Later, aggressive large-cell lymphoma. Died aged 54

Wassermann reaction (WR) and perhaps, too, gave positive reactions in other serological tests for syphilis, has been known for many years. The finding has quite a large literature and is of considerable clinical importance because of the possibility of its leading to mistakes in diagnosis.

It is now realized that the positive STS (serum test for syphilis) reactions were a reflection in almost all cases of the patients' unusual immunological reactivity rather than an immune response to syphilis. They are now commonly referred to as biological false positive (BFP) reactions. BFP reactions have been observed with the sera of patients suffering from AIHA of either the warm- or cold-antibody type. The majority of reports, however, have dealt with warm-antibody AIHA. In Table 23.4 are listed case reports dating back as far as 1932. They deal, therefore, with some patients studied before the advent of the DAT: it is, however, highly likely that the patients referred to had in fact suffered from AIHA.

It seems from published data that the sera of somewhere between 6 and 18% of patients who develop AIHA give BFP reactions.

Wilkenson and Sequeira (1955), in their review of the value of the treponemal immobilization test (TPI) as a verification test in suspected latent syphilis, stated that they had examined the sera of 10 patients with AIHA: sera from six of these patients had reacted positively in one or more STS tests; one had given discordant results in STS tests over a 5-month period. All the patients' sera failed to react in the TPI test. In contrast, Wilkenson and Sequeira reported that the sera of five out of seven patients with paroxysmal cold haemoglobinuria, which had reacted positively in STS tests (usually to a high titre), reacted positively, too, in the TPI test. Sera from the remaining two patients failed to react in both the STS and TPI tests.

Letman (1957) reported that four out of 18 AIHA patients had given positive Wassermann reactions. Three of the patients had idiopathic AIHA, the fourth had had infectious mononucleosis.

Allgood and Chaplin (1967), in their review of 47 patients thought to be suffering from idiopathic AIHA, listed 'positive serology' as a feature of three of them (6.4%).

Pirofsky (1969, p. 53) reported that the sera of 17 out of 141 patients with AIHA (of all types) reacted positively (11.9%), and it is interesting to note that the percentage was higher in females (18.7%) than in males (4.4%). (The incidence of positive tests given by the general hospital population was less than 3%.) Three out of 26 patients judged to have idiopathic AIHA (11.5%) gave positive reactions.

Conley (1981) reported that the sera of six out of 33 personally studied patients gave BFP reactions and in a later review Conley and Savarese (1989) gave details of seven patients: in four of them the reactions were known to have been present before the advent of AIHA while in three the reactions were discovered after the onset of AIHA. [Conley and Savarese (1989) also described similar findings in patients who had ITP and reviewed the quite extensive literature dealing with the familial incidence of BFP reactions.]

Haemoglobinaemia

As already referred to (p. 16), haemoglobinuria may accompany acute haemolytic episodes in warm-antibody AIHA if these are especially acute. In such cases the plasma-haemoglobin concentration is markedly raised and the plasma will have an obvious red tinge. Fortunately, such occurrences are relatively rare (except in young children, see p. 25). Minor increases in plasma haemoglobin, however, occur more frequently. Crosby and Dameshek (1951), for instance, reported finding raised concentrations in a series of patients in the absence of overt haemoglobinuria.

Nine of Crosby and Dameshek's patients appeared to have been suffering from idiopathic warm-antibody AIHA: the plasma haemoglobin concentration was elevated in eight of them — from 6 mg/dl (just abnormal) to 166 mg/dl (grossly elevated). The highest values were found in association with marked spherocytosis, and haemosiderin was present in the urine in amounts paralleling the plasma haemoglobin levels. Clinical remission was associated with a fall in plasma haemoglobin; indeed this was the first sign of improvement in several cases.

Haptoglobins. These are likely to be absent if haemolysis is markedly increased. Brus and Lewis (1959) investigated 10 serum samples from seven patients: haptoglobulins were absent from six of the samples, present in traces in two and present in normal amounts in two. The haemoglobin turnover in the last two patients was, however, thought to be at least four times the normal. Schumm's test is often positive, and in patients in whom there is much intravascular haemolysis methaemalbumin is demonstrable spectroscopically.

Serum bilirubin

In the absence of gallstones and/or liver disease, the serum bilirubin seldom exceeds 5 mg/dl of which the greater part is indirect-reacting (unconjugated).

Tisdale, Klatskin and Kinsella (1959) estimated the total and direct-acting pigment in 10 AIHA patients in whom there was no evidence of liver disease. The total bilirubin ranged from 1.56 to 16.1 mg/dl; and in only seven of 24 serum samples did the total pigment exceed 5.0 mg/dl, five of the samples being derived from the same patient. The highest direct-reacting figure was 0.9 mg/dl (out of a total of 6.0 mg) and the highest direct-reacting: total pigment ratio was 0.30 (0.55 mg out of a total of 1.82 mg). Normally, the direct-reacting: total pigment ratio is 0.03 or less, and the higher values found in AIHA suggest that some conjugated bilirubin may be regurgitated into the blood stream from the bile when the excretion is high, even in the absence of overt liver disease.

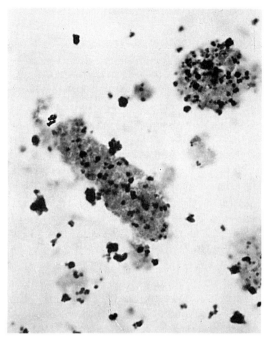

Fig. 23.27   Urine deposit stained by Perls's reaction to demonstrated haemosiderin.
From a patient with severe warm-antibody AIHA (Case 12 of Dacie, 1962, p. 684). x 1250.

Urine

A moderate excess of urobilinogen is generally found, and occasionally bile pigment also. As has also already been discussed (p. 25), haemoglobinuria is often a prominent sign in the most seriously ill patients. In severely anaemic patients there may be slight proteinuria, in the absence of haemoglobinuria, and a few casts may be found in the urinary deposit. According to Crosby and Dameshek (1951), haemosiderin is frequently found in small amounts; it may in fact be present in large amounts in patients in whom there is a major degree of persistent intravascular haemolysis (Fig. 23.27).

Oliguria and renal failure seldom occur, even in patients suffering from fulminating haemolysis with haemoglobinuria, but they have been reported, e.g. by Payne, Spaet and Aggeler (1955).

André, Dreyfus and Sultan (1963) reported the occurrence of mesobilifuchsinuria — causing brown to black discolouration of the urine — in an unusual and complicated case. The patient, a man aged 42, was found to have developed Hodgkin's disease, for which he received nitrogen mustard 2 years after the onset of warm-antibody AIHA. The following year he became acutely ill with severe anaemia, pyrexia and upper right abdominal pain, and passed dark urine containing mesobilifuchsin. Cholecystectomy was carried out, following which he went into remission and the urine became normally coloured. Liver biopsy revealed post-necrotic cirrhosis.

Faeces

Dark stools, a consequence of an increased excretion of stercobilin, are the rule, and the total daily excretion may exceed 1000 mg.

Pisciotta, Downer and Hinz (1956) reported the remarkably high figure of 20 000 mg per day in an AIHA patient receiving multiple transfusions in preparation for splenectomy! Previously, the maximum daily output in this patient had been 3000 mg. These findings illustrate the extraordinary rapidity with which transfused normal blood may be destroyed and also the remarkable latent capacity of the liver to excrete bilirubin.

ERYTHROCYTE METABOLISM

This is generally increased, in parallel with the reticulocyte count, in patients suffering from moderate to marked increases in haemolysis.

Brabec and co-workers (1965) measured glycolytic activity, the effect of methylene blue on erythrocyte respiration, ATP, ADP, 2,3-DPG, inorganic phosphate, GSH and its stability, and acetylcholinesterase and acid phosphatase activities in 20 patients with AIHA. Fourteen were suffering from moderate increases in haemolysis: their DATs were positive, their haemoglobin ranged from 8.2 to 12.4 g/dl, reticulocyte counts from 2.3 to 12.2% and ^{51}Cr T_{50} values from 11 to 19 days. Significant increases were found in the haemolysing patients in G6PD and acid phosphatase activities and in the increase in respiration brought about by methylene blue. The results of the other estimations were not significantly abnormal, as were all the observations made on the patients in clinical remission, irrespective of whether their DAT was positive. Patients giving a positive DAT were found to have reduced AChE activity, irrespective of whether haemolysis was increased (see also below).

Erythrocyte adenine nucleotides

Strong and co-workers (1985) measured erythrocyte ATP and ADP concentrations in 154 patients who had formed erythrocyte auto-antibodies. The mean concentration of ADP was significantly higher in the 96 patients who were actively haemolysing compared with the results in non-haemolysing patients and normal controls. The raised concentrations were thought mainly to reflect a decrease in mean cell age.

Acetylcholinesterase (AChE)

Interest in erythrocyte AChE activity in haemolytic anaemia stems from the discovery in 1956 by De Sandre, Ghiotto and Mastella that AChE activity might be markedly subnormal in patients with paroxysmal nocturnal haemoglobinuria. Low activity was subsequently noted in the erythrocytes of patients with AIHA and in ABO haemolytic disease of the newborn (HDN).

Tanaka, Valentine and Schneider (1964) reported in an abstract that the AChE activity was subnormal in eight out of 10 patients with AIHA, despite a raised reticulocyte count and increased G6PD activity. They suggested that the reduced activity was likely to be secondary to damage to the erythrocyte membrane. Choremis and co-workers (1965) likewise found significantly low activities in the erythrocytes of three children with AIHA compared with those of children suffering from other types of haemolytic anaemia. (There were no PNH patients in this series.) Subnormal values were subsequently reported from Japan, by Tsukada and Miwa (1969), i.e. in nine out of 27 patients with AIHA and in 14 out of 15 patients with PNH.

Sirchia and his co-workers (1970) reported in more detail on a large series of AIHA patients. Fifty-nine were studied: all gave a positive DAT; none had received drugs such as α-methyldopa or cephalothin. The results were compared with those obtained with the erythrocytes of 61 normal adults. Although there was considerable overlap with the normal, AChE activity tended to be significantly low in the patients whose erythrocytes were coated with IgG or IgG plus complement (C), despite raised reticulocyte counts

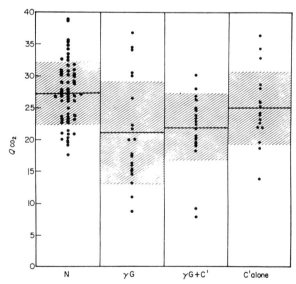

Fig. 23.28   Erythrocyte AChE activity in normal subjects (N) and in AIHA patients classified according to whether their erythrocytes were coated with γG(IgG), γG+C' or C' (complement) alone.
The horizontal lines and the hatched area indicate mean values ± 1 S.D. [Reproduced by permission from Sirchia et al. (1970).]

(Fig. 23.28). In contrast, in only one out of 17 patients whose cells were coated with C alone was the result below the lowest normal value. Sirchia et al. pointed out that the decrease in AChE activity was less marked and less constant than in ABO HDN and in PNH, that experimental deficiency brought about by AChE inhibitors does not accelerate erythrocyte destruction and that coating erythrocytes *in vitro* with antibodies does not seem to reduce the activity of the enzyme. They suggested that interaction between mononuclear cells and erythrocytes coated with antibodies might be responsible for the loss of AChE activity.

Scott and Rasbridge (1971) also reported on a large series of patients giving a positive DAT. Of 38 patients studied, 21 were forming IgG auto-antibodies; nine of

them were classified as having the idiopathic disease. A low AChE activity was found in some of the patients, particularly when related to erythrocyte age as assessed by the cells' creatine content. Density separation suggested an abnormal decline in enzyme activity associated with ageing (Fig. 23.29). Low values were found more frequently in patients whose DAT was of the anti-IgG type than in those whose erythrocytes only reacted with an anti-C serum. Scott and Rasbridge suggested that the low values found particularly in the IgG-reacting patients reflected a membrane lesion associated with spherocytosis and haemolysis and that 'intervention of the phagocytic cells of the reticulo-endothelial system is essential for these phenomena'. They noted, however, that the activity of ATPase, also a membrane enzyme, was affected to a lesser extent than that of AChE.

Herz, Kaplan and Scheye (1972) reported on erythrocyte AChE activity in 10 patients with AIHA (but gave no details of the patients). In only one of the patients was the enzyme's activity significantly reduced. In this patient density separation of the erythrocyte into 10 fractions showed that AChE activity was being lost as the cells aged at a rate approximately 5 times the normal (Fig. 23.30) — in striking contrast to that in a PNH patient in whom the enzyme's activity appeared to increase as the cells became older and denser. [In fact, in PNH the increase is apparent, not real — it reflects the fact that it is cells that have high AChE values initially (normal erythrocytes or cells with a minimal PNH lesion) that have a long life-span.]

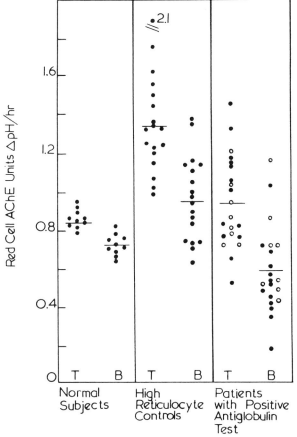

Fig. 23.29   Erythrocyte AChE activity in the top (T) and bottom (B) fractions of the blood of the normal subjects, 18 patients with high reticulocyte counts but negative DATs, and 21 patients with positive DATs.

● represents patients whose erythrocytes were agglutinated by anti-IgG sera and ○ patients whose erythrocytes were agglutinated by anti-C sera. The horizontal lines indicate mean values for each group. [Reproduced by permission from Scott and Rasbridge (1971).]

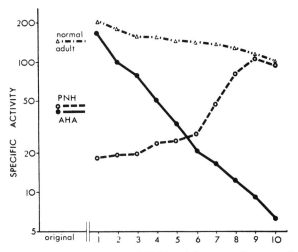

Fig. 23.30   Erythrocyte AChE activity according to cell density: a comparison between the blood of a normal adult subject and patients with auto-immune haemolytic anaemia (AHA) and paroxysmal nocturnal haemoglobinuria (PNH), respectively.

[Reproduced by permission from Herz, Kaplan and Scheye (1972).]

Erythrocyte membrane proteins

Gomperts, Metz and Zail (1973) submitted acetic-acid extracts of the erythrocyte membranes of six patients with AIHA (three of whom had the idiopathic disease) to electrophoresis in urea-starch gel. The pattern obtained differed from normal: one band ('band 1') was absent and an adjacent band ('band 2') was absent or only just discernible. The findings were similar to those previously obtained with the erythrocytes of HS patients, using the same technique (see Vol. 1, p. 190). Ten infants with haemolytic disease of the newborn (HDN) were also studied: the pattern produced by extracts from the erythro-cytes of five infants who had Rh HDN were similar to those of the AIHA patients, in contrast to the normal pattern given by five ABO HDN infants. Extracts prepared from erythrocytes exposed *in vitro* to IgG or IgM anti-D were similarly normal, and Gomperts, Metz and Zail suggested that the changes they had seen might have been caused *in vivo* by damage to the erythrocyte membrane as the result of interaction between macrophages and IgG-coated cells.

Tishkoff (1966) measured stromal protein, sialic acid and fucose concentrations in 11 patients suffering from miscellaneous types of haemolytic anaemia, and in 13 normal subjects and in seven patients with DAT-positive haemolytic anaemias. The stromal protein concentration was found to be higher in the anaemic patients in parallel with their reticulocyte count, irrespective of whether the DAT was positive or not. In the DAT-positive subjects, however, the fucose : protein ratio and, to a lesser extent, the sialic acid : protein ratio were decreased. The findings were interpreted as indicating an alteration in the carbohydrate moiety of the erythrocyte membrane, possibly brought about by activation of proteases secondary to antibody–antigen interaction.

Erythrocyte lipids

Brabec and co-workers (1969) estimated the cholesterol and the phospholipid content of the erythrocytes in 40 patients with AIHA: 24 were actively haemolysing at the time of the investigation; 16 were in remission, nine of whom had negative DATs. The cholesterol and phospholipid content per cell was found to be significantly subnormal in the patients whose erythrocytes were coated with IgG. The proportions of the individual phospholipid fractions were, however, normal. Brabec et al. suggested that the reduced content of erythrocyte lipids reflected the loss of surface resulting from sensitized-cell–mononuclear-cell interaction and were related to the development of spherocytosis and increased osmotic fragility.

REFERENCES

ALLGOOD, J. W. & CHAPLIN, H. JNR (1967). Idiopathic acquired autoimmune hemolytic anemia. A review of forty-seven cases treated from 1955 through 1965. *Amer. J. Med.*, **43**, 254–273.

ANDRÉ, R., DREYFUS, B. & SULTAN, C. (1963). Urines noires par mésobilifuchsine et anémie hémolytique acquise avec auto-anticorps. *Nouv. Rev. franç. Hémat.*, **3**, 189–193.

BAIKIE, A. G. & PIRRIE, R. (1956). Megaloblastic erythropoiesis in idiopathic acquired haemolytic anaemia. *Scot. med. J.*, **1**, 330–334.

BAKKER-V. AARDENNE, W. I. T., VERLOOP, M. C. & BOETZELAER, G. C. D. VAN (1958). Osmotic and mechanical fragility of erythrocytes in patients with idiopathic and symptomatic acquired hemolytic anemia. *Proc. 6th Congr. Europ. Soc. Haematol., Copenhagen, 1957*, p. 695–701. Karger, Basel.

BAXTER, E. H. & EVERHART, M. W. (1938). Acute hemolytic anemia (Lederer type). *J. Pediat.*, **12**, 357–362.

BEICKERT, A. (1956). Eine aregeneratorische Variante der chronischen erworbenen hämolytischen Anämie vom Typ Loutit. *Klin. Wschr.*, **34**, 195–197.

BERREY, B. H. & WATSON, J. D. (1951). Acquired hemolytic anemia. Report of a case in an infant with discussion of several etiological factors which may have been operative. *Arch. Pediat.*, **68**, 10–27.

BERTRAND, Y., LEFRÈRE, J. J., LEVERGER, G., COUROUCE, A. M., FEO, C., CLARK, M., SCHAISON, G. & SOULIER, J. P. (1985). Autoimmune haemolytic anaemia revealed by human parvovirus linked erythroblastopenia. *Lancet*, **ii**, 382 (Letter).

BETKE, K., RICHARZ, H., SCHUBOTHE, H. & VIVELL, O. (1953). Beobactungen zu Krankeitsbild, Pathogenese und Ätiologie der akuten erworbenen hämolytischen Anämie (Lederer-Anämie). *Klin. Wschr.*, **31**, 373–380.

BLAJCHMAN, M. A. (1971). Tissue antibodies in idiopathic autoimmune haemolytic anaemia. *Clin. exp. Immunol.*, **8**, 741–748.

BLAJCHMAN, M. A., DACIE, J. V., HOBBS, J. R., PETTIT, J. E. & WORRLEDGE, S. M. (1969). Immunoglobulins in warm-type autoimmune haemolytic anaemia. *Lancet*, **ii**, 340–344.

BONHAM CARTER, R. E., CATHIE, I. A. B. & GASSER. C. (1954). Aplastische Anämie (chronische Erythroblastophthise) bedingt durch Autoimmunisierung. *Schweiz. med. Wschr.*, **84**, 1114–1116.

BOUSSER, J., CHRISTOL, D., DAUSSET, J., RAMPON, S., JALLUT, H. & MERY, J. P. (1955). Épisode érythroblastopénique prolongé ayant marqué le début d'une anémie hémolytique chronique avec auto-anticorps. *Sang*, **26**, 804–810.

BOWMAN, J. M. (1955). Acquired hemolytic anemia. Use of replacement transfusion in a crisis. *Amer. Dis. Child.*, **89**, 226–232.

BRAAKER, J. (1960). Zur Klinik der durch Autoantikörper bedingten erworbenen hämolytischen Anämien. *Praxis*, **49**, 209–214.

BRABEC, V., BICANOVÁ, J., FRIEDMANN, B., KOUT, M., MIRČEVOVÁ, L., PALEK, J., VOPATOVÁ, M. & VOLEK, V. (1965). Stoffwechselveränderungen in Erythrozyten bei der autoimmunen hämolytischen Krankheit. *Acta haemat. (Basel)*, **34**, 88–100.

BRABEC, V., MICHALEC, Č., PALEK, J. & KOUT, M. (1969). Red cell lipids in autoimmune hemolytic anemia. *Blood*, **34**, 414–420.

BRITTIN, G. M., BRECHER, G., JOHNSON, C. A. & STUART, J. (1969). Spurious macrocytosis of antibody-coated red cells. *Amer. J. clin. Path.*, **52**, 237–241.

BRUS, I. & LEWIS, S. M. (1959). The haptoglobin content of serum in haemolytic anaemia. *Brit. J. Haemat.*, **5**, 348–355.

BURSTON, J., HUSAIN, O. A. N., HUTT, M. S. R. & TANNER. E. I. (1959). Two cases of acute auto-immune haemolysis and aplasia. *Brit. med. J.*, **i**, 83–86.

CARAPELLA DE LUCA, E. C., STEGAGNO, M., MORINO, G., BALLATI, G. & LORENZINI, F. (1984). Prolonged reticulocytopenia and transient erythroid hypoplasia in a child with autoimmune haemolytic anaemia. *Haematologica*, **69**, 315–320.

CASTEX, M. R., STEINGART, K., POLETTI, R. (1932). Hémoglobinurie: anémie aiguë à régéneration érythroblastique intense. *Sang*, **6**, 589–594.

CELADA, A. (1984). Autoimmune haemolytic anaemia and aplastic crisis. *Brit. J. Haemat.*, **57**, 178–179 (Letter).

CELADA, A., FARQUET, J. J. & MULLER, A. F. (1977). Refractory sideroblastic anemia secondary to autoimmune hemolytic anemia. *Acta haemat. (Basel)*, **58**, 213–216.

CHANARIN, I., DACIE, J. V. & MOLLIN, D. L. (1959). Folic-acid deficiency in haemolytic anaemia. *Brit. J. Haemat.*, **5**, 245–256.

CHARBONNIER, A. & DAUSSET, J. (1953). Étude électrophorétique des protides sériques au cours des anémies hémolytiques avec auto-anticorps incomplets chauds. *Ann. Biol. clin.*, **11**, 22–29.

CHOREMIS, C., NICOLOPOULOS, D., MATAXOTOU, K. & MOSCHOS, A. (1965). Erythrocyte cholinesterase activity in hemolytic anemias. *Acta pediat. scand.*, **54**, 218–224.

CHRISTEN, J.-P. & JACCOTTET, M. (1958). Anémie hémolytique immunologique par auto-anticorps. 1e partie: clinique. *Helv. paediat. Acta*, **13**, 131–139.

CHRISTENSON, W. N. & DACIE, J. V. (1957). Serum proteins in acquired haemolytic anaemia (auto-antibody type). *Brit. J. Haemat.*, **3**, 153–164.

CONLEY, C. L. (1981). Immunologic precursors of autoimmune hematologic disorders. Autoimmune hemolytic anemia and thrombocytopenic purpura. *Johns Hopk. med. J.*, **149**, 101–109.

CONLEY, C. L., LIPPMAN, S. M. & NESS, P. (1980). Autoimmune hemolytic anemia with reticulocytopenia. A medical emergency. *J. Amer. med. Ass.*, **244**, 1688–1690.

CONLEY, C. L., LIPPMAN, S. M., NESS, P. M., PETZ, L. D., BRANCH, D. R. & GALLAGHER, M. T. (1982). Autoimmune hemolytic anemia with reticulocytopenia and erythroid marrow. *New Engl. J. Med.*, **306**, 281–286.

CONLEY, C. L. & SAVARESE, D. M. F. (1989). Biologic false-positive serologic tests for syphilis and other serologic abnormalities in autoimmune hemolytic anemia and thrombocytopenic purpura. *Medicine (Baltimore)*, **68**, 67–84.

COUTEL, Y., BRETAGNE, J. & MOREL, H. (1962). Anémie hémolytique aiguë idiopathique avec auto-anticorps chauds chez un enfant de 9 ans. Guérison. *Arch. franç. Pédiat.*, **19**, 253–261.

CROSBY, W. H. & DAMESHEK, W. (1951). The significance of hemoglobinemia and associated hemosiderinuria, with particular reference to various types of hemolytic anemia. *J. Lab. clin. Med.*, **38**, 829–841.

CROSBY, W. H. & RAPPAPORT, H. (1956). Reticulocytopenia in autoimmune hemolytic anemia. *Blood*, **11**, 929–936.

CROSBY, W. H. & RAPPAPORT, H. (1957). Autoimmune hemolytic anemia. I. Analysis of hematologic observations with particular reference to their prognostic value. A survey of 57 cases. *Blood*, **12**, 42–55.

DACIE, J. V. (1954). *The Haemolytic Anaemias: Congenital and Acquired*, 525 pp. Churchill, London.

DACIE, J. V. (1962). *The Haemolytic Anaemias: Congenital and Acquired, Part II—The Auto-immune Haemolytic Anaemias*, 2nd edn, 377 pp. Churchill, London.

DACIE, J. V. (1967). *The Haemolytic Anaemias: Congenital and Acquired. Part III—Secondary or Symptomatic Haemolytic Anaemias*, 2nd edn, 272 pp. Churchill, London.

DACIE, J. V. & DE GRUCHY, G. C. (1951). Auto-antibodies in acquired haemolytic anaemia. *J. clin. Path.*, **4**, 253–271.

DAMESHEK, W. & SCHWARTZ, S. O. (1938a). The presence of hemolysins in acute hemolytic anemia; preliminary note. *New Eng. J. Med.*, **218**, 75–80.

DAMESHEK, W. & SCHWARTZ, S. O. (1938b). Hemolysins as the cause of clinical and experimental hemolytic anemias. With particular reference to the nature of spherocytosis and increased fragility. *Amer. J. med. Sci.*, **196**, 769–792.

DAMESHEK, W. & SCHWARTZ, S. O. (1940). Acute hemolytic anemia (acquired hemolytic icterus, acute type). *Medicine (Baltimore)*, **19**, 231–327.

DAVID, J. K. JNR & MINOT, A. S. (1944). Acute hemolytic anemia in infancy. Report of a case with demonstration of hemolytic activity of serum. *Amer. J. Dis. Child.*, **68**, 327–329.

DAVIDSON, L. S. P. (1932). Macrocytic haemolytic anaemia. *Quart. J. Med.*, **25** (N.S.1.), 543–578.

DAVIS, L. J., KENNEDY, A. C., BAIKIE, A. G. & BROWN, A. (1952). Haemolytic anaemias of various types treated with ACTH and cortisone. Report of ten cases, including one of acquired type in which erythropoietic arrest occurred during a crisis. *Glasgow med. J.*, **33**, 263–285.

DE GRUCHY, G. C. (1954). The diagnosis and management of acquired haemolytic anaemia. *Aust. Ann. Med.*, **3**, 106–115.

DE SANDRE, G., GHIOTTO, G. & MASTELLA, G. (1956). L'acetilcolinesterasi eritrocitoria. II. Rapporti con le malattie emolitiche. *Acta med. patav.*, **16**, 310-335.

DOUGLAS, A. S. & DACIE, J. V. (1953). The incidence and significance of iron-containing granules in human erythrocytes and their precursors. *J. clin. Path.*, **6**, 307–313.

EISEMANN, G. & DAMESHEK, W. (1954). Splenectomy for 'pure red-cell' hypoplastic (aregenerative) anemia associated with autoimmune hemolytic disease. *New Eng. J. Med.*, **251**, 1044–1048.

EVANS, R. S. (1943). Acute hemolytic anemia with autoagglutination: a case report. *Stanford med. Bull.*, **1**, 178–182.

FAROLINO, D. L., RUSTAGI, P. K., CURRIE, M. S., DOEBLIN, T. D. & LOGUE, G. L. (1986). Teardrop-shaped red cells in autoimmune hemolytic anemia. *Amer. J. Hemat.*, **21**, 415–418.

GASSER, C. (1952). Akute erworbene hämolytische Anämien mit Immunkörpernachweis und Erythrocytenphagocytose im peripheren Blut. *Schweiz. med. Wschr.*, **82**, 42–43.

GASSER, C. (1954). Hämolyse und erworbene hämolytische Erkrankungen. *Helvet. paediat. Acta*, **9**, 135–175.

GASSER, C. (1955). Pure red cell anemia due to auto-antibodies. *Sang*, **26**, 6–13.

GASSER, C. & HOLLÄNDER, L. (1951). Anémie hémolytique acquise aiguë provoquée par des auto-anticorps, accompagnée de purpura thrombocytopénique, chez un nourrisson de 7 semaines. *Rev. Hémat.*, **6**, 316–333.

GATMAN, M. & HAMILTON, L. (1949). Haemolytic anaemia. *J. clin. Path.*, **2**, 225–229.

GOMPERTS, E. D., METZ, J. & ZAIL, S. S. (1973). Red cell membrane protein in antibody induced haemolytic anaemia. *Brit. J. Haemat.*, **25**, 421–428.

GREENBERG, J., CURTIN-COHEN, M., GILL, E. M. & COHEN, A. (1980). Prolonged reticulocytopenia in autoimmune hemolytic anemia of childhood. *J. Pediat.*, **97**, 784–786.

GREENWALD, H. M. (1938). Acute hemolytic anemia. *Amer. J. med. Sci.*, **196**, 179–188.

GRUELUND, S. (1950). Megaloblastic hemolytic anemia. *Acta med. scand.*, Suppl. **239**, 101–106.

HABIBI, B., HOMBERG, J.-C., SCHAISON, G. & SALMON, C. (1974). Autoimmune hemolytic anemia in children. A review of 80 cases. *Amer. J. Med.*, **56**, 61–69.

HAHN, F. & LÜTTGENS, W. (1949). Autoagglutinationphänomene beim hämolytischen Ikterus. *Dtsch. Arch. klin. Med.*, **194**, 586–605.

HANSEN, O. P., SØRENSEN, C. H. & ASTRUP, L. (1982). Evans' syndrome in IgA deficiency. Episodic autoimmune haemolytic anaemia and thrombocytopenia during a 10 years observation period. *Scand. J. Haemat.*, **29**, 265–270.

HANSSEN, P. (1943). Acute hemolytic anemia. *Acta med. scand.*, **113**, 251–261.

HARGRAVES, M. M., HERRELL, W. E. & PEARMAN, R. O. (1941). Erythrophagocytic anemia (Lederer's anemia ?). Report of a case with recovery. *Proc. Staff Meetings Mayo Clin.*, **16**, 107–112.

HARLEY, J. & DODS, L. (1959). Some acquired haemolytic anaemias of childhood. *Aust. Ann. Med.*, **8**, 98–108.

HAUKE, G., FAUSER, A. A., WEBER, S. & MAAS, D. (1983). Reticulocytopenia in severe autoimmune hemolytic anemia (AIHA) of the warm antibody type. *Blut*, **46**, 321–327.

HAWLEY, J. G. & GORDON, R. S. J. (1954). Anemia associated with cold agglutinins. *N. Y. St. J. Med.*, **54**, 1516–1518.

HEGDE, U. M., GORDON-SMITH, E. C. & WORLLEDGE, S. M. (1977). Reticulocytopenia and 'absence' of red cell autoantibodies in immune haemolytic anaemia. *Brit. med. J.*, **ii**, 1444–1447.

HEISEL, M. A. & ORTEGA, J. A. (1983). Factors influencing prognosis in childhood autoimmune hemolytic anemia. *Amer. J. ped. Hemat./Oncol.*, **5**, 147–152.

HENNEMANN, H. H. (1955). La formation d'anticorps multiples au cours d'anémies hémolytiques acquises. *Rev. Belg. Path. Méd. exp.*, **24**, 479–484.

HENNEMANN, H. H. & FALCK, I. (1957). Über kombinationen von aplastischen mit hämolytischen syndromen. *Acta haemat. (Basel)*, **18**, 219–228.

HERRADOR, M. S. & DE CASTRO, S. (1960).

Fagocitosis de células blancas en medule ósea en un caso de anemia hemolitíca adquirida. *Sangre*, **5**, 77–83.

HERZ, F., KAPLAN, E. & SCHEYE, E. S. (1972). Red cell acetylcholinesterase deficiency in autoimmune hemolytic anemia and in paroxysmal nocturnal hemoglobinuria. *Clin. chim. Acta*, **38**, 301–306.

ISSITT, P. D., GRUPPO, R. A., WILKINSON, S. L. & ISSITT, C. H. (1982). Atypical presentation of acute phase, antibody-induced haemolytic anaemia in an infant. *Brit. J. Haemat.*, **52**, 537–543.

JENKINS, W. J. & MARSH, W. L. (1961). Autoimmune haemolytic anaemia. Three cases with antibodies specifically active against stored red cells. *Lancet*, **i**, 16–18.

KAZNELSON, P. (1924). Erfahrungen über die Indickationen der Splenektomie und über deren Wirkungmechanismus. *Wien. Arch. inn. Med.*, **7**, 87–116.

KÖLBL, H. (1955). Klinik und Therapie der akuten erworbenen hämolytischen Anämien im Kindesalter. *Öst. Zschr. Kinderheilk.*, **11**, 27–51.

KRACKE, R. R. & HOFFMAN, B. J. (1943). Chronic hemolytic anemia with autoagglutination and hyperglobulinemia; report of a fatal case. *Ann. intern. Med.*, **19**, 673–684.

KRACKE, R. & RISER, H. JNR (1949). The problem of hypersplenism. *J. Amer. med. Ass.*, **141**, 1132–1139.

KRETSCHMER, V. & MUELLER-ECKHARDT, C. (1972). Autoimmune hemolytic anemias. II. Immunoglobulins and β1A-globulin in the serum with special regard to the immunochemical type of autoantibodies and the course of the disease. *Blut*, **25**, 159–168.

LANDOLT, R. F. (1946). Akute hämolytische Anämie (Lederer–Brill) mit ausgedehnter Erythrozytenphagozytose im peripheren Blut. *Helvet. paediat. Acta*, **1**, 335–340.

LASKI, B., WAKE, E. J., BAIN, H. W. & GUNSON, H. H. (1961). Autohemolytic anemia in young infants. *J. Pediat.*, **59**, 42–46.

LEDERER, M. (1925). A form of acute hemolytic anemia probably of infectious origin. *Amer. J. med. Sci.*, **170**, 500–510.

LEDERER, M. (1930). Three additional cases of acute hemolytic (infectious) anemia. *Amer. J. med. Sci.*, **179**, 228–236.

LEES, M. H., FISHER, O. D. & SHANKS, J. M. (1960). Case of immune aplastic haemolytic anaemia with thrombocytopenia. *Brit. med. J.*, **i**, 110–111.

LEFRÈRE, J.-J., COUROUCÉ, A.-M., BERTRAND, Y., GIROT, R. & SOULIER, J. P. (1986). Human parvovirus and aplastic crisis in chronic hemolytic anemias: a study of 24 observations. *Amer. J. Hemat.*, **23**, 271–275.

LETMAN, H. (1957). Auto-immune haemolytic anaemia. *Dan. med. Bull.*, **4**, 143–147.

LETTS, H. W. & KREDENSTER, B. (1968).

Thrombocytopenia, hemolytic anemia, and two pregnancies. Report of a case. *Amer. J. clin. Path.*, **49**, 481–486.

LIESVELD, J. L., ROWE, J. M. & LICHTMAN, M. A. (1987). Variability of the erythropoietic response in autoimmune hemolytic anemia: analysis of 189 cases. *Blood*, **69**, 820–826.

LILLIE, E. W., GATENBY, P. B. B. & MOORE, H. C. (1954). A survey of anaemia in 4,314 cases of pregnancy. *Irish J. med. Sci.*, **6th Series**, 304–310.

LINKE, A. (1952). Klinische und experimentelle Beobactungen über aplastische Krisen der Erythropoese bei hämolytischen Anämien. *Verh. dtsch. Ges. inn. Med.*, **58**, 724–727.

LUBINSKI, H. & GOLDBLOOM, A. (1946). Acute hemolytic anemia associated with autoagglutination with a thermal amplitude of 0 to 37 C. *Amer. J. Dis. Child.*, **72**, 325–333.

McFADZEAN, A. J. S. & DAVIS, L. J. (1947). Iron-staining erythrocyte inclusions with especial reference to acquired haemolytic anaemia. *Glasgow med. J.*, **28**, 237–279.

MALLARMÉ, J., AUZÉPY, P., BERCOVICI, J. P. & LÉVY, J. (1965). Un cas d'anémie hémolytique acquise, avec leucopenie et thrombopenie, de la grossesse. *Nouv. Rev. franç. Hémat.*, **5**, 765–768.

MANGAN, K. F., BESA, E. C., SHADDUCK, R. K., TEDLOW, H. & RAY, P. K. (1984). Demonstration of two distinct antibodies in autoimmune hemolytic anemia with reticulocytopenia and red cell aplasia. *Exper. Hemat.*, **12**, 788–793.

MARTIN, H. & KILIAN, P. (1960). Erythroleukämoide Reaktion bei autoimmunhämolytischer Anämie und Zustand nach Splenektomie. *Verh. dtsch. Ges. inn. Med.* (**66** Congress), 1033–1037.

MARTONI, L. & MUSIANI, S. (1956). Anemia emolitica acquisata idiopatica autoimmune complicata di mieloaplasia eritoblastica in un lattante di 6 mesi. *Clin. pediat. (Bologna)*, **38**, 483–506.

MASON, V. R. (1943). Acquired hemolytic anemia. *Arch. intern. Med.*, **72**, 471–493.

MEYER, L. M. & BERTCHER, R. W. (1960). Acquired hemolytic anemia and transient erythroid hypoplasia of bone marrow. *Amer. J. Med.*, **28**, 606–608.

MILLER, B. A. & BEARDSLEY, D. S. (1983). Autoimmune pancytopenia of childhood associated with multisystem disease manifestations. *J. Pediat.*, **103**, 877–881.

MILLICHAP, J. G. (1952). Acute idiopathic haemolytic anaemia. *Arch. Dis. Childh.*, **27**, 222–229.

MÜLLER, W. & WEINREICH, J. (1956). Immun-Pancytopenien. *Klin. Wschr.*, **34**, 505–509.

MUELLER-ECKHARDT, C., MÖHRING, F., KRETSCHMER, V., HÖBEL, W. & LÖFFLER, H. (1977). Reappraisal of the clinical and etiologic significance of immunoglobulin deviations in autoimmune hemolytic anemia ('warm type'). *Blut*, **34**, 39–47.

MUIR, R. & McNEE, J. W. (1912). The anaemia

produced by a haemolytic serum. *J. Path. Bact.*, **16**, 410–438.

NEIMANN, N., MICHON, P., PIERSON, M. & LASCOMBES, G. (1956). L'anémie hémolytique acquise par auto-anticorps chez le nourrisson. *Arch. franç. Pédiat.*, **3**, 247–255.

O'DONOGHUE, R. J. L. & WITTS, L. J. (1932). The acute haemolytic anaemia of Lederer. *Guy's Hosp. Rep.*, **82**, 440–456.

OKEN, M. M., GRIFFITHS, R. W., WILLIAMS, R. C. JNR & REIMANN, B. E. F. (1973). Possible NZB syndrome in man. *Arch. intern. Med.*, **132**, 237–240.

PARSONS, L. G. (1938). The haemolytic anaemias of childhood. *Lancet*, **ii**, 1395–1401.

PAYNE, R., SPAET, T. H. & AGGELER, P. M. (1955). An unusual antibody pattern in a case of idiopathic acquired hemolytic anemia. *J. Lab. clin. Med.*, **46**, 245–254.

PETTIT, J. E., SCOTT, J. & HUSSEIN, S. (1976). EDTA dependent red cell neutrophil rosetting in autoimmune haemolytic anaemia. *J. clin. Path.*, **29**, 345–346.

PIROFSKY, B. (1969). *Autoimmunization and the Autoimmune Hemolytic Anemias*, 537 pp. Williams and Wilkins, Baltimore.

PISCIOTTA, A. V., DOWNER, E. M. & HINZ, J. E. (1959). Clinical and laboratory correlation in severe autoimmune hemolytic anemia. *Arch. intern. Med.*, **104**, 264–276.

PISCIOTTA, A. V. & HINZ, J. E. (1956). Occurrence of agglutinogens in normoblasts. *Proc. Soc. exp. Biol. Med.*, **91**, 356–358.

RAPOPORT, A. P., ROWE, J. M. & MCMICAN, A. (1988). Life-threatening autoimmune hemolytic anemia in a patient with the acquired immune deficiency syndrome. *Transfusion*, **28**, 190–191.

RAVAULT, P. P., GIRARD, M. & JOUD, A. (1939). Anémie hémolytique mortelle d'allure primitive. *Lyon Med.*, **163**, 581–591.

REISNER, E. H. JNR & KALKSTEIN, M. (1942). Auto-hemolysinic anemia with auto-agglutination: improvement after splenectomy. *Amer. J. med. Sci*, **203**, 313–322.

REMY, D. (1952). Cytomorphologische Besonderheiten (atypische Megaloblastose und Siderozyten) bei erworbener hämolytischer Anämie vom Typ Loutit. *Klin. Wschr.*, **30**, 947–948.

RENNER, W. F. & MCSHANE, J. R. (1947). The role of autoagglutinins in hemolytic anemias. *Sth. med. J. (Bgham, Ala)*, **49**, 973–980.

REYNOLDS, G. P. (1930). A case of acquired hemolytic jaundice with unusual features and improved by splenectomy. *Amer. J. med. Sci.*, **179**, 549–553.

RITZ, N. D. & HABER, A. (1962). Autoimmune hemolytic anemia in a 6-week-old child. *J. Pediat.*, **61**, 904–910.

ROSENTHAL, F. & CORTEN, M. (1937). Über das Phänomen der Autohämagglutination und über die Eigenschaften der Kältehämagglutinine. *Folia haemat. (Lpz.)*, **58**, 64–90.

ROSENTHAL, M. C., KOMNINOS, Z. D. & DAMESHEK, W. (1953). Multiple antibody formation in auto-immune hemolytic anemia. Report of a case. *New Engl. J. Med.*, **248**, 537–541.

ROSSI, W., DIENA, F. & SACCHETTI, C. (1957). Demonstration of specific and non-specific agglutinogens in normal bone marrow erythroblasts. *Experientia*, **13**, 440–441.

RUBINSTEIN, M. A. (1948). Transient positive Wassermann test for syphilis in acute hemolytic anemia. *J. Lab. clin. Med.*, **33**, 753–756.

RUBIO, F. JNR & BURGIN, L. (1957). Hemolytic disease complicated by pernicious anemia. Report of two cases. *Bull. Tufts-New Engl. med. Cent.*, **3**, 77–85.

RUSSELL, N. H., KEENAN, J. P. & FRAIS, M. A. (1978). Thrombocytopathy associated with autoimmune haemolytic anaemia. *Brit. med. J.*, **ii**, 604.

RYDER, R. J. W. (1965). Megaloblastic erythropoiesis in acquired haemolytic anaemia. *Irish J. med. Sci.*, **6th Series**, 165–169.

SACCHETTI, C., DIENA, F. & ROSSI, V. (1957). Comportamento degli eritroblasti nella anemia emolitica acquisita. *Haematologica*, **42**, 895–909.

SALMON, C. & HOMBERG, J.-C. (1971). Les anticorps associés au cours des anémies hémolytiques acquises avec auto-anticorps. In *Les Anémies Hémolytiques*, pp. 83–91. Masson, Paris.

SANSONE, G. (1957). Anemie emolitiche acute idiopatiche a genesi autoimmunitaria nell'infanzia. *Minerva pediat. (Torino)*, **9**, 270–273.

SCHUBOTHE, H. & MÜLLER, W. (1955). Über die Anwendbarkeit des Ehrlichschen Fingerversuches als Nachweismethode intravitalar Hämolyse und Erythrophagocytose bei hämolytischen Erkrankungen. *Klin. Wschr.*, **33**, 272–276.

SCHWARTZ, R. S. & COSTEA, N. (1966). Autoimmune hemolytic anemia: clinical correlations and biological implications. *Seminars Hemat.*, **3**, 2–26.

SCOTT, G. L. & RASBRIDGE, M. R. (1971). Red cell acetylcholinesterase and adenosine-tripospatase (sic) activity in patients with a positive antiglobulin test. *Scand. J. Haemat.*, **8**, 53–62.

SEEWAN, H. L. (1979). Subakute idiopathische autoimmunhämolytische Anämie mit protrahierter aplastischer Phase und erythrämischer Reaktion. *Wien. med. Wschr.*, **129**, 180–183.

SEIP, M. (1955). Aplastic crisis in a case of immuno-hemolytic anemia. *Acta med. scand.*, **153**, 137–142.

SELWYN, J. G. (1953). Unpublished observations.

SHAUB, F. & MAIER, C. (1956). Zur klinischen Bedeutung der mechanischen Resistenz der roten Blutkörperchen. *Acta haemat. (Basel)*, **15**, 90–105.

SHULMAN, L. E. & HARVEY, A. M. (1964). Hashimoto's thyroiditis in false-positive reactors to the tests for syphilis. *Amer. J. Med.*, **36**, 174–187.

SIEVERS, K., LEHTINEN, M. & AHO, K. (1968). Development of immune haemolytic anaemia and thrombocytopenia in a chronic biologic false-positive reactor for syphilis. *Scand. J. Haemat.*, **5**, 264–270.

SIRCHIA, G., FERRONE, S., MERCURIALI, F. & ZANELLA, A. (1970). Red cell acetylcholinesterase activity in autoimmune haemolytic anaemias. *Brit. J. Haemat.*, **19**, 411–415.

SÖDERHJELM, L. (1959). Non-spherocytic haemolytic anaemia in mother and new-born infant. *Acta paediat. scand.*, **48**, Suppl. 117, 34–39.

STATS, D., WASSERMAN, L. R. & ROSENTHAL, N. (1948). Hemolytic anemia with hemoglobinuria. *Amer. J. clin. Path.*, **18**, 757–777.

STEFFEN, C. (1955). Untersuchungen über den Nachweis sessile Antikörper an Knockenmarkzellen bei erworbener hämolytischer Anämie. *Wien. klin. Wschr.*, **67**, 224–228.

STERNER, L.-G. (1940–1941). Ein Fall von akuter hämolytischer Anämie vom Ledererschen Typ. *Acta paediat. (Uppsala)*, **28**, 196–206.

STRONG, V. F., SOKOL, R. J., RODGERS, S. A. & HEWITT, S. (1985). Adenine nucleotide concentrations in patients with erythrocyte autoantibodies. *J. clin. Path.*, **38**, 585–587.

TAN, E. M. & CHAPLIN, H. JNR (1968). Antinuclear antibodies in Coombs-positive acquired hemolytic anemia. *Vox Sang.*, **15**, 161–170.

TANAKA, K. R., VALENTINE, W. N. & SCHNEIDER, A. S. (1964). Red cell cholinesterase in Coombs positive auto-immune hemolytic anemia (AHA). *Clin. Res.*, **12**, 110 (Abstract).

TEETER, C. E. (1907). Recovery from leukanemia. *J. Amer. med. Ass.*, **48**, 608–609.

TISDALE, W. A., KLATSKIN, G. & KINSELLA, E. D. (1959). Significance of the direct-reacting fraction of serum bilirubin in hemolytic jaundice. *Amer. J. Med.*, **26**, 214–227.

TISHKOFF, G. H. (1966). Erythrocyte mucoids in acquired autoimmune hemolytic anemia. *Blood*, **28**, 229–240.

TOSATTI, P. M. (1947). Contributo allo studio dell' anemia emolitica acuta tipo Lederer. *Haematologica*, **27**, 337–385.

TROISIER, J. & CATTAN, R. (1932). Ictère hémolytique avec leuco-érythroblastose. Splénectomie. Guérison. *Sang*, **6**, 426–435.

TSUKADA, T. & MIWA, S. (1969). Studies on erythrocyte acetylcholinesterase. *Acta haemat. jap.*, **32**, 353–360.

VAN LOGHEM, J. J. (1965). Some comments on autoantibody induced red cell destruction. *Ann. N.Y. Acad. Sci.*, **124**, 465–476.

VERAS, S. & MANIOS, S. (1956). Anémie hémolytique acquise par auto-immunisation ayant présenté dans son évolution une aplasie érythroblastique aiguë. *Arch. franç. Pédiat.*, **13**, 1096–1110.

VERLOOP, M. C. & BAKKER-V. AARDENNE, W. I. T. (1958). In vitro autohaemolysis in congential and acquired haemolytic disorders. *Proc. 6th Congr.*

Europ. Soc. Haematol., Copenhagen, 1957, pp. 683–691. Karger, Basel.

VERLOOP, M. C., BAKKER-V. AARDENNE, W. I. T. & RICCI, C. (1959). In vitro autohaemolysis in congenital and acquired haemolytic disorders. *Acta med. scand.*, **163**, 385–403.

VIDEBAEK, A. (1962). Primary (idiopathic) auto-immune haemolytic anaemia. *Acta med. scand.*, **171**, 449–462.

VON DEM BORNE, A. E. G. KR., ENGELFRIET, C. P., BECKERS, D. & VAN LOGHEM. J. J. (1971). Autoimmune haemolytic anaemias. IV. Biochemical studies of red cells from patients with autoimmune haemolytic anaemia with incomplete warm autoantibodies. *Clin. exp. Immunol.*, **8**, 377–388.

WAGNER, K. (1955). Durch inkomplete Autoantikörper bedingte akute, febrile, hämolytische argeneratorische Anämie. *Acta haemat. (Basel)*, **14**, 313–320.

WASASTJERNA, C. (1954). Leukocyte-agglutinins in a case of chronic granulocytopenia and hemolytic anemia. *Acta med. scand.*, **149**, 355–360.

WAUGH, T. R. (1932). Acquired haemolytic jaundice in a woman previously splenectomized for essential thrombocytopenia. *Folia haemat. (Lpz.)* **48**, 248–260.

WEISS, G. B. & BESSMAN, J. D. (1984). Spurious automated red cell values in warm autoimmune hemolytic anemia. *Amer. J. Hemat.*, **17**, 433–435.

WILKENSON, A. E., & SEQUEIRA, P. J. L. (1955). Studies on the treponemal immobilization test. III. Use of the TPI as a verification test in suspected latent syphilis. *Brit. J. ven. Dis.*, **31**, 143–154.

WILLOUGHBY, M. L. N., PEARS, M. A., SHARP, A. A. & SHIELDS, M. J. (1961). Megaloblastic erythropoiesis in acquired hemolytic anemia. *Blood*, **17**, 351–356.

WOLF, H. G. (1956). Zur Diagnostik und Therapie hämolytischer Erkrankungen. *Arch. Kinderheilk.*, **153**, 156–169.

YOUNG, L. E., IZZO, M. J., ALTMAN, K. I. & SWISHER, S. N. (1956). Studies on spontaneous in vitro autohemolysis in hemolytic disorders. *Blood*, **11**, 977–997.

YOUNG, L. E. & LAWRENCE, J. S. (1946). Atypical hemolytic anemia. Observations with particular reference to the use of transfusions in the study of hemolytic mechanisms. *Arch. intern. Med.*, **77**, 151–178.

YOUNG, L. E. & MILLER, G. (1953). Differentiation between congenital and acquired forms of hemolytic anemia. *Amer. J. med. Sci.*, **226**, 664–673.

YOUNG, L. E., MILLER, G. & CHRISTIAN, R. M. (1951). Clinical and laboratory observations on autoimmune hemolytic disease. *Ann. intern. Med.*, **35**, 507–517.

ZINKHAM, W. H. & DIAMOND, L. K. (1952). In vitro erythrophagocytosis in acquired hemolytic anemia. *Blood*, **7**, 592–601.

Auto-immune haemolytic anaemias (AIHA): warm-antibody syndromes III: serological findings I: introduction; the direct antiglobulin test and other ways of demonstrating erythrocyte sensitization

Main characteristics of erythrocyte auto-antibodies   94
  Significance of the effect of temperature on antibody
  activity   95
  'Unitary' nature of agglutinins and lysins   96
Antiglobulin reactions in auto-immune haemolytic
anaemia   97
  Early reports   97
Further details of the antiglobulin reaction   99
  Prozones in the antiglobulin test   99
  Neutralization of antiglobulin serum by γ globulin   100
Use of anti-γ and anti-non-γ antiglobulin sera   104
Nature of the non-γ antiglobulin reaction—role of
complement   105
Use of anti-IgG, -IgM, IgA, anti-κ, anti-λ and anti-
C (complement) sera and sera against IgG subclasses   106
  Gm allotypes in warm-antibody AIHA   109
Clinical significance of the different Ig classes and IgG
subclasses   109

IgG2 and IgG4 antibodies as possible causes of haemolysis
in AIHA   110
IgA auto-antibodies and AIHA   111
Incomplete IgM warm antibodies and AIHA   113
Nature of the complement components that give rise to
positive antiglobulin reactions   113
Other ways of demonstrating erythrocyte sensitization   114
Radioactive antiglobulin tests   114
Complement-fixing antibody consumption (CFAC)
test   115
Enzyme-linked immunosorbent assays (ELISA)   116
Enzyme-linked antiglobulin tests   116
Auto-agglutination in media of high protein content   117
Use of Polybrene and PVP   118
Auto-agglutination of enzyme-treated erythrocytes: the
bromelin test   119
Erythrocyte–antibody (EA) rosette formation   119

As already referred to (p. 6), serological observations on haemolytic anaemia in man date from the first decade of the present century, the pioneer observations of Widal, Abrami and Brulé (1908a,b) and Chauffard and Vincent (1909) being particularly noteworthy. In these publications were described two basic phenomena which may be observed if blood from patients suffering from AIHA is studied *in vitro*, namely, auto-agglutination of the patient's whole blood and the ability of his or her serum to agglutinate or even lyse erythrocytes of the same blood-group. Almost 40 years were to pass before a further important phenomenon, the agglutinability of patients' erythrocytes by antiglobulin sera, was discovered (Boorman, Dodd and Loutit, 1946). The present Chapter deals with the direct antiglobulin test (DAT), the chemical nature of the auto-antibodies, the use of antiglobulin sera specific for Ig classes and IgG subclasses, and for comple-

ment and its components, and other ways of demonstrating erythrocyte sensitization. The occurrence, detection and characteristics of auto-antibodies in patients' serum are described in Chapter 25, and the specificity of warm auto-antibodies in Chapter 26. DAT-negative AIHA and the occurrence of positive DATs in healthy subjects and in hospital patients not suffering from overt haemolytic anaemia are dealt with in Chapter 27.

MAIN CHARACTERISTICS OF ERYTHRO-CYTE AUTO-ANTIBODIES

The main characteristics of the two types of antibody, warm and cold, responsible for AIHA may be summarized as follows:

Warm auto-antibodies. The majority react *in vitro* as incomplete antibodies, i.e. they sensitize erythrocytes to agglutination by antiglobulin sera and/or agglutinate enzyme-treated cells or cells suspended in colloid-containing media. Occasionally the antibodies act as, or are accompanied by, in-saline-agglutinating antibodies. They are characteristically strongly active at 37°C. They very rarely lyse normal unmodified erythrocytes but sera containing warm antibodies not infrequently lyse enzyme-treated cells at 37°C.

Most warm auto-antibody molecules are IgG (7S) globulins; some, however, are IgA or IgM (19S) globulins.* Most IgG antibodies have anti-Rh or an anti-Rh-like specificity (see p. 162); other well-defined specificities are uncommon. Sera containing more than one chemical type of auto-antibody are quite commonly met with. Similarly, antibodies of more than one specificity may often be demonstrated in a single sample of serum.

Cold auto-antibodies. Their activity is markedly potentiated by a fall in temperature; usually they are only slightly active or completely inactive at 37°C. They are typically powerful agglutinins and they almost invariably lyse enzyme-treated and paroxysmal nocturnal haemoglobinuria (PNH) erythrocytes. They may lyse normal erythocytes, too, to a lesser extent, particularly if the serum is slightly acidified. The antibodies that are lytic also sensitize cells to agglutination by broad-spectrum antiglobulin sera. This type of antiglobulin reaction is thought to be due to the binding on of complement.

Most cold auto-antibody molecules are IgM γ globulins; a minority are IgG. The great majority have a specificity within the Ii system (see p. 250). An exception is the Donath–Landsteiner (D–L) antibody of paroxysmal cold haemoglobinuria (PCH). It has anti-P specificity and is notable also for being an IgG γ globulin (see p. 354).

It is remarkable, as pointed out by Dacie and de Gruchy (1951), how 'individual' are the reactions *in vitro* of any particular patient's auto-antibody.

Thus, if the behaviour of different patients' antibodies are subjected to close scrutiny by assessing the antibodies' ability to agglutinate, lyse or sensitize to antiglobulin sera normal, enzyme-treated or PNH erythrocytes, the pattern of reactions is very variable, and it is hardly an exaggeration to say that the reactions of no two antibodies are qualitatively and quantitatively the same.

The distinction between warm and cold antibodies has proved valuable and can usually be clearly made. It was the basis of the many extensive reports and reviews on the serological aspects of the AIHAs that followed in the late 1940s and 1950s as the result of the resurgence of interest generated by the application of the antiglobulin test to the investigation of patients suffering from acquired haemolytic anaemia. Included in these early reports are those of Dameshek (1951), Dacie and de Gruchy (1951), Bouroncle, Dodd and Wright (1951), Young, Miller and Christian (1951), Wiener et al. (1952), Baumgartner (1952), Dacie (1953, 1954, 1955), Hubinont and Massart-Guiot (1955), Evans (1955), Evans and Weiser (1957), Holländer (1957), Hennemann (1957), Pisciotta and Hinz (1957), van Loghem, van der Hart and Dorfmeier (1958), Schubothe (1958, 1959) and Dausset and Colombani (1958, 1959).

Significance of the effect of temperature on antibody activity

This has been a topic of discussion and speculation for many years and it has been a widely held view that amongst human allo-antibodies warm antibodies (e.g. anti-D) are 'immune' and cold antibodies (e.g. anti-P and anti-Le^a) are 'naturally-occurring' and that anti-A and anti-B exist in both forms, i.e. are usually 'naturally-occurring' but can be immune. In animals, too, the same distinction could be demonstrated. Thus in rabbits repeatedly inoculated with sheep or horse erythrocytes the thermal optimum for the agglutinins produced rose as immunity develops and eventually passed 37°C (Millet and Hubinont, 1946). With the auto-antibodies of man the same distinction can be made: the warm auto-antibodies are pathological and potentially

---

*At the WHO meeting on the Nomenclature of Human Immunoglobulins held in Prague in 1964 it was proposed that the immunoglobulins should be referred to as γG or IgG, γA or IgA and γM or IgM globulins, etc. (Ceppellini et al., 1964). Currently, the terms IgG, IgA and IgM, etc. are most generally used.

very harmful but fortunately relatively infrequent, while cold auto-antibodies in low concentrations are present in almost all sera and are harmless. Nevertheless, in man at least, cold antibodies develop in the course of what appears to be an immune response to infection (e.g. after mycoplasma pneumonia). Even so, it is the rise in their thermal range towards body temperature which is the cause of their pathogenicity. Weiner (1958) referred to the warm auto-antibody type as 'hyperimmune' and the cold type as 'simple'. Earlier, Wiener (1951) had suggested that cold antibodies are normally heterogenetic in origin and that in consequence the antibodies were less perfectly adapted to human antigens; he concluded that such imperfect antigen–antibody complexes might well dissociate as the temperature was raised.

Exactly how and why some antibodies dissociate from their corresponding antigens as the temperature rises is an interesting question. It is certainly not just a question of molecular size or specificity. Thus human anti-D antibodies can exist as IgG and IgM molecules and both react optimally at about body temperature, while cold antibodies, which typically dissociate from antigens completely at body temperature, can be IgG (DL antibody) or IgM (anti-I).

The effect of temperature on agglutination was subject to close scrutiny by Lalezari and Oberhardt (1971) and Oberhardt, Lalezari and Jiang (1973) using a very sensitive automated method in which Polybrene acted as an enhancer of agglutination (Lalezari, 1968). Antigen–antibody bonds were allowed to form at room temperature. Dissociation was then assessed at a range of temperatures between 15°C and 55°C, the result being recorded as a 'temperature gradient dissociation curve' which reflected both the thermal characteristics of the antigen–antibody reaction being studied and the concentration of the antibody. An anti-Rh antibody was shown to be minimally more active at 15°C than at 22°C or 37°C, but to be less active at 45°C and markedly less active at 55°C. In contrast, an anti-I antibody was shown to be 1000 times more active at 15°C than at 37°C, while an anti-M antibody behaved in an intermediate fashion.

Hughes-Jones (1975), in a review of erythrocyte antigen–antibody interaction, discussed briefly why auto-antibodies differ so markedly in their responses to temperature change. The reaction between antigen and antibody liberates energy, either in the form of heat (an exothermic reaction) or as a change in entropy. Which type of energy is liberated depends on the chemical nature of the antigen, e.g. the nature of the bonds at the combining site. Cold-antibody reactions are mainly exothermic in contrast to warm-antibody reactions which do not liberate heat.

'Unitary' nature of agglutinins and lysins

Early concepts of the nature of antibodies postulated that agglutinins and lysins (and opsonins) were separate substances (see Browning, 1931; Zinsser, Enders and Fothergill, 1939). Later, the view that the different manifestations of antibody action might be explained by a single immune substance acting under different environmental conditions gained ground (Dean, 1917). A good deal of evidence was adduced in support of the latter concept (see Marrack, 1938; Zinsser, Enders and Forthergill, 1939).

Now it is realized that differences between the ability of individual antibodies to cause erythrocytes to undergo agglutination or lysis by complement (and phagocytosis by macrophages) are related to the structure of the antibody — in particular, to the size of the molecule, e.g. IgG or IgM, its valency, i.e. the number of Fab sites, and chemical differences within its constant (C) and hinge regions.

The remarkable diversity in behaviour *in vitro* of the auto-antibodies of AIHA has already been referred to. For instance, although in the majority of patients with warm-antibody AIHA the auto-antibodies do not agglutinate the patient's erythrocytes in saline suspension or lyse them in the presence of complement, occasionally they do so. It is known that in the latter instances IgM molecules or a mixture of IgM molecules as well as IgG molecules are being produced.

The behaviour of cold auto-antibodies *in vitro* is of special interest. Anti-I antibodies are, for instance, normally (? always) potentially lytic, and at first sight it seems unlikely that the antibody molecules producing agglutination and those producing lysis are one and the same. For example, if cold antibodies are titrated using normal erythrocytes, the agglutinin and lysin titres will be found to be strikingly different. Thus normal cells may be agglutinated at 20°C by an antibody diluted 1 in 4000, yet undergo only a trace of lysis in the presence of complement by the antibody diluted 1 in 4 under apparently optimal conditions. This difference, however, may well be due to the natural insensitivity of human erythrocytes to lysis by anti-I antibodies in the presence of complement compared with their sensitivity to agglutination. It is less easily explained on the hypothesis that an agglutinin is present in high concentration and a lysin in low concentration,

for the insensitivity of normal cells can be overcome to some extent if the serum is suitably acidified. Moreover, abnormal erythrocytes such as PNH cells and trypsinized cells are lysed much more easily and quickly and it is probably especially significant that the lysin titre using PNH erythrocytes often approximates closely to the agglutinin titre (Table 24.1)

ANTIGLOBULIN REACTIONS IN AUTO-IMMUNE HAEMOLYTIC ANAEMIA

Early reports

As already referred to (p. 9), Boorman, Dodd and Loutit (1946) and Loutit and Mollison (1946) were the first to demonstrate by means of the antiglobulin test (Coombs's test or the Coombs test*) the presence of incomplete antibodies adsorbed to the erythrocytes of patients with acquired haemolytic anaemia. Their observations were soon confirmed by other workers throughout the world.

---

*In his Philip Levine Award address, Coombs (1970), in describing the history and evolution of the antiglobulin reaction, paid a generous tribute to Carlo Moreschi who unbeknown to him (Coombs) had described the principle of the antiglobulin reaction many years previously. In Coombs's words: 'it gives me the greatest pleasure to remind you of the wonderful researches of Carlo Moreschi who, in two publications in 1908, showed that red blood cells and bacteria, after reacting with an amount of a corresponding immune serum in a dose which by itself would not cause agglutination, could be made to agglutinate rapidly if they were washed thoroughly and exposed to a precipitating serum for the species of animal which furnished the immune serum.'

Mourant (1983), in an essay on the discovery of the antiglobulin test described how Coombs 'by a brilliant feat of intuition, had conceived the principle of the anti-globulin test. He states that he was travelling on an ill-lit wartime train from London to Cambridge, trying to read some papers by Ehrlich on the side-chain theory, and speculating idly (like Kékulé on the tetravalent carbon atom) on the behaviour of red cells and antibodies, when he visualized the cells, already coated with molecules of incomplete antibody, which was of course a globulin, but still floating free, becoming linked together by molecules of another antibody, an anti-globulin antibody!

He realized that this idea could be the basis of a practical test, and he formulated in some detail its possible applications—essentially as the direct and the indirect antiglobulin tests.'

Denys and van den Broucke (1947), for instance, reported a positive direct Coombs test in two patients, one of whom was an infant, and mentioned positive results in four others. They also demonstrated the presence of free antibody in their patients' sera by means of an indirect Coombs test and made interesting observations on the varying sensitivity of normal cells to the antibodies. Sturgeon (1947) also reported positive direct and indirect tests with the erythrocytes and serum of three patients. He showed that the antibody could be eluted from washed erythrocytes by incubating saline suspensions of the cells at 37°C or at 56°C.

Evans, Duane and Behrendt (1947) also carried out some noteworthy studies on two patients; both gave a positive direct, but a negative indirect, antiglobulin test. Evans and his colleagues demonstrated that the material coating the patients' erythrocytes could be eluted by heating a suspension of cells in saline at 56°C for 5 minutes and that the eluted material could then be transferred to normal cells. They also demonstrated that the erythrocytes of their patients underwent auto-agglutination when suspended in 30% bovine albumin or 2% acacia and stressed the similarity between the presumed immune body of acquired haemolytic anaemia and Rh 'blocking' antibody.

The validity of Boorman, Dodd and Loutit's observations was also confirmed by Singer and Motulsky (1949). Sixteen patients with spherocytic anaemia were investigated; seven were patients with acquired

Table 24.1 Relative sensitivity of erythrocytes to lysis by a high-titre cold antibody at 20°C

Type of cell	pH	Dilutions of serum								
		1 in 1	1 in 4	1 in 16	1 in 64	1 in 256	1 in 1024	1 in 4096	1 in 16000	Control (normal serum diluent)
Normal	8.0	–	Trace	–	–	–	–	–	–	–
Normal	6.5	Trace	+	±	Trace	–	–	–	–	–
Trypsinized normal	8.0	–	+++	++	+	±	–	–	–	–
PNH	8.0	++±	+++	+++	+++	+++	++	+±	+	–

+++ denotes marked lysis; + +±, + +, +±, + and ± denote lesser but definite degrees of lysis; — denotes no lysis.

haemolytic anaemia and all seven (including one patient whose disease was secondary to reticulo sarcoma) gave positive direct Coombs tests. Of the remaining patients — one with haemolytic anaemia secondary to sulphonamide sensitivity and six with hereditary spherocytosis (HS), only one patient (who had HS in a severe phase) gave a positive reaction. The term 'developing test' was introduced as a synonym for Coombs's test.

Evans and Duane (1949) described 11 patients with acquired haemolytic anaemia (in one associated with chronic lymphocytic leukaemia) whose erythrocytes gave positive Coombs tests. Using dilutions of antiglobulin serum, a fairly consistent correlation was found between the intensity of the reaction and the activity of the disease. They reported, however, that in one patient an increase in the degree of sensitization, as judged by the antigloblin test, was not associated with an immediate recurrence of haemolysis.

Jordan and Dingle (1949) studied 10 patients with acquired haemolytic anaemia of varying type and obtained positive Coombs tests in seven of them. Three patients with idiopathic acquired haemolytic anaemia gave higher 'Coombs' titers' than the four patients with secondary haemolytic anaemia whose erythrocytes were only agglutinated in low dilutions of antiglobulin serum.

Kidd (1949) investigated six patients with acquired haemolytic anaemia whose erythrocytes gave strongly positive direct antiglobulin tests. He showed that potent eluates of the antibodies could be prepared by elution from erythrocyte stromata at a low pH.

Hackett (1950) found that the washed erythrocytes of a patient suffering from a severe form of AIHA and normal erythrocytes sensitized *in vitro* with a potent anti-D antibody absorbed the same component from an antiglobulin serum.

Young, Miller and Christian (1951) discussed in detail the use of the antiglobulin test in the diagnosis of haemolytic anaemia of the auto-immune type and drew attention to the technical difficulties in carrying out the test quantitatively. The relationship between the laboratory tests for sensitization and the clinical course of the disease was illustrated by two case histories.

These early reports were followed by an ever-increasing number of publications concerning the antiglobulin reaction in acquired haemolytic anaemia. Papers and monographs published up to 1960 which dealt with data based on relatively large numbers of patients include those of Dacie (1954), Davidsohn and Spurrier (1954), Heni and Blessing (1954a), Evans and Weiser (1957), Hennemann (1957), Pisciotta and Hinz (1957), van Loghem, van der Hart and Dorfmeier (1958), Chaplin and Cassell (1958), Dausset and Colombani (1959) and Cassell and Chaplin (1960).

Early reviews dealing with technical aspects of the antiglobulin test and with its value as a diagnostic tool include those of Rosenfield, Vogel and Rosenthal (1951), Hill and Haberman (1954) and Haberman (1958).

FURTHER DETAILS OF THE ANTIGLOBULIN REACTION

Soon after it had been established that the antiglobulin test was positive in many patients suffering from acquired haemolytic anaemia, attention was focused on the reaction itself. Two aspects in particular were studied: the development of prozones when diluted antiglobulin sera were used and the effect on the reaction of the prior addition of γ globulin, or other globulins, to the antiglobulin serum before it was used in the test.

Prozones in the antiglobulin test

van Loghem (1950), van Loghem and his co-workers (1950) and van Loghem, Stallman and van der Hart (1951) reported that when the sensitized erythrocytes of three patients with acquired haemolytic anaemia were suspended in various dilutions of antiglobulin serum in saline the reaction was inhibited in the strongest concentration of the antiglobulin serum (Fig. 24.1). A similar pattern of reaction had been found with cells sensitized by the Rh antibody anti-D (see Fulton Roberts 1950). van Loghem, Stallman and van der Hart (1951) contrasted the prozone reaction with their finding in a patient suffering from acquired haemolytic anaemia associated with cirrhosis of the liver where maximal agglutination took place in the strongest concentration of antiglobulin serum.

These observations were extended by later workers. Dacie (1953), who reported on 11 patients with antibodies of the warm type, noted that although a prozone was marked in some cases this was not true of all, even though the same highly potent antiglobulin serum was used (Table 24.2). It appeared that the absence of a prozone

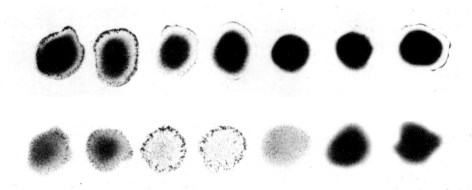

Fig. 24.1   Antiglobulin reactions carried out using various dilutions of an antiglobulin serum.
    Upper series: erythrocytes coated by complement. Lower series: erythrocytes sensitized with an IgG antibody. The dilutions of the antiglobulin serum ranged from 1 in 4 to 1 in 4096. The erythrocyte suspension on the extreme right is the control, with 9 g/1 NaCl substituted for antiglobulin serum.

could be correlated with the presence on the erythrocytes of protein other than γ globulin (Table 24.3).

Evans (1955) also studied the prozone phenomenon and recorded how in one instance this was abolished if the erythrocyte–antiglobulin serum suspension was immediately centrifuged. This was attributed to the centrifugation facilitating agglutination by bringing together cells before they became 'coated' with an excess of antiglobulin. Evans and Weiser (1957) reported further details of this phenomenon. However, in only one of their patients did a marked prozone develop with the three antiglobulin sera in use. They considered that this type of observation made it difficult to accept the hypothesis that antibody (antiglobulin) excess was the whole explanation of the phenomenon.

Chaplin and Cassell (1958, 1960) and Cassell and Chaplin (1960) described how they had used four different antiglobulin sera in studying the positive antiglobulin reactions given by the erythrocytes of 29 patients with various types of acquired haemolytic anaemia. One of the antisera was a conventional polyvalent antiglobulin serum, the other three were made using globulins eluted from erythrocytes sensitized *in vitro* by anti-D and from erythrocytes from patients with warm-antibody AIHA and paroxysmal cold haemoglobinuria, respectively. Broad cross-reactivity was observed when the four antisera were tested against a panel of sensitized erythrocytes. However, when the erythrocytes of the 29 patients were tested with all four sera, five different reaction patterns were noted, according to whether the patients' cells reacted with all four or with fewer than four of the sera and on whether prozones developed. Chaplin and

Cassel remarked on the striking heterogeneity of the reactions and on how almost every patient's erythrocytes reacted in a manner that was in some respects unique.

Neutralization of antiglobulin serum by γ globulin

In 1947, Coombs and Mourant demonstrated that the component in antiglobulin sera which reacted with erythrocytes coated with Rh antibody was in all probability an anti-γ globulin. They showed that the addition of a small amount of γ globulin to the antiglobulin serum rendered it incapable of agglutinating cells coated with Rh antibody, whereas the addition of α globulin or β globulin had only a slight effect which could be ascribed to contamination with traces of γ globulin. Wiener, Hyman and Handman (1949) carried out similar experiments and used the inhibition of the agglutination of erythrocytes sensitized with Rh antibody as a serological test for human serum globulin.

Dacie (1951) demonstrated that the agglutination of erythrocytes sensitized by auto-antibodies was affected in different ways if a human γ-globulin preparation was added to a potent rabbit antiglobulin serum. It was found when the test was carried out with the cells of two patients suffering from AIHA of the warm-antibody type

Table 24.2 The effect of diluting an antiglobulin serum on its ability to agglutinate the erythrocytes of patients suffering from acquired haemolytic anaemia

Case number or antibody	Type of antibody (W = warm) (C = cold)	Dilutions of antiglobulin serum					Control (saline)
		1 in 4	1 in 16	1 in 64	1 in 256	1 in 1024	
Anti-D	W	+	±	**++**	+	±	0
9	W	++	+++	**++++**	+++	+±	0
10	W	±	+	**+++**	++	±	0
Ki.	W	+±	**++**	+±	+	±	0
Ri.	W	++	**+++±**	++	±	0	0
Anti-H (normal incomplete cold antibody)	C	**++**	+	Trace	0	0	0
13	C	**++**	+	Trace	0	0	0
14	C	**+++**	+±	Trace	0	0	0
18	C	**++**	+±	±	Trace	0	0

++ denotes strong agglutination; +, + ±, ++ and + + ± denote intermediate grades of agglutination.
The optimum dilution of the serum is marked in bold.
Cases 9, 10, Ki. and Ri. were suffering from AIHA of the warm-antibody type, and Cases 13 and 14 from AIHA of the cold-antibody type. Case 18 was suffering from paroxysmal cold haemoglobinuria. The results with corpuscles sensitized by incomplete anti-D and incomplete anti-H, respectively, are shown for comparison.

Table 24.3 The effect of the addition of human γ globulin to a rabbit anti-human globulin serum on the ability of the latter to agglutinate the erythrocytes of patients suffering from acquired haemolytic anaemia

Case number or antibody	Type of antibody (W = warm) (C = cold)	Dilutions of 4% γ globulin solution					Control (saline)
		1 in 4	1 in 16	1 in 64	1 in 256	1 in 1024	
Anti-D	W	0	0	0	0	++	+++
9	W	0	0	0	0	+++	+++
10	W	0	0	0	0	Trace	++
Ki.	W	Trace	±	+±	+	+±	+++±
Ri.	W	Trace	+	+±	++	+++	+++
Anti-H (normal incomplete cold antibody)	C	±	++	+++	+++	+++	+++
13	C	±	+	++	++	++	++
14	C	+	++	++	++	++	++
18	C	++	++	++	++	++	++

+++ denotes strong agglutination; +, + ±, ++ and + + ± denote intermediate grades of agglutination.
Cases 9, 10, Ki. and Ri. were suffering from AIHA of the warm-antibody type, and Cases 13 and 14 from AIHA of the cold-antibody type. Case 18 was suffering from paroxysmal cold haemoglobinuria. The results with corpuscles sensitized by incomplete anti-D and incomplete anti-H, respectively, are shown for comparison.

Table 24.4 Effect of the addition to antiglobulin serum of human γ globulin in five cases of AIHA of the warm-antibody type and one case of the cold-haemagglutinin disease.

Patient	Dilutions of 3.8% human γ globulin						
	1 in 4	1 in16	1 in 64	1 in 256	1 in 1024	Control (saline)
Case 9 (Dacie, 1954)	–	–	–	–	+ + +	+ + +
Case 10 (Dacie, 1954)	–	–	–	–	Trace	+ +
Ki.	Trace	±	±	+	±	+ + ±
Ri.	Trace	+	+ ±	+ +	+ + +	+ + +
Mo.	+	+ +	+ +	+ +	+ +	+ + +
Mo. (eluate from erythrocytes)	–	–	–	–	±	+ + +
Case 9 (cold-haemagglutinin disease)	+ +	+ + +	+ + +	+ + +	+ + +	+ + +

+ + + denotes strong naked-eye agglutination; + + ±, + +, + ±, + and ± denote lesser degress of agglutination; – denotes no agglutination.

that the reaction was inhibited by very small amounts of γ globulin. Similar results were obtained with cells sensitized with the allo-antibody anti-D. In contrast, much more γ globulin was required to inhibit agglutination by antiglobulin serum in two further patients whose sera contained cold agglutinins in high titres. It was concluded that these results supported the concept that warm antibodies were γ globulins. The different type of reaction obtained with cells which had adsorbed cold antibodies was thought to indicate either that the antibodies were not γ globulins or that the antiglobulin serum was reacting with a component of fresh serum (not a γ globulin) adsorbed with the antibody. Crawford and Mollison (1951), using a different approach, also showed by absorption experiments that the erythrocytes of patients with AIHA, sensitized by warm or cold auto-antibodies, respectively, reacted with different components of antiglobulin sera. They concluded that several serologically distinguishable types of globulin may be adsorbed to human erythrocytes.

Dacie (1953, 1954, p. 235) described further studies. The observations originally made were confirmed, but in addition it was found, using cells coated apparently by warm antibodies, that inhibition of agglutination by antiglobulin serum was by no means always produced by the prior

Table 24.5 Reactions of the erythrocytes of patients suffering from idiopathic AIHA of the warm-antibody type with antiglobulin sera to which graded amounts of human γ globulin were added.

No. of patients studied	= 73
γ type	= 32
Intermediate type	= 28
Non-γ type	= 13

addition of very small amounts of γ globulin. The reaction might in fact be similar to that given by cells coated with cold antibodies, intermediate between the two, or inconstant (Tables 24.4 and 24.5). The term 'γ-globulin neutralization test' was coined to describe carrying out antiglobulin reactions with an antiglobulin serum to which graded amounts of γ globulin had been added (Table 24.4) (Fig. 24.2). Subsequently, antiglobulin sera reacting specifically with γ-globulin-coated cells or cells coated with globulins other than γ globulin were used. In the majority of instances where γ globulin in low concentration failed to inhibit agglutination of the patient's cells by antiglobulin serum it was found that the cells would nevertheless react with a specific anti-γ serum as well as with the 'anti-non-γ' serum, indicating that the cells were coated with antibody globulin as well as with other globulins (Dacie, 1960). The author's data on patients investigated in this way in the 1950s are shown in Table 24.6.

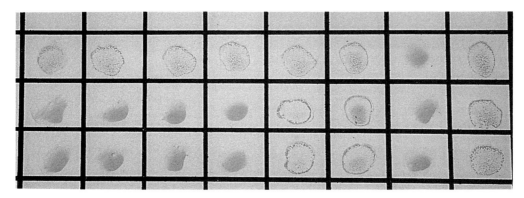

Fig. 24.2 Antiglobulin reactions carried out with a broad-spectrum antiglobulin serum to which diminishing concentrations of human γ globulin had been added.
Top row: erythrocytes from a patient with CHAD. Middle row: erythrocytes from a patient with warm-antibody AIHA. Bottom row: normal D-positive erythrocytes sensitized with allo-anti-Rh(D). The dilutions of γ globulin (in 9 g/1 NaCl) ranged (from left to right) from 1 in 4 to 1 in 4096. The two erythrocyte suspensions on the right are controls: those on the far right show agglutination brought about by antiglobulin serum, diluted 1 in 4, in the absence of γ globulin; those immediately to the left are the saline control, i.e. smooth suspensions in the absence of antiglobulin serum.

Table 24.6   Reactions of the erythrocytes of patients suffering from idiopathic AIHA of the warm-antibody type with anti-γ and anti-non-γ antiglobulin sera.

No. of patients studied	= 22
Agglutination by anti-γ serum alone	= 7
Agglutination by anti-non-γ serum alone	= 4
Agglutination by both sera	= 11

Vaughan and Waller (1954) and Vaughan (1955) also concluded that the proteins coating the erythrocytes of patients with acquired haemolytic anaemias might be composed of γ-globulin or non-γ-globulin components and that the latter globulins might be warm- or cold-reacting. Cutbush, Crawford and Mollison (1955) concluded that the incomplete cold antibody found in normal serum and the antibody bound to erythrocytes in cold-antibody haemolytic anaemia, and incomplete anti-Lewis antibody (anti-Le^a), were α or β globulins, as they reacted with rabbit antiglobulin serum containing only anti-α and anti-β globulins. They suggested, however, that all non-γ-globulin antibodies are only firmly bound to erythrocytes in the presence of normal serum factors which might be identical with complement.

Fudenberg, Barry and Dameshek (1958) described the results of a study into the nature of the material on the erythrocytes of patients with AIHA which reacted with antiglobulin sera. This they referred to as the 'erythrocyte-coating substance' (ECS). Eluates were prepared from the erythrocytes of 10 patients with warm-antibody AIHA and from four patients with cold-antibody AIHA. The erythrocyte life-span of the patients was also measured using ^{51}Cr. Antiglobulin inhibition tests, precipitin and precipitin inhibition tests indicated that the ECS in the warm-antibody cases was a γ globulin, or a substance that cross-reacted with γ globulin, and that the ECS in the cold-antibody cases, although a protein, lacked the characteristics of antibody. Fudenberg, Barry and Dameshek obtained evidence that suggested that the life-span of the patients' erythrocytes appeared to be inversely proportional to the concentration of ECS.

Firkin (1958) also reported on the nature of adsorbed antibody in acquired haemolytic anaemia. He prepared eluates from patients' erythrocytes and submitted the eluted material to possible precipitation in Ouchterlong plates. In six eluates a γ globulin was clearly identified; in two eluates two bands were formed, one indicating a γ globulin, one a β globulin.

Use of anti-γ and anti-non-γ antiglobulin sera

Vaughan (1956), using anti-γ and anti-non-γ sera, investigated 16 patients with miscellaneous types of primary or secondary acquired haemolytic anaemia. In nine instances the erythrocytes reacted with the anti-non-γ reagent only, in two with the anti-γ reagent only and in five with both reagents. Vaughan concluded that three sensitizing components were involved, γ globulin and warm and cold non-γ globulins. He prepared eluates by Kidd's (1949) method from the erythrocytes of four of his patients: he failed to detect eluted antibody in the two whose erythrocytes had reacted only with an anti-non-γ serum; he was, however, successful in the two patients whose cells had reacted both with an anti-γ and a non-γ serum. The eluted antibodies reacted only with the anti-γ serum. Pisciotta and Hinz (1957), too, using an antiglobulin serum to which γ globulin had been added, noted marked, moderate or failure of inhibition of agglutination.

Cassell and Chaplin (1960) used a γ-globulin neutralization test and obtained γ, 'mixed' or non-γ patterns in a series of 29 patients suffering from various types of acquired haemolytic anaemia. The majority of the reactions were of the 'mixed' or non-γ types.

Leddy and co-workers (1963) described the results of a study of 98 patients, observed over a 3-year period, whose erythrocytes had given positive reactions with antiglobulin sera. Of 24 patients with idiopathic AIHA, positive reactions with anti-γ sera alone had been obtained in ten, with anti-γ plus anti-non-γ sera in six and with anti-non-γ serum alone in six.

Yamada (1964) had studied 12 patients with idiopathic AIHA: five had given a γ-type DAT, four a non-γ result, two an intermediate result and in one patient the result, at one time non-γ, became γ later.

The fact that the results obtained using antiglobulin sera to which γ globulin had been added, although generally constant, might vary from time to time in a particular patient had been reported by Dacie (1953). Later, the author (Dacie, 1958) referred to another striking case where the erythrocytes of a patient, during a phase of severe haemolysis, appeared to be coated with globulins other than γ. During a remission, however, they reacted as if they were coated only with γ globulin, as did normal cells coated with an antibody eluted from the patient's cells during the period of active haemolysis. Similar observations, with the effect of the addition of γ globulin to antiglobulin serum varying at different stages in the patients' illness, were reported by Wuilleret (1958) and Konda and Yamada (1960).

Nature of the non-γ antiglobulin reaction—role of complement

The interesting observations quoted in the preceding paragraphs did not provide a certain answer as to the nature of the protein adsorbed to AIHA erythrocytes that gave 'intermediate' or non-γ antiglobulin reactions. Dacie (1957, 1959) (Table 24.4) had noted, as had Vaughan (1956), that when normal erythrocytes were exposed to antibodies eluted from corpuscles giving such reactions, the normal erythrocytes reacted with antiglobulin sera as if they were coated with γ globulin, and he concluded that in some cases at least the non-γ reaction was being brought about by protein adsorbed to erythrocytes in addition to the γ-globulin antibody. There seemed at the time to be three possible explanations for this: (1) that the additional protein was antibody not composed of γ globulin; (2) that the additional protein was a fraction or fractions of complement, or (3) that it was protein 'non-specifically' adsorbed to antibody-damaged erythrocytes. The evidence then available was insufficient for a firm conclusion to be reached. There seemed to be no real evidence that the antibody might be composed of, say, β globulin. Morever, it would then have to be accepted that β-globulin antibody did not withstand elution procedures, whereas γ-globulin antibody did.

The second possibility that the non-γ protein adsorbed to erythrocytes was complement appeared, too, to lack supporting evidence. The author had found that eluates prepared from cells coated with globulins other than γ failed to fix complement (or other serum proteins) on to normal erythrocytes *in vitro* when the test cells were exposed to the eluate plus fresh normal serum or the patient's fresh serum. Adsorption of complement, however, seemed to be the likely mechanism when the antibody was of the rare in-saline-agglutinating type. Konda and Yamada (1960), however, reported only partial inhibition in the γ-globulin neutralization test when eluates

from three cases were dissolved in fresh normal serum and normal erythrocytes then sensitized in the mixture.

The third alternative—that protein was being non-specifically adsorbed by antibody-damaged erythrocytes — appeared to have no direct evidence to support it. However, it was known that damage to the erythrocytes' surface by chemicals could lead to the adsorption of protein (Jandl and Simmons, 1957), and it was conceivable, therefore, that a variety of types of damage to the cell surface occurring *in vivo*, including that due to immune antibodies, might similarly lead to adsorption of protein and a positive antiglobulin reaction.

It is now realized that the non-γ antiglobulin reaction is in fact a reaction between anti-complement antibodies in the antiglobulin serum and complement adsorbed to erythrocytes along with the (γ) auto-antibodies. Proof of this stemmed from work carried out to elucidate the nature of 'incomplete' cold antibodies (see also p. 276). In relation to warm antibodies, it is now known, too, that the reactions they give rise to in the antiglobulin test reflect the ability of the antibodies to fix complement to the erythrocytes and that this in turn depends on their chemical nature. In brief, most warm anti-erythrocyte antibodies are IgG γ globulins and these typically do not fix complement. Not infrequently, however, the IgG molecules are accompanied by IgM antibody molecules that do fix complement, and it is the amount of complement that is then fixed that determines whether the antiglobulin reaction is γ, intermediate or non-γ in type. Rarely, complement-fixing anti-IgM molecules are present and IgG antibodies absent. The antiglobulin reaction is then of the non-γ type. IgA antibody molecules are sometimes formed; they do not, howver, fix complement, and the antiglobulin reaction they give rise to is of the γ type.

Proof that the non-γ reaction between sensitized erythrocytes and antiglobulin sera depended on the adsorption of complement components was provided by Dacie, Crookston and Christenson (1957). They used erythrocytes from patients suffering from warm- or cold-antibody AIHA and erythrocytes sensitized *in vitro* by a variety of antibodies, including anti-D and anti-K (as representative of warm allo-antibodies) and the cold antibodies, anti-Le^a, anti-H and the D–L antibody of paroxysmal cold haemoglobinuria, as well as sheep erythrocytes sensitized by rabbit anti-sheep sera. The complement components C1, C2 and C4 (but not C3) appeared to be necessary for the non-antiglobulin reaction to be positive, and it was concluded that the reaction was being brought about by the antiglobulin serum reacting with sublytic amounts of complement adsorbed with the antibody rather than by the antiglobulin serum reacting with the antibody. This conclusion was confirmed by Rosenfield, Haber and Gilbert (1960) and Leddy et al. (1962) in detailed studies. Rosenfield, Haber and Gilbert suggested that the term 'complement antiglobulin test' was appropriate for the reaction.

Leddy, Bakemeier and Vaughan (1965) reported that they had tested concentrated eluates, made from the erythrocytes of three patients, which had been agglutinated by anti-γG (IgG) and anti-C sera. These eluates induced *in-vitro* sensitization of normal erythrocyte to both anti-IgG and anti-C sera, and Leddy, Bakemeier and Vaughan suggested that complement components had been carried 'piggyback' by the auto-antibody on to the normal cells.

Identical experiments carried out with the erythrocytes of three similar patients led, however, to the transference of IgG alone, as did experiments with the cells, derived from other patients, which had been coated *in vivo* only with IgG. Leddy, Bakemeier and Vaughan concluded that some IgG auto-antibodies are responsible for complement fixation to erythrocytes *in vivo* and that in some cases, but not in all, complement components are firmly fixed to the sensitizing antibody.

The next steps in the story of the role of complement in the non-γ antiglobulin reaction were directed towards finding out exactly which complement components were involved. This is discussed on p. 280.

The more recent history of the use of the antiglobulin reaction in AIHA is of the progressive use of antiglobulin sera of increasing specificity. This had become possible because of the substantial advances in understanding of the chemistry of the human globulins, in particular the demonstration in the 1950s that there were a number of distinct classes of γ globulin which differed in structure and molecular size.

At first, the antiglobulin sera that had been used were made by immunizing animals, usually rabbits, against whole human serum or crude globulin preparations. Such sera were essentially anti-human globulin in specificity — later they were referred to often as 'broad-spectrum' sera. The specific anti-γ sera that became available were made as the result of the use of γ globulin of high purity as immunizing agent or by adding to a potent broad-spectrum serum sufficient electrophoretically separated α_2 globulin to inhibit completely the agglutination of erythrocytes sensitized by the incomplete cold antibody that exists in normal serum (see p. 278). Similarly, useful anti-non-γ sera had been made by adding to a broad-spectrum serum sufficient γ globulin to inhibit completely the agglutination of D-positive erythrocytes sensitized by the Rh antibody anti-D.

Use of anti-IgG, -IgM, -IgA, anti-κ, anti-λ and anti-C (complement) sera and sera against IgG subclasses

Next, sera directed against the main classes of the heavy chains of γ globulin, i.e. anti-IgG, anti-IgM and anti-IgA sera, and against the light chain types, κ and λ, became available, and later still antisera directed against subclasses of IgG, i.e. anti-IgG1–4. In parallel, animals were immunized to produce polyclonal antisera specific for human complement and for specific complement components, e.g. C3d. More recently, highly specific monoclonal antibodies have become available (Voak, 1989). The increasing availability of the above sera provided an excellent opportunity for the more detailed study of the antiglobulin reaction in warm-antibody AIHA, and in the 1960s and 1970s particularly the results of many such studies were published. In summary, the erythrocytes of rather more than half of the patients suffering from warm-antibody AIHA were found to react with specific anti-γ (IgG) sera as well as with anti-complement (anti-C) sera — they all reacted with anti-broad-spectrum sera, and rather less than half reacted only with specific anti-γ sera; a small percentage reacted (apparently) only with anti-C sera.

Published data from individual sources have varied rather widely, reflecting presumably the use of different reagents and perhaps differences in the patient populations studied. According to Issitt (1985), the data of Worlledge and Blajchman (1972), Issitt et al. (1976) and Petz and Garratty (1980), based on studies of 309 patients with warm-antibody AIHA, yielded when taken together the following mean percentages: positive reactions with anti-IgG sera plus anti-C sera 56%, with anti-IgG sera alone 35% and with anti-C sera alone 9%.

Only a small percentage of patients have erythrocytes that react with anti-IgA and anti-IgM sera; usually, although not invariably, such cells react with anti-IgG sera also, i.e., more than one IgG class has been formed.

Tests with antisera against the subclasses of IgG, namely, IgG1, IgG2, IgG3 and IgG4, have shown that more than 90% of patients form IgG1 auto-antibodies, usually (about 70%) as the sole subclass. Other subclasses are rarely formed by themselves; when present at all, they are usually found in association with IgG1.

Leddy and Bakemeier (1964) described how they had used antiglobulin sera directed against the two light-chain types, I(κ) or II (λ), of human 7S globulin (IgG). Eluates from the erythrocytes of 12 AIHA patients had been tested: eight reacted with anti-type-I sera, two with anti-type-II sera and two with both sera. (Similar tests carried out on erythrocytes sensitized with anti-D antibodies resulted in positive reactions with both types of antisera.) Leddy and Bakemeier reported that auto-antibodies possessing apparently only one type of light chain had been produced in both idiopathic and symptomatic types of AIHA.

Leddy and Bakemeier (1965) subsequently reported that of the 20 patients they had by then studied, 12 had formed auto-antibodies with only one light chain type, eight with both types; of six Rh allo-antibodies, both types of light chain were present in five, in one a single type. Leddy's (1966) review was an able summary of contempory knowledge.

Bakemeir and Leddy (1976a, b), in further detailed studies of several warm IgG auto-antibodies, reported that apparent homogeneity in relation to light-chain type was in some cases associated with the presence of multiple heavy-chain types. They discussed the connection between homogeneity and heterogeneity of the population of antibody molecules and the number of antibody specificities that could be demonstrated. Their data were considered to cast doubt on the concept of a monoclonal origin of the antibodies in most patients.

Ando (1965) reported on 32 patients with warm-antibody AIHA: the direct antiglobulin reaction was of the γ type in five and of the mixed (γ plus non-γ) in 27. Jeannet (1965, 1966) had studied 13 patients with idiopathic AIHA. Excluding four patients whose sera contained high-titre cold agglutinins, the direct antiglobulin tests indicated coating with IgG alone in one patient, with IgG plus complement in two patients and with complement alone in five.

Eyster and co-workers (1966) reported on the agglutination reactions of the erythrocytes of 18 patients with AIHA not associated with a raised cold-agglutinin titre, when tested with antisera prepared against an anti-heavy chain γG serum, an anti-γA serum, an anti-complement (C) serum and antisera prepared against κ and λ light chains. γG was demonstrated on the erythrocytes of five patients, γG plus C in nine patients and C alone in four patients. The erythrocytes of nine patients were tested with the anti-κ and anti-λ sera: all nine samples were agglutinated by both sera, but the relative strengths of the reactions varied, indicating a heterogeneous mixture of γG molecules.

Gerbal and co-workers (1967, 1968a,b) reviewed the results of serological studies based on a large number of patients. Five different types of direct antiglobulin reactions were recorded and correlated with the responsible antibody (Gerbal et al., 1968a): Type I [cold γM plus C, anti-I, 39 patients (16.5%)]; Type II [complement, γM, anti-I, 74 patients (31.5%)]; Type III [complement, unknown specificity, 15 patients (6.5%)]; Type IV [γG, anti-Rh, 39 patients (16.5%)], and Type V [mixed, anti-Rh plus anti-I, 63 patients (27.7%) and anti-Rh alone, 3 patients (1.3%)].

André and Najman (1967) also reported on patients studied in Paris: the DAT of 40 idiopathic AIHA patients was of the IgM type in two, IgG type in 19 and of the mixed (IgG plus complement) type in 17.

Engelfriet and co-workers (1968a) reviewed the serological findings in 186 patients with warm-antibody AIHA. The erythrocytes of 146 of them (89%) reacted with anti-IgG sera; only four reacted specifically with anti-IgM sera. The erythrocytes of an unspecified number of patients of both categories also reacted with anti-C sera.

Engelfriet and co-workers (1968b) described how they had prepared reagents specific for IgG, IgM, IgA and complement (C) and illustrated their use in the investigation of four patients suffering from AIHA of unknown origin. The auto-antibodies differed in each case: one was an incomplete IgM antibody, the second an incomplete IgA antibody and the third a mixture of IgG, IgM and IgA antibodies. The fourth patient's antibody lysed enzyme-treated cells at 37°C, particularly at pH 6.5; her erythrocytes were, however, not agglutinated by the anti-IgG serum but were strongly agglutinated by the anti-C serum.

Eyster and Jenkins (1969) reported further data based on 116 patients, the majority (99 patients) suffering from some underlying disease. Seventy-two had presented with signs of increased haemolysis: in 17 (24%) the erythrocytes were shown to be coated with γG, in 22 (31%) with γG plus complement (C), in 18 (25%) with C alone (cold-agglutinin titre normal) and in 15 (20%) with C alone (cold-agglutinin titre raised). The erythrocytes of the 17 patients with idiopathic AIHA were shown to be coated with γG in seven, with γG plus C in four and with C alone in six. Complement alone was the most frequently found coating material in 24 patients (all with some underlying disease) who did not present with overt haemolysis: the erythrocytes were coated with γG in five patients, with γG plus C in four patients and with C alone in 15 patients.

The results of studies on the DAT carried out by the author and his associates on AIHA patients studied at the Royal Postgraduate Medical School in the 1950s, 1960s and 1970s are summarized below:

Dacie (1962) stated that of 73 patients with idiopathic AIHA the DAT had been of the γ type in 32 (44%), intermediate type in 28 (38%) and non-γ type in 13 (18%). Worlledge (1967) was able to report on the DAT of 98 cases: in 58% the reaction indicated IgG on the erythrocytes, in 29% IgG plus complement (C) and in 13% C only.

Dacie and Worlledge (1969) reported on the use of specific anti-IgG, anti-IgM and anti-IgA sera, as well as anti-complement (C) sera, in 29 patients with warm-antibody AIHA: IgG alone was demonstrated on the erythrocytes of 16 (55%), IgG plus C in nine (31%), IgG plus IgM plus C in one, IgG plus IgM plus IgA in one, and C alone in two.

Worlledge and Blajchman (1972) reviewed the serological findings in 323 AIHA patients, 105 of whom were classified as having the idiopathic disease. Seventy-four had formed warm auto-antibodies: IgG alone was demonstrated on the erythrocytes in 28 (38%), IgA alone in two, IgG plus IgA in three, IgG plus complement (C) in 29 (39%), IgG plus IgM plus C in two, and C only in 10.

Dacie (1975) reported on 121 idiopathic warm-antibody patients. In addition to listing the percentages reacting with the anti-IgG, anti-IgA, anti-IgM and anti-C sera [which were similar to those of Worlledge and Blajchman (1972)], data based on the use in 57 patients of specific anti-IgG1, -IgG2, -IgG3 and -IgG4 sera were presented. IgG1 alone was demonstrated in 24 patients, 1 plus 2 in eight patients, 1 plus 3 in eight patients, 1 plus 4 in three patients, 1 plus 2 plus 3 in one patient, 2 alone in one patient, while in 12 patients

the results were unclear with the antisera then available.

In her last report, Worlledge (1982) recorded the DATs of 291 patients with warm-antibody AIHA. Of 178 patients judged to have the idiopathic disease, 64 (36%) had given positive results with anti-IgG sera and 68 (38%) with anti-C sera as well as anti-IgG sera; eight other combinations had been much less common. Over 86% of the samples had been agglutinated by anti-IgG sera and 48% by anti-C sera; 10% had been agglutinated by anti-C sera alone.

Further data from France were reported by Homberg, Cartron and Salmon (1971), based on studies on 461 patients forming warm auto-antibodies. Their disorder was classified in 151 as 'non-γ' (γMC) (26%), in 36 as C (complement) (6.2%), in 134 as γG (23.2%) and in 138 as 'mixed' (γG plus γMC) (23.8%).

In a more recent review of 593 patients forming warm auto-antibodies, Salmon, Homberg and Habibi (1975) recorded that their erythrocytes had reacted with anti-IgG sera in 192 cases (32%), with anti-IgG sera plus anti-C sera in 166 cases (28%) and with anti-C sera alone in 235 cases (40%)

Mueller-Eckhardt and Kretschmer (1972) reported on 21 AIHA patients who had been studied repeatedly over a period of 1–36 months. Twelve suffered from idiopathic (irreversible), and nine from symptomatic, AIHA. IgG auto-antibodies were detected in every patient; in nine they were associated with IgA and/or IgM auto-antibodies, but there were no instances of isolated IgA or IgM (or IgD or IgE) auto-antibody formation. IgG was present in eluates prepared from the erythrocytes of 10 patients, IgA in three eluates and IgM in seven eluates. κ and λ light chains were detected together in 14 patients; in the remainder only κ chains. Complement fixation was demonstrated in 10 patients. Mueller-Eckhardt and Kretschmer pointed out that the immunological picture varied in individual patients if they were followed throughout the course of their disease, and they illustrated this in a Table based on the data of seven patients. They pointed out, too, that this serological heterogeneity and variability made a monoclonal origin of the auto-antibodies unlikely and also that a classification of the AIHAs based solely on immunochemical criteria had little serological and clinical relevance because of the extent to which the antibody might vary during the course of a patient's disease.

Bell, Zwicker and Sacks (1973) reviewed the serological findings in 88 AIHA patients of whom 57 had formed warm auto-antibodies. The disorder was idiopathic in 18 and was associated with α-methyldopa therapy also in 18: the DAT of the idiopathic cases was of the IgG type in 14 and of the IgG plus complement (C) type in four; it was of the IgG type in all of the 18 α-methyldopa cases.

Rosse (1975), in his succinct review of the antiglobulin test in AIHA, discussed how the four types of reactions—IgG alone, IgG plus complement (C), C alone, and neither IgG nor C detectable on the erythrocyte membrane—were related to pathogenetic mechanisms and disease processes. In relation to the last category (Coombs-negative AIHA), Rosse pointed out that failure of agglutination could result from there being too few antibody molecules on the erythrocytes for them to be detected by antiglobulin sera used in the usual way and/or that low-affinity antibody molecules might be eluted from the cell surfaces while the cells were being washed in preparation for the antiglobulin test.

Issitt and co-workers (1976) gave details of the DAT in 87 cases of AIHA: IgG was present alone on the erythrocytes in 38 (44%), IgG plus complement (C) in 41 (47%), IgG plus IgM and/or IgA in one, and IgG plus IgM and/or IgA plus C in seven (8%). In contrast, in all 33 patients whose AIHA was associated with α-methyldopa therapy, only IgG could be demonstrated on their erythrocytes.

Petz and Garratty (1980, p. 193) listed the results of using monospecific antiglobulin sera in carrying out DATs in 104 patients with warm-antibody AIHA. There had been 13 reaction patterns: IgG alone or with other proteins (Igs + complement) in 85.6% of the patients, C3 alone or with other Igs in 78.9%, IgA alone or with other proteins in 21.2% and IgM alone or with other proteins in 7.7%. IgG alone had been recorded in only 18.3%, C alone in 10.6%; the most frequent association had been IgG plus C3 (46.2%).

A more recent development has been the use of radioimmune assay to demonstrate the terminal complex of complement (C5b-C9) on erythrocytes. Salama and co-workers (1983) used this technique in investigating 70 patients suffering from various types of warm- and cold-antibody AIHA and compared the results with more conventional tests for lysis. The results with the radioimmune assay paralleled those for lysis, but the former technique was found to be more sensitive in demonstrating the presence on the erythrocyte membrane of the terminal complex of complement than was the occurrence of visible lysis.

Gm allotypes in warm-antibody AIHA

Le Petit and Brizard (1971) and Le Petit et al. (1976) reported on IgG subclass and Gm genetic markers (allotypes) in 19 AIHA patients. They concluded that the antibodies were polyclonal and that antibodies of a different subclass, characterized by different genetic markers, might co-exist in the same patient. In 10 of the patients, IgG1, with or without IgG3 or IgG4, was the predominant subclass, and there was a preference, too, for the Gm1 allotype.

Litwin, Balaban and Eyster (1973) similarly investigated the IgG auto-antibodies of six AIHA patients for the genetic markers on the antibodies' heavy chains. They concluded that the auto-antibodies might be restricted with respect to Gm genetic characters, with a preference for the Gm(a) (Gm1) allotype. In three patients Gm(a) was the only allotype demonstrable.

Heterogeneity of warm auto-antibodies as assessed by isoelectric focusing

Andrzejewski and co-workers (1991) reported that they had separated by isoelectric focusing serum fractions from 28 patients with various forms of AIHA and from two non-anaemic individuals whose DAT was positive and that they had estimated erythrocyte binding quantitatively by a radio-immune assay. They found that the antibodies were present in a restricted number of fractions in the sera of some of the patients and that, moreover, the patterns varied in different patients. Their findings suggested that, although polyclonal, the antibodies were the product of a limited number of clones.

CLINICAL SIGNIFICANCE OF THE DIFFERENT Ig CLASSES AND IgG SUBCLASSES

The possible clinical significance of the different Ig classes and IgG subclasses and of the formation of multiple subclasses by individual patients is a matter of considerable interest. There are indications that haemolysis is usually more severe when more than one type of Ig class or IgG subclass is present and that multiple types of antibody are formed more frequently in idiopathic than in secondary cases.

Early observations, summarized by Swisher et al. (1965), had indicated that the occurrence of haemolysis in idiopathic cases was similar irrespective of whether the DAT test had been of the γ, non-γ or both varieties.

Chaplin (1973), in a valuable review, considered the clinical usefulness of the specific antiglobulin reagents available up to that time. In particular, he discussed the production and standardization of the reagents, how direct and indirect antiglobulin tests might be carried out, their sensitivity, false-negative and false-positive results, classifications based on patterns of antiglobulin reactivity, the fixation of complement, and the relationship between the strength of the reactions and the clinical severity of haemolysis in vivo, with particular reference to the subtypes of IgG and the fixation of complement. He pointed out that the available evidence indicated that IgG antibodies that were associated with in-vivo haemolysis were generally made up of IgG1 and IgG3 subclasses, less likely to be of IgG2 and rarely of IgG4 (see also p. 110).

Engelfriet and his co-workers (1974) reported on the incidence of Ig class and subclass in warm-antibody AIHA: in 86% of the patients IgG was present, in 8% IgM and in 6% IgA. The data from 226 patients were presented in relation to the subclass of their IgG: twelve possible combinations were recorded: IgG1 was present in 216 cases (in 160 cases by itself; in 56 cases with IgG of one or more of the other subclasses). The erythrocytes of 29 patients were not agglutinated by any of the anti-subclass IgG sera despite being agglutinated strongly by (polyvalent) anti-IgG serum.

Petz and Garratty (1980, p. 193), in summarizing their early experience with anti-IgG, anti-IgA, anti-IgM and anti-C sera, concluded that their use had not been of much clinical value. Later, however, Nance and Garratty (1983) reported that haemolysis had been more frequently present when multiple subclasses of IgG rather than a single subclass (i.e. IgG1) had been present: thus 39 % of patients with overt AIHA had formed more than one subclass compared with 13% of healthy blood donors or patients without evidence of haemolysis.

Kemppinen and co-workers (1981) reported on their experience with monospecific antiglobulin sera in 15 idiopathic and 59 secondary cases of AIHA. Multiple specificities were identified more frequently and haemolysis was more severe in the idiopathic than in the secondary cases. Thromboembolic complications and a fatal outcome were more frequent, too, in association with multiple specificities. (A positive reaction with anti-C sera was included as one component of multiple specificity.)

Engelfriet and his co-workers (1983) summarized their extensive experience based on 2000 patients with AIHA investigated in Amsterdam since 1961. Of these patients 869 (64%) had IgG on their erythrocytes and a further 449 (33%) IgG plus complement (C). IgA (30 cases) and IgM (27 cases) were detected relatively rarely: IgA was present alone in 11 cases and IgM alone in 13 cases; in the remaining cases they were present in addition to IgG. Engelfriet et al. also presented the results of testing for IgG subclasses. IgG1 was by far the commonest subclass, being present alone in 416 (72%) of 572 patients and in combination with subclasses 2–4 in a further 133 patients (23%). In all, 12 different combinations of IgG 1–4 were encountered.

Further data on IgG subclasses were recorded by Engelfriet et al. (1987), by then based on a study of 746 patients. Excluding 14 patients in whom no subclass had been detected, 12 reaction patterns had again been identified: IgG1 had been present in 702 patients, by itself in 552 and in combination with other IgG subclasses in 150 patients: IgG1 plus IgG2 had been present in 65 patients and IgG1 plus IgG3 in 57. Subclasses other than IgG had been rarely present alone: IgG2 only in five patients, IgG3 in 16 and IgG4 in seven.

Ben-Izhak, Shechter and Tatarsky (1985) had studied 25 idiopathic and 60 secondary cases: severe haemolysis had been a feature in seven out of 23 patients in whom the DAT had been of the anti-IgG type and in three out of 22 patients in whom the DAT had been of the anti-IgG plus anti-C type, while none of the patients in whom the DAT had been of the anti-C only type had experienced severe haemolysis. In striking contrast, 12 out of 14 patients whose erythrocytes had been coated with IgA ± IgM in addition to IgG plus complement had suffered from severe haemolysis. Ben-Izhak, Shechter and Tatarsky pointed out that multiple antibodies had been more frequent in idiopathic than in secondary cases.

In a recent report Sokol and his co-workers (1990) recorded the erythrocyte-bound IgG subclass in 304 patients with warm-antibody AIHA. IgG1 had been identified in almost all the patients (98%); it was the sole IgG in 64%. Multiple subclasses were present in 34.5%: the most frequent combinations were IgG1 plus IgG2 (10.2%), IgG1 plus IgG3 (10.2%) and IgG1 plus IgG4 (7.2%).

The results in 58 patients who had been tested three or more times were reviewed for possible change of subclass with time. In 25 there was evidence for this: an increase in subclass number in 11, a decrease in seven, an increase, then a decrease in six, and in one case a change from IgG3 to IgG1. Sokol and co-workers (1990) also reported that total cell-bound IgG, expressed as the number of molecules of IgG per erythrocyte, is strongly correlated with the presence of multiple subclasses of IgG. This observation fits in well with the reported association of multiple subclasses and severe haemolysis.

IgG2 and IgG4 antibodies as possible causes of haemolysis in AIHA

IgG2. The occurrence of IgG2-mediated AIHA appears to be a great rarity. Nance, Bourdo and Garratty (1983), however, described such a case.

Their patient, a 28-year-old female, had a haemoglobin of 6.2 g/dl and 22% reticulocytes. The DAT was strongly positive (4+) with an anti-IgG serum and moderately positive (2+) with an anti-C serum. Eluates reacted with all erythrocytes tested. Subclass testing revealed anti-IgG2 only and monocyte/monolayer assay revealed positive adherence and phagocytosis.

IgG4. von dem Borne and co-workers (1977) described an AIHA patient whose IgG antibodies were mainly IgG4; IGgl antibodies were, however, present at a lower concentration and also traces of IgG3 antibodies. The patient, who earlier had suffered from sarcoidosis, developed moderately severe haemolysis and a strongly positive DAT. Later, all clinical signs of increased haemolysis disappeared and the ^{51}Cr T$_{50}$ (21 days) was only just subnormal. The DAT remained, however, strongly positive, and it was at this time that the auto-antibodies were found to be largely of IgG4 subtype. von dem Borne et al. postulated that the virtual disappearance of increased haemolysis had been the result of the patient forming predominantly inactive (i.e. Ig4) rather than 'active' (i.e. IgG1 and IgG3) antibodies.

IgA AUTO-ANTIBODIES AND AIHA

Some interesting descriptions are available of patients in whom IgA auto-antibodies appear to have been responsible for the increased haemolysis.

Engelfriet and co-workers (1968b) described a 60-year-old man who had a severe acquired haemolytic anaemia of unknown origin. The DAT was apparently negative with an anti-IgG serum but positive with an anti-C serum. There was no auto-agglutination. Reinvestigation revealed a strongly positive DAT using an anti-IgA serum as well as a positive reaction with an anti-C serum. A weak reaction with an anti-IgG serum was shown to be due to the presence of contaminating anti-IgA antibodies. The DAT with an anti-IgM serum was negative, and the fixation of complement was unexplained. No free auto-antibodies could be demonstrated in the patient's serum. An eluate from his erythrocytes was shown to contain an IgA antibody of anti-e specificity incapable of fixing complement. Engelfriet et al. also described a 58-year-old patient with severe idiopathic AIHA who gave strongly positive reactions with anti-IgG, -IgA and -IgM sera and also with an anti-C serum. No free auto-antibodies could be demonstrated in the patient's serum. Eluates were found to contain both IgG and IgA antibodies of unidentifiable specificity. Again, the fixation of complement could not be explained.

Fagiolo and Laghi (1970) reported on the results of positive DATs in 19 patients with AIHA, 13 of the cases being of the idiopathic type. Using antisera specific for IgG, IgA, IgM and C, they recorded nine reaction patterns. In nine of the cases tests with the anti-IgA serum were positive, in eight in combination with positive tests with one or more of the other sera.

Wager and co-workers (1971) described five patients aged between 25 and 63 years who had formed IgA warm auto-antibodies; four had suffered from severe haemolysis and two had died. The DATs, which were positive with anti-IgA sera, had been positive, too, with anti-IgG sera in four of them. In the fifth patient the DAT had been positive with an anti-M serum as well as with an anti-IgA serum. In four of the patients the DAT had been positive with anti-C sera also. IgA antibody had been demonstrated in an eluate from the erythrocytes of one of the patients, but had not been demonstrated in their sera. Wager et al. remarked that as far as they knew IgA auto-antibodies had so far been described in 11 patients. Their own series of five patients had been identified out of a total of 150 patients in whom the DAT had been positive.

Stratton and co-workers (1972) described a 45-year-old woman who had developed a chronic but severe AIHA. Her haemoglobin was 5.6 g/dl and she had 34% reticulocytes. The DAT was strongly positive with a broad-spectrum antiglobulin serum and with an anti-IgA serum; it was negative with other anti-Ig sera and with anti-C sera. Anti-e was eluted from the patient's erythrocytes and was the only abnormal antibody detected in her serum. Her clinical state improved gradually when she was treated with prednisolone and cyclophosphamide.

Sturgeon and his co-workers (1979) described a 9-year-old boy who, after an illness lasting about 1 week, was found to have a haemoglobin of 6.2 g/dl, with 31% reticulocytes. AIHA was diagnosed, and he was treated with prednisone and responded slowly. The DAT was strongly positive, but only with an anti-IgA serum. An abnormal antibody in his serum was shown to have Rh specificity — it reacted with all cells tested with the exception of Rh_{null} cells — and an antibody of similar specificity was eluted from the boy's erythrocytes. In a review of 772 cases of AIHA described in the literature, Sturgeon et al. found that sensitization with an IgA auto-antibody had been reported in 41 of the patients (5.3%). However, in only five had the auto-antibodies been exclusively IgA in type; in their own experience of about 300 cases, the present patient was the only one of this type that they had encountered.

Suzuki and co-workers (1981) gave details of a 26-year-old woman who had developed a very severe acquired haemolytic anaemia. Blood transfusions were of transient benefit, but she eventually responded satisfactorily to prednisolone therapy (Fig. 24.3). Initially the DAT using a polyspecific serum was weakly positive. Subsequently the test was found to be strongly positive with anti-IgA and anti-C3 sera. Tests using anti-IgG and anti-IgM sera were negative. The indirect antiglobulin test (IAT) was positive only with the anti-IgA serum. IATs in the presence of fresh human AB serum were positive using an anti-C3 serum under circumstances that suggested that the IgA antibody was activating complement via the alternative pathway. The concentrations of the serum complement components Factor B and C3 were significantly decreased. In vitro, erythrophagocytosis by monocytes was demonstrated, and it was thought that this was likely to have been brought about mainly by interaction between C3-coated erythrocytes and the C3 receptors on monocytes.

Wolf and co-workers (1982) described a 71-year-old woman with a moderately severe recently developing haemolytic anaemia. Microspherocytes were noted in blood films. However, the DAT was negative on three successive days using a broad-spectrum antiglobulin serum. Nevertheless, her erythrocytes were found to auto-agglutinate in PVP or Polybrene, and subse-

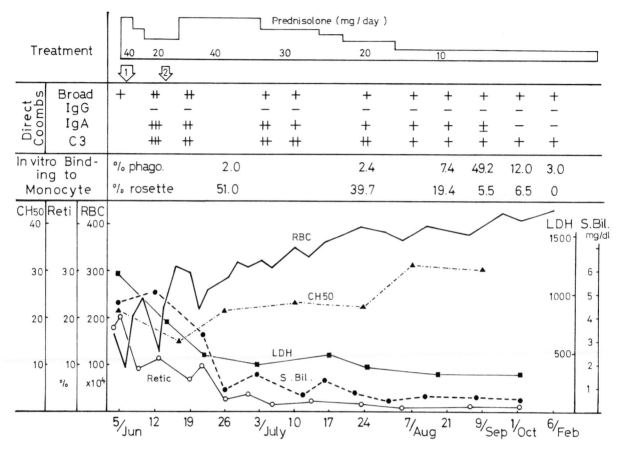

Fig. 24.3   Haematological and serological findings in a 26-year-old woman with an IgA idiopathic warm-antibody AIHA.

[Reproduced by permission from Suzuki et al. (1981).]

quently a DAT using a specific anti-IgA serum was found to be strongly positive. In addition, using specific reagents, her erythrocytes were found to be coated with small amounts of IgG, IgM and complement components. She eventually responded well to prednisone therapy.

A further elderly patient, a man aged 71, was described by Clark et al. (1984). For 7 years he had been suffering from chronic thrombocytopenic purpura which had been treated intermittently with low doses of prednisone. Suddenly he became anaemic and jaundiced and had haemoglobinuria. The DAT was weakly positive with polyspecific and anti-C3 sera: it was negative, however, with an anti-IgG serum. Serum haemolytic complement and total C3 were decreased. Subsequently the DAT was found to be strongly positive with an anti-IgA serum. An eluate from his erythrocytes was found to contain an IgA antibody, but abnormal antibodies were not demonstrated in his

serum. He continued to suffer from compensated haemolysis during the next 20 months, exacerbations of haemolysis being controlled by an increased dosage of prednisone. Eventually he went into complete remission following splenectomy. *In vitro*, the eluted antibody did not seem to fix complement. However, normal erythrocytes exposed to the antibody were lysed by normal human peripheral-blood monocytes in a system designed to demonstrate antibody-dependent cell-mediated cytotoxicity. Monocytes also ingested antibody-sensitized cells.

An account of a rather similar patient, a women aged 51, was given by Reusser et al. (1987). She had had repeated episodes of superficial thrombophlebitis of leg veins and had become increasingly weak during the 4 months prior to admission to hospital. She was found to have a well-compensated haemolytic anaemia, with a haemoglobin of 10.6 g/dl, 28% reticulocytes and spherocytes in blood films. The DAT and IAT using a broad-spectrum antiglobulin serum were negative and HS was considered as a possible diagnosis. Reinvestigation, however, showed that the DAT was weakly positive with anti-IgG and anti-C3d sera and strongly positive with an anti-IgA serum. An eluate yielded an antibody which gave a strongly positive IAT with an anti-IgA serum but not with other monospecific sera. Haemolysis was controlled only with high doses of steroids. Splenectomy, however, resulted in clinical remission, although the DAT remained positive with an anti-IgA serum and became positive once again with an anti-C3d serum.

INCOMPLETE IgM WARM AUTO-ANTIBODIES AND AIHA

Auto-antibodies formed of IgM globulins that fail to cause direct agglutination but which may be detected by anti-IgM antiglobulin sera have rarely been reported. Engelfriet and co-workers (1968b), however, described a 78-year-old woman with haemolytic anaemia who gave a 4-month history of increasing lassitude. The haemoglobin was 9.3 g/dl and osmotic fragility was increased. There was no auto-agglutination. The DAT was strongly positive with anti-IgM and anti-C sera, but negative with anti-IgG and -IgA sera. No abnormal antibodies were present in her serum. An IgM auto-antibody was, however, detected in an eluate prepared from the patient's erythrocytes by means of the IAT using an anti-IgM serum. Although complement had been detected on the patient's erythrocytes by means of the DAT, the eluted antibody could not be shown to be able to fix complement. Engelfriet et al. also mentioned their report at the 11th Congress of the International Society of Haematology held in Sydney in 1966 (Engelfriet et al. 1968a), in which they had referred briefly to four patients who had apparently formed incomplete IgM antibodies: as well as erythrocyte-bound IgM, incomplete IgM had been detected in the serum of two of these patients.

Kay and co-workers (1975) described a most unusual combination of auto-antibodies in a 49-year-old patient who had hypogammaglobulinaemia, hepatosplenomegaly and haemolytic anaemia. The serum concentrations of IgG and IgA were markedly subnormal but she had a raised monoclonal IgM level, initially 1250 mg/dl: about half of this was 19S IgM and half low molecular weight IgM. The DAT was positive, but only with an anti-IgM serum; it was negative with anti-IgG and anti-C3 and -C4 sera. Her serum contained an anti-I antibody, which directly agglutinated normal erythrocytes; its thermal optimum was most unusual, being 37°C. Slight lysis of normal erythrocytes was noted when they were incubated in the patient's serum in the presence of fresh normal serum: IATs on the residue of unlysed cells revealed agglutination by both anti-IgM and anti-IgG sera.

Shirey and co-workers (1989) reported that they had identified IgM auto-antibodies in five out of 115 patients with warm-type AIHA. In three of the patients the disease appeared to be idiopathic; in two, SLE and Waldenström's disease had been the primary diagnoses. In all the patients the erythrocytes were sensitized with IgG and complement; two eluates contained both IgM and IgG auto-antibodies. The sera of four of the patients agglutinated all cells tested at room temperature. In three of the patients the IgM antibody failed to react at 37°C; they responded to steroid therapy. In two patients the IgM antibody was active at 37°C; they failed to respond to steroids, splenectomy and cytotoxic drugs. Shirey et al. called attention to the poor prognosis associated with high-thermal-amplitude IgM auto-antibodies.

NATURE OF THE COMPLEMENT COMPONENTS THAT GIVE RISE TO POSITIVE ANTIGLOBULIN REACTIONS

The early work on the role of complement in the non-γ antiglobulin reaction has already been described (p. 105). Some more recent work that has defined more precisely the complement components involved is described below.

Gandini (1959) and Jenkins, Polley and Mollison (1960), using erythrocytes sensitized with complement-fixing anti-Lewis antibody (anti-Le^a), concluded that the adsorption of C2 is not necessary for a positive antiglobulin reaction. According to Jenkins, Polley and Mollison, the reaction was between C4 adsorbed to the cells and a corresponding anti-β_1 globulin in the antiglobulin serum. Pondman and co-workers (1960) concluded that the agglutination of sensitized erythrocytes that had bound complement (EAC$_{142}$) is independent of the decay of both bound C2 and C4 and is associated with the presence of the EAC$_{14}$ intermediate complex; they concluded, too, that agglutination is not necessarily associated with lytically active bound complement but may occur with (or perhaps only occurs with) EAC$_{14}$ that has decayed.

Harboe and co-workers (1963) experimented with erythrocytes sensitized with complement-binding anti-Le^a antibodies and an unusual complement-binding anti-Rh antibody and also with the erythrocytes of patients with AIHA that had bound complement *in vivo*. The cells were shown to be agglutinated by antibodies specifically directed against two components of the complement system that had recently been isolated, namely, β_{1c} (the hydrazine-sensitive portion of C3) and β_{1E} (C4). The agglutination of the cells by broad-spectrum antiglobulin sera was markedly inhibited by purified β_{1E} and β_{1c} globulins. In some experiments, however, a trace of agglutination remained after the addition of the two globulins, the cause of which could not be determined. Later studies by Kerr, Dalmasso and Kaplan (1971) suggested that the sera may have been reacting with erythrocyte-bound C5 and C6.

Engelfriet and co-workers (1970) prepared antisera specific for the β1E, β1A, β1C and α2D components of complement. [α2D globulin (C3d) is a product of the degradation of C3.] They found that erythrocytes sensitized by normal 'incomplete' cold antibody were agglutinated by the anti-β1E serum but not by the anti-β1C serum. However, erythrocytes sensitized *in vivo*, as in cold-antibody AIHA, were agglutinated only by the anti-α2D serum and they concluded that no β1E (C4) is present on circulating cells that have adsorbed cold antibodies *in vivo* and only the α2D part of the β1C (C3) molecule. Erythrocytes sensitized *in vitro* by anti-

Le[a] were agglutinated by all three specific anti-β1E, -β1A and -α2D sera.

Lachmann and co-workers (1983) used monoclonal anti-C3 antibodies to characterize the fragments of C3 that are found on erythrocytes. They showed that in chronic cold haemagglutinin disease (CHAD) patients the erythrocytes carry C3d,g (the final product of in-vivo C3 activation) rather than C3d and that this is the component that reacts with anti-α2D globulin sera.

Chaplin and Monroe (1986) compared in AIHA patients the reactions of in-vivo sensitized erythrocytes with a polyclonal rabbit anti-human C3d serum and four monoclonal mouse anti-human C3d sera. They found that the monoclonal anti-C3d sera caused agglutination more slowly than the polyclonal serum and that this was associated with striking prozones.

OTHER WAYS OF DEMONSTRATING ERYTHROCYTE SENSITIZATION

Following the demonstration in 1946 by Boorman, Dodd and Loutit that the antiglobulin reaction could be used as a simple but most valuable laboratory tool in the investigation of patients suffering from acquired haemolytic anaemias, attempts have been made to improve the test so as to increase its specificity and sensitivity and to enable it to provide a more accurate quantitative assessment of the degree to which the target erythrocytes are coated with auto-antibodies. The use that has been made of antisera specifically directed against individual IgG classes and subclasses (and against complement components) has been described earlier in this chapter. Three different approaches designed to improve the sensitivity of the reaction are briefly described below, namely, radioactive antiglobulin tests, a complement-fixing antibody consumption (CFAC) test and enzyme-linked immunosorbent assays or tests (ELISA and ELAT). A detailed account of the use and development of the above-mentioned techniques was given by Schreiber (1985).

In addition, some tests will be described based on the property of antibody-coated erythrocytes to undergo auto-agglutination in media of high

protein content or in media containing Polybrene or PVP or when enzyme-treated. Finally, mention will be made of a test based on the property of antibody-coated erythrocytes to adhere to cells containing abundant antibody Fc receptors.

RADIOACTIVE ANTIGLOBULIN TESTS

The use of radioactive antiglobulin sera in the detection of erythrocyte sensitization was reported by Costea et al. (1962) and an improved method for using [125I]anti-IgG was described by Jenkins, Moore and Hawiger (1977).

Coatea and his co-workers (1962), who used [131I]antiglobulin serum were able to demonstrate a clear correlation between the uptake of radioactivity and the strength of the DAT, as assessed from 0–4+, in 14 AIHA patients (Fig. 24.4). They also reported a small uptake of radioactivity (after allowing for non-specific uptake by normal erythrocytes) in four patients whose DAT was negative when read visually, as well as an increased uptake in two patients at the time of a haemolytic crisis and a diminution in uptake in two patients who had responded to treatment.

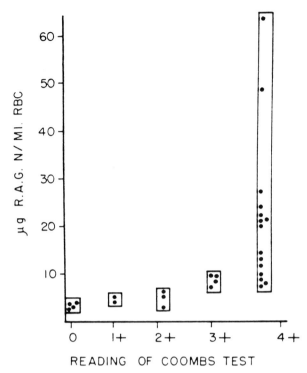

Fig. 24.4   Relationship between the strength of the antiglobulin (Coombs) test assessed visually and the uptake of ^{131}I-labelled antiglobulin serum.
[Reproduced by permission from Costea et al. (1962).]

Schmitz and co-workers (1981) also compared in a series of 125 patients, 66 with AIHA and 59 with a haemolytic anaemia of non-immune origin, the results of testing their erythrocytes with a conventional anti-IgG serum and a radioactive [^{125}I]anti-IgG serum. [Cell bound radioactivity was expressed as a percentage of the total radioactivity to which the cells were exposed: 2.09% was the upper limit in a series of control normal blood samples.] The radioactive test was clearly positive in all the patients who had given positive conventional anti-IgG DATs; it was positive, too, in 13 patients whose erythrocytes were agglutinated by anti-C sera but not by anti-IgG sera, and it was also positive in four out of six patients thought to have Coombs-negative haemolytic anaemia. It is interesting to note, however, that the test was negative in seven patients with cold haemagglutinin disease whose cells were strongly agglutinated by anti-C sera, and it was negative, too, in nine patients (six with multiple myeloma) who had hypergammaglobulinaemia.

COMPLEMENT-FIXING ANTIBODY CONSUMPTION (CFAC) TEST

Gilliland, Leddy and Vaughan (1970) used a CFAC test based on that of Moulinier (1956) as a means of increasing the sensitivity of the antiglobulin reaction. The test measures the quantity of unconsumed anti-IgG (γG) antibody by quantitative complement fixation using sensitized sheep erythrocytes as indicator. The erythrocytes of 16 patients with various types of AIHA (ten of whom had SLE, four idiopathic AIHA) were tested: in each case their erythrocytes had previously been shown to be coated with complement but not with IgG (as tested for by standard methods). The CFAC test demonstrated that the cells of 13 of the 16 patients were in fact coated with increased amounts of IgG (more than 35 molecules per cell) in addition to complement components. Eluates were made from the erythrocytes of seven of the patients, and when the eluates were sufficiently concentrated they were found to be able to sensitize normal erythrocytes to agglutination by an anti-IgG serum; six of the eluates fixed complement to the normal cells, too. Gilliland, Leddy and Vaughan concluded that the use of the sensitive CFAC test indicated that many patients with AIHA whose erythrocytes appear to be coated with complement only are in fact forming low concentrations of warm-reacting IgG antibodies and that it is these antibodies that lead to complement fixation *in vivo*. It is interesting to note, in view of the antibodies' ability to fix complement, that none of the antibodies appeared to have Rh specificity.

Gilliland, Baxter and Evans (1971) reported further details of the application of the CFAC test to the investigation of patients suspected of suffering from AIHA, with particular reference to cases in which the conventional DAT tests using anti-IgG and anti-C sera were negative. The erythrocytes of five out of six such patients were in fact found to be coated with increased amounts of IgG (70–434 molecules per cell), and in two patients whose positive DAT test with an anti-IgG serum was reversible (i.e., it was immediately positive but became negative on standing) 160 and 700 molecules of IgG per cell were demonstrated. Gilliland, Baxter and Evans stated that patients varied with respect to the number of IgG molecules per erythrocyte necessary for the DAT to be visibly positive: the cells of some patients were agglutinated with as little as 150 molecules per cell whereas the cells of other patients had required more than 475. In their experience patients with AIHA in whom the DAT had been clearly positive with anti-IgG sera had had from 150 to 2000 molecules of IgG per cell.

Fischer, Petz and Garratty (1973) reported their early experience of the use of the CFAC test of Gilliland, Leddy and Vaughan (1970). Patients whose erythrocytes had given positive DATs had 331–1060 molecules of IgG per cell, while normal subjects and patients suffering from a congenital haemolytic anaemia had less than 60 molecules per cell. Three patients suspected of having AIHA but in whom the DAT using a range of anti-Ig and anti-C sera had been negative, and in whom tests for auto-antibodies in their sera using enzyme-treated cells had been negative, too, had 127–290 molecules of IgG per cell, according to the CFAC test.

ENZYME-LINKED IMMUNOSORBENT ASSAYS (ELISA)

The use of ELISA in the investigation of patients suspected of suffering from AIHA has provided a relatively simple and sensitive quantitative means of detecting auto-antibodies adsorbed to erythrocytes and free in serum and of determining the average number of IgG molecules coating the patients' erythrocytes. The application of the ELISA principle to antiglobulin tests (ELAT) dates from the early 1980s and has also been widely used in the detection of blood-group antibodies in blood transfusion practice.

Osborne and Giblett (1980) used alkaline phosphatase coupled to a rabbit anti-human globulin serum and fluorescent 4-methylumbelliferyl phosphate as substrate and found that the method was about four times as sensitive as that in routine use in detecting anti-c and anti-D allo-antibodies; it was shown, too, to be able to discriminate clearly, using anti-c, between the reactions of cells of Rh genotypes *cde/cde* and *CDe/cde*.

Leikola and Perkins (1980) used a rabbit anti-human IgG antibody conjugated with alkaline phosphatase and *p*-nitrophenyl phosphate as substrate. Using a variety of allo-antibodies, e.g. anti-D, anti-Fy[a] and anti-Jk[a], they demonstrated that the optical density of the coloured product read at 405 nm was linearly proportional to the concentration of antibodies to which the test erythrocytes had been exposed.

Bodensteiner and co-workers (1983) reported on six AIHA patients, four with a positive and two with a negative DAT, as well as on a control group of normal subjects and patients suffering from a variety of anaemias not caused by immune haemolysis. The erythrocytes of the controls had, according to ELISA, less than 54 molecules of IgG per cell, with the exception of a sample with 150 molecules per cell derived from a patient with myeloma. The four AIHA patients in whom the DAT was positive were calculated to have erythrocytes coated with 1100–26000 molecules of IgG per cell and the cells of the two patients in whom the DAT was negative 650–850 molecules per cell. Bodensteiner et al. concluded that there was a good correlation between the clinical picture, haemoglobin level and reticulocyte count and the number of IgG molecules per cell as estimated by ELISA and that the results reflected, too, the effect of treatment. The presence of more than 950 molecules of IgG per cell was usually associated with brisk haemolysis. Nonspecific binding of IgG did not usually interfere with the estimation, even in patients with raised serum IgG levels.

ENZYME-LINKED ANTIGLOBULIN TESTS (ELAT)

Leach (1984) tested an enzyme-linked DAT (ELAT), using alkaline phosphatase as enzyme, alongside a standard DAT in a study of 52 patients referred for investigation of possible AIHA. The ELAT was positive in 24 patients compared to 22 positive results with a DAT using an anti-IgG serum.

Lown and co-workers (1984) compared the efficiency of an ELAT, using alkaline phosphatase as the enzyme label, with a low ionic strength conventional antiglobulin test in the detection and quantitative assessment of 222 anti-erythrocyte antibodies of varying specificities. While a general correlation was found to exist between the ELAT results and agglutination in conventional antiglobulin tests, a wide range of ELAT readings were found to correspond to each agglutination grading. Rigal and co-workers (1984) described how they had used a modified ELAT in which glucose oxidase was used as the enzyme label. They reported that the technique was 10 times more sensitive than the ordinary indirect antiglobulin test and could detect allo-anti-D at a concentration of 1 ng/ml.

Sokol and co-workers (1985) reported their extensive experience in the application of an ELAT, using alkaline phosphatase (AP) as label, in the investigation of 219 patients suspected of suffering from AIHA. A comparison was made between the results obtained using monospecific anti-IgG, -IgA, -IgM, -C3c, -C3d, -C4 and broad-spectrum antiglobulin sera and AP-linked anti-IgG, -IgA, -IgM goat antiglobulin sera (Sigma). In 61 patients both the (conventional) DAT and ELAT were positive and detected the same Ig classes; in 43 patients both tests were positive, but additional Ig classes (e.g. IgM ± IgA) were detected by the ELAT; in 33 patients in whom the DAT was positive with anti-C reagents only, the ELAT detected in 22 of them IgM, IgG ± IgA or IgM in addition, and in 16 patients in whom the DAT was negative with all antisera, the ELAT was positive. There were 66 patients in whom both the DAT and ELAT were negative: in 61 there was no evidence of increased haemolysis, while in five in whom haemolysis was present, this was being produced by a non-immune mechanism. Based on a comparison with the results of quantitative radioimmune assays, Sokol et al. calculated that the ELAT would be positive if erythrocytes were coated with more than 100–120 molecules of IgG per cell. Sokol et al. also concluded that other Ig classes, e.g. IgM and IgA, were quite commonly bound to erythrocytes in amounts too small to be detected by conventional DATs; they, nevertheless, appeared to act synergistically with cell-bound IgG in bringing about haemolysis. Sokol et al. concluded, too, that in AIHA in which the patients' erythrocytes appeared to be coated with complement only, active haemolysis could often be correlated with IgM detected on their cells by ELAT.

Sokol and co-workers (1987) reported that they had used both an ELAT and a radioimmune antiglobulin test—of similar sensitivity—in the investigation of 585 patients referred to a reference centre: 158 of these patients were shown to have up to 200 molecules of IgG coating their erythrocytes and in these cases a highly significant association was found between the amount of bound IgG, IgA and IgM and the presence or absence of increased haemolysis. These results thus confirmed the clinical value of sensitive tests designed to demonstrate small amounts of cell-bound IgG in patients in whom the results of the DAT carried out conventionally would be negative or doubtful; the tests, too, detected previously unsuspected bound IgA and IgM.

Sokol et al. (1988) described a modified ELAT, using an alkaline-phosphatase-linked goat anti-human globulin serum and p-nitrophenylphosphate as substrate. This enabled them to demonstrate small amounts of IgG, IgM and IgA bound to the erythrocytes of healthy individuals and to establish a normal range.

Enzyme-linked antiglobulin consumption assay (ELACA)

Kiruba and Han (1988) used an enzyme-linked antiglobulin consumption assay (ELACA) for the detection and estimation of IgG, IgM and C3 bound to erythrocytes. This was a modification of one developed for the study of platelets; it uses microplates and commercially available reagents and peroxidase as enzyme. The ELACA test was found to be able to provide estimates for the small amounts of IgG, IgM and C3 found on normal erythrocytes, namely, 106 ± 60 molecules of IgG, 4.5 ± 3 molecules of IgM and 37 ± 29 molecules of C3. Higher than normal values of all three components were demonstrated on the erythrocytes of hospital patients suffering from a variety of illnesses, mostly severe infections, and it is interesting to note that in these patients the conventional DAT was negative. 1% normal rabbit serum added to the assay system markedly diminished the amount of IgG, IgM and C3 that had been demonstrable, suggesting that the immunoproteins bound to the erythrocyte of the hospital patients had not been bound to the cell membrane by their Fab portion but had been bound non-specifically as immune complexes via C3b or C4b receptors. Two patients with AIHA were also studied and very large numbers of IgG molecules were demonstrated on their erythrocytes. However, in these patients, in contrast to those suffering from severe infections, the number of molecules present was relatively little reduced by the introduction of rabbit serum into the assay system.

AUTO-AGGLUTINATION IN MEDIA OF HIGH PROTEIN CONTENT

The auto-agglutination of erythrocytes coated by incomplete antibodies when suspended in whole plasma or serum, as in whole blood, has already been commented on (p. 58). This is without doubt an important sign of sensitization, but it seems likely that a relatively heavy coating of antibody is required. It suffers, too, sometimes as a practical test because it may be difficult to distinguish true auto-agglutination from rouleaux formation.

Wiener (1945) reported that by using the 'conglutination technique' he was able to demonstrate that the blood of a patient with acquired haemolytic anaemia underwent auto-agglutination in vitro at 37°C, and this technique or modifications of it was at one time widely used as a direct test of erythrocyte sensitization. Such tests are on the whole, however, less satisfactory than the very sensitive direct antiglobulin reaction, although a case can be made for applying the two types of test side by side (see below).

Neber and Dameshek (1947) reported that the erythrocytes of five patients with 'idiopathic acquired hemolytic anemia' underwent auto-agglutination when the patients' cells, previously washed in saline, were resuspended as a 2% suspension in 20% bovine serum albumin.

Brüggemann and Hahn (1949) pointed out that incomplete warm antibodies needed the presence of a thermostable non-specific serum factor for auto-agglutination to take place and Braunsteiner, Reimer and Speiser (1951) showed, as had Neber and Dameshek (1947), that suspension in 20% albumin would bring this about. Later, Michon, Lochard and Chamaly (1954) reported that this could be brought about very effectively and rapidly if the patient's own serum, concentrated by freezing and thawing, was used.

Blessing and Heni (1953) and Heni and Blessing (1954b) had earlier reported that the washed erythrocytes of two patients with 'Loutit-type' AIHA and a positive DAT had undergone unusually rapid sedimentation when suspended in 6% dextran.

Evans (1955) and Evans and Weiser (1957) used a mixture of 30% bovine albumin and serum (? equal volumes of each) and the patient's cells in 5% suspension. The mixture was centrifuged at 1000 rpm for 1 minute and then inspected for agglutination. The cells of 18 out of 41 patients underwent agglutination in this way — as many as 37 out of the 41 samples were, however, agglutinated by antiglobulin serum, and Evans and Weiser concluded that the test was of little diagnostic value as the reactions were often weak or equivocal. However, in two cases the serum-albumin test was positive although the cells were not agglutinated by antiglobulin serum.

Jandl and Castle (1956), using erythrocytes sensitized with incomplete anti-D, compared the agglutination-enhancing property of various human plasma protein fractions as well as that of macromolecular substances such as carboxymethylcellulose, polyvinylpyrrolidone (PVP) and dextran. Concentration for concentration, fibrinogen was the most effective, PVP almost as effective and albumin the least effective! Seven patients with acquired haemolytic anaemia were investigated in different stages of activity. Auto-agglutination in 5% PVP occurred more readily than in 25% human albumin. The test appeared to be even more sensitive than agglutination by antiglobulin serum. In one case it was clearly (2+) positive when the antiglobulin test was negative and in another the test remained strongly positive (3–4+) at a time when three or more washings with saline had rendered the patient's cells inagglutinable by antiglobulin serum.

USE OF POLYBRENE AND PVP

Lalezari (1968) introduced into serological practice the use of Polybrene (hexadimethrine bromide), a synthetic positively charged polymer, that causes erythrocytes to agglutinate by neutralizing the cells' negative charge. This non-specific agglutination is reversed in hypertonic salt solutions. Cells that are coated by antibodies, however, remain agglutinated. Exposing erythrocytes to an antibody diluted appropriately in a low-ionic strength medium containing Polybrene is the basis of Lalezari's Polybrene test. If the reaction is allowed to take place in an AutoAnalyser, agglutination, if it persists after the cells are suspended in a hypertonic solution (0.2 mol/l trisodium citrate), can be recorded quantitatively. The cells that are agglutinated sediment and are discarded; those that remain in suspension are eventually lysed and the reduction in the optical density of the lysed suspension provides a quantitative measure of any agglutination that has taken place.

Lalezari and Oberhardt (1971) described how they had used the Polybrene technique to study in detail the effect of temperature on antibody activity. Working mainly with anti-Rh_0 (D), anti-M and anti-I, they obtained interesting and characteristic temperature gradient dissociation curves, representing the consequence of the dissociation of already established immunological bonds. Further details of the Polybrene test were given by Lalezari in his 1976 review 'Serologic profile in autoimmune hemolytic disease'.

Burkart and co-workers (1974) demonstrated the value of the AutoAnalyser in detecting and recording quantitatively agglutination brought about by a range of antiglobulin sera, as well as by antisera against κ and λ light chains and against the C3 and C4 complement components. The addition of K-90 polyvinylpyrrolidone (PVP) to the antisera was found to increase the sensitivity of the AutoAnalyser results.

Hsu and co-workers (1974) used the above technique in the investigation of 34 patients who had given positive DATs and had been diagnosed as, or suspected of, suffering from idiopathic or secondary AIHA. There were three categories of patients: 16 in whom there was no evidence of active haemolysis at the time they were studied; 13, forming warm antibodies, who were actively haemolysing; and five, forming cold antibodies, who were also actively haemolysing. In general, the results obtained by the PVP-augmented automated technique paralleled those of the conventional visually read manual method. Sometimes, however, there were significant differences. The automated technique, however, had the advantage that degrees of agglutination were expressed quantitatively as percentages. Hsu et al. were thus able to obtain a profile of fascinating immunological data, based on the use of a range of antisera, for each of the patients they had studied; and they were able, too, to relate the data to the clinical state of the patients and in a few patients to their response to treatment.

Górska and co-workers (1978) adapted an AutoAnalyser system as a simple screen for erythrocytes coated by warm auto-antibodies. The optical density of a 20% suspension of test erythrocytes was compared with that of a control solution of saline. A solution of bromelin and methylcellulose was then introduced into the system and any change in the optical density of the cell suspension recorded. The erythrocytes of 38 patients with warm-antibody AIHA were tested in this way and significant reductions in optical density occurred in each case. The manual DAT was clearly positive in 23 of these patients but it was negative or doubtful at the time of testing in 15 patients.

AUTO-AGGLUTINATION OF ENZYME-TREATED ERYTHROCYTES: THE BROMELIN TEST

van Loghem, van der Hart and Dorfmeier (1958) reported on the results they had obtained with a battery of direct tests; namely, the antiglobulin, albumin, papain and trypsin tests, the latter two tests being designed to demonstrate auto-agglutination of the patients' cells when trypsinized or papainized. The direct antiglobulin test proved by far the most sensitive: in 30 out of 62 patients this test alone was positive, but in one patient the antiglobulin test was negative and all others positive and in a further patient the papain test alone was positive. van Loghem and his co-workers made the point that a positive albumin test was a pointer to the antibody being a specific Rh auto-antibody.

Pirofsky (1960) and Osgood (1961) used a bromelin test. (Bromelin is a mixture of proteolytic enzymes obtained from pineapple stem.) Pirofsky described his results in 42 patients with auto-immune haemolytic anaemia, all of whom gave positive antiglobulin tests of the warm-antibody type. The results ran parallel, with the bromelin test being sometimes more sensitive; occasionally the reverse was true. Two false-positives due to the presence of cold agglutinins were noted in 441 control tests in which the DAT was negative, while in three patients with myeloma the presence of rouleaux made it impossible to carry out the test satisfactorily.

By 1961 Pirofsky and his co-workers were able to report on over 100 000 blood specimens that had been tested for allo- and auto-antibodies by both the bromelin and antiglobulin tests. In the case of warm auto-antibodies, 57 had been detected by the bromelin test and one had not; using antiglobulin sera, 52 had been detected and six not detected. Pirofsky et al. stressed the value of using more than one test, e.g. the antiglobulin test and an enzyme test, in screening for antibodies. They stressed that up to the time of their report they had not encountered a single antibody, undetected by the antiglobulin and bromelin tests, that had given a positive albumin test.

ERYTHROCYTE–ANTIBODY (EA) ROSETTE FORMATION

Galili, Manny and Izak (1981) used the K-562 cell line (an erythro-myeloid line obtained from a chronic granulocytic leukaemia patient in blast crisis), which possesses Fc receptors in abundance, to detect subagglutinating amounts of antibodies attached to erythrocytes. According to Galili, Manny and Izak, it is possible in this way to increase the sensitivity of the antiglobulin test up to 50-fold without loss of specificity. The binding of at least five erythrocytes to a K-562 cell constitutes a positive test. Of 50 normal blood samples, 41 formed no positive rosettes and nine formed not more than 4% of positive rosettes. Six patients with DAT-negative AIHA were studied. The EA DAT test was positive in all six, with from 13% to 50% of the K-562 cells forming rosettes.

REFERENCES

ANDO, S. (1965). Clinical studies on autoimmune hemolytic anemia. I. Serological studies on free autoantibodies in serum. *Acta haemat. jap.*, **28**, 623–630.

ANDRÉ, R. & NAJMAN, A. (1967). Aspects actuels des anémies hémolytiques acquises à auto-anticorps. *Presse méd.*, **75**, 2703–2708.

ANDRZEJEWSKI, C. JNR, YOUNG, P. J., CINES, D. B. & SILBERSTEIN, L. E. (1991). Heterogeneity of human red cell autoantibodies assessed by isoelectric focusing. *Transfusion*, **31**, 236–244.

BAKEMEIER, R. F. & LEDDY, J. P. (1967a). Heavy chain: light chain relationships among erythrocyte autoantibodies. *J. clin. Invest.*, **46**, 1033 (Abstract).

BAKEMEIER, R. F. & LEDDY, J. P. (1967b). Structural characteristics of erythrocyte autoantibodies: recent studies and implications. *Blood*, **30**, 869 (Abstract).

BAUMGARTNER, W. (1952). Zur Klinik der serologisch bedingten hämolytischen Anämie. *Helv. med. Acta*, **19**, 71–94.

BELL, C. A., ZWICKER, H. & SACKS, H. J. (1973). Autoimmune hemolytic anemia: routine serologic evaluation in a general hospital population. *Amer. J. clin. Path.*, **60**, 903–911.

BEN-IZHAK, C., SHECHTER, Y. & TATARSKY, I. (1985). Significance of multiple types of antibodies on red blood cells of patients with positive direct antiglobulin test: a study of monospecific antiglobulin reactions in 85 patients. *Scand. J. Haemat.*, **35**, 102–108.

BLESSING, K. & HENI, K. (1953). Senkung gewaschener roter Blutkörperchen in Dextran als Nachweis gesteigerter Ballungsbereitschaft durch Aufladung mit inkompletten Antikörpern. *Medizinische*, **38**, 1229–1236.

BODENSTEINER, D., BROWN, P., SKIKNE, B. & PLAPP, F. (1983). The enzyme-linked immunosorbent assay: accurate detection of red blood cell antibodies in autoimmune hemolytic anemia. *Amer. J. clin. Path.*, **78**, 182–185.

BOORMAN, K. E., DODD, B. E. & LOUTIT, J. F. (1946). Haemolytic icterus (acholuric jaundice) congenital and acquired. *Lancet*, **i**, 812–814.

BOURONCLE, B. A., DODD, M. C. & WRIGHT, C.-S. (1951). A study of cold hemagglutinins for normal and typsinized red blood cells in the serum of normal individuals and of hemolytic anemias. *J. Immunol.*, **67**, 265–279.

BRAUNSTEINER, H., REIMER, E. E. & SPEISER, P. (1951). Schwere hämolytische Anämie mit blockierenden inkompletten Antikörpern. *Wien. Z.inn. Med.*, **32**, 157–162.

BROWNING, C. H. (1931). General properties of antigens and antibodies. In *A System of Bacteriology in Relation to Medicine*, Vol. 6, p. 220. Medical Research Council. His Majesty's Stationary Office, London.

BRÜGGEMANN, W. & HAHN, F. (1949). Über unvollständige Autoagglutinine ('Warmeagglutinine') bein hämolytischen Ikterus. *Ärztl. Wschr.*, **4**, 403–406.

BURKART, P., ROSENFIELD, R. E., HSU, T. C. S., WONG, K. Y., NUSBACHER, J., SHAIKH, S. H. & KOCHWA, S. (1974). Instrumental PVP-augmented antiglobulin tests. I. Detection of allogeneic antibodies coating otherwise normal erythrocytes. *Vox Sang.*, **26**, 289–304.

CASSELL, M. & CHAPLIN, H. JNR (1960). Studies on anti-eluate sera. II. Comparison of a conventional antiglobulin serum with three anti-eluate sera in the study of 70 patients with acquired hemolytic anemia. *Vox Sang.*, **5**, 43–52.

CEPPELLINI, R. et al. (14 authors) (1964). Nomenclature for human immunoglobulins. *Bull. Wld Hlth Org.*, **30**, 447–450.

CHAPLIN, H. JNR (1973). Clinical usefulness of specific antiglobulin reagents in autoimmune hemolytic anemia. *Progr. Hemat.*, **8**, 25–49.

CHAPLIN, H. JNR & CASSELL, M. (1958). The heterogeneity of positive antiglobulin reactions in acquired hemolytic anemia. *J. Lab. clin. Med.*, **53**, 803 (Abstract).

CHAPLIN, H. JNR & CASSELL, M. (1960). Studies in anti-eluate sera. I. The production of antiglobulin (Coombs) sera in rabbits by the use of antibodies eluted from sensitized red blood cells. *Vox Sang.*, **5**, 32–42.

CHAPLIN, H. JNR & MONROE, M. C. (1986). Comparisons of pooled polyclonal rabbit anti-human C3d with four monoclonal mouse anti-human C3ds. II. Quantitation of RBC-bound C3d, and characterization of antiglobulin agglutination reactions against RBC from 27 patients with autoimmune hemolytic anemia. *Vox Sang.*, **50**, 87–93.

CHAUFFARD, M. A. & VINCENT, C. (1909). Hémoglobinurie hémolysinique avec ictère polycholique aigu. *Sem. méd.*, **29**, 601–604.

CLARK, D. A., DESSYPRIS, E. N., JENKINS, D. E. JNR & KRANTZ, S. B. (1984). Acquired immune hemolytic anemia associated with IgA erythrocyte coating: investigation of the hemolytic mechanisms. *Blood*, **64**, 1000–1005.

COOMBS, R. R. A. (1970). History and evolution of the antiglobulin reaction and its application in clinical and experimental medicine (Philip Levine Award Address). *Amer. J. clin. Path.*, **53**, 131–135.

COOMBS, R. R. A. & MOURANT, A. E. (1947). On certain properties of antisera prepared against human serum and its various protein fractions: their use in the detection of sensitisation of human red cells with "incomplete" Rh antibody, and on the nature of this antibody. *J. Path. Bact.*, **59**, 105–111.

COSTEA, N., SCHWARTZ, R., CONSTANTOULAKIS, M. &

DAMESHEK. W. (1962). The use of radioactive antiglobulin for the detection of erythrocyte sensitization. *Blood*, **20**, 214–232.

CRAWFORD, H. & MOLLISON, P. L. (1951). Demonstration of multiple antibodies in antiglobulin sera. *Lancet*, **ii**, 955–957.

CUTBUSH, M., CRAWFORD, H. & MOLLISON, P. L. (1955). Observations on anti-human globulin sera. *Brit. J Haemat.*, **1**, 410–421.

DACIE, J. V. (1951). Differences in the behaviour of sensitized red cells to agglutination by antiglobulin sera. *Lancet*, **ii**, 954–955.

DACIE, J. V. (1953). Acquired hemolytic anemia. With special reference to the antiglobulin (Coombs') reaction. *Blood*, **8**, 813–823.

DACIE, J. V. (1954). *The Haemolytic Anaemias: Congenital and Acquired*, 525 pp. Churchill, London.

DACIE, J. V. (1955). The auto-immune haemolytic anaemias. *Amer. J. Med.*, **18**, 810–821.

DACIE, J. V. (1957). The cold haemagglutinin syndrome. *Proc. roy. Soc. Med.*, **50**, 647–650.

DACIE, J. V. (1958). Auto-immune haemolytic anaemias. *Acta haemat. (Basel)*, **20**, 131–136.

DACIE, J. V. (1959). Acquired haemolytic anaemia. In *Lectures on the Scientific Basis of Medicine, Vol. 7 (1957–58)*, pp. 59–79. University of London, Athlone Press, London.

DACIE, J. V. (1960). Acquired haemolytic anaemia. In *Lectures on Haematology*, pp. 1–17. University Press, Cambridge.

DACIE, J. V. (1962). *The Haemolytic Anaemias: Congenital and Acquired. Part II – The Auto-immune Haemolytic Anaemias*, 2nd edn, 377 pp. Churchill, London.

DACIE, J. V. (1975). Autoimmune hemolytic anemia. *Arch. intern. Med.*, **135**, 1293–1300.

DACIE, J. V., CROOKSTON, J. H. & CHRISTENSON, W. N. (1957). 'Incomplete' cold antibodies: role of complement in sensitization to antiglobulin serum by potentially haemolytic antibodies. *Brit. J. Haemat.*, **3**, 77–87.

DACIE, J. V. & DE GRUCHY G. C. (1951). Auto-antibodies in acquired haemolytic anaemia. *J. clin. Path.*, **4**, 253–271.

DACIE, J. V. & WORLLEDGE, S. M. (1969). Auto-immune hemolytic anemias. *Progr. Hemat.*, **6**, 82–120.

DAMESHEK, W. (1951). Acquired hemolytic anemia: Physiopathology with particular reference to autoimmunization and therapy. *Proc. 3rd Congr. int. Soc. Hemat., Cambridge*, pp. 120–133. Grune and Stratton, New York.

DAUSSET, J. & COLOMBANI, J. (1958). Étude statistique et pronostique de 100 cas d'anémie hémolytique immunologique. *Acta haemat. (Basel)*, **20**, 137–146.

DAUSSET, J. & COLOMBANI, J. (1959). The serology and the prognosis of 128 cases of autoimmune hemolytic anemia. *Blood*, **14**, 1280–1301.

DAVIDSOHN, I. & SPURRIER, W. (1954). Immunohematological studies in hemolytic anemia. *J. Amer. med. Ass.*, **154**, 818–821.

DEAN, H. R. (1917). The mechanism of the serum reactions. *Lancet*, **i**, 45–50.

DENYS, P. & VAN DEN BROUCKE, J. (1947). Anémie hémolytique acquise et réaction de Coombs. *Arch. franç. Pédiat.*, **4**, 205–217.

ENGELFRIET, C. P., BECKERS, TH. A. P., VAN'T VEER, M. B., VON DEM BORNE, A. E. G. KR. & OUWEHAND, W. H. (1983). Recent advances in immune haemolytic anaemia. In *Recent Advances in Haematology, Immunology and Blood Transfusion* (ed. by S. R. Hollán, I Bernát, G. Füst, G. Gárdos & B. Sarkadi), pp. 235–252. John Wiley and Akademiai Kiado, Budapest.

ENGELFRIET, C. P., OUWEHAND, W. H., VAN'T VEER, M. B., BECKERS, D., MAAS, N. & VON DEM BORNE, A. E. G. KR. (1987). Autoimmune haemolytic anaemias. *Baillieres Clin. Immunol. Allergy*, **1**, 251–267.

ENGELFRIET, C. P., PONDMAN, K. W., WOLTERS, G., VON DEM BORNE, A. E. G. KR., BECKERS, D., MISSET-GROENVELD, G. & VAN LOGHEM J. J. (1970). Autoimmune haemolytic anaemias. III. Preparation and examination of specific antisera against complement components and products, and their use in serological studies. *Clin. exp. Immunol.*, **6**, 721–732.

ENGELFRIET, C. P., VON DEM BORNE, A. E. G. KR., BECKERS, D. & VAN LOGHEM, J. J. (1974). Autoimmune haemolytic anaemia; serological and immunochemical characteristics of the autoantibodies; mechanisms of cell destruction. *Ser. Haemat.*, **7**, 328–347.

ENGELFRIET, C. P., VON DEM BORNE, A. E. G. KR., MOES, M. & VAN LOGHEM. J. J. (1968a). Serological studies in autoimmune haemolytic anaemia. *Proc. 11th Congr. int. Soc. Blood Transf., Sydney, 1966. Bibl. haemat.*, No. 29, Part 2, pp. 473–478. Karger, Basel.

ENGELFRIET, C. P., VON DEM BORNE, A. E. G. KR., VAN DEN GIESSEN, M., BECKERS, D. & VAN LOGHEM. J. J. (1968b). Autoimmune haemolytic anaemia. I. Serological studies with pure anti-immunoglobulin reagents. *Clin. exp. Immunol.*, **3**, 605–614.

EVANS, R. S. (1955). Autoantibodies in hematologic disorders. *Stanford med. Bull.*, **13**, 152–166.

EVANS, R. S. & DUANE, R. T. (1949). Acquired hemolytic anemia. I. The relation of antibody activity to activity of the disease. II. The significance of thrombocytopenia and leukopenia. *Blood*, **4**, 1196–1213.

EVANS, R. S., DUANE, R. T. & BEHRENDT, V. (1947). Demonstration of antibodies in acquired hemolytic anemia with anti-human globulin serum. *Proc. Soc. exp. Biol. Med.*, **64**, 372–375.

EVANS, R. S. & WEISER, R. S. (1957). The serology of autoimmune hemolytic disease: observations on forty-one patients. *Arch. intern. Med.*, **100**, 371–399.

EYSTER, M. E. & JENKINS, D. E. JNR (1969). Erythrocyte coating substances in patients with positive direct antiglobulin reactions. Correlation of γG globulin and complement coating with underlying diseases, overt hemolysis and response to therapy. *Amer. J. Med.*, **46**, 360–371.

EYSTER, M. E., NACHMAN, R. L., CHRISTENSON, W. N. & ENGLE, R. L. JNR (1966). Structural characteristics of red cell autoantibodies. *J. Immunol.*, **96**, 107–111.

FAGIOLO, E. & LAGHI, V. (1970). Caratterizzazione immunochimica degli anticorpi eritocitari nelle anemie emolitiche autoimmuni (Test di Coombs diretto con antisieri specifici). *Progresso medico (Roma)*, **26**, 280–283.

FIRKIN, B. G. (1958). The nature of the adsorbed antibody in acquired haemolytic anaemia. *Austr. J. exp. Biol.*, **36**, 359–364.

FISCHER, J., PETZ, L. D. & GARRATTY, G. (1973). Characterization of immune hemolytic anemias with negative direct antiglobulin (Coombs') test. *Clin. Res.*, **21**, 265 (Abstract).

FUDENBERG, H., BARRY, I. & DAMESHEK, W. (1958). The erythrocyte-coating substance in autoimmune hemolytic disease: its nature and significance. *Blood*, **13**, 201–215.

FULTON ROBERTS, G. (1950). The anti-globulin reaction. *Proc. int. Soc. Hemat., Cambridge, 1950*, pp. 147–154. Grune and Stratton, New York.

GALILI, U., MANNY, N. & IZAK, G. (1981). EA rosette formation: a simple means to increase sensitivity of the antiglobulin test in patients with anti red cell antibodies. *Brit. J. Haemat.*, **47**, 227–233.

GANDINI, E. (1959). Comportamento dei siere anti-globuline nell' emoagglutinazione del tipo cosiddetto non gamma-globulinico. *Proc. 7th Congr. int. soc. Blood Transf.*, pp. 516–519. Karger, Basel.

GERBAL, A., HOMBERG, J. C., ROCHANT, H., LIBERGE, G., DELARUE, F. & SALMON, CH. (1967). Nouvelle classification immunologique des anémies hémolytiques avec auto-anticorps. *Nouv. Rev. franç. Hémat.*, **7**, 401–406.

GERBAL, A., HOMBERG, J. C., ROCHANT, H., PERRON, L. & SALMON, CH. (1968a). Les auto-anticorps d'anémies hémolytiques acquises. I. Analyse de 234 observations. *Nouv. Rev. franç. Hémat.*, **8**, 155–178.

GERBAL, A., HOMBERG, J. C., ROCHANT, H., PERRON, L. & SALMON CH. (1968b). Les auto-anticorps d'anémies hémolytiques acquises. II. Nature, spécificité, intérêt clinique et mécanisme de formation. *Nouv. Rev. franç. Hemat.*, **8**, 351–368.

GILLILAND, B. C., BAXTER, E., & EVANS, R. S. (1971). Red-cell antibodies in acquired hemolytic anemia with negative antiglobulin serum tests. *New Engl. J. Med.*, **185**, 252–256.

GILLILAND, B. C., LEDDY, J. P. & VAUGHAN, J. H.

(1970). The detection of cell-bound antibody on complement-coated human red cells. *J. clin. Invest.*, **49**, 898–906.

GÓRSKA, B., MICHAEL-ARASZKIEWICZ, P., SEYFRIED, H. & ZUPÁNSKA, B. (1978). Automated screening of red cells for the detection of autoantibodies. *Vox Sang.*, **35**, 248–250.

HABERMAN, S. (1958). On the specificity and reactivity of Coombs' antiglobulin sera. *Blood*, **13**, 688–693.

HACKETT, E. (1950). Coombs test in acute acquired haemolytic anaemia. *Lancet*, **i**, 998–999.

HARBOE, M., MÜLLER-EBERHARD, H. J., FUDENBERG, H., POLLEY, M. J. & MOLLISON P. L. (1963). Identification of the components of complement participating in the antiglobulin reaction. *Immunology*, **6**, 412–420.

HENI, F. & BLESSING, K. (1954a). Die Bedeutung der Glutinine für die erworbenen hämolytischen Anämien. *Dtsch. Arch. klin. Med.*, **201**, 113–135.

HENI, F. & BLESSING, K. (1954b). Beschreibung zwier schwerer erworbener idiopathischer hämolytischer Anämien. *Klin. Wschr.*, **32**, 481–485.

HENNEMANN, H. H. (1957). *Erworbene hämolytische Anämien: Klinik und Serologie*, 198 pp. Georg Thieme, Leipzig.

HILL, J. M. & HABERMAN, S. (1954). The Coombs (antiglobulin test): indications and technics. *Amer. J. clin. Path.*, **24**, 305–320.

HOLLÄNDER, L. (1957). Die erworbenen hämolytischen Anämien. A. Serologie der erworbenen hämolytischen Anamien. In *Immunopathologie in Klinik und Forschung und das Problem der Autoantikörper* (ed. by P. Miescher and K. O. Vorländer) pp.180–259. Georg Thieme, Stuttgart.

HOMBERG, J. -C., CARTRON, J. & SALMON, CH. (1971). Intérêts pratiques de l'étude immunologique des anémies hémolytiques auto-immunes. *Rev. Prat. (Paris)*, **21**, 1357–1375.

HSU, T. C. S., ROSENFIELD, R. E., BURKART, P., WONG, K. Y. & KOCHWA, S. (1974). Instrumental PVP-augmented antiglobulin tests. II. Evaluation of acquired hemolytic anemia. *Vox Sang.*, **26**, 305–325.

HUBINONT, P. O. & MASSART-GUIOT, T. (1955). La sérologie de l'autoimmunisation dans ses rapports avec les anémies hémolytiques. *Acta clin. belg.*, **10**, 20–32.

HUGHES-JONES, N. C. (1975). Red-cell antigens, antibodies and their interaction. *Clinics Haemat.*, **4**, 29–43.

ISSITT, P. D. (1977). Autoimmune hemolytic anemia and cold hemagglutinin disease: clinical disease and laboratory findings. In *Progress in Clinical Pathology, Vol. VII* (ed. by M. Stefanini et al.), pp. 137–163. Grune and Stratton, New York.

ISSITT, P. D. (1985). Serological diagnosis and characterization of the causative autoantibodies. In *Immune Hemolytic Anemias (Methods in Hematology,*

Vol. 12) (ed. by H. Chaplin Jnr), pp. 1–34. Churchill Livingstone, New York.

ISSITT, P. D., PAVONE, B. G., GOLDFINGER, D., ZWICKER, H., ISSITT, C. H., TESSEL, J. A., KROOVAND, S. W. & BELL, C. A. (1976). Anti-Wr[b], and other autoantibodies responsible for positive direct antiglobulin tests in 150 individuals. *Brit. J. Haemat.*, **34**, 5–18.

JANDL, J. H. & CASTLE, W. B. (1956). Agglutination of sensitized red cells by large anisometric molecules. *J. Lab. clin. Med.*, **47**, 669–685.

JANDL, J. H. & SIMMONS, R. L. (1957). The agglutination and sensitization of red cells by metallic cations: interactions between multivalent metals and the red-cell membrane. *Brit. J. Haemat.*, **3**, 19–38.

JEANNET, M. (1965). Observations sur la spécificité du test de Coombs direct dans les anémies hémolytiques 'auto-immunes'. *Schweiz. med. Wschr*, **95**, 1442–1444.

JEANNET, M. (1966). Specificity of the antiglobulin test in 'auto-immune' hemolytic anemias. *Helv. med. Acta*, **33**, 151–163.

JENKINS, D. E. JNR, MOORE, W. H. & HAWIGER, A. (1977). A method for radioactive antiglobulin testing with ^{125}I labeled anti-IgG. *Transfusion*, **17**, 16–22.

JENKINS, G. C., POLLEY, M. J. & MOLLISON, P. L. (1960). Role of C'$_4$ in the antiglobulin reaction. *Nature (Lond.)*, **186**, 482–483.

JORDAN, W. S. JNR & DINGLE, J. H. (1949). Coombs titer variations in acquired hemolytic anemia. *J. Lab. clin. Med.*, **34**, 1614–1615 (Abstract).

KAY, N. E., DOUGLAS, S. D., MOND, J. J., FLIER, J. S., KOCHWA, S. & ROSENFIELD, R. E. (1975). Hemolytic anemia with serum and erythrocyte-bound low-molecular-weight IgM. *Clin. Immunol. Immunopath.*, **4**, 216–225.

KEMPPINEN, E., VUOPIO, P., SANDSTRÖM, P. & WAGER, O. (1981). Significance of monospecific antisera in the diagnosis and prognosis of autoimmune haemolytic anaemias. *Ann. clin. Res.*, **13**, 85–90.

KERR, R. O., DALMASSO, A. P. & KAPLAN, M. E. (1971). Erythrocyte-bound C5 and C6 in autoimmune hemolytic anemia. *J. Immunol.*, **107**, 1209–1210.

KIDD, P. (1949). Elution of an incomplete type of antibody from the erythrocytes in acquired haemolytic anaemia. *J. clin. Path.*, **2**, 103–108.

KIRUBA, P. & HAN, P. (1988). Quantitation of red cell-bound immunoglobulin and complement using enzyme-linked antiglobulin consumption assay. *Transfusion*, **28**, 519–524.

KONDA, S. & YAMADA, A. (1960). Characteristics of the auto-antibody attached to erythrocytes of the patient with auto-immune hemolytic anemia. *Acta haemat. Jap.*, **23**, 879–886.

LACHMANN, P. J., VOAK, D., OLDROYD, R. G., DOWNIE, D. M. & BEVAN, P. C. (1983). Use of monoclonal anti-C3 antibodies to characterise the fragments of C3 that are found on erythrocytes. *Vox Sang.*, **45**, 367–372.

LALEZARI, P. (1968). A new method for detection of red blood cell antibodies. *Transfusion*, **8**, 372–380.

LALEZARI, P. (1976). Serologic profile in autoimmune hemolytic disease: pathophysiologic and clinical interpretations. *Seminars Hemat.*, **13**, 291–310.

LALEZARI, P. & OBERHARDT, B. (1971). Temperature gradient dissociation of red cell antigen–antibody complexes in the Polybrene technique. *Brit. J. Haemat.*, **21**, 131–146.

LEACH, M. (1984). A direct enzyme-linked antiglobulin test for detection of red cell autoantibodies in auto-immune haemolytic anaemia. *Med. lab. Sciences*, **41**, 232–237.

LE PETIT, J. -C. & BRIZARD, C. P. (1971). Allotypie et isotypie des auto-anticorps des anémies hémolytiques auto-immunes type IgG. *Nouv. Rev. franç. Hémat.*, **11**, 255–260.

LE PETIT, J. C., RIVAT, L., FRANCOIS, N., ROPARTZ, C. & BRIZARD, C. P. (1976). Expression of genetic markers of erythrocyte immunoglobulin G autoantibodies in autoimmune hemolytic anemia. *Vox Sang.*, **31**, 183–190.

LEDDY, J. P. (1966). Immunological aspects of red cell injury in man. *Seminars Hemat.*, **3**, 48–73.

LEDDY, P. & BAKEMEIER, R. F. (1964). The L-chain types of erythrocyte autoantibodies. *J. clin. Invest.*, **43**, 1300 (Abstract).

LEDDY, J. P. & BAKEMEIER, R. F. (1965). Structural aspects of human erythrocyte autoantibodies. I. L chain types and electrophoretic dispersion. *J. exp. Med.*, **121**, 1–17.

LEDDY, J. P., BAKEMEIER, R. F. & VAUGHAN. J. H. (1965). Fixation of complement components to autoantibody eluted from human RBC. *J. clin. Invest.*, **44**, 1066 (Abstract).

LEDDY, J. P., HILL, R. W., SWISHER, S. N. & VAUGHAN, J. H. (1963). Observations on the immunochemical nature of red cell autosensitization. In *Immunopathology, Third int. Symp.* (ed. by P. Grabar and P. A. Miescher), pp. 318–331. Grune and Stratton, New York.

LEDDY, J. P., TRABOLD, N. C., VAUGHAN, J. H. & SWISHER, S. N. (1962). The unitary nature of 'complete' and 'incomplete' pathologic cold hemagglutinins. *Blood*, **19**, 379–396.

LEIKOLA, J. & PERKINS, H. A. (1980). Enzyme-linked antiglobulin test: an accurate and simple method to quantify red cell antibodies. *Transfusion*, **20**, 138–144.

LITWIN, S. D., BALABAN, S. & EYSTER, M. E. (1973). Gm allotype preference in erythocyte IgG antibodies of patients with autoimmune hemolytic anemia. *Blood*, **42**, 241–246.

LOUTIT, J. F. & MOLLISON, P. L. (1946). Haemolytic icterus (acholuric jaundice), congenital and acquired. *J. Path. Bact.*, **58**, 771–778.

LOWN, J. A. G., DAVIS, R. E., KELLY, A., BARR, A. L. & GIBSON, D. L. (1984). Evaluation of an enzyme-linked antiglobulin test for the detection of red cell antibodies. *Vox Sang.*, **47**, 157–163.

MARRACK, J. R. (1938). *The Chemistry of Antigens and Antibodies*. Medical Research Council Special Report, series No. 230. His Majesty's Stationary Office, London.

MICHON, P., LOCHARD, & CHAMALY, P. (1954). Anémie hémolytique acquise transitoire avec auto- et iso-anticorps. *Sang*, **25**, 521–524.

MILLET, M. & FINCLER, L. (1946). Remarques sur les affinités de l'auto-agglutinine (cold agglutinin) du sérum humain. *C. R. Soc. Biol. (Paris)*, **140**, 1226–1227.

MILLET, M. & HUBINOUT, P. O. (1946). Modification de l'optimum thermique de certaines agglutinines naturelles sous l'influence de l'immunisation. *C. R. Soc. Biol. (Paris)*, **140**, 1227–1228.

MOULINIER, J. (1956). Technique de la réaction de consommation d'antiglobuline. *Rev. franç. Ét. clin. biol.*, **1**, 355–364.

MOURANT, A. E. (1983). The discovery of the anti-globulin test. *Vox Sang.*, **45**, 180–183.

MUELLER-ECKHARDT, C. & KRETSCHMER, V. (1972). Autoimmune hemolytic anemias. I. Investigations on immunoglobulin type and complement fixation of cell-fixed and eluable autoantibodies. *Blut*, **25**, 63–76.

NANCE, S., BOURDO, S. & GARRATTY, G. (1983). IgG2 red cell sensitization associated with autoimmune hemolytic anemia. *Transfusion*, **23**, 413 (Abstract).

NANCE, S. & GARRATTY, G. (1983). Subclass of IgG on red cells of donors and patients with positive direct antiglobulin tests. *Transfusion*, **23**, 413 (Abstract).

NEBER, J. & DAMESHEK, W. (1947). The improved demonstration of circulating antibodies in hemolytic anemia by the use of bovine albumin. *Blood*, **2**, 371–380.

OBERHARDT, B. J., LALEZARI, P. & JIANG, A. F. (1973). A physicochemical approach to the characterization of red cell antigen–antibody systems. *Immunology*, **24**, 445–453.

OSBORNE, W. R. A. & GIBLETT, E. R. (1980). Enzyme-linked immunosorbent assay for the indirect anti-human globulin test. *Acta haemat. (Basel)*, **63**, 124–127.

OSGOOD, E. E. (1961). Antiglobulin-positive hemolytic anemias. *Arch. intern. Med.*, **107**, 313–323.

PETZ, L. D. & GARRATTY. G. (1980). *Acquired Immune Hemolytic Anemias*, 458 pp. Churchill Livingstone, New York.

PIROFSKY. B. (1960). A new diagnostic test for antiglobulin positive ('auto-immune') haemolytic anaemia. *Brit. J. Haemat.*, **6**, 395–401.

PIROFSKY, B., NELSON, H., IMEL, T. & CORDOVA, M. (1961). The present status of the antiglobulin and bromelin tests in demonstrating erythrocyte antibodies. *Amer. J. clin. Path.*, **36**, 492–499.

PISCIOTTA, A. V. & HINZ, J. E. (1957). Detection and characterization of autoantibodies in acquired auto-immune hemolytic anemia. *Amer. J. clin. Path.*, **27**, 619–634.

PONDMAN, K. W., ROSENFIELD, R. E., TALLAL, L. & WASSERMAN, L. R. (1960). The specificity of the complement antiglobulin test. *Vox Sang.*, **5**, 297–319.

REUSSER, P., OSTERWALDER, B., BURRI, H. & SPECK, B. (1987). Autoimmune hemolytic anemia associated with IgA—diagnostic and therapeutic aspects of a case with long-term follow-up. *Acta haemat. (Basel)*, **77**, 53–56.

RIGAL, D., MONESTIER, M., LAFONT, S., RAFFIN, T., GOT, A., MEYER, F. & JOUVENCEAUX, A. (1984). Improvement of enzyme-linked antiglobulin test by using an antiglobulin linked to glucose oxidase: description of the technique. *Vox Sang.*, **46**, 349–354.

ROSENFIELD, R. E., HABER, G. V. & GILBERT, H. S. (1960). Complement and the antiglobulin test. *Vox Sang.*, **5**, 182–200.

ROSENFIELD, R. E., VOGEL, P. & ROSENTHAL, N. (1951). The antiglobulin test. Technic and practical applications. *Amer. J. clin. Path.*, **21**, 301–318.

ROSSE, W. F. (1975). The antiglobulin test in autoimmune hemolytic anemia. *Ann. Rev. Med.*, **26**, 331–336.

SALAMA, A., BHAKDI, S., MUELLER-ECKHARDT, C. & KAYSER. W. (1983). Deposition of the terminal C5b-9 complement complex on erythrocytes by human red cell autoantibodies. *Brit. J. Haemat.*, **55**, 161–169.

SALMON, C., HOMBERG, J. C. & HABIBI, B. (1975). Immunologie des anémies hémolytiques auto-immune (Première partie). *Rev. franç. Transf. Immuno-hémat.*, **18**, 301–320.

SCHMITZ, N., DJIBEY, I., KRETSCHMER, V., MAHN, I. & MUELLER-ECKHARDT, C. (1981). Assessment of red cell autoantibodies in autoimmune hemolytic anemia of warm type by a radioactive anti-IgG test. *Vox Sang.*, **41**, 224–230.

SCHREIBER, A. (1985). Quantitation of RBC-bound immunoglobulin and complement components. In *Immune Hemolytic Anemias* (ed. by H. Chaplin Jnr), pp. 155–175. Churchill Livingstone, New York.

SCHUBOTHE, H. (1958). *Serologie und klinische Bedeutung der Autohämantikörper*, 284 pp. Karger, Basel.

SCHUBOTHE, H. (1959). Die Serologie der erworbenen hämolytischen Erkrankungen. *Proc. 7th Congr. int. Soc. Blood Transf.*, Rome, Sept. 3–6, 1958, pp. 827–835. Karger, Basel.

SHIREY, R. S., McCANN, E. L., KICKLER, T. S. & NESS, P. M. (1989). IgM autoantibodies in warm autoimmune hemolytic anemia. *Transfusion*, **29**, Suppl, 17S (Abstract S47).

SINGER, K. & MOTULSKY, A. G. (1949). The developing (Coombs) test in spherocytic hemolytic anemias. Its significance for the pathophysiology of spherocytosis and splenic hemolysis. *J. Lab. clin. Med.*, **34**, 768–783.

SOKOL, R. J., HEWITT, S., BOOKER, D. J. & BAILEY, A. (1990). Erythrocyte autoantibodies, subclasses of IgG and autoimmune haemolysis. *Autoimmunity*, **6**, 99–104.

SOKOL, R. J., HEWITT, S., BOOKER, D. J., & STAMPS, R. (1985). Enzyme linked direct antiglobulin tests in patients with autoimmune haemolysis. *J. clin. Path.*, **38**, 912–914.

SOKOL, R. J., HEWITT, S., BOOKER, D. J. & STAMPS, R. (1987). Small quantities of erythrocyte bound immunoglobulins and autoimmune haemolysis. *J. clin. Path.*, **40**, 254–257.

SOKOL, R. J., HEWITT, S., BOOKER, D. J., STAMPS, R. & BOOTH, J. R. (1988). An enzyme-linked direct antiglobulin test for assessing erythrocyte bound immunoglobulins. *J. Immun. Methods*, **106**, 31–35.

STRATTON, F., RAWLINSON, V. I., CHAPMAN, A., PENGELLY, C. D. R. & JENNINGS, R. C. (1972). Acquired hemolytic anemia associated with IgA anti-e. *Transfusion*, **12**, 157–161.

STURGEON, P. (1947). A new antibody in serum of patients with acquired hemolytic anemia. *Science*, **106**, 293–294.

STURGEON, P., SMITH, L. E., CHUN, H. M. T., HURVITZ, C. H., GARRATTY, G. & GOLDFINGER, D. (1979). Autoimmune hemolytic anemia associated exclusively with IgA of Rh specificity. *Transfusion*, **19**, 324–328.

SUZUKI, S., AMANO, T., MITSUNAGA, M., YAGYU, F. & OFUJI, T. (1981). Autoimmune hemolytic anemia associated with IgA autoantibody. *Clin. Immunol. Immunopath.*, **21**, 247–256.

SWISHER, S. N., TRABOLD, N., LEDDY, J. P. & VAUGHAN, J. (1965). Clinical correlations of the direct antiglobulin reaction. *Ann. N. Y. Acad. Sci.*, **124**, 441–447.

VAN LOGHEM, J. J. (1950). Serological investigations of the anti-human globulin serum (serum of Coombs) with special reference to the pathogenesis of erythroblastosis foetalis. *Maandschr. Kindergeneesk.*, **18**, 115–126.

VAN LOGHEM, J. J., KRESNER, M., COOMBS, R. R. A. & FULTON ROBERTS, G. (1950). Observations on a prozone phenomenon encountered in using the anti-globulin sensitization test. *Lancet*, **ii**, 729–732.

VAN LOGHEM, J. J., STALLMAN, H. F. & VAN DER HART, M. (1951). Anémie hémolytique et anticorps froid incomplets. *Rev. Hémat.*, **6**, 286–298.

VAN LOGHEM, J. J. JNR, VAN DER HART, M. & DORFMEIER, H. (1958). Serologic studies in acquired hemolytic anemia. *Proc. 6th int. Congr. int. Soc. Hemat., Boston, 1956*, pp. 858–868. Grune and Stratton, New York.

VAUGHAN, J. H. (1955). Antibody characteristics in acquired hemolytic anemias. *Clin. Res. Proc.*, **3**, 67 (Abstract).

VAUGHAN, J. H. (1956). Immunologic features of erythrocyte sensitization. I. Acquired hemolytic disease. *Blood*, **11**, 1085–1096.

VAUGHAN, J. H. & WALLER, M. V. (1954). Nature of the 'coating' globulins in the Coombs reaction of erythroblastosis fetalis and of acquired hemolytic anemia. *Clin. Res. Proc.*, **2**, 114 (Abstract).

VOAK, D. (1989). Monoclonal antibodies in immunohematology and their potential role in understanding autoimmune hemolytic anemia. *Transfusion*, **29**, 191–192.

VON DEM BORNE, A. E. G. KR., BECKERS, D., VAN DER MEULEN, F. W. & ENGELFRIET, C. P. (1977). IgG4 autoantibodies against erythrocytes, without increased haemolysis: a case report. *Brit. J. Haemat.*, **37**, 137–144.

WAGER, O., HALTIA, K., RÄSÄNEN, J. A. & VUOPIO, P. (1971). Five cases of positive antiglobulin test involving IgA warm type autoantibody. *Ann. clin. Res.*, **3**, 76–85.

WEINER, W. (1958). Serological pattern in auto-immune haemolytic anaemia. Result of investigation of sera and eluates in 30 cases. *Proc. 7th Congr. Europ. Soc. Haemat., Copenhagen, 1957*, pp. 675–680. Karger, Basel.

WIDAL, F., ABRAMI, P. & BRULÉ, M. (1908a). Les ictères d'origine hémolytique. *Arch. Mal. Coeur*, **1**, 193–231.

WIDAL, F., ABRAMI, P. & BRULÉ, M. (1908b). Auto-agglutination des hématies dans l'ictère hémolytique acquis. *C. R. Soc. Biol. (Paris)*, **64**, 655–657.

WIENER, A. S. (1945). Conglutination test for Rh sensitization. *J. Lab. clin. Med.*, **30**, 662–667.

WIENER, A. S. (1951). Origin of naturally occurring hemagglutinins and hemolysins: a review. *J. Immunol.*, **66**, 287–295.

WIENER, A. S., HYMAN, M. A. & HANDMAN, L. (1949). A new serological test (inhibition test) for human serum globulin. *Proc. Soc. exp. Biol. Med.*, **71**, 96–99.

WIENER, A. S., SAMWICK, A. A., MORRISON, M. & LOEWE, L. (1952). Acquired hemolytic anemia. *Amer. J. clin. Path.*, **22**, 301–312.

WOLF, C. F. W., WOLF, D. J., PETERSON, P., BRANDSTETTER, R. D. & HANSEN, D. E. (1982). Autoimmune hemolytic anemia with predominance of IgA autoantibody. *Transfusion*, **22**, 238–240.

WORLLEDGE, S. (1967). Auto-immunity and blood diseases. *Practitioner*, **199**, 171–179.

WORLLEDGE, S. (revised by HUGHES JONES, N. C. & BAIN, D.). (1982). Immune haemolytic anaemia. In *Blood and its Disorders*, 2nd edn (ed. by R. M. HARDISTY and D. J. WEATHERALL), pp. 479–513. Blackwell Scientific Publications, Oxford.

WORLLEDGE, S. M. & BLAJCHMAN, M. A. (1972). The autoimmune haemolytic anaemias. *Brit. J. Haemat.*, **23**, Suppl., 61–69.

WUILLERET, B. (1958). L'anémie hémolytique acquise par auto-anticorps de l'enfant C. P. étudiée à la lumière des tests immunohémolytiques érythrocytaires. *Helv. paediat. Acta*, **13**, 140–149.

YAMADA, A. (1964). Investigations on clinical observation of autoimmune hemolytic anemia and characteristics of the warm autoantibody obtained from patients' red cells. *Acta haemat. jap.*, **27**, 19–52.

YOUNG, L. E., MILLER, G. & CHRISTIAN, R. M. (1951). Clinical and laboratory observations on autoimmune hemolytic disease. *Ann. intern. Med.*, **35**, 507–517.

ZINSSER, H., ENDERS, J. F. & FOTHERGILL, L. D. (1939). *Immunity. Principles and Application in Medicine and Public Health*, p. 175. Macmillan, New York.

Auto-immune haemolytic anaemia (AIHA): warm-antibody syndromes IV: serological findings 2: auto-antibodies in serum

Auto-agglutination   127

Warm auto-agglutinins   128

Auto-antibodies in serum detectable by antiglobulin sera and/or by enzyme-treated erythrocytes   129
   Early reports   129
   Use of enzyme-treated erythrocytes   130
   DAT-negative cases, with positive indirect enzyme tests   133
   DAT-positive cases, with negative indirect enzyme tests   133

Demonstration of allo-antibodies in sera containing auto-antibodies   135

Auto-antibodies detectable in serum by use of albumin or serum–albumin mixtures   135

Auto-antibodies bringing about lysis in vitro   136

Studies on eluted antibodies   142

Transference of antibody from cell to cell in vitro   143

Effect of temperature, pH and heat on the activity in vitro of warm auto-antibodies   143

Effect of heparin on antibody activity in vitro   144
Inhibition of lysis or agglutination by normal sera   144

Factors in normal human sera agglutinating and/or lysing enzyme-treated or otherwise altered erythrocytes at 37°C   145
   The reversible agglutination of trypsinized erythrocytes   145
   Factors in normal human sera agglutinating and/or lysing erythrocytes treated by enzymes other than trypsin   147

Factors in normal sera causing erythrocytes to be agglutinated by antiglobulin sera   147

Some unusual auto- and pan-agglutinins   148
   Auto-agglutinins inhibited by ionized calcium   148
   'Albumin agglutinins'   148
   Antibodies active against stored erythrocytes   149
   Auto-antibodies agglutinating erythrocytes washed in saline   151
   Other unusual auto-agglutinins   151

AUTO-AGGLUTINATION

One possible consequence of the formation of erythrocyte auto-antibodies is auto-agglutination, as already referred to (p. 58). The phenomenon can frequently be seen in stained blood films. Where auto-agglutination is massive, this is most likely to be due to the presence of high-thermal-amplitude cold auto-antibodies. Warm auto-antibodies, however, can also provoke auto-agglutination, in which case clumps of erythrocytes are visible in blood films even if they are made at 37°C (See Fig. 23.5). It is quite common, too, for auto-agglutination to be visible to the naked eye if undiluted anticoagulated or defibrinated whole blood is allowed to stand for 5–15 minutes at room temperature or 37°C; occasionally, the agglutination becomes visible almost immediately.

There appear to be two ways in which auto-antibodies can bring about auto-agglutination at 37°C: the more frequent cause is the coating of erythrocytes with IgG (incomplete) antibodies leading to their mutual adhesion in undiluted human plasma, a phenomenon equivalent to the 'albumin agglutination' of cells sensitized by incomplete anti-D antibodies; less frequently, agglutination is brought about by genuine warm agglutinins, e.g. by IgM antibodies capable of causing agglutination even if the serum containing the antibodies is diluted in saline ('in-saline agglutinins').

Occasionally when viewed microscopically, the 'agglutination' can be seen to be due to marked rouleaux formation; in most instances, however, at least when the 'agglutination' is visible macroscopically, it will be seen to be genuine.

WARM AUTO-AGGLUTININS

The early literature on acquired haemolytic anaemia in which reference was made to auto-agglutination was reviewed by Dameshek and Schwartz (1940). Unfortunately, most of the cases referred to were incompletely investigated and the nature and thermal range of the causal antibodies were not established. In the 1940s and 1950s, however, descriptions of several cases were published in which it seems clear that warm auto-agglutinins were being formed.

Wiener (1942) referred to a child aged 16 months who was suffering from haemolytic anaemia and staphylococcal sepsis. The child's own erythrocytes were auto-agglutinated and the serum agglutinated cells of all the types tested at 37°C to a titre of 64.

Lubinski and Goldbloom (1946) described an auto-antibody in the serum of a child aged $11\frac{1}{2}$ years, of blood-group A, who died of acute haemolytic anaemia. This antibody agglutinated the child's own erythrocytes and also normal group-A and group-O cells to a titre of 4 in saline dilution at 0°C, room temperature and 37°C.

Kuhns and Wagley (1949) described the presence of apparently two distinct antibodies in the serum of a patient, also acutely ill. One antibody was a non-specific cold antibody with a titre at 2°C of 2048, but not active at 37°C, the other was a warm antibody which agglutinated in saline the patient's own erythrocytes to a titre of 64 and 63% of a panel of normal erythrocytes apparently irrespective of their blood groups as far as was known at the time. The auto-antibody of Wiener, Gordon and Gallop (1953) was also an in-saline agglutinin.

Michon, Lochard and Chamaly (1954) investigated a male aged 26 who had developed sudden acute haemolysis. The DAT was positive: auto-agglutination, noted at 4°C, persisted at 37°C. The patient's serum, when concentrated by conserving the serum at the bottom of the tube after freezing, caused extremely rapid auto-agglutination at 37°C.

Evans (1955) observed one instance of a bivalent antibody (in-saline agglutinin) active at 37°C out of 34 patients studied and van Loghem, van der Hart and Dorfmeier (1958) reported finding five warm agglutinins when testing the serum of 122 patients forming warm antibodies. Pisciotta and Hinz (1957) found in-saline agglutinins in the serum of three out of 33 patients studied, but in significant amounts in only one patient. Pisciotta, Downer and Hinz (1959) reported finding during the course of detailed studies carried out on a severely affected patient that the patient's serum diluted in saline agglutinated autologous as well as normal erythrocytes to a titre of 8 at 37°C. This antibody had lytic potency as well.

In 1962 the present author summarized his own observations made on patients he had investigated in the late 1940s and 1950s (Dacie, 1962, p. 433). In only four out of 85 sera specifically tested for the phenomenon was it possible to demonstrate unequivocally that normal erythrocytes were agglutinated in undiluted patients' serum at 37°C and in dilutions of it in saline. The serum of a further patient agglutinated normal cells weakly. All five patients were severely ill. Four died of their disease; the fifth, a child aged 3 years, was also suffering from acute haemolysis but her further history is unknown. Of the four other patients, one had developed in-saline agglutinating specific Rh auto-antibodies at high titre (Case 12 of Dacie, 1954, p. 202); two others had formed a remarkable and apparently similar type of auto-antibody, active at 37°C, but potentiated to some extent at lower temperatures as well as by fall in pH, which readily agglutinated and also lysed normal corpuscles *in vitro* [Case S. B. of Dacie (1949) and Case 7 of Dacie (1962, p. 439)]. The history of the fourth patient, who also suffered from thrombocytopenic purpura, was given by Dacie (1962, Case 4, p. 389).

Recent reports

Schanfield, Pisciotta and Libnock (1978) reported that they had investigated five patients with AIHA associated with the presence of IgM warm-reacting auto-antibodies. Auto-agglutination in four of them was severe enough to cause difficulty in blood grouping. The DAT was positive with broad-spectrum and anti-C3 and C3d reagents but negative with anti-IgG sera. Adding 2-mercaptoethanol (2-ME) to sera and eluates markedly reduced their ability to cause agglutination. Agglutination was enhanced if the target erythrocytes were enzyme-treated; lysis resulted in two cases.

Freedman and co-workers (1987) described in detail the serological findings in the case of a male aged 49 who suddenly developed an episode of acute haemolysis associated with haemoglobinuria. He had previously been in good health except for long-standing polyarthritis and atrial fibrillation. He had, however, undergone splenectomy for a ruptured spleen 19 years previously and had been transfused at the time. His haemoglobin on admission was 5.3 g/dl and his blood was noted to auto-agglutinate after withdrawal. His serum contained a powerful auto-agglutinin which agglutinated normal adult erythrocytes to the remarkably high titre of 128 at 37°C and papainized erythrocytes to a titre of 512. The antibody was less active at 22°C and much less active at 4°C. The DAT was strongly positive with anti-C3d and -C4d sera and weakly positive with an anti-IgM serum. It was negative with anti-IgG and -IgA sera. The patient's serum failed to lyse normal or papainized erythrocytes at 37°C. Eluates of the patient's erythrocytes, however, did lyse, in the presence of normal serum, normal erythrocytes weakly, particularly if the serum and eluates were acidified to pH 6.8; papainized cells were lysed a little more strongly. Treatment of the patient's serum with 2-ME, as well as column chromatography, demonstrated that the abnormal agglutinin was IgM and also confirmed the absence of any IgG antibody. Extensive tests failed to reveal any clear specificity. The patient died despite all attempts at treatment, including plasmapheresis. At necropsy, the findings were consistent with systemic lupus; the immediate cause of death was pulmonary infarction secondary to multiple bilateral pulmonary thromboemboli.

AUTO-ANTIBODIES IN SERUM DETECTABLE BY ANTIGLOBULIN SERA AND/OR BY ENZYME-TREATED ERYTHROCYTES

The demonstration by Boorman, Dodd and Loutit in 1946 by means of the antiglobulin reaction that certain patients with acquired haemolytic anaemia have erythrocytes that are coated by auto-antibodies was soon followed by finding in the serum of some of the patients abnormal auto-antibodies in equilibrium with the molecules of antibody coating the erythrocytes. Because, however, the molecules of auto-antibody in warm-type AIHA are adsorbed to the corresponding antigens on the surface of the erythrocytes at body temperature, the presence of antibody molecules free in the serum will depend not only on the amount of antibody that is being formed but also on its affinity for the corresponding erythrocyte antigens. In practice, too, whether an antibody can be demonstrated in serum also naturally depends upon the sensitivity, as well as the suitability, of the method or methods used in testing for its presence. Thus the sera of some patients can only be shown to contain abnormal auto-antibodies by the use of modified, e.g. enzyme-treated, erythrocytes. While the presence of auto-antibodies in serum only demonstrable by the use of enzyme-treated erythrocytes may not be important in relation to in-vivo haemolysis — such antibodies may, for instance, be present in high titre in patients in whom there is no clinical evidence of increased haemolysis — the presence of auto-antibodies that agglutinate or lyse normal erythrocytes at 37°C or that readily sensitize at 37°C normal erythrocytes to agglutination by antiglobulin sera, is associated usually with markedly increased haemolysis.

Early reports

The majority of early studies were concerned with the incidence of positive tests for free auto-antibodies, with the relative sensitivity of the methods used to detect them, and with the relationship between the presence of antibodies free in the serum and the severity of *in-vivo* haemolysis. The methods used — the indirect antiglobulin test (IAT), titration in serum-albumin mixtures and titration using enzyme-treated erythrocytes — were those then generally employed in the demonstration of allo-antibodies. [Abnormal allo-antibodies, as may have been provoked by past transfusions were, and still are, a potential cause of confusion in studies designed to demonstrate auto-antibodies free in serum (see p. 490)].

Denys and van den Broucke (1947), using the IAT, demonstrated free antibody in the serum of two severely ill patients, one an infant. They noted that normal erythrocytes varied in their sensitivity to the patients' antibodies, and showed in one of the patients that the titre of free antibody, as estimated by the IAT, diminished in parallel with the patient's clinical improvement.

Sturgeon (1947) described how he had demonstrated incomplete antibodies in the serum of three patients with acquired haemolytic anaemia by the 'indirect developing test'. He also had succeeded in eluting antibodies from the patients' erythrocytes by suspending them in saline for 30 minutes at 37°C or at 56°C. He showed that more antibody eluted at the higher temperature.

Gardner's (1949) observations were also important. He found that at a pH of 6.5–6.7 normal erythrocytes or the patient's own cells were agglutinated by the sera of 13 out of 15 patients. When the pH was raised to 8.0, agglutination was abolished but not sensitization to antiglobulin serum. In only three instances did sensitization result when normal cells were exposed to the patients' unacidified sera.

USE OF ENZYME-TREATED ERYTHRO-CYTES

Trypsinized cells were first used in the detection of allo-antibodies by Morton and Pickles (1947, 1951).* They were soon found to be a potent tool in the demonstration of auto-antibodies in cases of AIHA.

The mechanism by which enzymes such as trypsin and papain alter the surface of erythrocytes so that they are agglutinable by antibodies that do not agglutinate unmodified erythrocytes has been the subject of considerable debate and experiment.

Wheeler, Luhby and Scholl (1950) suggested that trypsin modified the erythrocyte surface in such a way

as 'to produce both a diminished "suspension stability" and a "rearrangement" or "uncovering" of portions of the antigenic moiety'.

Ponder (1951) reported that as the result of trypsin treatment erythrocyte volume was slightly increased, ghosts became unusually rigid, osmotic and mechanical fragilities were increased and electrophoretic mobility was reduced. He attributed the changes to 'effects on protein components of the red cell surface ultrastructure'.

Wright, Dodd and Bouroncle (1949) used trypsinized erythrocytes as well as the IAT in the investigation of 20 cases of acquired haemolytic anaemia. One or both tests were positive in 16 patients, 14 with trypsinized cells, 14 with antiglobulin serum. However, although 255 normal sera failed to agglutinate trypsinized cells, positive results were obtained in eight out of 21 cases of congenital haemolytic anaemia, six with trypsinized cells and four with antiglobulin serum. Wright, Dodd and Bouroncle observed that the avidity and titres in the acquired cases were generally greater with trypsinized cells than with the IAT.

Dacie and de Gruchy (1951) reported on 12 patients with idiopathic AIHA. The DAT was positive in all of them. The IAT at 37°C was only positive in three using unacidified patient's serum; it was, however, positive in nine if their serum had been previously acidified to approximately pH 6.5. Nine sera agglutinated trypsinized erythrocytes at 37°C.

Dausset and Vidal (1951) reported on 12 patients suffering from idiopathic AIHA. A variety of techniques was used, including the DAT and IAT, auto-agglutination in plasma-albumin, and antibody titration using normal erythrocytes suspended in plasma-albumin and trypsinized cells suspended in saline. They concluded that the use of trypsinized cells was the most sensitive method of detecting antibodies in patients' sera. Dausset (1951) referred to eight cases in which the test with trypsinized cells was the only one that was positive. Eyquem (1951) had compared the efficiency of the trypsinized-cell technique with titration in albumin and the indirect antiglobulin test and concluded that the results did not run parallel.

Rosenthal, Dameshek and Burkhardt (1951), who

---

*Dr. Pickles has recently (1989) described how early experiments on the possible effect of *Vibrio cholerae* filtrate on the agglutinability of erythrocytes by antiglobulin sera led to the discovery that enzyme-treated cells might be agglutinated by dilute anti-Rh antisera. Early in 1947 Dr. Robb-Smith returned from a trip to the U.S.A. with a sample of crystalline trypsin (Armour Laboratories). While this was found to destroy some blood-group antigens, the agglutinability of other antigens appeared to be enhanced in as much as erythrocytes bearing them were agglutinated by incomplete antibodies diluted in saline. Thus D-positive cells treated with the crystalline trypsin were found to be agglutinable by 20 samples of incomplete anti-D sera.

Cook, Heard and Seaman (1960) reported that trypsin liberates a sialomucopetide, thus diminishing the charge at the surface of the erythrocyte and reducing mutual repulsion (Eylar et al., 1962; Pollack et al., 1965). Aho and Christian (1966) listed four possible mechanisms by which papain enhances agglutination by incomplete antibodies: an increase in the number of receptor sites after enzyme treatment; the uncovering of antigens different from those that react with agglutinating antibodies; the removal of surface material which prohibits the linking of two erythrocytes by the antibody, and alteration of the surface in a way that lessens mutual repulsion between erythrocytes.

studied five AIHA patients, used trypsinized cells at three temperatures, 37°C, 22°C and 3°C, and compared the results with those obtained by titrating the antibodies with normal erythrocytes suspended in saline, and in albumin, at the three different temperatures. Whilst the results using the trypsinized cells and those obtained with normal erythrocytes suspended in albumin were of the same order, Rosenthal, Dameshek and Burkhardt thought that the trypsinized cells were less strongly agglutinated at 37°C than were the normal (not trypsinized) cells suspended in albumin; at 22°C, the intensity of agglutination was about the same by the two methods, but at 3°C the trypsinized cells were much more strongly agglutinated than were the normal cells in albumin.

Unger (1951), in experiments on trypsinized D-positive erythrocytes and anti-D sera, carried out IATs on trypsinized cells in each serum dilution that had failed to produce discernible agglutination. The antibody titre estimated in this way was at least twice as high as the titre obtained with the IAT using unmodified cells and four or more times as high as the titre obtained with trypsinized cells not subjected to the IAT.

Wright and his co-workers (1951), using trypsinized erythrocytes, compared the antibody titres in serum from peripheral blood and in serum obtained from splenic blood at the time of splenectomy. Twenty-three patients with either idiopathic or secondary AIHA accompanied by splenomegaly had been submitted to splenectomy. In 23 patients antibodies were demonstrated in blood from the spleen compared with 18 in whom antibodies were found in the peripheral blood, and even when antibodies were demonstrated in serum from both sources the titres and intensity of agglutination were greater in blood from the spleen.

Dausset (1952a) referred to four patients suffering from acquired haemolytic anaemia and cirrhosis of the liver in whom reactions using trypsinized cells were positive although the direct and indirect antiglobulin tests were negative. The patients' own erythrocytes, when trypsinized, underwent marked agglutination in their own plasma to which a one-fourth volume of 20% albumin had been added. Normal erythrocytes, when trypsinized, were also agglutinated by the patients' plasma, particularly in the presence of bovine albumin. Dausset believed that his patients had formed 'doubly incomplete antibodies' which he suggested might have two non-reactive valencies.

Davidsohn and Oyamada (1953) reported they had titrated the sera of 26 patients with AIHA (18 being idiopathic cases) for the presence of abnormal antibodies using four varieties of test erythrocytes—the patient's own cells, cells of homologous ABO and Rh group, group-O cells and cells of Rh(D) group opposite to that of the patient. The cells were used fresh or papainized and the titrations were carried out at 2°C and at 37°C using saline or albumin as diluents. In 11 cases there were no significant differences between the sensitivity of the test cells; in several instances, however, papainized cells were more strongly agglutinated than were the untreated cells. The sera of four patients agglutinated the patient's own cells to higher titres than the other test cells, while in 11 patients the patient's cells were alone agglutinated.

Foster and Hutt (1953) reported some interesting observations on an antibody in the serum of a patient suffering from Hodgkin's disease and haemolytic anaemia. The DAT was strongly positive and the patient's blood underwent auto-agglutination. Normal group-O erythrocytes were agglutinated at 37°C in both saline and albumin dilutions of the patient's serum to approximately the same titres. However, when trypsinized corpuscles were used, it was found that although strong agglutination followed the use of crystalline trypsin, no agglutination took place when comparable amounts of crude trypsin or chymotrypsin were used instead of the crystalline variety. This was thought to be due to the antigen sites being destroyed by the chymotrypsin. The exact specificity of the antibody was not determined.

Komninos and Rosenthal (1953) tested the eluates they had made from the erythrocytes of 16 AIHA patients by the IAT, by their ability to agglutinate trypsinized cells and by a combined IAT trypsinized-cell test. Eluted antibodies were detected in 13 cases. The IAT and the combined test seemed to be slightly more sensitive than were trypsinized cells alone in detecting the antibodies.

Ruggieri and Eyquem (1953) compared the efficiency of treating erythrocytes with trypsin and papain, as well as with *Vibrio cholerae* filtrate and potassium iodate, in the detection of auto-antibodies in cases of AIHA. Papain appeared to be the most effective of the agents tested.

Davidsohn and Spurrier (1954) reported on 35 patients with idiopathic AIHA and on 21 patients with secondary AIHA using three techniques. Free auto-antibody was demonstrated in the sera of approximately two-thirds of their patients in both series. They concluded that antibody appeared in the serum only after the erythrocytes had become saturated. They mentioned, however, five patients with antibody in their sera in whom the DAT was negative.

Evans and Weiser (1957) stated that the IAT was positive in eight out of 15 patients who had not been transfused, and had never been pregnant, and in 18 out of 26 patients who had been transfused or had been pregnant. They were cautious in interpreting the significance of their results, bearing in mind the difficulty in distinguishing auto-antibodies from allo-antibodies. Evans and Weiser, made, however, several additional points: namely, that the degree to which an auto-antibody dissociates has probably a bearing on the concentration of free antibody in the serum, that this might depend on the speed of reaction between antibody and the receptors on the cell surface, that a high rate of formation should result in an overspill into the plasma and that free auto-antibody might be derived from destroyed cells or eluted from cells about to be destroyed.

Pisciotta and Hinz (1957) reported on the sera of 33 patients (the majority forming warm antibodies) which they had tested with autologous erythrocytes and normal cells, using the saline, albumin and trypsinized-cell techniques. Sixteen out of 25 sera agglutinated trypsinized cells at 37°C, albeit some only weakly. Using 20% bovine albumin and normal (not trypsinized) cells, the titres were not so high and the end-points more difficult to read.

Heller, Nelken and Gurevitch (1958) had tested 164 sera from patients suffering from acquired haemolytic anaemia (AHA), ITP, pancytopenia, leukaemia or SLE. Papainized erythrocytes were agglutinated by 51 (31%) of the sera, whereas the IAT was positive in only four of the patients (2.4%). Eighteen patients had AHA: papainized cells were agglutinated by eight sera, although the IAT was positive in only one; five sera contained in addition leuco-agglutinins or thrombo-agglutinins.

van Loghem, van der Hart and Dorfmeier (1958) reported on tests for free antibody in the sera of 37 patients with warm-antibody AIHA. They had used six methods of antibody detection: titration with normal erythrocytes in saline, the IAT, titration with trypsinized cells in saline, the IAT on trypsinized cells, titration with papainized cells in saline and the IAT on papainized cells. The IAT was positive in 22 patients, while antibody was detected by the use of trypsinized cells in 15 and by papainized cells in 33. Only once was the IAT positive when the results of all the other tests were negative. None of the sera agglutinated normal cells in saline. van Loghem, van der Hart and Dorfmeier calculated that allo-antibodies, generated by past transfusions, are likely to be present in about 10% of patients.

Dacie (1959) emphasized that free antibody was more often detectable in patients who were severely ill than in those in comparative remission (Fig. 25.1). Of 40 patients studied, 20 had given positive indirect antiglobulin tests thought to be due to free auto-antibody in the serum.

Dausset and Colombani (1959) reported on 83 patients. They, too, noted a correlation between free antibody in the serum and the severity of the disease: for instance, antibody detectable by the IAT was present in only 18.5% of patients who were 'cured' of their disease against 52% of patients who died. Again, the use of enzyme-treated (trypsinized) erythrocytes gave a higher percentage of positives, the percentage rising from

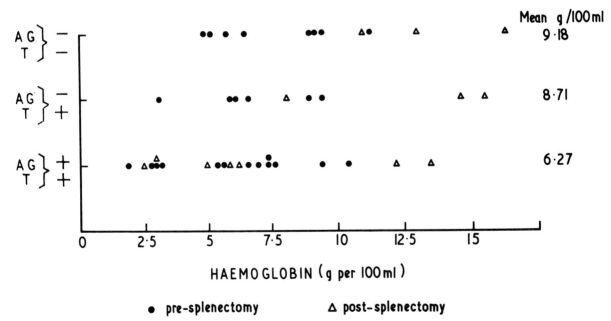

Fig. 25.1   Relationship between haemoglobin concentrations in g/dl and the presence or absence of auto-antibody free in the serum of 40 patients suffering from AIHA of the warm-antibody type.
AG = indirect antiglobulin test, either positive (+) or negative (−). T = test for agglutination of trypsinized normal erythrocytes at 37°C either positive (+) or negative (−). The mean haemoglobin concentrations are given; that of the AG−, T− series is significantly higher than that of the AG+, T+ series (P=0.02–0.05). (From Dacie, 1959.)

61.5 in the patients who recovered to 86 in those who died.

Dacie (1962, p. 434) reported that he had tested the sera of 84 warm-antibody AIHA patients and had found that 55 of them (65%) agglutinated trypsinized erythrocytes at 37°C. The tests had been carried out with cells of as near as possible the same phenotype as that of the patient or with a small panel of cells of different phenotypes. Other enzymes such as papain and ficin were not systematically employed. In some instances it was found that it was possible to increase the apparent antibody titre by substituting fresh normal compatible serum as diluent in the place of saline. The titre in one case was, too, increased by slight acidification of the serum used as diluent (Table 25.1). Prozones were not commonly met with, but in the striking example illustrated in Table 25.2 inhibition of agglutination in undiluted serum led to the antibody being originally almost missed.

Fukuoka and Ando (1965) reported on the serological studies that they had carried out on the sera of 37 Japanese patients with AIHA. The IAT was positive with 34 of the sera and 36 of the sera agglutinated normal erythrocytes treated with trypsin, ficin or bromelin. Two out of the three sera giving a negative IAT agglutinated ficinized cells.

DAT-negative cases, with positive indirect enzyme tests

Of particular interest are the reports of patients suffering from, or who have recently suffered from, acute haemolysis, in whom the DAT has

Table 25.1 Agglutination of trypsinized normal erythrocytes by the serum of a patient suffering from AIHA of the warm-antibody type (Case 9 of Dacie, 1954)

| Diluent | pH | Dilutions of patient's serum | | | | |
		1 in 2	1 in 4	1 in 8	1 in 16	Control (diluent only)
Saline	8.0	++	Trace	–	–	–
Normal serum	8.0	++	++	Trace	–	–
Acidified normal serum	6.5	++	++	+	Trace	–

++ denotes moderately strong naked-eye agglutination, and + a lesser degree of agglutination; – denotes no agglutination.

been repeatedly negative, yet indirect enzyme tests were clearly positive. Sometimes in fact trypsinized or papainized erythrocytes were agglutinated to high titres. Instances of this sort were recorded by Dausset (1952a), Dacie (1954, p. 233), Lemaire et al. (1954), Payne, Spaet and Aggeler (1955), Baikie and Pirrie (1956) and Sokal (1957). (See also p. 184, under DAT-negative AIHA.)

Dacie's (1954) case was a patient (To.) who on recovering from an acute haemolytic episode was found to have in his serum an apparently non-specific panagglutinin active at 37°C against trypsinized erythrocytes to high titres (256–1024), but which failed completely to sensitize the same cells, if untrypsinized, to agglutination by antiglobulin serum. The reactions of the serum, which also contained two immune allo-antibodies, anti-c and anti-E, were illustrated by Dacie (1954, p. 241) (Table 25.3). The patient described by Dacie (1962, p. 390) as Case 5 had also formed an antibody of this type.

The antibody demonstrated in patient To. is clearly most unusual. However, Dacie and Cutbush (1954), in investigating 10 patients, found that the antibodies of four of them ('non-specific' antibodies and anti-e) reacted preferentially with trypsinized erythrocytes and that anti-e and anti-D obtained from eluates of a further patient's erythrocytes could only be demonstrated using trypsinized cells.

Payne, Spaet and Aggeler's (1955) patient was also most unusual. She was a woman aged 59 who gave a history of previous minor haemolytic episodes. The occurrence of severe haemolysis with haemoglobinuria led to the discovery of an antibody in her serum that agglutinated trypsinized erythrocytes to a titre of 1024. Papainized cells were agglutinated, too, although less strongly. It was suggested that some common exogenous agent such as a viral or bacterial metabolite caused the erythrocytes to be sensitized to the action of the antibody. In contrast to the overt intravascular haemolysis that had occurred *in vivo*, the antibody did not cause lysis of the trypsinized cells *in vitro* in the presence of complement.

DAT-positive cases, with negative indirect enzyme tests

Rarely, the antibodies of warm-type AIHA,

Table 25.2 Agglutination of trypsinized normal erythrocytes by the serum of a patient suffering from AIHA of the warm–antibody type (Case 5 of Dacie, 1962)

Cells	Diluent	Dilutions of patient's serum							Control (diluent only)
		1 in 1	1 in 4	1 in 16	1 in 64	1 in 256	1 in 1,024	1 in 4,096	
Normal	Saline	–	–	–	–	–	–	–	–
Normal trypsinized	Saline	+	++	++++	+++	+	+	–	–
Patient's trypsinized	Saline	++	++	+++	++	++	+	–	–
Normal	Normal AB serum, cells in 20% albumin	+++	++	+	±	Trace	–	–	–

+ + + + denotes very strong naked-eye agglutination; + + +, + +, +, and ± denote lesser degrees of agglutination; – denotes no agglutination.

although sensitizing normal erythrocytes to antiglobulin serum, fail to agglutinate trypsinized cells. This was observed in three out of the 30 patients investigated by Dacie and de Gruchy (1951) using normal erythrocytes acted upon by crystalline trypsin. The reactions of one of these patients may be quoted as an example. Normal erythrocytes sensitized in her serum or in an eluate made from her own erythrocytes were agglutinated quite strongly by an antiglobulin serum, but the same cells when trypsinized were only very weakly agglutinated by the patient's serum and not agglutinated at all by the eluate made from the patient's cells. The antibody in this case appeared to be 'non-specific'.

DEMONSTRATION OF ALLO-ANTIBODIES IN SERA CONTAINING AUTO-AUTIBODIES

The occurrence of allo-antibodies, generated as the result (usually) of past blood transfusions, in the serum of patients with warm-antibody AIHA has already been referred to. Their possible presence is of practical importance if a patient is to be transfused, as they are a potential cause of serious blood transfusion reactions. Fortunately, it is not too difficult to demonstrate their existence in sera also containing free auto-antibodies, and several methods have been described by which this may be achieved (Morel, Bergren and Frank, 1978; Hanfland, 1982; James, Rowe and Tozzo, 1988). Basically, the methods depend on absorbing the serum with the

patient's own erythrocytes from which as much as possible of an adsorbed auto-antibody has been eluted.

The proportion of patients reported to have developed allo-antibodies has varied rather widely in different series—from the 10% of 122 patients, thought to be a 'rather high' figure, reported by van Loghem, van der Hart and Dorfmeier in 1958 to the 32% of the 41 patients of James, Rowe and Tozzo (1988). Of the 13 patients who had developed allo-antibodies in the latter series, multiple transfusions were thought to have been responsible in 11; in two, however, there appeared to be no easy explanation. Anti-E had been the most frequent allo-antibody, anti-K the next commonest.

AUTO-ANTIBODIES DETECTABLE IN SERUM BY USE OF ALBUMIN OR SERUM–ALBUMIN MIXTURES

The albumin or serum–albumin techniques already mentioned (p. 118) were used quite extensively in early studies but do not seem to have much to commend them. The methods are relatively insensitive compared with enzyme methods and agglutination is more difficult to read, and the results when positive may be expected to parallel those obtained by the IAT. Representative data are to be found in the studies of Neber and Dameshek (1947), Dameshek (1951), Davidsohn and Oyamada (1953) and Pisciotta and Hinz (1957). Lower titres were usually obtained if normal erythrocytes were

Table 25.3 The reactions *in vitro* of the serum of a patient (To.) with normal erythrocytes of the probable genotypes *CDe/CDe*, *cDE/cDE* and *cde/cde*.

Probable genotype of erythrocytes	Agglutination by antiglobulin serum	Agglutination in serum-albumin	Agglutination of trypsinized normal erythrocytes	
			(*Before* absorption with *CDe/CDe* corpuscles)	(*After* absorption with *CDe/CDe* corpuscles)
CDe/CDe	0	0	+++ (256)	0
cDE/cDE	+++	++ (16)	+++ (256)	++ (32)
cde/cde	++	+ (4)	++ (64)	+ (8)

The serum contained anti-E and anti-c as well as a non-specific antibody acting on trypsinized corpuscles. The figures in brackets refer to agglutinin titres.

substituted for the patients' own cells. This is probably due to the patients' erythrocytes having already adsorbed antibody *in vivo*, as shown by positive antiglobulin tests, and the consequent tendency to auto-agglutination in serum–albumin mixtures. Thus the use of the patients' own cells in the demonstration of free antibodies by these techniques gives results of uncertain significance.

Other macromolecular colloids such as dextran (Heni and Blessing, 1954a) were also used as substitutes for albumin, but it is doubtful whether they have any real advantages. Weiner (1958) used albumin-suspended enzyme-treated cells.

The phenomenon of 'albumin agglutination', i.e. agglutination in albumin-containing media in the absence of any evidence of increased haemolysis and a negative DAT, is discussed on p. 148.

AUTO-ANTIBODIES BRINGING ABOUT LYSIS *IN VITRO*

Reports of lysins in the sera of patients with AIHA have always excited interest. Such reports are rare, however, and some have been the cause of controversy. Unfortunately, many of the reports have been incomplete and deficient in detail. Also the mere demonstration of rapid autohaemolysis *in vitro* is no proof that the lysis is brought about by complement and antibody. Rapid autohaemolysis may be due, for instance, to the rapid lysis of spherocytes, as in Case 12 of Dacie (1954, p. 202). A distinguishing feature is that the lysis of spherocytes takes place even if complement is inactivated, as for instance when anticoagulants such as heparin are added to the blood. Nor can the presence of a warm lysin, as opposed to the cold variety of much more frequent occurrence, be considered to be proved unless the tests *in vitro* have been carried out with sera and erythrocyte suspensions that have been carefully warmed to 37°C before mixing, a point of technique that has seldom been mentioned. However, there is no doubt that warm lysins do exist. Their incidence is, however, very low. This is fortunate, as when present, haemolysis is likely to be hyperacute and the outlook for the patient uncertain, if not grave.

The concept that a 'lysin' is simply an antibody that has the ability to bring about the fixation of complement as the result of its interaction with antigen and that it is not a species of antibody molecule that is distinctly different from an agglutinin (or an opsonin) has been discussed briefly on p. 96.

Literature

The early literature was well reviewed by Dameshek amd Schwartz (1940) and by Dausset (1952b). The pioneer observations of Chauffard and Troisier (1908a,b) and Chauffard and Vincent (1909) have already been referred to. Chauffard and Vincent's patient was acutely ill, and had haemoglobinuria. During the acute phase of his illness an autolysin and isolysin were demonstrated in his serum. The lysin was most active at 37°C and it was no longer found in the patient's serum on his recovery.

Dausset (1952b) listed 11 additional reports dealing with lysins and haemolytic anaemia that were published in France within a few years of Chauffard's papers. None of the later descriptions appears, however, to be as convincing as that of Chauffard and Vincent, and nothing decisively new was discovered. It was not in fact until 1938 that the role of lysins in acute haemolytic anaemia with haemoglobinuria was re-emphasized by Dameshek and Schwartz (1938). Their report dealt with three patients: in the first patient isohaemolysis but not autohaemolysis was demonstrated; in the second only autohaemolysis; the antibody of the third patient, however, lysed the patient's erythrocytes *in vitro* as well as normal cells. Dameshek and Schwartz showed, as had Chauffard, that the antibodies were thermostable and needed complement for lysis, although they would fix antibody in the absence of thermolabile components of complement. Dameshek and Schwartz also reported that the lysins they studied were active both at 18°C and at 37°C and were inactivated by the addition of normal human serum. Another example of an abnormal lysin was

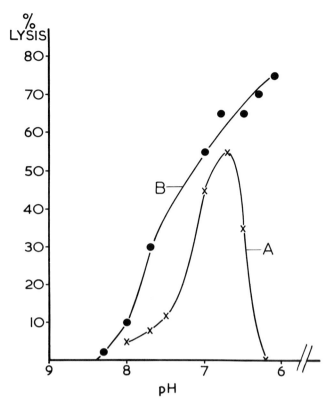

Fig. 25.2   Effect of pH on the lysis of normal erythrocytes by a 'warm lysin' in the serum of a patient suffering from fatal severe AIHA (Dacie, 1949).
A = effect on observed haemolysis; B = effect on the adsorption of the antibody.

reported by Farrar, Burnet and Steigman (1940). The activity of this lysin, too, was said to be inhibited by normal serum.

Effect of pH. In 1944, David and Minot described the presence of an abnormal lysin in the serum of an infant acutely ill with haemolytic anaemia. Normal erythrocytes, as well as those of the patient, were lysed *in vitro*, and it was noted that the amount of lysis was increased by the addition to the serum of a one-twentieth volume of 0.33N-HCl.

---

*According to Yachnin and Ruthenburg (1965), the optimum pH for the action of both human and guinea-pig complement is 6.5; at pH 6.0 its action is markedly inhibited. Human complement is more sensitive to pH alteration than is guinea-pig complement.
  Gardner and Harris (1950) also recorded briefly the demonstration in three patients of lysins most active at pH 6.3–6.8.

Dacie (1949) described in detail the presence of a lysin which lysed normal erythrocytes at 37°C in the serum of a girl fatally ill with AIHA, and showed that the lysin's activity was markedly influenced by pH; it was barely active in unacidified serum, but most strongly active at pH 6.5–7.2 (Fig. 25.2).

The optimum pH was about 6.8–7.0, with inhibition above 8.0 and below 6.0. Actually, the inhibition at pH 6.0 appeared to be due to inhibition of complement as the antibody itself seemed to be absorbed increasingly well as the serum was made more acid (Fig. 25.2).* The patient's serum lysed normal group-O erythrocytes to a titre of 8 at 37°C and lysed, even if unacidified, trypsinized normal erythrocytes to a titre of 256 and PNH erythrocytes to a titre of 64, also at 37°C. It also agglutinated normal erythrocytes at 37°C. Agglutination, like lysis, was enhanced by a fall in pH. At 37°C there was just perceptible auto-agglutination; at 20°C agglutination was more intense and when the serum was titrated with normal group-O erythrocytes the cold-agglutinin titre was 512. An important question that the author attempted to answer was whether the patient's serum contained a single cold auto-antibody—of high thermal amplitude and with a considerable lytic potential, or two antibodies—a cold agglutinin of moderate titre and a separate warm lytic antibody. The latter possibility seemed to be the more likely: thus the experiment recorded in Table 1, 2a–c (Dacie, 1949) indicates that progressively less lysis took place when the sensitizing temperature was reduced from 37°C to 16°C and finally to 2°C. It appeared, therefore, as if the patient was forming a genuine warm lysin. It is interesting to compare the findings in this case with those of the patient described by Dacie (1962, p. 439) as Case 7. In this case it seems likely, but was not proved, that a single auto-antibody was responsible for the very severe haemolysis from which he suffered (see p. 139).

Dacie and de Gruchy (1951) reported six additional examples of lysins apparently of the warm variety which they detected in the sera of patients suffering from idiopathic AIHA. These lysins, however, did not convincingly cause the lysis of normal erythrocytes at 37°C even at an acid pH; but normal cells when trypsinized or PNH erythrocytes were lysed to quite high titres in five out of the six cases. Subtle differences between the lytic antibodies in the sera of different patients were noted, for the lytic titres using trypsinized or PNH cells did not necessarily run parallel.

Subsequent case reports in which the presence of a warm lysin was mentioned include those of Tomek, Strasser and Speiser (1950), Dausset (1952b), van Loghem et al. (1952), Braunsteiner, Mannheimer and Reimer (1953) (an 'acid-lysin' in a patient with chronic lymphocytic leukaemia and haemolytic anaemia), Rosenthal, Komninos and Dameshek (1953), Verger et al. (1954), Heni and Blessing (1954b), Chevalier et al. (1954), Evans (1955), Baumgartner (1956), Martoni and Musiani (1956), Dausset et al. (1957) and Verger and Moulinier (1957). The experience of workers who had studied relatively large series of patients gives a good idea of the rarity of this type of antibody (see below).

Pisciotta and Hinz (1957) found evidence for warm lysins in three out of 26 patients investigated. However, lysis was repeatedly demonstrated in one case only; in the second, it occurred only when the patient's erythrocytes, after trypsinization, were exposed to fresh normal serum and in the third patient it was demonstrated only in a terminal crisis. Pisciotta, Downer and Hinz (1959) reported a further example in an adult suffering from severe haemolytic disease. This patient's erythrocytes also underwent lysis in fresh normal serum and her serum lysed normal cells, if trypsinized, at 37°C to a titre of 32.

Evans and Weiser (1957) were able to demonstrate a 'typical' warm lysin in only one of 11 patients investigated. This patient died of her disease, and her serum lysed normal group-O or -A cells *in vitro*. A further patient was described whose serum contained a 'unique' lytic factor. Autohaemolysis of the patient's blood on incubation occurred apparently only in the presence of anticoagulants and was demonstrable even if anticoagulants were added to heat-inactivated plasma or serum. The lysis was thought to be due to the presence of a heat-stable factor activated by the removal of Mg^{2+} or Ca^{2+} ions. The patient was treated with ACTH and cortisone and the strange lytic activity disappeared.

Letman (1957) had studied 18 patients. Lysins were sought for at 37°C by using trypsinized erythrocytes and by suspending normal (unmodified) cells in acidified serum. Four out of the 18 sera lysed the enzyme-treated cells and five sera the normal cells; two of these sera also brought about agglutination at 37°C. Two sera produced lysis by both techniques. The erythrocytes of one patient underwent lysis, when trypsinized, in fresh normal human serum.

Dausset and his colleagues published several further papers on warm lysins following Dausset's (1952b) review. In a paper dealing mainly with technique, Dausset, Colombani and Evelin (1957) emphasized that warm lysins occurred relatively frequently in acute or fulminating haemolytic anaemia in children, that the lysins were often demonstrable for a few days only at the height of the child's illness, and that the patient's serum was likely to be deficient in complement or even to be anticomplementary. Dausset and his colleagues concluded that the optimum pH requirements for lysins were variable but that slight acidification of the serum was a useful laboratory artifice. Dausset et al. (1957) described a case in which an 'acid-lysin' of the sort described in the review quoted above was clearly demonstrated. This patient's serum was in fact anticomplementary.

Dausset and Colombani (1959) summarized their experience. Warm lysins were demonstrated in four out of 83 idiopathic cases. Three of the patients were infants suffering from acute haemolytic anaemia with haemoglobinuria. Recovery took place within a few weeks aided by transfusion and steroids. In each case autologous and normal (untrypsinized) erythrocytes underwent lysis at 37°C and acidification of serum was unnecessary. In two cases the serum was depleted of complement; in one, the serum was anticomplementary. The fourth patient was an adult who died when uraemic.

van Loghem, van der Hart and Dorfmeier (1958) found only one convincing warm lysin amongst the sera of 122 patients who had formed warm antibodies; the antibody lysed normal cells only when trypsinized. Schubothe (1958) in his monograph *Serologie und klinische Bedeutung der Autohämantikörper*, which has in all 704 references, reviewed the occurrence of 'Warmeautohämolysine', but was not able to quote from personal experience.

Dacie (1962, p. 436), in the second edition of this book, reported that in only two out of a total of 89 patients he had studied up to that time had he been able to demonstrate unequivocally that their serum was capable of causing well-marked lysis of normal erythrocytes at 37°C. Two other sera, which actively lysed trypsinized and PNH cells, caused traces of lysis of normal cells.

Of the two patients whose sera lysed normal erythro-

Table 25.4 Agglutination of normal erythrocytes by the serum of a patient with acute AIHA (Case 7 of Dacie, 1962)

Approx. pH	Serum dilutions						
	1 in 2 (37°C)	1 in 8 (37°C)	1 in 32 (37°C)	1 in 8 (20°C)	1 in 32 (20°C)	1 in 128 (20°C)	1 in 512 (20° C)
8.0	−	−	−	+	−	−	−
7.8	±	−	−	+ + +	±	−	−
7.4	+	±	−	+ + + +	+ + +	+ +	−
7.0	+	±	−	+ + + +	+ + + +	+ + +	±
6.5	+	+	−	+ + + +	+ + + +	+ + +	±

+ + + + denotes very strong naked-eye agglutination; + + +, + +, + and ± denote lesser degrees of agglutination; − denotes no agglutination.

cytes, one, described by Dacie (1949), has already been referred to (p. 137). The other [Case 7 of Dacie (1962, p. 439)] was a boy aged 11 years who died of Evans syndrome after an illness that had lasted 8 years (see p. 35). In the last phase of his illness he developed an auto-antibody that agglutinated and also lysed his own erythrocytes at 37°C, both agglutination and lysis being enhanced as the pH of the cell-serum suspension was reduced from pH 8 to 6.5 (Tables 25.4 and 25.5). The nature of this antibody, the activity of which was enhanced by reduction in temperature, and its specificity, could not be determined. It was noted that the antibody's temperature requirement appeared to be intermediate between that of typical warm and cold antibodies.

Twenty-two out of the 89 sera lysed trypsinized and/or PNH cells: trypsinized cells were lysed in 15 out of 84 cases (18%) and PNH cells in 17 out of 89 cases (19%); in 10 cases both types of cells were lysed (Table 25.6). There was, however, no strict parallelism between the lysin titres for each type of cell, and although in most instances both types of cell were lysed this was not always so.

The effect of pH on the lysis of trypsinized erythro-cytes by the serum of one of these patients [Case 13 of Dacie (1954, p. 205)] is illustrated in Fig. 25.3: the optimum is approximately 6.5.

Dacie and Worlledge (1975) reported that 58 (40%) of 146 sera from patients with warm-

Table 25.5 Lysis of normal erythrocytes by the serum of a patient with acute AIHA (Case 7 of Dacie, 1962)

Approx. pH	Serum dilutions					
	1 in 2 (37°C)	1 in 8 (37°C)	1 in 32 (37°C)	1 in 8 (20°C)	1 in 32 (20°C)	1 in 128 (20°C)
8.0	Trace	−	−	−	−	−
7.8	Trace	−	−	Trace	−	−
7.4	+	−	−	+	−	−
7.0	+ + +	±	−	+ ±	+	−
6.5	+ + +	±	−	+ ±	+ +	Trace

+ + + denotes marked lysis, + +, + ±, + and ± lesser degrees of lysis; − denotes no lysis.

Table 25.6 Incidence of lysis at 37°C of trypsinized normal (TN) erythrocytes or PNH erythrocytes by sera of patients with AIHA of the warm-antibody type

No. of cases	Lysis of TN cells alone	Lysis of PNH cells alone	Lysis of PNH cells and TN cells	Total no. of cases with serum lytic activity
89	5	7	10	22

Lysis of trypsinized cells at 37°C	15 out of 84 = 18%
Lysis of PNH cells at 37°C	17 out of 89 = 19%

antibody AIHA lysed enzyme-treated erythrocytes *in vitro* at 37°C. As is shown in Table 25.7, the percentage of sera causing lysis differed according to the immunochemical nature of the auto-antibodies; in particular, lysis was particularly frequent in patients whose DAT indicated that the antibodies were complement-fixing.

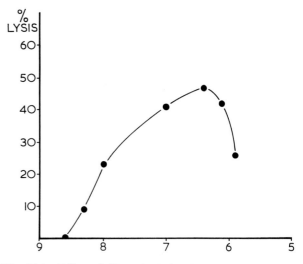

Fig. 25.3 Effect of pH on the lysis of trypsinized normal erythrocytes by a warm lysin (Case 13 of Dacie, 1954).

Table 25.7 Correlation between the type of direct antiglobulin reaction and the presence or absence of warm lysins active against enzyme-treated erythrocytes in the serum of 146 patients suffering from warm-antibody AIHA.

| Proteins on the erythrocyte surface | Lysis of enzyme-treated erythrocytes at 37°C | | | |
	Present	Absent	Total	% lysins
IgG	9	45	54	16
IgA	0	3	3	0
IgG + IgA	1	4	5	20
IgG + C	29	34	63	45
IgG + IgM + C	8	0	8	100
C	11	2	13	95
Totals	58	88	146	

From Dacie and Worlledge (1975).

von dem Borne and co-workers had described in 1969 the results of an important investigation into the incidence and nature of serum lysins in a large series of patients with warm-antibody AIHA. They reported that although they had demonstrated warm lysins active at 37°C against enzyme-treated cells in 87 AIHA patients their sera had never shown any activity against non-enzyme-treated cells; also that the antibodies were not absorbed by unmodified cells.

The warm lysins were the sole auto-antibody present in 24 patients; they were present in addition to an IgG incomplete antibody in 36 patients, with an incomplete IgM antibody in three patients, with incomplete IgG and IgM antibodies in five patients and with incomplete IgG and IgA antibodies in one patient. Warm lysins were never associated (in the experience of von dem Borne et al.) with high-titre cold auto-agglutinins or biphasic lysins. The temperature optimum for lysis was 30°C in the case of seven sera, 37°C with four sera (Fig. 25.4). The optimum pH was generally about 6.5; but it was 7.0–7.5 in the case of a serum containing an IgG lytic antibody (Fig. 25.5).

von dem Borne et al. (1969) reported the results of detailed serological studies on seven sera: in each patient the DAT had been positive using anti-complement (C) sera; their sera agglutinated enzyme-treated cells if complement was absent from the system, the agglutination titre being generally higher than the lysis titre at 37°C; acidifying the sera increased both lysis and agglutination; more lysis took place at 37°C than at 16°C and could be demonstrated (although less strongly) by a two-step as well as by a one-step procedure (complement present throughout); the indirect antiglobulin reaction was positive with enzyme-treated cells.

The sera were tested against erythrocytes pre-treated with a variety of enzymes—ficin, trypsin, bromelin and papain. Ficinized cells were most sensitive to lysis, trypsinized cells the least sensitive, while papainized cells were lysed as well as, if not better than, bromelin-treated cells. von dem Borne et al. pointed out that

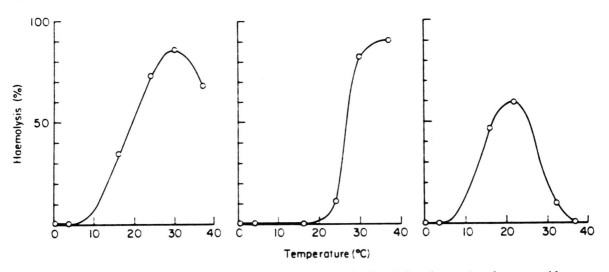

Fig. 25.4 Effect of temperature on lysis by two warm auto-antibodies (left and centre) and on one cold auto-antibody (right).
[Reproduced by permission from von dem Borne et al. (1969).]

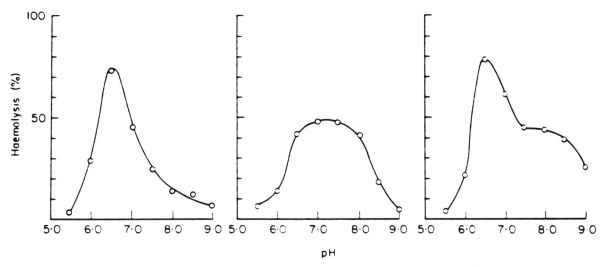

Fig. 25.5   Variable effect of pH on lysis by three warm auto-antibodies.
[Reproduced by permission from von dem Borne et al. (1969).]

as the sera varied in their ability to lyse erythrocytes pre-treated by the different enzymes it was advisable to use more than one enzyme in testing for lytic activity.

Ten sera were pre-treated with 2-ME: the activity of eight sera against enzyme-treated cells was abolished; it was not quite eliminated in the case of one serum and the activity of one other serum was hardly affected. Column chromatography confirmed that the antibodies were usually IgM in type and also confirmed the IgG nature of the antibodies in the sera the activity of which had been partially affected, or virtually not affected, by 2-ME. Column chromatography also conclusively demonstrated that the lytic antibody and an incomplete IgG antibody, often present in the same serum, were distinct and different entities.

Fresh rabbit and guinea-pig sera were compared with fresh human sera for their ability to bring about lysis of enzyme-treated cells: guinea-pig serum produced less lysis than human serum and rabbit serum hardly any lysis at all.

The sera were tested for their specificity against a panel of human erythrocytes. None of the antibodies showed any specificity within the Rh system; lysis was, however, often stronger with adult ii cells or cord cells than with adult I cells; one serum had typical IH specificity.

^{51}Cr erythrocyte auto-survival studies carried out on patients whose sera contained demonstrable lysins (against enzyme-treated cells) but were apparently free from incomplete IgG auto-antibodies gave T_{50} values of 21–22 days. The antibodies, although apparently incapable of lysing normal erythrocytes *in vitro* thus

caused, nevertheless, appreciable lysis *in vivo*, a finding concordant with that of positive DAT reactions with anti-C sera.

Later, Engelfriet and co-workers (1983) reported further data based on their large Amsterdam experience. The sera from 1680 patients forming warm auto-antibodies had been investigated: 168 sera (8.4%) contained warm haemolysins, 165 of which were designated incomplete (i.e. had lysed enyzme-treated cells only) and three complete (i.e. had had lysed normal unmodified cells); 138 sera (6.9%) contained warm haemolysins in addition to incomplete warm auto-antibodies.

A further example of a warm auto-antibody leading to the patient's rapid death has more recently been described by Araguas et al. (1990). A 42-year-old woman had suffered for 2 weeks from malaise, lumbar pain, chills, fever and probable haemoglobinuria. On admission to hospital, the haemoglobin was 4.7 g/dl and the DAT strongly positive. She developed disseminated intravascular coagulation and acute renal failure and died within 24 hours, despite all attempts at treatment, including high-dose corticosteroids and heparin. The auto-antibody agglutinated all erythrocytes tested at 4°C and 22°C and caused lysis at 37°C; inactivation by dithiothreitol showed that it was an IgM.

STUDIES ON ELUTED ANTIBODIES

Aside from providing material for studying antibody specificity (described in Ch. 26), eluates have provided important information on other aspects of antibody activity.

Several methods of antibody elution, varying in their complexity and efficiency have been employed. Landsteiner's useful and simple heat-elution method (Landsteiner and Miller, 1925) has to some extent been supplanted by more elegant, but also more time-consuming methods, e.g., those of Kidd (1949), Vos and Kelsall (1956), Greenwalt (1956), Weiner (1957), van Loghem, Mendes de Leon and van der Hart (1957). Jensen (1959), who published an interesting comparative study of elution methods, concluded that, although Landsteiner's method was the quickest and gave relatively good eluates, those of Weiner and van Loghem, Mendes de Leon and van der Hart were the best of those tried, although more time-consuming.

Methods described more recently include those of Rubin (1963), Mantel and Holtz (1976), Jenkins and Moore (1977), Rekvig and Hannestad (1977), Chan-Shu and Blair (1979), Massuet and Armengol (1980), Bueno, Garratty and Postoway (1981) and Branch, Sy Sion Hian and Petz (1982). Howard (1981), in a discussion on the principles of antibody elution, pointed out that they comprise disrupting antigen–antibody bonds by alteration in ionic strength or pH, thermal agitation or the use of organic solvents, and that because of the heterogeneity of the physical forces involved in binding, no single elution technique would be likely to be universally applicable. Panzer and co-workers (1984), who had compared xylene and chloroform with ether and heat as eluting agents, finding that no single method produced the strongest eluates with all the allo- and auto-antibodies tested, came to the same conclusion.

The results of some early studies carried out on antibodies eluted from the erythrocytes of AIHA patients are summarized below.

Komninos and Aksoy (1954) and Komninos and

Désy (1955) studied 29 eluates and made satisfactory high-titre antiglobulin sera by immunizing rabbits with some of them. These antisera cross-reacted with cells coated by anti-Rh. The eluted antibodies agglutinated trypsinized normal erythrocytes and gave positive indirect antiglobulin tests, and were shown to react better with, and to be absorbed better by, erythrocytes at 37°C than at 22°C or at 3°C. The titres at 3°C were $\frac{1}{4}$ or $\frac{1}{8}$ those at 37°C.

Roth and Frumin (1957) reported on studies made on 27 eluates derived from 17 patients with AIHA. The speed of absorption of the eluted antibodies by normal erythrocytes was found to be independent of the titre or blood type, but it could be varied by changes in the suspending medium and increased by the action of enzymes such as trypsin. Undiluted normal serum (or most samples of patients' serum) was thought to inhibit the coating of the test cells.

Evans and Weiser (1957) studied eight eluates. All were as active at 37°C as at lower temperatures and five were more active. Three were considered, on the basis of the γ-globulin neutralization test, not to be γ globulins; they were the ones whose activity was not influenced by temperature changes within the range 5–37°C.

Fudenberg, Barry and Dameshek (1958) reported on studies on 10 eluates made from the erythrocytes of patients suffering from primary or secondary warm-type AIHA. Rabbits were immunized with eluates made from both types of patients and comparable titres obtained. Moreover, erythrocytes 'coated' with eluates derived from either type of patient were agglutinated by the antisera irrespective of whether the sera had been formed against an eluate derived from a primary or secondary case. Fudenberg, Barry and Dameshek were able to demonstrate an inverse correlation between the survival times *in vivo* of the patients' erythrocytes and the quantity of 'coating substance' in the eluates, as determined by making serial dilutions of the eluate and using a constant amount of antiglobulin serum. They suggested that a quantitative estimation of the activity of the eluates provided a more reliable guide to the degree to which the patients' cells were sensitized by auto-antibody than an attempt to assess this directly by means of an antiglobulin reaction carried out on intact cells. Fudenberg and his colleagues also demonstrated by a precipitation-inhibition technique that the eluates did in fact contain γ globulin, and they showed that only a small proportion of the nitrogen present in the eluates reacted with antiglobulin sera, i.e. was clearly antibody nitrogen. The nature of the non-reacting material was unclear: its failure to react could have been due either to loss of immunological reactability during the elution or to the non-reacting material not being antibody at all.

Pirofsky (1958) made eluates by Kidd's method from the erythrocytes of four patients. The eluates acted as panagglutinins and were compared with the Rh antibody anti-D. It was found that whereas the mixing of anti-D with antiglobulin sera resulted in loss of potency of both the anti-D and antiglobulin antibody, the addition of eluted erythrocyte-coating material from a patient with AIHA did not result in loss in potency until normal group-O Rh-negative cells were added to the mixture. Agglutination of the cells and loss of antiglobulin activity then occurred. It was suggested that by 'coating' the erythrocyte surfaces, the coating material was altered so as to expose globulin groups not previously available for combination with antiglobulin antibody.

Chaplin and Cassell (1958, 1960) and Cassell and Chaplin (1960) reported further studies of antiglobulin sera prepared against eluted Rh antibody and eluted auto-antibodies derived from cases of primary or secondary AIHA. These antisera were compared with conventional antiglobulin sera prepared against whole human serum or its globulin fractions. Erythrocytes from 70 patients suffering from various types of acquired haemolytic anaemia were used as test cells. This work confirmed the broad cross-reactivity of sera prepared against eluted antibodies derived from primary and secondary cases of AIHA and against anti-D allo-antibody, respectively. For instance, the antiserum prepared against eluted anti-D reacted with all the cells tested including cells sensitized with the Donath–Landsteiner antibody. Chaplin and Cassell were also able to prepare antisera against eluates devoid of antibody activity demonstrable *in vitro*, and even against stroma derived from strictly normal erythrocytes.

Konda and Yamada (1960) reported on studies carried out on three patients with AIHA. Eluates were made and subjected to immuno-electrophoretic analysis. Two of the eluates gave detectable arcs in the region of normal γ globulin; these arcs were thought to be nearer the cathode than normal γ globulin or the arc produced by eluted anti-D. They, nevertheless, demonstrated that the eluates would absorb from antiglobulin serum components reacting with normal serum and anti-D antibody.

Transference of antibody from cell to cell *in vitro*

Selwyn and Hackett (1949) had demonstrated that when auto-antibody-coated erythrocytes were transfused to normal recipients some of the antibody became transferred to the normal cells so that they, too, gave a positive antiglobulin test. The same process can be demonstrated *in vitro*.

Evans (1955) and Evans and Weiser (1957) showed in five out of six experiments that antibody from patients' cells would transfer to normal cells. They pointed out that every patient's antigen–antibody reaction must have a dissociation constant and that this in all probability varied greatly from case to case.

EFFECT OF TEMPERATURE, pH AND HEAT ON THE ACTIVITY *IN VITRO* OF WARM AUTO-ANTIBODIES

Some experiments carried out on eluted antibodies to ascertain the effect of temperature on their absorption by normal erythrocytes have already been mentioned (p. 142). Schubothe (1958) made similar observations, using serum containing free auto-antibody: in three instances the thermal optimum (40°C) was the same as that for anti-D but in two other cases the optimum was 10–20°C. The pH curve for antibody binding showed a general increase as the pH was reduced from 9 to 6, exactly as found with anti-D. Gardner (1949) had earlier reported that acidifying patients' serum to pH 6.5–6.7 increased the chances of demonstrating the agglutination of normal erythrocytes or the patients' own erythrocytes (see p. 130).

Dacie (1953) similarly studied the effect of acidification to approximately pH 6.5 on indirect antiglobulin tests (IATs); whereas marked increases in agglutination were often observed with cells sensitized with cold antibodies, the effect with warm antibodies was less marked and might not be discernible. The enhancing effect that reduction in pH may have on the agglutination of trypsinized cells is illustrated in Table 25.1 (p. 133). Evans and Weiser (1957) reported on more detailed studies. Observations on the effect of lowering pH from 8.0 to 6.6 were made on 17 sera in which free auto-antibodies were demonstrable and on 12 antibody-containing eluates. In only one serum did change in pH enhance significantly the sensitization of cells suspended in it, as demonstrated by the IAT; in this instance sensitization at pH 7.4 was greater than at pH 8.0 or 6.6. In no instance was spontaneous agglutination of cells in serum at pH 6.6 observed, as had

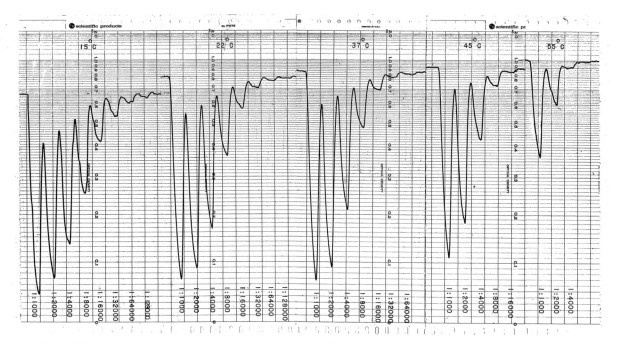

Fig. 25.6 Effect of temperature on the titre of a warm (anti-Rh_0) antibody, as demonstrated by the Polybrene technique.

A high optical density corresponds to deaggregation, i.e. lack of antibody activity. [Reproduced by permission from Lalezari and Oberhardt (1971).]

been reported by Gardner (1949). These discrepant results underline the marked patient-to-patient differences that exist. The effect of pH on the lytic activity of warm antibodies has already been discussed (p. 137).

Dacie (1953) showed that heating patients' serum to 56°C for 30 minutes did not affect its power of sensitizing normal cells to agglutination by antiglobulin serum. Schubothe (1958) confirmed these observations; he reported, however, that antibody activity was reduced if the temperature was raised to 60°C. He also studied the time needed for the binding on of auto-antibody to normal cells; some binding was demonstrable in 1 minute and almost maximal binding in 10 minutes; the results were the same with anti-D allo-antibody.

More recently, Lalezari and Oberhardt (1971) have used an automated Polybrene technique to study in detail the effect of temperature on a range of erythrocyte antigen–antibody reactions. Fig. 25.6. records titration values obtained with a high-titre anti-Rh_0 antibody at temperatures ranging from 15°C to 55°C. At 15°C there was a minimal increase in sensitivity; at 45°C, and especially at 55°C, sensitivity was markedly inhibited. [Their Fig. 3 records a similar experiment

carried out with a high-titre anti-I antibody. With this antibody there was a 1000-fold increase in sensitivity at 15°C compared with that at 37°C.]

Effect of heparin on antibody activity *in vitro*

Roth (1954) reported on experiments carried out on blood samples from three patients with AIHA which appeared to show that heparin, if present in sufficient concentration, interfered in some way with the agglutination of normal cells by the patients' serum or the agglutination of the patients' sensitized cells by antiglobulin serum. No such effect was demonstrable with Rh antibodies or with the sensitized erythrocytes of infants with haemolytic disease of the newborn. Roth and Frumin (1954) also experimented with protamine which they found agglutinated antibody-coated cells. Again, differences in behaviour were demonstrated between auto-antibodies and the allo-antibody anti-D.

Inhibition of lysis or agglutination by normal sera

There are some references in the early literature to the inhibition by normal serum of the lytic activity of the serum of several patients suffering from acute haemolytic anaemia likely to have been induced by auto-antibodies. Dameshek and Schwartz (1938) and Farrar, Burnet and Steigman (1940) reported instances of this phenomenon. The significance of these reports is uncertain: it is not likely that the normal sera were anticomplementary; simple dilution may possibly have been a factor. The present author has not observed any inhibition by normal serum of the lysis by warm auto-antibodies of trypsinized erythrocytes; fresh normal serum has in fact been used regularly as a source of complement in titrations.

There are also some references to normal human serum inhibiting agglutination. The significance of these reports is, too, uncertain.

Denys and van den Brouke (1947) mentioned that the agglutination by antiglobulin serum of normal erythrocytes exposed to the serum of their patients was slightly diminished by the presence of normal serum. Here again, dilution may have been a factor.

Martin du Pan (1948) referred to a more remarkable instance. An auto-agglutinin was present in the serum of a patient suffering from subacute AIHA which agglutinated normal group-O as well as the patient's erythrocytes at 37°C. The serum of many normal subjects was found to inhibit the agglutination and after a transfusion of normal serum it was found possible to select erythrocytes which were no longer agglutinated *in vitro* and to transfuse them to the patient.

Roth and Frumin (1957) reported that undiluted normal serum might inhibit the sensitization of normal erythrocytes by eluted auto-antibodies.

FACTORS IN NORMAL HUMAN SERA AGGLUTINATING AND/OR LYSING ENZYME-TREATED OR OTHERWISE ALTERED ERYTHROCYTES AT 37°C

There are in the serum of apparently normal individuals a number of factors (antibodies) that have the ability to agglutinate, and perhaps to lyse in the presence of complement and at the appropriate pH, human erythrocytes that have been altered (modified) by a variety of agents. Trypsinized erythrocytes, alone among the altered cells, however, have been observed to undergo reversible agglutination. Unaltered cells are not affected, and the antigens with which the antibodies react appear to be distinct from those determining the known blood groups. Except for the antibodies reacting with cells that have undergone T transformation (see p. 201), the antibodies, fortunately, are of little or no clinical significance, except in as much as they may under certain circumstances complicate cross-matching procedures or be confused with the auto-antibodies that lead to AIHA.

The cause of the development of the antibodies is not known for certain. It seems likely that they represent immune responses to external antigens, e.g. those of infective agents. If this is true, the antibodies should be regarded as cross-reacting hetero-antibodies rather than as auto-antibodies primarily developed against erythrocyte antigens. What proportion of human sera contain antibodies of the type under discussion is unclear. The author suspects that as the methods for demonstrating their presence are refined and become more sensitive, more and more sera will be found to react positively.

The reversible agglutination of trypsinized erythrocytes

Rosenthal and Schwartz (1951a, b) reported that normal human sera often had the property of agglutinating trypsinized erythrocytes at 37°C if agglutination was looked for by immediate certrifugation. They also reported that this type of agglutination disappeared (reversed) on incubation. Rosenthal and Schwartz demonstrated that agglutination and agglutination reversal were brought about by distinct factors. That causing agglutination was non-dialysable, destroyed by heating at 65°C for 1 hour and only weakly active at 'extremes of pH', whereas the factor causing the agglutination reversal was lost through dialysis, was thermostable, and was still active in markedly alkaline serum.

Rosenthal and Schwartz's observations were confirmed and extended by Spaet and Ostrom (1952), who showed that reversal of agglutination was accompanied by elution of the agglutinin and that this took place more rapidly in serum than in saline.

Hoyt and Zwicker (1953) pointed out that whereas trypsin treatment led to reversible agglutination, treatment with papain failed to do so. This and other evidence led them to suggest that the phenomenon was related to trypsin–anti-trypsin activity rather than to submerged antigens in the cells and pre-existing specific antibody in the serum.

Hurley and Dacie (1953) described the presence in the serum of a patient—in complete remission following treatment for pernicious anaemia—of a factor which lysed trypsinized normal erythrocytes rapidly within a relatively narrow pH range, 6.6–8.5. When heat-inactivated, the serum was found to contain large amounts of reversible agglutinin (titre 256). That the serum factor was probably a complement-binding antibody could be shown by demonstrating that the erythrocytes were agglutinated strongly, after agglutination had reversed, by antiglobulin sera, the reaction being of the non-γ type (Table 25.8). Coffield and Spaet (1959), too, provided evidence that the agglutinating factor was distinct from the normal serum trypsin inhibitor.

Heistø, Harboe and Godal (1965) reported studies on healthy blood donors: 95 out of 990 (9.6%) of donors were found to have sera that lysed trypsinized erythrocytes at 37°C and at 'physiological pH' (probably not the optimum for haemolysis). When heat-inactivated, the positively-reacting sera were found to agglutinate the test cells, often with a prozone—the possible reversibility of the agglutination was not discussed. Heistø, Harboe and Godal noted that the positively-reacting sera did not agglutinate or lyse papainized cells. Investigation of the families of four of the sera suggested a familial incidence.

Heistø, Jensen and Knuds (1971) tested a large number of different preparations of trypsin for their ability to render normal erythrocytes agglutinable by Rh allo-antibodies and to cause them to lyse in normal sera at 37°C. Whereas all the preparations of trypsin seemed to be equivalent with regard to promoting Rh agglutination, some samples of trypsin caused the cells to be lysed by the majority of human sera, other samples by only a very few, if any, of the sera. Heistø, Jensen and Knuds suggested that different trypsin preparations might be detecting lysins of different specificities.

Camoens and Berg (1973) reported detailed studies on the serum of a healthy adult which contained a lytic and agglutinating antibody in high titre which was thought to be similar, if not identical, to the warm lysins described by Heistø in some normal sera. The lysis titre was 32 and the agglutination titre as high as 130 000. There was a marked prozone, agglutination commencing in a serum dilution of 1 in 64. Remarkably, when normal human serum was used as diluent there was partial lysis but no agglutination. [There was no mention of the possible reversibility of agglutination which could have contributed to the prozone and have explained the complete inhibition of agglutination when normal serum was used as diluent.]

The mechanism of the reversible agglutination of trypsinized erythrocytes had been studied in detail by Mellbye (1965, 1966, 1969a,b). The agglutinin was shown to be γM globulin (Mellbye, 1965) and to be synthesized from early in life onwards, i.e. first by the fetus (Mellbye, 1966). The reversing factor was identified as histidine, which if added to dialysed serum was shown to be capable of restoring the serum's reversing capacity (Mellbye, 1967). The possibility that there were other reversing substances was, however, not ruled out. The 'trypsin agglutinin' receptor was reported to be a glycoprotein (Mellbye, 1969a).

The agglutinins active against erythrocytes altered by trypsin or other agents were considered not to cross-react one with another, and the uniqueness of the 'trypsin agglutinin'—in partic-

Table 25.8   The agglutination of trypsinized normal erythrocytes by patient C's serum.

| Diluent | Final dilution of fresh patient's serum | | | | | Time |
	1 in 4	1 in 16	1 in 64	1 in 256	Control (saline)	
Normal serum						
Agglutination	+	+++	+++	++	0	Immediately centrifuged
Agglutination	0	+	+	+	0	10 minutes at 37°C
Agglutination	0	0	0	0	0	20 minutes at 37°C
Lysis	+++	±	0	0	0	20 minutes at 37°C
Saline						
Agglutination	+±	+++	+++	++	0	Immediately centrifuged
Agglutination	0	+++	+±	±	0	30 minutes at 37°C
Agglutination	0	+	±	0	0	2 hours at 37°C
Agglutination	0	0	0	0	0	3 hours at 37°C
Reaction with antiglobulin serum	+++	+++	+++	0	0	

From Hurley and Dacie (1953).

ular its presence in cord serum and the reversibility of the agglutination — was emphasized (Mellbye, 1969b).

Factors in normal human sera agglutinating and/or lysing erythrocytes treated by enzymes other than trypsin

Auto-agglutinins active against papainized erythrocytes at 37°C were described in the sera of apparently normal subjects by Stratton and Renton (1958) and Whittingham, Lowy and Lind (1961).

Yachnin and Gardner (1961) compared the reactions of erythrocytes exposed *in vitro* to bromelin, cholera vibrio culture filtrate, ficin, influenza virus, iodate, papain and trypsin, respectively. They stressed the widely different capacity of the sera they tested to agglutinate or lyse the altered cells and the narrow pH range (with the optimum on the acid side of neutrality) required for lysis. The serum factors appeared to be more or less specific for each type of altered cell and in Yachnin and Gardner's words: 'These factors have many of the properties commonly associated with classical antibody.'

Dybkjaer and Kissmeyer-Nielsen (1967) described the results of a detailed study of the sera of 19 individuals — some normal, some suffering from a variety of conditions but none showing any signs of increased haemolysis — all of which contained auto-antibodies causing the agglutination of papainized erythrocytes. The unusual feature of the antibodies was that they appeared to have a definite specificity. This was within the Rh system, except for one serum which contained anti-Jk[a]. Anti-E was the commonest antibody, being present in 11 sera. In 11 patients the antibodies were found to be still present 1–2 years after they were first identified; in six they were found to be no longer present when their sera were retested. Treatment of the sera with 2-ME (2-mercaptoethanol) or streptomycin, and DEAE column chromatography, showed that the antibodies were IgM in type or, in two cases, IgA; none appeared to be IgG. Dybkjaer and Kissmeyer-Nielsen made the point that their study provided no evidence that the enzyme-reacting auto-antibodies were a precursor of a clinically more important auto-antibody.

Bell, Zwicker and Nevius (1973) experimented with erythrocytes treated with papain. Over a 13-year period 130 000 sera were screened for the ability to lyse papainized cells at 37°C. Lysis was produced by 0.1% of the sera and was most marked with cells that had

been stored for 4–7 days before being papainized. Trypsinized cells were lysed less strongly and variably by the sera causing lysis of the papainized cells. The sera did not lyse cells treated with bromelin or neuraminidase. The presence of the lysins could not be correlated with any specific condition, and 23 of the patients whose serum had given positive tests were transfused without any ill effect.

Randazzo, Streeter and Nusbacher (1973) reported that normal sera might contain a factor that agglutinated bromelin-treated erythrocytes but failed to agglutinate cells treated with papain, ficin or trypsin. The agglutinin had been identified in the serum of 2% of 15 000 blood donors, irrespective apparently of their blood group. It reacted best at 4°C, but some sera caused agglutination at 37°C, too. It did not fix complement, although its activity was destroyed by exposure to 2-ME.

Factors in normal sera causing erythrocytes to be agglutinated by antiglobulin sera

Hurley and Dacie (1953) had observed that normal erythrocytes, after trypsinization and incubation at 37°C in some apparently normal sera, were agglutinable by antiglobulin sera. The intensity and titre of agglutination was, however, far less than with the serum, referred to above, that contained a factor that reversibly agglutinated to a high titre, as well as lysed, trypsinized cells.

An apparently similar factor in normal serum was referred to by Janković (1954) as an 'incomplete warm antibody'. Two hundred normal sera were found to cause trypsinized erythrocytes to be agglutinated by antiglobulin sera after the cells had been incubated in the normal sera for 1 hour at 37°C. The sera did not agglutinate the trypsinized cells directly when suspended in saline or albumin. Agglutination took place best in slightly diluted antiglobulin sera or even in sera diluted to react well with anti-D-sensitized cells. The specificity of the antibody could not be established: the reactions appeared to be independent of the cells' ABO, Rh and MN groups, and the fact that the addition of H substance to the sera did not affect their ability to sensitize the cells distinguished the antibody from the incomplete cold antibody present in normal sera.

Evans (1955), in discussing the significance of positive tests for free antibodies given by the sera of patients with AIHA, reported that he and his colleagues had detected univalent antibodies in some normal sera capable of producing weak sensitization of erythrocytes *in vitro* at 37°C.

Delage and Simard (1958) described further observations along the same lines. Positive antiglobulin reactions were obtained when normal erythrocytes at concentrations of less than 10% were incubated at 37°C in strong concentrations of autologous or compatible homologous serum for periods of 2–5 hours. The results were negative at 1 hour and the strongest agglutination occurred in high concentrations of potent antiglobulin sera. The results were uniformly negative using neonatal serum but positive with the serum of 14- or 16-month-old babies. The reaction was abolished by pre-heating the serum to 56°C for 30 minutes; anticoagulants were also inhibitory.

In a more recent study Amsel, Ssebabi and Nzaro (1974) reported that approximately one-third of the sera of Ugandan villagers and medical and malarial patients contained auto-antibodies that gave positive antiglobulin tests after their erythrocytes had been exposed to bromelin. It is interesting that the test was negative in all of 33 medical students; on the other hand, it was positive in six out of 10 patients with haemolytic anaemia and tropical splenomegaly syndrome and in nine out of 11 patients suffering from haemolytic anaemia in pregnancy. Amsel, Ssebabi and Nzaro referred to earlier publications in which antibodies of varying nature had been shown to be present in the sera of an unusually high percentage of those living in tropical countries, compared to their incidence outside the tropics. It seems likely, as they pointed out, that the antibodies were formed 'either [as] a result of numerous infections, a sequel to the tissue damage caused by the infections, or [are] a non-specific concomitant of increased immunoglobulin production'.

SOME UNUSUAL AUTO- AND PAN-AGGLUTININS

A number of sera have been described in which antibodies have been detected that react *in vitro* only under particular (and unexpected) circumstances. Although their presence is interesting, they appear to be of little, if any, clinical significance. However, because they may be confused with pathogenic auto-antibodies and have been a source of difficulty in blood-transfusion practice, they are referred to briefly below.

Auto-agglutinins inhibited by ionized calcium

An interesting cold agglutinin was described by Parish and Macfarlane (1941) in the serum of a healthy man aged 27. This antibody agglutinated normal group-O erythrocytes as well as the patient's own cells at room or lower temperatures but only in the absence of ionized calcium. For instance, erythrocytes suspended in solutions of citrate or oxalate were agglutinated if added to the serum but not cells suspended in saline alone. Calcium chloride added to mixtures of serum and cells suspended in citrate inhibited agglutination.

Jacobowicz and Bryce (1949), in describing the reactions of anti-O agglutinins that they had identified in the serum of two healthy women, reported that the activity of one of them, which had persisted unchanged in the serum for 2 years, was inhibited by the presence of calcium. The reaction of the serum versus group-O, -A_2 and cord cells suggested that its specificity was anti-H. The serum acted strongly at room temperature but was still active at 37°C (titre 8). An additional unusual requirement of the antibody was that not only had calcium to be absent but sodium, as provided in normal saline, seemed to have to be in excess.

A further agglutinin present in the serum of a healthy blood donor, which reacted only in the absence of calcium, was described by Gunson (1969); it differed from the agglutinin described by Jacobowicz and Bryce (1949) only in not seeming to require an excess of sodium ions to react. Gunson reported that agglutination was reversed by the presence of either calcium ions or of metallic ions, e.g. those of zinc chloride and cadmium chloride, both of which release calcium from EDTA complexes. The agglutinin was shown to be anti-H and to be a 19S γM globulin. Gunson suggested that the calcium ions combine with the agglutinin molecules at their erythrocyte binding sites but are removed by salts which are able to chelate calcium.

'Albumin agglutinins'

An interesting phenomenon described originally under the title '"Albumin" auto-agglutinating property in three sera. "A pitfall for the unwary"' by Weiner and his co-workers (1956) at one time aroused considerable interest. The serum from three patients, who presented no evidence of any blood disorder, strongly agglutinated their own cells at 37°C, and all normal cells tested, when the cells were suspended in 20% or 30% bovine albumin. The cells were not, however, agglutinated in saline suspension and the IAT was negative in each case. Other similar reports soon followed (Weiner and Hallum, 1957; Moore, Linins and McIntyre, 1959; Marsh and Jenkins, 1961). Crowley and Hyland (1962) noted that the agglutination took place in the presence of commercially available bovine or human albumin and suggested that it resulted from the presence of denatured proteins in the preparations. Later, Golde, McGinniss and Holland (1969) suggested that the agglutination was brought about by the non-specific adsorption of antigen–antibody complexes on to the erythrocytes, the antibody being a γ globulin directed at albumin that had been altered by the addition to the preparation of acetyl tryptophanate or caprylate that had been added as stabilizers. Spence, Jones and Moore (1971) concluded that the ability to convert a non-reactive albumin preparation to one that would react with a patient's serum is a general property of short-chain fatty acids (3–8 carbon atoms in length — caprylic acid has 7 carbon atoms).

Golde, Greipp and McGinniss (1973), who studied four albumin-agglutinating sera, all causing pan- and auto-agglutination, concluded that although most sera reacted only with albumin stabilized by short-chain fatty acids, other specificities may exist. Subsequent work (Beck et al., 1976) has indicated that the 'albumin agglutinins' in human sera are in fact antibodies directed against sodium caprylate or other fatty acid salts and not against albumin. The human antibodies are usually IgM but may be IgG, which presumably explains the reported presence of 'albumin agglutinins' in cord sera (e.g. by Weiner and Hallum, 1957).

In none of the reports cited above has there been any suggestion that 'albumin agglutinins' have been responsible for increased haemolysis. This is true also of the report by Hossaini, Burkhardt and Hooper (1965). Their patient was a 7-year-old girl who developed an acute transient haemolytic anaemia (Hb 5 g/dl) of obscure origin, but possibly associated with the inhalation of DDT. The DAT and IAT were negative. However, her serum strongly agglutinated her own erythrocytes and normal group-O cells in the presence of 15% and 30%, but not of 7%, commercial bovine albumin at 4°C, 22°C and 37°C. On the other hand, it failed to agglutinate the cells in the presence of 25% human albumin. The child was successfully transfused despite the presence of the 'albumin agglutinins' and soon recovered completely. Hossaini, Burkhardt and Hooper concluded that the 'albumin agglutinins' were of no clinical significance. However, in this case at least, their detection in vitro under, admittedly, wholly unphysiological conditions is perhaps a pointer to the development of other auto-antibodies which, although not demonstrated in vitro, were of pathogenic significance in vivo and were responsible for the acute haemolysis.

A further example of a caprylate-dependent 'albumin auto-agglutinin' was described by Dube, Zoes and Adesman (1977). Their patient had sustained severe injuries following a car accident, including a retroperitoneal haematoma. The antibody was remarkable in that it had anti-e specificity.

Antibodies active against stored erythrocytes

Several unusual antibodies have been described which have reacted strongly with erythrocytes that have been stored but have failed to react, or only reacted weakly, with the same cells when fresh.

Hougie, Dandridge and Bobbit (1958) described an 80-year-old man suffering from haemolytic anaemia and Hodgkin's disease whose serum contained an unusual panagglutinin. The DAT was negative. The patient was group B, Rh+, and at first it was thought that his serum, while agglutinating at 37°C all B Rh+ samples tested, did not agglutinate his own erythrocytes. Later it was realized that all the cells tested except his own had been stored at 4°C for 72 hours. Further investigation showed that while storage at 4°C or 28°C for 24 hours failed to cause agglutination, storage for 48 hours resulted in all the samples tested, including the patient's cells, becoming agglutinable. Agglutination occurred irrespective of the presence of anticoagulants, but was delayed by EDTA and heparin; it was most marked with cells stored in their own serum.

Stratton, Renton and Rawlinson (1960) had investigated a woman aged 71 with anaemia and Hodgkin's disease. Her serum agglutinated a wide range of erythrocytes of different phenotypes, without any obvious blood-group specificity. The strength of agglutination increased progressively as the test cells were stored (Fig. 25.7). Agglutination was stronger when serum-albumin rather than saline was used as the

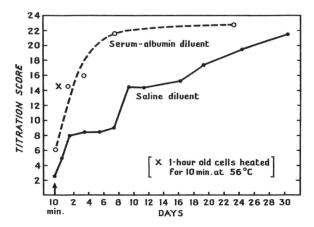

Fig. 25.7   Effect of the storage of erythrocytes on agglutination by an unusual auto-antibody.
[Reproduced by permission from Stratton, Renton and Rawlinson (1960).]

diluent in titrations, and the cells were more strongly agglutinated at 37°C than at 16°C. The agglutinated cells, when examined under the microscope, presented as a 'mixed field', and differential centrifugation indicated that it was the older (denser) erythrocytes that were mainly agglutinated (Fig. 25.8 a,b). Stratton, Renton and Rawlinson considered that the change towards increased agglutinability that could be produced *in vitro* by storage was probably taking place *in vivo*, too.

Jenkins and Marsh (1961) described three patients, women aged between 43 and 58, who had haemolytic anaemia associated probably with biological false-positive reactions for syphilis. In each case an unusual anti-erythrocyte antibody was present in their serum, the specificity of which could not be determined. In two of the patients the serum reacted with saline-suspended stored cells; in the third patient the IAT was positive with stored cells. In all three cases fresh cells from the same donors failed to react. One of the patients was investigated in detail. She had a severe haemolytic anaemia and had earlier been treated by X-irradiation and oophorectomy for carcinoma of the breast and ovaries. The DAT was positive (non-γ type) and there was auto-agglutination. In initial tests 25 out of 50 group-O erythrocyte samples, stored for various periods at −20°C in glycerol, were agglutinated at 37°C in saline or albumin to a titre of 128. Fresh samples from the same donors were not agglutinated. Enzyme-modified cells from all the donors tested — irrespective of whether the cells were stored or fresh—were agglutinated. Jenkins and Marsh concluded that the antigen with which the antibody was reacting arose during storage as the result of intracellular enzymes acting on a precursor substance and that during the patient's haemolytic crisis the antigen was present in an activated form. The possibility was considered that the antibody was an unusual form of an anti-T [known rarely to be responsible for haemolytic anaemia (see p. 203)]. Absorption experiments indicated, however, that this was not so.

Ozer and Chaplin (1963) described the results of a major study into the nature of an unusual agglutinin that, while failing to agglutinate normal compatible erythrocytes when they were fresh, agglutinated the

(a)   (b)

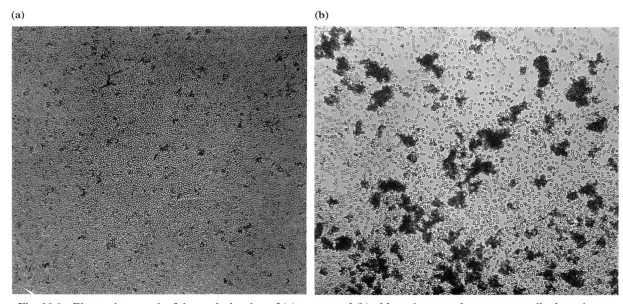

Fig. 25.8   Photomicrograph of the agglutination of (a) young and (b) old erythrocytes by an auto-antibody active against stored cells.
[Reproduced by permission from Stratton, Renton and Rawlinson (1960).]

same cells with progressively increasing strength as the cells were stored at 4°C for 5–21 days or for up to 24 hours at 37°C. The agglutinin was found in the serum of an elderly patient with splenomegaly and haemolytic anaemia associated with macroglobulinaemia.

The agglutinin was itself shown to be a macroglobulin; its activity was not affected by change in pH between 5.6 and 8.0, and it was as active at 37°C as it was at 4°C. Agglutination was demonstrable, using stored cells, up to serum dilutions of 1 in 100 000 or even higher. It appeared likely that the change to the surface of the erythrocytes that allowed them to be agglutinated when they had been stored was in some way linked with loss of intracellular glucose and high-energy phosphate compounds. In-vivo experiments, using ^{51}Cr, revealed a close relationship between agglutinability in vitro and shortened survival in vivo. A study carried out with ^{59}Fe indicated that the development of agglutinability during storage was unrelated to in-vivo chronological cell age.

Easton, Priest and Giles (1965) described a 60-year-old woman with hepatic cirrhosis. The DAT was positive with an anti-non-γ antiglobulin serum and her serum contained a wide-thermal-amplitude cold auto-antibody which lysed ficin-treated erythrocytes at 37°C. However, glycerol- or ACD-stored cells, or cells heated to 56°C for 30 minutes, reacted better than did fresh cells. The antigen with which the antibody reacted appeared to be present in varying degrees in all stored cell samples tested and no specificity could be established. Routine tests for syphilis were positive, too, but the reaction seemed likely to be a biologically false one.

Arndt and co-workers (1989) described a patient with AIHA whose serum contained an unusual antibody that caused a mixed field IAT and weakly lysed normal erythrocytes (and strongly lysed enzyme-treated cells). The DAT was positive: i.e. 3+ with an anti-C3 serum and 1+ with an anti-IgG serum. The antibody in the serum acted preferentially on stored erythrocytes and on old (dense) erythrocytes separated from whole blood by centrifugation. It was suggested that the antigen with which the antibody reacted was the senescent cell antigen thought to play a part in physiological erythrocyte destruction.

Auto-antibodies agglutinating erythrocytes washed in saline

Freisleben and Jensen (1960) described under the title 'An antibody specific for washed red cells' three sera, two from normal blood donors and one from a patient with fibroids, which agglutinated all erythrocytes tested, including the patient's own cells, provided the cells had been freshly washed in saline before being added to the serum. The antibody reacted strongly at 4°C, less strongly at room temperature and was inactive at 37°C. The agglutinin could be removed from the sera by absorption with freshly washed cells, the absorbing cells then being agglutinated by an anti-non-γ antiglobulin serum. No blood-group specificity could be demonstrated.

Allan and co-workers (1972) described four sera which contained antibodies similar to, although not apparently identical with, those described by Freisleben and Jensen (1960). In each case the sera agglutinated all the erythrocytes tested, provided the cells had been first washed in saline. Agglutination was strongest at 25°C but still occurred at 37°C. If, however, the washed cells were allowed to stand for 5–30 minutes before being added to the serum, agglutination failed to occur. (The time necessary for ⌐⌐ inactivation differed from serum to serum).

Other unusual auto-agglutinins

Harboe and co-workers (1961) described the formation by a man aged 66 who died of chronic pyelonephritis of an auto-antibody 'with peculiar haemagglutinating properties'. The patient was group A and his erythrocytes, and the cells of normal group-A individuals, were strongly agglutinated when washed in saline after having been exposed to the serum. The agglutinin in the serum was a high molecular weight γ globulin which was thought to have some of the characters of the rheumatoid factor. The antibody was present at high titre (512) and appeared to be equally active at 4°, 20° and 37°C. Harboe et al. concluded that the type of antibody they had investigated must be rare for it would be shown up whenever an IAT was attempted. Compared with washing in saline, agglutination was partially prevented if the cells were washed in EDTA or 3.1% trisodium citrate solution. The patient had a mild compensated haemolytic anaemia but this seems likely to have been associated with his chronic renal disease. The DAT was negative.

A further unusual auto-agglutinin was described by Dorner, Parker and Chaplin (1968) in the serum of a man aged 23 who died of renal cortical necrosis. He had sustained major trauma in a car accident, including massive intraperitoneal haemorrhage and received in all 38 units of blood over a 5-week period. Forty-four days after the accident his erythrocytes were found to auto-agglutinate in all media and his serum agglutinated all cells exposed to it. The agglutinin was present at a very high titre (2048) at 37°C and was slightly less active at 25°C and less active still at 4°C. It was inactivated by exposure to 2-ME. A remarkable feature of the case was that there was no evidence of in-vivo auto-agglutination. Dorner, Parker and Chaplin suggested that this was consistent with the fact that in-vitro agglutination was observed to take place only slowly: it was but weak after 1 minute and took 4–5 minutes to become intense. Attempts to carry out DATs were unsatisfactory as the cells in the saline control were strongly agglutinated.

REFERENCES

AHO, K. & CHRISTIAN, C. L. (1966). Studies of incomplete antibodies. I. Effect of papain on red cells. *Blood*, 27, 662–669.

ALLAN, C. J., LAWRENCE, R. D., SHIH, S. C., WILLIAMSON, K.R., SWEATT, M. A. & TASWELL, H. F. (1972). Agglutination of erythrocytes freshly washed with saline solution. Four saline-autoagglutinating sera. *Transfusion*, 12, 306–311.

AMSEL, S., SSEBABI, E. C. T. & NZARO, E. (1974). Red cell autoantibodies in Ugandan sera. *Clin. exp. Immunol.*, 16, 657–663.

ARAGUÁS, C., MARTÍN-VEGA, A., MASSAGUÉ, I. & DE LATORRE, F. J. (1990). 'Complete' warm hemolysins producing an autoimmune hemolytic anemia. *Vox Sang.*, 59, 125–126.

ARNDT, P., O'HOSKI, P., MCBRIDE, J. & GARRATTY, G. (1989). Autoimmune hemolytic anemia associated with an antibody reacting preferentially with 'old' red cells. *Transfusion*, 29, Suppl., 48S (Abstract S172).

BAIKIE, A. G. & PIRRIE, R. (1956). Megaloblastic erythropoiesis in idiopathic acquired haemolytic anaemia. *Scot. med. J.*, 1, 330–334.

BAUMGARTNER, W. (1956). Maladie par autoagression. Akute hämolytische Anämie, thrombocytopenische purpura und granulocytopenie. *Helv. med. acta*, 23, 324–330.

BECK, M. L., EDWARDS, R. L., PIERCE, S. R., HICKLIN, B. L. & BAYER, W. L. (1976). Serologic activity of the fatty acid dependent antibodies in albumin-free systems. *Transfusion*, 16, 434–436.

BELL, C. A., ZWICKER, H. & NEVIUS, D. B. (1973). Nonspecific warm haemolysins of papain-treated cells: serologic characterization and transfusion risk. *Transfusion*, 13, 207–213.

BOORMAN, K. E., DODD, B. E. & LOUTIT, J. F. (1946). Haemolytic icterus (acholuric jaundice) congenital and acquired. *Lancet*, i, 812–814.

BRANCH, D. R., SY SIOK HIAN, A. L. & PETZ, L. D. (1982). A new elution procedure using chloroform, a noninflammable organic solvent. *Vox Sang.*, 42, 46–53.

BRAUNSTEINER, H., MANNHEIMER, E. & REIMER, E. E. (1953). Erworbene hämolytische Anämie mit zeitweisen Auftreten eines pH-abhängigen Hämolysins. *Dtsch. Arch. klin. Med.*, 200, 316–322.

BUENO, R., GARRATTY, G. & POSTOWAY, N. (1981). Elution of antibody from red cells using xylene—a superior method. *Transfusion*, 21, 157–162.

CAMOENS, H. & BERG, K. (1973). Studies on naturally occurring warm haemolysins and haemagglutinins active against trypsinized red cells. Reproduction of the phenomena. *Vox Sang.*, 24, 283–286.

CASSELL, M. & CHAPLIN, H. JNR (1960). Studies on anti-eluate sera. II. Comparison of a conventional antiglobulin serum with three anti-eluate sera in the study of 70 patients with acquired hemolytic anemia. *Vox Sang.*, 5, 43–52.

CHAN-SHU, S. A. & BLAIR, O. (1979). A new method of antibody elution from red blood cells. *Transfusion*, 19, 182–185.

CHAPLIN, H. JNR & CASSELL, M. (1958). The heterogeneity of positive antiglobulin reactions in acquired hemolytic anemia. *J. Lab. clin. Med.*, 52, 803 (Abstract).

CHAPLIN, H. Jnr & Cassell, M. (1960). Studies on anti-eluate sera. I. The production of antiglobulin (Coombs) sera in rabbits by the use of antibodies eluted from sensitized red blood cells. *Vox Sang.*, 5, 32–42.

CHAUFFARD, M. A. & TROISIER, J. (1908a). Anémie grave avec hémolysine dans le sèrum; ictère hémolysinique. *Sem. méd. (Paris)*, 28, 345.

CHAUFFARD, M. A. & TROISIER, J. (1908b). Contributions à l'étude des hémolysines dans leurs rapports avec les anémies graves. *Bull. Mém. Soc. méd. Hôp. Paris*, 26, 94–105.

CHAUFFARD, M. A. & VINCENT, C. (1909). Hémoglobinurie hémolysinique avec ictère polycholique aigu. *Sem. méd. (Paris)*, 29, 601–604.

CHEVALIER, P., BILSKI-PASQUIER, G., EYQUEM, A., SAINT-PAUL, M. & VELEZ, E. (1954). Étude immuno-hématologique d'une anémie hémolytique acquise (co-existence d'anticorps multiples: auto- et iso-hémagglutinines, auto- et iso-hémolysines, leuco-agglutinines, thrombo-agglutinines, et hetero-agglutinines, donnant une réaction de Paul et Bunnell positive). *Sém. Hôp. Paris*, 30, 4351–4354.

COFFIELD, K. J. & SPAET, T. H. (1959). Studies on the normal serum panagglutinin active against trypsinated human erythrocytes. V. The nonidentity of the agglutinin with serum trypsin inhibitor and the components of complement. *J. Lab. clin. Med.*, 54, 871–875.

COOK, G. M. W., HEARD, D. H. & SEAMAN, G. V. F. (1960). A sialomucopeptide liberated by trypsin from the human erythrocyte. *Nature (Lond.)*, 188, 1011–1012.

CROWLEY, L. V. & HYLAND, F. R. (1962). The albumin autoagglutination phenomenon. *Amer. J. clin. Path.*, 37, 244–247.

DACIE, J. V. (1949). Hemolysins in acquired hemolytic anemia. Effect of pH on the activity in vitro of a serum hemolysin. *Blood*, 4, 928–935.

DACIE, J. V. (1953). Acquired hemolytic anemia. With special reference to the antiglobulin (Coombs') reaction. *Blood*, 8, 813–823.

DACIE, J. V. (1954). *The Haemolytic Anaemias: Congenital and Acquired*, pp. 164–216. Churchill, London.

DACIE, J. V. (1959). Acquired haemolytic anaemia. In *Lectures on the Scientific Basis of Medicine, Vol. 7 (1957–58)*, pp. 59–79. University of London, Athlone Press, London.

DACIE, J. V. (1962). *The Haemolytic Anaemias: Congenital and Acquired. Part II—The Auto-immune Haemolytic Anaemias*, 2nd edn, 377 pp. Churchill, London.

DACIE, J. V. & CUTBUSH, M. (1954). Specificity of auto-antibodies in acquired haemolytic anaemia. *J. clin. Path.*, 7, 18–21.

DACIE, J. V. & DE GRUCHY, G. C. (1951). Auto-antibodies in acquired haemolytic anaemia. *J. clin. Path.*, 4, 253–271.

DACIE, J. V. & WORLLEDGE, S. (1975). Auto-allergic blood diseases. In *Clinical Aspects of Immunology*, 3rd edn (ed. by P. G. H. Gell, R. R. A. Coombs and P. J. Lachmann), pp. 1149–1182. Blackwell Scientific Publications, Oxford.

DAMESHEK, W. (1951). Anémie hémolytique acquise. Physiopatholoque. Considerations sur l'auto-immunisation et le traitment. *Rev. Hémat.*, 6, 255–266.

DAMESHEK, W. & SCHWARTZ, S. O. (1938). The presence of hemolysins in acute hemolytic anemia. *New Engl. J. Med.*, 218, 75–80.

DAMESHEK, W. & SCHWARTZ, S. O. (1940). Acute hemolytic anemia (acquired hemolytic icterus, acute type). *Medicine (Baltimore)*, 19, 231–327.

DAUSSET, J. (1951). Note sur l'agglutination des hématies trypsinisées. *Rev. Hémat.*, 6, 382–384.

DAUSSET, J. (1952a). The agglutination mechanism of trypsin modified red cells. *Blood*, 7, 816–825.

DAUSSET (1952b). Les hémolysines dans les anémies hémolytiques et les hémoglobinuries. *Sem. Hôp., Paris.* 28, 814–824.

DAUSSET, J. & COLOMBANI, J. (1959). The serology and the prognosis of 128 cases of autoimmune hemolytic anemia. *Blood*, 14, 1280–1301.

DAUSSET, J., COLOMBANI, J. & EVELIN, J. (1957). Technique de recherche des auto-hémolysines immunologiques. *Rev. franç., Ét. clin. biol.*, 2, 735–745.

DAUSSET, J., COLOMBANI, J., JEAN, R. G., CANLORBE, P. & LELONG, M. (1957). Sur un cas d'anémie hémolytique aiguë de l'enfant avec présence d'une hémolysine immunologique et d'un pouvoir anticomplémentaire du serum. *Sang*, 28, 351–363.

DAUSSET, J. & VIDAL, G. (1951). Étude sérologique de douze cas d'anémie hémolytique acquise avec auto-anticorps. *Rev. Hémat.*, 6, 369–382.

DAVID, J. K. JNR & MINOT, A. S. (1944). Acute hemolytic anemia in infancy. Report of a case with demonstration of hemolytic activity of serum. *Amer. J. Dis. Child.*, 68, 327–329.

DAVIDSOHN, I. & OYAMADA, A. (1953). Specificity of auto-antibodies in hemolytic anemia. *Amer. J. clin. Path.*, 23, 101–115.

DAVIDSOHN, I. & SPURRIER, W. (1954). Immunohematological studies in hemolytic anemia. *J. Amer. med. Ass.*, 154, 818–821.

DELAGE, J. -M. & SIMARD, J. (1958). A natural warm 'auto-antibody'. *Canad. med. Ass. J.*, 78, 113–117.

DENYS, P. & VAN DEN BROUCKE, J. (1947). Anémie hémolytique acquise et réaction de Coombs. *Arch. franç. Pédiat.*, 4, 205–217.

DORNER, I. M., PARKER, C. W. & CHAPLIN, H. JNR (1968). Autoagglutination developing in a patient with acute renal failure: characterization of the autoagglutinin and its relation to transfusion therapy. *Brit. J. Haemat.*, 14, 383–394.

DUBE, V. E., ZOES, C. & ADESMAN, P. (1977). Caprylate-dependent auto-anti-e. *Vox Sang.*, 33, 359–363.

DYBKJAER, E. & KISSMEYER-NIELSEN, F. (1967). Enzyme reacting specific auto-antibodies in individuals showing no signs of auto-immune haemolytic anaemia. *Vox Sang.*, 12, 429–442.

EASTON, J. A., PRIEST, C. J. & GILES, C. M. (1965). An antibody against stored blood associated with cirrhosis of the liver and false-positive serological tests for syphilis. *J. clin. Path.*, 18, 460–461.

ENGELFRIET, C. P., BECKERS, TH. A. P., VAN'T VEER, M. B., VON DEM BORNE, A. E. G. KR. & OUWEHAND, W. H. (1983). Recent advances in immune haemolytic anaemia. In *Recent Advances in Haematology, Immunology and Blood Transfusion* (ed. by S. R. Hollán, I. Bernét, G. Füst, G. Gárdos and B. Sarkadi), pp. 235–252. John Wiley and Akadémiai Kiadó, Budapest.

EVANS, R. S. (1955). Autoantibodies in hematologic disorders. *Stanford med. Bull.*, 13, 152–166.

EVANS, R. S. & WEISER, R. S. (1957). The serology of autoimmune hemolytic disease: observations on forty-one patients. *Arch. intern. Med.*, 100, 371–399.

EYLAR, E. H., MADOFF, M. A., BRODY, O. V. & ONCLEY, J. L. (1962). The contribution of sialic acid to the surface charge of the erythrocytes. *J. biol. Chem.*, 237, 1992–2000.

EYQUEM, A. (1951). Problèmes immunologiques liés au diagnostic et au traitement des anémies hémolytiques acquises. *Rev. hémat.*, 6, 334–348.

FARRAR, G. E. JNR, BURNETT, W. E. & STEIGMAN, A. J. (1940). Hemolytic anemia and hepatic degeneration cured by splenectomy. *Amer. J. med. Sci.*, 200, 164–172.

FOSTER, W. D. & HUTT, M. S. R. (1953). Observations on the behaviour of enzyme-treated red cells in a case of haemolytic anaemia. *J. Path. Bact.*, 66, 383–389.

FREEDMAN, J., WRIGHT, J., LIM, F. C. & GARVEY, M. B. (1987). Hemolytic warm IgM autoagglutinins in autoimmune hemolytic anemia. *Transfusion*, 27, 464–467.

FREISLEBEN, E. & JENSEN, K. G. (1960). An antibody specific for washed red cells. In *Proc. 7th Congr. Europ. Soc. Haemat. London, 1959; Part II*, pp. 1156–1158. Karger, Basel.

FUDENBERG, H., BARRY, I. & DAMESHEK, W. (1958). The erythrocyte-coating substance in autoimmune hemolytic disease: its nature and significance. *Blood*, 13, 201–215.

FUKUOKA, T. & ANDO, S. (1965). Clinical studies on autoimmune hemolytic anemia. I. Serological studies on free autoantibodies in serum. *Acta haemat. jap.*, **28**, 623–630.

GARDNER, F. H. (1949). Transfer to normal red cells of an agglutinin demonstrable in the acidified sera of patients with acquired hemolytic jaundice. *J. clin. Invest.*, **28**, 783–784 (Abstract).

GARDNER, F. H. & HARRIS, J. W. (1950). The demonstration of hemolysins in acquired hemolytic anemia. *J. clin. Invest.*, **29**, 814–815 (Abstract).

GOLDE, D. W., GREIPP, P. R. & MCGINNISS, M. H. (1973). Spectrum of albumin auto-agglutinins. *Transfusion*, **13**, 1–5.

GOLDE, D. W., MCGINNISS, M. H. & HOLLAND, P. V. (1969). Mechanism of the albumin agglutination phenomenon. *Vox Sang.*, **16**, 465–469.

GREENWALT, T. J. (1956). A method of eluting antibodies from red-cell stromata. *J. Lab. clin. Med.*, **48**, 634–635.

GUNSON, H. H. (1969). A serum agglutinin inhibited by ionized calcium. *Vox Sang.*, **17**, 514–524.

HANFLAND, P. (1982). A simple method for the rapid and selective absorption of warm-reactive erythrocyte autoantibodies from serum. *Vox Sang.*, **43**, 310–320.

HARBOE, M. T., REINSKOU, T., HEISTÖ, H. & BJÖRNSTAD, P. (1961). Studies on a serum with peculiar haemagglutinating properties. *Vox Sang.*, **6**, 409–428.

HEISTØ, H., HARBOE, M. & GODAL, H. C. (1965). Warm haemolysins active against trypsinized red cells: occurrence, inheritance and clinical significance. *Proc. 10th Congr. int. Soc. Blood Transfusion, Stockholm 1964*, pp. 787–789. Karger, Basel.

HEISTØ, H., JENSEN, L. & KNUDS, F. (1971). Studies on trypsin treatment of red cells with special reference to differences between trypsin preparations. *Vox Sang.*, **21**, 115–125.

HELLER, I., NELKEN, D. & GUREVITCH (1958). Études sérologiques sur les anticorps antiérythrocytaires, antileucocytaires et antiplaquettaires dans différentes affections hématologiques. *Sang*, **29**, 17–22.

HENI, F. & BLESSING, K. (1954a). Die Bedeutung der Glutinine für die erworbenen hämolytischen Anämien. *Dtsch. Arch. klin. Med.*, **201**, 113–135.

HENI, F. & BLESSING, K. (1954b). Beschreibung zwier schwerer erworbener idiopathischer hämolytischer Anämien. *Klin. Wschr.*, **32**, 481–485.

HOSSAINI, A. A., BURKHART, C. R. & Hooper, G. S. (1965). A further example of the non-immune auto-agglutinating property of serum. *Transfusion*, **5**, 461–464.

HOUGIE, C., DANDRIDGE, J. & BOBBIT, A. B. (1958). A new autoagglutinin against stored erythrocytes. *Proc. 7th Congr. int. Soc. Blood Transfusion (Bibliotheca haemat., 10)*, 252–254. Karger, Basel.

HOWARD, P. L. (1981). Principles of antibody elution. *Transfusion*, **21**, 477–482.

HOYT, R. E. & ZWICKER, H. (1953). The role of enzyme in reversible agglutination of red cells. *J. Immunol.*, **71**, 325–330.

HURLEY, J. H. & DACIE, J. V. (1953). Haemolysis and reversible agglutination of trypsinized normal red cells by a normal human serum. *J. clin. Path.*, **6**, 211–214.

JACOBOWICZ, R. & BRYCE, L. M. (1949). Some observations on anti-O agglutinins. *Med. J. Aust.*, **ii**, 373–376.

JAMES, P., ROWE, G. P. & TOZZO, G. G. (1988). Elucidation of alloantibodies in autoimmune haemolytic anaemia. *Vox Sang.*, **54**, 167–171.

JANKOVIĆ, B. D. (1954). An incomplete warm antibody in normal human serum. *Acta med. iugoslavica*, **8**, 174–176.

JENKINS, D. E. JNR & MOORE, W. H. (1977). A rapid method for the preparation of high potency auto and alloantibody eluates. *Transfusion*, **17**, 110–114.

JENKINS, W. J. & MARSH, W. L. (1961). Autoimmune haemolytic anaemia. Three cases with antibodies specifically active against stored red cells. *Lancet*, **ii**, 16–18.

JENSEN, K. G. (1959). Elution of incomplete antibodies from red cells. A comparison of different methods. *Vox Sang.*, **4**, 230–239.

KIDD, P. (1949). Elution of an incomplete type of antibody from the erythrocytes in acquired haemolytic anaemia. *J. clin. Path.*, **2**, 103–108.

KOMNINOS, Z. D. & AKSOY, M. (1954). Studies on antibodies eluted from erythrocytes in autoimmune hemolytic anemia. *J. clin. Invest.*, **33**, 949 (Abstract).

KOMNINOS, Z. D. & DÉSY, L. (1955). Thermal range of activity of antibodies eluted from the red cells in autoimmune hemolytic anemia. *J. Lab. clin. Med.*, **46**, 74–79.

KOMNINOS, Z. D. & ROSENTHAL, M. C. (1953). Studies on antibodies eluted from red cells in autoimmune hemolytic anemia. *J. Lab. clin. Med.*, **41**, 887–894.

KONDA, S. & YAMADA, A (1960). Characteristics of the auto-antibody attached to erythrocytes of the patient with auto-immune hemolytic anemia. *Acta haemat. jap.*, **23**, 879–886.

KUHNS, W. J. & WAGLEY, P. F. (1949). Hemolytic anemia associated with atypical hemagglutinins. *Ann. intern. Med.*, **30**, 408–423.

LALEZARI, P. & OBERHARDT, B. (1971). Temperature gradient dissociation of red cell antigen–antibody complexes in the Polybrene technique. *Brit. J. Haemat.*, **21**, 131–146.

LANDSTEINER, K. & MILLER, C. P. JNR (1925). Serological studies on the blood of primates. II. The blood groups in anthropoid apes. *J. exp. Med.*, **42**, 853–862.

LEMAIRE, A., LOEPER, J., BOIREN, M. & DAUSSET, J. (1954). Anémie hémolytique aiguë avec auto-anticorps actif seulement sur les hématies traitées par un enzyme proteolytique. Étude d'une étiologie virale possible. *Bull. Mém. Soc. méd. Hôp. Paris*, **70**, 997–1007.

LETMAN, H. (1957). Auto-immune haemolytic anaemia. *Dan. med. Bull.*, **4**, 143–147.

LUBINSKI, H. & GOLDBLOOM, A. (1946). Acute hemolytic anemia associated with autoagglutination with a thermal amplitude of 0 to 37°C. *Amer. J. Dis. Child.*, **78**, 325–333.

MANTEL, W. & HOLTZ, G. (1976). Characterisation of autoantibodies to erythrocytes in autoimmune haemolytic anaemia by chloroquine. *Vox Sang.*, **30**, 453–463.

MARTONI, L. & MUSIANI, S. (1956). Anemia emolitica acquisata idiopatica autoimmune complicata di mieloplasia eritoblastica in un lattante di 6 mesi. *Clin. pediat. (Bologna)*, **38**, 483–506.

MARSH, W. L. & JENKINS, W. J. (1961). A possible specificity of albumin auto-antibodies. *Nature (Lond.)*, **190**, 180.

MARTIN DU PAN, R. (1948). L'ictère hémolytique, les 'hémagglutinines' et les 'antiagglutinines.' *Schweiz. med. Wschr.*, **78**, 34–37.

MASSUET, L. & ARMENGOL, R. (1980). A new method of antibody elution from red blood cells using organic solvents. *Vox Sang.*, **39**, 343–344.

MELLBYE, O. J. (1965). Reversible agglutination of trypsinised red cells by normal human sera. Identification of the agglutinating factor as a γM-globulin. *Scand. J. Haemat.*, **2**, 318–330.

MELLBYE, O. J. (1966). Reversible agglutination of trypsinised red cells by a γM-globulin synthesized by the human foetus. *Scand. J. Haemat.*, **3**, 310–324.

MELLBYE, O. J. (1967). Reversible agglutination of trypsinised red cells by normal human sera. Identification of the reversing factor as an amino acid. *Scand. J. Haemat.*, **4**, 135–144.

MELLBYE, O. J. (1969a). Properties of the trypsinised red cell receptor reacting in reversible agglutination by normal sera. *Scand. J. Haemat.*, **6**, 139–148.

MELLBYE, O. J. (1969b). Specificity of natural human agglutinins against red cells modified by trypsin and other agents. *Scand. J. Haemat.*, **6**, 166–172.

MICHON, P., LOCHARD, & CHAMALY, P (1954). Anémie hémolytique acquise transitoire avec auto et iso-anticorps. *Sang*, **25**, 521–524.

MOORE, B. P. L., LININS, I. & McINTYRE, J. (1959). A serum with an albumin-active, autoagglutinating property. *Blood*, **14**, 364–368.

MOREL, P. A., BERGREN, M. O. & FRANK, B. A. (1978). A simple method for the detection of alloantibody in the presence of warm autoantibody. *Transfusion*, **18**, 388 (Abstract, S-53).

MORTON, J. A. & PICKLES, M. M. (1947). Use of trypsin in the detection of incomplete anti-Rh antibodies. *Nature (Lond.)*, **159**, 779–780.

MORTON, J. A. & PICKLES, M. M. (1951). The proteolytic enzyme test for detecting incomplete antibodies. *J. clin. Path.*, **4**, 189–199.

NEBER, J. & DAMESHEK, W. (1947). The improved demonstration of circulating antibodies in hemolytic anemia by the use of bovine albumin. *Blood*, **2**, 371–380.

OZER, F. L. & CHAPLIN, H. JNR (1963). Agglutination of stored erythrocytes by a human serum. Characterization of the serum factor and erythrocyte changes. *J. clin. Invest.*, **42**, 1735–1752.

PANZER, S., SALAMA, A., BÖDEKER, R. H. & MUELLER-ECKHARDT, C. (1984). Quantitative evaluation of elution methods for red cell antibodies. *Vox Sang.*, **46**, 330–335.

PARISH, H. J. & MACFARLANE, R. G. (1941). Effect of calcium in a case of autohaemagglutination. *Lancet*, **ii**, 477–479.

PAYNE, R., SPAET, T. H. & AGGELER, P. M. (1955). An unusual antibody pattern in a case of idiopathic acquired hemolytic anemia. *J. Lab. clin. Med.*, **46**, 245–254.

PICKLES, M. M. (1989). The discovery of the enzyme test for Rh antibodies. *Vox Sang.*, **57**, 223–224.

PIROFSKY, B. (1958). Immunologic differences between iso-antibodies and auto-antibodies. *Amer. J. clin. Path.*, **29**, 120–127.

PISCIOTTA, A. V., DOWNER, E. M. & HINZ, J. E. (1959). Clinical and laboratory correlation in severe autoimmune hemolytic anemia. *Arch. intern. Med.*, **104**, 264–276.

PISCIOTTA, A. V. & HINZ, J. E. (1957). Detection and characterization of autoantibodies in acquired auto-immune hemolytic anemia. *Amer. J. clin. Path.*, **27**, 619–634.

POLLACK, W., HAGER, H. J., RECKEL, R., TOREN, D. A. & SINGHER, H. O. (1965). A study of the forces involved in the second stage of hemagglutination. *Transfusion*, **5**, 158–183.

PONDER, E. (1951). Effects produced by trypsin on certain properties of the human red cell. *Blood*, **6**, 350–356.

RANDAZZO, P., STREETER, B. & NUSBACHER, J. (1973). A common agglutinin reactive only against bromelin-treated red cells. *Transfusion*, **13**, 345 (Abstract).

REKVIG, O. P. & HANNESTAD, K. (1977). Acid elution of blood group antibodies from intact erythrocytes. *Vox Sang.*, **33**, 280–285.

ROSENTHAL, M. C., DAMESHEK, W. & BURKHARDT, R. (1951). Trypsin-modified erythrocytes. Their use as test cells in acquired hemolytic anemia. *Amer. J. clin. Path.*, **21**, 635–639.

ROSENTHAL, M. C., KOMNINOS, Z. D. & DAMESHEK, W. (1953). Multiple antibody formation in autoimmune hemolytic anemia. Report of a case. *New Engl. J. Med.*, **248**, 537–541.

ROSENTHAL, M. C. & SCHWARTZ, L. I. (1951a). Reversible agglutination of trypsin modified erythrocytes by normal human sera. *Fed. Proc.*, **19**, 332–333 (Abstract).

ROSENTHAL, M. C. & SCHWARTZ, L. I. (1951b). Reversible agglutination of trypsin treated erythrocytes by normal human sera. *Proc. Soc. exp. Biol. Med. N.Y.*, **76**, 635–638.

ROTH, K. L. (1954). Interaction of heparin with auto-agglutinins in idiopathic acquired hemolytic anemia. *Proc. Soc. exp. Biol. Med. N.Y.*, **86**, 352–356.

ROTH, K. L. & FRUMIN, A. M. (1954). In vitro differentiation between auto- and iso-immune antibodies by protamine and trypsin. *Science*, **120**, 945–946.

ROTH, K. L. & FRUMIN, A. M. (1957). Acquired hemolytic anemia: properties of eluted agglutinins and their interaction with red blood cells and Coombs' serum. *Blood*, **12**, 217–237.

RUBIN, H. (1963). Antibody elution from red blood cells. *J. clin. Path.*, **16**, 70–73.

RUGGIERI, P. & EYQUEM, A. (1953). Contribution à l'étude des anticorps décelés à l'aide des globules rouges traités par un enzyme proteolytique. *Ann. Inst. Pasteur*, **84**, 994–1000.

SCHANFIELD, M. A., PISCIOTTA, A. & LIBNOCK, J. (1978). Seven cases of hemolytic anemia associated with warm IgM autoantibodies. *Transfusion*, **18**, 623 (Abstract).

SCHUBOTHE, H. (1958). *Serologie und klinische Bedeutung der Autohämantikörper*, 284 pp. Karger, Basel.

SELWYN, J. G. & HACKETT, W. E. R. (1949). Acquired haemolytic anaemia: survival of transfused erythrocytes in patients and normal recipients. *J. clin. Path.*, **2**, 114–120.

SOKAL, G. (1957). Hypersplénisme hémolytique. Présence d'un anticorps au caractères inhabituels. *Rev. belge. Path.*, **26**, 95–105.

SPAET, T. H. & OSTROM, B. W. (1952). Studies on the normal serum panagglutinin active against trypsinated human erythrocytes: mechanism of agglutination reversal. *J. clin. Path.*, **5**, 332–335.

SPENCE, L., JONES, D. & MOORE, B. P. L. (1971). Effect of fatty acid salts on reactivity of albumin preparations with sera containing albumin auto-agglutinating factor. *Transfusion*, **11**, 193–195.

STRATTON, F. & RENTON, P. H. (1958). *Practical Blood Grouping*, 331 pp. Blackwell Scientific Publications, Oxford.

STRATTON, F., RENTON, P. H. & RAWLINSON, V. I. (1960). Serological differences between old and young cells. *Lancet*, **i**, 1388–1390.

STURGEON, P. (1947). A new antibody in serum of patients with acquired hemolytic anemia. *Science*, **106**, 293–294.

TOMEK, S., STRASSER, U. & SPEISER, P. (1950). Hämolytische Anämien in Verbindung mit Hämolysinen und Autoagglutininen. *Wien. klin. Wschr.*, **62**, 806–811.

UNGER, L. J. (1951). A method for detecting Rh_0 antibodies in extremely low titer. *J. Lab. clin. Med.*, **37**, 825–827.

VAN LOGHEM, J. J. JNR, MENDES DE LEON, D. E., FRENKEL-TIETZ, H. & VAN DER HART, M. (1952). Two different serologic mechanisms of paroxysmal cold hemoglobinuria, illustrated by three cases. *Blood*, **7**, 1196–1209.

VAN LOGHEM, J. J., MENDES DE LEON, D. E. & VAN DER HART, M. (1957). Recherches sérologiques dans les anémies hémolytiques acquises. *Congr. franç. Méd., 30ᵉ Session, Alger, 1955*. Masson, Paris. [quoted by Jensen (1959).]

VAN LOGHEM, J. J. JNR, VAN DER HART, M. & DORFMEIER, H. (1958). Serologic studies in acquired hemolytic anemia. *Proc. 6th int. Congr. int. Soc. Hemat. Boston, 1965*, pp. 858–868. Grune and Stratton, New York.

VERGER, P. & MOULINIER (1957). Anémie hémolytique du nourrisson avec auto-anticorps. Trois observations nouvelles. *Arch. franç. Pédiat.*, **14**, 606–614.

VERGER, P., MOULINIER, MARTIN & DANAN (1954). Anémie hémolytique acquise d'évolution chronique chez l'enfant. *Presse méd.*, **65**, 1091–1093.

VON DEM BORNE, A. E. G. KR., ENGELFRIET, C. P., BECKERS, D., VAN DER KORT-HENKES, G., VAN DER GIESSEN, M. & VAN LOGHEM, J. J. (1969). Autoimmune haemolytic anaemias. II. Warm haemolysins—serological and immunochemical investigations and ^{51}Cr studies. *Clin. exp. Immunol.*, **4**, 333–343.

VOS, G. H. & KELSALL, G. A. (1956). A new elution technique for the preparation of specific immune anti-Rh serum. *Brit. J. Haemat.*, **2**, 342–344.

WEINER, W. (1957). Eluting red-cell antibodies: a method and its application. *Brit. J. Haemat.*, **3**, 276–283.

WEINER, W. (1958). Serological pattern in auto-immune haemolytic anaemia. Result of investigation of sera and eluates in 30 cases. *Proc. 6th Congr. Europ. Soc. Haemat., Copenhagen, 1957*, pp. 675–680. Karger, Basel.

WEINER, W. & HALLUM, J. L. (1957). A further 'albumin' agglutinating serum. *Vox Sang.*, **2**, 38–42.

WEINER, W., TOVEY, G. H., GILLESPIE, E. M., LEWIS, H. B. M., & HOLLIDAY, T. D. S. (1956) 'Albumin' auto-agglutinating property in three sera. 'A pitfall for the unwary'. *Vox Sang.*, **1**, 279–288

WHEELER, W. E., LUHBY, A. L. & SCHOLL, M. L. L. (1950). The action of enzymes in hemagglutinating systems. II. Agglutinating properties of trypsin-modified red cells with anti-Rh sera. *J. Immunol.*, **65**, 39–46.

WHITTINGHAM, S., LOWY, H. & LIND, P. (1961). A serum from a group O woman containing an autoagglutinin to papainized cells, a 'hidden' anti-A antibody and a saline agglutinating anti-E (anti-rh") antibody. *Med. J. Aust.*, **i**, 320–322.

WIENER, A. S. (1942). Hemolytic transfusion reactions. I. Diagnosis, with special reference to the method of differential agglutination. *Amer. J. clin. Path.*, **12**, 189–199.

WIENER, A. S., GORDON, E. B., & GALLOP, C. (1953). Studies on autoantibodies in human sera. *J. Immunol.*, **71**, 58–65.

WRIGHT, C. S., DODD, M. C. & BOURONCLE, B. A. (1949). Studies of hemagglutinins in congenital and acquired hemolytic icterus. *J. Lab. clin. Med.*, **34**, 1768 (Abstract).

WRIGHT, C. S., DODD, M. C., BOURONCLE, B. A.,

DOAN, C. A. & ZOLLINGER, R. M. (1951). Studies of hemagglutinins in hereditary spherocytosis and in acquired hemolytic anemia: their relationship to the hypersplenic mechanism. *J. Lab. clin. Med.*, **37**, 165–181.

YACHNIN, S. & GARDNER, F. H. (1961). pH-dependent hemolytic systems. II. Serum factors involved in red cell lysis. *Blood*, **17**, 474–490.

YACHNIN, S. & RUTHENBERG, J. M. (1965). pH optima in immune hemolysis: a comparison between guinea-pig and human complement. *J. clin. Invest.*, **44**, 149–158.

Auto-immune haemolytic anaemia (AIHA): warm-antibody syndromes V: serological findings 3: specificity of the auto-antibodies

Early studies on specificity   *158*
    Incidence of specific auto-antibodies: early data   *161*
    'Non-specific' antibodies; early concepts   *161*
Recent studies on specificity   *162*
Anti-Rh auto-antibodies   *162*
    Reviews: 1964–1986   *165*
    Some noteworthy case reports   *165*
    Change in specificity of anti-Rh auto-antibodies with time   *166*
    Anti-Rh auto-antibodies with mimicking specificity   *166*
Anti-Wr^b (Wright) auto-antibodies   *169*
Uncommon or rare specific auto-antibodies   *169*
Anti-En^a auto-antibodies   *169*
Anti-Fy (Duffy) auto-antibodies   *170*

Anti-Ge (Gerbich) auto-antibodies   *170*
Anti-Jk (Kidd) auto-antibodies   *171*
Anti-K (Kell) auto-antibodies   *172*
Anti-Lu (Lutheran) auto-antibodies   *173*
Anti-S auto-antibodies   *174*
Anti-Sc3 (Scianna) auto-antibodies   *174*
Anti-U auto-antibodies   *174*
Anti-Vel auto-antibodies   *174*
Anti-Xg^a auto-antibodies   *175*
An auto-antibody against erythrocyte membrane protein 4.1   *175*
Anti-dl auto-antibodies   *175*
    'Non-specific' auto-antibodies   *176*
Species specificity of human warm auto-antibodies   *176*

An interesting and important question that has exercised the minds of those interested in AIHA from the late 1940s onwards—indeed up to the time of writing—has been the specificity of the auto-antibodies, i.e. the nature of the antigen or antigens on the erythrocyte surface with which the auto-antibodies react and the relationship between these antigens and those that determine the patients' blood-groups and react with the blood-group allo-antibodies. A subsidiary question for which an answer was at one time also sought was the extent to which the auto-antibodies of AIHA react with the erythrocytes of species other than man.

EARLY STUDIES ON SPECIFICITY

Until 1953, the auto-antibodies of AIHA were generally considered to be 'non-specific' or 'un-specific', i.e. they were thought to react with antigens or an antigen present on the surface of all human erythrocytes, which were distinct from the antigens that determined the patients' blood-groups.

Thus Wiener, Gordon and Gallop (1953) summarized contemporary views as follows:

'Red cell autoantibodies react not only with the individual's own red cells but also with the erythrocytes of all other human beings. The substances on the red blood cell envelope with which the autoantibodies combine are agglutinogens like the agglutinogens of A–B–O, M–N, and Rh–Hr systems, except that in the former case the blood factors with which the autoantibodies react are not type specific but are shared by *all* human beings. To a certain extent, therefore, the term "autoantibody" is misleading since the antibodies react with all human bloods as well as that of the person from whom the serum is derived, but once the full meaning of the term is learned this should cause no confusion. At any rate, from the clinical point of view, the prefix "auto" describes the most important attribute of the antibody, because the capacity to react with blood cells from other individuals becomes important only when blood transfusions are needed.'

It was because auto-antibodies were considered to react with all human erythrocytes that group-O cells had been used as a rule as a matter of convenience in seeking to detect *in vitro* antibodies free in the patient's serum or in eluates made from his or her erythrocytes. Nevertheless, in early work there had been indications that the sensitivity of normal group-compatible erythrocytes to the patients' auto-antibodies might vary considerably. However, the significance of this in relation to a possible definable specificity of the antibodies had not been fully appreciated. Some early work indicating differences in sensitivity is summarized below.

Denys and van den Broucke (1947) described how blood from 32 subjects was tested for compatibility with their patient's serum by means of the IAT. Twenty-six of the samples reacted positively, four gave weak reactions whilst two samples did not react at all. The reactions with a more active serum from a second patient were similar. However, the exact specificity of the antibodies in relationship to known blood-group antigens could not be determined; moreover, it appeared that all the samples of blood which reacted weakly or failed to react were from females. Kuhns and Wagley (1949) found an unidentifiable antibody in their patient's serum which agglutinated the patient's erythrocytes as well as 63% of a panel of normal erythrocytes apparently irrespective of their blood groups as far as they were then known.

Subsequently, it was suggested that antibodies reacting only with the patient's own erythrocytes might sometimes be formed. Davidsohn and Oyamada (1953) reported that when the sera of patients suffering from acquired haemolytic anaemia were tested for warm agglutinins, using 20% bovine albumin as a diluent, three consistent reaction patterns were observed: (1) in which antibodies in the patients' sera agglutinated normal erythrocytes to approximately the same titre as the patients' own cells; (2) in which the patients' cells were agglutinated to significantly higher titres than were the normal cells, and (3) in which the patients' cells were agglutinated but normal cells were not agglutinated ('auto-specific' antibodies). Dameshek (1951) had previously made similar observations, but concluded tentatively that the stronger reactions with the patients' erythrocytes were due to the cells being already 'coated' with antibody and that the presence of serum and albumin led to their agglutination. The DAT was in fact positive in both Damesheks's and Davidsohn and Oyamada's cases. Dameshek's interpretation seems likely to have been the correct one.

In addition to the differences referred to above in the sensitivity of erythrocytes to antibodies present in the serum of patients with AIHA, evidence was being accumulated at about the same time pointing to similarities between the auto-antibodies of AIHA and Rh allo-antibodies. Wiener as early as 1945 had reported, using the conglutination technique, auto-agglutination *in vitro* at 37°C of the erythrocytes of a case of acquired haemolytic anaemia, and Evans, Duane and Behrendt (1947) stressed the similarity of the behaviour of the immune antibody of acquired haemolytic anaemia and Rh blocking antibody in several in-vitro tests. Hackett (1950) compared the results of antiglobulin tests using erythrocytes from a case of acute AIHA and cells sensitized *in vitro* with the Rh antibody anti-D and showed that each type of cell adsorbed the same component out of the antiglobulin serum.

In 1953, Wiener and Gordon, and Wiener, Gordon and Gallop suggested that the auto-antibodies in AIHA might be directed against the 'nucleus of the Rh-Hr substance'. This hypothesis was based on finding that erythrocytes maximally sensitized with anti-D and AIHA auto-antibodies, respectively, reacted to the same titre with antiglobulin sera, and also on the observed reactions with erythrocytes of various species (see p. 176). Heni and Blessing (1954), too, put forward some interesting speculations. They suggested that as the antigenicity or antigen strength of antigens on the erythrocyte surface diminished so did the amount of antibody free in the plasma increase in relation to that found on cells. They also suggested that when antibodies were developed against strong antigens they were likely to be only slightly specific (panagglutinins), and that they would be more specific when formed against weaker antigens and that against the weakest antigens they might react solely with the patient's own erythrocytes.

With the observations mentioned in the previous paragraphs as a background, the stage was set for the demonstration of specificity.

Dr. Ruth Sanger in 1953 seems to have been the first to have recognized that an auto-antibody in the serum of a patient who had died of AIHA had a clearly definable specificity, namely against the Rh antigen e. Details of this finding were later briefly described in the second edition of Race and Sanger's book (1954). In their own words 'This beautifully clear investigation [that of

Weiner et al. (1953), referred to below] made the present authors realize that a curious result obtained by one of them in Australia had, after all, been true; the serum of a man, who had died of haemolytic anaemia 3,000 miles away, contained anti-e; his cells were clearly *CDe/cde*. However, since this ultimate sample of blood had been frozen, in error, three weeks previously, it was not taken as seriously as it deserved to be.'

The patient described by Weiner et al. (1953) also formed anti-e. The DAT was positive and eluates were found to contain an antibody reacting only with e-positive erythrocytes. As the patient's probable genotype was *CDe/CDe*, there seemed no doubt that the anti-e was acting as an auto-antibody and was presumably responsible for the patient's haemolytic anaemia. Holländer (1953) also reported finding a specific auto-antibody in a patient of probable Rh genotype *CDe/cde* suffering from AIHA. The patient's serum contained anti-c, whilst anti-c and a 'non-specific' component were eluted from his erythrocytes.

Dacie (1953) and Dacie and Cutbush (1954) reported on the specificity of the warm antibodies developed by 10 patients suffering from idiopathic AIHA. Several interesting facts emerged. Only one patient out of the 10 had failed to develop 'non-specific' antibodies. Instead, she formed both anti-e and anti-C; as her probable genotype was known to be *CDe/cde*, these antibodies clearly appeared to be specific auto-antibodies. The patient died of a fulminating haemolytic anaemia [see Dacie (1954, Case 12)]. The other nine patients had formed apparently 'non-specific' antibodies; in addition, however, three of them had formed anti-e, and one patient anti-e and anti-D (at different times). As the probable Rh genotype of the latter four patients was in each instance *CDe/cde*, it was clear that these antibodies, too, were auto-antibodies. Indeed, in two cases anti-e was successfully demonstrated in eluates. The 'non-specific' antibodies were equally interesting. In three it was possible to show that the 'non-specific' antibody consisted of two components: (1) 'non-specific' antibody in the 'strict' sense, i.e. an antibody reacting with and adsorbed by erythrocytes of all groups and types tested, including *–D–/–D–* cells, and (2) an

unidentified component reacting with and adsorbed by all erythrocytes tested except *–D–/–D–* cells, the *–D–/–D–* cells presumably being deficient in some antigen common to other types of erythrocytes in addition to being deficient in Cc and Ee.

Subsequently, van Loghem and van der Hart (1954a) reported the results of studies also carried out on 10 patients with AIHA, the antibodies being of the warm type in six of them. Specific auto-antibodies were identified in five of the six cases, the specificities being anti-D, anti-c, anti-c + e (two cases) and anti-Jk[a], respectively.

These early observations were soon confirmed by many workers in different parts of the world (Holländer, 1954; van Loghem and van der Hart, 1954b; Flückiger, Ricci and Usteri, 1955; Ruggieri and Puglisi, 1955; Crowley and Bouroncle, 1955, 1956; Kissmeyer-Nielsen, Bichel and Bjerre Hansen, 1956; Spielmann, 1956; Weiner, Whitehead and Walkden, 1956; Kissmeyer-Nielsen, 1957a, b; Komiya, Namihisa and Kato (1957); Meuli, 1957; Speiser, 1957; van Loghem, Mendes de Leon and van der Hart (1957); Wiener, Gordon and Russow, 1957; Ley, Mayer and Harris, 1958; van Loghem, van der Hart and Dorfmeier, 1958; Cicala, D'Onofrio and Paolucci, 1959; Dausset and Colombani, 1959; Högman, Killander and Sjölin, 1960; and Weiner, 1960).

With the exception of anti-K, twice reported (Flückiger, Ricci and Usteri, 1955; Dausset and Colombani, 1959), and anti-Jk[a] reported by van Loghem and van der Hart (1954a), all the specific auto-antibodies described in the papers listed in the foregoing paragraph belonged to the Rh system: anti-e occurred most frequently, but anti-D, anti-c, anti-C and anti-E had all been identified, either singly or in combination. In at least two of the published cases (Weiner, Whitehead and Walkden, 1956; Speiser, 1957) adsorbed auto-antibody 'blocked' the corresponding antigen sites, E and D, respectively, on the erythrocytes, with the result that the cells appeared to be E-negative and D-negative when first tested, and the free antibody in the serum an allo-antibody rather than a specific auto-antibody.

Holländer and Batschelet (1957) pointed out that the incidence of specific types of Rh auto-antibodies (with anti-e the most frequent, followed by anti-D) corresponded closely with the incidence of the Rh antigens in the English population.

Di Piero (1959) described a most unusual finding in the case of a boy aged 4 years. This was that an antibody detectable in his serum by means of the IAT reacted with his father's erythrocytes but failed to react with 20 other blood samples of known but varied antigenic constitution.

Another interesting point that had been noticed was that the antibodies did not always have the typical characters of Rh antibodies, although having apparently their specificity. Dacie and Cutbush (1954), for instance, noted that in one of their patients the antibody reacted with trypsinized cells only. Weiner (1958) used enzyme-treated cells suspended in albumin to detect antibodies in eluates, while Whittingham, Jakobowicz and Simmons (1961) reported that an auto-antibody of anti-e specificity was demonstrable in eluates but only by carrying out an antiglobulin test using trypsinized cells.

In several cases, too, antibodies were eluted off erythrocytes of a specificity not corresponding to the apparent genotype of the cells. Thus Spielmann (1956) reported demonstrating anti-D activity in an eluate made from Rh-negative erythrocytes; in this case anti-D was also present in the serum. Meuli (1957), too, described four interesting examples in three of which anti-E, anti-C plus anti-D, and anti-D, respectively, were present in the serum as apparent allo-antibodies and also identified in eluates. In the fourth case anti-E was eluted from cells of apparent R_1R_1 genotype. Similar observations were reported by Fudenberg, Rosenfield and Wasserman (1958) in two cases. In their first case anti-E was demonstrated in an eluate (also containing anti-D) from *CDe/cde* cells and in the second case anti-D was demonstrated in an eluate from *cde/cde* cells. Fudenberg and his colleagues suggested that the antibodies perhaps reacted in reality with some basic Rh structure but might also develop some specificity demonstrable often only after suitable absorptions.

Stratton and Renton (1958) similarly described a case in which an antibody of predominantly anti-C specificity was eluted from erythrocytes later shown to be of genotype *cDE/cde*, and Hubinont and co-workers (1959) described how an antibody of apparent anti-E specificity was eluted repeatedly from cells of genotype *cDe/cde*.

INCIDENCE OF SPECIFIC AUTO-ANTIBODIES: EARLY DATA

The information that had been published up to 1960 which has been summarized in the foregoing pages established without any possible doubt that in many cases of warm-antibody AIHA the auto-antibodies were directed against identifiable antigens. The data also showed, remarkably, that in nearly all cases in which a definite specificity could be established this had been within the Rh system. The proportion of patients forming specific antibodies was, however, uncertain. An important reason for this uncertainty was that interesting cases in which specific antibodies had been demonstrated were more likely to have been described than cases in which attempts to demonstrate specificity had failed.

The data available up to 1960, when the second edition of this book was being written, suggested that specific antibodies were being formed by about one-third of patients. Thus combining the experience of several groups of workers (Crowley and Bouroncle, 1955, 1956; Kissmeyer-Nielsen, 1957b; Meuli, 1957; van Loghem, van der Hart and Dorfmeier, 1958; Dausset and Colombani, 1959; and Weiner, 1960), specific auto-antibodies were demonstrated in 52 out of a total of 154 patients, an incidence of 34%. The author (Dacie, 1962, p. 449) recorded a similar figure—10 out of 33 patients (30%).

'Non-specific' antibodies; early concepts

The nature of the 'non-specific' antibodies apparently present in the majority of patients could not be defined in the 1950s; it had been demonstrated, moreover, e.g. by Dacie and Cutbush (1954), that 'non-specific' antibodies might sometimes consist of more than one component. Dacie (1962, p. 449) pointed out, too, that even when specific Rh auto-antibodies had been identified, unidentifiable 'non-specific' antibodies were almost always present at the same time, a finding that suggested rather strongly that the latter type of antibody was also related to the Rh system, recalling the suggestion of Wiener, Gordon and Gallop (1953) of an antibody directed against the 'nucleus of the Rh-Hr substance'.

The concept (widely held in the 1950s) of a 'non-specific' auto-antibody was criticized by Weiner (1959,

1960) on the grounds that every antibody must react with a corresponding 'specific' antigen. He suggested that 'non-specificity' might be explained by there being in the Rh system, and possibly in other blood-group systems, too, antigens of extreme frequency ('very public antigens') against which allo-antibodies were extremely unlikely to be produced but against which auto-antibodies might be formed. This hypothesis was very near to that of Wiener, Gordon and Gallop (1953), already referred to (p. 159). It seemed to the author at the time the second edition of this book was being written (Dacie, 1962, p. 450) that there was no reason to suppose that antigens, capable of being acted on by auto-antibodies, might not be present on the erythrocytes of *all* mankind, and that antibodies reacting with these hypothetical antigens might legitimately be referred to as 'non-specific', in contrast to the antibodies reacting with identifiably distinct, i.e. specific, blood-group antigens (see also p. 176).

RECENT STUDIES ON SPECIFICITY

The descriptions that have been given so far in this chapter brought the story of the unravelling of the specificity of the warm auto-antibodies of AIHA up to the time (1960) when the 2nd edition of *The Haemolytic Anaemias* (Part II) was being written. In the remaining sections are summarized what has been learnt in the subsequent three decades. As might have been expected, the early discoveries have been greatly expanded and elaborated, and the dominance of specificity within the Rh blood-group system has been confirmed. It is now known, too, that it is common (at least in relation to antibodies directed against Rh antigens) for several antibodies of different specificities to be present at the same time. Also, that antibodies of complicated specificity may mimic an antibody of apparent simple specificity. It is also realized that it is not rare for antibodies of a definable specificity to be eluted from the erythrocytes not carrying the corresponding antigen.

The incidence and specificity of the auto-antibodies that react with Rh antigens will be dealt with first, and this is followed by a description of the discovery and occurrence of the specific auto-antibody that has been next most frequently identified, namely anti-Wr[b]. Following this, there are brief sections devoted to the reports of the quite large number of auto-antibodies of

other specificities, of infrequent or rare occurrence, that have been identified. Finally, the auto-antibodies reacting with Rh_{null} erythrocytes as well as with cells of the common Rh phenotypes (anti-dl antibodies), and the one-time vexed question of 'non-specific' warm auto-antibodies, will be reconsidered in the light of recent discoveries.

ANTI-Rh AUTO-ANTIBODIES

Some studies based on relatively large series of patients will be reviewed first, with particular reference to the percentage of patients in whom the auto-antibodies had been shown to have Rh specificity. Several interesting facts have emerged. One is that cases in which the auto-antibodies have had a clear-cut specificity against simple Rh antigens such as e and D are rather rare—despite being relatively frequently reported; also that even when the antibodies such as anti-e and anti-D have been identified these specific antibodies are often accompanied by antibodies directed against other antigens. Another fact that has emerged is that antibodies that act apparently non-specifically fall into two broad categories: those that react with all cells bearing the common Rh antigens but do *not* react with cells whose Rh antigens have been deleted, e.g. *D--/D--* and *---/---* cells, and those that react as well with cells with deleted antigens as with cells of common Rh phenotypes. The former antibodies clearly react with 'basic' Rh antigens not present in the deleted cells; the latter react with antigens outside the Rh system.

Weiner and Vos (1963) investigated the specificity of the antibodies in 66 eluates that had been prepared from the erythrocytes of 56 patients with AIHA and 10 apparently normal blood donors in all of whom the DAT had been positive. The panel of cells used comprised erythrocytes with common Rh phenotypes as well as single samples of the rare *Dc–/Dc–*, *D--/D--* and *---/---* cells. Six of the eluates were found to contain specific Rh antibodies; the remaining 60 samples contained antibodies which were 'panagglutinating' and 'unspecific' when tested with the cells of the common Rh phenotypes. However, when the eluates were tested in addition with the cells with deleted Rh antigens three reaction patterns emerged.

Nine of the eluates agglutinated all the normal cells but failed to agglutinate the $D--/D--$ and $---/---$ samples, i.e. the eluates were reacting with an antigen or antigens common to cells with normal Rh antigens, but failed to react with cells in which some or all of these normal antigens had been deleted.

Twenty eluates reacted with $D--/D--$ cells but less well than with normal cells; six of these eluates reacted less strongly with $---/---$ cells and 11 eluates failed to react with the $---/---$ cells.

Thirty-one eluates reacted equally strongly with $D--/D--$ cells as with the normal cells; five of these eluates reacted less strongly with $---/---$ cells and an additional 11 eluates failed to react with the $---/---$ cells.

The antibodies that reacted with the normal (nl) cells but failed to react with the deleted cells were designated anti-nl, while those that reacted with the partly deleted ($D--/D--$) cells as well as with the normal cells, but failed to react with the $---/---$ cells, were designated anti-pdl (partly deleted). Antibodies that reacted with the normal cells and with both the partly deleted and $---/---$ cells were referred to as anti-dl (deleted). (Table 26.1). Weiner and Vos concluded that their eluates had contained anti-nl, anti-pdl and anti-dl antibodies singly or in combination.

Leddy and Bakemeier (1967) had investigated 31 AIHA patients with particular reference to the relationship between the DAT and the specificity of the auto-antibodies. The DAT had been positive with anti-γG sera in 17 patients: eluates from the erythrocytes of 10 of them failed to react with Rh_{null} cells; in two patients

the reaction was weaker than with cells with normal (non-deleted) Rh phenotypes and in five the Rh_{null} cells and normal cells reacted equally strongly. In 14 patients the DAT had been positive with both anti-γG and anti-C sera: in 13 of them the eluted antibodies reacted with Rh_{null} cells as strongly as with normal cells. The specificity of the antibodies that reacted with normal cells, but failed to react with Rh_{null} cells, was designated 'Rh-related': they behaved as panantibodies but absorption indicated the presence also of anti-e or anti-c in some of them. The specificity of the antibodies that reacted with Rh_{null} cells was designated 'non-Rh-related'. Antibodies with this specificity were thought to be heterogeneous, too.

Leddy and his co-workers (1970) had included LW-negative and $K^{o}K^{o}$ cells in a similar study. Eluates from 46 patients were tested. Twenty-six eluates were derived from erythrocytes coated with γG globulin alone: 12 failed to react with Rh_{null} cells, eight reacted in an intermediate fashion and six reacted strongly with the Rh_{null} cells. Twenty eluates were derived from erythrocytes coated with γG globulin and complement components: 16 reacted strongly with Rh_{null} cells and four gave intermediate reactions.

Eyster and Jenkins (1970) prepared eluates from the erythrocytes of 35 AIHA patients. Twelve were from cells coated with γG globulins only: the antibodies in six (50%) of these failed to react with Rh_{null} cells and were judged to be Rh-specific. Twenty-three eluates were from cells coated with γG globulins and complement components: a smaller percentage, six (26%), of the eluted antibodies appeared to be Rh-specific. However, after absorption with Rh_{null} cells, one of the eluates from the cells coated with γG alone and seven eluates from cells coated with γG globulins and complement were found to contain Rh-specific antibodies, the presence of which, before the absorptions, had been obscured by antibodies of other specificities.

Vos, Petz and Fudenberg (1970) had studied eluates from the erythrocytes of 24 patients with warm-antibody AIHA. Thirteen (54%) contained anti-nl antibodies (reacting with cells of normal Rh phenotypes but failing to react with Rh_{null} cells); three contained anti-dl antibodies (reacting with cells of normal Rh phenotypes *and* with Rh_{null} cells), and eight eluates

Table 26.1   **Reactions of anti-Rh auto-antibodies and anti-dl with erythrocytes of five Rh genotypes.**

Auto-antibodies	Erythrocytes				
	CDe/CDe	cDE/cDE	cde/cde	$D--/D--$	$---/---$ (Rh_{null})
Anti-e	+	−	+	−	−
Anti-c	−	+	+	−	−
Anti-D	+	+	−	+	−
Anti-nl	+	+	+	−	−
Anti-pdl	+	+	+	+	−
Anti-dl	+	+	+	+	+

were judged to contain both anti-nl and anti-dl antibodies. In all, 21 eluates were thought to contain antibodies against common Rh phenotypes and 11 eluates antibodies against antigens other than Rh. The use of ficinized cells was found to be better than the IAT in demonstrating anti-nl antibodies, while the reverse seemed to be true when testing for anti-dl antibodies with Rh$_{null}$ cells.

A larger series of similar patients was reported on by Vos, Petz and Fudenberg (1971). Anti-nl antibodies alone were demonstrated in 24 eluates (43%), anti-pdl antibodies alone in five eluates (9%) and anti-dl alone in six eluates (11%). Twenty eluates (37%) were thought to contain anti-nl, anti-pdl and anti-dl in various combinations. Complement had been demonstrated on the erythrocytes of 18 patients: eluates from these cells were all shown to contain antibodies of more than one specificity; 13 were thought to contain anti-nl, anti-pdl and anti-dl antibodies. In this series only three eluates were found to contain antibodies against well-defined Rh antigens, e.g. CDEce, in addition to anti-nl or anti-pdl. Vos, Petz and Fudenberg pointed out that

Table 26.2   Specificity of auto-antibodies eluted from the erythrocytes of patients with warm-antibody AIHA, with particular reference to the incidence of Rh antibodies.

Authors	No. of patients	Specificity
Weiner and Vos (1963); Weiner (1965)	60	At least 70% within the Rhesus system
Leddy and Bakemeier (1967)	(a) 17 DAT: anti-γG pos	12 Rh-related* (71%); 5 'non-Rh-related'
	(b) 14 DAT: anti-γG and anti-C pos	1 Rh related* (7%) 13 'non-Rh-related'.
Eyster and Jenkins (1970)	(a) 12 DAT: anti-γG pos	6 Rh-specific (50%)
	(b) 23 DAT: anti-γG and anti-C pos.	6 Rh-specific (26%)
Leddy et al. (1970)	(a) 26 DAT: anti-γG pos	20 Rh-related* (77%)
	(b) 20 DAT: anti-γG and anti-C pos	4 Rh-related* (20%)
Vos, Petz and Fudenberg (1970)	24	13 anti-nl* (61%) 3 anti-dl†; 8 anti-dl† + anti-nl*
Vos, Petz and Fudenberg (1971)	55	24 anti-nl* (44%); 6 anti-dl†
Issitt et al. (1976a)	87	4 'simple' anti-Rh; 33 'simple' anti-Rh with other auto-antibodies 4 anti-nl*; 20 anti-nl*, with other auto-antibodies 13 anti-dl†; 49 anti-dl†, with other auto-antibodies
Sokol, Hewitt and Stamps (1981)	573	459 incomplete auto/pan antibodies (80%) 71 anti-e (12%) 7 anti-e and other anti-Rh antibodies (1%) 29 anti-Rh (not anti-e) (5%) 8 auto-antibody only (1%)

*Anti-nl: eluates failed to react with – – –/– – – erythrocytes.
†Anti-dl: eluates reacted with – – –/– – – erythrocytes.

their data indicated that antibodies of a single specificity were more often composed of IgG than IgM or IgA and that multiple specificities were frequently associated with more than one Ig type, e.g., IgG with IgM and perhaps IgA, too, and usually with complement fixation also.

Lalezari (1973, 1976), described and illustrated how, using a Polybrene-enhanced AutoAnalyzer continuous flow system and mixing antibody-coated erythrocytes in different proportions with indicator cells of known Rh phenotypes, it was possible to determine the specificity of an auto-antibody and the relative sensitivity to it of cells of different Rh phenotypes.

Lalezari and Berens (1977) reported that they had studied several anti-Rh auto-antibodies in which both specific and panagglutinin activities had been demonstrated. Analysis by the AutoAnalyzer technique had revealed that the 'seemingly independent activities were properties of single antibody molecules reacting with complex antigens'.

Issitt and co-workers (1976) reported on the results of a large study on the specificity of the auto-antibodies of AIHA, with particular reference to the relationship between anti-Wr^b antibodies and anti-dl antibodies that reacted with Rh_{null} erythrocytes, as well as with cells of normal Rh genotypes. Sixty-four out of 87 patients had formed anti-dl antibodies: two were anti-Wr^b and a further 32 patients had formed anti-Wr^b in addition to antibodies of other specificities, an incidence of auto-anti-Wr^b of 39% (34 out of 87 patients) (see also p. 169). [Issitt et al. also reported on the incidence of auto-Wr^b in 30 haematologically normal blood donors (an incidence of 27%) and in 33 patients being treated with α-methyldopa (an incidence of 12%).] Details of the specificity in each of the 87 AIHA patients were tabulated: auto-antibodies of more than one specificity were present in 63 of them (72%), and it is especially interesting to note the rarity of specific anti-Rh antibodies, i.e. anti-c, anti-e, and anti-c and anti-E, which were present in only three of them. However, if anti-nl and anti-pdl are included as anti-Rh antibodies, 49 of the 87 AIHA patients (56%) had formed anti-Rh-specific antibodies.

Sokol, Hewitt and Stamps (1981) reported data based on a very large series of patients who had been investigated at the Blood Transfusion Centre in Sheffield between 1961 and 1980. Of 573 patients who had formed warm auto-antibodies, 459 (80%) were classified as having formed incomplete auto/pan antibodies, 71 anti-e (12.4%), seven anti-e plus other anti-Rh antibodies and 29 anti-Rh antibodies other than anti-e.

Worlledge (1982) summarized her data on specificity in 93 patients with warm-type AIHA. Of 61 patients whose erythrocytes were coated with IgG only, 87% were judged to have formed antibodies directed against Rh antigens. In contrast, of those patients whose erythrocytes were coated with IgG and complement, only 27% (7 out of 26) had a similar (anti-Rh) specificity. One-third of the eluates made from the erythrocytes of the whole series of 93 patients reacted at least equally strongly with Rh_{null} cells as with cells of normal Rh phenotypes. The antibodies in these eluates were considered to have anti-En^a or anti-Wr^b specificity or to be 'non-specific', or to be mixtures of these antibodies with antibodies of Rh specificity.

Data extracted from the foregoing reports are summarized in Table 26.2.

Reviews: 1964–1990*

Valuable reviews on the serology of AIHA which include discussions on the specificity of warm auto-antibodies include those of Salmon (1964), Gerbal et al. (1968), Pirofsky (1969, p. 458), Bell, Zwicker and Sachs (1973), Salmon, Homberg and Habibi (1975), Habibi (1977), Issitt (1977), Isbister (1978), Petz and Garratty (1980, p. 232), Salmon, Goudemond and Habibi (1984), Issitt (1985a,b), Issitt (1986) and Rosse (1990).

Some noteworthy case reports

The accounts summarized below that were published in the 1960s include particularly interesting features.

---

*Two additional reviews that should be mentioned (although not strictly speaking concerned with erythrocyte auto-antibodies) are those by Lewis et al. (1985) on the terminology of erythrocyte surface antigens (the Munich report) and by Issitt (1989) on recent observations on the biochemistry and genetics of the Rh blood-group antigens. Both reviews illustrate the complexity of the human blood groups and the multiplicity of antigens.

Weiner, Gordon and Kidd (1962) described a female aged 17 who had developed acute haemolytic anaemia with haemoglobinuria. The DAT was weakly positive: eluates, however, contained potent auto-antibodies of anti-E and anti-c specificity, best demonstrated with enzyme-treated erythrocytes.

Oski and Abelson's (1965) patient was a female infant aged 8 weeks who had developed acute haemolytic anaemia preceded by diarrhoea and vomiting. At first the DAT and IAT were negative; later they became positive and an apparent panagglutinin was found to consist of four components — anti-M, anti-E, anti-c and a 'non-specific' antibody.

Shapiro (1967) described a female infant who developed acute haemolytic anaemia when aged 3 months. An auto-antibody of anti-D specificity was demonstrated in her serum and in eluates from her erythrocytes. The particular interest in this case is that the child was the eighth child in a family, in which five children appear to have developed AIHA as part of a syndrome resembling runt disease; three had AIHA (see Table 22.2, p. 13).

Meara, Hoffman and Hewlett (1967) described a 60-year-old woman who had developed a moderately severe haemolytic anaemia, possibly precipitated by an injection of an influenza vaccine following which an influenza-like syndrome had developed. Her Rh genotype was cde/cde. The DAT and IAT were positive. Allo-anti-C and allo-anti-D antibodies were demonstrated in her serum, probably the result of immunization following a pregnancy and transfusions many years earlier. Eluates from her erythrocytes were found to contain an auto-antibody of anti-F specificity (thought to react with C and e antigens on the same chromosome).

The following more recently described case illustrates the 'individuality' of the auto-antibodies a patient may form. Kennedy, Waheed and Marsh (1981) described briefly a most unusual high-thermal-amplitude auto-agglutinin in the serum of a 37-year-old man who died within 72 hours of acute haemolysis associated with haemoglobinuria. The antibody which was powerfully active at 37°C reacted equally strongly with I and i (adult) erythrocytes and less strongly with i(cord) cells. Its activity was enhanced by enzyme treatment. It reacted strongly with all cells tested except Rh_{null} cells which were not agglutinated, and $-D-$ and other Rh-deletion cells, which were agglutinated less strongly. It was, however, neutralized by Sd^{a+} human urine and by guinea-pig urine, but not by Sd^{a-} urine, findings pointing to some relationship also with the Sd blood-group system.

Change in specificity of anti-Rh auto-antibodies with time

Dacie and Cutbush (1954) had shown that if eluates are prepared from the erythrocytes of patients with warm-antibody AIHA more than one auto-antibody component may be demonstrable. This was so in three out of five eluates they had studied: in one, as many as four components — anti-e, anti-D and two 'non-specific' — appeared to be elutable from a patient whose Rh genotype was CDe/cde. Gerbal and co-workers (1968), in a similar study, showed that the specificity of eluted antibodies might vary with time and illustrated this with data from three patients. In one, anti-nl plus anti-pdl, anti-e plus anti-nl, anti-nl, anti-nl plus anti-c, anti-e plus anti-nl plus anti-c, and anti-e, were demonstrated at different times during a 2-year and 3-month period. Similar observations have subsequently been reported by Bird and Wingham (1972), Dixon, Beck and Oberman (1969) and Kanra et al. (1987). In the case of the patient described by Adams, Moore and Issitt (1973), an anti-D auto-antibody was later found to be accompanied by an antibody that reacted with D-negative LW-positive cells, i.e. it was anti-LW.

Anti-Rh auto antibodies with mimicking specificity

A most interesting recent development in connection with the unravelling of the specificity of the auto-antibodies has been the realization that, although the antibodies appear to be specific for certain antigens, in reality they are reacting with more basic antigens, although showing a preference for certain specific antigens. In short, 'specific' auto-antibodies are commonly less specific than are their allo-antibody counterparts.

The fact that it was possible sometimes to demonstrate in eluates antibodies of a specificity not apparently corresponding to the antigenic make-up of the erythrocytes from which the eluates had been prepared has been known since the 1950s. Spielmann (1956) had reported finding an anti-D antibody in an eluate prepared from the erythrocytes of an Rh-negative patient who had anti-D in his serum. Meuli (1957) reported four similar occurrences. In three patients, anti-E, anti-C plus anti-D, and anti-D, respectively, were present in serum as allo-antibodies and also identified in eluates, while in the fourth case anti-E had apparently been eluted from *CDe/CDe* erythrocytes.

Fudenberg, Rosenfield and Wasserman (1958) described two patients in whom the findings were similar. The first patient, who had chronic lymphocytic leukaemia and AIHA, was of *Cde/cde,kk* genotype. Anti-D, anti-E and anti-K were present in his serum while eluates appeared to contain a panantibody; after absorption, however, anti-D and anti-E were identified. Their second patient, who had myeloid leukaemia and AIHA, was of *cde/cde* genotype, and anti-D, anti-C and anti-E were present in serum. Again, eluates appeared to contain a panantibody; after absorption, however, anti-D was identified. Fudenberg, Rosenfield and Wasserman suggested that one possible explanation was immunization to an Rh structure common to all Rh antigens and that 'such an antibody, although capable of reacting with all antigens containing the basic Rh structure, might nevertheless react preferentially with one or more specific Rh blood factors'.

Stratton and Renton (1958, p. 245) described a similar case in which an antibody, predominantly anti-C in specificity, was eluted from erythrocytes later shown to be of genotype *cDE/cde*; and Hubinont and co-workers (1952) described a patient of genotype *cDe/cde* in whose serum anti-C and anti-E were present and from whose erythrocytes anti-E, considered to be a cross-reacting antibody, was repeatedly eluted.

A major step forward in the understanding of the phenomenon of the elution of apparently specific antibodies from erythrocytes not thought to carry the corresponding antigen was the finding that in such cases the antibodies may be absorbed *in vitro* by cells apparently lacking the corresponding antigen, if the antibody-containing eluates are exposed to repeated absorptions. These observations have led to the concept of 'mimicking' antibodies.

In 1977, Issitt and his co-workers described as 'mimicking' auto-antibodies 'anti-E and anti-c' antibodies eluted from the erythrocytes of a man aged 76 of genotype *CDe/CDe* with myelofibrosis and a positive DAT (although no evidence of increased haemolysis). The eluted antibodies were shown to be completely absorbable by E-negative and c-negative cells, and Issitt et al. concluded that they were more closely related to the series of allo-antibodies referred to as 'anti-Hr' (Rosenfield et al., 1962) than to genuine anti-E or anti-c. The patient's serum contained anti-E, an allo-antibody, and also at various times 'auto-anti-

E', anti-nl and 'auto-anti-c', corresponding to the antibodies that could be eluted from erythrocytes.

The paper referred to above (Issitt et al., 1977) was followed in the same issue of *Transfusion* by a description of a 'mimicking' auto-antibody in a pregnant woman and in her newborn infant (Henry et al., 1977). Neither, however, appeared to suffer from increased haemolysis. The mother's genotype was *cDE/cde* and her DAT was positive. Eluates from her erythrocytes and from those of her infant (whose DAT was negative) were found to react with C-positive cells. Although the antibody contained in the eluates appeared initially to be anti-C, further tests indicated that it was more closely related to anti-Hr or anti-Rh34.

The apparent occurrence of mimicking antibodies, as described by Issitt and his co-workers in the publications cited in the two preceding paragraphs, led to a major reinvestigation of supposedly specific auto-anti-Rh antibodies in AIHA patients and in apparently normal individuals giving positive DATs. The results of this study were described by Issitt and Pavone (1978).

Forty-eight auto-antibodies with what had appeared to be 'simple' anti-Rh specificity, i.e. anti-e, -c, -E, -D, -C, -Ce and -G, were subjected to multiple absorptions. In 34 (71%) the antibodies were found to be absorbable by erythrocytes lacking the antigens the antibodies had apparently defined and it appeared in these cases that the antibodies that had seemed to be directed against e, E or c antigens most often had anti-Hr or anti-Hr$_0$ specificity. Of these 34 antibodies, 24 could be absorbed 'to exhaustion' by all erythrocytes bearing normal Rh antigens, regardless of the apparent specificity of the antibodies, although not by D--/D-- or Rh$_{null}$ cells; 10 antibodies, in contrast, were only partially absorbed by cells bearing 'wrong' (inappropriate) antigens. The remaining 14 antibodies were absorbed 'to exhaustion' by erythrocytes bearing the antigens they appeared to define; but they could not be absorbed by cells bearing inappropriate antigens. These antibodies thus possessed the specificity that preliminary tests had indicated.

Issitt and Pavone discussed possible explanations for the phenomenon they had so clearly demonstrated. They concluded, as already mentioned, that many auto-antibodies of apparent simple specificity are in reality anti-Hr or anti-Hr_0 antibodies produced by Hr-positive or Hr_0-positive individuals. [Hr and Hr_0 are Rh antigens of very high frequency, i.e. >99% (Rosenfield et al., 1962)]. Anti-Hr and anti-Hr_0 define [in Issitt's and Pavone's words] 'a portion of the Hr or Hr_0 agglutinogen that is either present in greater quantities, or in a sterically more acceptable form, on e-positive than on e-negative cells'; they are 'able to bind more firmly (or in greater quantity) to e-positive than to e-negative red cells with the result that in indirect antiglobulin tests, e-positive cells give positive reactions while e-negative samples fail to react'. The possibility that the presence in eluates of antibodies not corresponding to the erythrocytes' antigenic make-up could be explained by the Matuhasi–Ogata phenomenon, i.e. the binding on of antibodies of any specificity to antigen–antibody complexes (see Allen et al., 1969; and Bove, Holburn and Mollison, 1973) was considered to be a less likely explanation.

Some further noteworthy case reports of mimicking antibodies are summarized below.

The patient of Rand et al. (1978), a male aged 20 with a short history of haemolytic anaemia, had a negative DAT. Despite an R_1R_1 genotype, an antibody which reacted only with E-positive cells was eluted from his erythrocytes. A similar antibody was present in serum. Rand et al. concluded that their patient's antibody in reality was an auto-anti-Hr.

Weber and co-workers (1979) described the development of an allo-anti-C by a woman of Rh genotype cDE/cde, probably as the result of immunization occurring during her third pregnancy. She was the patient who had been described earlier by Henry et al. (1977) as forming an auto-anti-c of unusual (mimicking) type during her previous pregnancy. This antibody eventually disappeared, and Weber et al. suggested that the change from auto- to allo-antibody had been prompted by the introduction into her circulation of additional foreign immunogen carried on fetal erythrocytes.

Cheng (1985) described the occurrence of a similar mimicking auto-anti-C in eluates prepared from the erythrocytes of a 70-year-old man with chronic AIHA. The antibody was readily absorbed by R_1R_1 cells; in addition, however, it could be absorbed by R_2r cells if submitted to three absorptions.

Vengelen-Tyler and Mogck (1991) described two patients who had formed "hr^B-like" auto-antibodies which at first were thought to be allo-antibodies. The first patient had a severe haemolytic anaemia; the second patient was not anaemic. The antibodies were initially thought to be anti-e, but they were found not to react with (e + hr^B −) erythrocytes. The DAT was negative in both patients, and in the case of the first patient it was established when he was first studied that his erythocytes failed to react with the antibody. Later, when he was no longer haemolysing, his cells reacted positively, suggesting that the antigen corresponding with the antibody had been temporarily weakened.

Issitt (1986) summarized his conclusions as to the occurrence and role of mimicking antibodies in AIHA in his Emily Cooley Lecture which he had delivered to the American Association of Blood Banks. He emphasized that the most common situation in which mimicking antibodies are found on a patient's erythrocytes is when a true allo-antibody of the specificity mimicked is present in the patient's serum. As for the frequency of mimicking antibodies, i.e. antibodies wholly or partially absorbed by antigen-negative erythrocytes, his data indicated that about 70% of warm-antibody AIHA patients, 83% of α-methyldopa patients giving a positive DAT, and 43% of persons with a positive DAT who were apparently otherwise normal, had formed mimicking antibodies.

As for which apparently specific auto-antibodies are most likely to be mimics, Issitt's data (based it is true on rather small numbers) indicated that this was likely to be true of 33% of anti-D, 83% of anti-e, 100% of anti-c, 80% of anti-E, 75% of anti-C and 50% of anti-Ce.

Issitt summarized his findings by suggesting that if an auto-antibody appeared to have anti-e specificity there was a greater than 80% chance that it was really anti-Hr or anti-Hr_0, with a preference for e-positive cells; and if the antibody appeared to be anti-D, there was a greater than 60% chance that it really was auto-anti-D and not absorbable by D-negative cells.

The significance of mimicking antibodies in relation to the cause and mechanism of auto-antibody formation remains an intriguing problem. An even more basic problem is why the specificity of auto-Rh antibodies is usually so much 'broader' than that of allo-Rh antibodies, the specificity of which is characteristically 'narrow' and specific.

From the practical clinical point of view it is probably irrelevant whether an auto-antibody has true anti-Rh specificity or mimics a specific Rh antibody. Issitt quotes Mollison's (1959) demonstration that e-positive erythrocytes survived in an AIHA patient far less well then e-negative cells. The patient's antibody had been thought to be anti-e: Issitt demonstrated subsequently that the antibody could be absorbed by R_2R_2 cells and thus had been mimicking anti-e.

ANTI-Wr^b (WRIGHT) AUTO-ANTIBODIES

Goldfinger and co-workers (1975) reported that they had identified an auto-antibody formed by a 56-year-old woman with chronic AIHA having the specificity anti-Wr^b. The patient had a haemoglobin of 6.1 g/dl and 15% reticulocytes and was fairly well controlled by a daily dose of 5 mg of prednisone. The DAT was strongly positive with anti-IgG sera and weakly positive with anti-C sera. The auto-antibody was detected in her serum and in eluates from her erythrocytes: it reacted by the indirect antiglobulin and enzyme-treated cell techniques with all erythrocytes tested (including cells lacking rare high-incidence antigens such as Rh$_{null}$, U-negative and Vel-negative), but failed to react with the only known cell sample having the Wr (a+b−) phenotype. Goldfinger et al. noted, too, that the antibody reacted weakly with En(a−) cells and found that such cells, when tested with an anti-Wr^b antiserum, typed as Wr(b−). This led them to conclude that the anti-En^a specificity recorded in patients with warm AIHA might have been due to the presence of anti-Wr^b (see also p. 170).

The identification of anti-Wr^b by Goldfinger et al. (1975) as the apparent causal auto-antibody in a patient with warm-antibody AIHA, referred to in the previous paragraph, led Issitt and his co-workers (1976a) to test eluates that had been made from 150 individuals whose DAT had been found to be positive. Sera, too, were tested when known to contain auto-antibodies. The main thrust of this important study was to ascertain the frequency of anti-Wr^b antibodies in patients with AIHA (and also in patients under treatment with α-methydopa and in normal individuals who had

been found to give a positive DAT). Of the 150 eluates available, 87 had been from patients with AIHA, and 64 of the 87 (74%) had reacted with Rh$_{null}$ erythrocytes and thus had the specificity referred descriptively as anti-dl. These anti-dl antibodies were first absorbed with Wr(a+b−) cells and then retested to ascertain the percentage of residual unabsorbed antibodies that could be identified as anti-Wr^b. Two of the anti-dl antibodies were found to be anti-Wr^b and 32 of the 64 (50%) included anti-Wr^b in a mixture with antibodies of a different specificity. In relation to the whole series of 87 patients, auto-anti-Wr^b was present in 34, a high incidence of 39%. This incidence was second only to that of antibodies of anti-Rh specificity (anti-e, -E, -c, -C or -D or anti-nl or -pdl). Anti-Wr^b is thus a common antibody in warm-type AIHA.

UNCOMMON OR RARE SPECIFIC AUTO-ANTIBODIES

Their role in warm-antibody AIHA will be considered in alphabetical order as a matter of convenience.

Anti-En^a auto-antibodies

Worlledge (1972) reported at the 13th International Congress of the International Society of Blood Transfusion held in Washington in 1972 that approximately 33% of anti-dl auto-antibodies fail to react with cells of the rare En(a−) phenotype and deduced that one type of anti-dl was anti-En^a in specificity. Subsequent work by Issitt et al. (1975, 1976b) showed, however, that En(a−) cells are phenotypically Wr(a−b−) and that the only blood then known to be Wr (a+b−) was En(a+). This led them to suggest that Worlledge's antibodies were anti-Wr^b in specificity rather than anti-En^a.

Bell and Zwicker (1978) described the results of further tests that they had carried out on two of the eluates that had been shown by Issitt et al. (1976) to contain anti-Wr^b as well as an unidentified anti-dl antibody. These two eluates were shown to agglutinate En(a−) erythrocytes less strongly than En(a+) cells and further absorption of the eluates confirmed the presence of a second antibody that reacted with En(a+), Wr(a+b−) cells but not with En(a−) cells. Bell and Zwicker thus were able to demonstrate that some anti-dl antibodies may contain a component of apparent anti-En^a specificity in addition to anti-Wr^b. They pointed out, however, that En(a−) cells lack M and N and Wr^a and Wr^b antigens as well as En^a, and possibly other antigens, and that 'anti-En^a' 'may be, or may contain, an antibody to another antigen not present on En(a−) cells'; they also pointed out that of the 150 eluates studied by Issitt et al. (1976), it was only in the two eluates that they themselves had studied, and in possibly one other, that it had seemed at all likely that anti-En^a was present. These studies thus indicated that anti-En^a, although it does occur as an auto-antibody in AIHA, is rarely formed.

Pavone and co-workers (1981) described a further example of an auto-anti-En^a which differed apparently from previously described antibodies of similar specificity. The antibody had been detected in the serum of a 47-year-old woman, as well as in eluates prepared from her erythrocytes. She was suffering from a steroid-responsive, apparently idiopathic, chronic AIHA. The DAT was strongly positive with an anti-IgG serum and positive but less strongly so with an anti-C serum. The antibody reacted with all cells tested except En(a−) cells; it differed from previously studied anti-En^a antibodies in that, although inhibited by MN sialoglycoprotein (SGP), it reacted strongly with trypsinized cells, despite failing to react with cells that had been exposed to ficin or papain. Pavone et al. concluded that anti-En^a antibodies comprise a heterogeneous group of similar but not identical antibodies.

Anti-Fy (Duffy) auto-antibodies

van't Veer and co-workers (1984) described the presence of an auto-antibody that mimicked anti-Fy^b specificity in a 49-year-old woman suffering from menorrhagia. She had been transfused, and subsequently the DAT had been found to be positive with anti-IgG and anti-C sera. At first this was attributed to a transfusion reaction; later it became clear that she was suffering from mild compensated AIHA. In her serum, and in eluates from her erythrocytes, an antibody was present which appeared to react only with Fy(b+) cells. The antibody was found, however, to be totally absorbable by Fy(a+b−) cells, and elution and

absorption experiments showed that it was recognizing a determinant that was absent on Fy(a−b−), weakly expressed on Fy(b−) cells and strongly expressed on Fy(b+) cells. Later, an antibody of pure anti-Fy^b specificity was shown to have been formed.

Harris and Lukasavage (1989) briefly reported investigating two further patients who had formed mimicking anti-Fy auto-antibodies. As in the case of the patient described by van't Veer et al. (1984), both had presented with a history of a possible delayed transfusion reaction.

Anti-Ge (Gerbich) auto-antibodies

Reynolds, Vengelen-Tyler and More (1981) described a 14-year-old male suffering from acute AIHA in whose serum and erythrocyte eluate an anti-Ge antibody was identified. The DAT was strongly positive with anti-IgG and anti-C sera. Treatment with 2-ME showed that the antibody consisted of both IgG and IgM; it agglutinated and sensitized to antiglobulin sera cells of all types tested, including Rh$_{null}$ cells, with the exception of Ge-negative cells. The patient himself was Ge-positive. Ficin-treated Ge(+) cells did not react with the patient's serum. The patient mother had suffered from relapsing severe AIHA and she also had had Graves disease; her auto-antibody had the specificity anti-pdl.

Shulman and co-workers (1985, 1990) described a further case of AIHA attributed to an anti-Ge auto-antibody. Their patient was a 26-year-old woman with severe anaemia: haemoglobin 4.6 g/dl and reticulocyte count 1.9%. She was Ge-positive. The DAT and IAT were positive. Anti-Ge was identified in her serum and in an erythrocyte eluate. A transfusion with Ge(+) erythrocytes led to their rapid destruction and haemoglobinuria; in contrast, Ge(−) cells were subsequently shown to survive well. In vitro, tests with mononuclear monolayers showed that Ge(+) cells, sensitized with the patient's serum, were significantly phagocytosed.

Beattie and Sigmund (1987) described a further patient in whom an anti-Ge antibody had been identified. She was a 61-year-old woman with rheumatoid arthritis who had been treated with gold salts for over 4 years. She was severely anaemic: haemoglobin 5.4 g/dl, with 3.4–6.4% reticulocytes, but she was not leucopenic or thrombocytopenic. The DAT was negative and at first the anti-Ge antibody in her serum was considered to be an allo-antibody. However, it was shown that her serum strongly agglutinated her own erythrocytes when withdrawn 12 months later, and it became clear that the antibody was in fact an auto-antibody. It seemed likely, therefore, that the Ge antigen on her erythrocytes had been temporarily depressed. Treatment with prednisone was followed by a rise in haemoglobin and an increase in reticulocyte count to 13.7%. An interesting finding was an apparent deficiency of erythrocyte membrane β-SGPs: when tested for by SDS–PAGE during the acute phase of the patient's illness they were clearly reduced compared with SGPs in an erythrocyte sample procured 2 years later when she had recovered. An additional interesting finding was that of elliptocytes in the peripheral blood in the acute and convalescent phases of the patient's illness; on recovery, the anti-Ge antibody was found to have disappeared and the elliptocytosis was no longer present. Beattie and Sigmund suggested that gold toxicity 'may have caused alteration of the patient's red cell antigen synthesis and her immune system, leading to production of an autoantibody that transitorily masqueraded as an alloantibody'.

Reid and co-workers (1988) tested the erythrocytes of two patients with AIHA associated with anti-Ge auto-antibodies (Reynolds, Vengelen-Tyler and More, 1981; Shulman et al., 1985) to determine whether the erythrocyte β-SGPs were in any way abnormal. They found that the auto-anti-Ge2 produced by the patient of Reynolds et al. had a unique SGP specificity: it reacted with normal β-SGP but not with abnormal β-related SGPs associated with Ge-negative erythrocytes of the Gerbich and Yus types.

Göttsche, Salama and Mueller-Eckhardt (1990) described a further patient who had formed an anti-Ge auto-antibody. A man aged 42 developed severe haemolysis with haemoglobinuria. He had undergone splenectomy when 7 years old for a haemolytic anaemia (of unspecified type) and when aged 28 he had suffered from Hodgkin's disease but had achieved a complete remission following irradiation and chemotherapy. His present haemolytic anaemia, too, remitted following treatment with prednisone and cyclophosphamide. The DAT was positive with anti-C sera only, but an antibody in his serum agglutinated all normal erythrocytes tested at 37°C; it did not, however, agglutinate the patient's own cells. Eluates reacted strongly by the IAT using anti-IgA antiglobulin sera but only weakly with anti-IgG sera. The specificity of the antibody was eventually identified as being anti-Ge2, and it was suggested that the corresponding erythrocyte antigen had been markedly weakened during the acute phase of haemolysis.

Anti-Jk (Kidd) auto-antibodies

A small number of auto-antibodies of Jk specificity have been described. van Loghem and van der Hart (1954a) listed five specific auto-antibodies that had been identified in cases of warm-antibody AIHA: one was an anti-Jk[a], the others were anti-D, anti-c or anti-c plus anti-e.

Holmes, Pierce and Beck (1976) referred briefly to a normal blood donor, a young woman aged 17, whose DAT was weakly positive with an anti-IgG serum. Anti-Jk[a] was identified in eluates, but no atypical antibodies were found in her serum. Her Kidd phenotype was Jk(a+b+).

Patten and co-workers (1977) described a 53-year-old woman receiving Aldomet who had developed severe AIHA. The DAT was positive with a broad spectrum antiglobulin serum and weakly positive with a 'non-gamma' reagent. Anti-Jk[a] was identified in her serum and in an eluate from her erythrocytes. She rapidly improved after being taken off the Aldomet and being treated with prednisone. Eight months later the DAT was negative and the anti-Jk[a] was no longer detectable in her serum.

Ellisor and co-workers (1981, 1983) described the occurrence of auto-antibodies mimicking anti-Jk[b] plus anti-Jk3 in a 25-year-old woman who had developed a compensated AIHA in her first pregnancy. The DAT was strongly positive with anti-IgG, -IgGl, -C3 and -C3d sera and weakly positive with an anti-C4c serum. Antibodies, first identified as anti-Jk[b] plus anti-Jk3, were present in her serum and in eluates from her erythrocytes. Her Kidd phenotype was Jk(a−b+), Jk3. However, the antibodies were later found to be mimics, as in both serum and eluate they could be completely absorbed with Jk(a+b−), Jk(a−b+) and Jk(a−b−) cells. A healthy child was eventually delivered, whose DAT on cord blood was negative. The patient herself continued for at least 5 months after delivery to have a compensated haemolytic anaemia and a strongly positive DAT when her erythrocytes were tested with anti-IgG and anti-C3d sera.

Judd, Steiner and Cochran (1982) reported finding in the serum of three patients auto-anti-Jk[a] antibodies, but only when their sera were tested using low-ionic strength saline containing parabens as preservative (i.e. methyl and propyl esters of p-hydroxybenzoate). In none of the patients was there evidence of haemolytic anaemia; in one patient, however, the DAT was weakly positive with anti-IgG and anti-C sera. Eluates from the erythrocytes from all three patients failed to react with Jk(a−b+) cells. The parabens in some way seem to have enhanced the reactivity of the anti-Jk[a] antibody with its corresponding antigen, but how exactly this is brought about is unclear.

Strikas, Seifert and Lentino (1983) reported that they had identified an auto-antibody of anti-Jk[a] specificity in the serum of a patient who had developed a transient haemolytic anaemia associated with a *Legionella pneumophila* infection. The DAT and IAT were both positive.

O'Day (1987) described a further example of an auto-anti-Jk3 antibody. His patient was a 31-year-old woman in her first pregnancy. Thrombotic thrombocytopenic purpura (TTP) had been diagnosed in the first trimester and she had been transfused with three units of packed erythrocytes and fresh frozen plasma and had received, too, 24 single-unit platelet concentrates. Five months later anti-Le^a and anti-Le^b and anti-I, active at room temperature, were present in her serum, and also anti-Jk^b active at 37°C. The DAT was positive with an anti-IgG serum, and eluates from her erythrocytes reacted with all cells tested, including a Rh$_{null}$ sample. The eluates, however, failed to react with 14 samples of Jk(a−b−) cells. The patient's Kidd phenotype was Jk(a+b−)Jk3. A viable male infant was born at term. His DAT was weakly positive and cord serum reacted weakly with Jk(b+) cells. The baby's Kidd phenotype was Jk(a+b+).

Anti-K (Kell) auto-antibodies

Anti-K was first recognized as a possible, but rare, auto-antibody by Dausset and Colombani (1959). They had reviewed the history and haematological findings in 83 patients with idiopathic AIHA, and in 18 had attempted to define the specificity of the auto-antibodies. In seven, specific Rh antibodies were identified and in one of these an anti-Kell antibody was also present. This patient was a man aged 19 with severe AIHA who had died of his disease.

A second example of an auto-anti-K antibody was recognized by Flückiger, Ricci and Usteri (1955). It was present in the serum and in eluates from the erythrocytes of a woman aged 36 who suffered from AIHA and thrombocytopenia. She was group O, Rh-negative; and anti-e, and possibly a third unidentified antibody, were also present as auto-antibodies.

Further cases of AIHA associated with the formation of auto-anti-K antibodies were described in the 1970s; and in several of these, antigens of the Kell blood-group system were found to be depressed. Seyfried and co-workers (1972) described one such case. Their patient, a young man, developed quite suddenly a severe haemolytic anaemia: his haemoglobin fell to 2.3 g/dl, and there was leucopenia and severe thrombocytopenia, too. The DAT, at first negative, became weakly positive during the second week of his illness. During the acute phase, anti-Kp^b was identified in his serum: it did not, however, react with his erythrocytes. The K, Kp^a and Js^a antigens were absent and the antithetical antigens, k and Kp^b, were but weakly expressed. Kp(b−) erythrocytes were transfused and found to survive quite well (^{51}Cr T$_{50}$ 19 days), and aided by azathioprine and prednisone therapy he eventually recovered. At the same time the expression of his K and Kp^b antigens became normal.

Marsh, DiNapoli and Øyen (1978, 1979) reported that they had identified anti-K13 as the causal auto-antibody in a man aged 59 who suffered from chronic AIHA. (K13 is a high-incidence antigen related to the Kell blood-groups.) The DAT was positive with anti-IgG and anti-C sera. An auto-antibody eluted from the patient's erythrocytes reacted strongly with several panels of extensively typed erythrocytes, including cells lacking the common Kell antigens; it did not, however, react with K$_0$ or K13-negative cells. The patient's own Kell antigens did not seem to be reduced in antigenicity.

Beck and co-workers (1979) described another case in which the presence of an auto-anti-Kp^b was associated with weakening of the Kell blood-group antigens. Their patient was an 84-year-old woman who had suffered a gastrointestinal haemorrhage. The DAT was positive with anti-IgG and anti-C sera. Anti-Kp^b was identified in her serum as well as in eluates from her erythrocytes. The strength of the K$_x$ (precursor) Kell antigen was increased; otherwise, the reactions with a variety of anti-Kell antibodies, as measured by the use of antiglobulin serum, indicated reduced antigen strength.

Marsh and his co-workers (1979) reviewed the occurrence of auto-antibodies with specificity in the Kell blood-group system and described a further case of their own. Their patient was a man aged 19 who had been admitted to hospital as the result of a car accident. (He had been transfused 4 months earlier for blood loss sustained by falling through a window.) Following the car accident routine investigation prior to a possible blood transfusion had shown that the DAT was positive and that his serum contained an antibody which reacted with all cells tested. There was, however, no evidence of increased haemolysis. Further investigation indicated that the antibody appeared to be defining a 'new' high-incidence antigen related to the Kell blood-group system. Allo-anti-K, too, was identified in his serum. The patient's Kell blood-group antigens were depressed and it was postulated that 'the reduced antigenicity [was] caused by enzymatic degradation, possibly of bacterial origin, and that the acquired loss of Kell antigens, and the Kell-specific autoimmune state and the serum allo-anti-K [were] all related aspects of one phenomenon'.

According to Marsh et al. (1979) auto-antibodies against Kell blood-group antigens are formed by approximately 1 in 250 of those who form auto-antibodies against erythrocytes.

Garratty and co-workers (1980) described briefly a female patient, a carrier of chronic granulomatous disease, who had developed AIHA with a positive DAT.

An anti-Kell antibody and another antibody that was unidentified were present in her serum. Although the patient was Kell-negative, an anti-Kell antibody was eluted from her erythrocytes, and it was suggested that the eluted antibody was 'an auto-antibody with some Kell-type reactivity'.

Hare and co-workers (1981) described briefly another highly unusual anti-Kell antibody which had been formed by a patient with a brain tumour and AIHA. Two units of blood had been transfused 3 months previously. The DAT was positive with anti-IgG and anti-C3d. The patient's Kell phenotype was K−, k+, Kp(b+), Js(b+), and the expression of the antigens was normal. Nevertheless, anti-K was identified in serum and in eluates, and it was found that this antibody, although absorbed to 'exhaustion' with K+ cells, could also be absorbed although not completely by K− cells; it thus appeared to be directed against a high-incidence Kell receptor and to have at the same time a preference for K+ cells.

A further auto-anti-K antibody of the mimicking type was described by Viggiano, Clary and Ballas (1982). Their patient was a 68-year-old man with pancytopenia and a cellular bone marrow. The DAT was at first negative, but became positive later. The patient's Kell phenotype was K−, k+, Kp(b+), Js(b+). Eluates from his erythrocytes apparently contained anti-K, but this could be absorbed by, and eluted from, K− as well as K+ cells.

Another example of an auto-anti-Kp^b antibody was described by Manny et al. (1983). The patient, a woman aged 23, had been admitted to hospital for a therapeutic abortion. The DAT and IAT were positive, but there was no evidence of increased haemolysis. Anti-Kp^b was demonstrated in her serum and in eluates from her erythrocytes. Remarkably, the patient was Kp(a+), had weak k and Js^b antigens and had either depressed Kp^b antigens or was Kp(b−). The serological findings thus provide a further example of the phenomenon of the elution of a specific antibody from erythrocytes lacking the genetically determined corresponding antigen.

A further auto-antibody mimicking anti-Kp^b was described by Puig, Carbonell and Marty (1986) in a 74-year-old man who had a carcinoma of the larynx. The DAT was positive with anti-IgG, -IgM, -IgA and -C3 sera and his serum contained an antibody that reacted with all cells tested. Further investigation showed that the antibody in his serum, and in eluates from his erythrocytes, had anti-Kp^b specificity, despite the fact that the patient's Kell phenotype was Kp(a+b−).

Effect of AET on Kell antigens

Antigens of the Kell blood-group system are known to be inactivated if the erythrocytes bearing them are treated with AET (2-aminoethylisothiouronium bromide) (Advani et al., 1982). Marsh, Mueller and

Johnson (1982) reported that they had confirmed this inactivation in 17 blood samples suspected of containing Kell-related auto-antibodies.

Later, however, Marsh and co-workers (1985) reported that they had come across an auto-antibody that reacted with random erythrocyte samples and K_0 cells, and with cells treated with dithiothrietol–papain solution (ZZAP), but did not react with AET cells or with Rh_{null} cells. The pattern of activity was, however, unlike that of IgG antibodies that fail to react only with Rh_{null} cells. Marsh et al. concluded that the reactive antigen was not part of either the Kell or Rh systems but was 'probably modified by the membrane anomaly present in Rh_{null} red cells'. The antibody had been formed by an 83-year-old woman who died of fulminating AIHA. The DAT was strongly positive with anti-IgG sera but negative with an anti-C serum.

Anti-Lu (Lutheran) auto-antibodies

Fitzsimmons and Caggiano (1981) reported that they had identified an auto-antibody formed by a 42-year-old patient with an ovarian carcinoma as having anti-Lutheran specificity. The DAT was positive with anti-IgG and anti-C3d sera. The patient was Lu(a−b+) and her serum and erythrocyte eluate reacted with all cells tested except those of Lu(a−b−) phenotype. The auto-antibody was thus considered to be directed against a Lutheran antigen of high frequency. Her serum also contained anti-Wr^a as an allo-antibody.

Anti-LW (Landsteiner, Wiener) auto-antibodies

This specificity was demonstrated by Celano and Levine (1967) in six patients with AIHA who had been investigated within a 2-year period. The sera and eluates when first tested with a panel of cells of different phenotypes reacted non-specifically. Further tests with Rh-positive and Rh-negative, LW-negative cells indicated the presence of anti-LW. Anti-Rh antibodies were present also.

Vos and co-workers (1973) had studied with a panel of cells of extremely rare phenotypes eight eluates that had been found to contain multiple antibodies. They had been prepared from the erythrocytes of an unspecified number of AIHA patients. Anti-LW was identified in six eluates: in five cases Rh antibodies, i.e., anti-pdl, anti-dl or anti-e, were also present, and in one case anti-U.

Anti-LW, notwithstanding the two reports cited above, is a rare auto-antibody. Thus it was not found in a series of 93 eluates referred to by Worlledge and Blajchman (1972).

Anti-S auto-antibodies

Johnson and co-workers (1978) described briefly the formation of an auto-antibody of anti-S specificity by an adult male with severe AIHA. Sixteen years previously he had developed a nephrotic syndrome associated with SLE. The DAT and IAT were positive and anti-S was demonstrated in both his serum and in eluates from his erythrocytes. The possibility of an anti-U antibody reacting only against S-positive cells was excluded. Splenic sequestration was demonstrated and splenectomy carried out. Following this, despite the tapering off of steroids, he gradually recovered and the haematocrit rose to 47%.

Anti-Sc3 (Scianna) auto-antibodies

Peloquin and co-workers (1989) described briefly the presence of anti-Sc3-like antibodies in the serum of two patients with a lymphoma and Hodgkin's disease, respectively. The DAT was weakly positive with an anti-IgG serum in the first patient but more strongly positive with an anti-C serum, and was negative with an anti-IgG serum but strongly positive with an anti-C serum in the second patient. The common Scianna antigens, Sc1 and Sc3 were weak in both patients.

Anti-U auto-antibodies

Blajchman and his co-workers (1971), in reporting the occurrence of AIHA in a mother and her daughter, referred to the specificity of the antibody as anti-U; and Nugent, Colledge and Marsh (1971) described an 89-year-old woman who had suffered from severe anaemia for 5 months whose auto-antibody had a similar specificity.

The DAT was positive and she had been referred for further investigation with the aim of finding compatible blood for transfusion. Her serum was found to contain anti-U, not inactivated by 2-ME, and eluates from her erythrocytes contained anti-U also. The antibody reacted less strongly with $-D-/-D-$, U-positive cells than with U-positive cells of normal Rh phenotypes. It did not react with Rh_{null} cells, a finding consistent with previous observations indicating that Rh_{null} cells react weakly or not at all with anti-U sera (Schmidt et al., 1967). Nugent, Colledge and Marsh concluded that auto-antibodies of 'complex Rh' specificity that do not react with Rh_{null} cells may sometimes in reality have anti-U specificity.

Beck and co-workers (1972) described the formation of an anti-U auto-antibody by a 23-year-old man who had been admitted for thymectomy for myasthenia gravis. The DAT was positive with broad-spectrum antiglobulin sera, the reaction being inhibited by the prior addition of γ globulin. Anti-U and an unidentified antibody absorbed by U-negative cells were identified in eluates. Rh_{null} cells were acted upon less strongly than cells of normal Rh phenotypes. Despite the presence of the antibodies, the patient was not anaemic and the reticulocyte count was normal.

Marsh, Reid and Scott (1972) studied the auto-antibodies formed by 50 patients with warm-antibody AIHA, seeking particularly evidence of U, S or s specificity. Anti-U plus an unidentified non-specific antibody (reacting with Rh_{null} cells) were identified in one patient and anti-U, anti-e and a non-specific antibody identified in two other patients; all three were Caucasians. (In none of the 50 patients could auto-anti-S or auto-anti-s be identified.)

Kessey and co-workers (1973) reported, without giving details, that they had identified anti-U in a patient suffering from AIHA attributed to α-methyldopa therapy, and Vos et al. (1973), in their paper primarily directed to the identification of auto-anti-LW in patients with AIHA, reported the finding of anti-U in three patients: in one this was associated with anti-pdl, in one with anti-LW and in the third with anti-dl.

Bell and Zwicker (1980) described how they had identified an auto-anti-U in the serum of a man aged 91 with neurosyphilis and chronic lymphocytic leukaemia. He was anaemic: haemoglobin 5.4 g/dl, with 8% reticulocytes. The DAT was positive with broad-spectrum and anti-C sera, but negative with monospecific anti-IgG, -IgA and -IgM reagents. The anti-U antibody in his serum was only demonstrable if the serum had been acidified to pH 6.5 and the anti-C reagent used in antiglobulin tests.

Sacher and co-workers (1982) described a 74-year-old man suffering from a myelodysplastic syndrome who became severely anaemic. The DAT was strongly positive with anti-IgG sera and weakly positive with an anti-C3 serum. An anti-U antibody was identified in his serum and in an eluate from his erythrocytes; $-D-/-D-$ cells (expressing the U antigen weakly) were not agglutinated in IATs. No other auto-antibodies appeared to be present. D-positive, U-negative cells were transfused without any reaction. Following prednisone therapy the DAT became less strongly positive and ^{51}Cr-labelled U-positive cells were shown to survive well, compared with the rapid elimination of similar cells before the steroid had been given.

Anti-Vel auto-antibodies

A small number of patients have been described who have formed auto-antibodies of Vel specificity.

Szalóky and van der Hart (1971) identified an anti-Vel antibody in the serum of a patient with aplastic anaemia. He had not been transfused and the DAT was negative using anti-IgG, -IgM, -IgA, -IgD and -C sera. His serum weakly agglutinated

Vel-positive erythrocytes in saline at 37°C and strongly agglutinated and lysed bromelin-treated Vel-positive (but not Vel-negative) cells. The patient's own cells when bromelin-treated were agglutinated and lysed by his serum and also by two other anti-Vel sera. The reactions between the patient's serum and Vel-positive cells were inhibited by prior treatment of the serum with 2-ME. Despite the presence of an apparent auto-antibody, the survival of ^{51}Cr-labelled Vel-positive cells was normal, as was that of the patient's own cells.

Herron, Hyde and Hillier (1979) described a second anti-Vel auto-antibody. This was identified in the serum of a 76-year-old woman suffering from follicular lymphoma and AIHA. Her haemoglobin was 4.9 g/dl and she was moderately thrombocytopenic. The DAT was strongly positive with anti-C sera but negative with anti-IgG and -IgM sera. The antibody in her serum reacted with Vel-positive erythrocytes, and with the patient's own cells, at 37°C and 16°C; it was most active between 4°C and 16°C. It lysed Vel-positive cells weakly, if untreated, and papainized cells strongly, and was identified as an IgM antibody, being inactivated by DTT (dithiothreitol).

A further example of an anti-Vel auto-antibody that was apparently responsible for a severe and ultimately fatal AIHA was described by Becton and Kinney (1986). Their patient was an infant girl who when 9 weeks of age quite suddenly became febrile and anaemic and thrombocytopenic. The DAT and IAT were negative with polyspecific and monospecific reagents. Her serum, however, agglutinated (1+) at room temperature all cells tested including the infant's own cells; inactivation by DTT showed that it was formed of IgM. Seven samples of Vel-negative cells were not agglutinated. An initial transfusion with 'least incompatible', but Vel-positive, cells led to haemoglobinuria and disseminated intravascular coagulation. A short-term study with ^{51}Cr-labelled Vel-negative cells showed that they survived normally. There was no evidence that the infant was suffering from a collagen disease, an immunodeficiency syndrome or malignant disease.

Anti-Xg^a auto-antibodies

Yokoyama, Eith and Bowman (1967) described the occurrence in the serum of a 33-year-old woman in the course of her 6th pregnancy of anti-Xg^a as well as anti-S. The patient was severely anaemic, with a haemoglobin of 3.5 g/dl. The DAT was positive, and anti-Xg^a was identified in an eluate from her erythrocytes. The patient was Xg(a+),S−. The anti-Xg^a thus

appeared to be an auto-antibody and the anti-S an allo-antibody.

An auto-antibody against erythrocyte membrane protein 4.1

Wakui and co-workers (1988) reported the formation by a 61-year-old woman with chronic AIHA of a 'new' auto-antibody which reacted with a 78 kd erythrocyte membrane protein, protein 4.1. An anti-En^a-like antibody and anti-S were also identified in her serum. The DAT was positive with anti-IgG sera but negative with anti-IgA and -IgM sera and with anti-C sera. The anti-protein 4.1 was also identified in the serum of the patient's brother, but not in other patients with non-immune haemolytic anaemias or in normal subjects. In discussion, Wakui et al. referred to other reported occurrences of anti-cytoskeletal antibodies, e.g. in SLE, in chronic active hepatitis and in normal subjects; they also referred to the suggestion that anti-cytoskeletal membrane protein antibodies may play a physiological role in clearing the debris of lysed cells from the circulation.

ANTI-dl AUTO-ANTIBODIES

Anti-dl antibodies react with Rh$_{null}$ erythrocytes as well as with cells of the common Rh phenotypes. They thus appear to react with antigens outside the Rh blood-group system. In the preceding pages auto-antibodies of 12 specificities that react in this way have been described: of these, only anti-Wr^b has been found to be a common specificity. The reactions of the erythrocytes of the (rare) phenotypes required for the identification of anti-Wr^b, anti-En^a, anti-LW and anti-U are summarized in Table 26.3.

Table 26.3   Reactions of anti-dl, anti-Wr^b, anti-En^a, anti-LW and anti-U auto-antibodies with erythrocytes of five rare phenotypes

Auto-antibodies	Erythrocytes				
	En(a+), Wr(b−)	En(a−)	LW(a−)	U−	Rh$_{null}$
Anti-dl	+	+	+	+	+
Anti-Wr^b	−	−	+	+	+
Anti-En^a	+	−	+	+	+
Anti-W^a	+	+	−	+	−
Anti-U	+	+	+	−	−*

* The majority

'Non-specific' auto-antibodies

The original concept of a 'non-specific' auto-antibody was of an antibody the antigen of which was common to *all* human erythrocytes. The increasing availability of cells of rare phenotypes, i.e. cells lacking a very common antigen to which the antibody was in fact directed, has in the case of anti-En[a], anti-LW, anti-U and anti-Wr[b] antibodies enabled them to be identified and removed from the category of 'non-specific' antibodies (Table 26.3). It is possible that the identification of cells lacking other as yet unidentified very common antigens will enable other auto-antibodies, apparently reacting with all cells tested, to be similarly detected. It would be rash, however, to exclude the possibility of truly 'non-specific' antibodies. Certainly, at least when Issitt and his co-workers (1976) studied 87 eluates made from AIHA erythrocytes, there were 62 eluates (71%) in which anti-dl antibodies were present, the specificity of which could not be defined because they reacted with all the cells that were then available including those with rare phenotypes. Anti-dl was the only auto-antibody identified in 13 of these 62 eluates; in 49 eluates, antibodies of other defined specificities were present in addition to anti-dl.

In a later report, Issitt and co-workers (1980) listed 10 very common erythrocyte antigens that had been identified as targets for anti-dl antibodies: namely, in the Rh system, Hr, Hr_0, Rh34, Rh29 and LW; in the MN and Wright system, En[a], U and Wr[b]; and in the Kell system, Kp[b] and K13. (Jk3 had not up to that time been identified, which they considered surprising.) Issitt et al. also made the point that virtually every specific auto-antibody known to cause auto-immune haemolysis had also been identified as a benign antibody in individuals with a positive DAT but no evidence of disease.

SPECIES SPECIFICITY OF HUMAN WARM AUTO-ANTIBODIES

At one time the possibility of reactions between human erythrocyte auto-antibodies and mammalian erythrocytes other than those of man aroused considerable interest. Early data indicated in fact that the antibodies often reacted quite strongly with the cells of some primate species but failed to react, or reacted only weakly, with the cells of non-primate species.

Sturgeon (1947) reported that he had obtained negative results with both Rhesus-monkey and sheep cells. Kidd (1949), on the other hand, using the IAT, found that eluates from the erythrocytes of four patients with AIHA agglutinated Rhesus-monkey cells but failed to react with mouse, guinea-pig, rabbit, sheep and horse cells. Komninos and Rosenthal (1953) similarly failed to obtain positive reactions with rabbit, guinea-pig and sheep cells; in addition, the results of testing 12 eluates with *Macacus rhesus* (*mulatta*) cells, both unmodified and trypsinized, were negative.

Wiener, Gordon and Gallop (1953) tested the serum of one patient against the erythrocytes of various species using cells which had been acted upon by the enzyme ficin. Chimpanzee and Rhesus-monkey erythrocytes were agglutinated to slightly lower titres than were human cells; spider-monkey, cow, horse and sheep erythrocytes were agglutinated to far lower titres. Wiener, Gordon and Gallop pointed out that in this respect the behaviour of the antibody of their patient paralleled that of Rh antibodies.

Evans and Weiser (1957) tested three eluates containing warm antibodies against a variety of animal erythrocytes; only the cells of Rhesus monkeys became weakly agglutinable by antiglobulin serum.

Pirofsky and Pratt (1966) tested the erythrocytes of nine primate species and six non-primate species against eluates prepared from the erythrocytes of four patients suffering from AIHA associated with chronic lymphocytic leukaemia, ulcerative colitis or SLE, respectively. The cells of six of the primate species — ringtail lemur, squirrel monkey, Celebes ape, Rhesus monkey, baboon and chimpanzee — reacted positively, as they did in parallel tests with human anti-Rhesus allo-antibodies; in contrast, the cells of the tree shrew, fulvus lemur and woolly monkey failed to react with either the AIHA eluates or human anti-Rhesus allo-antibodies. The erythrocytes of the six non-primate species tested — rabbit, guinea-pig, dog, mouse, pigmy goat and grey whale — all failed to react.

Leddy (1969) compared the reactivity of the erythrocytes of two species of monkey, *Macaca mulatta* and *Macaca speciosa* against eluates prepared from the erythrocytes of six AIHA patients. Three of the eluates were designated 'non-Rh' as they reacted with Rh_{null} cells: one eluate reacted with the monkey cells, two failed to do so. Three further eluates were designated 'Rh-related' as they failed to react with Rh_{null} cells: all three eluates failed to react with the monkey cells.

REFERENCES

ADAMS, J., MOORE, V. K. & ISSITT, P. D. (1973). Autoimmune hemolytic anemia caused by anti-D. *Transfusion*, **13**, 214–218.

ADVANI, H., ZAMOR, J., JUDD, W. J., JOHNSON, C. L. & MARSH, W. L. (1982). Inactivation of Kell blood group antigens by 2-aminoethylisothiouronium bromide. *Brit. J. Haemat.*, **51**, 107–115.

ALLEN, F. H. JNR, ISSITT, P. D., DEGNAN, T. J., JACKSON, V. A., REIHART, J. K., KNOWLIN, R. J. & ABEBAHR, M. E. (1969). Further observations on the Matuhasi–Ogata phenomenon. *Vox Sang.*, **16**, 47–56.

BEATTIE, K. M. & SIGMUND, K. E. (1987). A Ge-like autoantibody in the serum of a patient receiving gold therapy for rheumatoid arthritis. *Transfusion*, **27**, 54–57.

BECK, M. L., BUTCH, S. H., ARMSTRONG, W. D. & OBERMAN, H. A. (1972). An antibody with U-specificity in a patient with myasthenia gravis. *Transfusion*, **12**, 280–283.

BECK, M. L., MARSH, W. L., PIERCE, S. R., DiNAPOLI, J., ØYEN, R. & NICHOLS, M. E. (1979). Auto-anti-Kp[b] associated with weakened antigenicity in the Kell blood-group system: a second example. *Transfusion*, **19**, 197–202.

BECTON, M.L. & KINNEY, T.R. (1986). An infant girl with severe autoimmune hemolytic anemia: apparent anti-Vel specificity. *Vox Sang.*, **51**, 108–111.

BELL, C. A. & ZWICKER, H. (1978). Further studies on the relationship of anti-En[a] and anti-Wr[b] in warm autoimmune hemolytic anemia. *Transfusion*, **18**, 572–575.

BELL, C. A. & ZWICKER, H. (1980). pH-dependent anti-U in autoimmune hemolytic anemia. *Transfusion*, **20**, 86–89.

BELL, C. A., ZWICKER, H. & SACKS, H. J. (1973). Autoimmune hemolytic anemia. Routine serologic evaluation in a general hospital population. *Amer. J. clin. Path.*, **60**, 903–911.

BIRD, G. W. G. & WINGHAM, J. (1972). Changes in specificity of erythrocyte autoagglutinins. *Vox Sang.*, **22**, 364–365.

BLAJCHMAN, M. A., HUI, Y. T., JONES, T. E. & LUKE, K. H. (1971). Familial autoimmune hemolytic anemia demonstrating U specificity. *Proc. 24th Annual Meeting American Ass. Blood Banks*, Chicago, p. 82.

BOVE, J. R., HOLBURN, A. M. & MOLLISON, P. L. (1973). Non-specific binding of IgG to antibody-coated red cells (the Matuhasi-Ogata phenomenon). *Immunology*, **25**, 793–801.

CELANO, M. J. & LEVINE, P. (1967). Anti-LW specificity in autoimmune acquired hemolytic anemia. *Transfusion*, **7**, 265–268.

CHENG, M. S. (1985). Anti-C as a sole autoantibody in autoimmune hemolytic anemia. *Transfusion*, **25**, 88 (Letter).

CICALA, V., D'ONOFRIO, F. & PAOLUCCI, D. (1959). Richerche immunoematologiche in due casi di anemia emolitica. *Proc. 7th Congr. int. Soc. Blood Transfusion, Rome, Sept. 3–6, 1958*, pp. 877–881. Karger, Basel.

CROWLEY, L.V. & BOURONCLE, B. A. (1955). Studies on the specificity of autoantibodies in acquired hemolytic anemia. *J. Lab. clin. Med.*, **46**, 805–806 (Abstract).

CROWLEY, L. V. & BOURONCLE, B. A. (1956). Studies on the specificity of autoantibodies in acquired hemolytic anemia. *Blood*, **11**, 700–707.

DACIE, J. V. (1953). Serology of acquired haemolytic anaemia. *4th Congr. Europ. Soc. Haemat., Amsterdam, Sept. 8–12, 1953*.

DACIE, J. V. (1954). *The Haemolytic Anaemias: Congenital and Acquired*, 525 pp. Churchill, London.

DACIE, J. V. (1962). *The Haemolytic Anaemias: Congenital and Acquired. Part II—The Auto-immune Haemolytic Anaemias*, 2nd edn, 377 pp. Churchill, London.

DACIE, J. V. & CUTBUSH, M. (1954). Specificity of auto-antibodies in acquired haemolytic anaemia. *J. clin. Path.*, **7**, 18–21.

DAMESHEK, W. (1951). Acquired hemolytic anemia. Physiopathology with particular reference to autoimmunization and therapy. *Proc. 3rd int. Congr. int. Soc. Hemat., Cambridge, England, Aug. 21–25, 1950*, pp. 120–133. Grune and Stratton, New York.

DAUSSET, J. & COLOMBANI, J. (1959). The serology and the prognosis of 128 cases of autoimmune hemolytic anemia. *Blood*, **14**, 1280–1301.

DAVIDSOHN, I. & OYAMADA, A. (1953). Specificity of auto-antibodies in hemolytic anemia. *Amer. J. clin. Path.*, **23**, 101–115.

DENYS, P. & VAN DEN BROUCKE, J. (1947), Anémie hémolytique acquise et réaction de Coombs. *Arch. franç. Pédiat.*, **4**, 205–217.

DI PIERO, G. (1959). Su una nuova osservazione di anemia emolitica acquisati in età pediatrica. *Haematologica*, **44**, 489–500.

DIXON, J., BECK, M. & OBERMAN, H. A. (1969). Variation in antibody specificity in a patient with autoimmune hemolytic anaemia. *Transfusion*, **9**, 290 (Abstract).

ELLISOR, S. S., REID, M., O'DAY, T. & SWANSON, J. (1981). Autoantibodies mimicking anti-Jk[b] plus anti-Jk3 associated with autoimmune hemolytic anemia in a primipara. *Transfusion*, **21**, 631 (Abstract).

ELLISOR, S. S., REID, M. E., O'DAY, T., SWANSON, J., PAPENFUS, L. & AVOY, D. R. (1983). Autoantibodies mimicking anti-Jk[b] plus anti-Jk3 associated with autoimmune hemolytic anemia in a primipara who delivered an unaffected infant. *Vox Sang.*, **45**, 53–59.

EVANS, R. S., DUANE, R. T. & BEHRENDT, V. (1947). Demonstration of antibodies in acquired hemolytic anemia with anti-human globulin serum. *Proc. Soc. exp. Biol. Med.*, **64**, 372–375.

EVANS, R. S. & WEISER, R. S. (1957). The serology of autoimmune hemolytic disease. Observations on forty-one patients. *Arch. intern. Med.*, **100**, 371–399.

EYSTER, M. E. & JENKINS, D. E. JNR (1970). γG erythrocyte autoantibodies: comparison of *in vivo* complement coating and *in vitro* 'Rh' specificity. *J. Immunol.*, **105**, 221–226.

FITZSIMMONS, J. & CAGGIANO, V. (1981). Autoantibody to a high-frequency Lutheran antigen associated with immune hemolytic anemia and a hemolytic transfusion episode. *Transfusion*, **21**, 612 (Abstract).

FLÜCKIGER, P., RICCI, C & USTERI, C. (1955). Zur Frage der Blutgruppenspezifität von Autoantikörpern. *Acta haemat. (Basel)*, **13**, 53–56.

FUDENBERG, H. H., ROSENFIELD, R. E. & WASSERMAN, L. R. (1958). Unusual specificity of auto-antibody in auto-immune hemolytic disease. *J. Mt Sinai Hosp.*, **25**, 324–329.

GARRATTY, G., SATTLER, M. S., PETZ, L. D. & FLANNERY, E. P. (1980). Immune hemolytic anemia with anti-Kell and a carrier state for chronic granulomatous disease. *Transfusion*, **20**, 737 (Abstract).

GERBAL, A., HOMBERG, J. C., ROCHANT, H., PERRON, L. & SALMON, C. H. (1968). Les auto-anticorps d'anémies hémolytiques acquises. I. Analyse de 234 observations. *Nouv. Rev, franç. Hémat.*, **8**, 155–178.

GOLDFINGER, D., ZWICKER, H., BELKIN, G. A. & ISSITT, P. D. (1975). An antibody with anti-Wr[b] specificity in a patient with warm autoimmune hemolytic anemia. *Transfusion*, **15**, 351–352.

GÖTTSCHE, B. M., SALAMA, A. & MUELLER-ECKHARDT, C. (1990). Autoimmune hemolytic anemia associated with a IgA autoanti-Gerbich. *Vox Sang.*, **58**, 211–214.

HABIBI, B. (1977). Antigènes cibles des autoanticorps antiérythrocytaires. *Rev. franç. Transf. Immuno-hémat.*, **20**, 205–211.

HACKETT, E. (1950). Coombs test in acute acquired haemolytic anaemia. *Lancet*, **i**, 998–999.

HARE, V., WILSON, M. J., WILKINSON, S. & ISSITT, P. D. (1981). A Kell system antibody with highly unusual characteristics. *Transfusion*, **21**, 613 (Abstract).

HARRIS, T. & LUKASAVAGE, T. (1989). Two cases of autoantibodies which demonstrate mimicking specificity in the Duffy system. *Transfusion*, **29**, Supp., 49 S (Abstract S 174).

HENI, F. & BLESSING, K. (1954). Die Bedeutung der Glutinine für die erworbenen hämolytischen Anämien. *Dtsch. Arch. klin. Med.*, **201**, 113–135.

HENRY, R. A., WEBER, J., PAVONE, B. G. &

ISSITT, P. D. (1977). A 'normal' individual with a positive direct antiglobulin test. Case complicated by pregnancy and unusual autoantibody specificity. *Transfusion*, **17**, 539–546.

HERRON, R., HYDE, R. D. & HILLIER, S. J. (1979). The second example of an anti-Vel auto-antibody. *Vox Sang.*, **36**, 179–181.

HÖGMAN, C., KILLANDER, J. & SJÖLIN, S. (1960). A case of idiopathic autoimmune haemolytic anaemia due to anti-e. *Acta paediat. (Uppsala)*, **49**, 270–280.

HOLLÄNDER, L. (1953). Specificity of antibodies in acquired haemolytic anaemia. *Experientia (Basel)*, **9**, 468.

HOLLÄNDER, L. (1954). Study of the erythrocyte survival time in a case of acquired haemolytic anaemia. *Vox Sang.*, **4**, 164–165.

HOLLÄNDER, L. & BATSCHELET, E. (1957). Beitrag zur Frage der Spezifität antierythrocytärer autoantikörper. *6th Congr. Europ. Soc. Haemat., Copenhagen, 1957*, Abstract 191 (p. 139).

HOLMES, L. D., PIERCE, S. R. & BECK, M. (1976). Autoanti-Jk[a] in a healthy blood donor. *Transfusion*, **16**, 521 (Abstract S-15).

HUBINONT, P. O., MASSART-GUIOT TH., BRICOULT, A. & GHYSDAD, P. (1959). Immunological specificity of eluates from 'Coombs positive' erythrocytes. (Preliminary note). *Vox Sang.*, **4**, 419–426.

ISBISTER, J. (1978). Autoantibodies to red cells—specificities and effects. *Proc. Symposium Recent Developments in Red Blood Cell Serology*, pp. 63–82. Australian Society of Blood Transfusion and Haematology Society of Australia, Sydney.

ISSITT, P. D. (1977). Autoimmune hemolytic anemia and cold hemagglutinin disease: clinical disease and laboratory findings. In *Progress in Clinical Pathology*, Vol. VII (ed. by M. Stefanini et al.), pp. 137–163. Grune and Stratton, New York.

ISSITT, P. D. (1985a). Serological diagnosis and characterization of the causative autoantibodies. In *Immune Hemolytic Anemias (Methods in Hematology)*, Vol. 12 (ed. by H. Chaplin Jnr), pp. 1–45. Churchill Livingstone, New York.

ISSITT, P. D. (1985b). *Applied Blood Group Serology*, 3rd edn, pp. 523–528. Montgomery Scientific Publications, Miami.

ISSITT, P. D. (1986). Some messages received from blood group antibodies. In *Red Cell Antigens and Antibodies* (ed. by G. Garratty), pp. 99–144. American Association of Blood Banks, Arlington, Virginia.

ISSITT, P. D. (1989). The Rh blood group system, 1988: eight new antigens in nine years and some observations on the biochemistry and genetics of the system. *Transf. Med. Rev.*, **3**, 1–12.

ISSITT, P. D. & PAVONE, B. G. (1978). Critical re-examination of the specificity of auto-anti-Rh antibodies in patients with a positive direct antiglobulin test. *Brit. J. Haemat.*, **38**, 63–74.

ISSITT, P. D., PAVONE, B. G., FROHLICH, J. A. &

McGUIRE MALLORY, D. (1980). Absence of autoanti-Jk3 as a component of anti-dl. *Transfusion*, **20**, 733–736.

ISSITT, P. D., PAVONE, B. G., GOLDFINGER, D. & ZWICKER, H. (1975). An En(a−) red cell sample that types as Wr (a−b−). *Transfusion*, **15**, 353–355.

ISSITT, P. D., PAVONE, B. G., GOLDFINGER, D., ZWICKER, H., ISSITT, C. H., TESSEL, J. A., KROOVAND, S. W. & BELL, C. A. (1976a). Anti-Wr[b], and other autoantibodies responsible for positive direct antiglobulin tests in 150 individuals. *Brit. J. Haemat.*, **34**, 5–18.

ISSITT, P. D., PAVONE, B. G., WAGSTAFF, W. & GOLDFINGER, D. (1976b). The phenotypes En(a−), Wr(a−b−) and En(a+), Wr(a+b−), and further studies on the Wright and En blood group systems. *Transfusion*, **16**, 396–407.

ISSITT, P. D., ZELLNER, D. C., ROLIH, S. D. & DUCKETT, J. B. (1977). Autoantibodies mimicking alloantibodies. *Transfusion*, **17**, 531–538.

JOHNSON, M. H., PLATT, M. J., CONANT, C. N. & WORTHINGTON, M. (1978). Autoimmune hemolytic anemia with anti-S specificity. *Transfusion*, **18**, 389 (Abstract S 57).

JUDD, W. J., STEINER, E. A. & COCHRAN, R. K. (1982). Paraben-associated autoanti-Jk[a] antibodies. Three examples detected using commercially prepared low-ionic-strength saline containing parabens. *Transfusion*, **22**, 31–35.

KANRA, T., DUNBAR, S., ERENER, G. & YAVUZ, H. (1987). A different example of autoimmune haemolytic anaemia caused by anti-D. *Brit. J. Haemat.*, **66**, 432–433 (Letter).

KENNEDY, M. S., WAHEED, A. & MARSH, W. L. (1981). A fatal case of autoimmune hemolytic anemia due to an unusual IgM antibody with possible Rh system specificity. *Transfusion*, **21**, 630 (Abstract).

KESSEY, E, C., PIERCE, S., BECK, M. L. & BAYER, W. L. (1973). Alpha-methyldopa induced hemolytic anemia involving autoantibody with U specificity. *Transfusion*, **13**, 360 (Abstract).

KIDD, P. (1949). Elution of an incomplete type of antibody from the erythrocytes in acquired haemolytic anaemia. *J. clin. Path.*, **2**, 103–108.

KISSMEYER-NIELSEN, F. (1957a). A case of auto-immune haemolytic anaemia with a very remarkable course. *Vox Sang.*, **2**, 88–93.

KISSMEYER-NIELSEN, F. (1957b). Specific auto-antibodies in immunohaemolytic anaemia, with a note on the pathogenesis of auto-immunization. In *P. H. Andresen. Papers in Dedication of His Sixtieth Birthday*, pp. 126–137. Munksgaard, Copenhagen.

KISSMEYER-NIELSEN, F., BICHEL, J. & BJERRE HANSEN (1956). Specific auto-antibodies in immunohemolytic anemia. *Acta haemat. (Basel)*, **15**, 189–201.

KOMIYA, M., NAMIHISA, T. & KATO, S. (1957). Autoimmune hemolytic anemia; their immunological and hematological features, and red cell survivals in 18 cases. *Acta haemat. jap.*, **20**, No. 3, Suppl., 1–12.

KOMNINOS, Z. D. & ROSENTHAL, M. C. (1953). Studies on antibodies eluted from the red cells in autoimmune hemolytic anemia. *J. Lab. clin. Med.*, **41**, 887–894.

KUHNS, W. J. & WAGLEY, P. F. (1949). Hemolytic anemia associated with atypical hemagglutinins. *Ann. intern. Med.*, **30**, 408–423.

LALEZARI, P. (1973). Direct determination of red cell bound antibody specificity. *Brit. J. Haemat.*, **24**, 777–792.

LALEZARI, P. (1976). Serologic profile in autoimmune hemolytic disease: pathophysiologic and clinical correlations. *Seminars Hemat.*, **13**, 291–310.

LALEZARI, P. & BERENS, J. A. (1977). Specificity and cross reactivity of cell-bound antibodies. Implications in autoimmune hemolytic diseases. In *Human Blood Groups. 5th int. Convoc. Immunol., Buffalo, N. Y.*, pp. 44–45. Karger, Basel.

LEDDY, J. P. (1969). Reactivity of human gamma G erythrocyte autoantibodies with fetal, autologous and maternal red cells. *Vox. Sang.*, **17**, 525–535.

LEDDY, J. P. & BAKEMEIER, R. F. (1967). A relationship of direct Coombs test pattern to autoantibody specificity in acquired hemolytic anemia. *Proc. Soc. exp. Biol. Med.*, **125**, 808–811.

LEDDY, J. P., PETERSON, P., YEAW, M. A. & BAKEMEIER, R. F. (1970). Patterns of serologic specificity of human γG erythrocyte autoantibodies. Correlation of antibody specificity with complement-fixing behavior. *J. Immunol.*, **105**, 677–686.

LEWIS, M. (Chairman) and 27 other authors (1985). ISBT Working Party on Terminology for Red Cell Surface Antigens: Munich report. *Vox Sang.*, **49**, 171–175.

LEY, A. B., MAYER, K. & HARRIS, J. P. (1958). Observations on a 'specific autoantibody'. *Proc. 6th Congr. int. Soc. Blood Transfusion, Boston, 1956*, (Bibliotheca haemat., 7), pp. 148–153. Karger, Basel.

MANNY, N., LEVENE, C., SELA, R., JOHNSON, C. L., MUELLER, K. A. & MARSH, W. L. (1983). Autoimmunity and the Kell blood groups: auto-anti-Kp[b] in a Kp(a+b−) patient. *Vox Sang.*, **45**, 252–256.

MARSH, W. L., DiNAPOLI, J. D. & ØYEN, R. (1978). Autoimmune hemolytic anemia caused by anti-K13. *Transfusion*, **18**, 623–624 (Abstract).

MARSH, W. L., DiNAPOLI, J. & ØYEN, R. (1979). Auto-immune hemolytic anemia caused by anti-K13. *Vox Sang.*, **36**, 174–178.

MARSH, W. L., DiNAPOLI, J., ØYEN, R., PACANOWSKI, L. & KESSLER, L. A. (1985). 'New' autoantibody specificity in autoimmune hemolytic anemia defined with red cells treated with 2-aminoethylisothiouronium bromide and a dithiothreitol solution. *Transfusion*, 25, 364–367.

MARSH, W. L., MUELLER, K. A. & JOHNSON, C. L. (1982). Use of AET-treated cells in the investigation of Kell related auto-immunity. *Transfusion*, 22, 419 (Abstract S 66).

MARSH, W. L., ØYEN, R., ALICEA, E., LINTER, M. & HORTON, S. (1979). Autoimmune hemolytic anemia and the Kell blood groups. *Amer. J. Hemat.*, 7, 155–162.

MARSH, W. L., REID, M. E. & SCOTT, E. P. (1972). Autoantibodies of U blood group specificity in autoimmune haemolytic anaemia. *Brit. J. Haemat.*, 22, 625–629.

MEARA, J. F., HOFFMAN, G. C. & HEWLETT, J. S. (1967). Autoimmune hemolytic anemia associated with anti-f: report of a case. *Transfusion*, 7, 48–50.

MEULI, H. C. (1957). Über blutgruppenspezifische antierythrocytäre Autoantikörper. *Blut*, 3, 270–275.

MOLLISON, P. L. (1959). Measurement of survival and destruction of red cells in haemolytic syndromes. *Brit. med. Bull.*, 15, 59–67.

NUGENT, M. E., COLLEDGE, K. I. & MARSH, W. L. (1971). Auto-immune hemolytic anemia caused by anti-U. *Vox Sang.*, 20, 519–525.

O'DAY, T. (1987). A second example of autoanti-Jk3. *Transfusion*, 27, 442 (Letter).

OSKI, F. A. & ABELSON, N. M. (1965). Autoimmune hemolytic anemia in an infant. Report of a case treated unsuccessfully with thymectomy. *J. Pediat.*, 67, 752–758.

PATTEN, E., BECK, C. E., SCHOLL, C., STROOPE, R. A. & WUKASCH, C. (1977). Autoimmune hemolytic anemia with anti Jk^a specificity in a patient taking Aldomet. *Transfusion*, 17, 517–520.

PAVONE, B. G., BILLMAN, R., BRYANT, J., SNIECINSKI, I. & ISSITT, P. D. (1981). An auto-anti-En^a, inhibitable by MN sialoglycoprotein. *Transfusion*, 21, 25–31.

PELOQUIN, P., MOULDS, M., KEENAN, J. & KENNEDY, M. (1989). Anti-Sc3 as an apparent autoantibody in two patients. *Transfusion*, 29, Suppl. 49 S (Abstract S 173).

PETZ, L. D. & GARRATTY, G. (1980). *Acquired Immune Hemolytic Anemias*, 458 pp. Churchill Livingstone, New York.

PIROFSKY, B. (1969). *Autoimmunization and the Autoimmune Hemolytic Anemias*, 537 pp. Williams and Wilkins, Baltimore.

PIROFSKY, B. & PRATT, K. (1966). The antigen in autoimmune hemolytic anemia. I. Reactivity of human autoantibodies and rhesus antibodies with primate and non-primate erythrocytes. *Amer. J. clin. Path.*, 45, 75–81.

PUIG, N., CARBONELL, F. & MARTY, M. L. (1986). Another example of mimicking anti-Kp^b in a Kp(a+b−) patient. *Vox Sang.*, 51, 57–59.

RACE, R. R. & SANGER, R. (1954). *Blood Groups in Man*, p. 361. Blackwell Scientific Publications, Oxford.

RAND, B. P., OLSON, J. D., GARRATTY, G. & PETZ, L. D. (1978). Coombs' negative immune hemolytic anemia with anti-E occurring in the red blood cell eluate of an E-negative patient. *Transfusion*, 18, 174–180.

REID, M. E., VENGELEN-TYLER, V., SHULMAN, I. & REYNOLDS, M. V. (1988). Immunochemical specificity of autoanti-Gerbich from two patients with autoimmune haemolytic anaemia and concomitant alteration in the red cell membrane sialoglycoprotein β. *Brit. J. Haemat.*, 69, 61–66.

REYNOLDS, M. V., VENGELEN-TYLER, V. & MORE, P. A. (1981). Autoimmune hemolytic anemia associated with autoanti-Ge. *Vox Sang.*, 41, 61–67.

ROSENFIELD, R. E., ALLEN, F. H. JNR, SWISHER, S. N. & KOCKWA, S. (1962). A review of Rh serology and presentation of a new terminology. *Vox Sang.*, 2, 287–312.

ROSSE, W. F. (1990). *Clinical Immunohematology: Basic Concepts and Clinical Applications*, pp. 457–460. Blackwell Scientific Publications, Boston.

RUGGIERI, P. & PUGLISI, G. (1955). Ricerche sierologiche nell'anemia emolitica acquisita. *Boll. Soc. ital. Emat.*, 3, No. 2 6pp.

SACHER, R. A., McGINNIS, M. M., SHASHATY, G. G., JACOBSON, R. J. & RATH, C. E. (1982). The occurrence of an auto-immune hemolytic anemia with anti-U specificity. *Amer. J. clin. Path.*, 77, 356–359.

SALMON, CH. (1964). La spécifité des auto-anticorps d'anemie hémolytique acquise. *Rev. franç. Ét. clin. biol.*, 9, 532–540.

SALMON, C., GOUDEMAND, M. & HABIBI, B. (1984). Autoimmunity. In *Human Blood Groups* (ed. by C. Salmon, J.-P. Cartron and P. Rouger), pp. 376–385. Masson Publishing USA, Inc., New York.

SALMON, C., HOMBERG, J.-C. & HABIBI, B. (1975). Immunologie des anémies hémolytiques auto-immunes. (Deuxieme partie). *Rev. franç. Transf. Immuno-hémat.*, 18, 497–513.

SCHMIDT, P. J., LOSTUMBO, M. M., ENGLISH, C. T. & HUNTER, O. B. JNR (1967). Aberrant U blood group accompanying Rh$_{null}$. *Transfusion*, 7, 33–34.

SEYFRIED, H., GÓRSKA, B., MAJ, S., SYLWESTROWICZ, T., GILES, C. M. & GOLDSMITH, K. L. G. (1972). Apparent depression of antigens of the Kell blood group system associated with autoimmune acquired hemolytic anemia. *Vox Sang.*, 23, 528–536.

SHAPIRO, M. (1967). Familial autohemolytic anemia and runting syndrome with Rh$_0$-specific autoantibody. *Transfusion*, 7, 281–296.

SHULMAN, I. A., THOMPSON, J. C., NELSON, J. M., VENGELEN-TYLER, V. & BRANCH, D. R. (1985). Autoanti-Gerbich causing severe autoimmune hemolytic anemia. *Transfusion*, 25, 447 (Abstract S 9).

SHULMAN, I. A., VENGELEN-TYLER, V., THOMPSON, J. C., NELSON, J. M. & CHEN, D. C. T. (1990). Autoanti-Ge associated with severe autoimmune hemolytic anemia. *Vox Sang.*, **59**, 232–234.

SOKOL, R. J., HEWITT, S. & STAMPS, B. (1981). Autoimmune haemolysis: an 18-year study of 865 cases referred to a regional transfusion centre. *Brit. med. J.*, **282**, 2023–2027.

SPEISER, P. (1957). Ueber eine beobachtete temporäre Ausnahme von Ehrlichschen Regel des Horror autotoxicus bei idiopathischer hämolytischer Anämie. *Wien. klin. Wschr.*, **69**, 149–154.

SPIELMANN, W. (1956). Spezifische autoantikörper bei hämolytischen Anämien. *Klin. Wschr.*, **34**, 248–253.

STRATTON, F. & RENTON, P. H. (1958). *Practical Blood Grouping*, p. 245. Blackwell Scientific Publications, Oxford.

STRIKAS, R., SEIFERT, M. A. & LENTINO, J. R. (1983). Autoimmune hemolytic anemia and *Legionella pneumophila* pneumonia. *Ann. intern. Med.*, **99**, 345.

STURGEON, P. (1947). A new antibody in serum of patients with acquired hemolytic anemia. *Science*, **106**, 293–294.

SZALÓKY, A. & VAN DER HART, M. (1971). An auto-antibody anti-Vel. *Vox Sang.*, **20**, 376–377.

VAN LOGHEM, J. J. JNR, MENDES DE LEON, D. E. & VAN DER HART, M. (1957). Recherches serologiques dans les anémies hémolytiques acquises. Étude spéciale sur la spécificité des auto-anticorps. *Proc. Congr. franç. Med. 30° Session, Alger, 1955*, pp. 79–108. Masson, Paris.

VAN LOGHEM, J. J. & VAN DER HART, M. (1954a). Varieties of specific autoantibodies in acquired haemolytic anaemia. *Vox Sang.*, **4**, 2–11.

VAN LOGHEM, J. J. & VAN DER HART, M. (1954b) Varieties of specific autoantibodies in acquired haemolytic anaemia (II). *Vox Sang.*, **4**, 129–134.

VAN LOGHEM, J. J. JNR, VAN DER HART, M. & DORFMEIER, H. (1958). Serologic studies in acquired hemolytic anemia. *Proc. 6th int. Congr. int. Soc. Hemat. Boston, 1956*, pp. 858–868. Grune and Stratton, New York.

VAN 'T VEER, M. B., VAN LEEUWEN, I., HAAS, F. J. L. M., SMELT, M., OVERBECKE, M. A. M. & ENGELFRIET, C. P. (1984). Red-cell auto-antibodies mimicking anti-Fy^b specificity. *Vox Sang.*, **47**, 88–91.

VENGELEN-TYLER, V, & MOGCK, N. (1991). Two cases of 'hr^B-like' autoantibodies appearing as alloantibodies. *Transfusion*, **31**, 254–256.

VIGGIANO, E., CLARY, N. L. & BALLAS, S. K. (1982). Autoanti-K antibody mimicking an alloantibody. *Transfusion*, **22**, 329–332.

VOS, G. H., PETZ, L. & FUDENBERG, H. H. (1970). Specificity of acquired haemolytic anaemia autoantibodies and their serological characteristics. *Brit. J. Haemat.*, **19**, 57–66.

VOS, G. H., PETZ, L. D. & FUDENBERG, H. H. (1971). Specificity and immunoglobulin characteristics of autoantibodies in acquired hemolytic anemia. *J. Immunol.*, **106**, 1171–1176.

VOS, G. H., PETZ, L. D., GARRATTY, G. & FUDENBERG, H. H. (1973). Autoantibodies in acquired hemolytic anemia with special reference to the LW system. *Blood*, **42**, 445–453.

WAKUI, H., IMAI, H., KOBAYASHI, R., ITOH, H., NOTOYA, T., YOSHIDA, K., NAKAMOTO, Y. & MIURA, A. B. (1988). Autoantibody against erythrocyte protein 4.1 in a patient with autoimmune hemolytic anemia. *Blood*, **72**, 408–412.

WEBER, J., CACERES, V. W., PAVONE, B. G. & ISSITT, P. D. (1979). Allo-anti-C in a patient who had previously made an autoantibody mimicking anti-C. *Transfusion*, **19**, 216–218.

WEINER, W. (1958). Serological pattern in auto-immune haemolytic anaemia. Result of investigation of sera and eluates in 30 cases. *Proc. 7th Congr. Europ. Soc. Haemat., Copenhagen, 1957*, pp. 675–680. Karger, Basel.

WEINER, W. (1959). To be or not to be an antibody: the 'agent' in autoimmune hemolytic anemia. *Blood*, **14**, 1057–1062.

WEINER, W. (1960). Probleme der autoimmunhämolytischen Anämien. *Klin. Wschr.*, **38**, 885–893.

WEINER, W. (1965). Specificity of antibodies in acquired haemolytic anaemias. *Proc. 10th Congr. int. Soc. Blood Transf., Stockholm 1964*, pp. 24–29. Karger, Basel.

WEINER, W., BATTEY, D. A., CLEGHORN, T. E., MARSON, F. G. W. & MEYNELL, M. J. (1953). Serological findings in a case of haemolytic anaemia, with some general observations on the pathogenesis of this syndrome. *Brit. med. J.*, **ii**, 125–128.

WEINER, W., GORDON, E. G. & KIDD, P. (1962). Haemolytic anaemias with unusual serology. *Vox Sang.*, **7**, 313–328.

WEINER, W. & VOS, G. H. (1963). Serology of acquired hemolytic anemias. *Blood*, **22**, 606–613.

WEINER, W., WHITEHEAD, J. P. & WALKDEN, W. J. (1956). Acquired haemolytic anaemia. Clinical and serological observations of two cases. *Brit. med. J.*, **1**, 73–77.

WHITTINGHAM, S., JAKOBOWICZ, R. & SIMMONS, R. T. (1961). Multiple antibodies imitating the presence of a panagglutinin in the serum of a patient suffering from haemolytic anaemia. *Med. J. Aust.*, **i**, 205–207.

WIENER, A. S. (1945). Conglutination test for Rh sensitization. *J. Lab. clin. Med.*, **30**, 662–667.

WIENER, A. S. & GORDON, E. B. (1953). Quantitative test for antibody-globulin coating human blood cells and its practical applications. *Amer. J. clin. Path.*, **23**, 429–446.

WIENER, A. S., GORDON, E. B. & GALLOP, C. (1953). Studies on auto-antibodies in human sera. *J. Immunol.*, **71**, 58–65.

WIENER, A. S., GORDON, E. B. & RUSSOW, E. (1957). Observations on the nature of the auto-antibodies in a case of acquired hemolytic anemia. *Ann. intern. Med.*, **47**, 1–9.

WORLLEDGE, S. M. (1972). Communication to the 13th International Congress of the International Society of Blood Transfusion, Washington.

WORLLEDGE, S. M. (1982). Immune haemolytic anaemia (Revised by Hughes Jones, N. C. and Bain, B.). In *Blood and its Disorders*, 2nd edn (ed. by R. M. Hardisty and D. J. Weatherall), pp. 479–513. Blackwell Scientific Publications, Oxford.

WORLLEDGE, S. M. & BLAJCHMAN, M. A. (1972). The autoimmune haemolytic anaemias. *Brit. J. Haemat.*, **23**, Suppl., 61–69.

YOKOYAMA, M., EITH, D. T. & BOWMAN, M. (1967). The first example of autoanti-Xg^a. *Vox Sang.*, **12**, 138–139.

Auto-immune haemolytic anaemia (AIHA): warm-antibody syndromes VI: Coombs-negative (DAT-negative) haemolytic anaemia; positive direct antiglobulin tests in normal subjects and in hospital patients; polyagglutinability and haemolytic anaemia

Coombs-negative (DAT-negative) auto-immune haemolytic anaemia   183

Effect of erythrocyte age on the binding of auto-antibodies   187
  Experimental studies on the resistance of reticulocytes to immune haemolysis   189

Positive direct antiglobulin tests in healthy people   189
  Modification of the MN blood-groups as a cause of a positive direct antiglobulin test   193

Estimations of the number of Ig and complement molecules coating erythrocytes   193

Significance and nature of erythrocyte-bound IgG   194

Complement components bound to normal erythrocytes   195

Positive direct antiglobulin tests in hospital patients   197
  Role of hypergammaglobulinaemia   198

Polyagglutinability and haemolytic anaemia   201
  Polyagglutination associated with severe infection in man   201

COOMBS-NEGATIVE (DAT-NEGATIVE) AUTO-IMMUNE HAEMOLYTIC ANAEMIA

The occurrence of Coombs-negative AIHA in pregnancy has already been discussed (p. 22). Clinically and haematologically similar cases of acquired haemolytic anaemia in which the DAT is negative, initially or persistently, and in which normal erythrocytes survive badly after transfusion and corticosteroid therapy is beneficial, have, however, been observed from time to time in non-pregnant patients. They comprise probably 3–6% of all patients in whom an auto-immune origin for their haemolytic anaemia is certain or seems highly likely.

Worlledge and Blajchman (1972) reported that of 323 patients with idiopathic or secondary AIHA studied at the Royal Postgraduate Medical School in London ten (3.1%) had had a negative DAT. Later Worlledge (1978) reported that of 184 patients with AIHA investigated between August 1972 and July 1974 eleven (6%) had had a negative DAT: 173 had presented with the full clinical and serological picture (including a clearly positive DAT), five with a negative DAT but with other evidence of serological abnormality, and six

with a negative DAT and no evidence of other serological abnormality.

Chaplin (1973) in his review concluded that in 2–4% of AIHA patients the DAT is likely to be negative. Boccardi and co-workers (1978) reported, however, a higher percentage of negative tests. They reviewed the results of the DAT in 98 patients diagnosed as suffering from warm-antibody AIHA: the test had been negative in five out of 47 patients (10.6%) with idiopathic AIHA and in six out of 40 patients (15%) with secondary AIHA, the majority suffering from a lymphoma. The sera of nine of the 11 patients giving negative DATs agglutinated papainized erythrocytes to low titres at 37°C and the two sera that had failed to cause direct agglutination caused positive results in indirect antiglobulin tests. Three of the sera lysed the papainized cells at 37°C.

Leaving aside falsely negative DATs due to errors in technique or impotent antiglobulin sera, a negative DAT in a case of genuine AIHA seems to result from there being too few antibody molecules on the erythrocyte surfaces for detection by conventional antiglobulin sera used in the usual way and/or to the affinity of the antibody molecules for the corresponding antigens on the erythrocyte surfaces being low, with the result that many of the molecules elute from the cells while they are being washed in preparation for testing.

One factor leading to too few antibody molecules on the erythrocyte surface for detection by antiglobulin sera used in the usual way is the presence in erythrocyte suspensions of a high proportion of reticulocytes, which appear to bind on certain IgG auto-antibodies less avidly than do more mature cells (see later, p. 188).

Chaplin (1973) had suggested, too, that occasionally an apparently negative reaction results from the causal auto-antibody being composed solely of IgA which would not be detected if an anti-IgG antibody had been used as the antiglobulin reagent in the DAT.

That patients apparently suffering from clinically typical AIHA might give unexpectedly weak or initially or persistently negative antiglobulin reactions has been known since the 1950s.

de Gruchy (1954) had, for instance, reported that in three out of 20 patients the DAT did not become positive until the patient's illness had lasted 2–4 weeks, and Davidsohn and Spurrier (1954) reported that the DAT was negative in five out of 38 patients although auto-antibodies were detectable in their serum. Heni and Blessing (1954) reported a similar case and suggested that the affinity of the antibody for the erythrocytes was weak.

Evans (1955) reported an exceptionally interesting observation: this was that in one patient the DAT was positive only with an antiglobulin serum obtained from a rabbit immunized with the patient's own serum proteins. Evans and Weiser (1957) reported still further variations. Negative tests were observed in four out of 41 patients. Weak reactions were observed in two children, both severely ill, and the erythrocytes of two further patients underwent auto-agglutination when centrifuged in a 30% bovine serum albumin–human serum mixture although the DAT was negative. The cells of a further patient were agglutinated by the antiglobulin serum if centrifuged immediately; on standing, however, the agglutination gradually reversed. Normal cells sensitized in an eluate from the patient's erythrocytes behaved in exactly the same way. The patient's cells, too, auto-agglutinated in the bovine serum albumin–human serum mixture. Later, in a further clinical relapse, agglutination in an antiglobulin serum became more normal and did not reverse.

Another possibly unique observation was reported by Miescher and Holländer (1956) who demonstrated a positive antiglobulin test using the 'build-up' or 'lattice' technique of Coombs, Gleeson-White and Hall (1951).

Miescher and Holländer's patient had an illness of uncertain nature (characterized by monocytosis and splenomegaly).

Cases which fall into a special category are those in which the DAT is negative, yet there is clear evidence of antibody formation in as much as an abnormal antibody can be demonstrated in serum by the use of enzyme-treated, e.g. trypsinized, erythrocytes. Lemaire and co-workers (1954), Payne, Spaet and Aggeler (1955) and Baikie and Pirrie (1956), for instance, all reported patients who developed acute haemolytic episodes but whose erythrocytes gave consistently negative DATs. The sera, however, contained a definite panagglutinin active against trypsinized erythrocytes. In two of these patients clinical recovery was associated eventually with the disappearance of the panagglutinin [see also Dacie (1962, p. 390, Case 5)]. Dacie and de Gruchy (1951) had reported a rather similar case (their Case 9) in which the DAT, positive at the onset of an acute haemolytic episode, became negative when the patient went into remission. A powerful panagglutinin active against trypsinized cells was nevertheless demonstrable in the patient's serum for at least 10 years after the attack.

More recently, the mechanism of Coombs-negative AIHA has been studied in detail, and in a high proportion at least of cases it has been shown that the patients' erythrocytes, although coated with auto-antibodies, have too few antibody molecules on their surfaces for detection by antiglobulin sera used in the usual way.

Early information bearing on the relationship between the number of antibody molecules bound to the surface of erythrocytes and agglutination by antiglobulin sera was reported by Dupuy, Elliott and Masouredis (1964), who had experimented with D-positive erythrocytes and radio-labelled [131I]anti-D. The most potent antiglobulin serum tested was found to cause visible agglutination of cells that had bound as little as 1% of the anti-D that could be bound to maximally sensitized cells, and it was calculated that the minimum number of adsorbed anti-D molecules that could be detected was about 100 per cell.

Gilliland, Baxter and Evans (1971) described in an important contribution how they had shown, using a sensitive complement-fixing antibody-consumption test (Gilliland, Leddy and Vaughan, 1970), that seven out of eight AIHA patients who had given persistently negative antiglobulin tests had, nevertheless, abnormal amounts of IgG on their surfaces. Normal controls were calculated to have less than 35 molecules of IgG per erythrocyte on their surface. The seven patients had 70–734 molecules; the eighth patient, in whom mild haemolysis had persisted following splenectomy, had less then 35 molecules of IgG per cell.

That the abnormal amounts of IgG on the erythrocyte surfaces was antibody globulin and not IgG non-specifically adsorbed was shown by the fact that eluates from large volumes of the patients' erythrocytes were able to coat normal erythrocytes sufficiently for them to be agglutinated by an anti-IgG serum. It is interesting to note that Gilliland, Baxter and Evans reported that in two of their patients the DAT was reversible: i.e. the test was positive only if the cell-serum suspension was centrifuged immediately after mixing; incubation for several minutes before or after centrifugation prevented or reversed the agglutination.

Later, Gilliland (1976), in a review, referred to a further nine patients with negative DATs whose erythrocytes had been shown to be coated with higher than normal amounts of IgG, namely, 76–350 molecules per cell. He also reported that the evidence then available as to the sensitivity of the DAT, performed manually using reliable reagents, indicated that the test should be positive with 300–500 molecules of IgG per cell. Six of Gilliland's nine patients had responded favourably to corticosteroid therapy, and this had been associated with a decrease in the amount of erythrocyte IgG. Gilliland stressed that the two groups of AIHA patients — with or without a positive DAT — suffered from clinically similar syndromes and that their anaemia might be idiopathic or secondary and might, too, be associated (as in DAT-positive cases) with thrombocytopenia, SLE or chronic lymphocytic leukaemia.

Parker, Habeshaw and Cleland (1972) had described the history of a 22-year-old man who developed a rapid-onset relapsing haemolytic anaemia which responded to corticosteroids and eventually to splenectomy. The DAT was negative and no abnormal antibodies could be demonstrated in his serum. However, the serum was shown to give a strongly positive phagocytosis test using the patient's and normal erythrocytes and mouse peritoneal macrophages (Stuart and Cumming, 1967).

Rosse (1974), in his review, considered the detection of small amounts of antibody on the erythrocyte surface in AIHA. He referred to AIHA patients with negative DATs that he and his colleagues (Rosse, Ebbert and Dixon, 1973, unpublished observations) had investigated by means of a modified antiglobulin adsorption test. They had 50–450 molecules of IgG per erythrocyte surface, compared to normal subjects whose cells were coated with less than 50 molecules.

Idelson and co-workers (1976), reporting from Moscow, stated that they had demonstrated antibodies in a large number of cases of AIHA in which the DAT was negative. They had used an 'aggregate-haemagglutination' test that was considered to be many times more sensitive than the DAT.

Petz and Garratty (1980) in their book *Acquired Immune Hemolytic Anemias* devoted a substantial part of a chapter to AIHA associated with a negative direct DAT. Their own data obtained by means of a complement-fixing antibody consumption (CFAC) test indicated that the DAT would be negative (in the case of an antibody of anti-D specificity) if there were less than 25 molecules of IgG on the erythrocyte surface; the test would become progressively positive as the number of molecules per cell increased, with 500 or more molecules giving 3–4+ positive tests. They described their experience with 27 patients suffering from acquired haemolytic anaemia: 22 had idiopathic AIHA (one with thrombocytopenia also); five had an associated disease. The erythrocytes of all but one of the patients gave a negative reaction in the DAT using an anti-IgG serum; eleven gave weak positive reactions with a potent anti-C3d serum. Auto-antibodies were detected in the sera of 11 patients (usually reacting only with enzyme-treated cells) or in concentrated eluates. The CFAC test revealed more than 25 molecules of IgG per erythrocyte in all the patients: 100–300 molecules in fifteen, more than 400 in five and more than 1400 (despite a negative DAT!) in one patient.

Information with respect to response to therapy and CFAC tests was available in seven patients: in six patients who had responded well to steroid therapy or splenectomy the CFAC test then indicated less than 25 molecules in five patients and 228 molecules in one patient despite clinical improvement. In a patient who did not respond to treatment the CFAC test indicated 607 molecules per erythrocyte, compared with 180 molecules before steroid therapy and splenectomy. Five patients were studied who had AIHA with a negative DAT and less than 25 molecules of IgG per erythrocyte; in four the DAT indicated C3d on their cells, although no antibodies could be detected in their sera or in eluates. Petz and Garratty also gave details of four particularly interesting patients.

Case 9.1 was a male aged 49 who had had recurrent attacks of severe haemolytic anaemia (and sometimes reticulocytopenia, leucopenia and thrombocytopenia) over a 12-year period. When tested in 1975 the CFAC test indicated 1400 molecules of IgG per erythrocyte while the patient's serum contained an antibody that reacted with enzyme-treated cells. The DAT was negative, using an anti-IgG serum but moderately strongly positive with an anti-C3d serum. Splenectomy — the spleen weighed 1164 g — led to clinical cure and the CFAC test then revealed less than 25 molecules of IgG per erythrocyte.

Case 9.2 was a man aged 20 who gave a 7-day history of increased haemolysis. The DAT was negative using a range of antiglobulin sera. The patient's Rh genotype was *CDe/CDe* and his serum contained an anti-E antibody reactive in the IAT, as well as an antibody with no obvious specificity that agglutinated enzyme-treated erythrocytes. Remarkably, eluates from the patient's erythrocytes reacted strongly with E-positive erythrocytes (although the patient's cells were E-negative). The patient responded satisfactorily to prednisone and the CFAC test was negative (< 25 molecules IgG per cell) when the patient was in remission. [This patient was also described by Rand et al. (1978).]

Case 9.3 was a man aged 17 who had a severe haemolytic anaemia associated with haemoglobinuria. A cold agglutinin was present in his serum (titre 512 at 4°C) but its thermal range extended only up as far as 22°C. The DAT was negative with anti-IgG, -IgA, -IgM and -C sera. The CFAC test demonstrated more than 400 IgG molecules per erythrocyte. He responded partially to steroid therapy but remitted after splenectomy.

Case 9.4 was a patient who had a relapsing haemolytic anaemia associated with pregnancy. Her illness was described in detail by Yam et al. (1980) (see p. 23).

Yam, Petz and Spath (1982) described how they had used a radio-isotopic method to detect erythrocyte IgG present in amounts below the threshold for detection by the antiglobulin reaction. The test was based on the adsorption of ^{125}I-labelled staphylococcal protein A, a protein that has an affinity for the Fc receptor of human IgG. Nine patients with acquired haemolytic anaemia of various types were investigated using this method. All had negative DATs. Increased amounts of erythrocyte IgG were detected in three of the patients; of the other six patients, one had formed a warm IgM lysin, in two the clinical findings suggested a non-immunological cause for the haemolysis, while in three the haemolytic mechanism was unclear — one of these patients had, however, responded to corticosteroids and one had a haemolytic anaemia associated with pregnancy.

Garratty and co-workers (1982) reported on a study of 40 patients with acquired haemolytic anaemia for which an immune basis was suspected as the cause, despite the DAT done conventionally being negative and tests on the patients' sera unhelpful. Using an enzyme-linked antiglobulin test (ELAT), the erythrocytes of 12 of the 40 patients were found to react positively, indicating increased amounts of IgG on their surfaces. In remission, however, the ELAT was negative. The erythrocytes of 15 of the patients were also subjected to five different tests—ELAT, a manual Polybrene test, a direct bromelin test, testing eluates after concentration, and a monocyte/mononuclear assay. Seven samples reacted positively, five in the ELAT and Polybrene tests, three in the bromelin test and two in the eluate test. Garratty et al. concluded that the ELAT was a satisfactory and convenient replacement for the CFAC assay.

Recently, evidence has been produced that indicates that the expression of the erythrocyte antigens with which the warm auto-antibodies of AIHA react may be reduced in some patients and result in negative DATs, despite the presence of active auto-antibodies in their serum.

van't Veer and co-workers (1981) described the history of a male child, aged 13, who had suffered from an AIHA since he was 1 year old. In 1980 he underwent a severe crisis. The DAT, which had previously been positive with anti-IgG and anti-C sera, became negative despite strongly reactive Rh antibodies (anti-C and anti-e) in his serum. These antibodies were readily absorbed by CcDee normal cells, but not by the patient's own cells, despite his Rh phenotype being CcDEe. van't Veer et al. concluded that the antigens recognized by the auto-antibodies were not identical with those recognized by allo-antibodies of apparently the same specificity. They suggested that in their patient the expression of antigens might vary within the erythrocyte population, and that the reactive population had been destroyed in the haemolytic crisis the patient had just experienced. In favour of this explanation was that after splenectomy (from which he had derived great benefit) the DAT became strongly positive and his erythrocytes reacted strongly with the antibodies in his serum.

Issitt and his co-workers (1982) described another remarkable case in which expression of the erythrocyte Rh antigens of a 22-month-old infant suffering from severe AIHA appeared to be so severely depressed that the DAT was negative. At the height of the infant's illness the anti-Rh antibodies in his serum, which reacted with most normal blood samples, appeared to be allo-antibodies rather than auto-antibodies. The infant responded to treatment but relapsed 10 weeks later. This time, however, the DAT was strongly positive, and tests then indicated that the earlier marked depression of Rh antigen expression no longer existed. Later, Issitt, Wilkinson and Gruppo (1983) reported that the DAT on the child's erythrocytes had eventually become negative after being positive for 2 years. They were then able to carry out titrations for Rh antigen strength using several of the antibodies present in the child's serum at the onset of his illness: they established that the strength of the D, e, hr^S and hr^B antigens were the same as in phenotype matched controls, confirming that the depression of Rh antigen strength originally observed was transient and directly related to his original acute haemolytic episode.

Gallacher and co-workers (1983) applied a quantitative in-vitro assay of monocyte macrophage interaction with erythrocytes in the investigation of 11 patients thought to have a DAT-negative AIHA. Seven of these patients produced positive erythrocyte association and phagocytosis indices, as did all 16 patients who

had given positive DATs and had presented with clinical evidence of increased haemolysis. [It is interesting to note that the phagocytosis test was negative in six patients with DAT-positive AIHA in whom there was no clinical evidence of increased haemolysis at the time they were tested.]

Hansen and co-workers (1984) reported on the use of an enzyme-linked immunosorbent assay (ELISA), using the erythrocytes themselves as solid phase, as a means of determining the amount of IgG on erythrocytes. Sixteen patients with various types of AIHA were studied—only three had idiopathic AIHA: 15 of them had abnormally high amounts of IgG on the erythrocyte surface, although only eight—those with the highest amounts of IgG on the cells—gave positive DATs. Thirteen rheumatoid arthritis patients were also studied—all had given negative DATs: 10 had increased amounts of IgG on the erythrocyte surface, a finding suggesting the binding on of circulating immune complexes to C3 receptors.

Szymanski and co-workers (1984) described a 75-year-old women who was investigated during an episode of acute haemolysis. The DAT and IAT were negative. However, when her erythrocytes were tested in a PVP-augmented automated system using a variety of diluted antiglobulin sera the cells were found to be strongly sensitized with non-agglutinating IgM molecules. The bound antibodies, after elution, were identified as warm-reacting monomeric IgM: they migrated with IgG molecules in an agarose column and were proved to be IgM not IgG by a sensitive haemagglutination inhibition assay.

Vengelen-Tyler and co-workers (1985) described a 72-year-old man with haemolytic anaemia, whose DAT using anti-IgG, anti-IgA, anti-IgM and anti-C3 sera was negative. His serum, however, contained an anti-D antibody that agglutinated albumin-suspended as well as ficinated erythrocytes; it also gave a 4+ positive IAT using an anti-IgA serum but only a weak reaction with an anti-IgG serum. An eluate from the patient's apparently unreactive erythrocytes reacted similarly, i.e., D-positive cells exposed to the eluate were strongly agglutinated by an anti-IgA serum but were only very weakly agglutinated by an anti-IgG serum.

EFFECT OF ERYTHROCYTE AGE ON THE BINDING OF AUTO-ANTIBODIES

It has been recently realized that cell age is an

important determinant of the ability of erythrocytes to bind IgG auto-antibodies to the cell surface. This difference in binding ability provides a part explanation, at least, for unexpectedly weak or negative DATs in some cases of AIHA.

Gray and Masouredis (1981) and Gray, Kleeman and Masouredis (1983), using [^{125}I] IgG anti-D and erythrocytes separated by centrifugation into fractions, reported that allo-anti-D was bound more avidly to mature erythrocytes than to reticulocytes, which had about 60% of D reactivity compared with more mature cells. They proceeded to make eluates from eight patients with AIHA (probably associated with α–methyldopa therapy). Their reticulocytes were found to have bound about 70% of the IgG bound to mature erythrocytes, as determined by the use of [^{125}I] staphylococcal protein A, and they considered that this indicated that the auto-antigen component defined by the auto-antibodies was incompletely expressed in reticulocytes. [Staphylococcal protein A has potential receptor sites for the Fc fragment of animal and human IgG: it binds to all human IgG subclasses with the possible exception of IgG3, and it will bind some IgA and IgM (see Gray and Masouredis, 1982).] Direct testing of DAT-positive cells, separated by density fractionation, also demonstrated a reduced amount of IgG on reticulocytes in four out of five patients; in the fifth, however, there appeared to be no difference in the amount of IgG auto-antibody bound by reticulocytes or mature erythrocytes.

Wallas, Tanley and Gorrell (1982) used mixtures of phthalate esters to provide a range of specific gravities from 1.078 to 1.114. Characteristic patterns of density distribution curves were obtained when the blood of AIHA patients was centrifuged in microcapillary tubes loaded with the ester mixtures. A DAT carried out on the top (lightest, reticulocyte-rich) fractions was generally less strongly positive compared with that of the bottom (heaviest) fractions, or compared with that of uncentrifuged blood: in two out of 12 cases the DAT of the lightest cells was negative. A different type of density distribution curve was given by the blood of patients who had developed a positive DAT as part of a delayed transfusion reaction, and in these patients a DAT carried out on the top (lightest) fractions (rich in newly formed reticulocytes) was negative in 10 out of 12 cases.

Branch, Sy Siok Hian and Petz (1982) and Branch and co-workers (1984), using standard quantitative antiglobulin reaction techniques, showed that warm auto-antibodies could be separated into two distinct categories—those that reacted preferentially with mature erythrocytes (Type I) and those that had apparently no preference for young or older cells (Type II). Of 24 blood samples from patients or apparently healthy subjects whose erythrocytes gave positive DATs, 19 could be classified as having erythrocytes coated with Type-I antibodies and five with Type-II. Of particular interest is the fact that the DAT was negative, using reticulocyte-enriched fractions, in seven out of the 19 Type-I samples. It is interesting to note, too, that the five Type-II patients, all of whom had strongly positive DATs, were severely anaemic (mean Hb 6.4 ± 2.4 g/dl). In contrast, six of the 19 Type-I patients were not anaemic and 11 were only slightly to moderately anaemic (mean Hb 10.2 ± 2.9 g/dl). Branch et al. suggested that the two types of antibodies recognized different antigenic determinants. There were, too, indications that the two types of antibodies might have different specificities, with Type-I antibodies reacting possibly with 'a cryptantigen closely associated with the Rh peptide but not yet fully expressed on very young red cells'. Branch et al. added that although the Rh(D) antigen was thought to be weaker in reticulocytes (see above), this did not in their experience interfere with the recognition of allo-antibody anti-D by means of the IAT. They hypothesized that the 'type I warm auto antibody may represent augmented production of the physiologic auto antibody reported to be responsible for the normal immune-mediated clearance of senescent red cells'.

[The possibility that the hypothetical physiological auto-antibody responsible for removing senescent erythrocytes from the circulation is an anti-galactosyl (anti-Gal) IgG was advanced by Galili et al. (1986). They reported that they had been able to demonstrate anti-Gal antibodies in every one of 400 normal human sera, and went on to suggest that the antibody reacted with cryptic α-galactosyl residues that become exposed normally as erythrocytes age. Earlier work in this field is referred to in Part 1 (p. 23) and Part 2 (p. 225.) of this book.]

Herron, Clark and Smith (1987) described serial observations on a patient who had AIHA associated with rheumatoid arthritis. The DAT was negative when she was actively haemolysing. Her Rh genotype was *rr* and an IgM anti-e was identified in her serum. This antibody agglutinated normal *rr* cells at 37°C in saline suspension. The patient's cells, in contrast, were only weakly agglutinated (at a time when her reticulocyte count was high). However, after she had responded favourably to prednisone (when her reticulocyte count was low) her cells were strongly agglutinated by serum samples taken when she was actively haemolysing. It was found, too, in experiments with density-fractionated normal *rr* cells, that suspensions of young cells were only weakly agglutinated by the serum (to the same extent as were the patient's cells when she was actively haemolysing); only suspensions of older cells of density greater than 1.09 were strongly agglutinated.

Magnani and co-workers (1988) reported data on erythrocyte-bound IgG as determined by flow cytometry, using an FITC-labelled affinity-purified antibody to human IgG. Normal human blood was separated into seven fractions by discontinuous Percoll density gradient centrifugation. The percentage of erythrocytes showing fluorescent intensity greater than background was found to increase progressively from the first (lightest and youngest) to the last (heaviest and oldest) fractions.

Experimental studies on the resistance of reticulocytes to immune haemolyisis

The observations quoted in the previous section concerning the effect of cell age on the sensitivity of human erythrocytes to immune haemolysis have their counterpart in earlier studies on the blood of laboratory animals.

Cruz and Junqueira (1952), in in-vitro experiments on the ability of immune sera to bring about the lysis of dog erythrocytes, compared the sensitivity of the cells of normal dogs with that of the cells of dogs previously treated with acetylphenylhydrazine so as to produce a high percentage of reticulocytes. In the latter group, 2–4 times as much immune serum was required to produce a similar amount of lysis. They also found that if an amount of immune serum was added to blood so as to bring about only partial lysis, the reticulocyte count in the unlysed residue of cells was considerably higher than that in the untreated blood.

Rice and Mathies (1960) compared the relative resistance to lysis by immune sera of the erythrocytes of the dog, guinea-pig, man and the rabbit. The reticulocytes and mature erythrocytes of the guinea-pig seemed to be approximately equally sensitive, the reticulocytes of the dog were found to be resistant to lysis by either concentrated or dilute immune sera, and in man and in the rabbit reticulocytes were relatively resistant to lysis only when the cells were exposed to concentrated immune sera.

POSITIVE DIRECT ANTIGLOBULIN TESTS IN HEALTHY PEOPLE

The antithesis of AIHA in the absence of a positive DAT is the occurrence of a positive DAT in the absence of any other evidence suggesting increased haemolysis caused by auto-immunization. The phenomenon is rare in strictly healthy people, but well documented; such positive reactions, on the other hand, are more frequent in hospital patients. Before, however, considering what is known of the occurrence and nature and mechanism of positive tests associated with auto-immunization in the apparent absence of increased haemolysis, the various causes of so-called 'false-positive reactions' will be briefly considered. Worlledge (1978) listed five possible causes:

1. Insufficiently absorbed antiglobulin sera containing in consequence anti-erythocyte antibodies;

2. Anti-T present in rabbit antiglobulin sera;

3. Antibodies against κ and λ light chains in antiglobulin sera;

4. Anti-transferrin in antiglobulin sera causing agglutination of reticulocytes;

5. Anti-albumin antibodies in antiglobulin sera.

She listed some references bearing on these possibilities, but concluded that they were unlikely in practice to have been a frequent cause of unexpectedly positive reactions.

An important reason for a genuinely positive antiglobulin test, not, however, associated with auto-immunization, is allo-immunization, as, for instance, in haemolytic disease of the new-born (HDN) and following the transfusion of incompatible blood or the administration of blood products containing antibodies active against a patient's erythrocyte antigens. These important causes of positive antiglobulin reactions will be considered in detail in Volume 4 of this book.

That the DAT might be positive in people who were apparently healthy has in fact been known since the late 1940s. Thus the author, referring to the interpretation of a direct antiglobulin test, wrote in the first edition of this book (Dacie, 1954, pp. 29–30):

'It cannot be assumed, for instance, that a positive direct antiglobulin test necessarily indicates that the patient is suffering from auto-immune haemolytic anaemia. Excluding false-positive tests due to the use of inadequately absorbed antiglobulin sera, positive tests may occasionally be given by the blood of patients suffering from a variety of diseases or even by that of a normal subject.'

'One type of positive reaction is due to sensitization occurring *in vitro*. If, for instance, clotted or defibrinated normal blood is allowed to stand in a refrigerator at 0° to 2°C. and the antiglobulin test subsequently carried out on corpuscles obtained from the chilled blood, the reaction may be positive due to adsorption of incomplete cold antibodies normally present in human sera (Dacie, 1950). Corpuscles obtained from chilled oxalated or heparinized blood are less likely to give this type of positive reaction as the presence of anticoagulants inhibits adsorption of the antibody. Sensitization by cold antibodies is not, however, the only cause of unexpected positive antiglobulin reactions. In some instances, the reaction will be found to be positive even if the possibility of chilling *in vitro* has been excluded by collecting the patient's blood directly into saline warmed at 37°C. The cause of this type of 'non-specific' reaction has not as yet been determined. It must be a very rare event with blood from a strictly healthy person; it is not, however, uncommon in diseases such as rheumatoid arthritis, disseminated lupus erythematosus, leukaemia, myelosclerosis, sarcoid, and aplastic anaemia, conditions in which abnormal amounts of globulins are often found in the serum. Nevertheless, it does not seem to be possible to correlate the incidence of positive reactions with the presence of abnormal amounts of any particular type of globulin. In particular, the reaction is usually negative in cases of hepatic cirrhosis and multiple myeloma despite great increases in gamma globulins.

'The "non-specific" reactions referred to in the preceding paragraph are usually weak ones; they are maximal in high concentrations of a potent antiglobulin serum. The reactions are relatively insensitive to the addition to the antiglobulin serum of small amounts of human γ globulin, a feature which distinguishes them from the reactions of most of the 'warm' antibodies found in cases of auto-immune acquired haemolytic anaemia.'

Dacie (1960, p. 49) had added: 'In connection with positive reactions given by normal cells it should be pointed out that slowly developing weak agglutination, occurring, as a rule, in well-diluted antiglobulin serum, is not uncommon. With suspensions on an opalescent tile this is not as a rule evident to the naked eye under at least 7 minutes, and for practical purposes is usually ignored. However, the agglutination is probably real and appears to represent an interaction between globulin (of uncertain nature), normally adsorbed to the erythrocyte surface, and the antiglobulin serum.'

In support of the contention that erythrocytes normally adsorb γ globulin and that this may be sufficient to give rise to positive antiglobulin reactions, some interesting observations of Boursnell, Coombs and Rizk (1953) and Stratton and Richardson Jones (1955) were cited.

Boursnell, Coombs and Rizk (1953), using antibodies tagged with ^{131}I, had shown that the amount of iodine non-specifically adsorbed might exceed that adsorbed as the result of the specific combination of Rh-positive cells and anti-D antibody, although the latter reaction alone gave a strongly positive antiglobulin test. Stratton and Richardson Jones (1955) showed that diluted antiglobulin serum would agglutinate normal erythrocytes in a capillary tube inclined at an angle of 45°, and that the agglutination could be abolished by either first absorbing the diluted serum with a large volume of normal cells or by adding γ globulin to it. They concluded that a globulin-like antigen is normally present on the surface of normal erythrocytes.

Positive DATs in blood donors

Studies of blood donors have provided interesting information on the frequency of positive DATs in apparently perfectly healthy people.

Mollison (1956) referred briefly to a blood donor whose erythrocytes gave a positive DAT of the γ type; their life-span estimated with ^{51}Cr was normal.

Darnborough (1958), in an early report, had described an interesting study on a regular male blood donor whose 25th donation was found to be unexpectedly incompatible. The DAT was positive; zoning was evident and the reaction was of the γ-globulin type. The patient's Rh genotype was *cde/cde* and anti-c was eluted from his erythrocytes. Despite these findings he was not anaemic and the reticulocyte count was less than 1%. A reduction in the serum haptoglobulins to 50% of normal suggested, however, the possibility of minimally increased haemolysis.

Stratton and Tovey (1959), commenting on Darnborough's report, stated that they had studied eight apparently healthy blood donors who had given positive DATs: two, however, had had virus pneumonia and one subsequently developed rheumatoid arthritis; the others had remained in good health.

Weiner (1965) stated that 21 blood donors, 17 males and four females, who had attended two Blood Transfusion Centres over a 6-year period, had given a positive DAT when their erythrocytes had been tested with a routine anti-human globulin serum containing predominantly anti-7S antibodies. The tests had remained positive in individual donors for periods of between 1 month and at least 3 years; they tended to become less strong as time passed and in the majority of donors eventually became negative. Eluted antibodies appeared to be 7S gammaglobulins, and their specificity within the Rh system was indistinguishable from that of antibodies of AIHA patients suffering from increased haemolysis. Weiner calculated that the incidence of positive DATs in the normal healthy population was probably between one and three per 10 000 people.

Speiser (1967) described positive DATs in three blood donors, in one of whom the test had been positive for 2 years.

Hennemann (1967, 1968), described in detail the history of a blood donor, aged 50, who had in the past given at least 70 donations. The DAT was strongly positive and of the γ type. The donor's haemoglobin was 15.8 g/dl, reticulocyte count 0.8%, and serum bilirubin 1 mg/dl. There was no clinical evidence of haemolysis and the ^{51}Cr T_{50} was 22 days (just subnormal). The patient was not taking any drugs. In discussion, Hennemann emphasized that unexplained

positive DATs in apparently healthy people sometimes become negative spontaneously but that this might take several years.

Schneider (1969) screened 200 000 apparently healthy blood donors and found abnormal auto-antibody reactions in 229 of them. Further investigation showed that 164 were suffering from some underlying disorder: chronic liver disease was the most frequent, infections were next frequent, and there were 19 donors who were being treated with α-methyldopa. Six patients had haemolytic anaemia.

Issitt and co-workers (1976) reported on the specificity of the auto-antibodies in 30 haematologically normal blood donors in whom the DAT had been positive. In 23 of them the antibody was classified as anti-dl (see p. 163): the antibody in two of the 23 was further identified as anti-Wr^b and six contained anti-Wr^b alongside other components. These findings in respect of specificity were similar to those of a larger series of AIHA patients.

Saleun and Baret (1977) gave details of seven apparently healthy blood donors who had given positive DATs and had been followed up for up to 6 months. The DAT had been positive with a polyspecific antiglobulin serum in all seven, with anti-IgG in six and with anti-C in six: it was negative in each case with an anti-IgM serum. Antibodies weakly reacting with enzyme-treated erythrocytes were demonstrated to be present in six sera. The donors appeared to be clinically and haematologically normal; their serum globulins and serum complement levels (C3 and C4), where tested, were normal, too. Tests for virus infections were negative also. Saleun and Baret estimated on the basis of their own experience that the frequency of positive DATs in blood donors was about 1 in 2000.

Worlledge (1978) reported an incidence of positive DATs in blood donors of approximately 1 in 9000. She gave details of the positive tests in seven donors: in three the reaction was positive with an anti-IgG serum, in two with an anti-complement (anti-C) serum and in two with both anti-IgG and anti-C sera.

Gorst and co-workers (1980), reporting from the Manchester Centre of the National Blood Transfusion Service, stated that they had come across 65 normal blood donors (41 male, 24 female) since 1964 whose erythrocytes had been found to give a positive DAT. Fifty-nine samples had been tested with anti-complement (C) serum as well as with anti-IgG sera: 23 were agglutinated by an anti-IgG serum, 28 had been agglutinated by anti-C sera and eight by both anti-IgG and anti-C sera. Thirty-two of the donors giving positive reactions had been recalled for further study: none presented any abnormal clinical findings and all were fit and well and their health fulfilled the criteria necessary for blood donation. All the donors except one (see below) remained healthy subsequently (for up to 18 years): the exception was a donor who, after having a positive DAT for 2 years, subsequently developed typical AIHA necessitating splenectomy for its control.

Gorst et al. estimated that the incidence of positive DATs in normal blood donors was approximately 1 in 14 000, and it is especially interesting to note that their data indicated an increasing liklihood of a positive reaction with increasing age. This point received support from the results of a collateral investigation on a small number of very old people—aged 90–105, one male, 14 females: the erythrocytes of eight of them gave positive reactions with anti-C sera.

Habibi and co-workers (1980), reporting from the Centre National de Transfusion Sanguine in Paris, stated that anti-erythrocyte auto-antibodies had been detected in 69 out of 892 000 blood donors aged between 20 and 60, an incidence of about 1 in 13 000. The donors had been followed up for up to 5 years. The antibodies were identified as IgG in 97% of the cases and various anti-tissue antibodies were also present in 41%. Twenty-five per cent of the donors had been receiving α-methyldopa; 10% were slightly anaemic, but in 72% there was subclinical evidence of an increase in erythrocyte destruction, e.g. a raised reticulocyte count and/or elevated serum bilirubin, and shortening of the erythrocyte life-span. The specificity of the auto-antibodies was established in 38 cases: it was anti-pdl in 34%, anti-nl in 30%, anti-dl in 26% and anti-D or anti-e in 10%.

In a later paper from Manchester, Stratton and his co-workers (1983) determined the subtypes of IgG on the erythrocytes of 22 normal blood donors giving positive DATs; they also estimated, using [^{125}I] anti-IgG sera, the number of molecules of IgG coating the cells and related the results to those obtained with the erythrocytes of four patients with clinically overt AIHA. Twenty of the normal donors had IgG1 on their erythrocytes and two IgG4, and the number of IgG molecules per cell was found to range from 110 (the DAT being positive but weak) to 950 (the DAT being strongly positive). Four patients with overt AIHA had from 2700 to 6000 molecules per cell, and the patient who had been a blood donor for 2 years and had had a positive DAT and who subsequently developed overt AIHA had 2000 IgG molecules on her erythrocytes at the time she was haemolysing. (One hundred and ten blood donors in whom the DAT was negative had 5–90 molecules of IgG per erythrocyte.)

The sera of the 22 normal donors giving positive DATs were investigated for the presence of auto-antibodies: nothing abnormal was found in 13 sera; weak non-specific reactions were given by four sera; weak cold auto-agglutinins were present in two sera and a weak auto-anti-D was identified in one serum. Stratton et al. concluded that the donors giving positive reactions with anti-IgG sera, but who remained in good health, had formed only low concentrations of circulating auto-antibodies and that their erythrocytes were in consequence coated with too few IgG molecules for there to be significant sequestration of the coated cells.

Bareford and co-workers (1985) reported further data on the incidence of positive DATs in healthy blood donors. Sixty-seven positive tests were encountered at the Yorkshire Regional Blood Transfusion Centre between 1962 and 1982, the donor population being about 500 000, i.e. an incidence of approximately 1 in 7500. During 1983, 26 of the donors, who had previously given positive reactions, were re-tested. The DAT was still positive in nine of them: of these, one had developed overt AIHA, one had had ulcerative colitis and one other mild arthritis. The test had become negative in 17, although in seven of them auto-antibodies could be detected in their serum by an enzyme technique employing papain. As in the donors described by Gorst et al. (1980), the incidence of a positive DAT increased with the age of the donor; but in contrast to the data of Gorst et al., IgG alone was detected on the donor's erythrocytes in the majority of cases; e.g., between 1977 and 1982 22 donors were found to have IgG alone on their cells, six IgG plus complement and two complement alone.

The interesting reports of Gorst et al. (1980), Stratton et al. (1983) and Bareford et al. (1985) certainly suggest that the finding of a positive DAT, using an anti-IgG serum, in an apparently healthy person is usually of little clinical significance and that overt AIHA, although it may develop, seldom does.

Positive DATs have occasionally been reported when the erythrocytes from normal blood donors have been deglycerolized after being stored frozen and then tested.

Moore, Dorner and Chaplin (1974) reported four such instances. When fresh samples of the donors' blood were obtained, the erythrocytes of one donor gave a strongly positive DAT and the sera of the other three were found to contain cold agglutinins. Subsequent screening of 109 random samples of frozen blood revealed six positive DATs (5.8%) when the erythrocytes were deglycerolized.

Reid, Ellisor and Avoy (1979) confirmed the important role of cold agglutinins (at relatively low titres) in causing the DAT to be positive by finding that if the donor's serum contained cold agglutinins at a titre of 16 or higher at 4°C, or if the serum caused agglutination at room temperature (22°C), the DAT was likely to be positive provided that the antiglobulin serum contained anti-C4. They demonstrated, too, that complement was being bound during the glycerolization procedure at room temperature and that its binding could be blocked by EDTA.

Modification of the MN blood-groups as a cause of a positive direct antiglobulin test

A rare and interesting cause of a positive DAT is genetic modification of the MN blood-groups. First, Jakobowicz, Bryce and Simmons (1949) described in Australia the co-existence of a positive DAT and a blood-group M variant in a mother and her child, neither of whom showed any signs of increased haemolysis. Later, Jensen and Freisleben (1962) in Denmark, and Jeannet, Metaxas-Bühler and Tobler (1963, 1964) in Switzerland described families in whom the DAT was positive and there was evidence for the presence of a modified (weakened) group-N antigen in the affected individuals. In none of them, however, were there any signs of increased haemolysis. It seemed as if the positively reacting erythrocytes were being agglutinated by n γ_{1M} (IgM) antibody. Presumably, modification to the MN antigen complex was facilitating adsorption of a naturally-occurring IgM 'auto-antibody'.

ESTIMATIONS OF THE NUMBER OF Ig AND COMPLEMENT MOLECULES COATING ERYTHROCYTES

In recent years it has become possible to determine with increasing accuracy the average number of Ig and complement molecules coating erythrocytes, and the results of this approach have been discussed earlier in relation to cases of DAT-negative AIHA (p. 185). The techniques have been applied, too, to clinically normal individuals, whose erythrocytes have given positive DATs and also to strictly normal individuals in whom the DAT is negative. These studies have shown not only that molecules of IgG and of complement components can be demonstrated bound to the erythrocytes of strictly normal individuals but also that the number of molecules bound increases progressively from small numbers in strictly normal individuals, to larger numbers in clinically normal individuals giving a positive DAT and to the largest numbers in patients with overt AIHA.

Freedman (1984) showed, using radiolabelled antiglobulin sera, that old (dense) erythrocytes separated from young (light) erythrocytes by centrifugation were coated with significantly more IgG, IgM and IgA than the young cells. The amount of bound C3d was also higher on old cells, and was shown to increase in erythrocytes stored at 4°C in plasma to which citrate-phosphate-dextrose had been added as anticoagulant.

Jeje and co-workers (1984) described how they had used an immunoradiometric technique to measure the amount of IgG on the erythrocytes of 20 healthy controls and 19 anaemic patients with AIHA. The IgG per 10^3 cells of the controls ranged from 3.7 to 16.0 fg (mean 7.23 fg) and that of the AIHA patients ranged from 7 to 1000 fg (mean 176 fg). Converting the results to molecules per cell gave a mean figure of 31 molecules in the controls and 760 molecules in the patients. There appeared to be no correlation between erythrocyte IgG and the haemoglobin level or reticulocyte count in the patients.

Merry and co-workers (1984) reported further data on the correlation between the number of IgG molecules bound to erythrocytes and the strength of the antiglobulin reaction. They used a radiolabelled anti-IgG serum and cells sensitized with a variety of allo-antibodies and also tested 234 blood samples that had been referred for study on account of the DAT being positive. The close correlation between agglutination strength and the number of bound IgG molecules is illustrated in Fig. 27.1. With 100–120 IgG molecules per cell, antiglobulin tests (using a spin technique) were negative; with over 1000 molecules agglutination was complete (5+). In 16 patients diagnosed as having DAT-negative AIHA the highest number of molecules was 260, the lowest 10; in 11 of these cases there were less than 100.

Nance and Garratty (1984, 1987) measured erythrocyte-bound IgG by flow cytofluorometry, using fluorescein-conjugated goat anti-human immunoglobulin. In a study of 50 patients and normal blood donors, all giving positive DATs, they confirmed that flow cytometry was far superior to a semi-quantitative antiglobulin test in assessing the amount of IgG bound to erythrocytes and that AIHA patients with overtly increased haemolysis had higher mean levels of IgG than AIHA patients not suffering from increased haemolysis. There was, too, despite considerable overlap between the groups, a progression in mean fluorescence from normal donors to patients taking α-methyldopa, to patients with AIHA without overt haemolysis, to babies with haemolytic disease of the newborn, and finally to patients with AIHA and overt haemolysis.

Schreiber (1985) reviewed the recent developments that have taken place in the quantitative measurement of erythrocyte-bound Ig and complement components. He concluded that while the newer assays have in common greater sensitivity and provide better information than the semi-quantitative data that can be obtained by the use of well-characterized monospecific antiglobulin sera, the tests generally fail to define precisely the number of Ig or complement molecules on the cell surface.

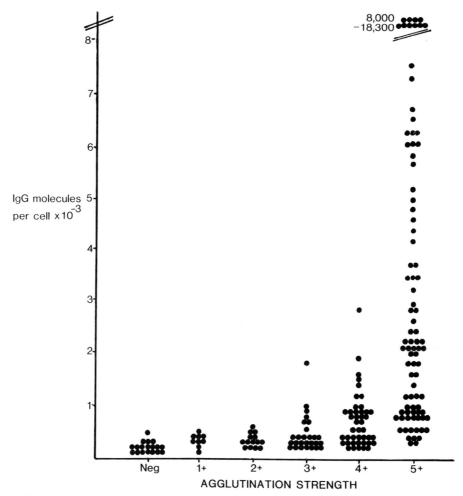

Fig. 27.1   Correlation between the strength of the DAT given by 234 blood samples referred to a transfusion centre and the estimated number of IgG molecules per erythrocyte.

[Reproduced by permission from Merry et al. (1984).]

SIGNIFICANCE AND NATURE OF ERYTHROCYTE-BOUND IgG

That IgG molecules can normally be shown to be present on the erythrocytes in health is a fact, as the reports summarized in the preceding pages substantiate. What is less certain is the nature of the globulin adsorbed and whether it plays an important, or indeed any, role in curtailing the life-span of erythrocytes in health.

According to Garratty (1987, 1988), in recent reviews, probably less than 50 IgG molecules are present per erythrocyte in health. The number

varies considerably between individuals — although it is relatively constant in any particular person. In a small minority of apparently healthy people 100 or more molecules are present: if so, the direct DAT is likely to be positive.

[The number of IgG (and C3) molecules estimated to be present in health has varied considerably in different reports. The discrepancies are likely to reflect differences and difficulties in technique rather than differences in the populations studied.]

Key questions are whether the IgG molecules bound to the erythrocyte surface in health are the same in nature and origin as the auto-antibody molecules responsible for AIHA and whether the only difference is that in health too few molecules are present to be of any significance in relation to the cells' life-span. Garratty (1987, 1988) concluded that two kinds of IgG are probably present normally: auto-antibody IgG, present particularly on older cells, and non-auto-antibody IgG (cytophilic antibody) present in amounts reflecting the concentration of IgG in the plasma (see also p. 198).

Another possibility is that some of the IgG coating the erythrocytes of DAT-positive individuals is IgG cross-reacting with IgG auto-antibody, i.e. anti-antibody. Masouredis, Branks and Victoria (1987) reported interesting data indicating that this is in fact sometimes the case. Eluates were prepared from the erythrocytes of 24 apparently healthy DAT-positive blood donors. Eight of the eluates, as well as containing IgG auto-antibodies, agglutinated three out of 10 samples of normal erythrocytes sensitized with anti-Rh(D) — a reaction which could be specifically inhibited by pre-incubating the antibody-containing eluates with anti-Rh(D). Masouredis, Branks and Victoria suggested that the Ig idiotype-anti-idiotype reaction that they had demonstrated might play a role in mitigating the effects of erythrocyte sensitization with IgG auto-antibodies and could help to explain the absence of haemolysis in some DAT-positive normal individuals.

[The role of erythrocyte-bound IgG in physiological erythrocyte destruction was considered briefly earlier in this book (Vol. 1, p. 23).]

COMPLEMENT COMPONENTS BOUND TO NORMAL ERYTHROCYTES

Rosenfield and Jagathambal (1978) subjected the well-washed erythrocytes of several hundred normal persons to possible agglutination in PVP-augmented automated antiglobulin tests. Without exception, all the samples were agglutinated by anti-C3, anti-C3d and anti-C4 sera. There were, however, marked differencies in agglutinability between individuals. Their cells were not agglutinated by anti-C3c sera, and this led Rosenfield

and Jagathambal to conclude that the C3 antigen detectable on normal erythrocytes is carried on the C3d fragment.

Hsu, Steinberg and Sawitsky (1979) reported similarly, i.e., they found that using an Auto-Analyser the erythrocytes of normal individuals were agglutinated by an anti-C3d serum but not by an anti-C3c serum. Treating the test samples with trypsin markedly reduced or abolished the agglutination by the anti-C3d serum. However, erythrocytes coated with C3d *in vivo* as in CHAD, or *in vitro* by exposure to serum in a low-ionic-strength medium, were found to be resistant to treatment with trypsin.

Chaplin, Nasongkla and Monroe (1980, 1981) used radiolabelled anti-C3d to measure quantitatively the number of C3d molecules bound to the erythrocytes of 174 normal blood donors. A wide range was found, i.e. 50–160 molecules in 98% of the donors—and there appeared to be no correlation with age or sex. The levels in individual donors appeared to be stable. Bound C3d was also estimated in 313 randomly selected hospital patients: 33% had values above the normal range and 8% had levels likely to be detected by a DAT using an anti-C3d serum. The great majority of the patients whose values were higher than normal were suffering from disorders ordinarily considered to be auto-immune in origin. Two patients had idiopathic AIHA: one (warm-antibody) patient had 3000 C3d molecules per erythrocyte, the other (cold-antibody) patient had 19 600.

Freedman and Barefoot (1982) also studied erythrocyte-bound C3d using a radiolabelled anti-antiglobulin technique. Like Chaplin, Nasongkla and Monroe (1981), they found that the amount bound normally was not related to age or sex and that it remained essentially unchanged in individuals. Cord-blood cells, however, carried less C3d than did cells from adults. Freedman and Barefoot's data are summarized in Fig. 27.2 in the form of frequency distribution curves. Thirty-nine per cent of 203 randomly selected hospital patients had C3d values above the normal range, the distribution curve being bimodal.

Chaplin, Coleman and Monroe (1983) described how they had used their radiolabelled technique to

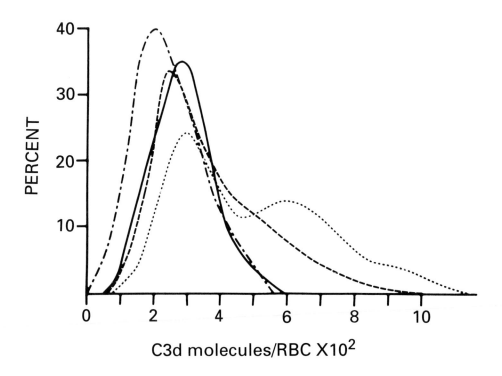

Fig. 27.2 **Frequency distribution of number of C3d molecules bound to erythrocytes obtained from several sources: staff (———), blood donors (-----), cord blood (-.-.-.-.), and hospital patients (excluding those with AIHA) (.......).**

[Reproduced by permission from Freedman and Barefoot (1982).]

study the in-vivo stability of C3d and C4d bound to erythrocytes. They infused three normal volunteers with their own erythrocytes which had been strongly coated *in vitro* with C3d and C4d and measured the concentration of the components on erythrocytes withdrawn from the circulation at intervals up to 21–34 days post-infusion. Immediate and long-term in-vivo survival of the infused erythrocytes was found not to be impaired by the complement coating. Of the bound C3d, 85–95% disappeared from the circulating erythrocytes within 5–8 days, the remainder more slowly. In contrast, C4d disappeared slowly, in two of the three subjects exponentially with half-times of 12–31 days.

Merry and co-workers (1983) used a monoclonal radiolabelled antiglobulin serum directed against a C3d determinant. With this serum they calculated that the mean number of C3 molecules bound to normal erythrocytes was 420 ± 140. Using cells sensitized with complement-fixing anti-Lewis or anti-Kell antibodies, agglutination by an anti-C3d serum increased from no agglutination to a $5+$ result as the number of C3 molecules that had been bound increased from 400 to 1250. A blood donor who had given a positive DAT had 4800 C3 molecules per cell while three patients with CHAD, who were actively haemolysing, had 15 000–52 020 molecules. Merry et al. reviewed earlier work and also discussed how many C3 molecules have to be bound so as to lead to increased haemolysis. While this was uncertain on the basis of the then available evidence, they concluded that many more molecules would be needed than are required to give rise to strongly positive antiglobulin tests.

POSITIVE DIRECT ANTIGLOBULIN TESTS (DATs) IN HOSPITAL PATIENTS

Although positive DAT tests are rarely met with in strictly healthy people, e.g. in blood donors, positive tests are quite frequent if the population tested comprises hospitalized patients tested at random. In the great majority of such cases the positive test will be found to be due to the presence of complement adsorbed to the erythrocyte surfaces, and there are good reasons to believe that in some instances at least the reaction is between adsorbed immune complexes and anti-complement components in antiglobulin sera.

Dacie and Worlledge (1969) and Worlledge (1978) reported that the erythrocytes from 40 out of 489 blood samples submitted for routine tests had been weakly agglutinated by anti-C sera, i.e. 8.2%; one sample only had been agglutinated by an anti-IgG serum and the patient from which this sample had been derived had been taking α-methyldopa.

Fischer and co-workers (1974), reporting on quantitative assays of erythrocyte-bound C3, stated that the antiglobulin tests with an anti-C3 serum became positive with 60–115 C3 molecules per cell and were strongly positive if there were as many as 1000 molecules per cell, and that the results correlated well with antiglobulin titres and scores. They had studied 25 patients suffering from a variety of disorders all of whose erythrocytes had been agglutinated by anti-C3 sera. Eight of 11 patients who had more than 1100 molecules of C3 per cell had overt haemolytic anaemia, compared with only two out of 14 patients whose erythrocytes had been coated with less than 1100 molecules. The presence or absence of haemolysis seemed, in the patients they studied, not to be correlated with the amount of IgG on the cells, and Fischer et. al. concluded that the amount of C3 bound had been an important determinant of haemolysis. The highest values for bound C3 (1910–7500 molecules per cell) had been found in three patients suffering from cold haemagglutinin disease (CHAD).

The data of Lau, Haesler and Wurzel (1976) had been based on the sole use of an anti-IgG antiglobulin serum. As expected, the tests were seldom positive. However, of 4664 erythrocyte samples derived from medical and surgical patients when first admitted to hospital (2225 male; 2439 female), 41 (0.9%) were agglutinated (+ to 4+ reactions). The patients from which the positively reacting samples had been obtained could be grouped into four categories — 13 patients who had been taking drugs (12 α-methyldopa, one cephalothin), seven with a malignant tumour, nine who had an immunological disorder (other than AIHA), and a miscellaneous group of 12 patients (including four who had had hip fractures). Only three of the patients presented any signs of increased haemolysis.

Freedman (1979) reported that 7–8% of erythrocyte samples from randomly selected patients were agglutinated by anti-C3d and anti-C4d anti-complement sera but not by anti-C3b/c or anti-C4c. None of Freedman's samples was agglutinated by an anti-IgG serum. The findings with the anti-C reagents were similar to those that were obtained in AIHA patients whose erythrocytes were agglutinated by anti-C sera only.

Judd and co-workers (1980) reported that 1830 out of 12 187 DATs carried out in a hospital blood bank had been positive, a high incidence. However, of the 1830 positive tests, 879 had been carried out on the blood of a group of patients who were perhaps especially likely to give positive tests — namely, on patients who were anaemic or had been recently transfused or whose serum had been found to contain unexpected antibodies when it was being screened prior to transfusion. Of these 879 positive tests, 10% were positive with anti-IgG sera only, 45% were positive with anti-IgG and anti-C3 sera and 44% with anti-C3 sera only.

Freedman, Ho and Barefoot (1982) provided more data on the incidence of raised levels of cell-bound complement in hospital patients. Estimating the number of molecules by a radioactive anti-antiglobulin technique using anti-C3d sera, 72 out of 227 randomly selected patients had moderately raised levels. None had AIHA; but they all were suffering from disorders in which complement was likely to have been activated. Twenty-six patients with AIHA were also investigated: all had given positive DATs, and in individual cases the estimates of the number of C3d molecules present correlated with the severity of their disease and their response to treatment (Fig. 27.3)

Huh and Lichtiger (1985) reported on the results of carrying out DATs in hospital patients prior to transfusion. The test was positive in 515 patients, an incidence of 3.5%. IgG was detected alone in 214 patients (41.6%), IgG plus complement (C3) in 132 (25.6%)

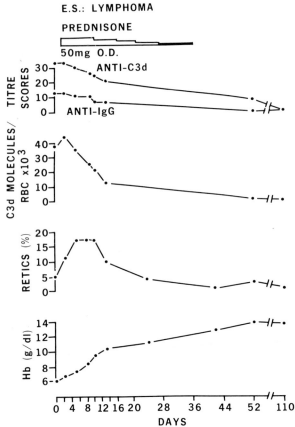

Fig. 27.3   Chart illustrating the response of a patient with AIHA and a lymphoma to treatment with prednisone, with especial reference to a diminution in the strength of the DAT (titre scores) and the number of C3d molecules coating erythrocytes.

[Reproduced by permission from Freedman, Ho and Barefoot (1982).]

and C3 alone in 97 (18.8%). Elutions carried out on 194 samples in which the cells were coated with IgG revealed non-reactive eluates in 114 and reactive (auto-antibody-containing) eluates in 18.

Judd and co-workers (1986) reported further data on the incidence of positive DATs, using anti-IgG sera, in patients tested prior to transfusion. Of 65 049 blood samples, 3570 (5.49%) were positive: 778 samples were investigated further; eluates were made and were found to be non-reactive in 66.6%.

Lepennec and co-workers (1989) carried out DATs on 185 symptomless individuals who had been shown to be HIV-1 seropositive. The test was positive in 7.5%, two with anti-IgG serum alone, two with anti-IgG plus anti-C sera, 10 with anti-C serum alone. Lepennec et al. contrasted the relatively low incidence of positive

tests with the much higher incidence (e.g. 55–60%) reported in AIDS patients.

Role of hypergammaglobulinaemia

As already referred to, it has been suggested that one component at least of the IgG present on normal erythrocytes is non-auto-antibody IgG and that the number of molecules on the cell surface reflects the concentration of IgG in the plasma (p. 195). Furthermore, if a relatively large number of molecules are present the DAT should be positive. There is some evidence that hypergammaglobulinaemia is in fact quite often associated with a positive DAT.

Szymanski and co-workers (1980) used the technique of Burkart et al. (1974) to enhance agglutination in a sensitive antiglobulin reaction using an AutoAnalyser, with Ficoll and PVP as enhancers of agglutination and an anti-IgG antiglobulin serum diluted (usually to 1 in 5000) in 0.5% bovine serum albumin. Washed suspensions of normal erythrocytes were strongly agglutinated in this system, and the fact that young cell suspensions (as separated by centrifugation) were less strongly agglutinated than older (denser) cell suspensions suggested that IgG accumulates on normal cells as they mature. The strength of agglutination was negatively correlated with the reticulocyte count in a series of patients with haemolytic anaemia [HS and non-spherocytic haemolytic anaemia in which the standard (manual) DAT was negative (Fig. 27.4)]. In contrast, agglutination was clearly positively correlated with the γ-globulin concentration in serum, being subnormal in hypogammaglobulinaemia and supranormal in hypergammaglobulinaemia (Figs. 27.4 and 27.5). Symanski et al. noted that the erythrocytes of three patients with haemolytic anaemia (two cases of unknown origin and one of PNH) were agglutinated 'normally' by the anti-IgG serum despite a young cell population, suggesting that higher than normal cell-bound IgG might be present in consequence of auto-antibody formation.

Further data supporting a link between hypergammaglobulinaemia and a positive DAT, in the absence of any evidence of abnormal auto-

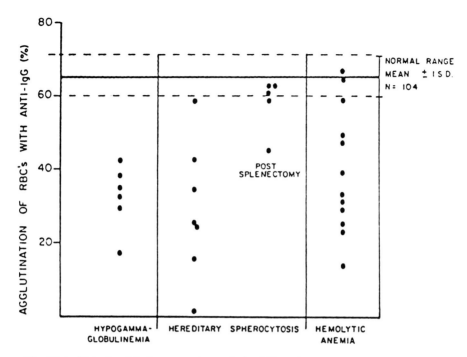

Fig. 27.4   Relationship between the agglutinability of erythrocytes by an anti-IgG serum and the presence of hypogammaglobulinaemia (left-hand data) or a raised reticulocyte count, as found in patients suffering from HS or non-spherocytic, DAT-negative, non-immune haemolytic anaemias (right-hand data).

[Reproduced by permission from Symanski et al. (1980).]

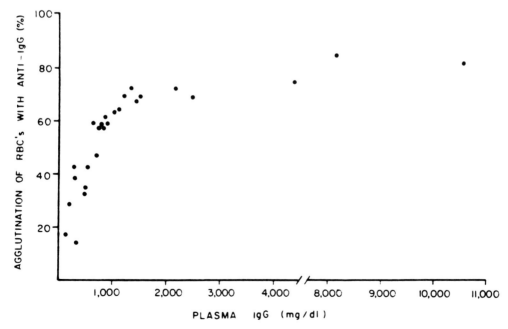

Fig. 27.5   Relationship between the agglutinability of erythrocytes by an anti-IgG serum and the concentration of plasma IgG.

[Reproduced by permission from Symanski et al. (1980).]

antibody formation and increased haemolysis, have more recently been reported.

Toy, Reid and Burns (1985) reported that they had found that the DAT carried out on 55 AIDS patients was positive in 10 (18%), compared with positive reactions in 0.6% of the general hospital population. Of the 10 positive reactions with the AIDS patients' samples, four were positive with an anti-IgG serum, four with anti-IgG and anti-C sera and two only with an anti-C serum. Eluates made from the positively reacting erythrocytes did not react with normal or penicillin- or cephalothin-treated erythrocytes and none of the patients appeared to be suffering from increased haemolysis. Toy, Reid and Burns suggested that the positive tests were associated with hypergammaglobulinaemia rather than with AIDS. In a follow-up study (on patients before transfusion), Toy et al. (1985) compared the incidence of elevated serum globulins in 76 patients giving positive DATs (none had AIDS) with 90 patients (none had AIDS) in whom the DAT was negative: 75% of the DAT-positive patients had elevated serum globulins compared with 29% of the DAT-negative patients, a statistically significant difference. It was interesting to note that 42% of the DAT-positive patients had a raised blood urea compared with 19% of the DAT-negative patients, also a statistically significant difference.

Heddle, Turchyn and Kelton (1985) and Heddle and co-workers (1988) described how they had investigated 74 patients who had been found to give a positive DAT: in 54, reactive eluates from their erythrocytes indicated auto-antibody formation; in 20, however, although the DAT was positive, the IAT was negative, eluates were non-reactive, and there was no evidence of haemolysis. A common feature, however, was hypergammaglobulinaemia (Fig. 27.6). Later, DATs were carried out on 44 consecutive hypergammaglobulinaemic patients; the test was positive in the three patients who had the highest serum IgG levels.

Garratty and Arndt (1987) set out to answer the question as to whether positive DATs demonstrated only by sensitive assays were likely to be explained by raised levels of serum IgG. In 'Coombs-negative' AIHA at least this did not seem to be so. The serum IgG levels in 46 patients whose erythrocytes had reacted positively in one or more sensitive tests (i.e. in the ELAT and Polybrene, polyethylene glycol and concentrated eluate tests) were compared with the serum IgG levels in 49 patients whose erythrocytes had given negative results in all four tests. The median serum IgG of the positively reacting patients was 900 mg/dl, compared with 800 mg/dl in the case of the negatively reacting patients, a difference that was not statistically significant. Garratty and Arndt concluded that erythrocyte-bound IgG detected by sensitive methods was likely to be associated with the presence of auto-antibodies rather than with the height of the serum IgG. However, it is noteworthy that the only two sera in which the IgG level exceeded 1800 mg/dl were derived from patients in the positively reacting group.

Huh and co-workers (1988) reported on studies carried out on 154 patients: (1) a group of 52 patients who had been found to give positive DATs when their blood was tested prior to transfusion; (2) a group of 52 patients who had given a negative DAT, and (3) a group of 50 patients found to have abnormally high serum IgG levels. Seventeen (33%) of the Group-1 patients had a high IgG level but a non-reactive eluate and no evidence of increased haemolysis; two only (4%) of the Group-2 patients had a high IgG level; while 25 (50%) of the Group-3 patients had a positive DAT, a non-reactive eluate and presented no evidence of increased haemolysis.

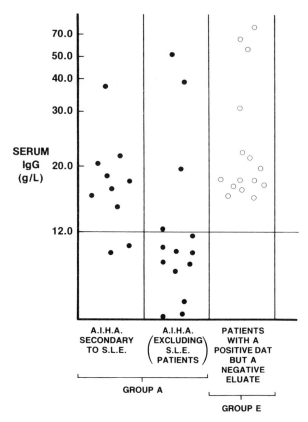

Fig. 27.6   Serum IgG levels in three series of patients: group A, patients with idiopathic AIHA or with AIHA associated with SLE; group E, patients giving a positive DAT but without demonstrable antibodies in eluates prepared from their erythrocytes.

[Reproduced by permission from Heddle et al. (1988).]

POLYAGGLUTINABILITY AND HAEMOLYTIC ANAEMIA

An unusual phenomenon is polyagglutinability, i.e. the agglutination of human erythrocytes by all (or almost all) adult human sera irrespective of blood groups, although not by the sera of new-born infants. Usually the polyagglutinability has been transient and associated with severe sepsis.

In vitro, it has been known for many years that suspensions of erythrocytes might become agglutinable by normal compatible human sera, if the cells were allowed to stand for hours at temperatures at which bacteria would grow. The phenomenon, which has been referred as that of Hübener–Thomsen–Friedenreich, is thought to be brought about by enzymes of bacterial origin (e.g. neuraminidase) acting on the surface of erythrocytes so as to unmask cryptantigens named T (after Thomsen) that are normally hidden. The cells then become agglutinable by antibodies (anti-T, anti-Tn, etc.) present in human sera as an immune response to bacteria (e.g. *E. coli* strains) present in the human colon (Springer and Tegtmeyer, 1981).

T is not the only cryptantigen that may be unmasked in the erythrocyte membrane by enzymes of bacterial origin. Tk is another such antigen, the responsible enzyme being endo-β-galactosidase. Tn is yet another antigen: this, however, is formed as the result of incomplete synthesis of the carbohydrate part of the MN blood-group antigens.

Both the T and Tn antigens can be readily detected by the use of plant lectins, proteins that have a selective affinity for simple sugars. In the case of T, a lectin from the seeds of the peanut (*Arachis hypogaea*) (Bird, 1964) is a most useful reagent, and for Tn a lectin from the seeds of the labiate *Salvia selarea* (Bird and Wingham, 1973).

According to Mollison, Engelfriet and Contreras (1987), polyagglutinable erythrocytes, as found in a patient suffering from severe sepsis, are not agglutinated by the patient's own serum. This is presumably because the anti-T antibodies are adsorbed to the patient's own erythrocytes. The question then arises as to whether polyagglutinability ever leads to increased haemolysis. There are in fact a series of published reports

suggesting that this may sometimes have happened (see below). There are also some experimental studies which support the concept.

According to Ejby-Poulsen (1954), haemolytic anaemia followed the T transformation of guinea-pig erythrocytes produced *in vivo* by the intravenous injection of a concentrated enzyme derived from *Str. pneumoniae*, type 19. An interesting haemolytic system, too, was described by Evans and his co-workers in young rabbits suffering from mucoid enteritis (Evans et al., 1959; Evans, Bingham and Weiser, 1963a, b). It was suggested that a bacterial product (? an enzyme) rendered the erythrocytes polyagglutinable by normally occurring potentially agglutinating and lytic plasma factors. Overt haemolytic anaemia was thought not to occur because of rapid depletion of the plasma factors.

Polyagglutination associated with severe infection in man

A possible example was described by Levine and Katzin (1938). Their patient was a child aged 4 years, suffering from a severe pneumococcal infection, whose group-O erythrocytes were agglutinated by the sera of approximately 15% of normal individuals irrespective of their blood groups. Agglutination took place at 25°C and more distinctly at 20°C, but not at 37°C. Four months later the child's erythrocytes were found to react normally.

Similar occurrences were reported by Gaffney and Sachs (1943), Basil-Jones, Sanger and Walsh (1946) and Boorman, Loutit and Steabben (1946). Boorman, Loutit and Steabben, experimenting with group-O erythrocytes that had been exposed to a culture of Friedenreich's M bacillus, obtained some evidence that suggested that the factor in normal serum that agglutinated the erythrocytes of their two patients was related to the anti-T of Friedenreich, e.g., normal sera absorbed with the patients' cells failed to agglutinate one suspension of the in-vitro transformed cells and agglutinated only weakly two other suspensions.

Engelson and Grubb (1949) described two

cases. The first patient, a female aged 28 with peritonitis, developed well marked temporary polyagglutinability: her erythrocytes were agglutinated by all sera tested at room temperature and weakly at 37°C; her own cells were, however, not agglutinated. The second patient, a 9-year-old boy, died with pyodermia and haemolytic anaemia. He seems possibly to have developed polyagglutinability as well as a high-thermal-amplitude cold auto-antibody.

Gasser and Holländer (1951) have been quoted as mentioning polyagglutinability as a feature of the blood picture of the 7-week-old infant they had described as suffering from a most severe and eventually fatal AIHA. The DAT was, however, strongly positive, and it is possible that the agglutination that was observed when the infant's erythrocytes were suspended in normal compatible sera was due to the auto-agglutination of antibody-coated cells in a medium of high protein content (see p. 127). (A more detailed account of this patient is given on p. 34.)

Hendry and Simmons (1955) described the occurrence of polyagglutinability in the case of a 30-year-old woman suffering from severe pelvic sepsis. She had been bleeding and needed transfusing. There was, however, no evidence of increased haemolysis. The phenomenon was still present 5 weeks later, but was less obvious and could then only be demonstrated at low temperatures (5–10°C).

van Loghem, van der Hart and Land (1955) described how the transfusion of plasma to an infant whose erythrocytes were polyagglutinable apparently precipitated a severe transfusion reaction.

Altmann, Nelson and Cusumano (1957) described a 45-year-old male who died of peritonitis, associated with jaundice thought to be secondary to haemolysis. His erythrocytes were polyagglutinable; this was most evident at 4°C, less marked at room temperature but still definite at 37°C.

Moreau and co-workers (1957) and Dausset, Moullec and Bernard (1959) reported the history of a patient who developed haemolytic anaemia following an acute infection of undetermined nature which had lasted 10 days. The patient's erythrocytes were found to be polyagglutinable and this persisted as an apparently permanent phenomenon for at least 9 years. The polyagglutinability was attributed to the presence of a 'new' antigen referred to as 'Tn'. Anti-Tn, which could be demonstrated in all of 490 sera tested, was considered to be distinct from anti-T. Whether Tn–anti-Tn interaction was responsible for the haemolysis is uncertain. The DAT was negative, although the erythrocytes were weakly auto-agglutinated. The patient's serum strongly agglutinated trypsinized Tn cells but only weakly agglutinated unmodified Tn cells; it also

contained a weak panagglutinin against trypsinized normal cells as well as an anti-E antibody and anti-platelet and anti-leucocyte antibodies.

Chorpenning and Hayes (1959) reviewed the occurrence of the 'Thomsen–Friedenreich' phenomenon in vivo and referred to a patient of their own, a 16-year-old female with abdominal sepsis. Polyagglutination developed. Her erythrocytes were, however, only slightly auto-agglutinated at 5°C. She became severely anaemic, but a major cause of this was found to be massive haemorrhage into the peritoneal cavity. Normal group-O erythrocytes experimentally altered by exposure to sterile culture filtrates of an organism isolated from the patient's blood were shown to remove the agglutinin from sera which had been shown previously to agglutinate the patient's erythrocytes.

van Loghem (1965) referred briefly to six patients who had developed polyagglutinability and haemolytic anaemia, the cryptantigen being T in four and Tn in two. Auto-agglutination was noted in one of the patients and weak auto-agglutination in two. The DAT was negative in five and positive in one. The bacterial infection was unidentified in three of the patients, but Cl. welchi, Staph. aureus and Str. pneumoniae were identified in the remaining patients, respectively.

Jørgensen (1967) described in detail the occurrence of polyagglutinability in a newborn infant who became severely jaundiced after birth (bilirubin 20 mg/dl on the 4th day). Both mother and infant were ABO and Rh (D) compatible. Approximately 10% of the child's erythrocytes were agglutinated by all adult sera or plasma samples tested, including those of the infant's mother, but not by cord plasma. The phenomenon, which had disappeared by the 16th day after delivery, appeared to be T polyagglutinability, but the cause remained uncertain. In particular, there was no evidence of infection in either mother or infant, and while it seems possible that the polyagglutinability had been responsible for the jaundice this did not appear to be likely.

Rickard, Robinson and Worlledge (1969) described a 14-month-old child with Down's syndrome who developed acute haemolytic anaemia as a complication of bronchopneumonia. Polyagglutinability became evident when the child's blood was grouped in preparation for a transfusion. The patient's erythrocytes were agglutinated by all the grouping sera, as well as by group-AB sera, but they were not agglutinated by cord sera. The cells were, too, strongly agglutinated by the anti-T in peanut extract; they were also agglutinated to a variable degree by rabbit sera irrespective of their content of antibodies against globulins or complement. No unusual antibodies were detected in the child's serum. The polyagglutination made ABO and Rh grouping impossible at room temperature; at 37°C, however, agglutination was less marked and it could be established that the child was group O Rh(D). The child responded well to two transfusions and to antibiotic therapy, and the polyagglutinability was no

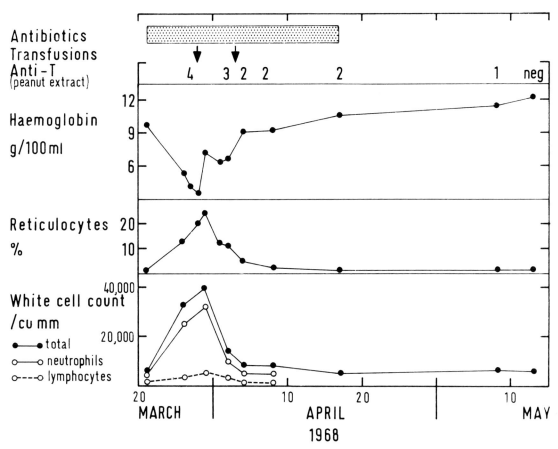

Fig. 27.7   Chart illustrating the occurrence of acute haemolytic anaemia in a 14-months-old child suffering from bronchopneumonia complicated by polyagglutinability.
[Reproduced by permission from Rickard, Robinson and Worlledge (1969).]

longer demonstrable 6 weeks or so after it had first been discovered (Fig. 27.7).

Gray, Beck and Oberman (1972) described a patient with peritonitis and an ileal perforation from whose blood *Cl. sporogenes* had been isolated. Her erythrocytes became polyagglutinable, blood tranfusions were relatively ineffective, and it was thought likely that anti-T in the donated plasma had been a cause of intravascular haemolysis.

Bird and Stephenson (1973) described a 7-week-old albino male infant who developed acute haemolysis following an operation for a strangulated inguinal hernia. The abdominal wound became infected following the operation; the infant became severely anaemic and his erythrocytes were found to have become polyagglutinable. They were agglutinated by 10 adult group-AB sera and anti-B sera (although the infant was A-positive) but not by three cord sera; the cells were agglutinated, too, by rabbit antiglobulin sera. Adult sera known to contain anti-T failed to agglutinate

the cells after the sera had been absorbed with adult cells 'activated' by *V. cholerae*.

Moores, Pudifin and Patel (1975) described a 38-year-old woman who had sustained a stab wound to her chest. She was febrile and had a neutrophil leucocytosis and rapidly became severely anaemic (haemoglobin 3 g/dl) and jaundiced. There was auto-agglutination, the DAT was positive and AIHA was diagnosed. The erythrocytes were strongly agglutinated by peanut anti-T and also by anti-T in the patient's own plasma, as well as by some but not all anti-M and anti-N sera. Incomplete T activation was postulated and the short episode of acute haemolysis was attributed to the presence of anti-T in the patient's plasma.

Graninger and co-workers (1977a,b) described a man aged 20 who had suffered apparently from a compensated haemolytic anaemia since infancy. His erythrocytes were agglutinated by almost all sera but there was no auto-agglutination and the DAT was negative. The polyagglutinability was distinguishable from that of T, Tn and Tk by the cells' reactions with various seed and snail extracts. In particular, the cells were not agglutinated by *Arachis hypogaea* (peanut) or *Dolichos biflorus* extracts and the cells' reactions with various anti-H reagents was variably, but mostly markedly, depressed. The polyagglutinability, which was believed to be a 'new' variety, was referred to as type 'VA' (Vienna).

Mullard and co-workers (1981) reported the occurrence of strong T-transformation and a severe haemolytic reaction in a 4-week-old infant following a transfusion of 80 ml of packed erythrocytes. He had been admitted to hospital uraemic and possibly septicaemic. He was transfused and following this there was a dramatic fall in haemoglobin, from 11.4 g/dl to 5.1 g/dl and he became deeply jaundiced. His erythrocytes were found to be polyagglutinable and the DAT was strongly positive, using anti-IgM and anti-complement reagents. The infant died, and at necropsy a large intraperitoneal abscess was found associated with a perforated appendix.

Levene and co-workers (1986) described a patient, a 16-year-old male, who suffered from post-operative intravascular haemolysis and acute renal failure which appeared to be aggravated by transfusions with fresh blood, platelets and fresh frozen plasma. Tests with lectins showed that his erythrocytes were T-transformed. Haemolysis ceased when he was transfused subsequently only with washed erythrocytes. The polyagglutination had disappeared when his erythrocytes were retested with lectins 4 months after surgery. The DAT had earlier been positive with a polyspecific antiglobulin serum and an anti-C3 serum, and weakly positive with an anti-IgG serum and in the saline control. It seemed likely that the aggravation of haemolysis following the transfusions had been brought about by the anti-T in the blood and plasma he had received.

Evidence that T-activation is in reality quite a common phenomenon in patients suffering from severe sepsis was provided by Lenz et al. (1987) in a systematic study of 53 adults with septicaemia being nursed in an intensive care unit. The presence of T-activation was sought by a direct test (agglutination by peanut extract) and by an indirect test employing a rabbit anti-peanut globulin. T-activation was established to have taken place in 17 patients (32%) and in two of the patients (4%) the degree of activation was strong enough for the direct test to be positive. Overt polyagglutination was, however, not detectable in any of the patients. The serum neuraminidase concentration was elevated in 12 out of 17 patients (71%), indicating the presence of neuraminidase-releasing bacteria. The serum haemoglobin concentration was found to be elevated in 12 out of 17 patients (71%) in whom there was evidence of T-activation and in five out of 36 patients (14%) in whom T-activation had not been demonstrated. In an analysis of their data Lenz et al. found significant correlations between T-activation and serum neuraminidase and between T-activation and serum haemoglobin; they concluded that their study 'tends to indicate' that neuraminidase T-activation in adults with severe infections can be a cause of haemolytic anaemia.

Despite suggestive case histories, as for instance those summarized above, the concept that T-inactivation *in vivo* can by itself lead to significant haemolysis has not been universally accepted. Issitt (1985), for instance, stated that he was 'not yet convinced that the hemolysis associated with in vivo T-activation in any of the reported cases can be absolutely attributed to anti-T'; he added that he leant 'towards the alternative explanation that toxins, enzymes or other products of infecting organisms cause both T-activation and in vivo red cell hemolysis without participation by anti-T.'

REFERENCES

ALTMANN, V., NELSON, M. S. & CUSUMANO, I. (1957). Polyagglutinability associated with hemolytic jaundice. Report of a case. *Amer. J. clin. Path.*, **27**, 433–437.

BAIKIE, A. G. & PIRRIE, R. (1956). Megaloblastic erythropoiesis in idiopathic acquired haemolytic anaemia. *Scot. med. J.*, **1**, 330–334.

BAREFORD, D., LONGSTER, G., GILKS, L. & TOVEY, L. A. D. (1985). Follow-up of normal individuals with a positive antiglobulin test. *Scand. J. Haemat.*, **35**, 348–353.

BASIL-JONES, B., SANGER, R. A. & WALSH, R. J. (1946). An agglutinable factor in red blood cells. *Nature (Lond.)*, **157**, 802.

BIRD, G. W. G. (1964). Anti-T in peanuts. *Vox Sang.*, **9**, 748–749.

BIRD, G. W. G. & WINGHAM, J. (1973). Seed agglutinin for rapid identification of Tn-polyagglutination. *Lancet*, **i**, 677.

BIRD, T. & STEPHENSON, J. (1973). Acute haemolytic anaemia associated with polyagglutinability of red cells. *J. clin. Path.*, **26**, 868–870.

BOCCARDI, V., GIRELLI, G., PERRICONE, R., CICCONE, F., ROMOLI, P. & ISACCHI, G. (1978). Coombs-negative autoimmune hemolytic anemia. Report of 11 cases. *Haematologica*, **63**, 301–310.

BOORMAN, K. E., LOUTIT, J. F. & STEABBEN, D. B. (1946). Polyagglutinable red cells. *Nature (Lond.)*, **158**, 446–447.

BOURSNELL, J. C., COOMBS, R. B. A. & RIZK, V. (1953). Studies with marked antisera. Quantitative studies with sera marked with iodine ^{131}I isotope and their corresponding red-cell antigens. *Biochem. J.*, **55**, 745–758.

BRANCH, D. R., SHULMAN, I. A., SY SIOK HIAN, A. L. & PETZ, L. D. (1984). Two distinct categories of warm autoantibody reactivity with age-fractionated red cells. *Blood*, **63**, 177–180.

BRANCH, D. R., SY SIOK HIAN, A. L. & PETZ, L. D. (1982). Evidence for two distinct categories of warm autoantibody activity when using reticulocyte-rich (RR) or reticulocyte poor (RP) red cell fractions. *Transfusion*, **22**, 430 (Abstract, S 109).

BURKART, P., ROSENFIELD, R. E., HSU, T. C. S., WONG, K. Y., NUSBACHER, J., SHAIKH, S. H. & KOCHWA, S. (1974). Instrumental PVP-augmented antiglobulin tests. I. Detection of allogeneic antibodies coating otherwise normal erythrocytes. *Vox Sang.*, **26**, 289–304.

CHAPLIN, H. JNR (1973). Clinical usefulness of specific antiglobulin reagents in autoimmune hemolytic anemia. *Progr. Hemat.*, **8**, 25–49.

CHAPLIN, H. JNR, COLEMAN, M. E. & MONROE, M. C. (1983). In vivo instability of red-cell-bound C3d and C4d. *Blood*, **62**, 965–971.

CHAPLIN, H., NASONGKLA, M. & MONROE, M. C. (1980). Quantitation of red blood cell-bound C3d (RBC-C3d) in normal subjects and random hospitalized patients. *Transfusion*, **20**, 646 (Abstract).

CHAPLIN, H., NASONGKLA, M. & MONROE, M. C. (1981). Quantitation of red blood cell-bound C3d in normal subjects and random hospitalized patients. *Brit. J. Haemat.*, **48**, 69–78.

CHORPENNING, F. W. & HAYES, J. C. (1959). Occurrence of the Thomsen–Friedenreich phenomenon in vivo. *Vox Sang.*, **4**, 211–244.

COOMBS, R. R. A., GLEESON-WHITE, M. H. & HALL, J. G. (1951). Factors influencing the agglutinability of red cells. II. The agglutination of bovine red cells previously classified as 'inagglutinable' by the building up of an 'antiglobulin: globulin lattice' on the sensitized cells. *Brit. J. exp. Path.*, **32**, 195–202.

CRUZ, W. O. & JUNQUEIRA, P. C. (1952). Resistance of reticulocytes and young erythrocytes to the action of specific hemolytic serum. *Blood*, **7**, 602–606.

DACIE, J. V. (1950). Occurrences in normal human sera of 'incomplete' forms of cold auto-antibodies. *Nature (Lond.)*, **166**, 36.

DACIE, J. V. (1954). *The Haemolytic Anaemias: Congenital and Acquired*, pp. 164–216. Churchill, London.

DACIE, J. V. (1960). *The Haemolytic Anaemias: Congenital and Acquired. Part I—The Congenital Anaemias*, 2nd edn, 339 pp. Churchill, London.

DACIE, J. V. (1962). *The Haemolytic Anaemias: Congenital and Acquired. Part II—The Auto-immune Haemolytic Anaemias*, 2nd edn, 377 pp. Churchill, London.

DACIE, J. V. & DE GRUCHY, G. C. (1951). Auto-antibodies in acquired haemolytic anaemia. *J. clin. Path.*, **4**, 253–271.

DACIE, J. V. & WORLLEDGE, S. M. (1969). Auto-immune hemolytic anemias. *Progr. Hemat.*, **6**, 82–120.

DARNBOROUGH, J. (1958). A unique case of auto-immune erythrocyte sensitization. *Brit. med. J.*, **ii**, 1451–1452.

DAUSSET, J., MOULLEC, J. & BERNARD, J. (1959). Acquired hemolytic anemia with polyagglutinability of red blood cells due to a new factor present in normal human serum (anti-Tn). *Blood*, **14**, 1079–1093.

DAVIDSOHN, I. & SPURRIER, W. (1954). Immunohematological studies in hemolytic anemia. *J. Amer. med. Ass.*, **154**, 818–821.

DE GRUCHY, G. C. (1954). The diagnosis and management of acquired haemolytic anaemia. *Aust. Ann. Med.*, **3**, 106–115.

DUPUY, M. E., ELLIOT, M. & MASOUREDIS, S. P. (1964). Relationship between red cell bound antibody and agglutination in the antiglobulin reaction. *Vox Sang.*, **9**, 40–44.

EJBY-POULSEN, P. (1954). Haemolytic anaemia produced experimentally in the guinea pig by T-transformation of the erythrocytes *in vivo* with purified concentrated enzyme. *Nature (Lond.)*, **174**, 929–930.

ENGELSON, G. & GRUBB, R. (1949). Abnormal agglutinability of red cells in pyogenic infections. Report of two cases. *Amer. J. clin. Path.*, **19**, 782–789.

EVANS, R. S. (1955). Autoantibodies in hematologic disorders. *Stanford med. Bull.*, **13**, 152–166.

EVANS, R. S., BINGHAM, M., HICKEY, M. & HASSETT, C. (1959). A hemolytic system associated with mucoid enteritis in rabbits. *Trans. Ass. Amer. Phycns*, **72**, 188–199.

EVANS, R. S., BINGHAM, M. & WEISER, R. S. (1963a). A hemolytic system associated with enteritis in rabbits. I. Nature of the cell change and the serum factors concerned. *J. exp. Med.*, **117**, 647–661.

EVANS, R. S., BINGHAM, M. & WEISER, R. S. (1963b). A hemolytic system associated with enteritis in rabbits. II. Studies on the survival of transfused red cells. *J. Lab. clin. Med.*, **62**, 559–570.

EVANS, R. S. & WEISER, R. S. (1957). The serology of autoimmune hemolytic disease. Observations on forty-one patients. *Arch. intern. Med.*, **100**, 371–399.

FISCHER, J. TH., PETZ, L. D., GARRATTY, G. & COOPER, N. R. (1974). Correlations between quantitative assay of red cell-bound C3, serologic reactions and hemolytic anemia. *Blood*, 44, 359–373.

FREEDMAN, J. (1979). False-positive antiglobulin tests in healthy subjects. *J. clin. Path.*, **32**, 1014–1018.

FREEDMAN, J. (1984). Membrane-bound immunoglobulins and complement components on young and old red cells. *Transfusion*, **24**, 477–481.

FREEDMAN, J. & BAREFOOT, C. (1982). Red blood cell-bound C3d in normal subjects and in random hospital patients. *Transfusion*, **22**, 511–514.

FREEDMAN, J., HO, M. & BAREFOOT, C. (1982). Red blood cell-bound C3d in selected hospital patients. *Transfusion*, **22**, 515–520.

GAFFNEY, J. C. & SACKS, H. (1943). Polyagglutinability of human red blood cells. *J. Path. Bact.*, **55**, 489–492.

GALILI, U., FLECHNER, I., KNYSZYNSKI, A., DANON, D. & RACHMILEWITZ, E. A. (1986). The natural anti-α-galactosyl IgG on human normal senescent red blood cells. *Brit. J. Haemat.*, **62**, 317–324.

GALLACHER, M. T., BRANCH, D. R., MISON, A. & PETZ, L. D. (1983). Evaluation of reticuloendothelial function in autoimmune hemolytic anemia using an in vitro assay of monocyte-macrophage interaction with erythrocytes. *Exper. Hemat.*, **11**, 82–89.

GARRATTY, G. (1987). The significance of IgG on the red cell surface. *Transf. Medicine Rev.*, **1**, 47–57.

GARRATTY, G. (1988). The clinical significance (and insignificance) of red-cell-bound IgG and complement. In *Current Applications and Interpretation of the Direct Antiglobulin Test* (ed. by M. E. Wallace and J. S. Levitt), pp. 1–24. American Association of Blood Banks, Arlington, Virginia.

GARRATTY, G. & ARNDT, P. (1987). Is there a correlation with RBC-bound IgG detected by sensitive assays, such as the enzyme-linked antiglobulin test (ELAT), and serum levels of IgG? *Transfusion*, **27**, 545 (Abstract S 155).

GARRATTY, G., POSTOWAY, N., NANCE, S. & BRUNT, D. (1982). The detection of IgG on the red cells of 'Coombs negative' autoimmune hemolytic anemias. *Transfusion*, **22**, 430 (Abstract S 108).

GASSER, C. & HOLLÄNDER, L. (1951). Anémie hémolytique acquise aiguë provoquée par des auto-anticorps, accompagnée de purpura thrombocytopénique, chez un nourrisson de 7 semaines. *Rev. Hémat.*, **6**, 316–333.

GILLILAND, B. C. (1976). Coombs-negative immune hemolytic anemia. *Seminars Hemat.*, **13**, 267–275.

GILLILAND, B. C., BAXTER, E. & EVANS, R. S. (1971). Red-cell antibodies in acquired hemolytic anemia with negative antiglobulin serum tests. *New Engl. J. Med.*, **285**, 252–256.

GILLILAND, B. C., LEDDY, J. P. & VAUGHAN, T. H. (1970). The detection of cell-bound antibody on complement-coated human red cells. *J. clin. Invest.*, **49**, 898–906.

GORST, D. W., RAWLINSON, V. I., MERRY, A. H. & STRATTON, F. (1980). Positive direct antiglobulin test in normal individuals. *Vox Sang.*, **38**, 99–105.

GRANINGER, W., POSCHMANN, A., FISCHER, K., SCHEDL-GIOVANNONI, I., HÖRANDNER, H. & KLAUSHOFER, K. (1977a). 'VA', a new type of erythrocyte polyagglutination characterized by depressed H receptors and associated with hemolytic anemia. II. Observations by immunofluorescence, electron microscopy, cell electrophoresis and biochemistry. *Vox Sang.*, **32**, 201–207.

GRANINGER, W., RAMEIS, H., FISCHER, K., PORSCHMANN, A., BIRD, G. W. G., WINGHAM, J. & NEUMANN, E. (1977b). 'VA', a new type of erythrocyte polyagglutination characterized by depressed H receptors and associated with hemolytic anemia. I. Serological and hematological observations. *Vox Sang.*, **32**, 195–200.

GRAY, J. M., BECK, M. L. & OBERMAN, H. A. (1972). Clostridial-induced type I polyagglutinability with associated intravascular hemolysis. *Vox Sang.*, **22**, 379–383.

GRAY, L. S., KLEEMAN, J. E. & MASOUREDIS, S. P. (1983). Differential binding of IgG anti-D and IgG autoantibodies to reticulocytes and red blood cells. *Brit. J. Haemat.*, **55**, 335–345.

GRAY, L. S. & MASOUREDIS, S. P. (1981). Expression of the D antigen during maturation of peripheral erythrocytes. *Transfusion*, **21**, 630 (Abstract).

GRAY, L. S. & MASOUREDIS, S. P. (1982). Interaction of ^{125}I-protein A with erythrocyte-bound IgG. *J. Lab. clin. Med.*, **99**, 399–409.

HABIBI, B., MULLER, A., LELONG, F., HOMBERG, J. C., FOUCHER, M., DUHAMEL, G. & SALMON, C. (1980). Auto-immunisation érythrocytaire dans la population 'normale'. *Nouv. Presse méd.*, **43**, 3253–3257.

HANSEN, O. P., HANSEN, T. M., JANS, H. & HIPPE, E. (1984). Red blood cell membrane-bound IgG: demonstration of antibodies in patients with autoimmune haemolytic anaemia and immune complexes in patients with rheumatic disease. *Clin. lab. Haemat.*, **6**, 341–349.

HEDDLE, N. M., KELTON, J. G., TURCHYN, K. L. & ALI, M. A. M. (1988). Hypergammaglobulinemia can be associated with a positive direct antiglobulin test, a nonreactive eluate, and no evidence of hemolysis. *Transfusion*, **28**, 29–33.

HEDDLE, N. M., TURCHYN, K. L. & KELTON, J. G. (1985). Hypergammaglobulinemia can be associated with a positive direct antiglobulin test, a non-reactive eluate, and no evidence of hemolysis. *Transfusion*, **25**, 451 (Abstract S 24).

HENDRY, P. T. A. & SIMMONS, R. T. (1955). An example of polyagglutinable erythrocytes, and reference to panagglutination, polyagglutination and autoagglutination as possible sources of error in blood grouping. *Med. J. Aust.*, **i**, 720–722.

HENI, F. & BLESSING, K. (1954). Die Bedeutung der Glutinine für die erworbenen hämolytischen Anämien. *Dtsch. Arch. klin. Med.*, **201**, 113–135.

HENNEMANN, H. H. (1967). Positive Coombs-Test bei klinisch Gesunden. *Dtsch. med. Wschr.*, **92**, 1179–1180.

HENNEMANN, H. H. (1968). Positive Coombs test in healthy people. *Germ. med. Monthly*, **13**, 212–213.

HERRON, R., CLARK, M. & SMITH, D. S. (1987). An autoantibody with activity dependent on red cell age in the serum of a patient with autoimmune haemolytic anaemia and a negative direct antiglobulin test. *Vox Sang.*, **52**, 71–74.

HSU, T. C. S., STEINBERG, J. & SAWITSKY, A. (1979). C3d antiglobulin haemagglutination of human red blood cells. A demonstration of two types of cell-bound C3d by means of trypsin digestion. *J. clin. Path.*, **32**, 1009–1013.

HUH, Y. O. & LICHTIGER, B. (1985). Evaluation of a positive autologous control in pretransfusion testing. *Amer. J. clin. Path.*, **84**, 632–636.

HUH, Y. O., LIU, F. J., ROGGE, K., CHAKRABARTY, L. & LICHTIGER, B. (1988). Positive direct antiglobulin test and high serum immunoglobulin G levels. *Amer. J. clin. Path.*, **90**, 197–200.

IDELSON, L. I., KOYFMAN, M. M., GORINA, L. G. & OLOVNIKOV, A. M. (1976). Application of a high sensitivity aggregate-haemagglutination test for the diagnosis of autoimmune haemolytic anaemia with a negative direct antiglobulin test. *Vox Sang.*, **31**, 401–407.

ISSITT, P. D. (1985). *Applied Blood Group Serology*, 3rd edn, p. 462. Montgomery Scientific Publications, Miami.

ISSITT, P. D., GRUPPO, R. A. WILKINSON, S. L. & ISSITT, C. H. (1982). Atypical presentation of acute phase, antibody-induced haemolytic anaemia in an infant. *Brit. J. Haemat.*, **52**, 537–543.

ISSITT, P. D., PAVONE, B. G., GOLDFINGER, D., ZWICKER, H., ISSITT, C. H., TESSEL, J. A., KROOVAND, S. W. & BELL, C. A. (1976). Anti-Wr[b], and other autoantibodies responsible for positive direct antiglobulin tests in 150 individuals. *Brit. J. Haemat.*, **34**, 5–18.

ISSITT, P. D., WILKINSON, S. L. & GRUPPO, R. A. (1983). Depression of Rh antigen expression in antibody-induced haemolytic anaemia. *Brit. J. Haemat.*, **53**, 688 (Letter).

JAKOBOWICZ, R., BRYCE, L. M. & SIMMONS, R. T. (1949). The occurrence of unusual positive Coombs reactions and M variants in the blood of a mother and her first child. *Med. J. Aust.*, **ii**, 945–948.

JEANNET, M., METAXAS-BÜHLER, M. & TOBLER, R. (1963). Anomalie héréditaire de la membrane érythrocytaire avec test de Coombs positif et modification de l'antigène de groupe N. *Schweiz. med. Wschr.*, **93**, 1508–1509.

JEANNET, M., METAXAS-BÜHLER, M. & TOBLER, R. (1964). Anomalie héréditaire de la membrane érythrocytaire avec test de Coombs direct positif et modification de l'antigène de groupe N. *Vox Sang.*, **9**, 52–55.

JEJE, M. O., BLAJCHMAN, M. A., STEEVES, K., HORSEWOOD, P. & KELTON, J. G. (1984). Quantitation of red cell-associated IgG using an immunoradiometric assay. *Transfusion*, **24**, 473–476.

JENSEN, K. G. & FREISLEBEN, E. (1962). Inherited positive Coombs' reaction connected with a weak N-receptor (N_2). *Vox Sang.*, **7**, 697–703.

JØRGENSEN, J. R. (1967). Prenatal T-transformation? A case of polyagglutinable cord blood erythrocytes. *Vox Sang.*, **13**, 225–232.

JUDD, W. J., BARNES, B. A., STEINER, E. A., OBERMAN, H. A., AVERILL, D. B. & BUTCH, S. H. (1986). The evaluation of a positive direct antiglobulin test (autocontrol) in pretransfusion testing revisited. *Transfusion*, **26**, 220–224.

JUDD, W. J., BUTCH, S. H., OBERMAN, H. A., STEINER, E. A. & BAUER, R. C. (1980). The evaluation of a positive direct antiglobulin test in pretransfusion testing. *Transfusion*, **20**, 17–23.

LAU, P., HAESLER, W. E. & WURZEL, H. A. (1976). Positive direct antiglobulin reaction in a patient population. *Amer. J. clin. Path.*, **65**, 368–375.

LEMAIRE, A., LOEPER, J., BOIREN, M. & DAUSSET, J. (1954). Anémie hémolytique aiguë avec auto-anticorps actif seulement sur les hématies traitées par un enzyme protéolytique. Étude d'une étiologie virale possible. *Bull. Mém. Soc. méd. Hôp. Paris*, **70**, 997–1007.

LENZ, G., GOES, V., BARON, D., SUGG, U. & HELLER, W. (1987). Red blood cell T-activation and hemolysis in surgical intensive care patients with severe infections. *Blut*, **54**, 89–96.

LEPENNEC, P.-Y., LEFRERE, J.-J., ROUZAUD, A.-M. & ROUGER, P. (1989). Red cell autoantibodies in asymptomatic HIV-infected subjects. *Transfusion*, **29**, 465–466 (Letter).

LEVENE, C., SELA, R., BLAT, J., FRIEDLAENDER, M. & MANNY, N. (1986). Intravascular hemolysis and renal failure in a patient with T polyagglutination. *Transfusion*, **26**, 243–245.

LEVINE, P. & KATZIN, E. M. (1938). Temporary agglutinability of red blood cells. *Proc. Soc. exp. Biol. Med.*, **39**, 167–169.

MAGNANI, M., PAPA, S., ROSSI, L., VITALE, M., FORNAINI, G. & MANZOLI, F. A. (1988). Membrane-bound immunoglobulins increase during red blood cell aging. *Acta haemat. (Basel)*, **79**, 127–132.

MASOUREDIS, S. P., BRANKS, M. J. & VICTORIA, E. J. (1987). Antiidiotypic IgG cross-reactive with Rh alloantibodies in red cell autoimmunity. *Blood*, **70**, 710–715.

MERRY, A. H., THOMSON, E. E., RAWLINSON, V. I. & STRATTON, F. (1983). The quantification of C3 fragments on erythrocytes: estimation of C3 fragments on normal cells, acquired haemolytic anaemia cases and correlation with agglutination of sensitized cells. *Clin. lab. Haemat.*, **5**, 387–397.

MERRY, A. H., THOMSON, E. E., RAWLINSON, V. I. & STRATTON, F. (1984). Quantitation of IgG on erythrocytes: correlation of number of IgG molecules per cell with the strength of the direct and indirect antiglobulin tests. *Vox Sang.*, **47**, 73–81.

MIESCHER, P. & HOLLÄNDER, L. (1956). Positiver modifizierter Antiglobulintest (Antiglobulin–Globulin–Kette) bei einem Fall von subakuter Splénomegalie. *Vox Sang.*, **1**, 265–273.

MOLLISON, P. L (1956). *Blood transfusion in Clinical Medicine*, 2nd edn, pp. 165 and 258. Blackwell Scientific Publications, Oxford.

MOLLISON, P. L., ENGELFRIET, C. P. & CONTRERAS, M. (1987). *Blood Transfusion in Clinical Medicine*, 8th edn, pp. 440–441. Blackwell Scientific Publications, Oxford.

MOORE, J. A., DORNER, I. & CHAPLIN, H. JNR (1974). Positive antiglobulin reactions with thawed deglycerolized red blood cells. *Vox Sang.*, **27**, 385–394.

MOORES, P., PUDIFIN, D. & PATEL, P. L. (1975). Severe hemolytic anemia in an adult associated with anti-T. *Transfusion*, **15**, 329–333.

MOREAU, R., DAUSSET, J., BERNARD, J. & MOULLEC, J. (1957). Anémie hémolytique acquise avec polyagglutinabilité des hématies par un nouveau facteur présent dans le sérum humain normal (anti-Tn). *Bull. Mém. Soc. méd. Hôp., Paris*, **73**, 569–587.

MULLARD, G. W., THOMPSON, I. H., LEE, D. & OWEN, W. G. (1981). Strong T-transformation associated with a severe haemolytic reaction in a young infant transfused with packed red cells. *Clin. lab. Haemat.*, **3**, 357–364.

NANCE, S. & GARRATTY, G. (1984). Correlates between in vivo hemolysis and the amount of RBC-bound IgG measured by flow cytofluorometry. *Blood*, **64** (Suppl. 1), 88a (Abstract 26).

NANCE, S. J. & GARRATTY, G. (1987). Application of flow cytometry to immunohematology. *J. immunol. Meth.*, **101**, 127–131.

PARKER, A. C., HABESHAW, T. & CLELAND, J. F. (1972). The demonstration of a 'plasmatic factor' in a case of Coombs' negative haemolytic anaemia. *Scand. J. Haemat.*, **9**, 318–321.

PAYNE, R., SPAET, T. H. & AGGELER, P. M. (1955). An unusual antibody pattern in a case of idiopathic acquired hemolytic anemia. *J. Lab. clin. Med.*, **46**, 245–254.

PETZ, L. D. & GARRATTY, G. (1980). *Acquired Immune Hemolytic Anemias.*, pp. 305–318. Churchill Livingstone, New York.

REID, M. E., ELLISOR, S. S. & AVOY, D. R. (1979). Positive direct antiglobulin test on thawed deglycerolized units of erythrocytes: prediction and prevention. *Amer. J. Hemat.*, **7**, 293–298.

RICE, J. D. JNR & MATHIES, L. A. (1960). Comparison of resistance of reticulocytes and mature erythrocytes to immune hemolysis. Studies in the guinea-pig, rabbit, dog and man. *Arch. Path.*, **70**, 435–440.

RICKARD, K. A., ROBINSON, R. J. & WORLEDGE, S. M. (1969). Acute acquired haemolytic anaemia associated with polyagglutination. *Arch. Dis. Childh.*, **44**, 102–105.

ROSENFIELD, R. E. & JAGATHAMBAL, K. (1978). Antigenic determinants of C3 and C4 complement components on washed erythrocytes of normal persons. *Transfusion*, **18**, 517–523.

ROSSE, W. F. (1974). The detection of small amounts of antibody on the red cell in auto-immune hemolytic anemia. *Ser. Haemat.*, **7**, 358–366.

SALEUN, J. P. & BARET, M. (1977). Test de Coombs direct positif chez des subjects apparemment normaux. *Rev. franç. Transf. Immuno-hémat.*, **20**, 667–669.

SCHNEIDER, W. (1969). Zur Bedeutung sogenannter erythrocytärer Autoantikörper bei Blutspendern. *Blut*, **19**, 564–569.

SCHREIBER, A. D. (1985). Quantitation of RBC-bound immunoglobulin and complement components. In *Immune Hemolytic Anemias (Methods in Hematology, Vol. 12)* (ed. by H. Chaplin Jnr), pp. 155–175. Churchill Livingstone, New York.

SPEISER, P. (1967). Some remarks on human erythrocytic autoantibodies. *Z. Immun-Forsch.*, **132**, 113–124.

SPRINGER, G. F. & TEGTMEYER, H. (1981). Origin of the anti-Thomsen–Friedenreich (T) and Tn agglutinins in man and in white leghorn chicks. *Brit. J. Haemat.*, **47**, 453–460.

STRATTON, F., RAWLINSON, V. I., MERRY, A. H. & THOMSON, E. E. (1983). Positive direct antiglobulin test and normal individuals. II. *Clin. lab. Haemat.*, **5**, 17–21.

STRATTON, F. & RICHARDSON JONES, A. (1955). The reactions between normal human red cells and antiglobulin (Coombs) serum. *J. Immunol.*, **75**, 423–429.

STRATTON, F. & TOVEY, J. H. (1959). Auto-immune erythrocyte sensitization. *Brit. med. J.*, **i**, 115 (Letter).

STUART, A. E. & CUMMING, R. A. (1967). A biological test for injury to the human red cell. *Vox Sang.*, **13**, 270–280.

SZYMANSKI, I. O., HUFF, S. R., SELBOVITZ, L. G. & SHERWOOD, G. K. (1984). Erythrocyte sensitization with monomeric IgM in a patient with hemolytic anemia. *Amer. J. Hemat.*, **17**, 71–77.

SZYMANSKI, I. O., ODGREN, P. R., FOSTIER, N. L. & SNYDER, L. M. (1980). Red blood cell associated

IgG in normal and pathologic states. *Blood*, **55**, 48–54.

Toy, P. T. C. Y., Chin, C. A., Reid, M. E. & Burns, M. A. (1985). Factors associated with positive direct antiglobulin tests in pretransfusion patients: a case-control study. *Vox Sang.*, **49**, 215–220.

Toy, P. T. C. Y., Reid, M. E. & Burns, M. (1985). Positive direct antiglobulin test associated with hyperglobulinemia in acquired immunodeficiency syndrome (AIDS). *Amer. J. Hemat.*, **19**, 145–150.

van Loghem, J. J. (1965). Some comments on auto-antibody induced red cell destruction. *Ann. N. Y. Acad. Sci.*, **124**, 465–476.

van Loghem, J. J., van der Hart, M. & Land, M. E. (1955). Polyagglutinability of red cells as a cause of severe haemolytic transfusion reaction. *Vox Sang. (Amst.)*, **5**, 125–128.

van't Veer, M. B., van Wieringen, P. M. V., van Leeuwen, I., Overbeeke, M. A. M., von dem Borne, A. E. G. Kr. & Engelfriet, C. P. (1981). A negative direct antiglobulin test with strong IgG red cell autoantibodies present in the serum of a patient with autoimmune haemolytic anaemia. *Brit. J. Haemat.*, **49**, 383–386.

Vengelen-Tyler, V., Choy, C. W., Ammerman, H. D. & Kasimian, D. (1985). An IgA autoanti-D associated with autoimmune hemolytic anemia. *Transfusion*, **25**, 471 (Abstract, S 106).

Wallas, C. H., Tanley, P. C. & Gorrell, L. P. (1982). Utilization of a cell separation technique to evaluate patients with a positive direct antiglobulin test. *Transfusion*, **22**, 26–30.

Weiner, W. (1965). 'Coombs positive' 'normal people'. *Proc. 10th Congr. int. Soc. Blood Transfusion, Stockholm 1964. Bibl. haemat.* **23**, 35–39. Karger, Basel.

Worledge, S. M. (1978). The interpretation of a positive direct antiglobulin test. *Brit. J. Haemat.*, **39**, 157–162 (Annotation).

Worledge, S. M. & Blajchman, M. A. (1972). The autoimmune haemolytic anaemias. *Brit. J. Haemat.*, **23**, Suppl., 61–69.

Yam, P., Petz, L. D. & Spath, P. (1982). Detection of IgG sensitization of red cells with ^{125}I staphylococcal protein A. *Amer. J. Hemat.*, **12**, 337–346.

Yam, P., Wilkinson, L., Petz, L. D. & Garratty, G. (1980). Studies on hemolytic anemia in pregnancy with evidence for autoimmunization in a patient with a negative direct antiglobulin (Coombs') test. *Amer. J. Hemat.*, **8**, 23–29.

Auto-immune haemolytic anaemia (AIHA): cold-antibody syndromes I: idiopathic types: clinical presentation and haematological and serological findings

Early observations on auto-agglutination   *210*

Recent reviews   *210*

Occurrence of high-titre cold agglutinins in haemolytic anaemia   *212*

Cold-haemagglutinin disease (CHAD)   *213*
  Early case reports   *213*

Clinical features of CHAD   *215*

Haematological findings in typical CHAD   *219*
  Serum proteins in CHAD   *223*

Serological findings in CHAD: a summary   *223*
  Direct antiglobulin test   *223*
  Cold-agglutinin titres   *223*
  Lysis of normal erythrocytes   *225*

Lysis of trypsinized erythrocytes   *226*

Resistance of erythrocytes that have survived lysis by cold auto-antibodies *in vivo* to lysis *in vitro*   *226*

Lysis of PNH erythrocytes   *228*

Differences in serological findings between individual patients   *228*

Atypical chronic cold-antibody AIHA   *228*

Concurrence of warm and cold auto-antibodies in AIHA   *230*

Acute cold-antibody AIHA in infants and children   *233*

Chronic cold-antibody AIHA in children   *234*

Cold-antibody AIHA in association with neoplasms (excluding lymphoproliferative disorders)   *234*

EARLY OBSERVATIONS ON AUTO-AGGLUTINATION

Autohaemagglutination of chilled blood was first described by Landsteiner in 1903 as occurring in various mammalian species, and Clough and Richter (1918) have been usually quoted as being the first to report on a raised content of auto-agglutinin in a human serum from a patient with a respiratory infection and to measure the titre.

Mino (1924) seems to have been the first to have used the term panhaemagglutinin (panemoagglutinina) and Amzel and Hirszfeld (1925) the phrase cold agglutination (Kälteagglutination). Since then the clinical significance of cold agglutination and the nature of the phenomenon have been extensively studied. Early reviews which reflected the state of knowledge at the time of writing include those of Bonnard (1933), Wiener (1935), Rosenthal and Corten (1937), Stats and Wasserman (1943), Young (1946), Savonen (1948), Benhamou, Zermati and Assus (1948), Hennemann (1951), Pisciotta (1955), Dacie (1957, 1962, 1964) and Schubothe (1958).

The early reports associated auto-agglutination and/or cold agglutination with a wide variety of pathological processes, but liver disease (Li Chen-Pien, 1926; Wyschegorodzewa, 1926; Debenedetti, 1919; Galli and Mussafia, 1939) and haemolytic anaemia (Rosenthal and Corten, 1937) were perhaps most frequently mentioned. An association with pregnancy (Kligler, 1922) and with pernicious anaemia (Koepplin, 1936) was also recorded. In more recent years it has been the association between raised titres of cold agglutinins and haemolytic anaemia of unknown causation or accompanying malignant lymphoproliferative diseases or following mycoplasma pneumonia or viral infections that has received the most attention.

RECENT REVIEWS

A great deal of progress has been made, too, in defining the immunochemical nature of the cold

Table 28.1   Cold-antibody auto-immune haemolytic anaemia: clinical syndromes.

Syndrome	Chronic or transient	Severity of haemolysis	Acrocyanosis	Haemoglobinuria
Cold-haemagglutinin disease (CHAD)	Chronic	Slight to moderate	Present	Usually present in cold weather
Atypical CHAD, includes 'mixed' cold and warm AIHA	Chronic	Moderate to severe	Not usually present	Seldom present
Cold-antibody AIHA in infancy and childhood (excluding PCH)	Almost always transient	Usually severe	Absent	May be present
Post-mycoplasma pneumonia haemolytic anaemia	Transient	Moderate to severe	Not usually present	May be present
Post-infectious mononucleosis haemolytic anaemia	Transient	Moderate	Absent	Rarely present
Paroxysmal cold haemoglobinuria (PCH)	Usually transient	Moderate to severe	Rarely present	Present
Cold AIHA associated with lymphoproliferative diseases	Chronic	Usually moderate	Absent	Not present

antibodies and their specificity. This aspect of cold auto-agglutination has been ably summarized in Roelcke's (1989) review. Other valuable reviews published between 1965 and 1991 include those of Evans, Turner and Bingham (1965), Schubothe (1965, 1966), Olesen (1966, 1967), Levin and Ritzmann (1966), Harboe (1971), Roelcke (1974), Frank, Atkinson and Gadek (1977), Pruzanski and Shumak (1977), Pruzanski and Katz (1984), Issitt (1985), Mollison, Engelfriet and Contreras (1987), Rosse (1990) and Nydegger, Kazatchkine and Miescher (1991).

It is now realized in fact that cold auto-antibodies lead to haemolysis in a number of clinical syndromes (Table 28.1). It is also known that the antibodies vary in their specificity and immunochemical nature (see Chapter 9). Thus the auto-antibody of CHAD is almost always anti-I in specificity, while anti-i is a relatively common cause of haemolysis in AIHA in lymphoproliferative diseases. Anti-i seems too, to be the characteristic antibody in infectious mononucleosis complicated by haemolytic anaemia. The antibodies are almost always IgM in nature: much less commonly they are IgG. However, the anti-P antibody of PCH is characteristically IgG.

OCCURRENCE OF HIGH-TITRE COLD AGGLUTININS IN HAEMOLYTIC ANAEMIA

Stats and Wasserman's (1943) review is a major and valuable work, and in their Table 1 they listed as many as 94 references to papers, published between 1890 and 1943, in which cold haemagglutination had been described. In 32 of the papers the patients described had suffered from haemolytic anaemia or haemoglobinuria, according to Stats and Wasserman's summaries. In all, 216 references were listed in the bibliography. Many of the earlier authors were in doubt as to the significance of their observations. Stats and Wasserman shared their doubt. However, although they felt that in the 'great majority' of cases cold haemagglutination was innocuous and 'may be looked upon as a laboratory curiosity', they concluded that 'in some cases of hemolytic

anemia, paroxysmal cold hemoglobinuria, Raynaud's syndrome, and peripheral gangrene the cold hemagglutination is of pathogenetic significance'. They stressed that cold agglutinins are constantly present in normal human and animal blood; also that in most instances the higher the titre the broader the thermal amplitude. They concluded that cold agglutinins in pathological sera differ from those in normal serum only in that the titres and thermal amplitude are likely to be greater.

By the late 1940s it was becoming apparent that there existed an obscure and rather rare syndrome, which affected almost exclusively elderly subjects, that was characterized by mild to moderate haemolytic anaemia and by the presence in the patient's serum of cold agglutinins at high titres, so that massive and rapid auto-agglutination took place if their blood, after withdrawal, was allowed to cool to room temperature. In cold weather the patients suffered from what was often described as Raynaud's phenomena* affecting the fingers, toes and ear-lobes and sometimes this led to local gangrene. Haemoglobinuria, too, often developed in cold weather. This is the condition now widely referred to as the cold-haemagglutinin disease or CHAD.

Cold auto-antibodies active at unusually high temperatures and/or present at moderately raised titres are not uncommonly present in the serum of patients forming well-defined warm IgG auto-antibodies. While in most instances they are probably not a cause of increased haemolysis, occasionally they may well contribute to this (p. 230). In other (unusual) cases, warm-acting

---

* Rosse (1990, p. 568) pointed out that describing the skin manifestations as Raynaud's phenomena is strictly speaking incorrect. Raynaud's disease, the consequence of vasoconstriction, leads in sequence to three phenomena: first, the affected part becomes white and perhaps numb; then it becomes swollen, stiff and livid, and finally, when the vasoconstriction passes off, the part becomes red due to reactive hyperaemia. In CHAD the changes, which Rosse refers to as acrocyanosis (literally 'blue extremity'), differ from those of Raynaud's disease in the absence of an initial white phase—there is in fact no vasoconstriction, and in that the blue cyanotic phase is more intense; the affected part may in fact become deep purple. There is, too, no final hyperaemic phase (see also p. 218). Both processes—vasoconstriction or arrest of the circulation due to auto-agglutination—can, however, lead to local gangrene.

antibodies, demonstrable by the use of enzyme-treated cells, may be present in the patient's serum in addition to cold auto-antibodies at raised titres acting on unmodified cells, and it seems likely, in some cases at least, that these warm antibodies, as well as the cold antibodies, play a part in bringing about haemolysis.

In this chapter will be reviewed the clinical presentation and haematological and serological findings of the first three syndromes listed in Table 28.1. Further details of the in-vitro behaviour, specificity and nature of the auto-antibodies are considered in Chapter 29. The haemolytic anaemias following mycoplasma pneumonia and infectious mononucleosis and other virus infections, and paroxysmal cold haemoglobinuria (PCH), are reviewed in Chapters 30–32.

COLD-HAEMAGGLUTININ DISEASE (CHAD)

Early case reports

Recognition that acrocyanosis might be associated with cold auto-agglutination dates at least as far back as the two reports on the aetiology of Raynaud's disease by Iwai and Mei-Sai (1925, 1926). Their 1925 account is particularly interesting.

Their patient was a 36-year-old Chinese giving a 6 years' history of Raynaud's disease. He did not apparently suffer from haemoglobinuria, nor was there any statement as to whether he was anaemic. His serum, however, contained a high-titre cold agglutinin (titre 1000 at 0°C after 10 minutes) which acted *in vitro* at temperatures up to 30°C on normal corpuscles as well as on those of the patient. Iwai and Mei-Sai demonstrated that the circulation of the patient's blood through fine tubes was impeded when the blood was cooled at 5°C and suggested that the Raynaud's phenomena were similarly the result of the capillaries in life being mechanically obstructed by auto-agglutinated corpuscles. They also reported that irrigation of the eye with saline cooled to 10°C arrested the flow of blood through the conjunctival capillaries as viewed through a corneal microscope. In their second case, a woman aged 78, Iwai and Meisai (1926) showed that cooling of the fingers was associated with breaking of the column of blood in the capillaries of the nail bed.

The association of acrocyanosis with intravascular haemolysis and haemoglobinuria and a raised titre of cold agglutinin seems to have been first recognized by Roth (1935), Ernstene and Gardner (1935) and Salén (1935).

Roth's (1935) patient was a man aged 59, who suffered from acrocyanosis affecting his hands, feet and nose when exposed to mild degrees of cold. General chilling had provoked haemoglobinuria. His blood underwent rapid auto-agglutination after withdrawal which was reversed by warming. Ernstene and Gardner's (1935) account was more complete: their patient, a man of 38, had attacks of haemoglobinuria and cyanosis of his ears, nose, fingers and toes on exposure to cold. His blood auto-agglutinated at room temperature, erythrocyte counts were difficult to carry out and the cold-agglutinin titre was reported as 1280. He was anaemic, with a haemoglobin of 10.5 g/dl.

Salén's (1935) case was also remarkable. His patient, a man aged 50, had repeated attacks of cyanosis affecting the ear-lobes, hands and feet, and also haemoglobinuria, in cold weather. His serum contained a high-titre cold agglutinin active to a titre of 1024 at 0°C; agglutinination reversed at temperatures greater than 30°C. A remarkable feature of this case was the way in which both the patient's erythrocytes and normal cells underwent haemolysis after exposure to the patient's serum.

There are many other accounts in the literature prior to 1935 in which high-titre cold agglutinins or auto-agglutination occurring at room temperature has been mentioned but they make rather baffling and unsatisfactory reading, at least from the point of view of trying to determine whether the patients described had been suffering from the syndrome under discussion.

The association of haemoglobinuria, apparently precipitated by cold, and acrocyanosis and/or gangrene of exposed parts of the body had also been reported in the earlier literature, even in that of the latter half of the nineteenth century. Unfortunately, these reports do not mention the vital point as to the presence or absence of auto-agglutination. In some, the result of an erythrocyte count was reported without comment (e.g. Henry, 1894). Most of these patients seem likely to have been suffering from paroxysmal cold haemoglobinuria (see Ch. 32 for references). However, in some instances the cold-haemagglutination disease is a possibility.

Druitt (1873), for instance, described in great detail the history, extending over 6 years, of a doctor aged 51 in whom cold or chilling brought on attacks of numbness of the feet and purplish-blue discolouration of the hands which were followed by the passage of bloody urine ('haematinuria'). The patient eventually obtained relief by living in India. Druitt believed that the nervous system was involved as well as the blood and wondered whether the latter was not undergoing 'a haemolysis, a decomposition or necrosis of blood globules'.

The reports of Roth, Ernstene and Gardner and Salén in 1935 were followed by a succession of papers, but the syndrome did not receive wide recognition until the early 1950s.

Relatively early reports, filling in details here and there, include those of McCombs and McElroy (1937), Formijne (1940), Benians and Feasby (1941), Stats and Bullowa (1943), Stats (1945), Heilmeyer and Schubothe (1946, 1948), Heilmeyer, Hahn and Schubothe (1947), Whittle, Lyell and Gatman (1947), Baumgartner (1948), Benhamou, Zermati and Assus (1948), Bateman (1949), Johnsson (1949), Malley and Hickey (1949), Schubothe and Altmann (1950), Bertoli and Baratta (1951), Ferriman et al. (1951), Gualandi and Lorenzini (1951), Chein, Chren Chiu and Hwan-Wen You (1952), van Loghem et al. (1952), Nelson and Marshall (1953), Bonnin (1954), Dacie (1954, p. 175), Goudemand and Ropartz (1954), Hawley and Gordon (1954), Rørvik (1954), André et al. (1955), Baumgartner (1955), Conn (1955), Mortara and Martinetti (1955), Pisciotta, Downer and Hinz (1955), Delage, Gauvreau and Simard (1956), Saita and Martelli (1956), Wiener et al. (1956), Dacie (1957), Gaddy and Powell (1958), Schubothe (1958) and Firkin, Blackwell and Johnston (1959). All the patients referred to in these papers were anaemic and had high-titre high-thermal-amplitude cold agglutinins in their serum; not all,

however, were reported as having haemoglobin-uria but most had suffered from varying degrees of acrocyanosis.

Stats's (1945) paper was particularly important for he stressed how easily the slightest manipulation of strong suspensions of agglutinated cells *in vitro* caused lysis of some of the cells and how, if the suspensions used were less than 4% in concentration, artefactual lysis could be avoided. He mentioned a serum with a titre at 4°C as high as 30 000. Heilmeyer, Hahn and Schubothe (1947) recorded a still higher titre, 131 072!, and noted that the upper limit of the antibody's activity was 33°C. Later, Heilmeyer and Schubothe (1948) reported that with three sera in-vitro agglutination actually took place at 37°C.

Johnsson (1949), too, reported an instance of cold agglutination stretching up to 37°C. His case was a remarkable one. The patient, who was suffering from anaemia of unknown causation, had a serum which was shown to agglutinate each of 80 blood samples to titres of 32 000 at 2°C and 2000 at 37°C. The patient's own erythrocytes, too, were also strongly agglutinated at 37°C, but they were far less sensitive, the titre at 37°C being 8.

Dacie (1950), in his description of the lytic activity of sera containing high-titre cold agglutinins, included observations on one of the patients (Case 3) whose clinical history was described by Ferriman et al. (1951). The interesting point that was established was that lysis *in vitro* of normal erythrocytes was greatly enhanced if the serum had been acidified before the addition of the suspension of erythrocytes: the optimum pH of the cell serum suspension was 6.6–6.9. It was also shown that it was the adsorption of the antibody that was enhanced by lowering the pH.

Ferriman and co-workers (1951) described three patients suffering from CHAD: their antibody titres were 32 000–128 000 at 2–5°C, with the upper thermal limit for the antibodies' activity 29–31°C.

Rørvik (1954) recorded a serum with an exceptionally high titre, 168 000 000! The likelihood of 'carry over' of serum in carrying out the titration must, however, be considered in this case.

Mortara and Martinetti's (1955) report is of particular interest because this contains a reference to the relative inagglutinability of neonatal erythrocytes (see p. 251).

Pisciotta, Downer and Hinz (1955) described the effect of albumin and trypsinization of the erythrocytes in raising the thermal range of cold antibodies and, in the case of trypsin, in increasing the titres at 3°C.

Schubothe's (1958) monograph contains further details on the effect of temperature and pH and on the speed of adsorption of antibody, which he found to be almost instantaneous. The use of albumin as diluent and trypsinization of the test cells were reported to increase the titre at 0°C fourfold.

Schubothe (1952) seems to have been the first to use of term *Kälteagglutininkranheit*.

By the end of the 1950s the detailed reports then available made it possible to describe with a fair degree of accuracy the clinical feature of the syndrome. The description given below is based on that given in the second edition of this book (Dacie, 1962, pp. 369–374).

CLINICAL FEATURES OF THE COLD-HAEMAGGLUTININ DISEASE (CHAD)

Age and sex. The disease seems particularly to affect relatively elderly subjects and both sexes are affected; the age distribution contrasts sharply with that of warm-antibody AIHA (see Fig. 22.1, p. 15). The ages of 21 patients investigated by the author are shown in Fig. 28.1: 16 of them

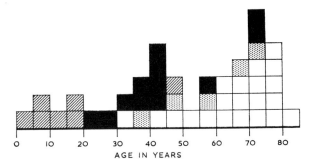

Fig. 28.1   Age distribution of 43 patients suffering from auto-immune haemolytic anaemia of the cold-antibody type.
Open squares = idiopathic cases; dotted squares = secondary cases; filled-in squares = post-mycoplasma pneumonia cases; diagonally ruled squares = paroxysmal cold haemoglobinuria.

were women and five were men. Later, Dacie and Worlledge (1969) reported that they had investigated 38 patients between 1948 and 1968: 22 were women and 16 men. Worlledge (1967) had stated that the average age of 29 patients had been 66.

General features. Anaemia is variable and not as a rule severe, and it is interesting to note that in only two of the 12 patients reviewed by Ferriman et al. (1951) was the haemoglobin reported as falling below 7.4 g/dl. Anaemia may be slight in warm weather, and most patients become definitely more anaemic in winter time (Fig. 28.2); some, at least, improve without treatment if kept warm in bed (Fig. 28.3). The disorder is typically a very chronic one. One of the

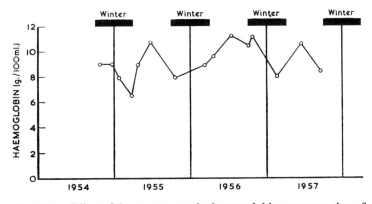

Fig. 28.2   Effect of the seasons on the haemoglobin concentration of a patient with cold-haemagglutinin disease.
[From Dacie (1957).]

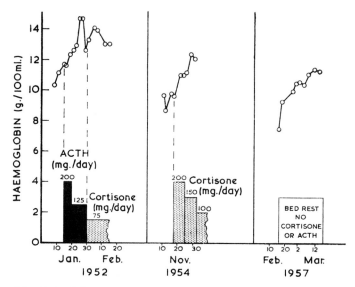

Fig. 28.3   Effect of treatment with steroids and bed rest on the haemoglobin concentration of a patient with cold-haemagglutinin disease.

[From Dacie (1957).]

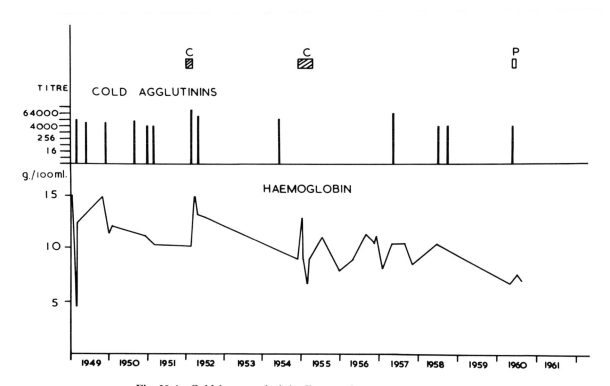

Fig. 28.4   Cold-haemagglutinin disease (Case 9 of Dacie, 1962).

Changes in haemoglobin and cold-agglutinin titre at 4°C in a patient observed between 1949 and 1961. C represents treatment with cortisone; P treatment with penicillamine.

patients described by Ferriman et al. was known to have been affected in 1938; she died of her disease in 1953, 15 years later. Another (Case 9 of Dacie, 1962, see below), a woman aged 79, had suffered from CHAD for at least 13 years (Fig. 28.4), and many other instances of a prolonged course can be found in the literature. The disorder at its best remains static; at its worst it typically only progresses slowly in intensity. The description by Gottlieb (1964) of a patient who spontaneously went into remission is thus most unusual.

Gottlieb's patient was a 40-year-old male who had suffered from symptoms typical of severe CHAD for 18 months. He then spontaneously and gradually improved so that 2 years after the onset of his illness his haemoglobin, at one time as low as 4.8 g/dl, had risen to 15.3 g/dl and the cold-agglutinin titre, at one time 2048, had fallen to 80.

The clinical history of Case 9 of Dacie (1962) is quoted below as typical of the syndrome.

A woman aged 66 first showed signs of CHAD in the winter of 1947, when she found that her hands, nose and ears became bluish purple in cold weather. In January 1949 a patch of gangrene appeared on her right thumb but this eventually healed. On particularly cold days she experienced haemoglobinuria.

She attended hospital at intervals up to December 1960. Her symptoms had not altered, except those associated with ischaemic heart disease which had become more serious in the last 2 years. Every winter she had been troubled with acrocyanosis, pallor and jaundice and haemoglobinuria, and had been forced to keep indoors in cold weather; in the warmer months of the year she had been generally free from symptoms and was able to lead a more or less normal life. Her blood picture had fluctuated correspondingly (Fig. 28.2), but the serological findings were remarkably constant. The effects of attempts at treatment with corticosteroids and of bed rest (and warmth) are shown in Fig. 28.3.

Physical signs. The patients' appearance is often dominated by acrocyanosis (described as Raynaud's phenomena by some authors). Their pallor and jaundice do not present any special features; as in warm-antibody AIHA the intensity of these signs depends upon the rate of haemolysis and the ability of the liver to excrete bilirubin.

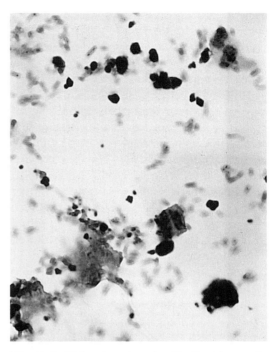

Fig. 28.5   Urine deposit stained by Perls's reaction to demonstrate haemosiderin.
From a patient with cold-haemagglutinin disease.

The spleen seems to be palpably enlarged only in a minority of patients. The liver may be slightly enlarged but this is not usually a conspicuous sign. The faeces are dark and contain excess stercobilin and the urine typically contains some excess of urobilin. As discussed below, haemoglobinuria often occurs in cold weather and haemosiderinuria may be conspicuous and is a more constant sign of intravascular haemolysis (see Fig. 28.5).

A tendency to easy bruising has been recorded (Firkin, Blackwell and Johnston, 1959) but this is an unusual symptom, as was the unusual tendency to venous thrombosis following venepuncture described by Heilmeyer and Schubothe (1948).

Acrocyanosis. Typically, the patients complain that in cold weather their fingers become cold and stiff, and become purplish in colour and slightly painful and numb, and that their toes, ear lobes and the tip of their nose may be similarly affected. An excellent colour photograph is to be found in Baumgartner's (1954) paper. The phenomena are quickly reversible in a warm environment and most patients are free from these symptoms in summer time.

Occasionally actual gangrene of a digit or digits develops (e.g. as described by Ferriman et al., 1951; Nelson and Marshall 1953; Gaddy and Powell, 1958; Mitchell, Pegrum and Gill, 1974). Rørvik (1954) reported even more serious effects: oedematous swelling and ulceration of the ears and weeping ulcers secondary to necrosis of the skin and subcutaneous tissues. He also noticed that pressure applied to the skin appeared to precipitate underlying necrosis. Saita and Martelli (1956) reported gangrene of the whole left hand; their patient had, however, worked with vibrating tools in the past and was known to have suffered from local angiospasm before the development of the cold agglutinins.

The association of actual tissue gangrene with the presence of a cryoglobulin, e.g. in the cases of Ferriman et al. (1951), Rørvik (1954) and Gaddy and Powell (1958), led to the idea that precipitation of cryoglobulin rather than auto-haemagglutination brings about the gangrene. In favour of this explanation is the observation that a similar clinical vascular syndrome may be produced by cryoglobulinaemia not associated with high-titre cold agglutinins (Berndt, 1956). A contributory factor may be local vascular degenerative changes. In some cases both cryoglobulins and high-titre cold agglutinins have been found to be present in the same serum, e.g. by Conn (1955). In some cases at least it is the cold agglutinin which is the cold-precipitable protein (see p. 243).

The pathogenesis of the acrocyanosis brought on by local chilling in patients whose blood contains high-titre high-thermal-amplitude cold agglutinins, but is free of cold-precipitable proteins, is now generally agreed to be due to auto-agglutination within the blood vessels bringing the circulation to a halt.

As already referred to (p. 213), this mechanism was first suggested by Iwai and Mei-Sai (1925, 1926) and demonstrated by them by observing the effect of chilling on the conjunctival and nail-bed capillaries. Good illustrations of the clumped erythrocytes and arrested circulation in conjunctival capillaries were given in the papers of Baumgartner (1948) and Harders (1958). Marshall, Shepherd and Thompson (1953) and

Hillestad (1959) showed that the blood-flow reactions to chilling are quite distinct from those in Raynaud's disease proper. No evidence of an abnormal vascular response could be obtained. Hillestad (1959) pointed out that the occurrence of local acrocyanosis depended on the titre and thermal amplitude of the cold agglutinins, the viscosity of the blood and the individual patient's vascular responses to cold. Peripheral vascular stasis can be diagnosed, according to Hillestad, by the absence of blanching in the cyanosed areas on pressure and by the failure of cold vasodilatation which normally should occur at temperatures below 15°C. The arrest in circulation is not simply confined to the superficial blood vessels; the circulation in whole parts may be arrested. For instance, Hillestad showed in one patient that when the ambient temperature was 17°C the circulation in his hand and feet rapidly decreased, while at 14°C it was arrested.

Haemoglobinuria. Most patients experience haemoglobinuria in particularly cold weather, but its frequency varies from patient to patient. In some, haemoglobinuria seems never to develop despite the fact that acrocyanosis is intense in cold weather (e.g. Case 2 of Ferriman et al., 1951); in others, such as the patient described by Bonnin (1954), haemoglobinuria was a striking and frequent symptom. It is possible that the presence or absence of haemoglobinuria is correlated with subtle differences in the ability of the antibodies to bring about lysis by complement (see p. 429). The haemosiderosis of the kidneys (Fig. 28.6), and the probable continuous occurrence of haemosiderinuria in patients not developing haemoglobinuria, is simply a reflection of less intense, but nevertheless intravascular, haemolysis.

Nephrotic syndrome. Poth, Sharp and Schrier (1970) described a most unusual occurrence—CHAD associated with the nephrotic syndrome. Their patient, a female aged 66, was moderately severely anaemic and suffered from acrocyanosis. Her serum contained a cryoprecipitable high-titre, high-thermal-amplitude and markedly lytic cold antibody. The dominant features of her illness were, however, the manifestations of the nephrotic syndrome; and Poth, Sharp and Schrier suggested that the IgM cold antibody, alone or in combination with complement, was aetiologically related to the nephrotic syndrome 'via attack on the glomerular basement membrane'.

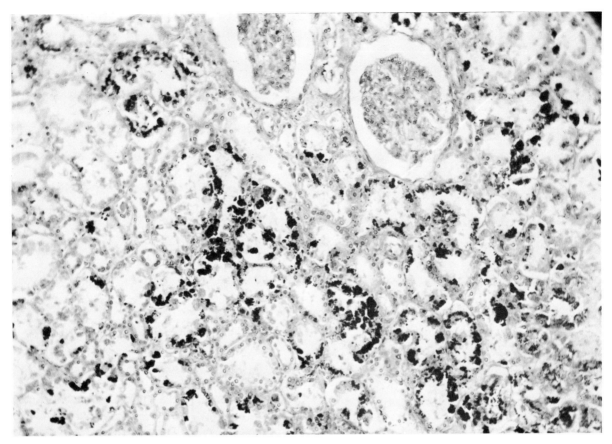

Fig. 28.6   Photomicrograph of a section of a kidney from a patient with cold-haemagglutinin disease (Case 2 of Ferriman et al., 1951).
Perls's reaction to demonstrate haemosiderin. × 175.

HAEMATOLOGICAL FINDINGS IN TYPICAL COLD-HAEMAGGLUTININ DISEASE (CHAD)

Auto-agglutination. A marked degree of macroscopic auto-agglutination occurring within a few seconds when blood samples are allowed to cool below body temperature is a characteristic sign, as is the rapidity with which the gross auto-agglutination reverses to give a smooth normal appearance when the blood sample is placed in a 37°C water-bath. Equally characteristic is the clumping observed in diluted blood prepared for manual blood counting unless the strictest care is taken to keep the blood, pipette and diluting fluid at or about 37°C. It is the ready reversibility and the grossness of the agglutination which distinguishes cold auto-agglutination from the finer irreversible auto-agglutination just visible to the naked eye which is characteristic of erythrocytes coated by warm antibodies.

Associated with, and in consequence of, the massive auto-agglutination is an abnormal tendency of concentrated cell-plasma or cell-serum suspensions to undergo lysis *in vitro*, as stressed by Stats (1945), and unless care is taken it is difficult to obtain unhaemolysed plasma or serum. If, however, the blood is delivered by means of a needle and a short piece of tubing into a container previously warmed to 37°C, or if a previously warmed syringe is used to withdraw the blood, unhaemolysed plasma or serum can be regularly obtained. Similarly, good films may be made if slides previously warmed to 37°C are used (see Fig. 28.7). Films made on slides not warmed above room temperature usually

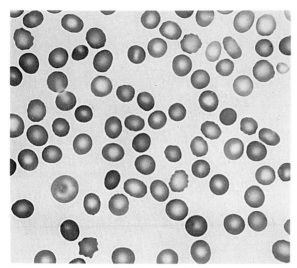

Fig. 28.7 Photomicrograph of a blood film of a patient with cold-haemagglutinin disease made at 37°C.
Auto-agglutination has completely dispersed. There is slight anisocytosis and spherocytosis. × 700.

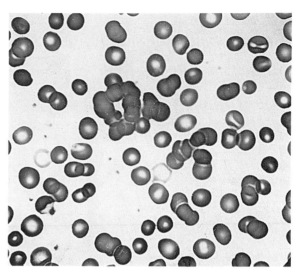

Fig. 28.9 Photomicrograph of a blood film of a patient with cold-haemagglutinin disease (Case 10 of Dacie, 1962).
Auto-agglutination has not completely dispersed. There is slight anisocytosis and spherocytosis. × 700.

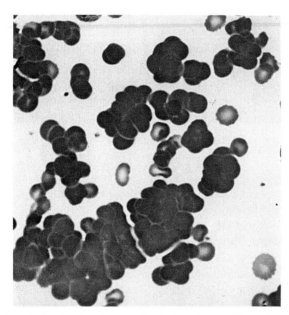

Fig. 28.8 Photomicrograph of a blood film of a patient with cold-haemagglutinin disease made at room temperature.
There is massive auto-agglutination but little spherocytosis. × 700.

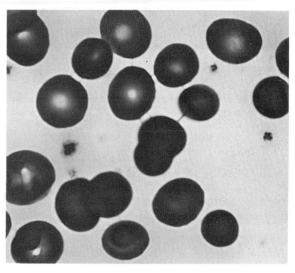

Fig. 28.10 Photomicrograph of the blood film shown in Fig. 28.8 at a higher magnification.
Fine filaments of cell membrane link adjacent cells. × 1700.

present the characteristic appearance shown in Fig. 28.8. Exceptionally, with a very high-thermal-amplitude antibody, agglutination fails to disperse completely at 37°C. In Fig. 28.9 is shown the appearance of a film, spread at 37°C, made from the blood of Case 10 of Dacie (1962). At a higher magnification (Fig. 28.10), fine threads of membrane can be seen still linking together cells in the process of being dissociated by warmth.

Whole-blood viscosity. In a careful study,

Girolami, Cella and Patrassi (1976) showed that the whole blood of a patient suffering from typical CHAD underwent a significant increase in viscosity when cooled from 37°C to 32°C compared to that of a patient with a chronic haemorrhagic anaemia who had a similar haematocrit. The patient's plasma viscosity was similar to that of a normal control both at 37°C and at 32°C.

Blood picture

The findings in five patients studied by the author (Dacie, 1962) are reproduced in Table 28.2. The erythrocyte count and haemoglobin data are in each case minimum values.

Erythrocytes. When looked at in films made on warmed slides, the erythrocytes usually appear to be less abnormal than in warm-antibody AIHA: anisocytosis and macrocytosis are less marked and poikilocytes are usually inconspicuous. Spherocytosis is less intense (Fig. 28.7). Polychromasia will be present according to the reticulocyte count. Nucleated erythrocytes are seldom present in large numbers. Erythrophagocytosis cannot usually be seen in films of freshly drawn blood but it has been described (Baumgartner, 1948): it can be seen more frequently in blood which has been incubated or in buffy-coat preparations (Fig. 3.30, Vol. 1). Schubothe and Müller (1955) showed that local erythrophagocytosis, as well as massive haemolysis, developed in the blood of a CHAD patient whose finger, to which a ligature had been applied, was immersed for 30 minutes in water at 20°C.

Erythrophagocytosis can, too, be readily demonstrated if normal erythrocytes are suspended at room temperature (20–22°C) in a CHAD patient's serum that is capable (after acidification to pH 6.5–6.8) of bringing about lysis under these conditions, if normal leucocytes are added to the mixture (Fig. 28.11).

Absolute values. The MCV is normal or slightly increased and the MCHC usually normal (Table 28.2).

It should be noted that the presence of high-titre cold auto-agglutinins may result in erroneous absolute

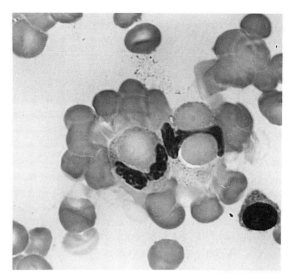

Fig. 28.11   Cold-haemagglutinin disease (Case 10 of Dacie, 1962).
Erythrophagocytosis resulting from adding a fresh suspension of leucocytes to normal I-positive erythrocytes suspended in the patient's acidified serum at 20°C in the presence of fresh human serum complement. × 1260.

values, if measured by automated means. Spurious macrocytosis was recorded by Hattersley et al. (1971) and Petrucci, Dunne and Chapman (1971) using model S Coulter counters, as well as high values for MCH and MCHC (>36 g/dl). These high figures result from erroneously low erythrocyte counts due to the persistence in the diluted blood suspension of agglutinates. Subsequent confirmatory reports include those of Komarmy and Barnes (1972), De Lange, Eernisse and Veltkamp (1972) and Bessman and Banks (1980).

Reticulocyte count. Slight to moderate increases are the rule (Table 28.2). There are some data, however, that suggest that erythropoiesis may sometimes be (perhaps often is) relatively ineffective.

Cazzola, Barosi and Ascari (1983) described two women aged 65 and 61, respectively, suffering from CHAD. Features of their illness were the low reticulocyte counts (33 and 54 × 10^9/l), despite low haemoglobin levels (6.2 and 7.7 g/dl), hyperplastic erythroid bone marrow and an only moderately reduced mean erythrocyte life-span (67 and 45 days, normal 88–141 days). Erythrokinetic studies using ^{59}Fe-transferrin indicated marked ineffective erythropoiesis, and it was suggested that the high-thermal-amplitude cold antibodies were damaging the erythrocyte precursors. Cazzola, Barosi and Ascari suggested that ineffective erythropoiesis may often be a

Table 28.2 Representative haematological data in cases of auto-immune haemolytic anaemia of the idiopathic cold-antibody type.

Patient	Erythrocytes (minimum) ($\times 10^{12}$/l)	Haemoglobin (minimum) (g/dl)	MCV (mean) (fl)	MCHC (mean) (%)	Reticulocytes (maximum) (%)	Leucocytes (range) (per µl)	Platelets (range) (per µl)	Bilirubin (maximum) (mg/dl)	Comment
Cold-haemagglutinin disease									
A.D. (Case 9)*	1.8	6.9	101	32	16	2800–11000	170000–320000	2.0	The cold-antibody formation has persisted for at least 14 years.
L.S. (Case 14)†	1.8	6.2	109	34	16	1800–8000	50000–150000	2.5	Died of an anaplastic carcinoma of pancreas. This was considered to be a coincidental disease
L.T. (Case 11)*	1.5	5.6	111	33	19	3000–17000	190000–570000	7.8	Patient died aged 76 of miliary tuberculosis and tuberculous osteitis, possibly exacerbated by steroid therapy
E.W. (Case 10)*	1.7	7.3	129	33	24	11000–13000	280000		A relatively young patient, aged 42, whose cold antibody has an exceptional thermal range
Atypical case, without acrocyanosis and haemoglobinuria									
L.R. (Case 13)†	2.1	8.7	113	34	8	1800–11000	40000–280000	2.5	Patient died aged 61 of heart failure due to pulmonary hypertension following multiple pulmonary emboli (see *Brit. med. J.*, 1960)

* = Described by Dacie (1962). † = Described by Dacie (1954).

significant factor in the production of anaemia in CHAD. They quoted the earlier data of Samson et al. (1976) who had included one patient with CHAD amongst 11 patients in whom the incorporation of [^{51}N]-aminolaevulinic acid and [^{15}N]glycine into haem and early labelled bilirubin had been measured. These techniques, too, had indicated that erythropoiesis in the CHAD patient was markedly ineffective (45% of the total erythropoiesis).

Leucocytes and platelets. The counts are usually normal, but both leucopenia and thrombocytopenia may be encountered (see Table 28.2).

Osmotic fragility. This may be normal but often it is slightly increased (Fig. 23.12, p. 64). The tests should ideally be carried out at 37°C and because rise in temperature increases osmotic resistance the normal standard range cannot then be used for comparative purposes.

Mechanical fragility. This test is inappropriate as auto-agglutinated whole blood undergoes marked haemolysis if manipulated in any way.

Serum proteins in CHAD

Amongst the 85 patients with AIHA whose serum proteins had been estimated by Christenson and Dacie (1957) were 10 patients suffering from idiopathic CHAD. Their total serum protein concentration (5.0–8.0 g/dl, mean 7.0 g/dl) did not differ from that of 41 normal controls. However, the γ-globulin concentration tended to be higher than normal — patients, range 1.10– 2.69 g/dl, mean 1.72 g/dl; normal controls, range 0.78–1.73 g/dl, mean 1.34 g/dl. Moreover, an abnormal γ_1 peak could be seen on paper electrophoresis in nine of the 10 cases. Later work (see p. 241) established that the γ_1 peak was caused by the presence of monoclonal (γM) cold agglutinin.

Harboe and Torsvik (1969) provided further quantitative data. The sera of 15 patients with chronic CHAD had been studied. Each serum contained a monoclonal γM (IgM) globulin: in the 10 sera in which γM peaks had been visible on agar electrophoresis the γM concentration was estimated to range from 0.31 to 2.45 g/dl. Serial observations were carried out for up to 3 years, during which time the serum γM concentrations, and the cold-agglutinin titres, were virtually unchanged.

SEROLOGICAL FINDINGS IN THE COLD-HAEMAGGLUTININ DISEASE: A SUMMARY

The description by the author of the serological findings in CHAD (Dacie, 1962, pp. 465–487) had been based on studies carried out on 16 patients. This description forms the basis of the following summary. Further details of the reactions of the antibodies *in vitro* and of their specificity and immunochemistry are given in Chapter 29 (pp. 241–273).

Direct antiglobulin test (DAT)

This is typically positive using anti-complement sera, even when care is taken to avoid chilling the blood after withdrawal by delivering blood taken in a warmed syringe directly into saline at 37°C. Reactions with anti-IgG and IgM sera are almost always negative.

Cold-agglutinin titres

In the great majority of patients the titres at 2–4°C will be found to range between 1024 and 512 000. In individual patients, however, the titres remain generally constant over long periods of time or may slowly increase. In patients receiving chemotherapy a fall in titre parallels any clinical response (see. p. 503).

The fall in titre on rise in temperature does not run strictly parallel from case to case. There is usually, however, a striking loss of activity as the temperature rises above 20°C (Fig. 28.12) and the upper thermal limit for the detection of definite agglutination using normal adult group-O erythrocytes ranges between 25 and 37°C; in most instances 30–32°C is the limit (Table 28.3). In one of the author's 16 patients normal erythrocytes were, however, agglutinated in undiluted serum at 37°C — the patient's own cells were, however, not agglutinated at this temperature.

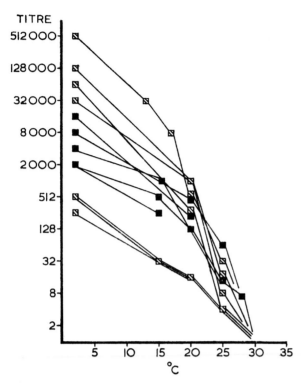

Fig. 28.12   The relationship between temperature and cold-agglutinin titre.

Diagonally ruled squares = cases of auto-immune haemolytic anaemia of the idiopathic cold-antibody type. Filled-in squares = cases of haemolytic anaemia of cold-antibody type following mycoplasma pneumonia.

Variation in pH between the range 6.0 to 8.5 makes little difference to the agglutinin titre. With most sera, however, agglutination in undiluted serum is less intense in serum acidified to pH 6.5–6.8.

Relative resistance to agglutination by cold agglutinins of patients' erythrocytes compared to normal erythrocytes

It has been recognized for many years that a patient's own erythrocytes are usually markedly less agglutinable by high-titre cold auto-agglutinins than those of normal adults. This difference is illustrated in Table 28.4, in which it is shown, too, that the differences in agglutinability were more marked at the higher temperatures than at 2–4°C in three out of the four cases. Dacie (1962, p. 468) suggested that the observed resistance to agglutination was likely to be due to the most sensitive cells, i.e. those that were acted on by the antibody at a relatively high temperature, being continually removed from the circulation, thus leaving behind a selected and relatively resistant population. In Case E. W. (Table 28.4), this relative resistance seems likely to have been of clinical value as normal cells were agglutinated by her serum at 37°C.

Table 28.3   Serological data on 16 patients suffering from the cold-haemagglutinin disease.

Case	Sex, age	Agglutination					Lysis						
		Normal cells		Upper thermal limit, °C	Trypsinized cells		Normal cells				Trypsinized cells, pH 8.0	PNH cells, pH 8.0	
							pH 6.5–7.0		pH 8.0				
		2–4°C (titre)	20°C (titre)		20°C (titre)	37°C (titre)	20°C	37°C	20°C	37°C	37°C	37°C	
B.R.	F. 61	64 000	256	29°	—	0	+ +	–	+	–	0	0	
–.H.	M. 78	128 000	1024	31°	—	0	+ +	–	–	–	0	0	
A.D.	F. 67	64 000	1024	32°	16 000	0	+ + +	–	–	–	0	0	
L.S.	F. 75	512 000	512	30°	—	0	+ +	±	–	–	0	4	
T.M.	M. 71	64 000	16 000	32°	256 000	0	+ +	–	+ +	–	64	>256	
A.S.	F. 73	64 000	256	30°	8000	0	+	–	±	–	0	4	
M.A.	F. 72	8000	128	—	16 000	0	+ +	–	–	–	0	0	
M.B.	F. 60	8000	16	—	512	0	+	–	–	–	0	0	
H.O.	M. 62	4000	1024	31.5°	16 000	0	+ + ±	–	+ +	±	1024	—	
J.K.	F. 68	64 000	1024	29°	4000	0	+	–	–	–	0	4	
L.C.	M. 56	1024	16	27.5°	512	0	+ +	–	–	–	0	4	
V.d.B.	M. 61	4000	256	—	4000	0	+ + +	–	+ +	–	16	256	
E.W.	F. 42	64 000	64 000	37°	64 000	32	+ + +	+	+ + +	+	>1024	>1024	
N.R.	F. 76	32 000	64	30°	4000	4	+	–	–	–	0	0	
E.S.	F. 80	4000	1024	26°	1024	0	+ +	–	+	–	0	1	
E.T.	F. 75	1024	4	25°	16	0	+ + +	–	+ +	–	0	0	

Table 28.4 Comparison of titrations of the serum cold agglutinin in four patients with the cold-haemagglutinin disease using patient's and normal erythrocytes.

| | Agglutinin titres | | | | | | | |
| | Patient's cells | | | | Normal cells | | | |
Patient	2–4°C	20°C	30°C	37°C	2–4°C	20°C	30°C	37°C
E.W.	2000	256	1	0	16 000	16 000	64	1
E.R.	16 000	4	1	0	32 000	64	1	0
E.S.	4000	16	0	0	4000	1024	0	0
E.T.	256	16	0	0	1024	4	0	0

It has also been shown that the erythrocytes of patients suffering from cold-antibody AIHA are less sensitive to lysis by high-titre cold antibodies than are normal adult erythrocytes. This, it has been suggested, is due to the accumulation of complement components blocking the further deposition of antibody and complement on cells that have been acted upon *in vivo* by complement-fixing antibodies but have escaped destruction.

Agglutination of enzyme-treated erythrocytes

Trypsinized (I) erythrocytes are typically agglutinated (by anti-I sera) to far higher titres than are unmodified cells. In the case of the 16 sera, the results with which are set out in Table 28.3, the titres at 20°C were 4–16 times greater and the thermal limit for detectable agglutination was raised. Two of the sera agglutinated trypsinized cells at 37°C.

For the effect of enzymes on agglutination by anti-Pr antibodies, see p. 265.

Lysis of normal erythrocytes

Sera containing high-titre cold agglutinins (of anti-I specificity) are characteristically able to lyse normal erythrocytes at 20°C in the presence of complement; often, however, the serum needs to be acidified for this to be demonstrable.

As is shown in Table 28.3, all 16 sera caused substantial lysis of normal erythrocytes when acidified to pH 6.5–7.0 before the cells were added. In eight of the 16 sera a lesser degree, and in two sera an almost maximal degree, of lysis took place in unacidified sera at pH 8.0. Several of the sera were able to bring about lysis at 30°C; one produced some lysis at 37°C, with or without acidification, and another a trace of lysis at 37°C in acidified serum only. There is a fairly close relationship between the upper thermal limit for the agglutination and lysis of normal cells.

By varying the pH of the serum to which the cells are added, it is possible to construct a pH–lysis curve; it will then be found that the optimum pH for lysis is 6.5–7.0 (measured after the addition of the cells to serum (Fig. 29.6, p. 275). Inhibition below pH 6.0 seems to be the result of the inhibition of complement (Fig. 29.7, p. 275). Although the pH range for lysis by an 'acid-lysin' is typically a narrow one (pH 6.0–8.0) (Fig. 29.6), exceptionally, sera produce lysis over a wider range (Fig. 29.6, curve B) (see also Table 28.5).

Prozones

In titrating sera to demonstrate lysis, the possibility of a prozone affecting the first tube or two of the titrations has to be kept in mind. One factor producing such prozones is deficiency or absence of complement in the patient's serum. Two examples of prozones are illustrated in Table 28.5. Serum L.S. is acting as a typical 'acid-lysin'; serum T.M. is a serum with which acidification

Table 28.5 The effect of pH on the lysis of normal erythrocytes by the sera of two patients suffering from the cold-haemagglutinin disease.

| | | Dilutions of patients' serum | | | | | | |
	pH	1 in 1	1 in 2	1 in 8	1 in 32	1 in 128	1 in 512	Control (normal serum diluent)
L.S.	8.0	–	–	–	–	–	–	–
	6.5	–	++	++	+	Trace	–	–
T.M.	8.0	–	–	++	+±	+	±	–
	6.5	–	–	++	+	Trace	–	–

+ + denotes a moderate amount of lysis; + ±, + and ± denote less marked but definite lysis; – denotes no lysis.

had relatively little effect on lysis, and in this titration more lysis in fact developed at pH 8.0 than at pH. 6.5.

Optimum temperature

Normal room temperature in Britain (20–22°C) seems to be about optimal for the occurrence of lysis. This temperature is well within the thermal range for antibody attachment and sufficiently warm for maximal lysis to be brought about by complement, if the preparation is allowed to stand for 1–2 hours. At lower temperatures, although antibody can presumably be attached more quickly, complement activity is inhibited and little lysis occurs. Little or no lysis results, too, if the suspension of cells in serum is chilled at, say, 0–4°C and then warmed at 37°C, i.e. under circumstances that result in maximum lysis when the antibody under test is the Donath–Landsteiner antibody of paroxysmal cold haemoglobinuria (see Table 28.6). It seems as if, in CHAD, the intense agglutination at low temperatures interferes in some way with the fixation of complement.

Lysis of trypsinized erythrocytes

The antibodies regularly bring about the lysis of trypsinized cells. Acidification of serum increases the lytic titre in most instances but lysis always occurs in unacidified sera. The lytic titre is generally considerably lower than the agglutination titre, if comparisons are made at 20°C, but always higher than the corresponding lytic titre obtained with normal cells. Typical results are shown in Table 28.7. Most sera lyse trypsinized cells at 30°C and some even at 37°C (Table 28.3).

Resistance of erythrocytes that have survived lysis by cold auto-antibodies *in vivo* to lysis *in vitro*

Evans, Turner and Bingham (1967) and Evans et al. (1968) reported that the erythrocytes of patients with cold-antibody AIHA that have been

Table 28.6 Differences in the lytic ability of sera containing cold auto-antibodies.

	Temperature (°C)	Serum A.D.*	Serum E.F.[†]	Serum B.C. (D-L antibody)
Agglutinin titre	30	0	2	0
Normal cells	18	4000	1000	4
	2	64 000	4000	16
Lysin titre	30	1	2	0
Normal cells,	18	16	64	1
pH 7.0	0→37	1	4	16
Lysin titre	30	32	256	1
PNH cells,	18	4000	4000	8
pH 8.0	0→37	8000	8000	32

*Cold-hæmagglutinin disease.
[†] Post-mycoplasma pneumonia haemolytic anaemia.

coated *in vivo* with the C4 and C3 components of complement, but have not undergone lysis, are abnormally resistant to lysis *in vitro* by complement-fixing cold antibodies. They found, too, that normal erythrocytes can be made *in vitro* similarly resistant to complement lysis by incubation with cold agglutinins at temperatures (e.g. 25°C, followed by 37°C) that allow transient interaction between cells and antibody. The development of resistance was found to be paralleled by an increasing uptake of ^{131}I-labelled antiglobulin serum containing anti-β_1c and anti-β_1e antibodies. There was, too, a decrease in the adsorption of ^{131}I-labelled cold antibody during the development of resistance to the antibody and a reduced susceptibility to agglutination. Evans, Turner and Bingham suggested that the resistance to adsorption of the cold antibody is the result of steric hindrance by accumulated incomplete complement complexes.

The resistance to agglutination and lysis of erythrocytes already coated by complement components was studied further by Engelfriet et al. (1972). They concluded that erythrocytes that are affected *in vivo* by complement-fixing cold antibodies, but escape destruction, lose the β_1E and β_1A components of complement from their membrane, and that fresh β_1E and β_1A molecules cannot be bound to sites where the original molecules had been attached. They further suggested that as the unreactive sites accumulate the cells become resistant to the lytic effect of the cold antibodies, not because the

Table 28.7 **Relative sensitivity of erythrocytes to lysis by a high-titre cold antibody at 20°C.**

Type of cell	pH	Dilutions of serum								Control (normal serum diluent)
		1 in 1	1 in 4	1 in 16	1 in 64	1 in 256	1 in 1024	1 in 4096	1 in 16000	
Normal	8.0	–	Trace	–	–	–	–	–	–	–
Normal	6.5	Trace	+	±	Trace	–	–	–	–	–
Trypsinized normal	8.0	–	+ + ±	+ +	+	±	–	–	–	–
PNH	8.0	+ + ±	+ + +	+ + +	+ + +	+ + +	+ +	+ ±	+	–

+ + + denotes marked lysis; + + ±, + +, + ±, + and ± denote lesser but definite degrees of lysis; – denotes no lysis.

antibodies are unable to react with the antigenic determinants, but because the antigen–antibody interaction is unable to lead to the fixation of activated β_1E and β_1C.

In relation to the protective effect of erythrocyte-bound C3d on the uptake of further cold-antibody–complement complexes, Chaplin, Coleman and Monroe (1983) referred to their own observation of the relatively rapid in-vivo turnover of the majority of acutely-bound C3d molecules. They pointed out that this would reduce the protection offered by erythrocyte-bound C3d, as the loss of C3d would provide opportunities for the deposition of new C3d molecules and in consequence continuation of haemolysis.

Lysis of paroxysmal nocturnal haemoglobinuria (PNH) erythrocytes

PNH erythrocytes are extremely sensitive to lysis by all potentially lytic antibodies and as was shown by Dacie (1950) they are lysed in very highly diluted sera containing high-titre cold antibodies. Their great sensitivity compared with normal cells is shown in Table 28.7. Almost maximal lysis occurs in unacidified serum, and the lysis titres using PNH cells at 20°C are generally comparable with the agglutination titres obtained with trypsinized cells: PNH cells are in fact far more sensitive to lysis by cold antibodies than are trypsinized cells (see Table 28.7). PNH cells are almost always lysed at 30°C and they were lysed at 37°C by eight of 15 sera studied by the author: in only three instances, however, did the lytic titre exceed 4 at that temperature.

DIFFERENCES IN SEROLOGICAL FINDINGS BETWEEN INDIVIDUAL PATIENTS SUFFERING FROM THE COLD-HAEMAGGLUTININ DISEASE

A striking feature of the data summarized in the foregoing summary has been the striking differences in findings between individual patients (see also Table 28.3). Not only are there major differences in the amount of antibody formed, as indicated by the wide range of cold-agglutinin titres at 2–4°C, but the effect of temperature on agglutination and the effect of pH on the ability of the sera to cause lysis vary considerably from patient to patient. Another interesting variable is the way that one serum is much more lytic than another in relation to its ability to bring about agglutination. On the assumption that lysis and agglutination are brought about by the same antibody molecules, the differences in antibody activity mentioned above seem to indicate subtle qualitative differences between one antibody and the next, differences that no doubt are manifestations of the uniqueness of the individual.

ATYPICAL CHRONIC COLD-ANTIBODY AIHA

In addition to the patients exhibiting the signs and symptoms of CHAD, which have been summarized on pp. 215–218, a minority of patients are met with whose symptoms and signs and serological picture are less typical. Thus both Forbes (1947) and Mellinkoff and Pisciotta (1949) described young men with Raynaud's phenomena or acrocyanosis without haemoglobinuria and without significant anaemia.

The serological findings in four patients, studied by the author (Dacie, 1962, p. 373) who had formed cold auto-antibodies of high thermal amplitude but had not suffered from acrocyanosis or haemoglobinuria and who had presented somewhat distinct and characteristic serological pictures, are summarized in Table 28.8. All were women, aged between 54 and 73, suffering from moderately severe to severe haemolysis.

A remarkable feature of each serum was its persistent ability to lyse trypsinized erythrocytes, or PNH cells, to quite high titres at 37°C. The low titres for the lysis of trypsinized cells at 20°C,

Table 28.8 Serological data on four patients suffering from idiopathic acquired haemolytic anaemia of the cold-antibody type, (?) distinct from the cold–haemagglutinin disease.

Case	Sex, age	Agglutination					Lysis								WR and Kahn test
		Normal cells			Trypsinized cells		Normal cells				Trypsinized cells		PNH cells		
							pH 6.5–7.0		pH 8.0		pH 8.0 (titre)		pH 8.0 (titre)		
		2–4°C (titre)	20°C (titre)	30°C (titre)	20°C (titre)	37°C (titre)	20°C	37°C	20°C	37°C	20°C	37°C	20°C	37°C	
L.R. (Case 13 of Dacie, 1954)	F. 54	1024	16	0	1024	16	–	Trace	–	–	4	128	512	512	+
M.J. (Case 12 of Dacie and de Gruchy,1951)	F. 73	512	32	0	...	0	–	–	–	–	...	32	...	16	+
M.G. (Case 5 of Dacie and de Gruchy, 1951)	F. 56	1024	32	0	...	2	+	Trace	–	–	...	32	...	32	...
O.G.	F.	256	2	0	256	4	–	–	–	–	0	64	8	256	+

– denotes no lysis; ... no observation.

compared with the much higher titres at 37°C, suggested that the lysis at 37°C may have been produced by a warm-acting antibody distinct from the cold agglutinin. In two of the patients traces of lysis of normal unmodified cells took place at 37°C. In two patients serum complement was measured and found to be significantly lowered (10–32 units, normal 70–150 units). The Wassermann and Kahn reactions were positive in the three patients tested; in two of them, at least, the reactions were probably false-positive.

Subsequently, Lie-Injo and Pillay (1964) described five patients with chronic cold-antibody AIHA whose clinical syndrome and serological findings deviated considerably from typical CHAD: three were Malays and two Chinese. Their ages ranged between 11 and 38 years. None had experienced acrocyanosis. In all five the DAT was of the non-γ type and cold agglutinins at moderately raised titres (128–2048 at 4°C), but of high thermal activity, were present in their sera. Trypsinized cells underwent lysis at 37°C. All five patients responded to treatment with prednisolone.

Lie-Injo also reported that she had investigated three patients with idiopathic AIHA in Indonesia; one was a Chinese man and two were Indonesian women. They, too, had formed cold auto-antibodies, and the serological findings were very similar to those of the patients that she had studied with Pillay in Malaya. These serological findings were considered to be typical of chronic AIHA in the tropics. Lie-Injo and Pillay concluded that the disorder was probably not rare.

Two rather similar patients were described by Schreiber, Herskovitz and Goldwein (1977): one was a woman aged 63, the other a man aged 55. Both had formed high-thermal-amplitude, complement-fixing antibodies of only moderate titres at 4°C. The first patient gave a 2-week history of a mild upper respiratory infection, and when examined had a haemoglobin of 6.5 g/l, with 7% reticulocytes and some spherocytes in the blood film. The DAT was strongly positive with anti-C3 sera, but negative with anti-IgG sera. Plasma complement components were subnormal or at the lower limits of normal. The cold-agglutinin titre was 256 at 4°C, 64 at 25°C and as high as 32 at 37°C; the antibody appeared to be an IgM and to have anti-I specificity. The second patient had noted a gradual onset of fatigue and when examined his haemoglobin was 6.8 g/dl. A few spherocytes were seen in his blood films, too; and the serological findings were almost identical with those of the first patient. Both patients responded to corticosteroid therapy but needed continuous therapy to maintain a haemoglobin of 10 g/dl.

CONCURRENCE OF WARM AND COLD AUTO-ANTIBODIES IN AIHA

Low-titre cold agglutinins active up to about 20°C, but not at temperatures above this, are quite commonly found in the sera of patients with otherwise typical warm-antibody AIHA. The reason for their presence is obscure but they probably play no part in the causation of the increased haemolysis. Less commonly, cold agglutinins at clearly raised titres at 4°C (> 64) are present. Rather rarely, but perhaps in 5–10% of patients, IgM cold agglutinins active up to 30°C, or even 37°C, may be present, in addition to warm-acting IgG auto-antibodies, and in these cases it seems probable, or at least possible, that the high-thermal-amplitude cold antibodies play a part in bringing about the haemolysis.

The clinical syndrome presented by patients forming both warm and cold antibodies conforms more closely to that presented by severely-affected patients forming warm antibodies alone than to the cold-haemagglutinin syndrome. Thus haemolysis has mostly been severe, exposure to cold seems to play no part in precipitating haemolysis, and acrocyanosis is not a feature. In some of the patients the disorder has appeared to be idiopathic; in other patients it has been secondary. Both sexes of a wide range of ages are affected.

The literature on 'mixed' warm- and cold-antibody AIHA is now quite extensive (see below) and, although the clinical and serological findings merge into those of severe warm-antibody AIHA and the cases are both clinically and serologically rather heterogeneous, they comprise an important group that deserves close attention.

Dacie and de Gruchy (1951) reported that the sera of seven out of 12 patients regarded as suffering from idiopathic AIHA (some severely ill, some in remission) contained cold agglutinins at clearly raised titres (256–1024 at 2–5°C). It is interesting to note that all seven patients were described as being severely ill or suffering from moderately active haemolysis. The DAT was positive in each case. The thermal range of the cold agglutinins was not determined, but the fact that the patients' sera agglutinated and lysed trypsinized erythrocytes to (mostly) high titres at 37°C suggested strongly that these patients were also forming warm auto-antibodies. The IAT was, too, positive at 37°C, and normal cells were agglutinated at 37°C by the patients' sera diluted in a serum–albumin mixture, as described by Neber and Dameshek (1947).

Fagiolo and Laghi (1970) reported on a serological investigation of 18 AIHA patients; in nine the DAT was positive with anti-IgG sera at 37°C and two of these patients were recorded as having a raised titre of cold agglutinins at 4°C—in one case the titre was 1024 and in the other 128.

Crookston (1975) described a patient, a 70-year-old man, suffering from 'small cell lymphosarcoma' and a severe grade of AIHA. Warm IgG and cold IgM auto-antibodies were both present, and the DAT was positive with both anti-IgG and anti-C3 sera. Anti-E and anti-K allo-antibodies were also present. The warm antibody reacted with all cells except Rh_{null} cells; the cold antibody had anti-i specificity reacting to a titre of 1024 with cord-blood cells at 4°C; it reacted with the patient's cells up to 33°C. Both antibodies were thought to have contributed to the patient's increased haemolysis.

Moake and Schultz (1975) described a 37-year-old woman suffering from severe extravascular haemolysis. This was associated with the formation of IgG warm auto-antibodies as well as cold-reactive IgG, IgA and IgM antibodies. The serum complement titre was reduced, particularly that of C4. The Monospot test was transitorily positive early in her illness and it is possible, but was not proved, that infective mononucleosis provided the stimulus for the formation of the multiple antibodies.

Kay, Gordon and Douglas (1978) described the case of a 50-year-old man who was suffering from a severe AIHA of 1 month's duration. The DAT was positive with anti-IgG and anti-C sera. A warm auto-antibody (of undetermined specificity) was present and in addition a monoclonal IgM (κ) antibody with anti-i specificity, active up to 10°C *in vitro* and which did not apparently fix complement. A subpopulation of the patient's lymphocytes formed rosettes with i (cord) erythrocytes but not with I (adult) cells, and the number of T cells present was diminished. Following splenectomy, the patient went into remission. The presence of a lymphoma was suspected but not proved. Sections of the spleen showed, however, lymphoid hyperplasia.

Joshi, Iyer and Bhatia (1980), writing from Bombay, reported on the serological findings in 55 patients with AIHA. Eighteen of the patients had formed cold auto-antibodies, five warm auto-antibodies and 32 were described as forming biphasic auto-antibodies which reacted at 37°C as well as at 6°C. The latter group of antibodies were considered to be heterogeneous; some at least appear to have been mixtures of warm and cold antibodies. Warm antibodies of Rh specificity were identified in two cases; in-saline-reacting cold antibodies were present in 17 cases, 14 of the antibodies having specificities within the Ii complex. Low-titre in-saline-reacting antibodies giving equivalent reactions at 6°C and 37°C were present in 11 patients.

Petz and Garratty (1980) described the results of a detailed investigation into the incidence of abnormal cold agglutinins in patients with warm-antibody AIHA. They found that 35% of 244 patients had had antibodies in their sera which brought about the agglutination of normal (not enzyme-treated) erythrocytes at 20°C. The specificity of the antibodies was anti-I (when determined) and the titres at 4°C were usually normal (<64) in spite of the antibodies' abnormal thermal range. The antibodies did not react at 30°C (even in albumin) and they were judged not to be significant in relation to the patients' increased haemolysis.

Petz and Garratty (1980) also referred to the rare occurrence of patients with AIHA in whom the serological findings indicated the presence of warm auto-antibodies and cold auto-antibodies at raised titres. They had studied four such patients (three females, one male, aged from 28 to 80): in three of the patients an associated lymphoma was present; in one there appeared to be no underlying disease. The DAT was positive with anti-IgG and anti-C3 sera in all four patients; it was also positive with an anti-IgA serum in one patient and with anti-IgM sera in two. The warm auto-antibody appeared to be non-specific; the cold antibodies (titres at 4°C 128–4096, with a thermal range extending up to 37°C) were identified as anti-i in three patients and the specificity was unidentified in one.

Vroclans-Deiminas and Boivin (1980), in a brief review of the serological findings in 341 patients giving positive DATs, recorded that in 46 of them the DAT had been positive with both anti-IgG and anti-C sera. Twenty-one patients had formed both warm and cold antibodies. Elution studies indicated the presence of warm-reacting antibodies of Rh type in some of them; their sera contained cold (anti-I) antibodies at raised titres (32 or higher).

Sokol, Hewitt and Stamps (1983) described 25 patients as suffering from AIHA of mixed warm- and cold-antibody type: in 12 of the patients the disease appeared to be idiopathic; in the remainder it was of the secondary type, SLE or a lymphoma being the most frequent underlying condition. The DAT was positive in all the patients: in 24 of the patients it was positive with anti-IgG sera and with anti-C3d or anti-C sera; in one patient the reaction was positive with anti-IgG and anti-IgA sera only. Most of the patients were over 60 years of age and haemolysis was severe in the majority. Although usually responding to treatment, the disorder generally ran a chronic course with intermittent exacerbations, making management difficult. The IgG and IgM components comprising the antibodies could be separated. The cold antibodies had a high thermal range, being active at 30°C or above. Study of eluates and sera revealed no definite specificity in the case of the warm antibodies, except in one patient in which Rh$_{null}$ cells failed to react. The cold antibodies mostly showed specificity within the Ii system: anti-I was present in 14 sera and anti-i in one serum; in nine cases the specificity could not be established. In Sokol, Hewitt and Stamps's experience mixed warm- and cold-antibody type AIHA had comprised 7% out of a total of 865 cases investigated; the male to female ratio was 1:1.5.

Freedman and co-workers (1985) described a 58-year-old man suffering from severe AIHA. Nine years previously ITP had been diagnosed and 7 years previously he had had a thyroidectomy; recently he had developed a deep-vein thrombosis in his right leg. He was found to be forming three distinct auto-antibodies: a low titre (64 at 4°C) IgM anti-I antibody, the thermal range of which just reached 37°C; an IgG warm antibody detectable by the IAT, and an IgM warm antibody which haemolysed and agglutinated papainized cells at 37°C, both reactions being enhanced at pH 6.8. The DAT was positive with anti-IgG, -C3d and -C4d sera. On admission the haemoglobin was 5.6 g/dl and the platelet count was as low as 27×10^9/l; spherocytes were present. Whilst in hospital the condition of his right leg worsened and eventually gangrene developed, necessitating amputation. He recovered from the operation, however, and responded well to prednisone, 100 mg daily, and was eventually discharged on a maintenance dose. Freedman et al. concluded that all three auto-antibodies may have contributed to the haemolysis.

Shulman and co-workers (1985) surveyed the serological data in 144 patients with AIHA and concluded that in twelve (8.3%) the findings satisfied criteria for both warm-antibody AIHA and [less clearly, see below] cold haemagglutinin disease; nine were females. Their sera contained IgM cold antibodies active up to 37°C as well as warm IgG antibodies. All the patients had suffered initially from severe haemolysis. Their haemoglobin at diagnosis ranged between 4.4 and 8.8 g/dl (mean 6.3 g/dl). They all responded dramatically to corticosteroid therapy. Six of the patients had idiopathic AIHA; five had SLE and one a non-Hodgkin's lymphoma; four had concomitant thrombocytopenia (Evans syndrome). The specificity of the warm antibodies could not be established and the same was true of the cold antibodies except in one case (anti-i). The sera lysed enzyme-treated cells at 20°C and 37°C. The titres of the cold antibodies at 4°C (64 or less) were barely abnormal; a striking abnormal feature, however, was that although weaker at 37°C they still reacted at this temperature. Shulman et al. pointed out that their patients did not suffer from classical CHAD: the cold-agglutinin titres were low, haemolysis *in vivo* was not related to cold, anaemia was profound and the initial response to corticosteroid therapy was dramatic. Nor did they suffer from classical AIHA (in which cold agglutinins active up to about 20°C are not infrequently present).

As for prognosis, increased haemolysis eventually ceased in four of the patients, but seven required continuous corticosteroid therapy for its control. One patient was lost to follow-up. Shulman et al. concluded that their twelve patients were suffering from a distinct category of AIHA.

Kajii, Miura and Ikemoto (1991) reported on the results of a detailed study of three patients, out of a total of 46 AIHA patients, who had formed both warm and cold auto-antibodies. Two of the patients were women aged 65 and 71, respectively, one a man aged 59. The woman aged 65 had had a T-cell lymphoma; in the other two patients their disease appeared to be idiopathic. All three patients were severely anaemic — haemoglobins 5.4–6.4 g/dl, with 5–39% reticulocytes. In each case the cold antibodies were shown to be IgMκ and the warm antibodies IgGκ. The specificity of the cold antibodies differed from case to case: one was anti-Om, one anti-I; that of the third patient was undetermined and unusual in that it reacted with her erythrocytes to a much higher titre than with cells of normal adults — titres 2048 and 64, respectively, at 4°C. The specificity of the warm antibodies was undefined; eluates reacted with I and i cells similarly. It was concluded that in each case the warm and cold antibody components reacted with different antigens.

ACUTE COLD-ANTIBODY AIHA IN INFANTS AND CHILDREN

Rather rarely, small children, even infants, suffer from acute haemolytic anaemia associated with the development of raised titres of cold auto-agglutinins and auto-agglutination. Anaemia may be very severe, but is typically transient. There may be haemoglobinuria. Usually there is evidence of a preceding viral infection. A variety of antibody specificities have been described — e.g. anti-I, anti-i, anti-Pr^a, anti-Sd^x (anti-Rx).

Early reports

Patterson and Stewart Smith (1936) described a child, a boy aged 7 years, who had become acutely anaemic, and noted that marked auto-agglutination disappeared at 37°C so that erythrocyte counts were possible in a warmed counting chamber. The leucocyte count reached 72×10^9/l. The child was transfused and recovered.

Unger, Wiener and Dolan (1952) described a newborn infant suffering from haemolytic anaemia and purpura. The DAT was positive and the infant's serum contained a cold agglutinin at a titre of 1000. There were also indications of encephalitis. An intra-uterine virus infection and antibody formation *in vivo* were postulated. No abnormal antibodies were detected in the serum of the infant's mother. The infant gradually recovered and the titre of cold agglutinins diminished gradually — at 11 months it was one-quarter of that at birth.

Bakx, van Loghem and Klomp-Magnée (1953) described an infant which became jaundiced and slightly anaemic 14 days after birth. The DAT was weakly positive and the serum contained cold agglutinins to a titre (in saline) of 256 at 16°C and at 4°C. The mother's serum contained cold agglutinins to a titre of 8 at 16°C and at 4°C. The child gradually recovered and it was postulated that it had suffered from viral hepatitis (as had the mother possibly, too), associated with cold-antibody formation, and a mild haemolytic syndrome.

Grislain, Mainard and de Berranger (1963) described the occurrence in a premature infant of what was considered to be a cold panantibody of maternal origin. (The exact nature of the antibody was not established.) The infant's mother had suffered from a very severe haemolytic anaemia which had developed during her third pregnancy. The DAT was strongly positive, but only in strong concentrations of antiglobulin serum, and the cold-agglutinin titre did not exceed 32. She did not respond to corticosteroid therapy and had received 27 blood transfusions. She died soon after the delivery of a premature infant. A DAT carried on the infant's erythrocytes was positive, but as with its mother's cells, only in strong concentrations of antiglobulin serum. It died after a second exchange transfusion.

More recent studies

Roelcke and co-workers (1971) described detailed serological studies carried out on two children, aged 11 months and 8 years, respectively, both of whom had suffered from transient haemolytic anaemia associated with transiently raised cold-agglutinin titres. The antibodies were shown to be formed of IgG and to be reacting with a hitherto undescribed antigen, referred to as Pr^a, immunochemically allied to Pr$_1$/Pr$_2$ (see p. 266).

Gerbal and co-workers (1971) described how three children in a family were found to give positive DATs. Two of them showed signs of mild haemolytic anaemia. Their mother's DAT was positive, too, and she had anti-i in her serum (at the time of the birth of her third child).

Habibi and co-workers (1974), in their review of 80 cases of AIHA in childhood, reported that cold agglutinins were present in raised titres in only four of them; one was an acute transient case, three were chronic cases. This gives an idea of the rarity of cold-antibody haemolytic anaemia in childhood.

Cregut and co-workers (1974) and Habibi and co-workers (1975) reported finding in the serum of a newborn an IgM anti-Pr^a at a titre of 500. It had a high thermal range and the DAT (with anti-C) was positive. The infant's blood underwent auto-agglutination at room temperature, but there was, however, no evidence of increased haemolysis. The cause of the antibody's formation was obscure; neither the mother nor the infant appeared to be suffering from an infection.

Zupánska and co-workers (1976), in a review of 44 cases of acute and chronic AIHA in childhood, reported that nine acutely ill children, most of whom were less than 5 years of age, had cold auto-antibodies (of unspecified titre) in their serum. In each case the haemolysis had followed an infection, and in one child this had been a mycoplasma pneumonia. The DAT had been positive in only two of the children, and most of them were said not to have become severely anaemic. All of them recovered within 1 month.

Eden and Innes (1978) referred briefly to five children, aged between 1 year and 7 months to 5 years, with cold-antibody AIHA. In four the onset was acute and anaemia severe; in the fifth the onset was more gradual and the haemoglobin did not fall below 10.2 g/dl—this child had suffered from a mycoplasma infection. The four other children had had upper respiratory tract infections, thought to be viral in origin. All five children gave positive DATs with anti-C sera; three had low reticulocyte counts (2.7–3.6%) in relation to their low haemoglobin levels (4.1–6.0 g/dl).

Marsh and co-workers (1980) described finding a 'new' cold auto-antibody in the serum of a 5-year-old girl with acute haemolytic anaemia which appeared to be related to the Sd^a blood group: the 'new' antibody was referred to as anti-Sd^x. The child was treated with prednisone and eventually recovered. (A similar antibody had been detected in the serum of a 69-year-old woman suffering from chronic AIHA).

O'Brien and co-workers (1988) described finding in the serum of a 3-year-old boy who had developed acute AIHA an IgM cold auto-antibody referred to as anti-Rx (previously called anti-Sd^x). The child made a good recovery as the antibody disappeared from his serum. Initially the antibody agglutinated adult I, adult ii and cord cells to a titre of 64 at 4°C and its activity stretched up to 30°C.

CHRONIC COLD-ANTIBODY AIHA IN CHILDREN

Chronic cold antibody AIHA occurs only very rarely in childhood.

Bonham-Carter, Cathie and Gasser (1954) described a 5-year-old boy who suffered from relapsing AIHA, associated with episodes of severe reticulocytopenia, which persisted for at least 18 months. The DAT and IAT were strongly positive and a high-thermal-amplitude cold agglutinin was present in his serum; no details, however, were recorded.

Seip, Harboe and Cyvin (1969) reported that two sisters had both suffered from chronic AIHA, when aged 4 and 12 years, respectively. The child aged 4 developed a cold-antibody AIHA, with cold-agglutinin titres of 256 at 4°C and 16 at 20°C. The DAT was positive with anti-C sera, but negative with anti-IgG and anti-M sera. The child aged 12 had developed warm-antibody AIHA. The course of the younger child was prolonged, lasting at least 5 years and, as in the case described by Bonham-Carter, Cathie and Gasser (1954), was interspersed with episodes of severe reticulocytopenia and erythroblastopenia.

COLD-ANTIBODY AIHA IN ASSOCIATION WITH NEOPLASMS (EXCLUDING LYMPHOPROLIFERATIVE DISORDERS)

The frequent association between cold-antibody AIHA and lymphoproliferative disorders is well known and generally accepted and will be discussed in Volume 4 of this book. Whether other types of neoplastic disorders occur more frequently in patients with cold-antibody AIHA than in patients of the same age who are not forming abnormal amounts of cold antibodies is a matter of debate. Wortman, Rosse and Logue (1979) described four patients with, respectively, a squamous carcinoma of the lung, metastatic adenocarcinoma of the adrenal, metastatic adeno-carcinoma of the colon, and a mixed parotid tumour as well as a basal cell carcinoma. All four were forming high-titre IgM anti-I cold antibodies —titres 800–25 000 at 4°C. Their ages were 50, 17, 56 and 77, respectively. In discussing these patients, Wortman, Rosse and Logue suggested three possible mechanisms whereby the association between the malignancies and the formation of the cold antibodies might not be fortuitous. These were: (1) that tumour-associated antigens might stimulate the production of antibodies which cross-reacted with erythrocyte antigens; (2) that dedifferentiated tumour cells might produce the antibodies; and (3) that a general immunodeficiency state might lead to failure of immunological recognition as well as to failure to control neoplastic growth.

Wortman, Rosse and Logue referred to three previously described cases: patients suffering from a carcinoid tumour of the ampulla of Vater, carcinoma of the larynx and a thoracic neurinoma, respectively. Earlier Søltoft and Lind (1968) had described a further patient, an 85-year-old man with CHAD and a metastasizing adenocarcinoma of the prostate. The cold-agglutinin titre was 128 000 at 4°C and his serum contained cryoglobulin. In discussion, Søltoft and Lind discussed the possible connection between Waldenström's macroglobulinaemia and CHAD and malignant disease and listed eight pertinent references. Their conclusion was that the data so far available seemed, however, to be insufficient to demonstrate any real connection.

An apparent cause-and-effect association between a uterine myoma and cold-antibody AIHA was described by Kornberg, Naparstek and Herschko (1980). Their patient was anaemic (haemoglobin 6.0 g/dl, with 3% reticulocytes); the spleen was palpable 6 cm below the left costal margin and the uterus was 'grossly enlarged'. The DAT was positive with anti-C3 and -C4 sera and serum complement was subnormal. An IgM anti-I cold agglutinin was present at a titre of 2048. Hysterectomy was carried out and a large benign myoma removed. Within 10 days of the operation the cold-agglutinin titre had fallen to 32 and the haemoglobin had risen to 12.0 g/dl. One year later the patient was in perfect health; her haemoglobin was 15 g/dl and the spleen was no longer palpable.

More recently, Lippman and co-workers (1987) described a 56-year-old woman who presented with back pain of 4 days' duration. She was found to have a severe haemolytic anaemia (haemoglobin 6.7 g/dl), with haemoglobinuria and moderate thrombocytopenia, and to have a high-thermal-amplitude cold autoantibody in her serum. Thought possibly to have had mycoplasma pneumonia, she was found actually to be suffering from disseminated oat-cell bronchial carcinoma. The cold-agglutinin titre in albumin was 128 at 4°C, with antibody activity extending up almost to 30°C. Lysis *in vitro* of normal erythrocytes took place biphasically or monophasically almost up to 35°C with an optimum of 25°C; it was not enhanced by acidification. The antibody was anti-I in specificity and an IgM. The DAT was positive with anti-C serum only. There was marked peripheral-blood spherocytosis. Her anaemia and platelet count responded temporarily to prednisone (80 mg/day).

REFERENCES

AMZEL, R. & HIRSZFELD, L. (1925). Ueber die Kälteagglutination der roten Blutkörperchen. *Z.Immun.-Forsch.*, **43**, 526–538.

ANDRÉ, R., DREYFUS, B., SALMON, C. & MALASSENET, R. (1955). Hémoglobinurie et acrocyanose paroxystiques avec agglutinines froides à un titre trés élevé. *Bull. Mém. Soc. Méd. Paris*, **71**, 146–159.

ANTONACI, B. (1955). Studi e considerazioni sulle autoemoagglutinine a freddo. *Minerva med. (Torino)*, **46**, 510–516.

BAKX, C. J. A., VAN LOGHEM, J. J. JNR & KLOMP-MAGNÉE, W. (1953). Acquired haemolytic anaemia in a newborn. *Vox Sang. (Amst.)*, **3**, 79–83.

BATEMAN, J. C. (1949). Symptoms attributable to cold hemagglutination. *Arch. intern. Med.*, **84**, 523–531.

BAUMGARTNER, W. (1948). Kälteagglutinine und periphere Zirkulationsstörungen. *Helv. med. Acta*, **15**, 411–416.

BAUMGARTNER, W. (1954). Die erworbenen hämolytischen Anämien und der hämolytische Transfusionszwischenfall. Pathogenese und Klinik unter dem Gesichtspunkt der serologischen Hämatogie. *Helv. med. Acta*, **21**, Suppl. 35, 1–192.

BAUMGARTNER, W. (1955). Die Kälteagglutininkrankheit. *Schweiz. med. Wschr.*, **85**, 1157–1162.

BENHAMOU, E., ZERMATI, M. & ASSUS, A. (1948). Les agglutinines froides (à propos de 56 cas observés). *Ann. Méd.* **49**, 499–543.

BENIANS, T. H. C. & FEASBY, W. R. (1941). Raynaud's syndrome with spontaneous cold haemagglutination. *Lancet*, **ii**, 479–480.

BERNDT, H. (1956). Die Kälteagglutininkrankheit. *Schweiz. med. Wschr.*, **86**, 443.

BERTOLI, R. & BARATTA, P. F. (1951). Anemia hemolytica cronica con emolisi da freddo. *Minerva med. (Torino)*, **42**(1), 628–630.

BESSMAN, J. D. & BANKS, D. (1980). Spurious macrocytosis, a common clue to erythrocyte cold agglutinins. *Amer. J. clin. Path.*, **74**, 797–800.

BONHAM-CARTER, R. E., CATHIE, I. A. B. & GASSER, C. (1954). Aplastische Anämie (chronische Erythroblastophthise) bedingt durch Autoimmunisierung. *Schweiz. med. Wschr.*, **84**, 1114–1116.

BONNARD, R. (1933). La grande auto-agglutination des hématies. *Sang*, 7, 807–820.

BONNIN, J. A. (1954). Chronic acquired hemolytic anemia associated with hemoglobinuria and Raynaud's phenomenon. *Blood*, **9**, 959–964.

BRITISH MEDICAL JOURNAL (1960). An obscure case; demonstrated at the Postgraduate Medical School of London, **ii**, 926–934.

CAZZOLA, M., BAROSI, G. & ASCARI, E. (1983). Cold haemagglutinin disease with severe anaemia, reticulocytopenia and erythroid bone marrow. *Scand. J. Haemat.*, **30**, 25–29.

CHAPLIN, H., COLEMAN, M. E. & MONROE, M. C. (1983). In vivo instability of rbc-bound C3d and C4d. *Transfusion*, **23**, 965–971.

CHEIN CHREN CHIU & HWAN-WEN YOU (1952). Reversible cold hemagglutination with peripheral vascular symptoms. Report of a case. *Chinese med. J.*, **70**, 10–16.

CHRISTENSON, W. N. & DACIE, J. V. (1957). Serum proteins in acquired haemolytic anaemia (autoantibody type). *Brit. J. Haemat.*, **3**, 153–164.

CLOUGH, M. C. & RICHTER, I. M. (1918). A study of an auto-agglutinin occurring in a human serum. *Johns Hopk. Hosp. Bull.*, **29**, 86–93.

CONN, H. O. (1955). Acute hemolytic anemia, cryoglobulinemia and cold agglutination. *New Engl. J. Med.*, **253**, 1011–1013.

CREGUT, R., HABIBI, B., BROSSARD, Y. & VERNON, P. (1974). A cold autoagglutinin in the newborn. *Lancet*, **ii**, 474 (Letter).

CROOKSTON, J. H. (1975). Hemolytic anemia with IgG

and IgM autoantibodies and alloantibodies. *Arch. intern. Med.*, **135**, 1314–1315.

DACIE, J. V. (1950). The presence of cold haemolysins in sera containing cold haemagglutinins. *J. Path. Bact.*, **62**, 241–257.

DACIE, J. V. (1954). *The Haemolytic Anaemias: Congenital and Acquired*, 525 pp. Churchill, London.

DACIE, J. V. (1957). The cold haemagglutinin syndrome. *Proc. roy. Soc. Med.*, **50**, 647–650.

DACIE, J. V. (1962). *The Haemolytic Anaemias: Congenital and Acquired. Part II—The Auto-immune Haemolytic Anaemias*, pp. 366–377 and pp. 458–505. Churchill, London.

DACIE, J. V. (1964). Das Kälte-Hämagglutinin-Syndrom. *Med. Klinik*, **59**, 371–374.

DACIE, J. V. & DE GRUCHY, G. C. (1951). Auto-antibodies in acquired haemolytic anaemia. *J. clin. Path.*, **4**, 253–271.

DACIE, J. V. & WORLLEDGE, S. M. (1969). Auto-immune hemolytic anemias. In *Progress in Hematology VI* (ed. by E. B. Brown and C. V. Moore), pp. 82–120. Grune and Stratton, New York.

DAMESHEK, W. & SCHWARTZ, S. O. (1940). Acute hemolytic anemia (acquired hemolytic icterus, acute type). *Medicine (Baltimore)*, **19**, 231–327.

DAVIDSON, L. S. P. (1932). Macrocytic haemolytic anaemia. *Quart. J. Med.*, **25** (N.S.1.), 543–578.

DE LANGE, J. A., EERNISSE, G. J. & VELTKAMP, J. J. (1972). Cold agglutinins and the Coulter Counter Model S. *Amer. J. clin. Path.*, **58**, 599–600 (Letter).

DEBENEDETTI, E. (1929). La grande auto-agglutination des hématies. *Presse méd.*, **37**, 1688–1692.

DELAGE, J.-M., GAUVREAU, L. & SIMARD, J. (1956). Les anémies hémolytiques par auto-anticorps. Étude clinique et expérimentale. *Union méd. Canad.*, **85**, 132–141.

DRUITT, R. (1873). Two cases of intermittent haematinuria. *Med. Tms Gaz. (Lond.)*, **i**, 408–411; 461–462.

EDEN, O. B. & INNES, E. M. (1978). Reticulocytopenia in immune haemolytic anaemias. *Brit. med. J.*, **i**, 111 (Letter).

ENGELFRIET, C. P., VON DEM BORNE, A. E. G. KR., BECKERS, D., REYNIERSE, E. & VAN LOGHEM, J. J. (1972). Autoimmune haemolytic anaemias. V. Studies on the resistance against complement haemolysis of the red cells of patients with chronic cold agglutinin disease. *Clin. exp. Immunol.*, **11**, 255–264.

ERNSTENE, A. C. & GARDNER, W. J. (1935). The effect of splanchnic nerve resection and sympathetic ganglionectomy in a case of paroxysmal hemoglobinuria. *J. clin. Invest.*, **14**, 799–805.

EVANS, R. S., TURNER, E. & BINGHAM, M. (1965). Studies with radioiodinated cold agglutinins of ten patients. *Amer. J. Med.*, **38**, 378–395.

EVANS, R. S., TURNER, E. & BINGHAM, M. (1967).

Chronic hemolytic anemia due to cold agglutinins: the mechanism of resistance of red cells to C' hemolysis by cold agglutinins. *J. clin. Invest.*, **46**, 1461–1474.

EVANS, R. S., TURNER, E., BINGHAM, M. & WOODS, R. (1968). Chronic hemolytic anemia due to cold agglutinins. II. The role of C' in red cell destruction. *J. clin. Invest.*, **47**, 691–701.

FAGIOLO, E. & LAGHI, V. (1970). Caratterizzazione immunochimica degli anticorpi eritrocitari nelle anemia emolitiche autoimmuni. (Test di Coombs diretto con antisieri specifici). *Progr. med. (Roma)*, **26**, 280–283.

FERRIMAN, D. G., DACIE, J. V., KELLE, K. D. & FULLERTON, J. M. (1951). The association of Raynaud's phenomena, chronic haemolytic anaemia, and the formation of cold antibodies. *Quart. J. Med.*, N. S. **20**, 275–292.

FIRKIN, B. G., BLACKWELL, J. B. & JOHNSTON, G. A. W. (1959). Essential cryoglobulinaemia and acquired haemolytic anaemia due to cold antibodies. *Aust. Ann. Med.*, **8**, 151–157.

FORBES, G. B. (1947). Autohaemagglutination and Raynaud's phenomenon. *Brit. med. J.*, **i**, 598–600.

FORMIJNE, P. (1940). Verschijnselen en vormen van paroxysmale haemoglobinurie. *Ned. T. Geneesk.*, **84**, 3394–3402.

FRANK, M. M., ATKINSON, J. P. & GADEK, J. (1977). Cold agglutinins and cold-agglutinin disease. *Ann. Rev. Med.*, **28**, 291–298.

FREEDMAN, J., LIM, F. C., MUSCLOW, E., FERNANDES, B. & ROTHER, I. (1985). Autoimmune hemolytic anemia with concurrence of warm and cold red cell autoantibodies and a warm hemolysin. *Transfusion*, **25**, 368–372.

GADDY, C. G. & POWELL, L. W. JNR (1958). Raynaud's syndrome associated with idiopathic cryoglobulinemia and cold agglutinins. Report of a case and discussion of classification of cryoglobulinemia. *Arch. intern. Med.*, **102**, 468–477.

GALLI, F. & MUSSAFIA, A. (1939). Su di un caso di grande autoagglutinazione. *Policlinico (sez. med.)*, **46**, 233–236.

GERBAL, A., LAVALLÉE, R., ROPARS, C., DIONEL, C., LACOMBE, M. & SALMON, CH. (1971). Sensibilisation des hématies d'un nouveau-né par un auto-anticorps anti-i d'origine maternelle de nature IgG. *Nouv. Rev. franç. Hémat.*, **11**, 689–700.

GIROLAMI, A., CELLA, G. & PATRASSI, G. (1976). Increased whole blood viscosity on cooling in a patient with cold hemagglutinin disease. *Vox Sang.*, **31** (Suppl. 1), 1–8.

GOTTLIEB, L. H. (1964). Cold agglutinin disease—a report of spontaneous remission. *Calif. Med.*, **101**, 120–123.

GOUDEMAND, M. & ROPARTZ, C. (1954). À propos d'un cas d'anémie hémolytique chronique avec crises d'hémoglobinurie 'a frigore'. Étude immunologique. Interprétation nosologique. *Sang*, **25**, 572–591.

GRISLAIN, J.-R., MAINARD, R. & DE BERRANGER, P. (1963). Ictère hémolytique néo-natal par pan-anticorps froids d'origine maternalle. *Arch. franç. Pédiat.*, 20, 853–856.

GUALANDI, G. & LORENZINI, R. (1951). Sindrome di Raynaud da grande autoagglutinazione 'a frigore' delle emazie. *Minerva med. (Torino)*, **42 (ii)**, 927–932.

HABIBI, B., HOMBERG, J.-C., SCHAISON, G. & SALMON, C. (1974). Autoimmune hemolytic anemia in children. A review of 80 cases. *Amer. J. Med.*, **56**, 61–69.

HABIBI, B., CREGUT, R., BROSSARD, Y., VERON, P. & SALMON, C. (1975). Auto-anti-Pr^a: a 'second' example in a newborn. *Brit. J. Haemat.*, **30**, 499–505.

HARBOE, M. (1971). Cold auto-agglutinins. *Vox Sang.*, 20, 289–305.

HARBOE, M. & TORSVIK, H. (1969). Protein abnormalities in the cold haemagglutinin syndrome. *Scand. J. Haemat.*, **6**, 416–426.

HARDERS, H. (1958). Der conjunctival-Kältetest. Eine Methode zum Studium 'Agglutininativer Kälteempfindlichkeit'. *Klin. Wschr.*, **36**, 74–78.

HATTERSLEY, P. G., GERARD, P. W., CAGGIANO, V. & NASH, D. R. (1971). Erroneous values on the model S Coulter counter due to high titer cold autoagglutinins. *Amer. J. clin. Path.*, **55**, 442–446.

HAWLEY, J. G. & GORDON, R. S. JNR (1954). Anemia associated with cold agglutinins. *N.Y. St. J. Med.*, **54**, 1516–1518.

HEILMEYER, L., HAHN, F. & SCHUBOTHE, H. (1947). Hämolytische Anämien auf der Basis abnormer serologischer Reaktionen. *Klin. Wschr.*, **24/25**, 193–205.

HEILMEYER, L. & SCHUBOTHE, H. (1946). Hämolytische Anaemie mit gleichzeitiger Kältehämoglobinurie, hervogerufen durch Autoagglutinine. *Med. Klin.*, **41**, 578–579.

HEILMEYER, L. & SCHUBOTHE, H. (1948). Anémies hémolytiques par l'agglutinine au froid. *Sang*, **19**, 473–480.

HENNEMANN, H. H. (1951). Untersuchungen über das Vorkommen und die klinische Bedeutung von Kälte-(Auto-)Agglutininen. *Z. ges. inn. Med.*, **6**, 385–398.

HENRY, F. P. (1894). Clinical report of two cases of Raynaud's disease. *Amer. J. med. Sci.*, **108**, 10–19.

HILLESTAD, L. K. (1959). The peripheral circulation during exposure to cold in normals and in patients with the syndrome of high-titre cold haemagglutination. II. Vascular response to cold exposure in high-titre haemagglutination. *Acta med. scand.*, **164**, 211–218.

ISSITT, P. D. (1985). *Applied Blood Group Serology*, pp. 540–548. Montgomery Scientific Publications, Miami.

IWAI, S. & MEI-SAI, N. (1925). Etiology of Raynaud's disease (a preliminary report). *Jap. med. World*, **5**, 119–121.

IWAI, S. & MEISAI, N. (1926). Etiology of Raynaud's disease (second report). *Jap. med. World*, **6**, 345–347.

JOHNSSON, S. (1949). On autoagglutinins active at body temperature. *Acta med. scand.*, **134**, 180–188.

JOSHI, S. R., IYER, Y. S. & BHATIA, H. M. (1980). Serological and immunoglobulin studies in autoimmune haemolytic anaemia with emphasis on the nature of biphasic antibodies. *Acta haemat. (Basel)*, **64**, 31–37.

KAJII, E., MIURA, Y. & IKEMOTO, S. (1991). Characterization of autoantibodies in mixed-type autoimmune hemolytic anemia. *Vox Sang.*, **60**, 45–52.

KAY, N. E., GORDON, L. I. & DOUGLAS, S. D. (1978). Autoimmune hemolytic anemia in association with monoclonal IgM(κ) with anti-i activity. *Amer. J. Med.*, **64**, 845–850.

KLIGLER, I. J. (1922). Autohemo-agglutination of human red blood corpuscles. *J. Amer. med. Ass.*, **78**, 1195–1196.

KOEPPLIN, F. (1936). Ein Fall von Autohämagglutination. Experimentelle Untersuchungen zur Aufklärung der Entstehungsweise des Phänomens. *Z. klin. Med.*, **129**, 512–531.

KOMARMY, L. & BARNES, M. G. (1972). Warming blood to correct erroneous Model S Coulter Counter values due to cold agglutinins. *Amer. J. clin. Path.*, **57**, 421–422 (Letter).

KORNBERG, A., NAPARSTEK, E. & HERSCHKO, C. (1980). Cryopathic haemolytic anaemia associated with uterus myomatosis. *Acta haemat. (Basel)*, **63**, 235 (Letter).

LANDSTEINER, K. (1903). Ueber Beziehungen zwischen dem Blutserum und den Körperzellen. *Münch. med. Wschr.*, **50**, 1812–1814.

LEVIN, W. C. & RITZMANN, S. E. (1966). Relation of abnormal protein to formed elements of blood: effects upon erythrocytes, leukocytes and platelets. *Ann. Rev. Med.*, **17**, 323–336.

LI CHEN-PIEN (1926). Investigation on 'cold' or auto-hemoagglutination. *J. Immunol.*, **11**, 297–318.

LIE-INJO LUAN ENG & PILLAY, R. P. (1964). Idiopathic auto-immune haemolytic anaemia in Malaya. *Acta haemat. (Basel)*, **31**, 282–288.

LIPPMAN, S. M., WINN, L., GRUMET, F. C. & LEVITT, L. J. (1987). Evans' syndrome as a presenting manifestation of atypical paroxysmal cold hemoglobinuria. *Amer. J. Med.*, **82**, 1065–1072.

McCOMBS, R. P. & McELROY, J. S. (1937). Reversible autohemagglutination with peripheral vascular symptoms. *Arch. intern. Med.*, **59**, 107–117.

MALLEY, L. K. & HICKEY, M. D. (1949). Paroxysmal cold haemoglobinuria of non-syphilitic type. *Lancet*, **i**, 387–390.

MARSH, W. L, JOHNSON, C. L., ØYEN, R., NICHOLS, M. E., DINAPOLI, J., YOUNG, H., BRASSEL, J.,

CUSUMANO, I., BAZAZ, G. R., HABER, J. M. & WOLF, C. F. W. (1980). Anti-Sd^x: a 'new' auto-agglutinin related to the Sd^a blood group. *Transfusion*, **20**, 1–8.

MARSHALL, R. J., SHEPHERD, J. T. & THOMPSON, I. D. (1953). Vascular responses in patients with high serum titres of cold agglutinins. *Clin. Sci.*, **12**, 255–264.

MELLINKOFF, S. M. & PISCIOTTA, A. V. (1949). Cold hemagglutination in peripheral vascular disease. *Ann. intern. Med.*, **30**, 655–662.

MINO, P. (1924). La panemoagglutinina del sangue umane. *Policlinico, Sez. prat.*, **31**, 1355–1359.

MITCHELL, A. B. S., PEGRUM, G. D. & GILL, A. M. (1974). Cold agglutinin disease with Raynaud's phenomenon. *Proc. roy. Soc. Med.*, **67**, 113–115.

MOAKE, J. L. & SCHULTZ, D. E. (1975). Hemolytic anemia associated with multiple autoantibodies and low serum complement. *Amer. J. Med.*, **58**, 431–437.

MOLLISON, P. L., ENGELFRIET, C. P. & CONTRERAS, M. C. (1987). *Blood Transfusion in Clinical Medicine*, 8th edn, pp. 415–425. Blackwell Scientific Publications, Oxford.

MORTARA, M. & MARTINETTI, L. (1955). Su di un caso di anemia emolitica cronica con sindrome de Raynaud e crioagglutinazione. *G. Clin. med.*, **36**, 1791–1801.

NELSON, M. G. & MARSHALL, R. J. (1953). The syndrome of high-titre cold haemagglutination. *Brit. med. J.*, **ii**, 314–317.

NYDEGGER, V. E., KAZATCHKINE, M. D. & MIESCHER, P. A. (1991). Immunopathologic and clinical features of hemolytic anemia due to cold agglutinins. *Seminars Hemat.*, **28**, 66–77.

O'BRIEN, D. A., MULLAHY, D. E., GARVEY, M. A. & JACKSON, J. F. (1988). Cold autoimmune haemolytic anaemia in a 3-year-old infant due to anti-Rx (previously anti-Sd^x). *Clin. lab. Haemat.*, **10**, 105–108.

OLESEN, H. (1966). On the cold agglutinin syndrome: biochemistry and physiology of cold agglutinins, thermodynamics of cold agglutinin reactions. 93 pp. Thesis. Munksgaard, Copenhagen.

OLESEN, H. (1967). The cold agglutinin syndrome. *Dan. med. Bull.*, **14**, 138–141.

PATTERSON, H. W. & STEWART SMITH, G. (1936). Acute haemolytic anaemia of Lederer in a child. *Lancet*, **ii**, 1096–1097.

PETRUCCI, J. V., DUNNE, P. A. & CHAPMAN, C. C. (1971). Spurious erythrocyte indices as measured by the model S Coulter counter due to cold agglutinins. *Amer. J. clin. Path.*, **56**, 500–502.

PETZ, L. D. & GARRATTY, G. (1986). *Acquired Immune Hemolytic Anemias*, pp. 345–348. Churchill Livingstone, New York.

PISCIOTTA, A. V., DOWNER, E. & HINZ, J. (1955). Cold hemagglutination in acute and chronic hemolytic syndromes. *Blood*, **10**, 295–311.

POTH, J. A., SHARP, G. S. & SCHRIER, S. C. (1970).

Cold agglutinin disease and the nephrotic syndrome. *J. Amer. med. Ass.*, **211**, 1990–1992.

PRUZANSKI, W. & KATZ, A. (1984). Cold agglutinins—antibodies with biological diversity. *Clin. immunol. Rev.*, **3**, 131–168.

PRUZANSKI, W. & SHUMAK, K. H. (1977). Biologic activity of cold-reacting autoantibodies (in two parts). *New Engl. J. Med.*, **297**, 538–545; 583–589.

ROELCKE, D. (1974). A review: cold agglutination. Antibodies and antigens. *Clin. Immunol. Immunopath.*, **2**, 266–280.

ROELCKE, D. (1989). Cold agglutination. *Transf. Med. Rev.*, **3**, 140–166.

ROELCKE, D., ANSTEE, D. J., JUNGFER, H., NUTZENADEL, W. & WEBB, A. J. (1971). IgG-type cold agglutinins in children and corresponding antigens. Detection of a new Pr antigen: Pr$_a$. *Vox Sang. (Basel)*, **20**, 218–229.

RØRVIK, K. (1954). The syndrome of high-titre cold haemagglutination. A survey and a case report. *Acta med. scand.*, **148**, 299–308.

ROSENTHAL, F. & CORTEN, M. (1937). Über das Phänomen der Autohämagglutination und über die Eigenschaften der Kältehämagglutinine. *Folia haemat. (Lpz.)*, **58**, 64–90.

ROSSE, W. R. (1990). *Clinical Immunohematology: Basic Concepts and Clinical Applications*. 677 pp. Blackwell Scientific Publications, Boston.

ROTH, G. (1935). Paroxysmal hemoglobinuria with vasomotor and agglutinative features. *Proc. Mayo Clin.*, **10**, 609–615.

SAITA, G. & MARTELLI, E. A. (1956). Emoglobinuria parossistica con sindrome di Raynaud e gangrena della mano sinistra da crioagglutininemia a titolo elevato in soggetto con crisi angiospastiche da strumento vibrante. *Med. d. Lavoro*, **47**, 630–638.

SALÉN, E. B. (1935). Thermostabiles, nicht Komplexes (Auto-)Hämolysin bei transitorischer Kältehämoglobinurie. *Acta med. scand.*, **86**, 570–592.

SAMSON, D., HALLIDAY, D., NICHOLSON, D. C. & CHANARIN, I. (1976). Quantitation of ineffective erythropoiesis from the incorporation of [^{15}N]delta-aminolaevulinic acid and [^{15}N]glycine into early labelled bilirubin. II. Anaemic patients. *Brit. J. Haemat.*, **34**, 45–53.

SAVONEN, K. (1948). Cold haemagglutination test and its clinical significance. *Ann. Med. exp. Fenn.*, **26** (Suppl. 3). 100 pp.

SCHREIBER, A. D., HERSKOVITZ, B. S. & GOLDWEIN, M. (1977). Low-titre cold-hemagglutinin disease. Mechanism of hemolysis and response to corticosteroids. *New Engl. J. Med.*, **296**, 1490–1494.

SCHUBOTHE, H. (1952). Antikörperbedingte hämolytische Anämien. *Verh. dtsch. Ges. inn. Med.*, **58**, 679–694.

SCHUBOTHE, H. (1958). *Serologie und klinische Bedeutung der Autohämantikörper*, pp. 56–236. Karger, Basel.

SCHUBOTHE, H. (1965). Current problems of chronic cold hemagglutinin disease. *Ann. N. Y. Acad. Sci.*, **124**, 484–490.

SCHUBOTHE, H. (1966). The cold hemagglutinin disease. *Seminars Hemat.*, **3**, 27–47.

SCHUBOTHE, H. & ALTMANN, H. W. (1950). Kältehämagglutine als Ursache chronischer hämolytischer Anämien. *Z. klin. Med.*, **146**, 428–479.

SCHUBOTHE, H. & MÜLLER, W. (1955). Über die Anwendbarkeit des Ehrlichschen Fingerversuches als Nachweismethode intravitaler Hämolyse und Erythrophagocytose bei hämolytischen Erkrankungen. *Klin. Wschr.*, **33**, 272–276.

SEIP, M., HARBOE, M. & CYVIN, K. (1969). Chronic autoimmune hemolytic anemia in childhood with cold antibodies, aplastic crises, and familial occurrence. *Acta paediat. scand.*, **58**, 275–280.

SHULMAN, I. A., BRANCH, D. R., NELSON, J. M., THOMPSON, J. C., SAXENA, S. & PETZ, L. D. (1985). Autoimmune hemolytic anemia with both warm and cold autoantibodies. *J. Amer. med. Ass.*, **253**, 1746–1748.

SOKOL, R. J., HEWITT, S. & STAMPS, B. K. (1983). Autoimmune haemolysis: mixed warm and cold antibody type. *Acta haemat. (Basel)*, **69**, 266–274.

SØLTOFT, J. & LIND, K. (1968). The cold haemagglutinin syndrome and carcinoma of the prostate. A case report. *Acta path. microbiol. scand.*, **73**, 13–18.

STATS, D. (1945). Cold hemagglutination and cold hemolysis. The hemolysis produced by shaking cold agglutinated erythrocytes. *J. clin. Invest.*, **24**, 33–42.

STATS, D. & BULLOWA, J. G. M. (1943). Cold hemagglutination with symmetric gangrene of the tips of the extremities; report of a case. *Arch. intern. Med.*, **72**, 506–517.

STATS, D. & WASSERMAN, L. R. (1943). Cold hemagglutination—an interpretive review. *Medicine (Baltimore)*, **22**, 363–424.

UNGER, L. J., WIENER, A. S. & DOLAN, D. (1952). Anémie auto-hémolytique chez un nouveau-né. *Rev. Hémat.*, 7, 495–504.

VAN LOGHEM, J. J. JNR, MENDES DE LEON, D. E., FRENKEL-TIETZ, H. & VAN DER HART, M. (1952). Two different serologic mechanisms of paroxysmal cold hemoglobinuria, illustrated by three cases. *Blood*, 7, 1196–1209.

VROCLANS-DEIMINAS, M. & BOIVIN, P. (1980). Analyse des résultats observés au cours de la recherche d'une auto-sensibilisation anti-érythrocytaire chez 2400 malades. *Rev. franç. Transf. Immunohémat.*, **23**, 105–117.

WHITTLE, C. H., LYELL, A. & GATMAN, M. (1947). Raynaud's phenomenon, with paroxysmal haemoglobinuria, caused by cold haemagglutination. *Proc. roy. Soc. Med.*, **40**, 500–501.

WIENER, A. S. (1935). *Blood Groups and Blood Transfusion*, p. 28. Bailliere, Tindall and Cox, London.

WIENER, A. S., UNGER, L. J., COHEN, L. & FELDMAN, J. (1956). Type-specific cold auto-antibodies as a cause of acquired hemolytic anemia and hemolytic transfusion reactions: biologic test with bovine red cells. *Ann. intern. Med.*, **44**, 221–240.

WORLLEDGE, S. (1967). Auto-immunity and blood diseases. *Practitioner*, **199**, 171–179.

WORTMAN, J., ROSSE, W. & LOGUE, G. (1979). Cold agglutinin autoimmune hemolytic anemia in nonhematologic malignancies. *Amer. J. Hemat.*, **6**, 275–283.

WYSCHEGORODZEWA, W. D. (1926). Zur Frage der Autohämagglutination. *Z. klin. Med.*, **104**, 524–529.

YOUNG, L. E. (1946). The clinical significance of cold hemagglutinins. *Amer. J. med. Sci.*, **211**, 23–39.

ZUPAŃSKA, B., LAWKOWICZ, W., GÓRSKA, B., KOZLOWSKA, J., OCHOCKA, M., ROKICKA-MILEWSKA, R., DERULSKA, D. & CIEPIELEWSKA, D. (1976). Autoimmune haemolytic anaemia in children. *Brit. J. Haemat.*, **34**, 511–520.

Auto-immune haemolytic anaemia (AIHA): cold-antibody syndromes II: immunochemistry and specificity of the antibodies; serum complement in auto-immune haemolytic anaemia

Chemical nature of cold auto-antibodies: early studies *241*

Chemical nature of cold auto-antibodies: recent studies *244*

Cold-antibody AIHA associated with more than one Ig class of antibody *244*

IgG cold auto-antibodies *244*
   Cold detectable 'warm' IgG auto-antibodies *245*

IgA cold auto-antibodies *246*

Light chains—kappa (K) and lambda (L) *246*
   Recent descriptions of IgM lambda (L) cold auto-antibodies *247*
   A low-molecular-weight IgM lambda anti-I auto-antibody *247*

Specificity of cold auto-antibodies *247*
   Species specificity: early studies *247*

Specificity in relation to human erythrocytes *249*
   Early studies *249*

The Ii system *250*
   Interaction between anti-I antibodies and isolated antigens *253*

Recent studies on the Ii blood-group system *253*
   Relationship with ABH(O) blood groups: anti-HI(OI), anti-AI and anti-BI *254*
   Relationship with the P blood groups *255*

Chemical nature of the Ii antigens *255*

Anti-I^{T} *256*
   Anti-I^{T} in Hodgkin's disease *256*

Other Ii variants *257*
   A cold agglutinin specifically active against stored erythrocytes *257*
   Cold agglutinins specifically active against 'cryptic' Ii antigens *257*
   Anti-I antibodies the activity of which is enhanced by added preservatives *258*

Technical factors affecting cold-agglutinin titres *258*
   Designation of antibodies as anti-I or anti-i *258*
   Enhancing effect of albumin-containing media *259*

Variation in disease in the agglutinability and lysis of patients' erythrocytes by anti-I antibodies *259*

Variation in disease in the agglutinability of patients' erythrocytes by anti-i antibodies *261*

Anti-I antibodies in the serum of healthy subjects *263*
   Range of anti-I in health *263*

Occurrence of anti-i in disease *264*

The Pr(SP$_1$) blood-group system *265*
   Anti-HD *265*
   Anti-Pr *266*
   Anti-Pr antibodies only demonstrable in low-ionic strength saline (LISS) *267*
   Occurrence of low-titre anti-Pr antibodies in routine serum samples *267*

Auto-anti-A and anti-B cold antibodies *268*
   Anti-A *268*
   Anti-B *268*

Auto-anti-H *269*

Auto-anti-M and -anti-N cold antibodies *269*
   Anti-M *269*
   Anti-N *270*
   Anti-N in patients undergoing chronic dialysis *270*
   Cross-reactivity of anti-M and anti-N *271*

Other rare specific cold auto-antibodies *271*
   Anti-P *271*
   Anti-Sd^{x} *272*
   Anti-Me *272*
   Anti-Om *272*
   Anti-D *272*

Fixation of complement by cold auto-antibodies *273*

Early reports of cold haemolysins *273*
   Effect of pH on lysis *in vitro*: 'acid haemolysins' *274*

'Incomplete' cold antibodies *276*
   Early observations *276*
   Later studies *276*
   Do 'incomplete' cold auto-antibodies exist? *277*

The 'incomplete' cold auto-autibody in normal serum: further details *278*
   Nature of the normal 'incomplete' cold auto-antibody *278*
   Relationship between the cold auto-agglutinins and the 'incomplete' cold auto-antibodies present in normal sera *279*

Clinical significance of 'incomplete' cold auto-antibodies *279*

Nature of complement components fixed to erythrocytes by 'incomplete' and lytic cold auto-antibodies *280*
   Early studies *280*
   Recent studies on the fixation of complement *281*

Serum complement in AIHA *282*
   Recent reports of serum-complement depletion in AIHA *283*

CHEMICAL NATURE OF COLD AUTO-ANTIBODIES: EARLY STUDIES

The development of techniques of electrophoresis and ultracentrifugation made it possible, first in the mid 1940s, but particularly in the 1950s, to investigate the nature of the high-titre cold auto-antibodies present in the sera of patients suffering from the chronic cold-haemagglutinin disease (CHAD). The concentration of γ globulin in the sera was found to be elevated, and it was not long before it was established that the excess γ globulin consisted of cold-antibody protein. It was found, too, that this protein if present in sufficient amounts formed a sharp peak distinct from that of normal γ globulin when subjected to electrophoresis. The mobility of this (γ_1) peak on paper electrophoresis at pH 8.6 was found to be typically faster than that of normal γ globulin and to occupy a position somewhere between normal γ (γ_2) globulin and β globulin (Fig. 29.1). Subsequently, the narrowness of the γ_1 peak was shown to reflect the monoclonality of the antibody protein.

Ultracentrifugation established that the cold-antibody protein was typically a macromolecular protein of the 19S class, i.e. was γM(IgM) in nature.

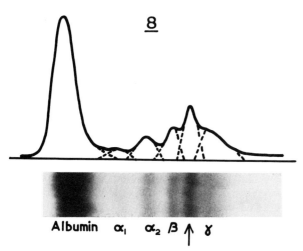

Fig. 29.1   Paper electrophoresis strip of the serum protein of a patient with CHAD.
The very high titre cold auto-antibody is responsible for the γ_1-globulin peak (marked with an arrow). [Reproduced by permission from Christenson and Dacie (1957).]

Stats and co-workers (1943) appear to be the first to report on electrophoretic studies carried out on a serum containing a high-titre cold agglutinin (titre 2560). Absorption of the serum with erythrocytes reduced the concentration of γ globulin by 16% and inspection of their figures suggests that the serum had given a small abnormal γ(γ_1) peak. Spaet and Kinsell (1953) also demonstrated the γ globulin nature of the cold agglutinin present in the serum of a patient with acquired haemolytic anaemia. Segments of the filter-paper electrophoretic strips of the patient's serum were tested for their content of cold agglutinins and only the γ globulin fraction was found to be active. Also, an eluate prepared from erythrocytes exposed to the cold agglutinins yielded a homogeneous band on electrophoresis which had the mobility of γ globulin.

Gordon (1953) studied the serum of a patient whose clinical history was subsequently recorded by Hawley and Gordon (1954). Cold-agglutinin activity was found in the euglobulin fraction of serum and relatively pure cold agglutinin was obtained by elution from erythrocyte stromata. On electrophoresis of the eluate, 75% of the protein was found to be concentrated in one peak and ultracentrifugation showed that 65% of the material flowed with a sedimentation coefficient of S_{20W} 18. By sampling the cell at the end of the run the cold-agglutinin activity was shown clearly to be associated with 18S component.

Schubothe (1954), too, subjected the serum of a patient suffering from CHAD to ultracentrifugation and found that it contained 12% of macroglobulin. He noted that electrophoresis of the patient's serum revealed an increase in β_2 globulin and raised the question as to the relationship between the presence of the abnormal serum component and the existence of the abnormal auto-antibody. Rørvik (1954) also described a protein abnormality demonstrable on electrophoresis: his patient, who also suffered from CHAD, had a serum which gave a 'split β'.

Vargues, Zermati and Labrosse (1955) used a chemical method of separation and were able to show a general increase in 'euglobulin I_1' (a γ globulin) up to six times the normal concentration in patients whose sera contained raised concentrations of cold agglutinins. They showed, too, that 'euglobulin I_1' extracted from serum containing cold agglutinins contained the agglutinins at higher titres than did the parent serum.

Weber (1956) studied five sera derived from patients suffering from CHAD and prepared eluates of their cold agglutinins from erythrocyte stromata. All the preparations were found to behave homogeneously in the ultracentrifuge and to give macroglobulin peaks with sedimentation constants ranging from S_{20W} 17.6 to 18.0, mean 17.8 S. The molecular weights of the antibodies were calculated to be in the range 330 000–350 000.

Christenson and Dacie (1957) reported on 38 patients suffering from various types of cold-antibody haemolytic anaemia. Their findings were as follows: in

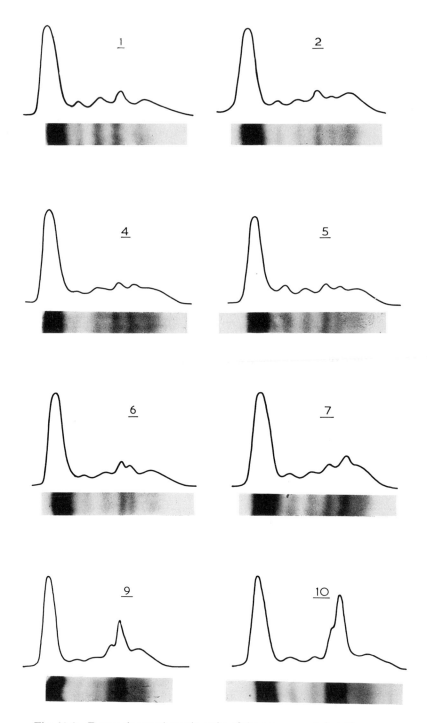

Fig. 29.2 Paper electrophoresis strip of the serum proteins of eight patients with CHAD.
   Their sera contained cold auto-antibodies at titres of 8000–256 000 at 4°C. Abnormal γ_1-globulin peaks were given by all the sera except that of Case 1. [Reproduced by permission from Christenson and Dacie (1957).]

nine out of ten patients suffering from CHAD and in whose serum cold agglutinins were present at titres exceeding 8000 at 4°C, paper electrophoresis of their serum showed abnormal γ_1 globulin peaks (Fig. 29.1). Three of the sera contained cryoglobulins which on concentration were shown to have the electrophoretic mobility of the γ_1 peak. Inspection of Christenson and Dacie's Fig. 2 shows that the γ_1 peak occupied a variable position in the β–γ region, being either midway between the β and γ_2 peaks or slightly nearer the β position (Fig. 29.2). The remaining patients studied, who were suffering from idiopathic haemolytic anaemia associated with relatively low-titre cold auto-agglutinins, 'post-virus pneumonia' haemolytic anaemia, secondary haemolytic anaemia or paroxysmal cold haemoglobinuria, had sera which gave less abnormal electrophoretic patterns. Only one serum, that of a patient with reticulosarcoma, gave an abnormal γ_1 peak.

Christenson and his colleagues (1957) described further studies of the abnormal γ_1 peaks. In three patients suffering from CHAD the peaks were shown to consist of cold-antibody protein by absorption of the serum with erythrocytes, by isolation of the protein by cellulose-column electrophoresis and by elution of cold antibody from erythrocytes. The cryoglobulin contained in one of the sera was shown to consist wholly, or at least very largely, of antibody protein. Studies in the ultracentrifuge showed that the antibody protein forming the γ_1 peaks consisted of macro-molecular protein of sedimentation coefficient (S_{20w}) approximately 16.

Fudenberg and Kunkel (1957) studied eight sera derived from patients suffering from acquired haemolytic anaemia of the cold-antibody type. The agglutinin titres varied from 512 to 40 000 and in four of the eight cases sufficient abnormal protein was present to form a visible peak on electrophoresis. In most instances the mobility of the abnormal protein corresponded to that of fast γ globulin, but it was in the centre of the γ globulin in one instance and in two instances the peak was in the β globulin region. The position of the abnormal peaks was found to correspond with the greatest cold agglutinin activity, and the titre could be positively correlated with the height of the peaks. Ultracentrifugal studies indicated that the cold agglutinins were macroglobulins of the 19S class.

Subsequent early studies of sera containing high-titre cold agglutinins in which abnormal peaks were demonstrated in the β–γ region include those of Wiener et al. (1958), Ess, Gramlich and Mohrung (1958), Firkin, Blackwell and Johnston (1959), Mehrotra and Charlwood (1960) and Wiedermann, Kubíková and Churý (1960).

Ess, Gramlich and Mohrung (1958) described serological and physiochemical observations made on the serum of a patient who had developed a remarkable cold agglutinin (titre 128 000 at 2°C) following a 'lymphotropic virus infection'. Studies of the γ_1 fraction of serum in an ultracentrifuge gave a sedimentation constant of S_{20} 11–14.8, but the authors calculated that the sedimentation constant of the cold agglutinin itself might have been as high as 52 ± 5.

Mehrotra and Charlwood (1960) studied seven samples of eluted antibodies prepared by dissociation of cold agglutinins from erythrocyte stromata. On ultra-centrifugation sedimentation coefficients (S_{20w}) ranging from 17.1 to 18.8 were obtained. In most instances the eluates contained as much as 1 g protein per 100 ml, and by using these concentrated eluates it was possible to show that all contained traces of material still heavier than S_{20w} 18. Mehrotra and Charlwood also studied the effect of mercapto-ethanol on the cold-agglutinin titre of 19 sera derived from patients with haemolytic anaemia of the cold-antibody type. As expected, the use of a reagent known to dissociate disulphide bonds and to cause macroglobulins to break up into units of S_{20} 6.5 produced a marked lowering of the agglutinin titres.

Cold auto-antibodies have also been studied by preparing antisera against purified antibody. Some early studies are referred to below:

Firkin and Blackburn (1956), Firkin (1958) and Firkin, Blackwell and Johnston (1959) studied several patients forming cold auto-antibodies and prepared antisera against the eluted antibodies. Using the Ouchterlony plate technique, Firkin and Blackburn (1956) obtained reactions of identity between the eluted material and crude β globulin eluted from paper electrophoresis strips. Firkin (1958) reported on further studies using the same technique. Eight patients were investigated; three of them had formed cold agglutinins; two adults had formed warm auto-antibodies and two infants suffered from haemolytic disease of the newborn. γ globulins were identified in the eluates in most instances; in one instance a second abnormal protein was demonstrated and in another a β globulin was identified. Firkin, Blackwell and Johnston (1959), in studies on a further patient suffering from cryo-globulinaemia and haemolytic anaemia, prepared an antiserum against the patient's cryoglobulin; the antiserum contained two antibodies, one reacting against the cryoglobulin and one against normal γ globulin.

Mehrotra (1960a) worked with eluted cold antibodies derived from six patients suffering from CHAD and one patient with a haemolytic anaemia associated with lymphosarcoma. The eluted antibodies were studied (1) by immuno-electrophoretic analysis, along with the parent serum, against an equine anti-human serum, and (2) by double diffusion in agar gel, along with electrophoretically separated γ_1 globulin, against anti-19S γ globulin rabbit sera. The protein acting as cold antibody was localized in the β_2M position in each instance on immuno-electrophoresis, and by double-diffusion it was found to be immunologically identical with the protein forming the γ_1 electrophoretic peak of the parent serum.

Mehrotra (1960b) described evidence which suggested that the high-titre cold auto-agglutinins present in the sera of patients with various types of haemolytic anaemia were immunologically distinguishable. He found that when sera from rabbits which had been immunized against human cold agglutinins were tested by double-diffusion in agar gel against autologous and homologous cold-agglutinin-containing sera and against a normal serum, the normal serum produced a single band while the sera containing high-titre cold agglutinins formed two bands. Moreover, when the rabbit sera were further absorbed with excess of normal serum or with γ_2 or γ_1 fractions of normal serum, they reacted with the autologous serum only, which suggested the presence of individually specific groupings in the autologous cold-agglutinin protein. In an extension of this work, Harris and Fairley (1962) demonstrated that a cryomacroglobulin that had been formed by a patient with CHAD possessed at least two antigenic determinants not found on normal serum globulins. One cross-reacted with other sera containing high-titre cold antibodies and with isolated cold antibodies; the other appeared to be patient-specific.

CHEMICAL NATURE OF COLD AUTO-ANTIBODIES IN AIHA: RECENT STUDIES

The fact that cold antibodies might be present in the sera of certain patients in very large amounts has greatly facilitated their study. Particular attention has been paid to the Ig class and light (L)-chain type of the antibodies, the relationship (if any) between Ig class and L-chain type and specificity, the chemical nature of the corresponding antigens on the erythrocyte surface, and the correlation, if any, between Ig class and L-chain type and the clinical condition of the patient forming the antibody. The important reviews of Roelcke, published in 1974 and 1989, illustrate the large amount of work that has been carried out in these fields.

Cold-antibody AIHA associated with more than one Ig class of antibody

It is now known that although the great majority of high-titre cold auto-antibodies are IgM, this is not invariably so. Occasionally, the antibody molecules are IgG, alone or in combination with IgM molecules; they are rarely IgA. The less common IgG and IgA variants seem to be associated relatively frequently with antibodies of specificity other than anti-I, the vast majority of which are IgM. It is interesting, too, to note (see below) that the IgG and IgA antibodies have been more frequently reported in patients suffering from a secondary type of cold-antibody AIHA, e.g. from an AIHA associated with a lymphoproliferative disorder or an infection, than in patients with idiopathic CHAD.

IgG cold auto-antibodies

Reports of patients in whom IgG cold auto-antibodies have been detected include those of Goldberg and Barnett (1967), Ambrus and Bajtai (1969); Capra et al. (1969), MacKenzie and Creevy (1969, 1970) Roelcke and Jungfer (1970), Roelcke et al. (1971), Mygind and Ahrons (1972), Ratkin, Osterland and Chaplin (1973), Freedman and Newlands (1977), Silberstein et al. (1985), Judd et al. (1986), Szymanski, Teno and Rybak (1986), Silberstein, Berkman and Schreiber (1987) and Curtis et al. (1990).

The clinical state of the patients who were the subjects of the case reports referred to above has varied: some of the patients have been very seriously ill, particularly those in whom the causal antibody has been exclusively IgG (see Curtis et al., 1990); in some the haemolysis has been acute and transient; other patients have suffered from a chronic illness.

Goldberg and Barnet's (1967) patient had infectious mononucleosis: the IgG component was the auto-antibody and the IgM component appeared to be a cold anti-antibody reacting with the IgG antibody. Both components had to be present for agglutination to take place.

Capra and co-workers (1969) had closely studied the sera of 50 patients who had developed infectious mononucleosis: 'incomplete' 7S anti-i cold agglutinins were identified in 90%, 'complete' 19S anti-i cold agglutinins in 35%, cold reactive 19S anti-γ-globulin in 72% and 'mixed' anti-i cold agglutinins (7S anti-i plus 19S anti-γ-globulin) in 66%.

The patients studied by Roelcke et al. (1971) were two children who had suffered from transient cold-antibody haemolytic anaemia.

Mygind and Ahrons's (1972) patients were two women, aged 31 and 30, respectively, with chronic CHAD, who had first trimester abortions. On fractionation of their sera, most of the cold antibody was found to be IgM, but IgG and IgA cold auto-antibody molecules were also present.

Ratkin, Osterland and Chaplin (1973) had estimated by radial immuno-diffusion the IgG, IgA and IgM concentration in eluates that had been prepared in a carefully standardized and controlled way from normal erythrocytes that had been sensitized at 0°C by exposure to 19 different high-titre cold antibodies, 14 of which had been derived from CHAD patients. As expected, the IgM concentrations were 32–4800 times the concentrations of residual Ig predicted to be present in the fluid in which the erythrocytes were suspended after the last washing. Seventeen of the 19 eluates contained 9–660 times the predicted concentration of IgG and six of the 19 eluates contained 12–226 times the expected concentrations of IgA. These findings certainly suggest that IgG cold antibodies are not infrequently present in sera containing high-titre cold antibodies alongside the characteristic and usually dominant IgM antibodies. Less commonly, IgA cold antibodies are present as well. Some recent reports of patients who had formed both IgG and IgM cold antibodies, i.e. biclonal antibodies, are referred to below.

Recent reports of biclonal cold-antibody AIHA

Freedman and Newlands (1977) had investigated two women, aged 23 and 20, respectively. The first gave a 10-year history of chronic AIHA, the onset of which had been acute; the second gave a 1-year history of AIHA, the onset of which had also been acute. The serological findings were similar in each of them: the DAT was positive with anti-C4d/C3d and anti-IgG sera, and in their sera were identified an IgM anti-I cold antibody, which was complement-binding, and in addition an IgG anti-I cold antibody the activity of which extended up to 37°C, which was not complement-binding.

The patient described by Silberstein et al. (1985) was a 40-year-old man giving a 3 years' history of CHAD. Recently he had become more anaemic and had had haemoglobinuria. The haemoglobin was 6.8 g/dl and reticulocyte count 14%. The DAT was positive with an anti-IgG serum. Serum contained a cold antibody which agglutinated I erythrocytes to a titre of 700 at 4°C and cord and adult i cells to a titre of 256; at room temperature the titre with I cells was 512. Heat eluates demonstrated both IgG kappa and IgM kappa antibodies at a ratio of 1.2 to 0.08. He was treated for 6 months with immunosuppressive drugs, but haemolysis persisted. Splenectomy was then undertaken, and for the subsequent 30 months no form of therapy was required.

Szymanski, Teno and Rybak's (1986) patient, a male aged 65, suffered from a severe haemolytic anaemia of 2 months' duration: the haemoglobin was 7.6 g/dl and

reticulocyte count 15%, and there had been transient thrombocytopenia. The DAT was positive with an anti-IgG serum. IgG and IgM auto-antibodies were present in his serum. Their thermal optimum was unusual, the titres with adult group-O cells being 16 at 4°C, 128 at 22°C and 1 at 37°C. The antibodies did not fix complement. Their specificity could not be determined; the titres with cold-blood cells were, however, half those with adult cells.

The patient described by Tschirhart, Kunkel and Shulman (1990) was a 65-year-old man under investigation for prostatic hypertrophy. His haemoglobin was 10.9 g/dl, with 4.8% reticulocytes. The DAT was weakly positive with an anti-C3d serum. His serum contained a high-thermal-amplitude anti-I agglutinin, the titre with autologous erythrocytes being 2048 at 4°C, 64 at room temperature, 4 at 30°C and zero at 37°C. Immunoelectrophoresis of antibody eluates showed the presence of monoclonal IgA, IgM and kappa light chains.

The patients described by Judd et al. (1986) and by Curtis et al. (1990), who had formed antibodies of Pr specificity, are referred to on p. 267.

An IgG cold antibody acting as a biphasic lysin

Shirey and co-workers (1986) described an unusual IgG antibody which acted in vitro as a biphasic haemolysin. It had anti-i specificity and was best demonstrated by the D-L 4–37°C procedure or by the IAT sensitizing at 4°C. Their patient, a male aged 71 giving a 12-year history of chronic lymphocytic leukaemia, became quite suddenly anaemic — his haematocrit fell from 40 to 28% without any evidence of haemorrhage. Haemoglobinuria was not observed, although haemosiderinuria was recorded. The maximum titre in a cold–warm titration was 64 with i erythrocytes and 8 with I erythrocytes; acidification of the serum did not enhance lysis. The DAT was positive with polyspecific and anti-C sera but negative with an anti-IgG serum.

Cold-detectable 'warm' IgG auto-antibodies

Mackenzie and Creevy (1969, 1970) described six patients in whom the DAT using an anti-IgG serum was negative or only weakly positive at 37°C but strongly positive when the test was carried out at 4°C. Two of the patients had AIHA associated with lymphosarcoma, three had idiopathic AIHA and one had AIHA associated with systemic lupus erythematosus (SLE). In two of the patients the DAT using an anti-IgA serum was positive at both 37°C and at 4°C and in one patient the DAT using an anti-IgM serum was also positive at both temperatures. The DAT using an anti-β1C serum was positive in all six patients, but in one only if the test was carried out at 4°C. Mackenzie and Creevy concluded that the temperature effect was probably due to a 'configurational' change affecting the antibody attached to the erythrocyte surface at temperatures above 10°C, which obscured available antigenic sites or interfered with lattice formation, with the result that the antiglobulin test appeared to be negative. They stressed that the antibodies, however, differed from most cold auto-antibodies in that they were IgG, and reacted with both anti-kappa and anti-lambda light chain sera, and did not elute readily at 37°C. Mackenzie and Creevy suggested that the formation of this type of IgG antibody provided an explanation for some of the cases of 'complement only' DATs. The specificity of the antibodies they had studied was not recorded.

IgA cold auto-antibodies

Angevine, Andersen and Barnett (1966) and Andersen (1966) studied a cold antibody present in the serum of a patient suffering from reticulosarcoma. He was not anaemic. The cold-agglutinin titre was 1024–4096 but there was no agglutination at 37°C. The antibody did not fix complement and appeared to be formed entirely of IgA, type-K molecules. It had a sedimentation coefficient of 10.5S and could be inactivated by 2-mercapto-ethanol. Its specificity was undetermined: it was not anti-I or anti-i.

LIGHT CHAINS—KAPPA AND LAMBDA

A characteristic feature of the high-titre anti-I IgM cold auto-antibodies of CHAD, in keeping with their monoclonal nature, is that the light chains of the antibody molecules are monotypic: most, but in not quite all cases, kappa chains (type-K molecules) are present and lambda chains (type-L molecules) are absent. In contrast, in the case of the high-titre cold antibodies formed transitorily in response to mycoplasma or viral infections, both types of chain are typically present. This is true also of the low-titre cold auto-antibodies present in normal sera.

As implied above, IgM cold auto-antibodies of exclusively lambda light-chain type are occasionally produced, and of particular interest is that in many of these cases the patients forming the antibodies have been suffering not from CHAD but from a chronic cold-antibody haemolytic anaemia associated with an underlying disorder

such as a lymphoma. In these cases, too, the specificity of the antibody has often been found to be atypical, i.e., other than anti-I. The significance of these interesting associations has been the subject of considerable debate and the topic of cold antibodies and their light chains has by now quite a large literature. Some of this is summarized below.

Reports on the exclusively kappa nature of the light chains in CHAD date from the early 1960s (Franklin and Fudenberg, 1961; Harboe et al., 1965; Harboe and Lind, 1966; Costea, Yakulis and Heller, 1966; van Furth and Diesselhoff-den Dulk, 1966; Cooper and Worlledge, 1967; Costea, Yakulis and Heller, 1967).

Harboe and co-workers (1965) studied the auto-antibodies of 37 patients with CHAD and found kappa light chains only. Harboe and Lind (1966) stated that 87 isolated monoclonal cold antibodies had yielded only kappa light chains. They had studied the light chains of the cold agglutinins in nine patients who had suffered from pneumonia; in four of these both kappa and lambda light chains were identified. The reactions with anti-L sera were always weak and lambda chains were apparently absent in five of the cases.

Costea, Yakulis and Heller (1966) detected, however, both K- and L-type light chains in the cold auto-antibodies formed by 15 patients who had developed mycoplasma pneumonia and by seven patients who had had infectious mononucleosis. This was true, too, of the cold-antibodies present in the sera of 10 normal individuals. In contrast, the antibodies formed by five CHAD patients yielded K-type light chains only. Costea, Yakulis and Heller (1967), reporting on the same patients, went on to suggest that K-type light chains might play a central role in determining antibody specificity to antigens belonging to the Ii system.

Cooper and Worlledge (1967) reported on the light chains of the antibodies formed by six CHAD patients and referred, too, to the specificity of the antibodies. Five of the antibodies yielded K-type light chains only; two were anti-I; three had specificities other than anti-I —one was described as 'Not-I$_1$', two as 'Not I$_2$'. One of the antibodies yielded L-type light chains only; its specificity was 'Not-I$_1$'.

Feizi (1967) reported that the cold auto-antibodies of three CHAD patients had yielded only L-type light chains. One of the antibodies was anti-I; two had specificities other than anti-I.

Cooper (1968) reported on studies carried out on the light chains of the antibodies of 18 CHAD patients— 17 were kappa, one lambda. When submitted to starch gel electrophoresis, they yielded patterns that were more homogeneous than those given by normal light chains. The banding was comparable with that of Bence-Jones light chains. However, the patterns given by individual patients varied, and Cooper concluded that cold agglutinins of similar specificity differed chemically, a finding consistent with their serological individuality.

Further evidence of chemical differences between individual cold agglutinins was provided by Cohen and Cooper (1968). They had studied the amino-acid composition of the kappa light chains and of the heavy (μ) chains of the auto-antibodies of four CHAD patients. Individual differences in composition were detected. These were similar in extent to those found with the M components in six cases of Waldenström's macroglobulinaemia.

Recent descriptions of IgM lambda (L-type) cold auto-antibodies

Noteworthy reports include those of Macris et al. (1970), Roelcke, Ebert and Feizi (1974), Pruzanski, Cowan and Parr (1974), Crookston (1975), Isbister et al. (1978), Kuenn et al. (1978), Lee et al. (1979) and Fingerle and Check (1982).

The patient described by Macris et al. and three of the patients referred to by Pruzanski, Cowan and Parr, and those described by Crookston, Isbister et al., Kuenn et al. and Lee et al. suffered from a lymphoproliferative disorder. The serum studied by Fingerle and Check was especially interesting as it contained two apparently distinct cold auto-antibodies: one was an IgM with kappa light chains and of anti-I specificity; the other was an IgM with lambda light chains and of an undefined ('not-I') specificity. The disorder — a diclonal gammopathy — was believed to be unique in that both pathological IgMs acted as cold antibodies. The patient's bone marrow resembled that in Waldenström's macroglobulinaemia: it contained an excess of lymphocytes (13%) and plasma cells (4%). Immunoperoxidase staining showed that two types of plasma cells were present, one forming kappa light chains, the other lambda light chains.

A low-molecular-weight IgM lambda anti-I auto-antibody

Kay and co-workers (1975) described a most unusual case. Their patient was a 49-year-old woman whose liver and spleen had been found to be enlarged 16 months previously. Splenectomy had been carried out, and histological examination revealed non-caseating granulomas in both liver and spleen. Later, she had suffered from persistent pyrexia with daily peaks up to 104°F. Her haemoglobin was 10 g/dl and the leucocyte count 22 × 10^9/l, with 57% neutrophils and a shift to the left. The DAT was positive with an anti-IgM serum, and a low-molecular-weight IgM antibody was present in eluates from her erythrocytes. The serum levels of IgG and IgA were markedly subnormal and the serum IgM was initially as high as 1250 mg/dl. Immunoelectrophoresis demonstrated a monoclonal IgM lambda protein in her serum, and lambda light chains were present in her urine. Ultracentrifugation showed that only 5–6% of the IgM in her serum was of the 19S type: the remainder had a low molecular weight (7S–4S). The serum contained an anti-I agglutinin; its titre was 64 and its thermal optimum 37°C. Normal erythrocytes underwent slight lysis in her serum, and the unlysed cells were agglutinated by both anti-IgM and anti-C sera, and also by an anti-IgG serum.

SPECIFICITY OF COLD AUTO-ANTIBODIES

Species specificity: early studies

Many studies have been carried out on the reactions between animal erythrocytes and the high-titre cold auto-antibodies found in the sera of patients suffering from various types of haemolytic anaemia as well as on the low-titre cold auto-antibodies found in normal sera. Early studies revealed no very clear pattern, but the antibodies were found to cross-react with certain animal species, particularly with rabbit, pig and monkey erythrocytes.

Clough and Richter (1918) studied a patient who almost certainly had suffered from a 'virus' pneumonia and found that the patient's serum contained cold agglutinins against rabbit, guinea-pig, hen, sheep, cat and pig erythrocytes as well as against human cells: absorption with either rabbit or human erythrocytes removed the agglutinins acting on both types of cell. Mino (1924) who had introduced the term 'panhaemagglutinin' also concluded that cold agglutinins did not distinguish between human and animal cells. Rosenthal and Corten (1937) described observations they had made on a patient suffering from acquired haemolytic anaemia in whom cold auto-agglutination was conspicuous. The cold agglutinins were eluted off the patient's erythrocytes and then shown to be capable of agglutinating rabbit cells and pig cells.

Turner and Jackson (1943) carried out an extensive study on the sera of seven patients who had developed high-titre cold agglutinins following 'virus' pneumonia. Cold agglutinins active against rabbit, mouse, guinea-pig, horse and sheep cells were present in each serum, but equally powerful hetero-antibodies were found in normal sera not containing high-titre cold agglutinins active against human erythrocytes. Eluates into warm saline, obtained from human cells sensitized by the patients' sera in the cold, were next tested for specificity: rabbit and human cells were found to be agglutinated to about the same titre, and guinea-pig and pig erythrocytes to low titres. On the other hand, absorption experiments showed that the anti-human agglutinins could be removed without affecting to any significant degree the agglutination of the heterologous erythrocytes, except possibly that of guinea-pig cells.

Further studies were described by Finland, Peterson and Barnes (1945). Like Turner and Jackson, they found that heterospecific agglutinins existed in many normal human sera and that, of the species they studied, rabbit erythrocytes were agglutinated to the highest titres. Finland, Peterson and Barnes also tested a panel of animal erythrocytes against human sera, known to contain cold agglutinins active against human cells at pathologically raised titres (128–2048), derived from patients who had suffered from 'virus' pneumonia. In most cases the titres against the animal cells seemed to be independent of the presence or absence of cold antibodies active against human cells. However, agglutination of monkey erythrocytes occurred more regularly and to higher titres in sera containing anti-human cold antibodies in raised concentrations; reversal at 37°C was usually incomplete. Absorption experiments showed that whereas absorption with rabbit erythrocytes resulted in a significant fall in the titres against human and guinea-pig cells, as well as against autologous cells, absorption with human or guinea-pig erythrocytes had little effect on the cold-agglutinin titres for heterologous cells.

These observations were extended by Millet and Fincler (1946), who found that it was impossible to absorb cold agglutinins against human erythrocytes from human serum by means of rabbit, guinea-pig or ox cells. They reported, however, that this specificity depended upon surface antigens, for if erythrocyte stromata were used instead of intact corpuscles, species specificity disappeared.

Wiener, Gordon and Gallop (1953) studied three patients whose sera contained cold antibodies in raised concentrations. All three patients had an acquired haemolytic anaemia; in two of them this was secondary to lymphoblastoma or lymphomatosis. The antibodies were found to react strongly with Rhesus-monkey, spider-monkey, pig and rabbit erythrocytes, but only weakly or not at all with chimpanzee, cow, horse or sheep cells.

Delage, Gauvreau and Simard (1956) experimented with the serum of a patient suffering from CHAD. This serum agglutinated both rabbit cells and sheep cells; when administered intravenously to rabbits severe haemolysis and haemoglobinuria resulted, irrespective of whether the animals were chilled. Delage, Gauvreau and Simard also reported that the antibody was absorbed by *Shigella dysenteriae*. Schubothe (1958) investigated six sera derived from patients suffering from CHAD and prepared eluates from group-O cells exposed to the antibodies. These eluates were tested against the erythrocytes of nine animal species. The highest titres were recorded against rabbit and pig cells, followed by guinea-pig and rat cells. Dog, mouse, horse and sheep cells were agglutinated to low titres or not at all. It is interesting to note that the results with four species whose cells were regularly agglutinated did not run exactly parallel when different sera were used: for instance, with the first serum pig cells were the most sensitive; with the second and third, rabbit and rat cells; with the fourth, pig cells; with the fifth, pig, guinea-pig and rabbit cells, and with the sixth, pig and rabbit cells. Schubothe's results underline how subtle are the differences which exist between individual human antibodies; they help to explain the many discrepancies to be found in the early literature on species specificity.

Further data on the species specificity of a high-titre anti-I antibody were recorded by Moor-Jankowski, Wiener and Gordon (1964). I reactivity was found to cut across taxonomic lines: it was absent or poorly developed in anthropoid apes and gibbons, although well developed in New World (Cebus) monkeys; in rabbits it was well developed; in sheep it was absent.

Further data on specificity were provided by Evans, Turner and Bingham (1965). Eluates containing ^{131}I trace-labelled cold agglutinins were prepared from erythrocytes exposed to the serum of seven patients: five of the sera were anti-I; two were anti-i. The adsorption at 5°C of the labelled antibodies by rabbit, dog, sheep, rat and human adult and cord-blood erythrocytes was compared. Rabbit cells adsorbed more agglutinin than adult human cells in three instances; dog, sheep and rat cells generally adsorbed much less. Of interest was the variability in the retention of the agglutinins on rabbit cells when the suspensions were warmed at 37°C: with one serum only 50% of the agglutinin was eluted, in another 99%. Sheep cells adsorbed more of the two anti-i agglutinins than did the other animal cells, and in the case of one serum more than human cord cells.

Tönder and Harboe (1966) reported on a comparison of the agglutinability of human and rabbit erythrocytes, respectively, by seven human sera containing high-titre cold auto-agglutinins. The titres with human cells ranged from 256 to 32 000 at 4°C. Whereas with the rabbit cells the titres were almost identical with those recorded with the human cells at 4°C, at 20°C the titres with the human cells were far less (< 8 to 128), while those with the rabbit cells were almost the same as at 4°C. At 37°C the titres with the human cells were all < 8, while those with the rabbit cells ranged from 16 to 32 000 — with one serum the titre with rabbit cells (32 000) was the same at 4, 20 and 37°C. Absorption and elution experiments showed that the human cells (at 4°C) and the rabbit cells (at 37°C) were being agglutinated by the same molecules. Tönder and Harboe's data illustrate the heterogeneity of human anti-I sera and also the importance of antigen differences in determining the effect of temperature on the activity of cold auto-agglutinins.

As is referred to later, anti-Pr cold auto-antibodies vary, too, in their reaction with animal erythrocytes. These differences have been used as a basis for classification. Thus, anti-Pr_{1h} is human-specific, while anti-Pr_{1d} is human- plus dog-specific, and anti-Pr_3 agglutinates cat and sheep erythrocytes.

SPECIFICITY IN RELATION TO HUMAN ERYTHROCYTES

This is now known to be a highly complex subject, for although the majority of pathological cold auto-antibodies have a well-defined specificity, namely, anti-I, antibodies of other specificities exist and, as has already been referred to, are found most frequently in the sera of patients suffering from cold-antibody haemolytic anaemias associated with infections or lymphoproliferative disorders.

Early studies

Mino (1924) is usually quoted as having introduced the concept of the 'non-specific' nature of cold agglutinins; he concluded that all human erythrocytes shared a common receptor and that no distinction could be made with regard to reactivity between cells of different ABO groups. Amzel and Hirszfeld (1925), on the contrary, concluded that there were in fact differences in the agglutinability of human cells by cold agglutinins, but they also concluded as the result of absorption experiments that there were no qualitative differences in the receptors on the cell surfaces. Kettel (1929) titrated 378 sera and demonstrated cold agglutinins in 360 of them. He reported that the titres tended to be lowest in group-O sera and highest in group-B sera and that the titres with autologous cells were usually relatively low.

Boxwell and Bigger (1931) reviewed the early literature and described an antibody which agglutinated group-O cells more strongly than group-AB, -A, or -B cells. Wheeler, Gallacher and Stuart (1939) reported on another case, possibly of 'virus' pneumonia, in which the cold agglutinin appeared to agglutinate group-O and -A_2 cells more strongly than group-A cells. However, eluates of the cold antibody seemed to lack any specificity. Stratton (1943) also reported observations indicating, in three out of five patients, an anti-O specificity or preferential agglutination of group-O cells; the antibodies of the other two patients (one with haemolytic anaemia) seemed, however, to lack specificity. Finland, Peterson and Barnes (1945) described the results of experiments carried out with nine sera derived from patients with 'virus' pneumonia. Group-O cells reacted more strongly than group-AB, -A or -B cells in the case of seven of the sera.

Bird (1951; 1953a,b), too, reported a complicated relationship between certain cold agglutinins and the ABO blood groups. Bird (1951) had investigated a patient with acquired haemolytic anaemia whose serum contained an apparently 'non-specific' cold agglutinin. He found that if this serum was absorbed with the patient's own (group-AB) erythrocytes, it then ceased to agglutinate O, A and B cells as well as autologous cells. However, when the serum was absorbed with group-O cells, so that it was no longer active against O cells, agglutinins persisted which still reacted with group-A, -B and the patient's cells. Bird's experiments in fact suggested that this particular serum was a mixture of anti-O, anti-A, anti-B and anti-patient's cell components. A similar combination of components was stated to be present in seven other group-AB sera studied in the same way. Bird (1953a), however, reported that absorption with group-O cells usually removes all the supposed components of a cold panagglutinin. In a further paper (Bird, 1953b) he stated that certain group-AB sera containing cold agglutinins reacted with various types of erythrocytes independently of their supposed H content.

Thus although some of the early work quoted above indicated a relationship between the ABO groups and agglutination by cold auto-antibodies, with group-O cells being perhaps the most sensitive, this had not been the general experience. Turner and Jackson (1943) and Young (1946), for instance, and Dacie (1954b), too, had found no relationship between ABO groups and agglutinability. Wiener, Gordon and Gallop (1953) concluded, however, that cold auto-antibodies were in fact 'directed against the nucleus of the A-B-O-substance'.

Dacie (1954b), who had prepared eluates of antibodies from group-O erythrocytes exposed to 10 sera derived from patients with cold-antibody haemolytic anaemia, had found that the antibodies agglutinated cells irrespective of their ABO groups.

Crookston, Dacie and Rossi (1956) later reported more elaborate studies. Sixty-four samples of erythrocytes derived from healthy adults were tested for their agglutinability by a single serum containing a high-titre cold antibody. This was found to vary considerably, but it seemed to be independent of the ABO, Rh, MNSs, P, Lutheran, Kell, Lewis, Duffy and Kidd groups. Moreover, the sensitivity of the different cells appeared to be a normally-distributed characteristic (Fig. 29.3). Absorption experiments using strongly reacting cells and weakly reacting cells showed that they were reacting with the same antigen. Fetal erythrocytes were not tested. Unger, Wiener and Dolan (1952) and Mortara and Martinetti (1955) had earlier found that fetal cord-blood cells might be poorly agglutinated by high-titre cold agglutinins.

THE Ii SYSTEM

Wiener and his co-workers (1956) tested a serum derived from a patient suffering from CHAD against 22 964 blood samples! Five samples only, as well as the patient's own cells, were not agglutinated at room temperature. The insensitive cells were designated 'i' or 'I-negative' and the serum

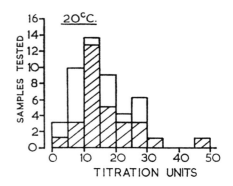

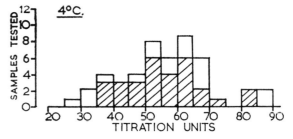

Fig. 29.3   Histograms illustrating the variability in agglutinability of 48 samples of normal adult (I) erythrocytes by a high-titre anti-I antibody in the serum of a patient (L.S.) with CHAD.
Hatched columns = group O; unhatched columns = group A. [Reproduced by permission from Crookston, Dacie and Rossi (1956).]

was said to contain 'anti-I'. The 'I factor' was considered to be unrelated to any blood-factor system known at that time. Normal human cells were designated I, and less strongly-reacting cells I_2 and I_3. It is interesting to note that the 'negative' cells were agglutinated at room temperature (24°C), if ficinated, and at 4°C even without enzyme treatment.

Subsequently, further I-negative cells were discovered—in Caucasians (Jenkins et al., 1960; Jakobowicz and Simmons, 1964) and in blacks (Tippett et al., 1960). The I-negative (i) cells of Tippett and her co-workers (1960) were slightly stronger-reacting than the cells of Jenkins's patient, and there were hints of some relationship with the ABO system. As described by Issitt (1967), the frequency of the i phenotype in adults is, according to different reports, somewhere between 1 in 3000 to less than 1 in 17 000.

Jenkins and his co-workers (1960) reported the finding of anti-I in the serum of an I-negative (i) apparently healthy English blood donor. The antibody was as active at 20°C as at 10°C (titre

16) and was weakly active at 37°C. It did not distinguish between group-O, -A or -A$_2$ cells and only agglutinated cord cells very weakly.

Jenkins et al. demonstrated, using the erythrocytes of their i patient, that the apparently non-specific weak cold agglutinins present in the sera of 50 individuals were of anti-I specificity. Jenkins et al. concluded, too, that the I antigen is a graded character and that its strength fits a curve of normal distribution. As mentioned above, this had been the conclusion, too, of Crookson, Dacie and Rossi (1956) who had assessed the agglutinability by a high-titre cold agglutinin (later shown to be anti-I in specificity) of 48 samples of normal erythrocytes (Fig. 29.3). Tippett and her co-workers (1960) concluded that anti-I antibodies were to be found in three different environments: in AIHA of the cold-antibody type: in [normal] sera containing 'non-specific' complete cold auto-agglutinin and in the sera of normal people whose erythrocytes have abnormally little antigen and are of the rare phenotype i.

Marsh and Jenkins (1960) and Marsh (1961) described some most interesting observations. Marsh and Jenkins studied two sera derived from patients with reticulum-cell sarcoma and anaemia, and 'reticulosis' and anaemia, respectively. The two sera behaved antithetically compared with anti-I sera in that they agglutinated normal adult cells weakly and cord-blood or adult I-negative cells very strongly. Marsh and Jenkins, therefore, designated the sera 'anti-i'. Marsh (1961) concluded that all infants at birth are of the phenotype i, and thus react very weakly with anti-I sera, and that normally the phenotype i changes to I within 18 months of birth (Fig. 29.4). The adult specimens of i blood which had been found he attributed to an abnormality in the development of the I antigen due to the absence of a genetically-determined factor. Marsh quoted the observations of Jenkins et al. and of Tippett et al. that cells which are weak in I are also weak in H; and he suggested that the factor that adult i cells lack may also be involved in the development of H (which is also weak in fetal cells). Concluding that all cells possess variable amounts of the two antigens involved, Marsh ranged the cells as I (normal adult cells), I$_{(int)}$ (weakly-reacting cells from adults possibly inheriting a

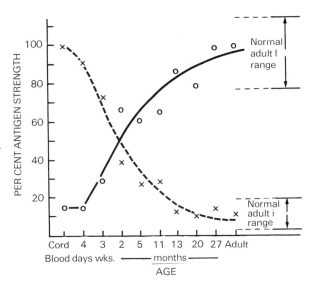

Fig. 29.4 Titration scores given by the erythrocytes of infants of selected ages when titrated in an anti-I serum and in an anti-i serum, calculated as percentages of the scores given by normal adult (I) and normal cord-blood (i) erythrocytes.
[Reproduced by permission from Marsh (1961).]

single dose of the I development factor), i$_{(cord)}$, i$_2$ and i$_1$. 'i' was reserved for cells completely lacking in I.

Later, Marsh, Nichols and Reid (1971) referred to the I antigen being formed of two main components I^F (I^{fetal}) and I^D (I^{developed}). I^F was considered to be present on all human erythrocytes including cord-blood i and adult i, and was also present on Rhesus monkey cells. In contrast, I^D developed slowly before birth and then more quickly up to 18 months *post partum*. Marsh, Nichols and Reid concluded that there were both qualitative as well as quantitative differences in the I antigen in adult I-positive cells.

Evans, Turner and Bingham (1965) described some interesting comparative data using adult I and cord-blood erythrocytes to titrate the cold agglutinins in 10 sera, five derived from patients who had suffered from 'viral' pneumonia or another infection and five from patients with CHAD. The ratio of the titres with the I and cord cells, respectively, varied widely, i.e. from 16:1 to 1:16 in the post-infection patients and from 2560:1 to 2:1 in the CHAD patients.

Olesen (1966), who had studied the reaction between erythrocytes and the high-titre cold agglutinins obtained from three patients, two with CHAD and one with Waldenström's macro-globulinaemia, estimated that the number of cold-agglutinin sites per erythrocyte was approximately 32 000 on I cells and 70 000–111 000 on i cells: he estimated, too, that at 5°C 50–500 molecules per erythrocyte were required for agglutination while at 37°C 10^4 or more molecules would be required. He pointed out, too, that for I and i erythrocytes the term 'specificity' has only relative significance, for both I and i cells are agglutinated by anti-I and anti-i antibodies; 'specificity' referred only to the observed differences in titres obtained with I and i cells. In his own study the difference had varied between a factor of 3 to 100.

Maas and Schubothe (1968) came to the same conclusion, namely, that the difference in agglutinability by high-titre anti-I sera of I and i erythrocytes varies widely. Fifty samples of cord-blood cells were tested for their agglutinability by an anti-I serum that agglutinated adult erythrocytes to a titre of 8000–16000 at 2–4°C. The titres with the cord-blood cells ranged from 4 to 2000, i.e. up to a titre one-quarter of that of the lowest adult titre.

Further data on the reaction between cold agglutinins and I-positive (I) cells and I-negative (i) cells were summarized in an abstract by Rosse, Borsos and Rapp (1967). Cold agglutinins were shown to differ in their affinity for I antigen, some antibodies being tightly bound, some more loosely, and the fixation of C1a was found to enhance binding: i cells fixed less antibody than I cells, the difference being greater with antibodies that were highly dissociable. If dissociability was decreased by papain, the amount of antibody fixed by I cells and i cells became more nearly the same. Rosse, Borsos and Rapp concluded that all human erythrocytes contain antigens that react with cold agglutinins and that the dissociability of the antibody varies with different cells and with different antibodies; they suggested that the degree of dissociability plays a role in determining whether a cell appears to be I-positive (I) or I-negative (i). Details of their observations on the enhancement of the fixation of anti-I cold antibodies by the first component of complement (C1a) were given by Rosse, Borsos and Rapp (1968).

Rosse and Sherwood (1970) employed the 'C'1a fixation and transfer test' of Borsos and Rapp (1965) to study the difference in behaviour of adult (I) and cord-blood (i) erythrocytes. A single molecule of antibody was found to be required for the fixation of one molecule of C1a to either I or i cells. Rosse and Sherwood concluded that the I antigen content in adult I cells is not as different from that of cord-blood or adult i cells as the nomenclature (I-positive or I-negative) suggests. The amount of anti-I antibody and C1a fixed by different adult erythrocytes differed markedly, and the same was true of cord-blood cells. The two ranges overlapped considerably, although the amount of antibody fixed by the cord-blood cells was generally less. The difference between the cord-blood cells and 'low-activity' adult I cells and 'high-activity' adult I cells appeared not to be due to the presence of different or extra antigens on the latter, as it was found that cord-blood (i) cells and 'low activity' adult I cells were able to absorb all the antibody that reacts with 'high-reactivity' I cells. The observable difference between adult I and cord-blood (i) and adult i cells was found to be less marked if the cells were pre-treated with papain or if the reactions were carried out at a higher temperature. Rosse and Sherwood concluded that the difference between I and i cells with regard to the fixation of cold agglutinins is due in large part to a difference in affinity between the antibody and antigen on the cell surface rather than to a major difference in the number of antigen sites. They suggested that the chemical structure of the antigen might be slightly different in the two types of cell and that the greater affinity of the I antigen is due to a better 'fit' of the antibody, or that the microenvironment around the antigen is different. (As previously discussed briefly, there is evidence that the I and i antigens *do* differ chemically.)

That the difference between I-positive and I-negative (i) cells is quantitative was clearly demonstrated by Cooper and Brown (1973). They had assessed the specificity of the cold agglutinins in the sera of 13 CHAD patients and in two normal sera by absorbing dilutions of the sera at 4°C with standardized suspensions of pooled adult group-O I cells and pooled group-O cord-blood (i) cells, respectively. The residual antibody in each serum was then measured in an AutoAnalyser, and the ratio of the percent absorption by the i cells and I cells determined—an index of the i to I specificity of each cold agglutinin. The ratio varied from 2.40 and 2.00 in the case of two sera previously designated as anti-i to 0.00 in the case of two of the CHAD sera. The ratio of the remaining 11 sera ranged widely—from 2.00 to 0.19.

A further interesting observation illustrating the complexity of the Ii antigen system was described by McGinniss, Grindon and Schmidt (1974). They reported that the erythrocytes of a healthy blood donor reacted strongly as I-positive when tested with the iso-anti-I obtained from five genetic I-negative adults or when tested with seven low-titre anti-I of miscellaneous origin; in contrast they were not agglutinated by the high-titre anti-I antibodies present in the sera of six CHAD patients or by a strong anti-I^T antibody. Thus the donor's cells, by being agglutinated strongly by polyclonal anti-I but not by monoclonal anti-I, were demonstrating the existence of at least two separate I determinants on adult I-positive erythrocytes.

Further evidence on the heterogeneity of anti-I sera was provided by Dzierzkowa-Borodej, Seyfried and Lisowska (1975), who had studied 12 sera, the titres of which ranged from 32 to 2×10^6. The sera could be grouped into three categories: five reacted weakly with i adult and I^F cells, three reacted strongly with i adult cells and weakly with I^F cells, and four reacted weakly with i adult cells and strongly with I^F cells. The conclusion was reached that anti-I sera often have more than one specificity: thus eight of the 12 sera appeared to have two or three specificities, e.g. anti-I^D plus anti-I^F plus anti-I^S (an anti-I inhibited by saliva) or anti-I^D plus anti-i.

Additional evidence of Ii antigen site heterogeneity was provided by Doinal, Ropars and Salmon (1976). They used several homogeneous (monoclonal) IgM cold agglutinins (two anti-I, two anti-i and one anti-Ii cross-reacting) to determine antigen site densities of I and i (adult) and i (cord) erythrocytes, as well as equilibrium and thermodynamic constants. The two anti-I antibodies recognized two different I determinants with different antigen site densities. The i erythrocytes appeared to be even more heterogeneous: one anti-i antibody reacted mainly with an anti-i component present on cord erythrocytes; the other anti-i reacted with a different i component present on adult i cells.

Subtypes of the i antigen

Feizi and Kabat (1972), using a quantitative precipitation technique, had postulated four subtypes, and further evidence of the heterogeneity of the i antigen was presented by Dzierżkowa-Borodej and Voak (1979): three subtypes were identified as the result of agglutination, absorption and elution studies, using several anti-i sera and atypical Ii erythrocytes; a fourth was identified by an inhibition method using i substance present in human serum and amniotic fluid.

Interaction between anti-I antibodies and isolated antigens

Lauf and Rosse (1969) and Rosse and Lauf (1970) showed that I antigen could be removed from the erythrocyte membrane in a water-soluble form. They found that the solubilized antigen reacts differently from the antigen attached to the cell membrane in that the dependence on temperature for the antibody–antigen reaction is lost, i.e. it occurs as well at 37°C as at 0°C. They concluded that the temperature effect observable with intact cells is due to a change in the antigen rather than in the antibody.

In a subsequent study, Lau and Rosse (1975) showed that the cold-reacting auto-antibodies, anti-I, anti-i and anti-P (the Donath–Landsteiner antibody) would react with their corresponding antigens on glycophorin, the major membrane glycoprotein, at 37°C, i.e., the reactions with glycophorin when isolated from the erythrocyte membrane were temperature-independent.

In relation to the difference in the effect of temperature on the reactions between cold antibodies and intact erythrocytes and between cold antibodies and antigens extracted from the cell membrane, it is interesting to recall the description by Millet and Fincler, published in 1946, of the reactions of a cold auto-agglutinin present in human serum. They reported that, although the antibody fixed to intact erythrocytes only at temperatures less than 5°C, if erythrocyte stroma was substituted for intact cells, antibody fixation then took place up to a much higher temperature, almost in fact up to 37°C.

RECENT STUDIES ON THE Ii BLOOD-GROUP SYSTEM

These have confirmed the considerable heterogeneity of the antibodies and the existence of a complex antigen system. The subject was extensively reviewed by Roelcke in 1974 and again in 1989. Chemical studies have provided evidence that the Ii antigens and ABH(O) antigens are closely related and it is therefore not surprising that certain anti-I antibodies have been found to react more strongly with, respectively, A_1, B or O erythrocytes than with erythrocytes of other ABH(O) phenotypes. These cold antibodies have been designated anti-IA, anti-IB, anti-IH and anti-HI, and presumably react with antigens determined by the combined action of the I and A, B or H genes.

Anti-I reacts with antigens only fully expressed on adult erythrocytes: in contrast, anti-i reacts with antigens already fully expressed on neonatal erythrocytes (and rarely on adult cells) (Fig. 29.4). Chemical studies have provided an explanation for this reciprocal relationship. The Ii antigens are formed of repeating N-acetyllactosamine units: anti-i reacts with a linear chain of these units; anti-I with a branched chain. A 'branching enzyme' converts the i (antigen) to I. The Ii antigenic determinants are bound in the erythrocyte membrane to glycolipids and glycoproteins.

A large number of antibodies recognizing naturally occurring variants of the Ii antigens have been described (see below). In the laboratory the antibodies have been characterized in the main by their reactions with adult I, cord-blood i and adult i cells, the cells being used untreated or treated with a protease enzyme, generally papain, or with sialidase (neuraminidase).

Relationship with the ABH(O) blood groups: anti-HI (OI), anti-AI and anti-BI

Early reports indicating a relationship in some cases have already been referred to. More recent reports include those of van Loghem et al. (1962), Gold (1964), Rosenfield et al. (1964), Voak (1964), Salmon et al. (1965), Schmidt and McGinniss (1965), Yokoyama (1965) and Bird (1966).

Voak (1964) reported that he had identified in the course of carrying out routine antenatal tests five sera that contained antibodies that appeared to have a conjoined anti-HI specificity. In particular, they failed to react with erythrocytes lacking H (OhI+) and erythrocytes lacking I (OiiH+). Three of the sera were tested with ABH secretor saliva: they were not neutralized. The sera gave graded responses according to the ABO group of the cells tested: i.e., with O cells, +; with A_2 cells, ±, and with A_1 cells, – or very weak.

Salmon and his co-workers (1965) reported on studies carried out on eluates prepared from the erythrocytes of six patients who had suffered from AIHA associated with the formation of γM auto-antibodies. Three of the eluates contained anti-I, one anti-HI; one contained what appeared to be a mixture of anti-HI and anti-AI, and one a mixture of anti-I, anti-HI, anti-AI and anti-BI. Salmon et al. concluded that their studies showed that the 'building of the I antigen is phenotypically related to the building of ABH specificities, and that there exists in particular a BI specificity'.

Bird (1966), in his review, concluded that while most high-titre cold auto-agglutinins have a specificity related to the Ii system, low-titre auto-agglutinins are sometimes specific for A, B, O(H), M, N or even P, and that mixtures of such agglutinins could appear to be non-specific.

Subsequent papers dealing with the association of the ABH(O) and Ii blood-group systems include those of Issitt (1967), Tegoli et al. (1967),

Chessin and McGinniss (1968), Drachmann (1968), Voak et al. (1968), Baumgarten and Curtain (1970), Doinel, Ropars and Salmon (1974), Boccardi, Girelli and Zappi (1975), Morel, Garratty and Willbanks (1975), Bird and Wingham (1977), Dodds et al. (1979) and Uchikawa and Tohyama (1986).

Most of the antibodies referred to in the above-mentioned publications were found in patients who were not anaemic or in whom there was no evidence of auto-immune haemolysis. However, there are a small number of reports in which complex anti-AI or anti-BI antibodies seemed to have been responsible for increased haemolysis.

Boccardi, Girelli and Zappi (1975) described an interesting auto-antibody which appeared to have a different specificity at 4°C than it had at 22°C. It had been found in the serum of a 72-year-old woman suffering from chronic CHAD. Her ABO group was A_1. At 4°C the antibody agglutinated strongly erythrocytes of all ABO groups as well as cord-blood cells (titres 1024–2048); at 22°C it failed to agglutinate cord cells while still agglutinating O cells and A_1 cells quite strongly (titre 128), i.e. it behaved as an anti-I antibody. The antibody's activity at 4°C and at 22°C was enhanced if the target cells were first treated with papain. Later, the antibody reacted at 22°C as an anti-A_1 antibody rather than as anti-I. The antibody lysed weakly group-O, -A_1 and -A_2 cells at 22°C but failed to lyse cord-blood cells; lysis was enhanced if the serum was acidified. More lysis took place if the suspensions were placed first at 4°C, then at 37°C. Under these circumstances cord cells were lysed quite as strongly as were the adult O, A_1 and A_2 cells, i.e. the pattern of reaction was the same as in agglutination tests.

Dodds and co-workers (1979) described a group-B woman aged 47 who developed severe anaemia associated with a poorly differentiated lymphocytic lymphoma. Her haemoglobin was 7 g/dl and reticulocyte count 2%, and marked auto-agglutination and a few spherocytes were noted in blood films. The DAT was positive with an anti-C serum. Her serum contained a high-titre IgM cold antibody with a marked preference for BI erythrocytes. The titres at 4°C were: with OI cells, 2; with A_1I cells, 256; with A_2I cells, 32; with BI cells, 8192; with O cord-cells, cells, 0; with B cord-blood cells, 512. The thermal amplitude of the antibody extended to 37°C, at which temperature the titre with normal BI cells was 4. (The titre at 37°C with her own cells was not recorded.)

Ciruzzi and co-workers (1983) described the case of a woman aged 52 who was suffering from a chronic illness characterized by attacks of haemoglobinuria and acrocyanosis brought on by exposure to cold. Her haemoglobin was 11 g/dl and reticulocyte count 0.7%.

The DAT was positive with anti-C sera. Her serum contained an unusual antibody able to bring about lysis *in vitro* biphasically, i.e. by exposing cell suspensions at 0–18°C, followed by incubation at 37°C. The titre of the antibody was recorded as 128 using I+ erythrocytes; in specificity it was considered to be anti-IH.

Uchikawa and Tohyama (1986) described a group-B patient who died of anaemia associated with acute lymphocytic leukaemia. Her haemoglobin was as low as 2.2 g/dl, and her serum agglutinated at 37°C all donor erythrocytes tested. It contained a potent IgM lambda cold antibody which agglutinated strongly at 37°C adult group OI and Oi erythrocytes; B erythrocytes were agglutinated, too, but less strongly. However, the serum failed to agglutinate Oh erythrocytes at 37°C and also the patient's own cells (perhaps, it was suggested, because the antigen sites were blocked by antibody).

Relationship with the P blood-groups

A small number of antibodies have been described the reactions of which suggest that they are the product of interaction between the I and P blood-group systems. Relevant reports include those of Tippett et al. (1965), Issitt et al. (1968), Booth (1970) and Allen et al. (1974).

CHEMICAL NATURE OF THE Ii ANTIGENS

Early work on the chemical nature of the I antigen complex (Feizi et al., 1971a,b; Feizi and Kabat, 1972) was summarized by Feizi (1981) and reviewed by Roelcke (1974, 1989). The finding that a glycoprotein from hydatid cyst fluid inhibited agglutination by certain anti-I sera (Tippett et al., 1960) and that bacterial filtrates rich in β-galactosidase and β-N-acetyl hexosamidase (Marcus, Kabat and Rosenfield, 1963) destroyed the I activity of erythrocytes were early indicators of the carbohydrate nature of the Ii antigens.

Another seminal discovery was the observation that a water-soluble inhibitor of anti-I is present in variable amounts in human saliva and in relatively high concentrations in human milk (Dzierżkowa-Borodej et al., 1970; Marsh, Nichols and Allen, 1970); it is also present in human amniotic fluid and urine (Cooper, 1970). Marsh and his co-workers (1972) were able, too, to identify water-soluble I substance in the saliva and milk of an i

adult woman, whose serum contained an iso-anti-I antibody. In 1973, Cooper and Brown were able to report that they had identified a glycoprotein in normal serum that inhibited agglutination by anti-i antibodies.

Glycoproteins derived from ovarian cyst fluid were also found to be capable of inhibiting anti-I sera, which suggested that the antibodies were reacting with antigenic determinants expressed on the blood-group precursor chains of the glycoproteins (Feizi et al., 1971a,b). As already referred to, further research has established that the i antigen is formed of a straight chain glycolipid—a lacto-*N-nor*hexaosyl ceramide (Niemann et al., 1978) and that the I antigen is formed of a branched chain glycolipid — a lacto-*N*-iso-octaozyl ceramide (Feizi et al., 1979). These Ii determinants are internal structures of the ABH(O) antigens (Roelcke, 1989).

Issitt (1985), on p. 194 of his valuable review *Applied Blood Group Serology*, pointed out that the heterogeneity of the I system antibodies, as shown by their reactions with intact erythrocytes, was 'amplified at the biochemical level'; he stressed that I and i are 'not distinct entities, each with an immunodominate carbohydrate and each defined by an antibody of relatively straightforward specificity, but rather represent a whole series of 'different determinants'. The antibodies referred to as anti-I and anti-i he described as representatives of two groups of antibodies with related but far from identical specificities which 'define a series of (probably proximal) determinants on the inner regions of the red cell ABH-bearing chains'. Issitt referred to the biochemical research that had demonstrated the correlation between the lack of branched oligosaccharide chains on the erythrocytes of embryos and fetuses and their high content of i: it is the lack of branched chains on both the cord-blood erythrocytes and those of adults with the rare i phenotype that results in the structures with which anti-i antibodies combine being readily accessible; as the branched chains with which anti-I antibodies react increase in numbers, however, the access of anti-i becomes more and more restricted, and eventually the i antigens become almost inaccessible and the cells react as I-positive. This is the process that underlies the change from i-positivity to I-positivity which occurs in the first 18 months or so of life (Fig. 29.4).

ANTI-I^T

A variant of anti-I, referred to as anti-I^T, has been found commonly in the serum of certain Melanesian populations.

It had been noted that, while collecting blood for transfusion in Rabaul, in the island New Britain, a high proportion of the blood samples stored at 4°C underwent auto-agglutination and that the great majority of the samples showing this phenomenon had been derived from people of the Kuana (Tolai) linguistic group. This observation led Curtain and co-workers (1965) to undertake a comprehensive investigation into the incidence of cold auto-agglutinins in the sera of a large number of different linguistic groups in New Britain. They found that as many as 18 out of 140 sera derived from the Tolai people agglutinated normal group-O erythrocytes at 4°C at titres exceeding 50 and that two of these sera reacted at 20°C and one at 37°C. The sera were unusual, too, in their specificity: thus 39 out of 45 sera that agglutinated adult cells also agglutinated fetal cells and cells from an I-negative donor. Curtain et al. concluded that a single specificity might not be involved and that the majority of the antibodies 'are directed against i or one or more undetermined antigens present at high frequency'.

Further studies on Melanesian sera were described by Booth, Jenkins and Marsh (1966). They coined the term I^T to describe the specificity of the antibodies — T standing for an antigen 'transitional' between i and I with which the antibodies were thought to react. 364 sera, mostly from antenatal patients were screened for cold auto-antibodies: in 278 there was auto-agglutination at 4°C and 32 reacted at 20°C. Six of the sera were studied in detail: one appeared to be a typical anti-I, but five reacted preferentially with cold-blood (i) cells, although reacting (to a lower titre) with adult (I) cells; they reacted weakly with adult i cells and very weakly with Cyanmolgus monkey cells. The antibodies thus did not have anti-i specificity, and it was concluded that although the specificity appeared to be within the Ii system the antibodies were reacting with a transitional antigen present in maximal amounts in the erythrocytes of newborn infants.

Layrisse and Layrisse (1968) reported that anti-I^T was present also at a high incidence (84%) in the sera of a group of Indians living in the upper Orinoco region in Venezuela. The antibody was absent, on the other hand, from the sera of 30 Indians living in the Orinoco delta and from the sera of 50 blood donors living in Caracas.

Layrisse and Layrisse (1972) reported further data. The cold agglutinins were shown to be IgM and to be of both kappa and lambda light chain types. Most were anti-I^T in specificity. Although it seemed likely that their presence was a response to microbial infection it was not possible to establish any clear linkage.

Booth (1972) reported that Melanesians belonging to certain ethnic groups have erythrocytes that react outstandingly weakly with anti-I^T sera. Family studies confirmed that this weakness had a genetic basis.

Anti-I^T in Hodgkin's disease

Garratty and co-workers (1972) detected an anti-I^T in the serum of a Caucasian American suffering from Hodgkin's disease. Using the antiglobulin technique they showed that the antibody reacted well with fetal erythrocytes but only weakly with adult I cells and adult i cells. The antibody, an IgG, reacted optimally at 37°C; the DAT was, however, negative and there was no auto-agglutination.

Garratty and co-workers (1974) described three more IgG anti-I^T auto-antibodies, which had been formed by patients with AIHA associated with Hodgkin's disease. The DAT was strongly positive, using anti-IgG and anti-C sera, in all three patients. Their sera contained low-titre anti-I detectable at 4°C and an antibody—an IgG anti-I^T — demonstrable by the IAT at 37°C. Eluates prepared from the patients' erythrocytes reacted strongly with cord-blood i cells, weakly with adult I cells and still more weakly with adult i cells. Aside from the three examples of anti-I^T described in their report, no further examples of anti-I^T were found by Garratty et al. in a large survey which included 50 patients with Hodgkin's disease in whom the DAT was negative, three patients with Hodgkin's disease in whom the DAT was positive, but who presented no evidence of overt haemolysis, and in 70 patients with AIHA which was idiopathic or associated with other types of lymphoma.

Schmidt and co-workers (1974) referred in an abstract to an elderly woman who had a mild haemolytic anaemia. There was no evidence of Hodgkin's disease. Her serum contained an IgM anti-I^T antibody. Attempts to find compatible blood for transfusion failed, and when a ^{51}Cr-labelled test dose of the least incompatible blood was transfused, 75% of the erythrocytes were eliminated within 1 hour.

A further case of anti-I^T causing AIHA was reported by Freedman, Newlands and Johnson (1977). Their patient was a 56-year-old man who had a moderately severe haemolytic anaemia which was apparently of the idiopathic type. Many spherocytes were seen in blood films. The DAT was positive with anti-C4d and anti-C3 sera, but was negative with anti-IgG, -IgA and -IgM sera. The antibody, which was an IgM, reacted most strongly at 37°C: the titre with i cord blood cells was 512, with adult I cells 32 and with adult i cells 4. The patient's own cells were not agglutinated at 37°C.

OTHER Ii VARIANTS

Roelcke (1989) listed 12 distinct antigens within the Ii system against which antibodies had been developed and summarized the reactions of the antibodies with untreated, sialidase-treated and papainized erythrocytes derived from normal adults (I), newborn infants (i) and i adults. Amongst the specificities listed were anti-Gd (Roelcke et al., 1977), 'anti-cryptic' (Roelcke, Meiser and Brücher, 1979), anti-Sa (Roelcke et al., 1980), anti-F1 (Roelcke, 1981a; König, Kather and Roelcke, 1984; Roelcke and Weber, 1984), anti-Lud (Roelcke, 1981b), anti-Vo (Roelcke, Kreft and Pfister, 1984) and anti-Li (Roelcke, 1985).

Cold agglutinin anti-Sa (an IgMK) had been formed by a 77-year-old man with CHAD, cold agglutinin anti-F1 by a female patient with an immunoblastoma, and cold agglutinin anti-Vo (an IgML) by a 60-year-old woman with AIHA associated with a non-Hodgkin's lymphoma.

König, Kather and Roelcke (1984) described a patient who had had an atypical pneumonia of unknown causation complicated by cold-antibody AIHA. Cold agglutinins of both anti-I and anti-F1 specificity were present. Roelcke and Weber (1984)

described a further patient who had developed a transient haemolytic anaemia in whom the same combination of antibodies, anti-I and anti-F1, was present. In this patient, too, tests for *Mycoplasma pneumoniae*, cytomegalovirus and Epstein–Barr and rubella viruses were negative.

Suzuki and co-workers (1985) described a 65-year-old man with symptoms of CHAD whose serum contained a high-titre IgM kappa cold antibody. Lymph-node biopsy revealed a poorly differentiated follicular lymphoma. The specificity of the antibody, tentatively referred to as anti-Om resembled, but was not quite identical with, that of anti-Sa.

A cold agglutinin specifically active against stored erythrocytes

Brendemoen (1952) described the presence of an unusual cold antibody in the serum of an elderly woman who suffered from anaemia [of unspecified type], splenomegaly and subsequently hepatitis. Serum reactions for syphilis were reported to be positive. The DAT was positive—this was thought to be due to the presence of an incomplete cold antibody. Her serum failed to agglutinate at 5°C erythrocytes that had been stored at 5°C for 48 hours: however, if the cells had been stored at 37°C for 48 hours they were agglutinated at 5°C to a titre of 32 and at 15°C to a titre of 8. Fresh normal erythrocytes became agglutinated after treatment with typsin for 30 minutes or after heating at 56°C for 5 minutes. Brendemoen suggested that a 'new' agglutinogen developed as the result of storage, or treatment with trypsin, and that the antibody in the patient's serum was reacting with it. The specificity of the antibody was not determined; it appeared to be independent of the ABO, MN, P, Rh and Lewis systems.

Cold agglutinins specifically active against 'cryptic' Ii antigens

Perhaps not very different from the antibody described by Brendemoen (1952) (see above), are the two cold antibodies studied by Roelcke, Meiser and Brücher (1979). They were present in the sera of two women aged 66 and 65, respectively, one of whom suffered from chronic lymphocytic leukaemia and severe AIHA, the other from Waldenström's macroglobulinaemia and severe AIHA. The antibodies failed to react completely, or almost completely, with unmodified normal erythrocytes in the cold; however, they reacted with papainized cells to a titre of 64, and with neuraminidase-treated cells to titres of 32 and 128, respectively. Remarkably, unmodified erythrocytes from a patient with a congenital dyserythropoietic anaemia were agglutinated in the cold by both sera, to titres of 128 and 4, respectively, and to titres of 1000 and 16 when the cells were papainized. It was suggested that this type of antibody, although directed against cryptic antigens, may lead to haemolysis *in vivo*.

Pruzanski and co-workers (1987) tested 120 sera containing monoclonal macroglobulins ('without conventional cold agglutinin activity') for their ability to agglutinate enzyme-treated erythrocytes. Twenty-five of the sera agglutinated papain-treated and/or neuramidase-treated cells at 4°C to titres exceeding 32. Three patterns of behaviour were noted with respect to I or i specificity, some sera reacting as anti-I, others as anti-i or anti-not Ii. The sera had been derived from 13 men and 12 women aged between 42 and 85 years. Sixteen had suffered from Waldenström's macroglobulinaemia, six from benign monoclonal gammopathy, one from primary amyloidosis, one from multiple myeloma, and the diagnosis in one patient was unknown. None of the patients was recorded as suffering from increased haemolysis:

Cold agglutinins the activity of which is enhanced by added preservatives

Rarely, it seems that for ill-understood reasons the activity of certain cold auto-agglutinins is enhanced in the presence of preservatives. Two examples of this phenomenon are quoted below.

Thimerosal. Shirey, Harris and Moore (1979) reported that an anti-I antibody present in the serum of a 78-year-old man suffering from chronic myeloid leukaemia agglutinated normal I-positive erythrocytes at temperatures up to 25°C, but only if the test cells had been washed and suspended in saline to which thimerosal had been added as preservative. There was no agglutination if the cells had been suspended in ordinary or low-ionic-strength saline or had been pre-papainized. The antibody was inactivated by 2-ME and by human milk; it was absorbed by the patient's own cells at 4°C, and for this the presence of thimerosal was unnecessary.

Sodium azide. Reviron and co-workers (1984) described the unusual reactions of an anti-I auto-agglutinin present in the serum of a healthy woman aged 25. The antibody was unusual in that its activity was markedly enhanced in the presence of sodium azide (NaN_3). With autologous erythrocytes the titre at 5°C was 64 in the absence of NaN_3; with NaN_3 the titre was 256: At 22°C the titre without NaN_3 was zero, with NaN_3 128. The effect of NaN_3 on 20 other anti-I sera was explored: none of the sera was potentiated. Reviron et al. pointed out that it is well established that erythrocyte–antibody reactions can be modified by additives–acting in a variety of ways (see also p. 118). In relation to cold agglutinins, they referred only to the observations of Shirey, Harris and Moore (1979) on the enhancing effect of thimerosal, summarized above.

TECHNICAL FACTORS AFFECTING COLD-AGGLUTININ TITRES

It has been realized for many years that in titrating cold agglutinins the end-point recorded (the titre —the reciprocal of the serum dilution) depends considerably on how the test has been carried out: for example, on how the serum has been obtained and how dilutions have been prepared, on the cells selected for the titration and their concentration, on the ratio of cell suspension to serum dilutions, on the duration of the test and on how the end-point has been read. Early papers dealing with these technical factors include those of Finland et al. (1945), Ellenhorn and Weiner (1953) and Issitt and Jackson (1968). More recently, cold agglutinins have been described the activity of which *in vitro* has been shown to be dependent to a major degree on the medium with which the antibody-containing serum has been diluted or on the age of the cells used for the titrations.

Designation of antibodies as anti-I or anti-i

With most sera there is little difficulty in determining whether a cold auto-antibody is anti-I or anti-i in specificity. This is illustrated in Table 29.1. The difference in agglutinability between the I-positive and I-negative cells is obvious and unmistakable. It is interesting to note, however, that the I-negative cells were, nevertheless, agglutinated at 4°C to a moderately high titre and agglutinated to a much higher titre when trypsinized. Issitt (1985, p. 196) stressed the importance of titrations in determining specificity; he illustrated this point with data from three sera, all of which strongly agglutinated I, i (cord) and

Table 29.1   Comparative sensitivity of normal I-positive and 'I-negative' erythrocytes to agglutination by a high-titre cold antibody.

Type of erythrocyte	Titres	
	19°C	4°C
Normal I-positive	256	16 000
Trypsinized normal I-positive	4096	16 000
'I-negative'	1	512
Trypsinized 'I-negative'	16	8000

adult i cells when the sera were undiluted. When titrated, however, the specificity became clear: with an anti-I serum the titres with adult I, i cord and adult i cells were, respectively, 2048, 16 and 8; with an anti-i serum and the same cells, the titres were 16, 1024, 2048, and with an anti-I^T serum, 32, 512 and 8.

Enhancing effect of albumin-containing media

Haynes and Chaplin (1971) described finding that the serum of a patient with hypogammaglobulinaemia contained cold agglutinins which agglutinated erythrocytes to the modest titre of 128 when diluted in saline but agglutinated the same cells to the extraordinary high titre of 131 000 when diluted in 22% albumin. The patient suffered from severe, acute AIHA and the DAT was strongly positive with anti-C3 and anti-C4 antiglobulin sera. This observation led Haynes and Chaplin to study the effect of albumin as a diluent in the titration of other cold-agglutinin-containing sera, both from normal individuals and from patients. Modest enhancement of titre (but up to 6 times in one case) was observed with three out of 13 normal sera and with seven out of 24 patients' sera. Haynes and Chaplin suggested that the striking enhancement of the cold-agglutinin titre by albumin in the case of their original patient might have been of clinical significance, as the severity of in-vivo haemolysis seemed to be out of proportion to the apparent modest titre of the antibody when conventionally titrated in saline.

Bird and Wingham (1973) described an anti-I antibody which agglutinated in cross-matching tests at 37°C normal group O I-positive blood samples in albumin but which failed to agglutinate the same cells in saline suspension, whether papainized or unmodified, and which failed to give positive IAT tests. The serum, however, weakly agglutinated normal I-positive cells in saline at 4°C. The antibody was shown to be an IgM, being inactivated by 2-ME. Bird and Wingham tested other anti-I sera and found that some had their titre clearly enhanced, others only slightly, but none to the extent that they had observed with the serum they had originally investi-

gated. Bird and Wingham showed that the enhancement of agglutination took place irrespective of whether the albumin preparation used contained caprylate (see also p. 149).

Garratty, Petz and Hoops (1973, 1977) described the results of titrating cold agglutinins in the sera of patients whose DAT had been positive as the result of the adsorption of complement. Twenty-eight of the 32 patients investigated by Garratty, Petz and Hoops (1977) had haemolytic anaemia, and all except one had cold-agglutinin titres (in saline at 4°C) ranging from 64 to 10 240. Fifteen of the sera agglutinated normal adult erythrocytes suspended in saline at 30°C; in contrast, as many as 28 of the sera reacted at 30°C when 0.06 ml of 30% bovine albumin had been added to 0.2 ml of saline in each titration tube. At 37°C, only two of the sera agglutinated normal cells suspended in saline, while 19 caused agglutination in the presence of the albumin. At 4°C, the titrations were similar in both media. Of the four patients whose sera failed to agglutinate the test cells in albumin at 30°C, none had haemolytic anaemia. Garratty, Petz and Hoops concluded that cold-agglutinin titres and thermal amplitude were better correlated with the clinical state of the patients when the titrations were carried out in a saline medium to which albumin had been added rather than in saline alone.

A further example of an interesting cold agglutinin the activity of which was markedly enhanced in the presence of albumin was described by Sniecinski et al. (1988). This had been formed by a 52-year-old man who had suffered from acrocyanosis and urticaria for 4 years. His blood auto-agglutinated at room temperature but not at 37°C and he was not anaemic, and the reticulocyte count was only 1.1–2.0%. The DAT was weakly positive with anti-C sera; the IAT at 37°C was negative. The cold-agglutinin titre at 4°C was 4096 in saline dilutions but zero at 22°C and upwards. In albumin, however, the titre at 22°C was 128; at 30°C it was 32 and at 37°C it was 1.

VARIATION IN DISEASE IN THE AGGLUTINABILITY AND LYSIS OF PATIENTS' ERYTHROCYTES BY ANTI-I ANTIBODIES

The agglutinability of erythrocytes by anti-I sera is

commonly but variably increased in blood diseases characterized by dyserythropoiesis. The cause of the increase is obscure but presumably abnormalities at the erythrocyte surface are able to increase the availability of I antigens or to facilitate antigen–antibody interaction in some other way. The increased agglutinability varies considerably from case to case and does not seem to be confined to any particular type of disease. Lysis by anti-I and complement tends to be augmented in a similar way, although there is no close parallelism between the agglutinability and sensitivity to lysis.

Lewis, Dacie and Tills (1961) tested 334 samples of erythrocytes for their agglutinability at 20°C by a high-titre anti-I antibody derived from a patient suffering from typical CHAD: 100 of the samples were from patients suffering from a variety of blood diseases (exclusive of PNH), 100 of the samples were from 'medical' patients not suffering from a blood disease, 100 of the samples were from normal adults, 25 were from newborn infants, and nine samples were from PNH patients. The results of this study are reproduced in Table 29.2. Statistical analysis showed that the difference between the means for the medical patients and normal subjects was not significant;

in contrast, the difference between the blood-disease patients (and the PNH patients) and the normal subjects was highly significant ($P < 0.001$). Although the abnormalities were not confined to any particular disease, the highest values (agglutination 'scores' and percentage lysis) were found in megaloblastic anaemia, myelosclerosis, aplastic anaemia and leukaemia. It is particularly interesting to note that the sensitivity to agglutination and lysis reverted towards normal in megaloblastic anaemia under treatment. In the series as a whole, although there was a tendency, supported by statistical analysis, for increases in agglutinability to be accompanied by increases in lysis, there was no close parallelism. For example, some highly agglutinable cells underwent little lysis, although the converse did not seem to be true — except in PNH. An additional interesting feature of the data summarized in Table 29.2 is the wide range of agglutinability and lysis within each category. This is in conformity with the concept that I-positivity is a graded character (see p. 252).

McGuinniss, Schmidt and Carbone (1964) described some interesting observations on the agglutinability by an anti-I serum of normal erythrocytes and the erythrocytes of patients who were suffering from a

Table 29.2 Comparison of the sensitivity to agglutination and lysis by a high-titre cold antibody of the erythrocytes of patients with blood diseases, paroxysmal nocturnal haemoglobinuria (PNH), 'medical' patients, normal subjects and newborn infants.

Group and no. of subjects in group	Agglutination score		Lysis (% lysis in 1 in 10 serum)	
	Range	Mean ± S.E.	Range	Mean
Blood diseases (100)	0–140	61 ± 3.3	0–40	13.0
PNH patients (9)	45–105	67 ± 6.5	19–95	57.5
'Medical' patients (100)	2–140	36 ± 2.6	0–28	2.9
Normal subjects (100)	0–140	38 ± 3.1	0–24	3.0
Newborn infants (25)	0–12	0.1 ± 0.5	0	0

Statistical analysis of these data for agglutination show (1) that the difference between the means for the normal and 'medical' subjects is not significant ($0.7 > P > 0.6$); (2) that the difference between the means for the normal and blood-disease subjects is highly significant ($P < 0.001$); and (3) that the difference between the means for the blood-disease and PNH subjects is not significant ($0.4 > P > 0.3$). Because of the skew deviation of the data for lysis the standard errors of the means have not been estimated. A χ^2 test on these results confirms that there is no significant difference between the means of lysis for the normal and 'medical' subjects whereas there is a highly significant difference between the means for the normal and blood-disease subjects and between the means for the blood-disease and PNH subjects.
[From Lewis, Dacie and Tills (1961).]

variety of illnesses including blood diseases. The antibody they used was unusual in that it was present in the serum of an I-negative individual, and was regarded as being a 'natural' antibody. While it agglutinated, as expected, without exception the erythrocytes of 333 presumably healthy blood donors, a surprising number of samples of patients' erythrocytes (14 out of 116) appeared to be I-negative; in addition, six samples were judged to have given intermediate reactions. Ten of the 'I-negative' patients and five of the 'I-intermediate' patients suffered from leukaemia.

Ducos and co-workers (1965) reported that they had failed to confirm McGuinniss, Schmidt and Carbone's observations, referred to above. Using an anti-I antibody obtained from an apparently healthy person, only one out of 10 000 blood donors was classified as I-negative, while of 56 leukaemia patients and 2 250 patients suffering from other disorders, none was I-negative. In retrospect, the discrepancy between the two sets of data may well have been due to a difference in the antibodies used for the tests rather than in the patients' I antigens.

Rochant and co-workers (1973) assayed the I and i antigens of 250 and 273 patients, respectively, most of whom suffered from a malignant blood disease, using an electronic cell counter to assess agglutination. Their data indicated that the I antigen was very often increased, and very seldom decreased, in acute leukaemia and in myeloproliferative syndromes and marrow failure, and also in most lymphomas and chronic lymphocytic leukaemia; it was not, however, increased in 'refractory anaemias'. An excess of i antigen was found to be typical of malignant and benign myeloproliferative diseases; in lympho-proliferative disorders the i antigen was, however, normal.

VARIATION IN DISEASE IN THE AGGLU-TINABILITY OF PATIENTS' ERYTHRO-CYTES BY ANTI- i ANTIBODIES

As with anti-I, the agglutinability by anti-i of the erythrocytes of patients with blood diseases is often increased.

The phenomenon was first reported by Giblett and Crookston (1964) in the case of a 15-year-old boy with thalassaemia major. Subsequently, a further 17 patients, all with thalassaemia major, were tested and in all but one of them (who had been transfused several days previously) the titration scores were found to be significantly increased and to be only a little lower than those given by cord-blood erythrocytes. There appeared to be no correlation between the anti-i score and the ABO groups, or with the severity of the patient's anaemia or the Hb-F percentage.

The same anti-i serum was next used to test the erythrocytes of 145 normal adults, 120 patients not suffering from a blood disorder and 160 patients suffering from a variety of blood disorders. Many of the erythrocyte samples from these patients were also tested with a second anti-i serum, with similar results. It was found that the erythrocytes of most patients with aplastic anaemia and of many with leukaemia reacted abnormally strongly with the sera and that this was true of some patients with thalassaemia minor. High scores were found, too, in the four PNH patients tested. Increased agglutinability was sometimes present, too, in cases of chronic haemolysis, as in Hb-S disease and HS. On the other hand, increased agglutinability was not observed in acute blood loss, polycythaemia, megaloblastic anaemia, myelosclerosis, thrombo-cytopenia, and SLE. A moderate increase was found in a few patients with chronic myelogenous or lymphocytic leukaemia and in multiple myeloma. In all these patients there appeared to be no correlation with Hb-F percentage, and an increase in anti-i score was not associated with any diminution in anti-I score. Giblett and Crookston speculated that 'proliferative stress' might be a factor in causing the apparent increase in the i antigen; proliferative activity alone did not seem to be a possible explanation.

In a further report on the association of increased erythrocyte agglutinability by anti-i and marrow stress, Hilman and Giblett (1965) described the results of a detailed study of the results of treating an iron-overloaded patient with haemochromatosis by repeated phlebotomy. Before phlebotomy the erythrocyte i score was zero; it, however, gradually increased over a period of several months and eventually the score was 23. In contrast the erythrocyte I and H scores remained unaltered. Two weeks after the last phlebotomy the score had fallen to 15; 2 months later it was again zero. Hilman and Giblett concluded that in blood disorders the increased agglutinability by anti-i is correlated with rapid marrow transit, rather than with the severity of the anaemia or with the reticulocyte count or Hb-F percentage; they suggested that the i reactivity of prematurely released erythrocytes represented the retention of a property which normally disappears at an early developmental stage, and Hilman and Giblett reiterated that an increased i agglutinability score had been noted in cases where there was impaired marrow proliferation, as in marrow hypoplasia and myelofibrosis, in decompensated haemolytic disease and in ineffective erythropoiesis.

Cooper, Hoffbrand and Worlledge (1968) described how they had tested the anti-I and anti-i agglutinability of the erythrocytes of a series of patients suffering from sideroblastic, megaloblastic or iron-deficiency anaemia and compared their agglutinability with that of the erythrocytes of normal adults and of cord-blood cells. Raised titres with anti-i sera were found with the erythrocytes of 13 out of 15 sideroblastic anaemia patients (titre range 32–1000) and with the cells of seven out of eight pernicious anaemia patients (titre range 32–512). In 16 out of 17 pernicious anaemia patients in remission the titres with their erythrocytes were normal, as they also were in eight iron-deficiency anaemia patients. Anti-I titres using patients' erythrocytes were usually raised in those patients whose erythrocytes had given raised titres with the anti-i serum. The anti-

i titre in a pernicious anaemia patient was closely followed during his response to therapy and was shown to decrease steadily within a 3-month period, indicating that the increased sensitivity to agglutination probably persisted for the life-span of the erythrocyte (Fig. 29.5). In relation to the cause of the increased agglutinability, Cooper, Hoffbrand and Worlledge concluded that it probably depended upon membrane alterations resulting from disordered erythropoiesis; the concept that a shortened maturation time within the bone marrow might be the explanation they thought unlikely. They pointed out that in pernicious anaemia, in which they had found increased agglutinability to both anti-i and anti-I, the maturation time has been shown to be normal or prolonged.

Another disorder in which the erythrocytes are more than normally agglutinable by anti-i sera is the rare congenital dyserythropoietic anaemia, CDA type II (HEMPAS) (Crookston et al., 1969; Crookston, Crookston and Rosse, 1969; Verwilghen et al., 1973). With anti-i, the erythro-

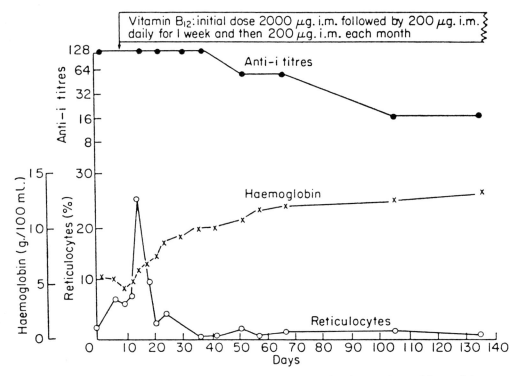

Fig. 29.5 **Haematological response and change in anti-i titre in a patient with pernicious anaemia following treatment with vitamin B$_{12}$.**
[Reproduced by permission from Cooper, Hoffbrand and Worlledge (1968).]

cytes of five patients were found to be as agglutinable as the cells of newborn infants, and they were unusual, too, in undergoing some lysis. In contrast, the patients' cells were not unusually agglutinable by anti-I sera, although they did undergo more lysis than the cells of normal adults.

Increased sensitivity to agglutination by anti-i sera has also been described in acanthocytosis associated with abetalipoproteinaemia (Bassen–Kornzweig syndrome). The erythrocytes of the patient described by Berrebi and Levene (1976) were as sensitive as cord-blood cells to agglutination; there was, however, no increase in anti-I agglutinability.

The agglutinability of the erythrocytes in sickle-cell (Hb-SS) disease and sickle-cell (Hb-AS) trait by anti-i and anti-I sera was studied in detail by Maniatis, Frieman and Bertles (1977) and Maniatis, Papayannopoulou and Bertles (1979). The results of their studies have already been summarized in Volume 2 of this book (p. 86). Briefly, they concluded that the expression of both the i and I antigens are increased in sickle-cell disease and in the trait. The agglutinability by anti-i of Hb-SS cells was intermediate between that of cord-blood cells and normal adult cells, and that of Hb-AS cells was slightly greater than that of normal cells, with some overlap. Again, there appeared to be no correlation between the percentage of Hb F and reactivity to anti-i. Subsequently, Basu and co-workers (1984), using an immuno-electron-microscopic technique, demonstrated that both i and I antigens are present at an unusually high density on the surface of Hb-SS cells.

COLD AUTO-ANTIBODIES IN THE SERUM OF HEALTHY SUBJECTS

It has been known for many years that the sera of normal animals commonly agglutinate their own erythrocytes at low temperatures, e.g. $0-4°C$ (Landsteiner, 1903). Later, Landsteiner and Levine (1926) showed that this was true of human blood, too. Cold auto-agglutinins are present in fact at low titres (most commonly at titres ranging from 2 to 32) in the serum of almost all individuals. Their thermal range is limited, however, not extending above $15-20°C$, and in consequence they are of no clinical significance. Almost always I-positive erythrocytes are agglutinated much more strongly, and to higher titres, than are i cells, i.e. the antibodies typically have

anti-I specificity. There are, however, a few reports of the occurrence of other specificities. Thus low-titre anti-i antibodies (Signal and Booth, 1976) or anti-Pr antibodies (Marsh and Jenkins, 1968; Roelcke and Kreft, 1984) have been encountered in apparently healthy individuals, as well as anti-i and anti-I existing together (Jackson et al., 1968).

According to Adinolfi (1965b), cold agglutinins are commonly present in the cord-blood serum of newborn infants. Using strongly reacting O I-positive erythrocytes, agglutinins active at $0°C$ were demonstrated in 14 out of 23 cord sera and in 20 out of 23 of the corresponding maternal sera. The anti-I antibody in the cord sera did not as a rule react with the autologous cord cells; in three out of the 10 sera, however, there was a weak positive reaction. Inactivation by 2-ME showed that the anti-I antibody was a γM globulin and thus likely to be of fetal rather than of maternal origin.

The blood donor described by Signal and Booth (1976) as having an anti-i antibody in his serum appeared to be in good health but the serum concentrations of IgA and IgM were abnormally high and an immunofluorescence test for anti-nuclear factor was weakly positive. Subclinical liver damage was considered to be a possibility.

Range of cold-antibody titres in health

Favour (1944) reported a detailed study of student nurses in Boston. In March, April, June and July (1943) the sera of groups of 25 student nurses were found to be free from cold agglutinins. Subsequently, in September, October and November, 73 serum samples from a group of 27 student nurses were tested on several occasions: 46 of the samples then contained cold agglutinins at a titre between 5 and 40, and in two samples the titres were 80 and 160, respectively. It is interesting to note (and probably significant) that ten of the nurses had had colds and 13 tracheobronchitis during the period they had been studied. Favour also observed that individuals who had apparently developed cold agglutinins during an infection might gradually lose their agglutinins on recovery from the infection.

Savonen (1948), who investigated 437 normal subjects, found titres of 32 or above in only 4.5%. Janković (1955) titrated the cold agglutinins in the sera of 100 adult blood donors and of 100 patients not suffering from blood diseases. In only two of the 100 normal sera did the cold-agglutinin titre reach 64, but if trypsinized cells were used the normal range extended to 512. Three of the patients' sera gave titres of 256 with normal cells, which were extended to 2048 when trypsinized cells were used. No zoning was observed with the normal cells but this was not uncommon with the trypsinized cells and in ten cases it was very marked.

Schubothe (1958, p. 114), basing his report on the cold-agglutinin titres of 50 healthy adults between the ages of 20 and 30, stated that the titres in most of them lay between 8 and 32; he instanced 0–128 as the extreme range.

More recently, Dube, Zuckerman and Philipsborn (1978) described studies on the sera of 120 individuals—blood donors and children in the United States undergoing routine examination. The mean titre for unmodified cells was 8.7 ± 1.1 and for ficin-treated cells 18.7 ± 1.1. When the titres were correlated with age, they appeared to be at their highest in the 9–16 year age-group and they were found to be statistically significantly higher in those aged between 11 and 25 years compared with those aged between 26 and 64. The titres in females were found to be significantly higher than those in males. The titres were not correlated with the ABO blood group.

The cause of the formation of cold antibodies in health remains uncertain. They appear to be polyclonal and to be of both kappa and lambda light-chain types. The most likely explanation for their presence is that they represent immune responses to exogenous stimuli, most likely derived from infectious agents affecting the respiratory tract. The fact that the highest titres are found in relatively young subjects is in accord with this hypothesis.

Under the title 'Epidemic autoimmunity: cold auto-agglutinins in Melanesia', Baumgarten and co-workers (1968) reported a high incidence (up to 94% positive) of cold auto-agglutinins in several populations living in New Britain. The titres, 10 to 640, appeared to be higher than those found in western populations. Most were anti-I but a few were identified as anti-I^T or anti-AI. Two hundred of the antibodies were tested for kappa and lambda light chains: both chains were identified in 160, kappa alone in 24 and lambda alone in 16.

OCCURRENCE OF ANTI-i IN DISEASE

As already referred to (p. 251), anti-i was first described in the sera of two anaemic patients suffering from reticulum-cell sarcoma and 'reticulosis', respectively (Marsh and Jenkins, 1960; Marsh, 1961). Subsequently it was identified as the causal antibody in other patients suffering from various types of lymphoma and as *the* characteristic auto-antibody in patients who develop AIHA in association with infectious mononucleosis (see p. 318). As already mentioned (p. 263), the cold auto-antibody present at low titres in the serum of strictly normal individuals is almost always anti-I rather than anti-i in specificity. It may, however, be more common in the serum of hospital patients. Even so, the data of Bell, Zwicker and Sacks (1967) give an idea of its rarity. They reported that they had identified anti-i in the sera of only eight patients during a 2-year period while carrying out a routine hospital transfusion service. Two of the patients had a lymphoproliferative disease, the others suffered from carcinoma of the colon, carcinoma of the breast, uterine fibroids, ulcerative colitis, pregnancy and Caesarean section, and trauma and amputation, respectively. The antibody titres, using cord-blood erythrocytes, ranged from 4 to 64. The erythrocytes of four of the patients underwent auto-agglutination at 4°C ($\pm$ to +++).

In the tropics anti-i may be less rare. Pitney, Thomas and Wells (1968), for instance, reported that cold agglutinins at raised titres (i.e. > 64) were commonly present in the sera of individuals, suffering from massive splenomegaly, who were resident in the Watut Valley in New Guinea. Their sera contained macroglobulins at raised concentrations, of which 16–33% was cold agglutinin. Testing the sera with I and i erythrocytes, and with the erythrocytes of Cynamolgus monkeys (rich in i antigen), indicated that the majority of the antibodies had anti-i specificity. Pitney, Thomas and Wells concluded that tropical splenomegaly was another disorder in which anti-i is developed in association with hyperplasia of reticulo-endothelial tissue.

In the absense of a lymphoma or other underlying disease, anti-i has rarely been found at a high titre. The author is unaware of it ever being identified as the causal antibody in typical idiopathic CHAD. It has, however, been described as a monoclonal antibody in association with an IgG warm panagglutinin in a patient suffering from severe AIHA who responded to splenectomy, and in whom there was no evidence of a lymphoma or SLE (see below).

Kay, Gordon and Douglas's (1978) patient was a 50-year-old man who gave a month's history of progressive illness before admission to hospital. His haemoglobin was then 5.5 g/dl and reticulocyte count 20%. The DAT was positive with anti-IgG and anti-C3 sera. His serum contained a monoclonal IgM kappa cold antibody which agglutinated i erythrocytes to a titre of 1024 at 4°C and I erythrocytes to a titre of 32. The thermal range of the antibody extended only up to 10°C. A subpopulation of the patient's lymphocytes formed rosettes with i cells but not with I cells.

THE Pr (Sp$_1$) BLOOD-GROUP SYSTEM

Marsh and Jenkins in 1968 described studies on the serological behaviour and specificity of a type of cold antibody which appeared to be quite distinct from the anti-I and anti-i antibodies which they were also studying. They had tentatively referred to the unusual antibodies—which appeared to be a homogeneous group, as anti-'Not-I', a title which they admitted was unsatisfactory. They suggested as a more appropriate title anti-Sp$_1$, reflecting the fact that the antibody appeared to be directed against a basic antigen present in all human erythrocytes but absent in animal erythrocytes. They had found that blood samples derived from 20 300 blood donors were, without exception, strongly agglutinated when exposed to the anti-Sp$_1$ at a low temperature. A major difference between anti-I and anti-Sp$_1$ was the way the antibodies reacted against normal

erythrocytes treated with proteolytic enzymes. Whereas with anti-I agglutination was strengthened and the titre increased, with anti-Sp$_1$ the reactions were markedly reduced, sometimes almost completely suppressed. Anti-Sp$_1$ antibodies had not been identified in the sera of healthy individuals, and in pathological sera they were found to be relatively rare, two examples only being identified amongst 268 consecutive cold antibodies investigated.

That auto-antibodies of pathogenic importance existed that failed to react with enzyme-treated erythrocytes had been reported as far back as 1953. Wiener, Gordon and Gallop then reported that they had investigated the serum of a 70-year-old woman who was dying from a fulminating haemolytic anaemia. Her serum contained a potent auto-agglutinin which was almost as active at 37°C as it was at 5°C—the titres were 190 and 380, respectively. Ficinized cells were, however, not agglutinated at either temperature, even in undiluted serum. Wiener, Gordon and Gallop pointed out that the effect of the enzyme paralleled its action on the M–N–S system of agglutinogens and inferred that the patient's antibody had been directed against 'the M–N–S substance, but against that portion of that molecule which is alike in all human beings'.

Anti-HD

Roelcke (1969) described under the title anti-HD (anti-Heidelberg) two high-titre cold antibodies—γA kappa and γM kappa, respectively, the activity of which could be abolished completely, or almost completely, by treating the target erythrocytes with the proteases papain, trypsin, bromelin and ficin or with RDE (neuraminidase). Additionally, it was found that the specificity of the antibodies was quite distinct from that of antibodies of the Ii system. Roelcke, Uhlenbruck and Bauer (1969) subsequently reported that the antibodies could be separated into two categories, HD$_1$ and HD$_2$, on the basis of different reactions with human and animal erythrocytes: the HD$_1$ receptor was found to be present on human erythrocytes only, the HD$_2$ receptor on rat and guinea-pig cells in addition.

Anti-Pr

Roelcke and Uhlenbruck (1970) in a Letter to *Vox sanguinis* proposed that the antigens for cold antibodies, which were susceptible to inactivation by proteases, should be referred to as Pr (Pr_1 and Pr_2) in preference to Sp_1, as suggested by Marsh and Jenkins, or HD, as had been suggested by Roelcke (1969). This suggestion has been generally accepted, and the corresponding antibodies have been termed anti-Pr. The literature on anti-Pr is quite extensive, and antibodies of IgA, IgM and IgG class and anti-Pr specificity have been implicated rather rarely as the causal monoclonal antibodies in cases of chronic AIHA or formed very rarely transitorily.

Homberg and co-workers (1971) found in a retrospective survey of 143 sera containing cold agglutinins at a raised titre two giving the reactions of an anti-Sp_1 antibody. One of the sera had been derived from a patient with chronic lymphocytic leukaemia and cirrhosis.

Roelcke and co-workers (1971) described the finding in the serum of two children, aged 11 months and 8 years, respectively, of cold auto-antibodies of anti-Pr specificity. The children had suffered from transient haemolytic anaemia, that in the younger child following a *Mycoplasma pneumoniae* infection. The antibodies, which were of the IgG class, differed from anti-Pr_1 and anti-Pr_2 in that, although they failed to agglutinate protease-treated erythrocytes, they nevertheless agglutinated erythrocytes that had been treated with neuraminidase. The term anti-Pr_a was suggested as a title for the 'new' type of antibody.

Garratty and co-workers (1973) described a patient with long-standing 'CHAD' whose cold antibody had a specificity that was not within the Ii system. The antibody failed to react with erythrocytes that had been treated with papain or neuraminidase. The pattern of reaction, however, differed from that previously described for anti-Pr_1 or anti-Pr_2. The patient's bone marrow contained 10% or more of plasma cells and electrophoresis revealed a monoclonal IgA kappa protein; multiple myeloma was suspected but not proved.

Roelcke (1973a,b) described how anti-Pr antibodies can be separated into anti-Pr_1 and Pr_2 according to their reactions with human and dog erythrocytes. Anti-Pr_{1h} is human-specific; anti-Pr_{1d} is human- plus dog-specific. Anti-Pr_2 also reacts with both human and dog erythrocytes but papain only inactivates the human antigen; papainized dog cells are still agglutinated.

Roelcke (1973b) called attention to the possible association between antibody class and specificity, pointing out that all three IgA kappa cold agglutinins that had been described had had anti-Pr_1 specificity.

Roelcke, Ebert and Feizi (1974) described the studies they had carried out on two monoclonal cold antibodies that had lambda light chains. One had anti-I specificity; the other was an anti-Pr_1.

Tonthat and co-workers (1976) described a further example of a monoclonal IgA kappa cold agglutinin of anti-Pr_{1d} specificity that had been formed by a patient with persistent HB antigen cirrhosis.

Roelcke, Ebert and Geisen (1976) described as anti-Pr_3 a 'new' anti-Pr antibody that had been formed by a 19-year-old man who had suffered from rubella. The serum was differentiated from other anti-Pr antibodies by its ability to agglutinate cat and sheep erythrocytes. A further example of an anti-Pr_3 antibody was identified by Birgens, Dybkjaer and Roelcke (1982).

Dellagi and co-workers (1981) described a most unusual cold antibody in the serum of a 33-year-old woman who had suffered from a rapidly progressing anaemia. Her haemoglobin was 5 g/dl and reticulocyte count 13%. The DAT was initially positive with anti-C sera, but negative subsequently. Her blood auto-agglutinated after collection. The cold-agglutinin titre was low (16 at 4°C), but the antibody had a high thermal range—titres 8 at 22°C, 4 at 32°C and 1 at 37°C. The antibody was identified as being IgG and of anti-Pr specificity.

Roelcke and co-workers (1982) identified in the serum of a 58-year-old man with CLL an anti-Pr cold antibody the reactions of which did not conform to those of anti-Pr_{1h}, -Pr_{1d}, -Pr_2 or -Pr_3. The antibody was tentatively referred to as anti-Pr Ad.

Roelcke and Kreft (1984) reported on the studies they had carried out on 41 sera containing cold antibodies of anti-Pr specificity. The antibody titres varied from 4 to 32 000. The great majority of the antibodies were of the IgM class with kappa light chains; only one was an IgG. One was an IgM with lambda light chains. Three of the antibodies were identified as anti-Pr_2, five as anti-Pr_3 and three as anti-Pr_a. Twenty-four of the anti-Pr_1 sera were sub-classified on the basis of their reactions with human and dog erythrocytes; six were identified as anti-Pr_{1h}, 16 as anti-Pr_{1d} and two sera were unclassifiable.

Rose and Kwaan (1985) reported that they had investigated a patient presenting with a 'diffuse reticular pattern of skin mottling on the trunk and extremities, which did not blanch with gentle pressure but faded on rubbing and rapidly reappeared'. This was considered to be livedo reticularis.[*] The patient was a 62-year-old man. His haemoglobin was 9.8 g/dl and there were 4–7% reticulocytes, and blood films revealed marked auto-agglutination. An anti-Pr IgM cold agglutinin was identified in his serum.

Judd and co-workers (1986) described a further variant anti-Pr antibody. This had been formed by a 32-year-old woman who had developed a persistent haemolytic anaemia following a viral infection. The DAT was negative, but rosettes of erythrocytes were found around neutrophils and a Donath–Landsteiner (D–L) test was positive. The patient, however, never had had haemoglobinuria and haemolysis *in vivo* did not seem to be exacerbated by cold. The antibody giving the positive D–L test was an IgG but its specificity was not anti-P. Unexpectedly, it was found that protease-treated and neuraminidase-treated erythrocytes were not lysed in the D–L test. The antibody thus appeared to be anti-Pr-like and acted as a biphasic lysin.

Roelcke, Dahr and Kalden (1986) described a further variant antibody that had been formed by a 60-year-old woman suffering from chronic Raynaud's phenomena. Her haemoglobin was 9.8 g/dl, but the DAT was negative. The cold-agglutinin titre was 32 000. The antibody was an IgM kappa monoclonal protein. It acted like an anti-Pr antibody at low temperatures and like an anti-M at a higher temperature (e.g. 25°C); it was designated as anti-Pr^M.

Northoff, Martin and Roelcke (1987) reported that they had investigated a 43-year-old woman who had developed a transient haemolytic anaemia associated with varicella. The DAT was positive with anti-C sera. The antibody was shown to be IgG and appeared to be monotypic with kappa light chains. Its specificity was identified as anti-Pr$_{1h}$.

Johnson and co-workers (1989) referred to a life-threatening occurrence. Their patient was a 6-week-old infant who developed acute haemolysis shortly after being injected with DPT vaccine. The antibody reacted at 37°C with all erythrocytes tested except ficinized cells and the rare M^kM^k cells; in specificity it was thought probably to be anti-Pr. The infant eventually recovered after immunosuppressive therapy and many transfusions, including exchange transfusions.

Curtis and co-workers (1990) described another remarkable case. Their patient, a 21-year-old man, also suffered from a life-threatening haemolytic anaemia associated with haemoglobinuria. He was sufficiently ill to require 54 transfusions within 10 days, having failed to respond to corticosteroids, cyclophosphamide and multiple plasma exchanges. Eventually, as a ^{51}Cr

study had revealed predominantly splenic sequestration, splenectomy was carried out. He steadily improved following the operation and made a complete recovery within 6 months. The DAT and IAT carried out at 22°C were negative with both polyspecific and anti-C3d sera: at 0–4°C, however, both tests were strongly positive. His serum contained a high-thermal-amplitude cold antibody, titre 80–256 at 4°C, the activity of which extended just up to 37°C. The antibody failed to fix complement; it was an IgG1κ, and its specificity was shown to be that of anti-Pr$_a$.

Another antibody with an unusual specificity (anti-Ju) was described by Göttsche, Salama and Mueller-Eckhardt (1990). This had been formed by a 63-year-old man who was suffering from mild compensated haemolytic anaemia. I and i (cord) cells were equally sensitive to agglutination by the antibody, the titres being 256 at 0°C, 256 at 16°C, 64 at 22°C and 2 at 37°C. Papainized cells were less sensitive, the titre at 22°C being 32, and neuraminidase (RDE)-treated cells were less sensitive still, the titre at 22°C being 16. The antibody was more potentially lytic, as judged by C5b-9 deposition on unmodified erythrocytes, than a control anti-I serum.

Anti-Pr antibodies only demonstrable in low-ionic-strength saline (LISS)

O'Neill and co-workers (1986) described the reactions of two sera containing cold auto-antibodies of anti-Pr$_1$ specificity that were only demonstrable in LISS media. They were present in the serum of a 57-year-old woman suffering from an iron-deficiency anaemia and in the serum of a 61-year-old man admitted to hospital for cystectomy. The serum of the first patient agglutinated LISS-suspended erythrocytes to a titre of 16 at 4°C. Agglutination was also strong at room temperature and also occurred at 37°C; the IAT was positive at 37°C using LISS-suspended cells. There was, however, no evidence of in-vivo haemolysis. The antibody in the serum of the second patient was more powerful: the titre at 4°C was 256, and the antibody reacted up to 37°C. The IAT at 37°C was positive with LISS-suspended cells but not with cells suspended in albumin. The DAT of the second patient was positive (2+) with anti-C sera and weakly positive with an anti-IgG serum. As in the first case, there appeared, however, to be no evidence of in-vivo haemolysis and he was transfused uneventfully with four units of blood.

Occurrence of low-titre anti-Pr antibodies in routine serum samples

Anti-Pr has but rarely been identified in sera being routinely tested for cold agglutinins. As already referred to (p. 265), Marsh and Jenkins (1968) had found only two examples of anti-Sp$_1$ in 268 consecutive sera tested. Subsequently, Roelcke, Ebert and Anstee

---

*The term *livedo reticularis* has been used by dermatologists to describe a mottled violet discoloration of the skin brought about by local causes rather than by cyanosis of central origin. Champion (1965) and Copeman (1975), in reviews, stressed that the condition has many causes. Champion mentioned cryoglobulinaemia but not AIHA or CHAD; Copeman mentioned cryofibrinogens, cryoglobulins and macroglobulinaemia under the heading 'Hyperviscosity of blood and blood stasis in capillary-venules'. Livedo *reticularis* has also been referred to as livedo *annularis* (see p. 18).

(1974) reported a very similar incidence. They had tested 301 sera. Only one contained anti-Pr (in addition to anti-I). Of the remaining sera, 292 contained anti-I, four anti-i and four anti-I plus (?) anti-i.

AUTO-ANTI-A AND ANTI-B COLD ANTIBODIES

Rarely haemolytic anemia results from the development of antibodies directed against the A or B antigens

Anti-A

Rochant and co-workers (1972) described a group-A_1 61-year-old woman, suffering from reticulosarcoma, who had relapsed after splenectomy. The DAT was positive, but there was no clinical evidence of haemolysis. Her serum contained an anti-A_1 antibody at a titre of 256 at 4°C, but inactive at 22°C. The antibody was shown to be an IgM monoclonal protein with lambda light chains; its activity was completely inhibited by A substance in saliva.

Szymanski, Roberts and Rosenfield (1976) described a group-A man aged 73 who had developed a fatal multisystem syndrome — obstructive lung disease, glomerulonephritis, and cirrhosis, associated with acute haemolytic anaemia accompanied by haemoglobinuria. The haematocrit was 21%, the platelet count 110 × 10^9/l and many spherocytes were visible in blood films, as well as erythrophagocytosis by monocytes. The DAT was strongly positive with an anti-IgG serum but negative with an anti-C reagent. His serum contained an antibody which agglutinated A_1 and A_2 erythrocytes at 22°C and O cells weakly; its action was inhibited by porcine A substance. The IAT was positive at 37°C with A_1 cells and less strongly so with A_2 cells; O cells were not agglutinated. A heat eluate made from the patient's erythrocytes contained an antibody which reacted with A_1 cells, and weakly with A_2 cells, when tested by the IAT. It was speculated that the anti-A antibody might have reacted with A antigens in tissue cells and that this had led to his multisystem syndrome.

A further patient who developed acute haemolytic anaemia associated with an auto-anti-A antibody was described by Parker et al. (1978). She was a group-A little girl aged 2 who had had an upper respiratory tract infection. Her haemoglobin was 4.1 g/dl and there were 2.7% reticulocytes. The presence of haemosiderinuria and methaemalbuminaemia indicated intravascular haemolysis. The DAT was positive with an anti-C reagent. Her serum agglutinated A_1 and A_2 cells weakly at room temperature and more strongly at 4°C; there was no agglutination at 37°C. However, the IAT was positive at 37°C with both A_1 and A_2 cells, and antibodies agglutinating these cells at room temperature, and less strongly at 37°C, were demonstrated in eluates prepared from her erythrocytes. The activity of the antibody was not enhanced by enzymes; it was inhibited by A_1 secretor saliva. Inactivation by dithiothrietol indicated that it was an IgM antibody.

Anti-B

Auto-antibodies of anti-B specificity have rarely been described and in most cases, but not quite in all [e.g. the patients of Atichartakarn et al. (1985), see below] their presence has not been associated with obvious signs of increased haemolysis. This presumably has been due to the fact that the antibodies have generally not reacted at or near to body temperature, as in the cases described by Seyfried, Walewska and Giles (1963) and Finke et al. (1976).

van Loghem and co-workers (1963) reported, but without giving details, that they had identified an auto-anti-B antibody in one patient (out of 63) who had suffered from cold-antibody AIHA.

Lopez and co-workers (1975) described a 72-year-old man who had presented with chronic pulmonary insufficiency and heart failure. His erythrocyte count was 3.5 × 10^{12}/l but no further details were recorded. He was group AB and the DAT was positive with anti-C sera. His serum contained an anti-B antibody which gave a titre with adult B cells of 256 and with cord-blood B cells of 128. Its thermal range with adult B cells extended up to 30°C. It was shown to be an IgM antibody with kappa light chains, and its activity was inhibited by B substance in saliva. Lopez et al. concluded that it was a genuine anti-B antibody rather than an anti-BO.

Another interesting auto-anti-B antibody was described by McClelland et al. (1981). Their patient was a group B 81-year-old woman suffering from acute leukaemia. Her haemoglobin was 8.9 g/dl and there were 3.5% reticulocyes. Auto-agglutination was obvious in blood films and the DAT was positive with an anti-C3d serum. Her serum, in addition to anti-A, contained an antibody which agglutinated B cells at 4°C (+++), 22°C (++) and 37°C (+). Group-O cells were not agglutinated even at 4°C and cord-blood B cells were agglutinated at 4°C and 22°C, indicating anti-B specificity, not anti-BI.

The patients of Atichartakarn et al. (1985), referred to above, both developed transient acute haemolytic anaemia possibly precipitated by viral infections. They were a man aged 21 and a woman aged 20. Their haemoglobins were 4.9 g/dl and 5.3 g/dl, respectively. They both recovered after being transfused with group-O blood and receiving dexamethasone, penicillin and gentamycin. The serological findings in both patients were almost identical. They were group B. The DAT was positive with broad-spectrum antiglobulin sera and a low-titre, but high-thermal-range, anti-B was present in their serum: in Case 1 the titre at room temperature and at 37°C was 4; in Case 2 the titre at room temperature was 2 and at 37°C the titre was 1.

Auto-anti-H

Crowley (1958) described the possibly unique occurrence of an incomplete high-thermal-amplitude cold auto-antibody with apparently an anti-H specificity. His patient was a severely anaemic middle-aged woman. Her history and the haematological and serological findings are summarized on p. 279.

AUTO-ANTI-M AND ANTI-N COLD ANTIBODIES

Anti-M

Although allo-anti-M is an antibody relatively commonly formed by NN individuals, auto-anti-M is a rare antibody. However, in most cases it has seemed not to have led to haemolysis *in vivo*, as in the reports of Fletcher and Zmijewski (1970), Tegoli et al. (1970), Hysell, Beck and Gray (1973), Lown, Barr and Kelly (1980) and Vale and Harris (1980). There are, however, at least four reports of its identification in patients who have suffered from cold-haemagglutinin disease (CHAD).

van Loghem and co-workers (1963) reported that an auto-anti-M antibody had been identified in one patient (out of 63) who had suffered from cold-antibody AIHA. However, no details of this case were given.

Bowes (1976) reported to the 8th Triennial Conference of the (British) National Transfusion Service how he had investigated a patient suffering from CHAD and identified the causal antibody as a monoclonal auto-anti-M with lambda light chains. The antibody titres with pooled adult M-positive erythrocytes were 6400 at 4°C, 2000 at 20°C and 64 at 30°C. Enzyme-treated cells were not agglutinated. MM cells were shown to be more strongly agglutinated than MN cells. NN cells were not agglutinated at 20°C but they were agglutinated at 4°C (titre 512). Agglutination was sensitive to pH: at pH 8.0, MM cells were not agglutinated at 30°C, compared with titres of 128 at pH 7.0 and 256 at pH 6.0.

Sangster and co-workers (1979) described a woman aged 63 with chronic CHAD who had suffered from Raynaud's phenomena and livedo reticularis. Her haemoglobin was 9.5 g/dl and polychromasia and auto-agglutination were noted in blood films. The DAT was weakly positive with an anti-C3 serum. Her serum contained a cold antibody which agglutinated MM, MN and NN cells at 17°C and at 30°C only MM and MN cells. Adult and cord-blood cells were agglutinated equally. The patient's own (MM) cells were agglutinated at 4°, 17°, 30° and 37°C, at titres of 2000, 2000, 32 and 1, respectively; the titres were appreciably higher when 20% albumin was used as diluent, i.e. 64 at 30°C and 8 at 37°C.

A further example of an auto-anti-M as the causal antibody in CHAD was described by Chapman, Murphy and Waters (1982). Their patient was an 85-year-old woman. Her minimum haemoglobin was 8.2 g/dl; there were 10.6% reticulocytes and her blood underwent gross auto-agglutination after withdrawal. The MCV was recorded as 170 fl in a Coulter count at room temperature and as 101 fl at 37°C (see p. 221). Bone-marrow aspiration showed that about 20% of the nucleated cells were small lymphocytes. The DAT was positive but only with an anti-C3d serum, and MM cells were shown, by means of the IAT, to bind on more complement than MN cells. The antibody was shown to be a monoclonal IgM kappa; it was inhibited by M substance but not by N substance. It agglutinated group-OMM, -OMN and -ONN erythrocytes to very high titres, i.e. to > 1 × 10^6 at 4°C, and at 20°C to titres of 6000, 2000 and 64, respectively. At 37°C it agglutinated OMM cells to a titre of 256 and OMN cells to a titre of 128; ONN cells were not agglutinated. Adult and cord-blood erythrocytes reacted similarly, and agglutination was almost totally abolished if the test cells had been enzyme-treated. The IAT with OMM cells was strongly positive with anti-C reagents and negative with ONN cells. Because of the strong reaction of the antibody with NN cells at a low temperature, implying that it reacted with a structure common to both the M and N antigens (although showing a preference for the M antigen), Chapman, Murphy and Waters referred to the specificity of the antibody as anti-M-like.

Anti-N

Like auto-anti-M, auto-anti-N antibodies have seldom been identified, and most have been found in the serum of healthy individuals, e.g., as described by Metaxas-Buhler, Ikin and Romanske (1961), Greenwalt, Sasaki and Steane (1966), Moores, Botha and Brink (1970) and Hysell, Gray and Beck (1974). But, as with auto-anti-M, a few patients have been studied, too, in whom an auto-anti-N has seemed to have played a significant pathogenic role.

Bowman and co-workers (1974) described finding an auto-anti-N antibody in the serum of a 18-year-old man who 3 weeks previously had developed symptoms suggestive of infectious mononucleosis. On admission to hospital, he was found to have a haemolytic anaemia of moderate severity: the haemoglobin was 6.9 g/dl, there were 4.4% reticulocytes and a few erythrophages were seen in blood films. Otherwise the blood picture and serological findings confirmed a diagnosis of infectious mononucleosis. The DAT was positive with anti-C3 and anti-C3,4 reagents, and antibody was present in his serum which agglutinated N erythrocytes to a titre of 512 at 4°C, 8 at 22°C and 1 at 37°C. M cells were agglutinated, too, at 4°C, but much more weakly than were N cells. The activity of the antibody was inhibited by 2-mercapto-ethanol (2-ME), indicating that it was an IgM. The serum complement concentration was slightly lower than normal. Bowman et al. pointed out that the antibody differed from previously described anti-N antibodies in that it had strong complement-binding properties.

Dube and co-workers (1975) described another example of an auto-anti-N which had been formed apparently also in response to a viral illness. Their patient was a 7-year-old boy who had given a 2-weeks' history of headache, nausea, vomiting, abdominal pain and high pyrexia. His haemoglobin was 6 g/dl and there were 23.4% reticulocytes; spherocytes were present in blood films. His blood group was ON. The DAT was positive with anti-IgG sera, but negative with anti-C3, anti-IgA and anti-IgM sera. Eluates from his erythrocytes reacted with N-positive cells only, as did an antibody in his serum, as judged by the IAT. A weak cold agglutinin was also present in his serum; this was inactivated by 2-ME. The 2-ME did not, however, affect the antibody which gave rise to the positive IAT. Dube et al. concluded that this was an IgG auto-anti-N; it failed to react with enzyme-treated cells.

A further example of an IgG auto-antibody with anti-N specificity was described by Cohen et al. (1979). Their patient was a 21-year-old woman who was suspected of suffering from systemic lupus erythematosus (SLE). Haemolysis was severe and there was, too, marked thrombocytopenia: the haemoglobin was

5.5 g/dl, with 37% reticulocytes, and the platelet count 3×10^9/l. Her erythrocytes underwent auto-agglutination when centrifuged at 37°C in her serum and also auto-agglutinated in group-AB serum as well as in 6% albumin or simply when suspended in saline. Her blood group was AB, M-negative, N-positive. The DAT was strongly positive with anti-IgG sera and positive, too, but less strongly so, with anti-C reagents. An antibody in her serum, and present also in eluates from her erythrocytes, agglutinated at 37°C N and MN cells in saline suspension, and some but not all samples of M cells, the reactions being stronger at room temperature than at 37°C. Exposure to 2-ME did not affect the activity of the antibody, which retained its ability to agglutinate N-positive cells in saline suspension or by the IAT.

Telen and co-workers (1989) described, in an abstract, their findings in a 21-year-old woman who was suffering from severe haemolysis accompanied by haemoglobinuria. She had previously suffered from thrombocytopenia during pregnancy. When studied, her haematocrit was 18%, despite eight transfusions during the previous week, and the reticulocyte count was less than 1%. The DAT was weakly positive with an anti-C3 serum only. Her serum contained an auto-anti-N antibody which consisted of both warm and cold components, both of which were IgG antibodies. The patient's phenotype was M-positive, N-positive. She eventually recovered after being transfused with N-negative blood and being treated with prednisone and azathioprine.

Auto-anti-N formed by patients undergoing chronic haemodialysis

A remarkable finding has been the discovery of auto-anti-N in the serum of a small but highly significant minority of patients undergoing chronic haemodialysis for various types of renal disease (Howell and Perkins, 1972; McLeish, Brathwaite and Peterson, 1975; Boettcher et al., 1976). The cause of the antibody development is obscure, but damage to the erythrocytes rendering them immunogenic as the result of exposure to the dialysis membranes or from residual formaldehyde used as a sterilizing agent has been suggested. The antibodies do not seem to have been responsible for significant in-vivo haemolysis.

Howell and Perkins (1972) found 12 examples of anti-N among 416 patients (approximately 3%) who were being treated by chronic haemodialysis: eight of the patients were N positive, three being homozygotes (NN). The antibodies appeared only after at least 14 months of treatment and decreased in titre or disappeared after cessation of the dialysis. Their presence was not related to blood transfusion. The titres in saline ranged from 2 to 16 at 21°C, and were less when ficinized cells were substituted for unmodified normal erythrocytes. The patient's own cells were agglutinated, if NM or NN.

McLeish, Brathwaite and Peterson (1975) identified anti-N in the sera of six out of 40 patients on chronic haemodialysis: four were NM, one MM and one NN. All the sera reacted best at 4°C but they reacted, too, at room temperature and two of the sera at 37°C also. The DAT was positive in each patient, using an anti-broad spectrum serum and it was positive, too, in three patients with an anti-IgG serum. There was, however, no evidence of significant in-vivo haemolysis. None of the patients gave a history suggestive of past auto-immune disease: their renal lesions were chronic glomerulonephritis or polycystic disease.

Boettcher and co-workers (1976) studied two anti-N sera that had been formed by patients undergoing chronic haemodialysis. They found that the antibody was directed against a precursor of the MN antigens, as all its activity could be removed by absorption with neuraminidase-treated M cells. The antibody reacted at 4°C with N cells only; formaldehyde-treated N cells were, however, acted on at 25°C and 37°C as well. Boettcher et al. concluded that the anti-N antibodies had been formed as an immune response to erythrocytes which had been exposed to residual formaldehyde during their passage through a dialysis unit that had been sterilized with formaldehyde.

Cross-reactivity of anti-M and anti-N

As has been recorded in the case records summarized above, both auto-anti-M and auto-anti-N antibodies, although preferentially reacting with M-positive and N-positive cells, respectively, commonly react more weakly with cells of the other phenotype, suggesting that they react with a structure or structures common to both M and N antigens.

This phemomenon had earlier been reported by Hirsch et al. (1957) in the case of allo-anti-M and allo-anti-N antibodies. Four antibodies of each specificity had been studied: the anti-M sera did not react with N cells under any circumstances; the anti-N sera, although definitely specific for N cells at certain temperatures, nevertheless agglutinated M cells at lower temperatures or when the cells had been treated with trypsin. The possibility that this cross-reactivity may sometimes be of clinical significance is suggested by the description by Hinz and Boyer (1963) of a 62-

year-old woman suffering from severe AIHA of unknown origin. Her haemoglobin was 4.5 g/dl and the reticulocyte count 35%. The DAT was positive with a non-γ antiglobulin serum. An agglutinin in her serum reacted with approximately 75% of donor cells. The patient's blood-group was OMM; the antibody, which appeared to be an allo-antibody, had anti-N specificity: it agglutinated N cells at 23°C to a titre of 256 and at 37°C to a titre of 64. M (adult) cells were, however, agglutinated by the antibody at 1°C as were M cord-blood cells. When the M cells were trypsinized they were agglutinated, however, as strongly as untreated N cells. The patient's own cells were weakly agglutinated in her own serum at 25°C and strongly at 4°C. In addition to the anti-N antibody, the patient's serum contained a γ_1M cryoglobulin, and electrophoresis showed a prominent α_1 peak and a reduced content of γ_2 globulins. Serum complement was subnormal, and the IAT using the patient's serum and N cells was positive if fresh normal serum was added to the patient's serum.

OTHER RARE SPECIFIC COLD AUTO-ANTIBODIES

Anti-P

Although P-specific cold auto-antibodies are well known to be responsible for paroxysmal cold haemoglobinuria, their occurrence in any other haemolytic syndrome seems to be of the utmost rarity. At least one such case has, however, been described (see below).

von dem Borne and co-workers (1982) had investigated a 54-year-old man with an immunoblastic non-Hodgkin's lymphoma and a severe haemolytic anaemia. The haemoglobin was 4.7 g/dl and there were 7.1% reticulocytes. The DAT was positive, but only with anti-C sera. A cold antibody was present, but agglutination was only demonstrable using albumin as diluent or with bromelin-treated (BT) erythrocytes. The titres were: at 4°C, in albumin 128 and with BT cells 4000; at 16°C, in albumin 64 and with BT cells 256. There was no agglutination at 37°C. Both normal unmodified cells and BT cells were lysed at 16°C (at pH 6.5): the titres were 512 with normal cells and 2000 with BT cells; the BT cells were, too, lysed at 37°C (titre 128). Tests for lysis by the two-stage Donath–Landsteiner procedure (4°C, then 37°C) were negative. Using the lysis of BT cells at 16°C as indicator, P1 and P2 cells were lysed to a high titre (3200–6400); there, was, however, no lysis of P1^k and pp cells, results clearly indicating P specificity. The antibody was shown to be a monoclonal IgM globulin with kappa light chains.

Anti-Sd[x]

Marsh and co-workers (1980b) described two patients who had developed haemolytic anaemia associated with the formation of an auto-antibody identified as anti-Sd[x], a 'new' antibody related to the Sd[a] group. The first patient was a 5-year-old girl who had developed a severe but transient haemolytic anaemia. Her haemoglobin was 8.6 g/dl and there were 32% reticulocytes. The DAT was strongly positive, but only with anti-C reagents. There was marked auto-agglutination. The second patient was a woman aged 69 who had had a persistent anaemia for many years. Her haematocrit was 35% and there were 3.2% reticulocytes, suggestive of mild compensated haemolysis. The DAT was weakly positive on one occasion only with anti-C reagents. The antibodies from both cases reacted similarly. Agglutination was most active at 12°C or 22°C but extended up to 37°C; it was pH-dependent, being maximal at pH 6.5 (titre 320) and minimal at pH 8.0 (titre 10). Both antibodies reacted with the erythrocytes of more than 5000 people, no non-reactors being found. The Sd[x] antigen was not denatured by neuraminidase or papain or ficin; it was present on some primate erythrocytes. The antibody was slightly inhibited by human saliva and milk and was inhibited by the urine of Sd(a+), but not by that of Sd(a–), individuals; it was strongly inhibited by guinea-pig urine.

Marsh and co-workers (1980a) referred in an abstract to the two patients described above and then to four additional patients in whom auto-anti-Sd[x] had been identified. They stressed that in four of the six patients the auto-antibody formation had followed upper respiratory tract infections, probably of viral origin. In each, the antibodies were most active at a low pH and were capable of lysing papainized cells, and they were all inhibited by Sd(a+) human urine but not by Sd(a–) urine.

A further patient who had formed anti-Sd[x] auto-antibodies was described by Denegri et al. (1983). He was a man aged 28 who had been admitted to hospital as possibly suffering from endocarditis. A cardiac murmur had been noted when he was aged 8, and when 26 he had contracted syphilis. His haemoglobin was 7.9 g/dl and he had 14% reticulocytes. The DAT was strongly positive with anti-IgG, anti-IgM and anti-C sera. His serum contained an IgM high-thermal-amplitude cold auto-antibody the activity of which extended up to 37°C; also, apparently, an IgG warm antibody of the same specificity. Treatment of the serum with DTT or 2-ME inhibited agglutination, but the IAT remained positive, indicating the presence of the IgG antibody. Tests with a range of rare blood types and with human and guinea-pig urine established that the antibody had Sd[x] specificity.

Anti-Me

A 'new' cold auto-antibody referred to as anti-Me (milk-enhanced) was described by Salama, Pralle and Mueller-Eckhardt (1985) in the serum of a 61-year-old woman suffering from Waldenström's macroglobulin-aemia and haemolytic anaemia. Her haemoglobin was 8.4 g/dl and there were 8% reticulocytes. The DAT was positive with an anti-C3d serum but negative with anti-IgG, -IgM or -IgA sera. The cold-agglutinin titre was 128 at 0°C and 4 at 30°C, and agglutination was found to be enhanced in the presence of defatted milk that had been heated in a boiling water-bath for 10 minutes. I and i cells were equally sensitive to agglutination. Agglutination was enhanced by treating the erythrocytes with papain and it was unaffected or slightly increased by treating them with neuraminidase. Papainized cells were strongly lysed at 20°C and at 37°C; unmodified cells were weakly lysed at 20°C. Lysis was affected by pH, but the optimum was comparatively wide (pH 6 to pH 8) and lysis occurred at pH 9.

Anti-Om

A cold agglutinin which reacted against a 'new' common erythrocyte antigen, designated Om, was described by Kajii and Ikemoto (1989) in the serum of a 59-year-old man suffering from CHAD. The DAT was positive with anti-C3d sera. The cold-agglutinin titre was 1024 at 4°C and 16 at 30°C. Agglutination was enhanced if the erythrocytes had been treated with papain or neuraminidase. I and i cells were agglutinated to similar titres. The activity of the antibody was markedly inhibited by human milk—in contrast to the activity of anti-Me which is increased by human milk (see above). (According to Kajii and Ikemoto anti-Me is the only other antibody that reacts with a neuraminidase-resistant antigen common to both I and i cells.)

Anti-D

Longster and Johnson (1988) described the presence of an IgM auto-antibody of anti-D specificity in the serum of a 59-year-old woman suffering from a non-Hodgkin's lymphoma complicated by haemolytic anaemia. Her haemoglobin was 5.2 g/dl and polychromasia and auto-agglutination were noted in blood films. The DAT was positive with anti-C reagents but negative with anti-IgG, -IgM and -IgA sera. Her blood group was O, and the Rh phenotype ccDEE. The anti-D in her serum reacted in saline and by enzyme techniques with all Rh(D)-positive cells tested. Agglutination was abolished by prior treatment of the serum with DTT. The activity of the antibody was affected by temperature: at 20°C the titre with D-positive cells (phenotype ccDEe) was 64: at 37°C it was 8. Ten weeks later the results were: at 4°C the titre was 64; at 20°C it was 16 and at 37°C it was 4. Another unusual feature (for an anti-D antibody) was the fact that the antibody appeared to fix complement as shown by the positive DAT with anti-C3c, -C3d and -C4 sera.

FIXATION OF COMPLEMENT BY COLD AUTO-ANTIBODIES

Many cold auto-antibodies fix complement to the surfaces of erythrocytes as the result of their reaction with antigen, and if sufficient complement is fixed lysis is the result. However, if the amount fixed is insufficient for lysis its presence on the erythrocyte surface can, nevertheless, be demonstrated by the cells being agglutinated by antiglobulin sera containing anti-complement components. Cold auto-antibodies which fix complement in this way and give a positive antiglobulin reaction, but which do not cause lysis or obvious agglutination when the antibody and erythrocytes in saline suspension react under optimum conditions, have been referred to as 'incomplete' cold antibodies by analogy with the common type of incomplete anti-Rh(D) warm antibody. Cold auto-antibodies which cause actual lysis by complement as the result of the reaction between antibody and antigen have been referred to as 'cold haemolysins'. This term is acceptable as long as it is remembered that the antibody molecule bringing about lysis is the same molecule that leads to agglutination if the target erythrocytes are exposed to the antibody in the absence of complement.

Many anti-I cold auto-antibodies can be shown to be capable of bringing about obvious lysis *in vitro*, particularly if the pH of the cell–serum suspension is adjusted to the acid side of neutrality, the optimum pH being 6.5–6.8. If the target erythrocytes are treated with enzymes such as trypsin or papain lysis is more easily produced; the effect of pH is then less important and the lysis titre is likely to be considerably increased. Paroxysmal nocturnal haemoglobinuria (PNH) erythrocytes are generally more sensitive still, and they are particularly useful in detecting an antibody's potential for bringing about lysis. The clinical importance of an anti-I antibody's lytic potential depends upon whether it readily causes lysis of normal erythrocytes at the natural pH of plasma (approximately pH 7.5) and, most importantly, on its thermal range. If lysis takes place *in vitro* at temperatures of 30°C or above, the patient is likely to suffer from very serious intravascular haemolysis.

EARLY REPORTS OF COLD HAEMOLYSINS

The early literature on lysis produced *in vitro* by sera containing high-titre cold auto-agglutinins was reviewed by Stats and Wasserman (1943) and by the author in 1950 (Dacie, 1950a). The accounts up to that time were somewhat unsatisfactory, being incomplete and the results inconstant, and the possibility of artefactual lysis due to working with too strong concentrations of erythrocytes, as stressed by Stats and Wasserman (1943) and Stats (1945), cannot, in some instances at least, be excluded.

Compared with the numerous reports of the demonstration *in vitro* of high-titre cold agglutinins, few workers described the coexistence of cold haemolysins. Wyschegorodzewa's (1926) patient suffered from moderate anaemia and enlargement of the liver and spleen: in the serum an autohaemolysin and isohaemolysin were said to be associated with a cold autohaemagglutinin (titre not given). In the patient described by Ernstene and Gardner (1935), exposure to cold resulted in cyanosis and attacks of haemoglobinuria. A cold agglutinin was present in his serum at a titre of 1280. The Donath–Landsteiner reaction was reported to be positive on four occasions. The observations of Salén (1935) are the most comprehensive. He described what he considered to be a thermostable non-complement-requiring lysin in the serum of a patient suffering from episodes of haemoglobinuria. The cold-agglutinin titre was 1024. Lysis occurred if the supernatant of a mixture of cold plasma and erythrocytes was removed and replaced by cold saline. It appeared as if the plasma protected the cells from lysing.

Stats and Wasserman (1943) and Stats (1945) described the results of experiments that they had carried out with two samples of oxalated plasma containing cold auto-agglutinins at titres at 4°C of 20 000 and 30 000, respectively. They compared the mechanism of the lysis produced by these two samples with that of the Donath–Landsteiner (D–L) antibody of paroxysmal cold haemoglobinuria and concluded that the two mechanisms were fundamentally different. The D–L antibody was described as causing lysis as the result of fixation of antibody and complement in the cold, followed by warming. In contrast, the lysis caused by the two high-titre cold agglutinins occurred in the cold (at 4°C) and was strictly dependent on the intensity of the agglutination, for slight dilution of the plasma (or serum) was found to prevent lysis. Moreover, if the concentration of erythrocytes was reduced, lysis was less, even although agglutination was intensified. Finally, mechanical trauma was found to be necessary for lysis to occur. Stats (1945) established this clearly by a number of elegant and revealing experiments.* His simplest experiment is reproduced below:

'A. Five tenths ml of whole oxalated blood [containing a high-titre cold agglutinin] was kept at 4°C for 30 minutes. During this time the tube was tapped 20 times every 5 minutes. Marked hemolysis was observed.

B. The same procedure as (A) but without tapping failed to show any hemolysis.

---

*To avoid the risk of artefactual (mechanical) lysis the present author recommends that the final concentration of erythrocytes in any serum dilution should not exceed 5%; also that the concentration of the washed cells to be added to the serum should not exceed 50%. The cell suspensions should be added directly to the serum in tubes without being allowed to make contact with the walls of the tubes. The cells should be mixed gently in the serum and then left undisturbed at the selected temperature and the cells allowed to sediment spontaneously. Finally, after inspection for lysis, the tubes should be centrifuged at a low speed after gently resuspending the sedimented cells in the serum.

C. The same procedure as (A) but carried out at 37°C failed to show any hemolysis.'

When the above experiment was repeated using heat-inactivated serum and added erythrocytes, the results were exactly the same, i.e. complement played no part in the lysis.

Heilmeyer, Hahn and Schubothe (1947) described four unusual cases of haemolytic anaemia. In one patient (Case 1b) a cold agglutinin was present at a very high titre (131 000). Slight lysis, noticed at 0°C, was attributed either to damage to the erythrocytes as the result of the intense agglutination or to the presence of a lysin which was considered not to be of the Donath–Landsteiner type.

Another unusual case of a man who experienced an episode of acute haemolytic anaemia with haemoglobinuria was reported by Ellis, Wollenman and Stetson (1948). The blood picture, in addition to showing evidence of erythrocyte regeneration, was suggestive of infectious mononucleosis. The Wassermann reaction was negative but the serum was reported to contain agglutinins against sheep cells at a titre of 1024, cold auto-agglutinins at a titre of 256 at 4–6°C and a cold auto- and iso-haemolysin.

Effect of pH on lysis *in vitro*; 'acid haemolysins'

Dacie (1950a), working with seven sera containing high-titre cold agglutinins, was able to show that each serum would cause the lysis of normal erythrocytes if the serum was suitably acidified beforehand; the optimum pH was found to be in the range 6.5–7.0 (Fig. 29.6), and more antibody was shown to be adsorbed progressively from pH 8.2 to 5.8 (Fig. 29.7). Without complement no lysis took place, and complement also seemed to be required for adsorption of the antibody at a low temperature as well as for bringing about actual lysis. Paroxysmal nocturnal haemoglobinuria (PNH) erythrocytes were shown to be extremely sensitive to lysis by the sera, much more so than normal cells. Lysis readily occurred at room temperature (20°C) and allowing the preparation to stand at this temperature produced

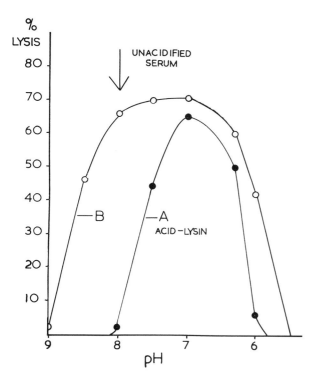

Fig. 29.6   Effect of pH on the lysis of normal erythocytes by two sera containing high-titre cold auto-antibodies.

A is the typical pH–lysis curve of an 'acid-haemolysin'; B is an exceptional curve showing almost maximal lysis in unacidified serum (pH 8.0). [Reproduced by permission from Dacie (1955).]

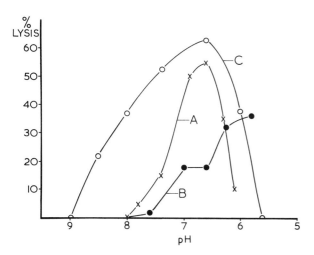

Fig. 29.7   Effect of pH on the lysis of normal erythrocytes by a high-titre cold auto-antibody.

A = effect on observed lysis; B = effect on the adsorption of the antibody; C = effect on the action of human serum complement.

more lysis than carrying out the cold–warm Donath–Landsteiner procedure.

Subsequently, 'acid haemolysins' in sera containing high-titre cold agglutinins were reported from many other laboratories, e.g. by Matthes and Schubothe (1951), van Loghem et al. (1952), Marcolongo (1953), Schubothe (1953), Bonnin (1954), Krauter and Rieder (1957), Pisciotta and Hinz (1957), Dausset, Colombani and Evelin (1957), Schubothe (1958), van Loghem, van der Hart and Dorfmeier (1958) and Dausset and Colombani (1959).

Further observations from the author's laboratory were reported by Ferriman et al. (1951), and Dacie (1954a, p. 250, 1955, 1957). Ferriman and his co-workers pointed out that the serum of their Case 1 was unusual in that lysis of normal erythrocytes took place without it being necessary to acidify the serum; lysis was, however, increased by acidification. Dacie (1954a, p. 251) mentioned another case in which slightly more lysis took place in unacidified serum (pH 8.0) than in serum acidified to pH 6.5 and a similar observation was made by Bonnin (1954). (Dacie 1955) in a paper in which the behaviour of the 'acid-haemolysins' in sera from patients suffering from CHAD and 'virus' pneumonia, respectively, were compared with the Donath–Landsteiner antibody, demonstrated how individual sera varied in their ability to cause lysis of normal and PNH erythrocytes, and in the thermal range of antibody activity and in the differing effects pH had on lysis (see also Table 28.3, p. 224).

Schubothe (1958) also described in detail the in-vitro behaviour of 'monothermische* Kältehämolysine'. He illustrated the effect of temperature on lysis, the maximum occurring between 20 and 25°C, the optimum 22°C, and stressed that the range 12.5–32°C depends upon the joint effect of temperature on antibody and complement. He illustrated, too, the progressive binding on of antibody as the pH was lowered from 9 to 6, and also time–lysis curves: lysis was rapid, most occurring within 10 minutes although maximum lysis was not reached for 60 minutes.

---

*The Donath–Landsteiner antibody has often been referred to, chiefly in Continental literature, as a 'bithermische Hämolysine'.

Schubothe also found, if lysis was carried out in two stages, that fresh complement-containing serum was not essential in the first (cold) stage; more lysis, however, occurred if active complement was present throughout.

Using ^{131}I trace-labelled anti-I and anti-i antibodies, Evans, Turner and Bingham (1965) confirmed that the adsorption of the antibodies increased progressively as the pH was lowered from 7.6 to 6.6. The optimum pH for lysis by complement was shown to be 6.6 to 6.8, with inhibition at pH 7.8 and 6.4.

The author's own observations on the ability of high-titre cold auto-antibodies to bring about the lysis of normal, enzyme-treated and PNH erythrocytes were described in Part II of the 2nd edition of this book (Dacie, 1962, pp. 468–478). They have been summarized earlier on p. 225 when the serological findings in CHAD were described.

Details were given, too, by Dacie (1962, p. 439) of two patients who died of a severe haemolytic anaemia associated with the formation of auto-antibodies which caused auto-agglutination and lysis at 37°C. Their activity was enhanced by a reduction in pH and also to a moderate extent by fall in temperature.

'INCOMPLETE' COLD ANTIBODIES

Early observations

Dacie (1950b) reported that an apparently 'incomplete' form of cold auto-antibody could be demonstrated to be present in many, if not in all, normal sera by means of the antiglobulin reaction. He showed that normal erythrocytes exposed to serum at 2–5°C subsequently undergo agglutination in strong concentrations of antiglobulin serum and that the agglutinable material adsorbed to the cell surface resists elution even if the corpuscles are repeatedly washed in saline at 37°C. He also showed that the reaction could only be obtained with fresh serum and that the presence of anticoagulants, as well as heat-inactivation, prevented sensitization. Later, Ferriman and his co-workers (1951) reported that strong direct and indirect antiglobulin reactions, suggestive of the presence of 'incomplete' cold

auto-antibodies, could readily be obtained using the erythrocytes or serum of patients suffering from the cold-haemagglutinin disease (CHAD). Dacie (1951) demonstrated that the reaction between antiglobulin serum and cells sensitized by 'incomplete' cold antibodies persisted even if relatively large amount of human γ globulin were first added to the antiglobulin serum.

'Incomplete' cold antibodies were next reported from Germany: Schubothe and Matthes (1951) described positive direct and indirect antiglobulin reactions in two patients suffering from CHAD whose sera contained high-titre cold antibodies.

The nature of the 'non-γ' antiglobulin reaction was considered by Dacie (1951) and it was concluded on the basis of the evidence then available that 'incomplete' cold antibodies were either not γ globulins or that the antiglobulin serum was reacting with a component of fresh serum (not a γ globulin) adsorbed with the antibody. It subsequently became clear that the second explanation was correct and that the agglutination was being brought about by the interaction of anti-complement components in the antiglobulin serum with complement adsorbed to the erythrocytes in association with the cold (and potentially lytic) antibody (Dacie, Crookston and Christenson, 1957, 1958; Leddy et al., 1962).

The involvement of complement provided an explanation for several puzzling features of the cold-antibody antiglobulin reaction: for instance, the thermolability of 'incomplete' cold antibodies, the inhibiting effect of anticoagulants, the pattern of reaction with diluted antiglobulin serum, the failure of added γ globulin to inhibit the antiglobulin reaction and the failure of attempts to elute 'incomplete' cold antibodies (e.g. by Vaughan, 1956; Evans and Weiser, 1957; and Fudenberg, Barry and Dameshek, 1958).

Later studies

The early work, outlined above, which demonstrated that complement played an important role in the agglutination by antiglobulin sera of erythrocytes exposed at low temperatures to the action of cold auto-antibodies, left several important questions unanswered. One was whether 'incomplete' forms of cold antibodies really existed; another was the nature of the complement components adsorbed to the erythrocytes with which the antiglobulin sera reacted.

Do 'incomplete' cold auto-antibodies exist?

The answer to this question seems to the author to depend on how an 'incomplete' antibody is defined. In their original description of the antiglobulin test, Coombs, Mourant and Race (1945) described antibodies, incapable of bringing about direct agglutination of erythrocytes in suspension in saline but detectable by means of antiglobulin sera, as 'weak and incomplete'. Earlier, Wiener (1944) and Race (1944) had independently described anti-Rh antibodies in human sera that had a blocking effect, i.e. the antibodies were capable of preventing agglutination by in-saline-agglutining antibodies. Race had referred to the antibody he had studied as being 'incomplete'. In 1945, Diamond and Denton had reported that the presence of albumin enhanced agglutination by anti-Rh antibodies; and in 1947 Morton and Pickles reported that incomplete Rh antibodies would bring about the direct agglutination of erythrocytes if the cells had first been treated with trypsin.

According to the criteria referred to above, which defined the basis for the description of certain (warm) anti-Rh antibodies as 'incomplete', 'incomplete' cold antibodies certainly exist.

The enhanced agglutination brought about by cold antibodies in some cases in the presence of albumin has already been mentioned (p. 259), as has the existence of cold antibodies only detectable if the target erythrocytes had been pre-treated with enzymes (p. 257). It is also possible to argue that the increased titres generally observed if anti-I antibodies are titrated using enzyme-treated cells means that among the population of antibody molecules there are some ('incomplete') molecules that react only on modified cells. On the other hand, describing cold auto-antibodies as 'incomplete' because they are able to fix complement to erythrocytes, so as to give positive antiglobulin reactions with anti-complement antisera, yet are apparently incapable of bringing about visible agglutination or lysis, now seems to the author to be less firmly justified. It seems reasonable to view some at least of such antibodies as being strongly complement-fixing but incapable of causing agglutination or lysis because they are present in too low concentrations. The data summarized in Table 29.3 illustrate this point: at low dilutions the antibody caused agglutination and complement fixation; at high dilutions, e.g. 1 in 1024, its presence was detectable only by the antiglobulin reaction.

Another example of an 'incomplete' antibody that is in reality probably not strictly 'incomplete' is the 'incomplete' cold auto-antibody described by the author as present in many normal sera (Dacie, 1950b) (see below): if tested with the exceptionally complement-sensitive PNH erythrocytes, some of the cells are lysed: on this

Table 29.3 Adsorption of complement by erythrocytes exposed to dilutions of a high-titre cold antibody, in the absence of lysis.

	Serum dilutions					
	1 in 16	1 in 64	1 in 256	1 in 1024	1 in 4096	Control (normal serum diluent)
Agglutination	++	+	trace	–	–	–
Lysis	–	–	–	–	–	–
Agglutination by antiglobulin serum	++	++	+±	+	±	–
Residual serum complement (%)	13	81	95	100	99	100

Agglutination was read first and then lysis. The sensitized cells were then washed and suspended in antiglobulin serum, and the residual complement content of the cold-antibody-containing serum was titrated.
++ denotes moderate and + ±, + and ± lesser amounts of agglutination, – denotes no agglutination or lysis.

criterion the antibody could be regarded as 'complete'.

The 'incomplete' cold auto-antibody in normal serum: further details

As already referred to on p. 276, the author (Dacie 1950b) reported that if the defibrinated blood of healthy normal individuals was allowed to stand for 1–2 hours at 2–5°C and the erythrocytes were subsequently washed several times in saline warmed to 37°C, the washed cells would be agglutinated by antiglobulin sera if the sera were used in strong concentrations. He also showed that stronger reactions could be obtained if weaker (0.5–5%) suspensions of washed cells were suspended in autologous serum and that such suspensions would sometimes give weak positive reactions even if sensitization had been carried out at room temperature; on the other hand, if the autologous serum had been heated at 56°C for 5–30 minutes before the cells were added to it, the cells were no longer agglutinable by the antiglobulin serum. Subsequently, as already mentioned, it became clear that the observed positive reactions were in reality brought about by a reaction between complement bound to the cell membranes and anti-complement antibodies in the antiglobulin serum. The possibility that the antibody present in human sera might have any particular specificity was not explored at the time, although it had been noted that the intensity of the positive reaction varied. In the original text it was, for instance, stated that incomplete cold antibodies could often — not always — be demonstrated in an individual's serum. Also, Dr. G. C. de Gruchy (G. C. de G.), who was working with the author at the time, had noted that his defibrinated blood gave very weak reactions compared with those given by the author's (J. V. D.) own blood (G. C. de G. was group A_1, J. V. D. group A_2). Subsequently, it was clearly established by Crawford, Cutbush and Mollison (1953), and confirmed by Leddy et al. (1962), that the 'incomplete' cold auto-antibodies present in human sera had an anti-H specificity. Thus group-O erythrocytes gave reactions that were stronger than those given by A_1 cells, while A_2 cells gave intermediate

reactions. Also, the antibody was found to be inhibited by human saliva obtained from secretors of H substance.

Nature of the normal 'incomplete' cold auto-antibody

It has proved difficult to determine exactly the nature of the normal, 'incomplete' antibody. According to Crawford and Mollison (1956) and Polley, Mollison and Soothill (1962), it is present in the serum of newborn infants, suggesting the possibility that it might be a 7S γ globulin. According, however, to Adinolfi, Daniels and Mollison (1963), fractionation by DEAE-cellulose chromatography showed that the antibody did not elute as a 7S γ globulin. It was also found that erythrocytes sensitized by the antibody were not agglutinated by potent anti-7S γ-globulin sera (or by anti-19S γ-globulin sera). The antibody, too, was identified in the serum of 10 out of 11 patients with hypogammglobulinaemia—in none of which sera could anti-A, anti-B or anti-I be demonstrated.

The results of further attempts to characterize the normal 'incomplete' antibody were described by Adinolfi (1965a,c). Its presence in cord-blood sera appeared to be independent of its presence in the corresponding maternal serum, which suggested that the antibody was being formed by the infant and had not been transferred through the placenta. Its titre was found, too, to be approximately constant in individual infants from a few weeks to 6 months of age, a finding also against the possibility of transplacental passage. By its interaction with certain polysaccharides and bacteria it resembled properdin, but it differed markedly from properdin in its specificity and in other serological characteristics. In relation to its specificity, it was found that the amount of the antibody in normal serum was related inversely to the amount of H substance carried by the erythrocytes: thus group-A_1B individuals had the most, followed by A_1, B, A_2B and A_2 individuals, with group-O individuals having the least. An interesting difference was demonstrated in relation to the thermolability of the antibody: it was relatively heat-labile at 56°C and destroyed rapidly at 63°F, whereas both anti-D (an IgG antibody) and anti-P_1 (an IgM antibody) were almost unaffected by heating at 56°C for up to 3 hours. Attempts to elute the normal 'incomplete' cold antibody from sensitized erythrocytes or their stroma by standard methods were generally unsuccessful, but partial elution was, however, achieved at 37°C by eluting into serum rather than into saline (Adinolfi, 1965c).

Relationship between the cold auto-agglutinins and the 'incomplete' cold auto-antibodies present in normal sera

The two types of antibodies appear to be distinct: the agglutinins are IgM globulins while the nature of the 'incomplete' antibodies is uncertain—they are not IgM (or IgG or IgA) globulins (see above). Also, the agglutinins are typically anti-I in specificity, while the 'incomplete' antibodies are anti-H. According to Schubothe (1955), too, the strengths of the antiglobulin reaction given by the antibodies and the cold-agglutinin titres do not run parallel.

Clinical significance of 'incomplete' cold auto-antibodies

There seems little doubt but that the 'incomplete' cold auto-antibodies found in normal sera are of no clinical significance. In disease, however, 'incomplete' cold antibodies, as distinct from complement-fixing complete (agglutinating) antibodies, seem likely to be sometimes responsible for in-vivo haemolysis. This was the view of Schubothe and Matthes (1951) who, in a brief report, described the occurrence of 'incomplete' cold antibodies in two patients with CHAD: the most significant finding was that their fresh serum gave positive indirect antiglobulin reactions with normal erythrocytes at 37°C, the titres being high, 256–512.

Crowley (1958) had investigated a middle-aged woman, who had suffered from AIHA of several years' duration that appeared to have been brought about by an 'incomplete' cold antibody of anti-H specificity. Her haemoglobin was 5.3 g/dl and reticulocyte count 20%, and macrocytosis and mild spherocytosis were present. The patient was group A_1. The DAT was positive and her blood underwent auto-agglutination after withdrawal. Her serum contained an antibody which agglutinated saline-suspended group-O cells at 4°C and at room temperature, but not at 37°C. Erythrocytes suspended in 22% bovine albumin were, however, strongly agglutinated at 37°C, and the IAT was positive at 37°C, too. Absorption and elution studies suggested that a single cold auto-antibody was present, and titration in albumin, or using trypsinized erythrocytes,

indicated that group-O cells were more sensitive than A_1 cells. The antibody could, too, be neutralized completely by saliva from known secretors of ABH substance. In addition to the 'incomplete' cold antibody, the patient's serum appeared to contain a low-titre cold agglutinin to which group-A cells were more sensitive than O cells. This latter antibody was thought to be innocuous: the 'incomplete' antibody, on the other hand, was looked upon as responsible for the patient's illness, and to be probably a pathological variant of the 'incomplete' cold auto-antibody present in many normal sera.

As referred to on p. 20, Capra and co-workers (1969), who had studied the sera of 50 patients with infectious mononucleosis, concluded that the majority (90%) of the sera contained γG 'incomplete' anti-i cold agglutinins, along with 19S 'complete' agglutinating antibodies in 35% of the sera. The 'incomplete' antibodies were maximally active at 0–5°C. That the positive antiglobulin reactions given by i cells sensitized in the cold were not due to adsorbed complement was demonstrated by: (1) failure of the sensitized cells to be agglutinated by an anti-B_1C (complement) serum; (2) by heat-inactivation not affecting the antibody titre, and (3) by the sensitized cells being agglutinated by an anti-γG antiglobulin serum.

Moore and Chaplin (1973), in a further interesting report, described a 16-year-old girl who was admitted to hospital severely anaemic: the haemoglobin was 3.9 g/dl and there were 31% reticulocytes. The DAT was positive both with anti-IgG and with anti-C3 sera. Her serum contained an IgM cold agglutinin, the titre of which was 256 at 4°C; but in addition it contained an IgG 'incomplete' cold antibody, with lambda light chains, at a titre of 64 at 4°C and 4 at 37°C. The IgG antibody did not require complement for binding to erythrocytes, but it could bind complement and lyse papainized cells. Its specificity could not be determined; in particular, it lacked Ii, P, Rh and ABH specificity. The patient responded well to steroid therapy and splenectomy, but mild compensated haemolysis persisted and the DAT was still strongly positive 10 months after the onset of her illness.

Possible transplacental passage of an 'incomplete' cold auto-antibody

Holländer (1952) reported that the DAT was positive in the case of an Rh-positive newborn infant who, nevertheless, showed no signs of increased haemolysis. The reaction was of the non-γ (complement) type, for it persisted even after γ globulin had been added to the antiglobulin serum. The reaction was thought to be the result of the transplacental passage of an 'incomplete' cold antibody that was present in the mother's serum at an abnormally high concentration: its titre at 4°C was 128, at 16°C, 32 and at 22°C, 8.

NATURE OF COMPLEMENT COMPONENTS FIXED TO ERYTHROCYTES BY 'INCOMPLETE' AND LYTIC COLD AUTO-ANTIBODIES

The discovery that the positive 'non-γ' antiglobulin reactions given by erythrocytes exposed to cold agglutinins were due to interaction between complement bound to the erythrocytes and anti-complement antibodies in the antiglobulin serum led to extensive investigations into the nature of the complement components bound to the erythrocytes' surface as the result of the antibody–antigen reaction. It is now known that the main complement component that can be detected on surviving erythrocytes as the result of in-vivo sensitization is a derivative of C3, C3d,g (an α-2D globulin), which is the final product of in-vivo C3 activation. *In vitro*, however, both C4 and C3 can be detected by the use of appropriate antisera when erythrocytes interact with complement-binding antibodies.

Early studies

In the course of their work that first established the role of complement in bringing about the agglutination by antiglobulin sera of erythrocytes that had been exposed to several types of potentially lytic antibodies, Dacie, Crookston and Christenson (1957) found that treating the human serum used as a source of complement with ammonia, so as to destroy C4, prevented agglutination by antiglobulin sera as well as lysis. In contrast, treating the serum with zymosan so as to inactivate C3, although it prevented lysis, did not prevent agglutination by antiglobulin sera. This was found to be so also in the case of sheep cells that had been sensitized with a rabbit anti-sheep cell serum. It thus appeared as if the C1, C2 and C4 components of complement, but not the C3 component, were required for the irreversible binding of complement to erythrocytes that were reacting with antibodies capable of causing lysis.

From 1960 onwards, the increasing knowledge of the complexity of the complement system and of the chemistry of the complement proteins, and improvements in immunological techniques, have enabled the more exact identification of the complement components involved when erythrocytes sensitized with complement-fixing antibodies are agglutinated by antiglobulin sera.

Jenkins, Polley and Mollison (1960) reported that the 'non-gamma globulin' Coombs reaction depended upon the interaction between C4 adsorbed to erythrocytes and a corresponding anti-β_1 globulin in the antiglobulin serum. Pondman and co-workers (1960) came to essentially the same conclusion: that the agglutination of optimally sensitized sheep erythrocytes by antiglobulin serum was the result of an interaction with bound and decayed C4.

In 1962, Polley, Mollison and Soothill and Adinolfi and co-workers described the results of classifying a wide range of blood-group antibodies as $\beta_2 M$ (IgM) or γ (IgG) antibodies based on their reactions with anti-$\beta_2 M$, anti-γ and anti-β_1 (complement) antiglobulin sera. Amongst the antibodies they tested was the anti-I antibody that had been formed by the normal i adult described by Jenkins et al. (1960). This antibody strongly agglutinated I cells up to 30°C but not at 37°C; it did, however, sensitize the cells to antiglobulin sera (anti-$\beta_2 M$ and anti-β_1) at 37°C. The serum did, therefore, appear to contain some non-agglutinating 'incomplete' antibody molecules which remained firmly fixed to erythrocytes at 37°C.

The isolation and characterization of the C3 and C4 components of complement, referred to, respectively, as β_{1C} globulin and β_{1E} globulin, and the development of antisera against these proteins, facilitated further advances. Both proteins, i.e. C3 and C4, were identified by Harboe et al. (1963) on erythrocytes sensitized by complement-binding antibodies, and the agglutination of the sensitized cells was found to be inhibited by adding β_{1C} and β_{1E} globulins to 'broad-spectrum' antiglobulin sera. The erythrocytes of a patient suffering from cold-antibody AIHA were found, too, to be agglutinated by anti-β_{1C} and anti-β_{1E} sera.

Harboe (1964) described experiments to determine whether, when cold agglutinins are eluted by warmth from erythrocytes sensitized by the antibody at a low temperature, any of the antibody remains on the erythrocyte surface in addition to complement. High-titre cold auto-agglutinins were obtained from two patients and trace-labelled with ^{131}I. The results indicated that more than 95% of the radioactivity adsorbed to the erythrocytes in the cold could be recovered in the saline used to wash the cells at 37°C. It was concluded, therefore, that complement persists on the erythrocyte surface without the presence of any antibody, once complement fixation has been achieved.

Evans, Turner and Bingham (1964, 1965) similarly showed that when erythrocytes were exposed to ^{131}I trace-labelled high-titre cold agglutinins at 5°C and subsequently washed at 37°C, up to 99% of the adsorbed radioactivity was recovered in the eluting fluid.

Further studies on the interaction between complement and cold agglutinins were described by Boyer and Hinz (1967) and by Boyer (1967). Boyer and Hinz reported that the 11S component of C1 (C1$_q$), C1 and C4, must react in sequence for the antiglobulin test to become positive. The 11S component and C1 reacted maximally at 1°C but failed to react at 37°C. In contrast, C4 failed to react at 1°C; it reacted maximally at 20°C but failed to react, or only reacted weakly, at 37°C. Calcium ions were required for the reaction of C1, but neither calcium nor magnesium ions were required for the reaction of the 11S component or that of C4.

Rosse, Borsos and Rapp (1968) presented evidence that the presence of Cla during the interaction at a low temperature of anti-I cold antibodies with human erythrocytes increases the adherence of the antibody to the cells.

Engelfriet and co-workers (1970) described the preparation and use of specific antisera against complement components. They reported that erythrocytes exposed *in vitro* to complement-binding allo- or auto-antibodies were agglutinated by anti-β1E, -β1A and -α2D sera while the cells of AIHA patients were agglutinated only by the anti-α2D serum. It was concluded, therefore, that *in vivo* the β1E and β1A components are lost.

Logue, Gockerman and Rosse (1971) and Logue, Rosse and Gockerman (1973) described how they had measured the amount of C3 attached to the erythrocytes of patients by a quantitative assay based on the fixation of C1 to erythrocyte C3–anti-C3 complexes. With this technique they were able to demonstrate that significant amounts of C3 were fixed to erythrocytes as the result of local or general cold stress. They concluded as the result of their experiments that most of the C3 on the erythrocyte membrane that they could detect by their assay was haemolytically harmless. This was because C3, if slowly but continuously deposited on the cell membrane, would be almost completely inactivated by an inactivator in plasma (C3b INA). However, if the number of C3 molecules on the erythrocyte membrane was abruptly increased as the result of sudden cold stress this would lead to haemolysis, as their inactivation could not proceed quickly enough to prevent some of the complement sequences from proceeding to completion.

Fischer and co-workers (1974) described the results of using an immunochemical method to determine the number of C3 molecules on erythrocytes, with the aim of assessing the significance of cell-bound C3 in immune haemolysis. They experimented with erythrocytes that had been sensitized *in vivo*, obtained from patients with various types of AIHA, including patients suffering from CHAD and PCH and cells sensitized *in vitro* with an anti-Le^a serum. They also related the number of molecules detected with the results of antiglobulin tests using a range of anti-complement sera. They found that the antiglobulin test, using an anti-C3 serum, became positive with 60–115 molecules of C3 per cell and was strongly positive if there were as many as 1000 molecules per cell. Applying quantitative measurements of the number of C3 molecules per cell to clinical problems, Fischer et al. found that only two of 14 patients with evidence of overt haemolytic anaemia had fewer than 1100 molecules of C3 per cell, whereas eight out of 11 patients with overt haemolytic anaemia had more than 1100 molecules. The presence or absence of haemolysis in these patients could not be explained by differences in the amount of IgG on the patient's cells.

Recent studies on the fixation of complement

Rosse, Adams and Logue (1977) reported on the time and temperature requirements for the fixation of complement components to erythrocytes exposed to anti-I cold auto-antibodies. The amounts of C4, C3 and C5 bound to the cell membranes were individually assayed. The experiments were carried out in two phases: a cold phase (15°C or below) and a warm phase during which the cell suspensions were warmed to 37°C. During the first (cold) phase only antibody and C1 are fixed; during the second (warm) phase C4 and C3 are fixed. The fixation of C4 begins at about 18°C; thereafter, the rate at which C4 is fixed rapidly diminishes as the temperature rises because antibody and C1 are eluted. The fixation of C4 depends, therefore, on the thermal amplitude of the antibody. If this is high, more C4 is fixed and hence more complement sequences can be completed. C2 is bound to C4 by the action of C1. This cannot happen until C4 is fixed and it must occur before C1 is eluted.

C3 is activated by the enzyme, $C\overline{42}$, formed by the combination of C2 and C4; its fixation cannot be accomplished until C2 and C4 have been fixed. The amount of C3 fixed increases very little at 37°C, because the enzyme $C\overline{42}$ is unstable at this temperature. C3 itself is unstable and is rapidly degraded by the enzyme C3b inactivator. C5 is attached to C3 and is enzymatically cleaved by C2 in the $C\overline{42}$ complex. Once C5 has been cleaved it initiates the terminal lytic complex; at first its fixation is rapid but this soon diminishes rapidly. Rosse, Adams and Logue's observations provide a logical basis for understanding why high-titre cold antibodies act as rather poor lysins. In their own words: 'The fastidious and contradictory temperature requirements for the fixation of antibody and for the activation of complement, the activity of the processes that normally inactivate the complement sequence, and the marked resistance of the normal red cell membrane to the lytic action of the complement all play a role in the inefficiency of lysis of these cells.'

Salama and co-workers (1983) described an immunoradiometric method for detecting the C5b-9 complex on erythrocytes that had been exposed to complement-fixing antibodies. In-vitro experiments demonstrated that deposition of radioactivity, indicating C5b-9 fixation, paralleled, and tended to be more sensitive than the visual appearance of lysis. *In vivo*, intact (surviving) erythrocytes from patients forming cold (or warm) complement-fixing auto-antibodies carried C3/C4 components but never detectable C5b-9.

In recent years monoclonal antibodies specific for complement components have become available. Their use has shown that the erythrocytes of CHAD patients are coated with C3d,g (α-2D globulin). C3d,g with C3c, are the final products of the splitting of C3bi, itself derived from C3b by the C3b inactivator (Lachmann et al., 1983). Voak and his co-workers (1983), using monoclonal antibodies, reported that the erythrocytes of four CHAD patients, suffering from active haemolysis, had erythrocytes that were strongly (+++) agglutinated by both anti-C3g and anti-C3d sera. The erythrocytes of four patients suffering from other types of cold-antibody AIHA gave negative to +++ reactions with the anti-C3g serum but strong reactions with the anti-C3d serum.

SERUM COMPLEMENT IN AIHA

In vitro, it is easy to demonstrate that complement is utilized in experimental systems when lysis takes place, and this is true even in the absence of lysis when fixation of complement can be demonstrated by means of the antiglobulin reaction (Table 29.3). The question arises as to how often and to what extent is serum complement demonstrably depleted in patients suffering from AIHA. In fact, abnormally low serum-complement levels are not infrequent in AIHA of both the warm- and cold-antibody types; occasionally, complement activity may appear to be absent or the serum may even be anticomplementary. There appear to be two circumstances that lead to lower serum-complement levels: (1) where a large amount of a complement-binding auto-antibody is being formed which leads to a severe grade of intravascular haemolysis and consequent rapid utilization of complement; and (2) where complement activity is lowered, for reasons which are obscure, in the absence of evidence for much intravascular haemolysis.

Most of the patients in the first category have been demonstrated to have formed actively lytic high-titre cold antibodies, e.g. Case 19 of Dacie and de Gruchy (1951), Cases 2 and 3 of van Loghem et al. (1952) and the patients studied by Jonsen and Kåss (1959), Case 13 of Dacie (1954a, p. 205) and the patient of Goudemand and Ropartz (1954). The serum of one of van Loghem's cases appeared to be anticomplementary, and Jonsen and Kåss were able to show a fall in titre of C2 and a smaller fall in C1 activity when their patient was deliberately exposed to cold.

Jonsen, Käss and Harboe (1961) reported on serum complement activity, and on C1, C2, C3 and C4 activity separately, in five patients suffering from typical chronic CHAD. The DAT was positive, the reaction being of the non-γ type, in each case. Only one of the patients had had attacks of overt haemoglobinuria. Serum complement activity was, however, subnormal in each patient, C2 activity being particularly deficient.

Notable examples of 'warm haemolysins' with diminished or absent complement activity were described by Gardner and Harris (1950) and by Dausset (1954) and Dausset et al. (1957), the serum of the first patient being anticomplementary. The patient described as Case 7 (Dacie 1962, p. 439) also suffered from serum-complement depletion, probably secondary to intravascular haemolysis.

Raeder (1955), van Loghem, Mendes de Leon and van der Hart (1955), van Loghem, van der Hart and Dorfmeier (1958) and Jordan (1958) all reported data on the incidence of lowered serum-complement levels in patients forming warm antibodies.

Raeder found subnormal levels in seven out of 15 patients suffering from miscellaneous types of haemolytic anaemia; in three patients the levels were low throughout their illness, while in four the loss in activity was only transitory. In the chronic cases the low complement levels may, Raeder suggested, have been due to failure of regeneration as well as to increased utilization. van Loghem, van der Hart and Dorfmeier summarized their experience by stating that low complement levels were found in 20% of patients forming incomplete warm antibodies and in 50% of those forming cold agglutinins. Jordan reported low complement values in three patients with immunohaemolytic anaemia forming warm antibodies as well as in one patient with 'hyper-splenism'; normal values were found in the remaining 26 patients studied (excluding four with paroxysmal cold haemoglobinuria).

The present writer's experience up to 1962 is

Table 29.4 Serum complement concentrations in patients suffering from idiopathic auto-immune haemolytic anaemia.

Type of antibody	Complement concentration		
	Normal	Subnormal	Absent
Warm	8	4	1*
Cold	0	7†	2

*Case 7 of Dacie (1962).
†Normal concentrations were recorded on other occasions in three patients.

summarized in Table 29.4. It is particularly noteworthy that in the patient described as Case 13 by Dacie (1954a, p. 205), the serum-complement levels remained reduced and unaltered although the rate of haemolysis was substantially diminished by splenectomy (Fig. 29.8). Later, this patient went into almost complete haematological remission without, however, any corresponding rise in complement titre. This type of observation focuses attention on deficiencies in complement synthesis or the continuous formation of anticomplementary substances as factors which are important in some cases in relation to low serum-complement activity.

The low serum complement levels which are so characteristic of active paroxysmal cold haemoglobinuria are referred to in Chapter 32 (p. 355).

Recent reports of serum-complement depletion in AIHA

Wager and co-workers (1971) gave details of five patients with AIHA who had formed IgA warm auto-antibodies in addition to IgG auto-antibodies. Their serum Ig concentrations and those of C3 and C4 and C1-esterase inhibitor were recorded: two patients had low C3 levels, two low C4 levels and two low C1-esterase inhibitor levels.

Kretschmer and Mueller-Eckhardt (1972) reported on the serum immunoglobulin and β1A-globulin levels in 21 patients with AIHA who were forming incomplete warm antibodies. The serum β1A-globulin (taken as a measure of serum complement) was measured at the time of maximum haemolysis and also followed in some

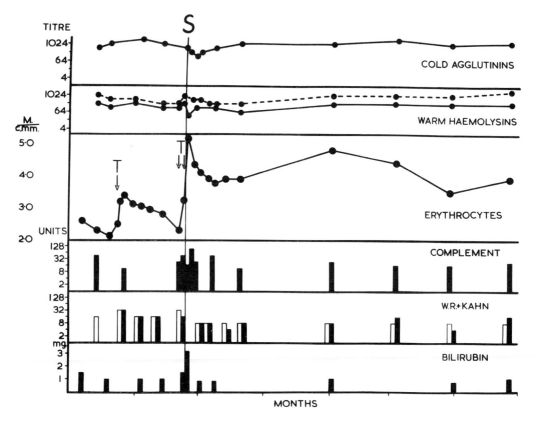

Fig. 29.8   Response of a patient with atypical CHAD [Case 13 of Dacie (1954, p. 207)] to splenectomy (S).
 T = blood transfusions, ●– – – –● = lysis titre at 37°C using PNH erythrocytes; ●——● = lysis titre using trypsinized normal erythrocytes. The (reduced) serum complement titre was not affected by splenectomy, despite a reduction in of in-vivo haemolysis.

patients during the course of their illness. At the time of maximum haemolysis the β1A-globulin was reduced in 15 out of 21 patients (71%). In 16 patients, in whom the β1A-globulin was estimated during the course of their illness, with one exception, the level tended to rise in parallel with clinical improvement.

Further information on serum-complement levels in AIHA of the warm-antibody type were reported by Kretschmer and Mueller-Eckhardt in 1977. Their data were by then based on the study of 79 patients, 35 with chronic idiopathic AIHA and 34 with symptomatic AIHA, and on seven patients whose DAT was positive but in whom there was no evidence of haemolysis. The levels of serum C3 and C4 were similar in both the idiopathic and symptomatic cases. Reduced levels were, however, more frequent in patients who had complement components fixed to their erythrocytes, as demonstrated by the DAT, than in those in which they were absent. Thus, of 17 patients with IgG alone fixed, none had decreased serum C3 or C4 levels; of 33 patients with IgG and C fixed, nine had decreased C3 and 14 decreased C4; and of 19 patients with C alone fixed, four had decreased C3 and nine decreased C4. In addition, Kretschmer and Mueller-Eckhardt's data indicated that the C4 levels were lower in patients in whom incomplete warm haemolysins were demonstrable than in patients in whom they were absent; also that the C3 and C4 concentrations, if followed throughout the course of a patient's illness, were closely correlated with the severity of haemolysis.

REFERENCES

ADINOLFI, M. (1965a). Some serological characteristics of normal incomplete cold antibody. *Immunology*, **9**, 31–42.

ADINOLFI, M. (1965b), Anti-I antibody in normal human newborn infants. *Immunology*, **9**, 43–52.

ADINOLFI, M. (1965c). Further attempts to characterize the normal incomplete cold antibody. *Immunology*, **9**, 365–375.

ADINOLFI, M., DANIELS, C. & MOLLISON, P. L. (1963). Evidence that 'normal incomplete cold antibody' is not a gamma-globulin. *Nature (Lond.)*, **199**, 389–390.

ADINOLFI, M., POLLEY. M. J., HUNTER, D. A. & MOLLISON, P. L. (1962). Classification of blood-group antibodies as β_2M or gamma globulin. *Immunology*, **5**, 566–579.

ALLEN, F. H. JNR, MARSH, W. L., JENSEN, L. & FINK, J. (1974). Anti-IP: an antibody defining another product of interaction between the genes of the I and P blood group systems. *Vox Sang.*, **27**, 442–446.

AMBRUS, M. & BAJTAI, G. (1969). A case of an IgG-type cold agglutinin disease. *Haematologia*, **3**, 225–235.

AMZEL, R. & HIRSZFELD, L. (1925). Ueber die Kälteagglutination der roten Blutkörperchen. *Z. Immun.-Forsch.*, **43**, 526–538.

ANDERSEN, B. R. (1966). Gamma-A cold agglutinin: importance of disulfide bonds in activity and structure. *Science*, **154**, 281–283.

ANGEVINE, C. D., ANDERSEN, B. R. & BARNETT, E. V. (1966). A cold agglutinin of the IgA class. *J. Immunol.*, **96**, 578–586.

ATICHARTAKARN, V., CHIEWSILP, P., RATANASIRIVANICH, P. & STABUNSWADGAN, S. (1985). Autoimmune hemolytic anemia due to anti B autoantibody. *Vox Sang.*, **49**, 301–303.

BASU, M. K., LEE., M. M., MANIATIS, A. & BERTLES, J. F. (1984). Characteristics of I and i antigen receptors on the membrane of erythrocytes in sickle cell anemia. *J. Lab. clin. Med.*, **103**, 712–719.

BAUMGARTEN, A. & CURTAIN, C. C. (1970). A high frequency of cold agglutinins of anti-IA specificity in a New-Guinea highland population. *Vox Sang.*, **18**, 21–26.

BAUMGARTEN, A., CURTAIN, C. C., GOLAB, T., GORMAN, J. G. & RUTGERS, C. F. (1968). Endemic autoimmunity: cold auto-agglutinins in Melanesia. *Brit. J. Haemat.*, **15**, 567–577.

BELL, C. A., ZWICKER, H. & SACKS, H. J. (1967). Anti-i: identification of the 'non-specific' cold-agglutinin. *Vox Sang*, **13**, 4–6.

BERREBI. A. & LEVENE, C. (1976). Acanthocytes bearing the i antigen. *Vox Sang.*, **30**, 396–398.

BIRD, G. W. G. (1951). The nature of auto-agglutinins. *Lancet*, **i**, 997.

BIRD, G. W. G. (1953a). Observations on haemagglutinin 'linkage' in relation to iso-agglutinins and auto-agglutinins. *Brit. J. exp. Path.*, **34**, 131–137.

BIRD, G. W. G. (1953b). Specificity of complete cold auto-agglutinins. *Nature (Lond.)*, **172**, 734.

BIRD, G. W. G. (1966). Autohaemagglutinins. With special reference to cold autoagglutinins with ABO-blood group specificity. *Blut*, **12**, 281–285.

BIRD, G. W. G. & WINGHAM, J. (1973). Anti-I autoantibody acting preferentially in albumin. *Vox Sang.*, **25**, 162–165.

BIRD, G. W. G. & WINGHAM, J. (1977). Erythrocyte autoantibody with unusual specificity. *Vox Sang.*, **32**, 280–282.

BIRGENS, H. S., DYBKJAER, E. & ROELCKE, D. (1982). Identification of a cold agglutinin with anti-Pr$_3$ specificity. *Scand. J. Haemat.*, **29**, 207–210.

BOCCARDI, V., GIRELLI, G. & ZAPPI, P. (1975). Cold-haemagglutinin disease with an autoantibody exhibiting different specificities at different temperatures. *Scand. J. Haemat.*, **14**, 268–276.

BOETTCHER, B., NANRA, R. S., ROBERTS, T. K., MALLAN, M. & WATTERSON, C. A. (1976). Specificity and possible origin of anti-N antibodies developed by patients undergoing chronic haemodialysis. *Vox Sang.*, **31**, 408–415.

BONNIN, J. A. (1954). Chronic acquired hemolytic anemia associated with hemoglobinuria and Raynaud's phenomena. *Blood*, **9**, 959–964.

BOOTH, P. B. (1970). Anti-I^{T}P$_1$: an antibody showing a further association between the I and P blood group systems. *Vox Sang.*, **19**, 85–90.

BOOTH, P. B. (1972). The occurrence of weak I^T red cell antigens among Melanesians. *Vox Sang.*, **22**, 64–72.

BOOTH, P. B., JENKINS, W. J. & MARSH, W. L. (1966). Anti-I^T: a new antibody of the I blood-group system occurring in certain Melanesian sera. *Brit. J. Haemat.*, **12**, 341–344.

BORSOS, T. & RAPP, H. J. (1965). Hemolysis titration based on the fixation of the activated first component of complement: evidence that one molecule of hemolysin suffices to sensitize an erythrocyte. *J. Immunol.*, **95**, 559–566.

BOWES, A. (1976). Chronic cold agglutinin disease due to auto-anti-M. A paper given to the 8th Triennial Conference of the [British] National Transfusion Service.

BOWMAN, H. S., MARSH, W. L., SCHUMACHER, H. R., OYEN, R. & REIHART, J. (1974). Auto anti-N immunohemolytic anemia in infectious mononucleosis. *Amer. J. clin. Path.*, **61**, 465–472.

BOYER, J. T. (1967). Complement and cold agglutinins. II. Interactions of the components of complement and antibody within the haemolytic complex. *Clin. exp. Immunol.*, **2**, 241–252.

BOYER, J. T. & HINZ, C. F. JNR (1967). Complement and cold agglutinins I. Complement coating of normal human erythrocytes by cold agglutinins. *Clin. exp. Immunol.*, **2**, 229–239.

BOXWELL, W. & BIGGER, J. W. (1931). Autohaemagglutination. *J. Path. Bact.*, **34**, 407–417.

BRENDEMOEN, O. J. (1952). A cold agglutinin specifically active against stored red cells. *Acta path. microbiol. scand.*, **31**, 574–578.

CAPRA, J. D., DOWLING, P., COOK, S. & KUNKEL, H. G. (1969). An incomplete cold-reactive γG antibody with i specificity in infectious mononucleosis. *Vox Sang.*, **16**, 10–17.

CHAMPION, R. H. (1965). Livedo reticularis. A review. *Brit. J. Dermat.*, **77**, 167–179.

CHAPMAN, J., MURPHY, M. F. & WATERS, A. H. (1982). Chronic cold haemagglutinin disease due to an anti-M-like autoantibody. *Vox Sang.*, **42**, 272–277.

CHESSIN, L. N. & McGINNISS, M. H. (1968). Further evidence for the serologic association of the O(H) and I blood groups. *Vox Sang.*, **14**, 194–201.

CHRISTENSON, W. N. & DACIE, J. V. (1957). Serum proteins in acquired haemolytic anaemia (auto-antibody type). *Brit. J. Haemat.*, **3**, 153–164.

CHRISTENSON, W. N., DACIE, J. V., CROUCHER, B. E. E. & CHARLWOOD, P. A. (1957). Electrophoretic studies on sera containing high-titre cold haemagglutinins: identification of the antibody as the cause of an abnormal γ₁ peak. *Brit. J. Haemat.*, **3**, 262–275.

CIRUZZI, J., CARRERAS-VESCIO, L. A., REY, J. A., TERUYA, J. & MARLETTA, J. (1983). Hemoglobinuria paroxistica 'a frigore' por hemolisina bifasica de especificidad anti-IH. *Sangre (Barcelona)*, **28**, 775–781.

CLOUGH, M. C. & RICHTER. I. M. (1918). A study of an auto-agglutinin occurring in a human serum. *Johns Hopk. Hosp. Bull.*, **29**, 86–93.

COHEN, D. W., GARRATTY, G., MOREL, P. & PETZ, L. D. (1979). Autoimmune hemolytic anemia associated with IgG auto anti-N. *Transfusion*, **19**, 329–331.

COHEN, S. & COOPER, A. G. (1968). Chemical differences between individual human cold agglutinins. *Immunology*, **15**, 93–100.

COOMBS, R. R. A., MOURANT, A. E. & RACE, R. R. (1945). A new test for the detection of weak and 'incomplete' Rh agglutinins. *Brit. J. exp. Path.*, **26**, 255–266.

COOPER, A. G. (1968). Purification of cold agglutinins from patients with chronic cold haemagglutinin disease. Evidence of their homogeneity from starch gel electrophoresis of isolated light chains. *Clin. exp. Immunol.*, **3**, 691–702.

COOPER, A. G. (1970). Soluble blood group I substance in human amniotic fluid. *Nature (Lond.)*, **227**, 508–509.

COOPER, A. G. & BROWN, M. C. (1973). Serum i antigen: a new human blood-group glycoprotein. *Biochem. biophys. Res. Commun.*, **55**, 297–304.

COOPER, A. G., HOFFBRAND, A. V. & WORLLEDGE, S. M. (1968). Increased agglutinability by anti-i of red cells in sideroblastic and megaloblastic anaemia. *Brit. J. Haemat.*, **15**, 381–387.

COOPER, A. G. & WORLLEDGE, S. M. (1967). Light chains in chronic cold haemagglutinin disease. *Nature (Lond.)*, **214**, 799–800.

COPEMAN, P. W. M. (1975). Livedo reticularis: signs in the skin of disturbance of blood viscosity and of blood flow. *Brit. J. Dermat.*, **95**, 519–529.

COSTEA, N., YAKULIS, V. & HELLER, P. (1966). Light-chain heterogeneity of cold agglutinins. *Science*, **152**, 1520–1521.

COSTEA, N., YAKULIS, V. & HELLER, P. (1967). The dependence of cold agglutinin activity on K chains. *J. Immunol.*, **99**, 558–563.

CRAWFORD, H., CUTBUSH, M. & MOLLISON, P. L. (1953). Specificity of incomplete 'cold' antibody in human serum. *Lancet*, **i**, 566–567.

CRAWFORD, H. & MOLLISON, P. L. (1956). In Mollison (1956), *Blood Transfusion in Clinical Medicine*, p. 254. Blackwell Scientific Publications, Oxford.

CROOKSTON, J. H. (1975). Hemolytic anemia with IgG and IgM autoantibodies and alloantibodies. *Arch. intern. Med.*, **135**, 1314–1315.

CROOKSTON, J. H., CROOKSTON, M. C., BURNIE, K. L., FRANCOMBE, W. H., DACIE, J. V., DAVIS, J. A. & LEWIS, S. M. (1969). Hereditary erythroblastic multinuclearity associated with a positive acidified-serum test: a type of congenital dyserythropoetic anaemia. *Brit. J. Haemat.*, **17**, 11–26.

CROOKSTON, J. H., CROOKSTON, M. C. & ROSSE, W. F. (1969). Red cell membrane abnormalities in hereditary multinuclearity. *Blood*, **34**, 844 (Abstract).

CROOKSTON, J. H., DACIE, J. V. & ROSSI, V. (1956). Differences in the agglutinability of human red cells by the high-titre cold antibodies of acquired haemolytic anaemia. *Brit. J. Haemat.*, **2**, 321–331.

CROWLEY, L. V. (1958). Blood group specific autoantibodies in acquired hemolytic anemia. Incomplete cold antibody with anti-H specificity. *Amer. J. clin. Path.*, **29**, 426–429.

CURTAIN, C. C., BAUMGARTEN, A., GORMAN, J., KIDSON, C., CHAMPNESS, L., RODRIGUE, R. & GAJDUSEK, D. C. (1965). Cold haemagglutinins: unusual incidence in Melanesian populations. *Brit. J. Haemat.*, **11**, 471–479.

CURTIS, B. R., LAMON, J., ROELCKE, D. & CHAPLIN, H. (1990). Life-threatening, antiglobulin test-negative, acute autoimmune hemolytic anemia due to a non-complement-activating IgG1κ cold antibody with Pr_a specificity. *Transfusion*, **30**, 838–843.

DACIE, J. V. (1950a). The presence of cold haemolysins in sera containing cold haemagglutinins. *J. Path. Bact.*, **62**, 241–257.

DACIE, J. V. (1950b). Occurrences in normal human

sera of 'incomplete' forms of 'cold' auto-antibodies. *Nature (Lond.)*, **166**, 36.

DACIE, J. V. (1951). Differences in the behaviour of sensitized red cells to agglutination by antiglobulin sera. *Lancet*, **ii**, 954–955.

Dacie, J. V. (1954a). *The Haemolytic Anaemias: Congenital and Acquired*, 525 pp. Churchill, London.

DACIE, J. V. (1954b). The serology of acquired haemolytic anaemia. *Sang*, **25**, 675–678.

DACIE, J. V. (1955). The haemolytic activity of cold antibodies. *Proc. roy. Soc. Med.*, **48**, 211–215.

DACIE, J. V. (1957). The cold haemagglutinin syndrome. *Proc. roy. Soc. Med.*, **50**, 647–650.

DACIE, J. V. (1962). *The Haemolytic Anaemias: Congenital and Acquired. Part II— The Auto-immune Haemolytic Anaemias*, 377 pp. Churchill, London.

DACIE, J. V., CROOKSTON, J. H. & CHRISTENSON, W. N. (1957). 'Incomplete' cold antibodies: role of complement in sensitization to antiglobulin serum by potentially haemolytic antibodies. *Brit. J. Haemat.*, **3**, 77–87.

DACIE, J. V., CROOKSTON, J. H. & CHRISTENSON, W. N. (1958). Incomplete cold antibodies. *Proc. 6th Congr. int. Soc. Blood Transfusion, Boston, 1956*, pp. 145–147. *Bibliotheca haematologica, Fasc. 7*, Karger, Basel.

DACIE, J. V. & DE GRUCHY, G. C. (1951). Auto-antibodies in acquired haemolytic anaemia. *J. clin. Path.*, **4**, 253–271.

DAUSSET, J. (1954). Les hémolysines immunologiques aspécifiques. Conditions de leur recherche systématique. *Acta chir. belg.*, **53** (Suppl. 1), 67–76.

DAUSSET, J. & COLOMBANI, J. (1959). The serology and the prognosis of 128 cases of autoimmune hemolytic anemia. *Blood*, **14**, 1280–1301.

DAUSSET, J., COLOMBANI, J. & EVELIN, J. (1957). Technique de recherche des auto-hémolysines immunologiques. *Rev. franç. Ét. clin. biol.*, **11**, 735–745.

DAUSSET, J., COLOMBANI, J., JEAN, R.G., CANLORBE, P. & LELONG, M. (1957). Sur un cas d'anémie hémolytique aiguë de l'enfant avec présence d'une hémolysine immunologique et d'un pouvoir anticomplémentaire du sérum. *Sang*, **28**, 351–363.

DELAGE, J.-M., GAUVREAU, L. & SIMARD, J. (1956). Les anémies hémolytiques par auto-anticorps. Étude clinique et expérimentale. *Union méd. Canada*, **85**, 132–141.

DELLAGI, K., BROUET, J.C., SCHENMETZLER, C. & PRALORAN, V. (1981). Chronic hemolytic anemia due to a monoclonal IgG cold agglutinin with anti-Pr specificity. *Blood*, **57**, 189–191.

DENEGRI, J. F., NANJI, A. A., SINCLAIR, M. & STILLWELL, G. (1983). Autoimmune hemolytic anemia due to immunoglobulin G with anti-Sd^x specificity. *Acta haemat.*, **69**, 19–22.

DIAMOND, L. K. & DENTON, R. L. (1945). Rh agglutination in various media with particular

reference to the value of albumin. *J. lab. clin. Med.*, **30**, 821–830.

DODDS, A. J., KLARKOWSKI, D., COOPER, D. A. & ISBISTER, J. P. (1979). In-vitro synthesis of anti-BI cold agglutinin complicating a case of lymphoma. *Amer. J. clin. Path.*, **71**, 473–475.

DOINEL, C., ROPARS, C. & SALMON, C. (1974). Anti-I(A + B): an autoantibody detecting an antigenic determinant of I and a common part of A and B. *Vox Sang.*, **27**, 515–523.

DOINEL, C., ROPARS, C. & SALMON, C. (1976). Quantitative and thermodynamic measurements on I and i antigens of human red blood cells. *Immunology*, **30**, 289–297.

DRACHMANN, O. (1968). An autoaggressive anti-BI (O) antibody. *Vox Sang.*, **14**, 185–193.

DUBE, V. E., HOUSE, R. F. JNR, MOULDS, J. & POLESKY, H. F. (1975). Hemolytic anemia due to auto anti-N. *Amer. J. clin. Path.*, **63**, 828–831.

DUBE, V. E., ZUCKERMAN, L. & PHILIPSBORN, H. F. JNR (1978). Variation of cold agglutinin levels. *Vox Sang.*, **34**, 71–76.

DUCOS, J., RUFFIE, J., COLOMBIES, P., MARTY, Y. & OHAYON, E. (1965). I antigen in leukaemic patients. *Nature (Lond.)*, **208**, 1329–1330.

DZIERŻKOWA-BORODEJ, W., SEYFRIED, H. & LISOWSKA, E. (1975). Serological classification of anti-I sera. *Vox Sang.*, **28**, 110–121.

DZIERŻKOWA-BORODEJ, W., SEYFRIED, H., NICHOLS, M., REID, M. & MARSH, W. L. (1970). The recognition of water-soluble I blood group substance. *Vox Sang.*, **18**, 222–234.

DZIERŻKOWA-BORODEJ, W. & VOAK, D. (1979). Subtypes of i demonstrated by the use of atyptical Ii cell types and inhibition studies. *Brit. J. Haemat.*, **41**, 105–113.

ELLENHORN, M. J. & WEINER, D. (1953). Variables in the determination of cold hemagglutinins. *Amer. J. clin. Path.*, **23**, 1031–1039.

ELLIS, L. B., WOLLENMAN, O. J. & STETSON, R. P. (1948). Autohemagglutinins and hemolysins with hemoglobinuria and acute hemolytic anemia, in an illness resembling infectious mononucleosis. *Blood*, **3**, 419–430.

ENGELFRIET, C. P., PONDMAN, K. W., WOLTERS, G., VON DEM BORNE, A. E. G. KR., BECKERS, D., MISSET-GROENVELD, G. & VAN LOGHEM, J. J. (1970). Autoimmune haemolytic anaemia. III. Preparation and examination of specific antisera against complement components and products, and their use in serological studies. *Clin. exp. Immunol.*, **6**, 721–732.

ERNSTENE, A. C. & GARDNER, W. J. (1935). The effect of splenic nerve resection and sympathetic ganglionectomy in a case of paroxysmal hemoglobinuria. *J. clin. Invest.*, **14**, 799–805.

ESS, H., GRAMLICH, F. & MOHRUNG, D. (1958). Serologische und physikochemische Eigenshaften eines Kälteagglutinins. *Klin. Wschr.*, **36**, 852–856.

EVANS, R. S., TURNER, E. & BINGHAM, M. (1964). Studies with I^{131} tagged cold agglutinins. *Proc. 9th Congr. int. Soc. Blood Transfusion, Mexico 1962*, pp. 347–351. Karger, Basel.

EVANS, R. S., TURNER, E. & BINGHAM, M. (1965). Studies with radioiodinated cold agglutinins of ten patients. *Amer. J. Med.*, **38**, 378–395.

EVANS, R. S. & WEISER, R. S. (1957). The serology of autoimmune hemolytic disease. Observations on forty-one patients. *Arch. intern. Med.*, **100**, 371–399.

FAVOUR, C. B. (1944). Autohemagglutinins—'cold agglutinins'. *J. clin. Invest.*, **23**, 891–197.

FEIZI, T. (1967). Lambda chains in cold agglutinins. *Science*, **156**, 1111–1112.

FEIZI, T. (1981). The blood group Ii system: a carbohydrate antigen system defined by naturally [occurring] monoclonal or oligoclonal autoantibodies in man. *Immunological Commun.*, **10**, 127–156.

FEIZI, T., CHILDS, R. A., WATANABE, K. & HAKOMORI, S. I. (1979). Three types of blood group specificity among monoclonal anti-I autoantibodies revealed by analogues of a branched erythrocyte glycolipid. *J. exp. Med.*, **149**, 975–980.

FEIZI, T. & KABAT, E. A. (1972). Immunochemical studies on blood groups. LIV. Classification of anti-I and anti-i sera into groups based on reactivity patterns with various antigens related to the blood group A, B, H, Le^a, Le^b and precursor substances. *J. exp. Med.*, **135**, 1247–1258.

FEIZI, T., KABAT, E. A., VICARI, G., ANDERSON, B. & MARSH, W. L. (1971a). Immunochemical studies on blood groups. XLVII. The I antigen complex— Precursors in the A, B, H, Le^a and Le^b blood group system—Hemagglutination inhibition studies. *J. exp. Med.*, **133**, 39–52.

FEIZI, T., KABAT, E. A., VICARI, G., ANDERSON, B. & MARSH, W. L. (1971b). Immunochemical studies on blood groups. XLIX. The I antigen complex: specificity differences among anti-I sera revealed by quantitative precipitin studies; partial structure of the I determinant specific for one anti-I serum. *J. Immunol.*, **106**, 1578–1592.

FERRIMAN, D. G., DACIE, J. V., KEELE, K. D. & FULLERTON, J. M. (1951). The association of Raynaud's phenomena, chronic haemolytic anaemia, and the formation of cold antibodies. *Quart. J. Med.*, **20**, 275–292.

FINGERLE, R. E. & CHECK, I. J. (1982). Diclonal gammopathy in chronic cold agglutinin disease. *Amer. J. clin. Path.*, **78**, 867–870.

FINKE, M., SACHS, V., VOLLERT, B., LOPEZ, M., SALMON, C., HOPPE, H. H. & FISCHER, K. (1976). An auto-anti-B in an A$_1$B person. Serological studies. *Blut*, **32**, 371–374.

FINLAND, M., PETERSON, O. L. & BARNES, M. W. (1945). Cold agglutinins. III. Observations on certain serological and physical features of cold agglutinins in cases of primary atypical pneumonia and of hemolytic anemia. *J. clin. Invest.*, **24**, 474–482.

FINLAND, M., SAMPER, B. A., BARNES, M. W. & STONE, M. B. (1945). Cold agglutinins. IV. Critical analysis of certain aspects of a method for determining cold isohemagglutinins. *J. clin. Invest.*, **24**, 483–489.

FIRKIN, B. G. (1958). The nature of the absorbed antibody in acquired haemolytic anemia. *Aust. J. exp. Biol. med. Sci.*, **36**, 359–363.

FIRKIN, B. G., & BLACKBURN, C. R. B. (1956). Identification of a cold agglutinin as a β globulin. *Aust. J. exp. Biol. Med.*, **34**, 407–410.

FIRKIN, B. G., BLACKWELL, J. B. & JOHNSTON, G. A. W. (1959). Essential cryoglobulinaemia and acquired haemolytic anaemia due to cold agglutinins. *Aust. Ann. Med.*, **8**, 151–157.

FISCHER, J. T., PETZ, L. D., GARRATTY, G. & COOPER, N. R. (1974). Correlations between quantitative assay of red cell-bound C3, serologic reactions, and hemolytic anemia. *Blood*, **44**, 359–373.

FLETCHER, J. L. & ZMIJEWSKI, C. M. (1970). The first example of auto-anti-M and its consequences in pregnancy. *Int. Arch. Allergy*, **37**, 586–595.

FRANKLIN, E. C. & FUDENBERG, H. A. (1961). Antigenic heterogeneity of human Rh antibodies, rheumatoid factors, and cold agglutinins. *Arch. Biochem. Biophys.* **104**, 433–437.

FREEDMAN, J. & NEWLANDS, M. (1977). Autoimmune haemolytic anaemia with the unusual combination of both IgM and IgG autoantibodies. *Vox Sang.*, **32**, 61–68.

FREEDMAN J., NEWLANDS, M. & JOHNSON, C. A. (1977). Warm IgM anti-I^T causing auto-immune haemolytic anaemia. *Vox Sang.*, **32**, 135–142.

FUDENBERG, H., BARRY, I. & DAMESHEK, W. (1958). The erythrocyte coating substance in autoimmune hemolytic disease: its nature and significance. *Blood*, **13**, 201–215.

FUDENBERG, H. H. & KUNKEL, H. G. (1957). Physical properties of red cell agglutinins in acquired hemolytic anemia. *J. exp. Med.*, **106**, 689–702.

GARDNER, F. H. & HARRIS, J. W. (1950). The demonstration of hemolysins in acquired hemolytic anemia. *J. clin. Invest.*, **29**, 814–815 (Abstract).

GARRATTY, G., HAFFLEIGH, B., DALZIEL, J. & PETZ, L. D. (1972). An IgG anti-I^T detected in a Caucasian American. *Transfusion*, **12**, 325–329.

GARRATTY, G., PETZ, L. D., BRODSKY, I. & FUDENBERG, H. H. (1973). An IgA high-titre cold agglutinin with an unusual blood group specificity within the Pr complex. *Vox Sang.*, **25**, 32–38.

GARRATTY, G., PETZ, L. D. & HOOPS, J. K. (1973). The correlation of cold agglutinin titrations in saline and albumin with hemolytic anemia. *Transfusion*, **13**, 363 (Abstract).

GARRATTY, G., PETZ, L. D. & HOOPS, J. K. (1977). The correlation of cold agglutinin titrations in saline and albumin with haemolytic anaemia. *Brit. J. Haemat.*, **35**, 587–595.

GARRATTY, G., PETZ, L. D., WALLERSTEIN, R. O. & FUDENBERG, H. H. (1974). Autoimmune hemolytic anemia in Hodgkin's disease associated with anti-I[T]. *Transfusion*, **14**, 226–231.

GIBLETT, E. R. & CROOKSTON, M. C. (1964). Agglutinability of red cells by anti-i in patients with thalassaemia major and other haematological disorders. *Nature (Lond.)*, **201**, 1138–1139.

GOLD, E. R. (1964). Observations on the specificity of anti-O and anti-A$_1$ sera. *Vox Sang.*, **9**, 153–159.

GOLDBERG, L. S. & BARNETT, E. V. (1967). Mixed γG-γM cold agglutinin. *J. Immunol.*, **99**, 803–809.

GORDON, R. S. JNR (1953). The preparation and properties of cold hemagglutinin. *J. Immunol.*, **71**, 220–225.

GÖTTSCHE, B., SALAMA, A. & MUELLER-ECKHARDT, C. (1990). Autoimmune hemolytic anemia caused by a cold agglutinin with a new specificity (anti-Ju). *Transfusion*, **30**, 261–262.

GOUDEMAND, M. & ROPARTZ, C. (1954). À propos d'un cas d'anémie hémolytique chronique avec crises d'hémoglobinurie 'a frigore'. *Sang*, **25**, 572–591.

GREENWALT, T. J., SASAKI, T. & STEANE, E. A. (1966). Second example of anti-N in a blood donor, of group MN. *Vox Sang.*, **11**, 184–188.

HARBOE, M. (1964). Interactions between ^{131}I trace-labelled cold agglutinin, complement and red cells. *Brit. J. Haemat.*, **10**, 339–346.

HARBOE, M. & LIND, K. (1966). Light chain types of transiently occurring cold haemagglutinins. *Scand. J. Haemat.*, **3**, 269–276.

HARBOE, M., MULLER-EBERHARD, H. J., FUDENBERG, H., POLLEY, M. J. & MOLLISON, P. L. (1963). Identification of the components of complement participating in the antiglobulin reaction. *Immunology*, **6**, 412–420.

HARBOE, M., VAN FURTH, R., SCHUBOTHE, H., LIND, K. & EVANS, R. S. (1965). Exclusive occurrence of K chains in isolated cold haemagglutinins. *Scand. J. Haemat.*, **2**, 259–266.

HARRIS, G. & FAIRLEY, G. H. (1962). Immunological identification of a cryomacroglobulin in a patient with acquired haemolytic anaemia associated with a cold antibody. *Nature (Lond.)*, **194**, 1090–1091.

HAWLEY, J. G. & GORDON, R. S. J. JNR (1954). Anemia associated with cold agglutinins. *N. Y. St. J. Med.*, **54**, 1516–1518.

HAYNES, C. R. & CHAPLIN, H. JNR (1971). An enhancing effect of albumin on the determination of cold hemagglutinins. *Vox Sang.*, **20**, 46–54.

HEILMEYER, L., HAHN, F. & SCHUBOTHE, H. (1946–1947). Hämolytische Anämien auf der Basis abnormer serologischer Reaktion. *Klin. Wschr.*, **24/25**, 193–205.

HILMAN, R. S. & GIBLETT, E. R. (1965). Red cell membrane alteration associated with 'marrow stress'. *J. clin. Invest*, **44**, 1730–1736.

HINZ, C. F. JNR & BOYER, J. T. (1963). Dysgammaglobulinemia in the adult manifested as autoimmune hemolytic anemia. Serologic and immunochemical characterization of an antibody of unusual specificity. *New Engl. J. Med.*, **269**, 1329–1335.

HIRSCH, W., MOORES, P., SANGER, R. & RACE, R. R. (1957). Notes on some reactions of human anti-M and anti-N sera. *Brit. J. Haemat.*, **3**, 134–142.

HOLLÄNDER, L. (1952). Inkomplette Kälteantikörper als Ursache des positiven Antiglobulintestes beim neugeborenen Kinde. *Helv. paediat. Acta*, 7, 512–516.

HOMBERG, J. C., KRULIK, M., HABIBI, B. & DEBRAY, J. (1971). Une agglutinine froide anti-Sp$_1$, au cours d'une leucémie lymphoïde chronique compliquée de cirrhose hépatique. *Nouv. Rev, franç. Hémat.*, **11**, 489–495.

HOWELL, E. D. & PERKINS, H. A. (1972). Anti-N-like antibodies in the sera of patients undergoing chronic hemodialysis. *Vox Sang.*, **23**, 291–299.

HYSELL, J. K., BECK, M. L. & GRAY, J. M. (1973). Additional examples of cold autoagglutinins with M specificity. *Transfusion*, **13**, 146–149.

HYSELL, J. K., GRAY, J. M. & BECK, M. L. (1974). Auto anti-N—an additional example. *Transfusion*, **14**, 72–74.

ISBISTER, J. P., COOPER, D. A., BLAKE, H. M., BIGGS, J. C., DIXON, R. A. & PENNY, R. (1978). Lymphoproliferative disease with IgM lambda monoclonal protein autoimmune hemolytic anemia. *Amer. J. Med.*, **64**, 434–440.

ISSITT, P. D. (1967). I blood group system and its relation to other blood group systems. *J. med. lab. Tech.*, **24**, 90–97.

ISSITT, P. D. (1985). *Applied Blood Group Serology*, 683 pp. Montgomery Scientific Publications, Miami.

ISSITT, P. D. & JACKSON, V. A. (1968). Useful modifications and variations of technics in work on I system antibodies. *Vox Sang.*, **15**, 152–153.

ISSITT, P. D., TEGOLI, J., JACKSON, V., SANDERS, C. W. & ALLEN, F. H. JNR (1968). Anti-IP$_1$: antibodies that show an association between the I and P blood groups systems. *Vox Sang.*, **14**, 1–8.

JACKSON, V., ISSITT, P. D., FRANCIS, B. J., GARRIS, M. L. & SANDERS, C. W. (1968). The simultaneous presence of anti-I and anti-i in sera. *Vox Sang.*, **15**, 133–141.

JAKOBOWICZ, R. & SIMMONS, R. T. (1964). The identification of anti-I agglutinins in human serum: an atypical antibody which simulates a non-specific cold agglutinin. *Med. J. Aust.*, **i**, 194–195.

JANCOVIĆ, B. D. (1955). Reaction between incomplete cold auto-antibody and trypsin treated red cells. *Acta med. Jugoslav.*, **9**, 28–37.

JENKINS, G. C., POLLEY, M. J. & MOLLISON, P. L. (1960). Role of C'$_4$ in the antiglobulin reaction. *Nature (Lond.)*, **186**, 482–483.

JENKINS, W. J., MARSH, W. L., NOADES, J., TIPPETT,

P., SANGER, R. & RACE, R. R. (1960). The I antigen and antibody. *Vox Sang.*, 5, 97–106.

JOHNSON, S. T., MCFARLAND, J. G., CASPER, J. T., OSHIMA, J. L. & GOTTSCHALL, J. L. (1989). An unusual case of autoimmune hemolytic anemia following DPT vaccination. *Transfusion*, 29, Suppl. 50 (Abstract S178).

JONSEN, J. & KÅSS, E. (1959). Investigations on complement and complement components in a case of high-titre cold hemagglutination. *Acta med. scand.*, 165, 229–233.

JONSEN, J., KÅSS, E. & HARBOE, M. (1961). Complement and complement components in acquired hemolytic anemia with high titer cold antibodies. *Acta med. scand.*, 170, 725–729.

JORDAN, F. L. J. (1958), The role of complement in immunohemolytic disease. *Proc. 6th int. Congr. int. Soc. Hemat.*, Boston, 1956, pp. 825–832. Grune and Stratton, New York.

JUDD, W. J., WILKINSON, S. L., ISSITT, P. D., JOHNSON, T. L., KEREN, D. F. & STEINER, E. A. (1986). Donath–Landsteiner hemolytic anemia due to an anti-Pr-like biphasic hemolysin. *Transfusion*, 26, 423–425.

KAJII, E. & IKEMOTO, S. (1989). A cold agglutinin: Om. *Vox Sang.*, 56, 104–106.

KAY, N. E., DOUGLAS, S. D., MOND, J. J., FLIER, J. S., KOCHWA, S. & ROSENFIELD, R. E. (1975). Hemolytic anemia with serum and erythrocyte-bound low-molecular weight IgM. *Clin. Immunol. Immunopath.*, 4, 216–225.

KAY, N. E., GORDON, G. I. & DOUGLAS, S. D. (1978). Autoimmune hemolytic anemia in association with monoclonal IgM(κ) with anti-i activity. *Amer. J. Med.*, 64, 845–850.

KETTEL, K. (1920). Recherches sur les agglutinines au froid dans les sérums humains. *C. R. Soc. Biol. (Paris)*, 100, 371–373.

KÖNIG, A. L., KATHER, H. & ROELCKE, D. (1984). Autoimmune hemolytic anemia by coexisting anti-I and anti-F1 cold agglutinins. *Blut*, 49, 363–368.

KRAUTER, ST. & RIEDER, H. (1957). Bedeutung der Säurekältehämolysine im Verlaufe erworbener hämolytischer Anämien. *Wien. klin. Wschr.*, 69, 821–825.

KRETSCHMER, V. & MUELLER-ECKHARDT, C. (1972). Autoimmune hemolytic anemias. II. Immunoglobulins and β1A-globulin in the serum with special regard to the immunochemical type of autoantibodies and the course of the disease. *Blut*, 25, 159–168.

KRETSCHMER, V. & MUELLER-ECKHARDT, C. (1977). Significance of complement activities in autoimmune haemolytic anaemia of 'warm type'. *Blut*, 35, 447–455.

KUENN, J. W., WEBER, R., TEAGUE, P. O. & KEITT, A. S. (1978). Cryopathic gangrene with an IgM lambda cryoprecipitating cold agglutinin. *Cancer*, 42, 1826–1833.

LACHMANN, P. J., VOAK, D., OLDROYD, R. G., DOWNIE, D. M. & BEVAN, P. C. (1983). Use of monoclonal anti-C3 antibodies to characterise the fragments of C3 that are found on erythrocytes. *Vox Sang.*, 45, 367–372.

LANDSTEINER, K. (1903). Ueber Beziehungen zwischen dem Blutserum und den Körperzellen. *Münch. med. Wschr.*, 50, 1812–1814.

LANDSTEINER, K. & LEVINE, P. (1926). On the cold agglutinins in human serum. *J. Immunol.*, 12, 441–460.

LAU, F. O. & ROSSE, W. F. (1975). The reactivity of red blood cell membrane glycophorin with 'cold reacting' antibodies. *Immunol. Immunopath.*, 4, 1–8.

LAUF, P. K. & ROSSE, W. F. (1969). The solubilization of the 'I' and 'i' antigens in human red cells. *Blood*, 34, 841 (Abstract 51).

LAYRISSE, Z. & LAYRISSE, M. (1968). High incidence cold autoagglutinins of anti-I^T specificity in Yanomama Indians of Venezuela. *Vox Sang.*, 14, 369–382.

LAYRISSE, Z. & LAYRISSE, M. (1972). Cold reacting auto-antibodies in Venezuelan populations. *Vox Sang.*, 22, 457–468.

LEDDY, J. P., TRABOLD, N. C., VAUGHAN, J. H. & SWISHER, S. N. (1962). The unitary nature of 'complete' and 'incomplete' pathologic cold hemagglutinins. *Blood*, 19, 379–396.

LEE, C. H., CHERIAN, R., HUGHES, W. G. & NURBHAI, M. (1979). Lymphoproliferative disease with monoclonal IgM gammopathy and cold agglutinin. *Aust. N. Z. J. Med.*, 9, 602–603.

LEWIS, S. M., DACIE, J. V. & TILLS, D. (1961). Comparison of the sensitivity to agglutination and haemolysis by a high-titre cold antibody of the erythrocytes of normal adults and of patients with a variety of blood diseases including paroxysmal nocturnal haemoglobinuria. *Brit. J. Haemat.*, 7, 64–72.

LOGUE, G., GOCKERMAN, J. & ROSSE, W. (1971). Measurement of in vivo attachment of third component of complement (C3) to human red cells by cold agglutinin antibody. *Blood*, 38, 810. (Abstract No. 71).

LOGUE, G. L., ROSSE, W. F. & GOCKERMAN, J. P. (1973). Measurement of the third component of complement bound to red blood cells in patients with the cold agglutinin syndrome. *J. clin. Invest.*, 52, 493–501.

LONGSTER, G. H. & JOHNSON, E. (1988). IgM anti-D as auto-antibody in a case of 'cold' auto-immune haemolytic anaemia. *Vox Sang.*, 54, 174–176.

LOPEZ, M., BANOPOULOS, H., LIBERGE, G. & SALMON, C. (1975). A cold autoagglutinin of anti-B specificity in an A₁B patient. *Vox Sang.*, 28, 371–375.

LOWN, J. A. G., BARR, A. L. & KELLY, A. (1980). Auto anti-M antibody following renal transplantation. *Vox Sang.*, 38, 301–304.

MAAS, D. & SCHUBOTHE, H. (1968). Studies on the

quantitative range of agglutinability of cord red cells by high-titre cold agglutinins. *Vox Sang.*, **14**, 292–294.

McCLELLAND, W. M., BRADLEY, A., MORRIS, T. C. M., BURNSIDE, P. & ROBERTSON, J. H. (1981). Auto-anti-B in a patient with acute leukaemia. *Vox Sang.*, **41**, 231–234.

McGINNISS, H. H., GRINDON, A. J. & SCHMIDT, P. J. (1974). Evidence for two anomalous I blood group determinants. *Transfusion*, **14**, 257–260.

McGUINNISS. M. H., SCHMIDT, P. J. & CARBONE, P. P. (1964). Close association of I blood group and disease. *Nature (Lond.)*, **202**, 606.

MACKENZIE, M. R. & CREEVY, N. C. (1969). Hemolytic anemia with cold detectable IgG antibodies. *Blood*, **34**, 829 (Abstract 14).

MACKENZIE, M. R. & CREEVY, N. C. (1970). Hemolytic anemia with cold detectable IgG antibodies. *Blood*, **36**, 549–558.

McLEISH, W. A., BRATHWAITE, A. F. & PETERSON, P. M. (1975). Anti-N antibodies in hemodialysis patients. *Transfusion*, **15**, 43–45.

MACRIS, N. T., CAPRA, J. D., FRANKEL, G. J., IOACHIM, H. L., SATZ, H. & BRUNO, M. S. (1970). A lambda light chain cold agglutinin-cryomacroglobulin occurring in Waldenström's macroglobulinemia. *Amer. J. Med.*, **48**, 524–529.

MANIATIS, A., FRIEMAN, B. & BERTLES, J. F. (1977). Increased expression in erythrocytic Ii antigens in sickle cell disease and sickle cell trait. *Vox Sang.*, **33**, 19–36.

MANIATIS, A., PAPAYANNOPOULOU, T. & BERTLES, J. F. (1979). Fetal characteristics of erythrocytes in sickle cell anemia: an immunofluorescence study of individual cells. *Blood*, **54**, 159–168.

MARCOLONGO, F. (1953). Anemie emolitiche acquisite du auto-immunizzazione. *Recenti Progr. Med.*, **15**, 1, 137–239.

MARCUS, D. M., KABAT, E. A. & ROSENFIELD, R. E. (1963). The action of enzymes from Clostridium tertium on the I antigenic determinant of human erythrocytes. *J. exper. Med.*, **118**, 175–194.

MARSH, W. L. (1961). Anti-i: a cold antibody defining the Ii relationship in human red cells. *Brit. J. Haemat.*, 7, 200–209.

MARSH, W. L. & JENKINS, W. J. (1960). Anti-i: a new cold antibody. *Nature (Lond.)*, **188**, 753.

MARSH, W. L. & JENKINS, W. J. (1968). Anti-Sp₁: the recognition of a new cold auto-antibody. *Vox Sang.*, **15**, 177–186.

MARSH, W. L., JENSEN, L., DECARY, F. & COLLEDGE, K. (1972). Water-soluble I blood group substance in the secretions of i adults. *Transfusion*, **12**, 222–226.

MARSH, W. L., JOHNSON, C. L., DINAPOLI, J., OYEN, R., ALICEA, E., RAO, A. H. & CHANDRASEKARAN, V. (1980a). Immune haemolytic anaemia caused by auto anti-Sdˣ: a report of six cases. *Transfusion*, **20**, 647 (Abstract).

MARSH, W. L., JOHNSON, C. L., ØYEN, R., NICHOLS, M. E., DiNAPOLI, J., YOUNG, H., BASSEL, J., CUSUMANO, I., BAZAZ, G. R., HABER, J. M. & WOLF, C. F. W. (1980b). Anti-Sdˣ. a 'new' auto-agglutinin related to the Sdᵃ blood group. *Transfusion*, **20**, 1–8.

MARSH, W. L., NICHOLS, M. E. & ALLEN F. H. JNR (1970). Inhibition of anti-I sera by human milk. *Vox Sang.*, **18**, 149–154.

MARSH, W. L., NICHOLS, M. E. & REID, M. E. (1971). The definition of two I antigen components. *Vox Sang.*, **20**, 209–217.

MATTHES, M. & SCHUBOTHE, H. (1951). Hämolysine im Serum von Patienten mit hohem Kälteagglutinintiter. *Klin. Wschr.*, **29**, 263–264.

MEHROTRA. T. N. (1960a). Immunological identification of the pathological cold auto-antibodies of acquired haemolytic anaemia as β_2-M globulin. *Immunology*, **3**, 265–271.

MEHROTRA, T. N. (1960b). Individual specific nature of the cold auto-antibodies of acquired haemolytic anaemia. *Nature (Lond.)*, **185**, 323–324.

MEHROTRA, T. N. & CHARLWOOD, P. A. (1960). Physico-chemical characterization of the cold auto-antibodies of acquired haemolytic anaemia. *Immunology*, **3**, 254–264.

METAXAS-BUHLER, M., IKIN, E. W. & ROMANSKE, J. (1961). Anti-N in the serum of a healthy blood donor. *Vox Sang.*, **6**, 574–582.

MILLET, M. & FINCLER, L. (1946). Remarques sur les affinités de l'autoagglutinine (cold agglutinin) du sérum humain. *Compt. rend. Soc. Biol.*, **140**, 1226–1227.

MINO, P. (1924). La panemoagglutinina del sangue umano. *Policlinico Sez. prat.*, **31**, 1355–1359.

MOOR-JANKOWSKI, J., WIENER, A. S. & GORDON, E. B. (1964). Blood-group antigens and cross-reacting antibodies in primates, including man. III. Heterophile-like behavior of the blood factor I. *Exp. Med. Surg.*, **22**, 308–315.

MOORE, J. A. & CHAPLIN, H. JNR (1973). Autoimmune hemolytic anemia associated with an IgG cold incomplete antibody. *Vox Sang.*, **24**, 236–245.

MOORES, P., BOTHA, M. C. & BRINK, S. (1970). Anti-N in the serum of a healthy type MN person—a further example. *Amer. J. clin. Path.*, **54**, 90–93.

MOREL, P., GARRATTY, G. & WILLBANKS, E. (1975). Another example of anti-IB. *Vox Sang.*, **29**, 231–233.

MORTARA, M. & MARTINETTI, L. (1955). Su di un caso di anemia emolitica cronica con sindrome di Raynaud e crioagglutinazione. *G. Clin. med.*, **36**, 1791–1801.

MORTON, J. A. & PICKLES, M. M. (1947). Use of trypsin in the detection of incomplete anti-Rh antibodies. *Nature (Lond.)*, **159**, 779–780.

MYGIND, K. & AHRONS, S. (1972). IgG cold agglutinins and first trimester abortion. *Vox Sang.*, **23**, 552–560.

NIEMANN, H., WATANABE, K., HAKOMORI, S.-i, CHILDS, R. A. & FEIZI, T. (1978). Blood group i and

I activities of 'lacto-N-norhexaosylceramide' and its analogues: the structural requirements for i-specificities. *Biochem. biophys. Res. Commun.*, **81**, 1286–1293.

NORTHOFF, H., MARTIN, A & ROELCKE, D. (1987). An IgGκ-monotypic anti-Pr$_{1h}$ associated with a fresh varicella infection. *Europ. J. Haemat.*, **38**, 85–88.

OLESEN, H. (1966). Thermodynamics of the cold agglutinin reaction. *Scand. J. clin. lab. Invest.*, **18**, 1–15.

O'NEILL, P., SHULMAN, I. A., SIMPSON, R. B., HALIMA, D. & GARRATTY, G. (1986). Two examples of low ionic strength-dependent autoagglutinins with anti Pr$_1$ specificity. *Vox Sang.*, **50**, 107–111.

PARKER, A. C., WILLIS, G., URBANIAK, S. J. & INNES, E. M. (1978). Autoimmune haemolytic anaemia with an anti-A autoantibody. *Brit. med. J.*, **i**, 26.

PISCIOTTA, A. V. & HINZ, J. E. (1957). Detection and characterization of autoantibodies in acquired auto-immune hemolytic anemia. *Amer. J. clin. Path.*, **27**, 619–634.

PITNEY, W. R., THOMAS, H. N. & WELLS, J. V. (1968). Cold haemagglutinins associated with splenomegaly in New Guinea. *Vox Sang.*, **14**, 438–445.

POLLEY, M. J., MOLLISON, P. L. & SOOTHILL, J. F. (1962). The role of 19S gamma-globulin blood-group antibodies in the antiglobulin reaction. *Brit. J. Haemat.*, **8**, 149–162.

PONDMAN, K. W., ROSENFIELD, R. E., TALLAL, L. & WASSERMAN, L. R. (1960). The specificity of the complement antiglobulin test. *Vox Sang.*, **5**, 297–319.

PRUZANSKI, W., COWAN, D. H. & PARR, D. M. (1974). Clinical and immunochemical studies of IgM cold agglutinins with lambda type light chains. *Clin. Immunol. Immunopath.*, **2**, 234–245.

PRUZANSKI, W., JACOBS, H., SAITO, S., DONNELLY, E. M. & LUI, L. C. (1987). Cryptic cold agglutinin activity of monoclonal macroglobulins. *Amer. J. Hemat.*, **26**, 167–174.

RACE, R. R. (1944). An 'incomplete' antibody in human serum. *Nature (Lond.)*, **153**, 771–772.

RATKIN, G. A., OSTERLAND, C. K. & CHAPLIN, H. JNR (1973). IgG, IgA, and IgM cold-reactive immunoglobulins in 19 patients with elevated cold agglutinins. *J. Lab. clin. Med.*, **82**, 67–78.

READER, R. (1955). Complement in acquired haemolytic anaemia. *Aust. Ann. Med.*, **4**, 279–286.

REVIRON, M., JANVIER, D., REVIRON, J. & LAGABRIELLE, J. F. (1984). An anti-I cold auto-agglutinin enhanced in the presence of sodium azide. *Vox Sang.*, **44**, 211–216.

ROCHANT, H., TONTHAT, H., ETIEVANT, M. F., INTRATOR, L., SYLVESTRE, R. & DREYFUS, B. (1972). Lambda cold agglutinin with anti-A$_1$ specificity in a patient with reticulosarcoma. *Vox Sang.*, **22**, 45–53.

ROCHANT, H., TONTHAT, H., MAN, NGO, M.,

LEFANO, J., HENRI, A. & DREYFUS, B. (1973). Étude quantitative des antigènes érythrocytaire I et i en pathologie. *Nouv. Rev. franç. Hémat.*, **13**, 307–318.

ROELCKE, D. (1969). A new serological specificity in cold antibodies of high titre: anti-HD. *Vox Sang.*, **16**, 76–79.

ROELCKE, D. (1973a). Serological studies on the Pr$_1$/Pr$_2$ antigens using dog erythrocytes. Differentiation of Pr$_2$ from Pr$_1$ and detection of a Pr$_1$ heterogeneity: Pr$_{1h}$/Pr$_{1d}$. *Vox Sang.*, **24**, 354–361.

ROELCKE, D. (1973b). Specificity of IgA cold agglutinins: anti-Pr$_1$. *Europ. J. Immunol.*, **3**, 206–212.

ROELCKE, D. (1974). A review. Cold agglutination. Antibodies and antigens. *Clin. Immunol. Immunopath.*, **2**, 266–280.

ROELCKE, D. (1981a). A further cold agglutinin, F1, recognizing a N-acetylneuraminic acid-determined antigen. *Vox Sang.*, **41**, 98–101.

ROELCKE, D. (1981b). The Lud cold agglutinin: a further antibody recognizing N-acetylneuraminic acid-determined antigens not fully expressed at birth. *Vox Sang.*, **41**, 316–318.

ROELCKE, D. (1985). Li cold agglutinin: a further antibody recognizing sialic acid-dependent antigens fully expressed on newborn erythrocytes. *Vox Sang.*, **48**, 181–183.

ROELCKE, D. (1989). Cold agglutination. *Transf. Med. Rev.*, **3**, 140–166.

ROELCKE, D., ANSTEE, D. J., JUNGFER, H., NUTZENADEL, W. & WEBB, A. J. (1971). IgG-type cold agglutinins in children and corresponding antigens. Detection of a new Pr antigen: Pr$_a$. *Vox Sang.*, **20**, 218–229.

ROELCKE, D., DAHR, W. & KALDEN, J. R. (1986). A human monoclonal IgM K cold agglutinin recognizing oligosaccharides with immunodominant sialyl groups preferentially at the blood group M-specific peptide backbone of glycophorins: anti-Pr^m. *Vox Sang.*, **51**, 207–211.

ROELCKE, D., EBERT, W. & ANSTEE, D. J. (1974). Demonstration of low-titre anti-Pr cold agglutinins. *Vox Sang.*, **27**, 429–441.

ROELCKE, D., EBERT, W. & FEIZI, T. (1974). Studies on the specificities of two IgM lambda cold agglutinins. *Immunology*, **27**, 879–886.

ROELCKE, D., EBERT, W. & GEISEN, H. P. (1976). Anti-Pr$_3$: serological and immunochemical identification of a new anti-Pr subspecificity. *Vox Sang.*, **30**, 122–133.

ROELCKE, D., FORBES, I. J., ZALEWSKI, P. D., DÖRKEN, B. & LENHARD, V. (1982). A further subspecificity within human monoclonal anti-Pr cold agglutinins. *Blut*, **45**, 109–114.

ROELCKE, D. & JUNGFER, H. (1970). Kombinierte μ/γ-Antigenität von Paraprotein-Immunoglobulinen mit Kälteautoantikörper-Aktivität. *Klin. Wschr.*, **48**, 914–918.

ROELCKE, D. & KREFT, H. (1984). Characterization of

various anti-Pr cold agglutinins. *Transfusion*, **24**, 210–213.

ROELCKE, D., KREFT, H. & PFISTER, A.-M. (1984). Cold agglutinin Vo. An IgM λ monoclonal human antibody recognizing a sialic acid determined antigen fully expressed on newborn erythrocytes. *Vox Sang.*, **47**, 236–241.

ROELCKE, D., MEISER, R. J. & BRÜCHER, H. (1979). Human cold agglutinins against 'cryptic' erythrocyte antigens. *Blut*, **39**, 217–224.

ROELCKE, D., PRUZANSKI, W., EBERT, W., RÖMER, W., FISCHER, E., LENHARD, V. & RAUTERBERG, E. (1980). A new human monoclonal cold agglutinin Sa recognizing terminal N-acetylneuraminyl groups on the cell surface. *Blood*, **55**, 677–681.

ROELCKE, D., RIESEN, W., GEISEN, H. P. & EBERT, W. (1977). Serological identification of the new cold agglutinin specificity anti-Gd. *Vox Sang.*, **33**, 304–306.

ROELCKE, D. & UHLENBRUCK, G. (1970). 'Nomenclature of neuraminic acid containing receptors which correspond with cold antibodies'. *Vox Sang.*, **18**, 478–479 (Letter).

ROELCKE, D. & UHLENBRUCK, G. & BAUER, K. (1969). A heterogeneity of the HD-receptor, demonstrable by HD-cold antibodies: HD1/HD2. Immunochemical aspects. *Scand. J. Haemat.*, **6**, 280–287.

ROELCKE, D. & WEBER. M. T. (1984). Simultaneous occurrence of anti-F1 and anti-I cold agglutinins in a patient's serum. *Vox Sang.*, **47**, 122–124.

RØRVIK, K. (1954). The syndrome of high-titre cold agglutination. A survey and a case report. *Acta med. scand.*, **148**, 299–308.

ROSE, V. L. & KWAAN, H. C. (1985). Anti-Pr hemagglutinin associated with livedo reticularis. *Amer. J. Hemat.*, **19**, 419–421.

ROSENFIELD, R. E., SCHROEDER, R., BALLARD, R., VAN DER HART, M., MOES, M. & VAN LOGHEM, J. J. (1964). Erythrocytic antigenic determinants characteristic of H,I in the presence of H (IH), or H in the absence of i [H(−i)]. *Vox Sang.*, **9**, 415–419.

ROSENTHAL, F. & CORTEN, M. (1937). Über das Phänomen der autohämagglutination und über die Eigenshaften der Kältehämagglutinine. *Folia haemat. (Lpz.)*, **58**, 64–90.

ROSSE, W. F., ADAMS, J. & LOGUE, G. (1977). Hemolysis by complement and cold-reacting antibodies: time and temperature requirements. *Amer. J. Hemat.*, **2**, 259–270.

ROSSE, W. F., BORSOS, T. & RAPP, H. J. (1967). Reaction of cold agglutinin antibodies with I+ and I− red blood cells. *J. clin. Invest.*, **46**, 1111 (Abstract).

ROSSE, W. F., BORSOS, T. & RAPP, H. J. (1968). Cold-reacting antibodies: the enhancement of antibody fixation by the first component of complement (C'la). *J. Immunol.*, **100**, 259–265.

ROSSE, W. F. & LAUF, P. K. (1970). Reaction of cold agglutinins with I antigen solubilized from human red cells. *Blood*, **36**, 777–784.

ROSSE, W. F. & SHERWOOD, J. B. (1970). Cold-reacting antibodies: differences in the reaction of anti-I antibodies with adult and cord red blood cells. *Blood*, **36**, 28–42.

SALAMA, A., BHAKDI, S., MUELLER-ECKHARDT, C. & KAYER, W. (1983). Deposition of the terminal C5b-9 complement complex on erythrocytes by human red cell autoantibodies. *Brit. J. Haemat.*, **55**, 161–169.

SALAMA, A., PRALLE, H. & MUELLER-ECKHARDT, C. (1985). A new red blood cell cold autoantibody (anti-Me). *Vox Sang.*, **49**, 277–284.

SALÉN, E. B. (1935). Thermostabiles, nicht Komplexes (Auto-)Hämolysin bei transitorischer Kältehämoglobinurie. *Acta med. scand.*, **86**, 570–592.

SALMON, C., HOMBERG, J. C., LIBERGE, G. & DELARUE, F. (1965). Autoanticorps à spécificités multiples, anti-HI, anti-AI, anti-BI, dans certains éluats d'anémie hémolytique. *Rev. franç. Ét. clin. biol.*, **10**, 522–525.

SANGSTER, J. M., KENWRIGHT, M. G., WALKER, M. P. & PEMBROKE, A. C. (1979). Anti blood group-M antoantibodies with livedo reticularis, Raynaud's phenomenon, and anaemia. *J. clin. Path.*, **32**, 154–157.

SAVONEN, K. (1948). Cold haemagglutination test and its clinical significance. *Ann. Med. exp. Fenn.*, **26** (Suppl. 3), 100 pp.

SCHMIDT, P. J., McGURDY, P., HAVELL, T., JENKINS, A. & McGUINNIS, M. (1974). An anti-I^T of clinical significance. *Transfusion*, **14**, 507 (Abstract).

SCHMIDT, P. J. & McGINNISS, M. H. (1965). Differences between anti-H and anti-OI red cell antibodies. *Vox Sang.*, **10**, 109–112.

SCHUBOTHE, H. (1953). Serologische Besonderheiten unspezifischer Saurekältehämolysine. *Klin. Wschr.*, **31**, 814–815.

SCHUBOTHE, H. (1954). Kombination von Paraproteinämie und autoantikörperbildung. *Schweiz. med. Wschr.*, **85**, 1109 (in Discussion).

SCHUBOTHE, H. (1955). Comparative serologic studies on different types of incomplete haemantibodies. *Rev. belg. Path. Méd. exp.*, **24**, 337–343.

SCHUBOTHE, H. (1958). *Serologie und klinische Bedeutung der Autohämantikörper.* pp. 56–236. Karger, Basel.

SCHUBOTHE, H. & MATTHES, M. (1951). Inkomplette antikörper im serum von patienten mit hohem kälteagglutinintiter. *Klin. Wschr.*, **29**, 228.

SEYFRIED, H., WALEWSKA, I. & GILES, C. M. (1963). A patient with apparently normal A₁B cells whose serum contains anti-B. *Vox Sang.*, **8**, 273–280.

SHIREY, S., HARRIS, J. & MOORE, L. (1979). An autoanti-I greatly enhanced in the presence of thimerosal. *Transfusion*, **19**, 642 (Abstract).

SHIREY, R.S., PARK, K., NESS, P. D., KICKLER, T. S., RONES, J., DAWSON, R. B. & JIJI, R. (1986). An anti-i biphasic hemolysin in chronic paroxysmal cold hemoglobinuria. *Transfusion*, **26**, 62–64.

SIGNAL, T. & BOOTH, P. B. (1976). A New Zealand family with i members. *Vox Sang.*, **50**, 391–395.

SILBERSTEIN, L. E., BERKMAN, E. M. & SCHREIBER, A. D. (1987). Cold hemagglutinin disease associated with IgG cold-reactive antibody. *Ann. intern. Med.*, **106**, 238–242.

SILBERSTEIN, L. E., SHOENFELD, Y., SCHWARTZ, R. S. & BERKMAN, E. M. (1985). A combination of IgG and IgM autoantibodies in chronic cold agglutinin disease: immunologic studies and response to splenectomy. *Vox Sang.*, **48**, 105–109.

SNIECINSKI, I., MARGOLIN, K., SHULMAN, I., OIEN, L., MEYER, E. & BRANCH, D. R. (1988). High-titer, high-thermal-amplitude cold autoagglutinin not associated with hemolytic anemia. *Vox Sang.*, **55**, 26–29.

SPAET, T. H. & KINSELL, B. G. (1953). Studies on the normal serum panagglutinin active against trypsinated human erythrocytes. II. Relationship to cold agglutination. *J. lab. clin. Med.*, **42**, 205–211.

STATS, D. (1945). Cold hemagglutination and cold hemolysis. The hemolysis produced by shaking cold agglutinated erythrocytes. *J. clin. Invest.*, **24**, 33–42.

STATS, D., PERLMAN, E., BULLOWA, J. G. M. & GOODKIND, R. (1943). Electrophoresis and antibody nitrogen determinations of a cold hemagglutinin. *Proc. Soc. exp. Biol. Med. N. Y.*, **53**, 188–190.

STATS, D. & WASSERMAN, L. R. (1943). Cold hemagglutination—an interpretive review. *Medicine (Baltimore)*, **22**, 363–424.

STRATTON, F. (1943). Some observations on autohaemagglutination. *Lancet*, **i**, 613–614.

SUZUKI, S., MIURA, H., HIRAKAWA, S., SUNADA, M., AMANO, T., NISHIYA, K., OTA, Z. & ROELCKE, D. (1985). A monoclonal IgM^K cold agglutinin bearing a new anti-Sa specificity. *Acta haemat. jap.*, **48**, 1074–1082.

SZYMANSKI, I. O., ROBERTS, P. L. & ROSENFIELD, R. E. (1976). Anti-A autoantibody with severe intravascular hemolysis. *New Engl. J. Med.*, **294**, 995–996.

SZYMANSKI, I. O., TENO, R. & RYBAK, M. E. (1986). Hemolytic anemia due to a mixture of low-titre IgG lambda and IgM lambda agglutinins reacting optimally at 22°C. *Vox Sang.*, **51**, 112–116.

TEGOLI, J., HARRIS, J. P., ISSITT, P. D. & SAUNDERS, C. W. (1967). Anti-IB, an expected 'new' antibody detecting a joint product of I and B genes. *Vox Sang.*, **13**, 144–157.

TEGOLI, J., HARRIS, J. P., NICHOLS, M. E., MARSH, W. L. & REID, M. E. (1970). Autologous anti-I and anti-M following liver transplant. *Transfusion*, **10**, 133–136.

TELEN, M. J., COMBS, M. R., HALL, S. E. & ROSSE, W. F. (1989). IgG auto-anti-N as a cause of severe autoimmune hemolytic anemia. *Transfusion*, **29**, Suppl. 50S (Abstract S177).

TIPPETT, P., NOADES, J., SANGER, R., RACE, R. R., SAUSAIS, L., HOLMAN, C. A. & BUTTIMER, R. J. (1960). Further studies of the I antigen and antibody. *Vox Sang.*, **5**, 107–121.

TIPPETT, P., SANGER, R., RACE, R. R., SWANSON, J. & BUSCH, S. (1965). An agglutinin associated with the P and ABO blood group systems. *Vox Sang.*, **10**, 269–280.

TÖNDER, O. & HARBOE, M. (1966). Heterogeneity of cold haemagglutinins. *Immunology*, **11**, 361–368.

TONTHAT, H., ROCHANT, H., HENRY, A., LEPORRIER, M. & DREYFUS, B. (1976). A new case of monoclonal IgA kappa cold agglutinin with anti-Pr$_1$d specificity in a patient with persistent HB antigen cirrhosis (brief report). *Vox Sang.*, **30**, 464–468.

TSCHIRHART, D. L., KUNKEL, L. & SHULMAN, I. R. (1990). Immune hemolytic anemia associated with biclonal cold autoagglutinins. *Vox Sang.*, **59**, 222–226.

TURNER, J. C. & JACKSON, E. B. (1943). Serological specificity of an auto-antibody in atypical pneumonia. *Brit. J. exp. Path.*, **24**, 121–126.

UCHIKAWA, M. & TOHYAMA, H. (1986). A potent cold autoagglutinin that recognizes Type 2H determinant on red cells. *Transfusion*, **26**, 240–242.

UNGER, L. J., WIENER, A. S. & DOLAN, D. (1952). Anémie auto-hémolytique chez un nouveau-né. *Rev. Hémat.*, **7**, 495–504.

VALE, D. R. & HARRIS, I. M. (1980). An additional example of auto-anti-M. *Transfusion*, **10**, 133–136.

VAN FURTH, R. & DIESSELHOFF-DEN DULK, M. (1966). The formation in vitro of cold auto-hemagglutinins with anti-I specificity. *J. Immunol.*, **96**, 920–925.

VAN LOGHEM, J. J. JNR, MENDES DE LEON, D. E., FRENKEL-TIETZ, H. & VAN DER HART, M. (1952). Two different serologic mechanisms of paroxysmal cold hemoglobinuria, illustrated by three cases. *Blood*, **7**, 1196–1209.

VAN LOGHEM, J. J. JNR, MENDES DE LEON, D. E. & VAN DER HART, M. (1955). Bluttransfusionen bei hämolytischen Anämien. Serologische Ergebnisse. *Ergebnisse der Bluttransfusionsforshung (Bibliotheca haematologica, Fasc. 2)*, pp. 84–98. Karger, Basel.

VAN LOGHEM, J. J. JNR, VAN DER HART, M. & DORFMEIER, H. (1958). Serologic studies in acquired hemolytic anemia. *Proc. 6th int. Congr. int. Soc. Hemat., Boston, 1958*, pp. 858–868. Grune and Stratton, New York.

VAN LOGHEM, J. J., VAN DER HART, M., VEENHOVEN-VAN RIESZ, E., VAN DER VEER, M., ENGELFRIET, C. P. & PEETOOM, F. (1962). Cold auto-agglutinins and haemolysins of anti-I and anti-i specificity. *Vox Sang.*, **7**, 214–221.

VAN LOGHEM, J. J., PEETOOM, F., VAN DER HART, M., VAN DER VEER, M., VAN DER GIESSEN, M., PRINS, H. K., ZURCHER, C. & ENGELFRIET, C. P. (1963). Serological and immunochemical studies in haemolytic anaemia with high-titre cold agglutinins. *Vox Sang.*, **8**, 33–46.

VARGUES, R., ZERMATI, M. & LABROSSE, S. (1955). Une agglutinine froide chimiquement définie l'euglobuline I₁ de Sandor. *Sang.*, **26**, 294–305.

VAUGHAN, J. H. (1956). Immunologic features of erythrocyte sensitization. 1. Acquired hemolytic disease. *Blood*, **11**, 1085–1096.

VERWILGHEN, R. L., LEWIS, S. M., DACIE, J. V., CROOKSTON, J. H. & CROOKSTON, M. C. (1973). HEMPAS: congenital dyserythropoietic anaemia (Type II). *Quart. J. Med.*, **42**, 257–278.

VOAK, D. (1964). Anti-HI, a new cold antibody of the H.O.I. complex. A preliminary report. *Scand. J. Haemat.*, **1**, 238–239.

VOAK, D., LACHMANN, P. J., DOWNIE, D. M., OLDROYD, R. G. & BEVAN, P. C. (1983). Monoclonal antibodies—C3 serology. *Biotest Bull.*, **4**, 339–347.

VOAK, D., LODGE, T. W., HOPKINS, J. & BOWLEY, C. C. (1968). A study of the antibodies of the H'O'I-B complex with special reference to their occurrence and notation. *Vox Sang.*, **15**, 353–366.

VON DEM BORNE, A. E. G. KR., MOL, J. J., JOUSTRA-MAAS, N., PEGELS, J. G., LANGENHUIJSEN, M. M. A. C. & ENGELFRIET, C. P. (1982). Autoimmune haemolytic anaemia with monoclonal IgM(κ) anti-P cold autohaemolysins. *Brit. J. Haemat.*, **50**, 345–350.

WAGER, O., HALTIA, K., RÄSÄNAN, J. H. & VUOPIO, P. (1971). Five cases of positive antiglobulin test involving IgA warm type antibody. *Ann. clin. Res.*, **3**, 76–85.

WEBER, R. (1956). Molecular weight of cold hemagglutinins. *Vox Sang.*, **1**, 37–38.

WHEELER, K. M., GALLACHER, H. J. & STUART, C. A. (1939). An unusual case of autoagglutination. *J. Lab. clin. Med.*, **24**, 1135–1138.

WIEDERMANN, D., KUBÍKOVÁ, A. & CHURÝ, Z. (1960). Zur Frage der lokalisation der Kälteagglutinine im electrophoretischen Eiweissspektrum. *Schweiz. med. Wschr.*, **90**, 682–684.

WIENER, A. S. (1944). A new test (blocking test) for Rh sensitization. *Proc. Soc. exp. Biol. Med. (N.Y.)*, **56**, 173–176.

WIENER, A. S., BRIGGS, D. K., WEINER, L. & BURNETT, L. (1958). Studies on human gamma globulin. II. Observations in a case of acquired hemolytic anemia due to cold autoantibodies, in multiple myeloma, and in other clinical problems. *J. Lab. clin. Med.*, **51**, 539–545.

WIENER, A. S., GORDON, E. B. & GALLOP, C. (1953). Studies on the autoantibodies in human sera. *J. Immunol.*, **71**, 58–65.

WIENER, A. S., UNGER, L. J., COHEN, L. & FELDMAN, J. (1956). Type-specific cold auto-antibodies as a cause of acquired hemolytic anemia and hemolytic transfusion reactions. Biologic test with bovine red cells. *Ann. intern. Med.*, **44**, 221–240.

WYSCHEGORODZEWA, W. D. (1926). Zur Frage der Autohämagglutination. *Z. klin. Med.*, **104**, 524–529.

YOKOYAMA, M. (1965). Close relationship between A and I blood groups. *Nature (Lond.)*, **206**, 411–412.

YOUNG, L. E. (1946). The clinical significance of cold hemagglutinins. *Amer. J. med. Sci.*, **211**, 23–39.

Auto-immune haemolytic anaemia (AIHA): cold-antibody syndromes III: haemolytic anaemia following mycoplasma pneumonia

Early descriptions of high-titre cold agglutinins in primary atypical pneumonia 296

Descriptions in the 1960s of high-titre cold agglutinins in acute respiratory diseases 298

Identification of the infective agent of primary atypical pneumonia as *Mycoplasma pneumoniae* (the Eaton agent) 298

Early descriptions of mycoplasma pneumonia haemolytic anaemia 299
  Clinical features 299
  Gangrene 299
  Acrocyanosis and phlebothrombosis 301
  Renal involvement 301

Later case reports of mycoplasma pneumonia haemolytic anaemia of special interest 301

Laboratory findings in mycoplasma pneumonia haemolytic anaemia 302

Serological findings in mycoplasma pneumonia haemolytic anaemia 302
  Individual differences in the ability of the antibodies to bring about agglutination or lysis *in vitro* 304
  Specificity 305
  Specificities other than anti I: anti P 305
  Species specificity 305

Immunochemistry of cold agglutinins in *Mycoplasma pneumoniae* infection 305

Interaction between *Mycoplasma pneumoniae* and the I antigen 307

Prognosis of mycoplasma pneumoniae haemolytic anaemia 308

Treatment 308

EARLY DESCRIPTIONS OF HIGH-TITRE COLD AGGLUTININS IN PRIMARY ATYPICAL PNEUMONIA

The frequent development of cold auto-antibodies in high concentrations by patients suffering from 'virus' (primary atypical) pneumonia was first conclusively demonstrated by Peterson, Ham and Finland (1943), and subsequently reported in independent studies by Turner (1943), Turner and Jackson (1943) and Turner et al. (1943), and by Horstmann and Tatlock (1943) and Meiklejohn (1943). Shone and Passmore (1943) had, too, reported the occurrence of auto-agglutination in 54 Indian soldiers affected by an outbreak of 'pneumonitis' of unknown causation, which had developed after their arrival in the Middle East.

Confirmation of the association was soon forthcoming, based on additional studies of large numbers of patients suffering from primary atypical pneumonia, e.g. by the Commission on Acute Respiratory Diseases (1944), Favour

(1944), Streeter, Farmer and Hayes (1944), Finland et al. (1945a), McNeil (1945) and Springarn and Jones (1945). In fact, however, isolated instances of an unusual degree of auto-agglutination in patients suffering from respiratory infections had been noticed before this. Both Clough and Richter (1918) and Wheeler, Gallacher and Stuart (1939) had carried out detailed studies on their patients' sera, but the possible connection between the abnormal agglutinins and the preceding infection was not appreciated. Clough and Richter, finding cold agglutinins in the blood of a daughter of their patient, in fact erroneously concluded that the abnormality might have been inherited.

In 1943, Peterson, Ham and Finland, and Horstmann and Tatlock, referred briefly to instances of acute haemolytic anaemia amongst the patients of their series, and two other possible examples were reported by Dameshek (1943). Most of these patients had, however, received sulphonamide drugs also, and the relationship between the anaemia and the preceding infection was not immediately clear. Subsequently, however, cases were reported in patients who had not received chemotherapy and it was not long before it was realized that 'virus' pneumonia might rarely be complicated by acute haemolytic anaemia of characteristically sudden onset and short duration, quite independently of the possible haemolytic effects of drugs used in treatment.

A point of considerable interest in relation to the outbreaks of primary atypical pneumonia, referred to above, was the frequency with which this type of pulmonary infection led to a rise in cold-agglutinin titre. According to the data of Finland et al. (1945a), Florman and Weiss (1945) and Young (1946), the incidence of raised titres was greater than 50%. In later outbreaks, however, the reported incidence was substantially lower: according to Finland and Barnes, reporting in 1954, the mean incidence was 22%, range 14–30%. Even so, the incidence was far higher than that found in patients suffering from most other types of infection (see below and Savonen, 1948).

The finding of raised titres of cold agglutinins in patients suffering from atypical pneumonias naturally led to studies of the incidence of raised titres in other infections, particularly in respiratory infections. The incidence was found in fact to be generally far lower, and when the titre was raised this was almost always to a modest degree only.

Meiklejohn (1943) had tested sera from 133 patients suffering from various infections, including 22 with bacterial pneumonia: in every case the cold-agglutinin titre was less than 40, compared with 46 out of 74 primary atypical pneumonia patients in whom the titre exceeded 40.

The Commission on Acute Respiratory Diseases (1944), which had reported on the sera of 93 patients with primary atypical pneumonia and 121 patients suffering from other types of respiratory disease, found that 29 patients of the former group (31%) had a cold-agglutinin titre exceeding 32, while only one patient out of the 121 patients of the latter group had a titre exceeding 32.

Favour (1944) described, however, higher incidences in both primary atypical pneumonia patients and in control groups: 32 out of 46 patients of the former group had a cold-agglutinin titre exceeding 40 compared with 12 out of 27 patients with tracheobronchitis

and five out of 14 patients with 'colds'. 'Scattered' patients suffering from rubella, chicken-pox, mumps, ornithosis, trachoma, infectious mononucleosis, bacterial infections, hepatitis, leukaemia and 'allergy' were all reported to have had a titre of 40 or more. Favour reported, however, that a titre exceeding 160 was uncommon except in the primary atypical pneumonia patients.

Streeter, Farmer and Hayes (1944) found the cold-agglutinin titre to be 40 or more in 20 out of 50 patients with primary atypical pneumonia (40%). In contrast, two out of 104 patients with other types of respiratory illness (1.9%) had a raised titre. Included in the total were 33 patients with pneumococcal infections: only one patient had a raised titre.

Finland and his co-workers (1945a) reported on cold-agglutinin titres in 1069 patients: 200 had had primary atypical pneumonia and 137 of them had a titre in excess of 40 (68.5%). In contrast, only one out of 151 patients suffering from pneumococcal pneumonia and two out of 149 patients with other types of bacterial pneumonia had a raised titre.

Springarn and Jones (1945) reported a relatively high incidence of cold agglutinins in their control series. They had had 91 patients with atypical pneumonia of whom 56 had a titre of 112 or more. In contrast, six out of 24 patients with bacterial pneumonia (25%) had a similarly raised titre. Of 100 normal controls (hospital personnel), while 89 had a titre of 56 or lower, 11 had a titre of 112 or 224. (It is probably significant that Springarn and Jones had read the titrations after a relatively long exposure (16–20 hours) at 5°C and that the end-points were read microscopically).

Finland and Barnes (1951) discussed why the reported percentages of patients with acute respiratory disorders who had had a raised titre of cold auto-agglutinins varied so widely. They considered that this could be explained probably by differences in the patient populations and in technique and interpretation. They themselves reviewed the incidence of raised titres of cold auto-agglutinins in 123 patients who had suffered from pneumonia or other acute respiratory infections. Forty of these patients had had primary atypical pneumonia and nine had had probably the same disorder with complications: the incidence of raised titres of cold agglutinins was 75% and 100%, respectively. In striking contrast, only two out of 22 patients (9%) with pneumococcal pneumonia had a raised titre, and in 52 patients who had suffered from other types of acute respiratory disorder the titres were normal. Amongst these 52 patients were 26 who had suffered from proved or probable bacterial (but not pneumococcal) pneumonia and 18 who had been infected with an influenza virus.

Grobbelaar (1957) described some interesting data which indicated that primary atypical pneumonia as it then occurred in South Africa was seldom associated with a rise in cold-agglutinin titre. Thus of 79 patients who had been diagnosed as suffering from virus or primary atypical pneumonia only two (2.6%) had a raised titre (>16). In other patients suffering from respiratory diseases the incidences of a raised titre were similarly low: e.g., one patient only out of 33 with pulmonary tuberculosis (3%) and two patients out of 33 patients suffering from other types of respiratory disease (6%); the incidence in 445 patients not suffering from a respiratory disease was as low as 0.67%.

Descriptions in the 1960s of high-titre cold agglutinins in acute respiratory diseases

Reports published in the 1960s indicated that raised cold-agglutinin titres in patients with acute respiratory diseases were at that time by no means so confined to those suffering from primary atypical pneumonia as the data of Finland and Barnes (1951) had suggested.

Mufson and co-workers (1961) reported on another large series of patients with primary atypical pneumonia. Of 109 Marine Corps recruits diagnosed serologically as suffering from Eaton agent pneumonia, 49 (45%) had developed raised cold agglutinins compared with four out of 23 patients (17%) with adenovirus pneumonia and seven out of 122 patients (6%) with atypical pneumonia of unknown causation.

Jansson and Wager (1964) and Jansson et al. (1964) reported on studies in Helsinki on 246 patients with pneumonia: 102 (41%) were judged to have had raised cold-agglutinin titres, i.e. titres of 32 or higher. Of these, tests for the Eaton-agent (mycoplasma) were positive in only 26%.

In the United Kingdom, Andrews (1965) reported that 24 out of 63 patients (38%) thought to have had *Mycoplasma pneumoniae* infections had had a raised titre of cold agglutinins: in contrast, of 237 patients suffering from a variety of viral infections only three (1.3%) had had a raised titre.

Sussman and co-workers (1966) concluded, however, that in small children at least the presence of a raised titre of cold agglutinins in patients suffering from respiratory disorders was no help in arriving at an aetological diagnosis. Of 444 children less than 4 years of age, 28 had developed cold agglutinins at a raised titre: in none of them, however, were serological tests for the Eaton agent positive; in contrast, other pathological agents were identified in 16 out of the 28.

Data on the relationship between the occurrence of a raised titre of cold agglutinins, the DAT and serum Ig levels in *Mycoplasma pneumoniae* infection were described by Feizi et al. (1966) and Feizi (1967a). She had studied 113 patients suffering from an epidemic respiratory illness in Scotland. The diagnosis of *Mycoplasma pneumoniae* infection was based on a fourfold fall in complement fixation titre against mycoplasma antigen on follow-up: 14 patients had had undoubted infection, 26 patients probable infection and in 14 patients in whom antibodies were demonstrable but only at a low titre the diagnosis was thought to be uncertain. Cold agglutinins at a raised titre (>32) were present in half of the patients with undoubted infection. The DAT (anti-C only) was positive in all the patients with undoubted infection and in a minority of those with probable infection. No patient, however, had developed overt haemolytic anaemia. [The DAT was positive, although less frequently, in patients suffering from other viral illnesses, e.g. in two of three patients with measles and in one out of three patients with influenza B]. Patients with mycoplasma infection were found often to have raised levels of serum IgM, and some but not all the excess IgM was absorbable by erythrocytes at a low temperature.

As already referred to, a small minority of patients who had been diagnosed as suffering from primary atypical pneumonia developed transient acute haemolytic anaemia. These patients appear to have responded to the infection in an exaggerated way: i.e. they produced cold antibodies of unusually high titre, and which reacted at an unusually high temperature, and which by being strongly complement-fixing were potentially strongly haemolytic.

IDENTIFICATION OF THE INFECTIVE AGENT OF PRIMARY ATYPICAL PNEUMONIA AS *MYCOPLASMA PNEUMONIAE* (THE EATON AGENT)

At the same time as the serological and haematological consequences of primary atypical pneumonia were being elucidated, studies into the nature of the infective agent had been carried out. These led to the isolation by Eaton, Meiklejohn and van Herick (1944) and Eaton et al. (1945) of a filtrable agent transmissible to cotton rats, hamsters and chick embryos. This agent (the Eaton agent) was later shown to be capable of growing on artificial media (Chanock, Hayflick and Barile, 1962) and to be not a virus but a mycoplasma, a pleuropneumonia-like organism (a PPLO), which was eventually named as a 'new' species — *Mycoplasma pneumoniae* (Chanock et al., 1963).

It seems likely that most, if not practically all, of

the cases of 'primary atypical' or 'virus' pneumonia described in the 1940s, and subsequently, were in fact caused by this agent. It is for this reason that in the subsequent discussion the term mycoplasma pneumonia will be used in preference to virus or primary atypical pneumonia.

EARLY DESCRIPTIONS OF MYCOPLASMA PNEUMONIA HAEMOLYTIC ANAEMIA

The literature on acute haemolytic anaemia following mycoplasma pneumonia soon became quite extensive.

Amongst the cases described in the 1940s and 1950s are those of Dameshek (1943),* Finland et al. (1945b), Ginsberg (1946), Colmers and Snaveley (1947), Battaglia (1947), Besterman and Brigden (1949), Eyquem (1950), Neeley et al. (1951), Wiener et al. (1951), Siegenthaler (1952), Aaron (1952), Moeschlin et al. (1954), Pisciotta, Downer and Hinz (1955), Stewart and Friedlander (1957) and Evans and Weiser (1957).

Other possible examples can be found in the older literature, e.g. the second patient described by Giordano and Blum (1937), as suffering from an acute haemolytic anaemia of the Lederer type and the first patient described by Antopol, Applebaum and Goldman (1939) who had, however, received sulphanilamide.

The viral pneumonias and pneumonias of probable viral origin were the subject of a valuable and comprehensive review by Reimann (1947).

Dacie and de Gruchy (1951) described the serological findings in four patients, the clinical history of one of them having been recorded by Besterman and Brigden (1949), and this patient and a further patient were referred to in more detail by Dacie (1954, pp. 221–225). In all, up to 1960, the author studied the serology of 10 patients, over a period of 12 years (see Table 30.1).

---

*Dameshek's two patients had both received short courses of sulphonamide drugs.

Clinical features

When haemolysis occurs after mycoplasma pneumonia, it does so usually towards the end of the second week or during the third week of the patient's illness. The onset is usually sudden. The patient, who may have already recovered from his respiratory infection, becomes ill once more with increasing pallor and jaundice, and prostration. There may even be haemoglobinuria (Dameshek, 1943; Horstmann and Tatlock, 1943; Berlin, 1950; Neely et al., 1951; Stewart and Friedlander, 1957; Schubothe et al; 1970; Bell, Zwicker and Rosenbaum, 1973; Niejadlik and Lozner, 1974; Boccardi et al., 1977). The spleen often, but not invariably, becomes palpable. Both sexes are affected, and most of the patients have been adults (Fig. 28.1 p. 215).

Gangrene. In rare instances gangrene of the extremities has developed in the course of the illness.

Pepino (1942) had described a possible case. Extensive symmetrical gangrene followed a pulmonary infection in a woman aged 58. The urine was stated to contain much urobilin and the haemoglobin was 70%. The presence or absence of auto-agglutination was, however, not mentioned.

Platt and Ward (1945) described how a 30-year-old woman, who had suffered from primary atypical pneumonia complicated by severe haemolytic anaemia, had developed multiple phlebothromboses which led to extensive gangrene of the right leg necessitating amputation below the knee.

Carey, Wilson and Tamerin (1948) described how the feet of their patient, a woman aged 31, became gangrenous, and impending gangrene of the feet was reported by Stats, Wasserman and Rosenthal (1948). Rønnov-Jessen (1950) also mentioned that gangrene of the finger-tips developed in an elderly man aged 75. In these patients the gangrene was presumably due to thrombosis following intense intravascular auto-agglutination.

Kumar, Singh and Bhatia (1958) described the case of a 32-year-old woman who was admitted to hospital with severe bilateral gangrene affecting fingers and toes which had developed over a period of 10 days. She was found to be severely anaemic (haemoglobin 6.0 g/dl) and to be leucopenic (total count $2.5 \times 10^9/1$). Her blood underwent auto-agglutination at room temperature (30°C). The cold-agglutinin titre was 2048 at 4°C and 512 at 30°C. The DAT was positive. Her anaemia responded to prednisone therapy, but she slowly relapsed when the drug was withdrawn. Splenectomy was eventually carried out and was followed by a

Table 30.1 Serological data on ten patients suffering from haemolytic anaemia following 'virus' pneumonia.

Case	Sex age	Agglutination — Normal cells			Lysis										Indirect antiglobulin test — Normal cells			
					Normal cells				Trypsinized cells (titre)		PNH cells (titre)				pH 6.5–7.0		pH 8.0	
					pH 6.5–7.0		pH 8.0		pH 8.0		pH 8.0							
		2–4°C (titre)	20°C (titre)	30°C (titre)	20°C	37°C	20°C	37°C	20°C	37°C	20°C	37°C			20°C	37°C	20°C	37°C
A.S.	F. 33	4000	256	…	+	−	−	−	64	64	1024	0			…	−	…	−
E.M.	F. 73	4000	256	<4	+±	−	−	−	16	0	1024	16			+	+	±	−
I.P.	F. 22	16000	256	…	++	−	−	−	32	0	1024	16			++	−	±	−
–G.	M. 35	2000	…	…	+	−	−	−	4	0	512	16			++	+	++	−
M.A. (Case 15, Dacie, 1954)	M. 35	8000	512	…	++	−	−	−	64	0	2048	16			++	±	…	…
M.T. (Case 16, Dacie, 1954)	M. 41	4000	128	4	++	−	−	−	…	4	256	16			++	++	+±	+±
E.F.	F. 31	8000	1024	4	++	−	+	−	512	16	4000	64			++	+	++	+±
J.L.	F. 41	2000	64	…	+	−	−	−	64	0	…	…			+±	±	+±	…
L.V.	F. 41	2000	64	…	+	−	−	−	…	…	…	…			++	±	+±	−
G.A.	M. 72	4000	256	4	+	−	−	−	32	32	256	32			…	…	…	…

++, +±, + and ± denote intensities of lysis or agglutination; − denotes no lysis or agglutination; … denotes no observation.

remission which lasted for at least 5 months. The cold antibodies disappeared after the operation and the DAT became negative. The nature of this patient's illness is uncertain; it is possible that she had had mycoplasma pneumonia.

Kibukamusoke and Somers (1962) described three African patients who developed extensive and serious gangrene of the extremities associated with acute cold-antibody haemolytic anaemia. The precipitating cause of the haemolysis was uncertain. The cold-agglutinin titres were raised in two of the patients—256 and 512, respectively — and marked auto-agglutination was noted in the third; erythrophagocytosis was prominent in the peripheral blood of one of the patients. Whether mycoplasma infection was the cause of their illness is uncertain, but it seems possible. The Donath–Landsteiner test was reported to be positive in two of the patients; the Kahn test was negative. There was no evidence of malaria.

Acrocyanosis and phlebothrombosis. Helwig and Freis (1943) made an early and interesting observation: this was of intense acrocyanosis of the nose, ears and hands following a respiratory infection in a man of 38, diagnosed as suffering from atypical pneumonia. The cold-agglutinin titre was 5000 but there were apparently no overt signs of haemolytic anaemia. Peterson, Ham and Finland (1943) also mentioned that phlebothromboses and pulmonary emboli had occurred during the later part of the illness or during the convalescence of certain patients, but these occurrences, too, were not apparently associated with haemolysis.

Renal involvement. Renal involvement following mycoplasma pneumonia is a rare event but it has been recorded.

Corelli and Ruggieri (1951) reported that a 55-year-old man, who had developed severe haemolysis associated with haemoglobinuria 2 weeks after the onset of 'virus' pneumonia, had died with a blood urea of 277 mg/dl. His haemoglobin had fallen to 20%, and the leucocyte count was 60×10^9/l. The DAT was strongly positive and a cold agglutinin, the activity of which extended up to 37°C, was present.

Boulet and co-workers (1956) described the occurrence of transient acute glomerulonephritis accompanying severe haemolysis as a sequel to an atypical pneumonia.

Lawson and co-workers (1968) described transient acute renal failure and oliguria under similar circumstances. Their patient was a 54-year-old woman who had suffered from respiratory symptoms and pleuritic pain. Two weeks after the onset of her illness she developed oliguria and was found to have a haemoglobin of 6 g/dl. The urine contained haemoglobin but no erythrocytes. The blood urea was 270 mg/dl and the DAT was positive. She was treated by means of peritoneal dialysis and given prednisolone and eventually completely recovered after 7 days of oliguria. The cold-agglutinin titre had been 2560 at 4°C and 256 at 25°C. The anti-mycoplasma titre was shown to rise from 16 to 256. There was a notable leucocytosis of 55×10^9 cells per litre.

LATER CASE REPORTS OF MYCOPLASMA PNEUMONIA HAEMOLYTIC ANAEMIA OF SPECIAL INTEREST

In recent years post-mycoplasma haemolytic anaemia has been relatively seldom reported. For one thing, the disorder is no longer the novelty it was in the 1940s and 1950s; it seems likely, too, that effective antibiotic treatment of the causal infection has markedly diminished the incidence of the haemolytic complication.

The selected case reports that are summarized below contain features of special interest.

Walsh (1961) described a patient who developed severe haemolysis 2 weeks after the onset of a mild respiratory illness, diagnosed as possibly viral pneumonia. The haemoglobin fell to 3.1 g/dl with 49.6% reticulocytes. The DAT was positive; serum contained a high-thermal-amplitude antibody of apparently anti-I specificity but of relatively low titre—32 at 4°C, 16 at room temperature, still active at 37°C. The antibody agglutinated the blood of more than 500 donors irrespective of their blood group. Transfusion, thought essential as a life-saving measure, was followed by gross haemoglobinuria. The patient, nevertheless, recovered, aided probably by high doses of prednisolone (300 mg daily).

Copps (1964) reported that a 14-year-old boy who became moderately severely anaemic following primary atypical pneumonia also developed a skin rash diagnosed as erythema multiforme. His haemoglobin was 6.2 g/dl and the cold-agglutinin titre 2560.

Schneider (1967) described a 40-year-old patient who developed acute haemolysis following an illness diagnosed as virus pneumonia. The cold-agglutinin titre was reported at the height of his illness to be as high as 4 million at 4°C, 64 000 at 20°C and 128 at 37°C, falling rapidly on recovery to 250 000, 64 and <2, respectively on the 6th day, and to 16, 2 and <2 on the 16th day! Electrophoresis of the serum protein demonstrated a moderate rise in globulin which disappeared after absorbing the serum with erythrocytes.

Schubothe and his co-workers (1970) described in

detail the histopathological findings in a male aged 43 who had died of severe intravascular haemolysis. Many intact erythrocytes were visible in phagocytic cells in the liver and spleen.

The 17-year-old youth described by Bell, Zwicker and Rosenbaum (1973) presented with an illness resembling that of paroxysmal cold haemoglobinuria.

The report of Niejadlik and Lozner (1974) was noteworthy in that a mother aged 51 and her son aged 23 had both suffered from a *Mycoplasma pneumoniae* infection. They both had developed respiratory symptoms and later substantial rises in cold-agglutinin titre—in the mother to 8192 and in her son to 2048. Both had rises in anti-*Mycoplasma pneumoniae* titres to 16 and 32, respectively. The mother became acutely anaemic with a haematocrit of 15% and a leucocyte count of 52 × 10⁹/l; her son developed symptoms suggestive of the Stevens–Johnson syndrome, but he did not apparently suffer from overt haemolysis. The mother became hyperpyrexic (temperature 104°F), and treating this by means of a cooling mattress appeared to precipitate intravascular haemolysis and haemoglobinuria.

LABORATORY FINDINGS IN MYCOPLASMA PNEUMONIA HAEMOLYTIC ANAEMIA

Auto-agglutination *in vitro* at room temperature occurring immediately after withdrawal of blood is an invariable and striking finding. Anaemia is often severe and rapidly progresses, erythrocyte counts as low as 1×10^{12}/l having been recorded. Peripheral blood films show in addition to auto-agglutination a variable degree of polychromasia, depending upon the stage of the disease, and as a rule moderate to marked spherocytosis. There may be evidence of erythrophagocytosis (Pisciotta, 1955). Erythrocyte osmotic fragility is usually increased to a moderate degree.

The total leucocyte count may be markedly raised (Dameshek, 1943; Ginsberg, 1946; Parker, Joliffe and Finland, 1947; Neely et al., 1951; Aaron, 1952; Maisel, 1967; Lawson et al., 1968; Fiala et al., 1974; etc.), counts exceeding 40×10^9 cells per litre being not uncommon. Hortsmann and Tatlock (1943) recorded a count as high as 100×10^9/l in a fatal case. Most of the cells are neutrophils, but myelocytes may be present in small numbers. Auto-agglutination of leucocytes may be seen in blood films made at room temperature (Feizi et al., 1966) (Fig. 30.1).

The patient described by Moeschlin et al. (1954) was remarkable in that the haemolytic episode was followed by an episode of severe granulocytopenia and mild thrombocytopenia. The leucopenia, which was marked for 1 month and persisted for a year, was thought to be caused by incomplete auto-leuco-agglutinins.

The serum-bilirubin concentration is usually raised to between 1 and 3 mg/dl. The plasma-haemoglobin level is almost invariably above normal and methaemalbumin is usually demonstrable in the acute phase of the haemolysis. Haptoglobins are markedly lowered or absent.

SEROLOGICAL FINDINGS IN MYCOPLASMA PNEUMONIA HAEMOLYTIC ANAEMIA

Cold auto-antibodies. Cold-agglutinin titres at the time of onset of haemolysis typically range between 512 and 32 000 at 2–4°C, and it is interesting to note that the exceptionally high titre of 32 000 was found in the patient whose feet became gangrenous (Carey, Wilson and Tamerin, 1948). The rise and fall in the cold-agglutinin titre of the patient described by Dacie (1954, Case 15) is illustrated in Fig. 30.2. Early summarized data on serological findings were given by Dacie and de Gruchy (1951), Dacie, (1954, p. 219) and Dausset and Colombani (1959). The DAT is always positive but only with anti-C sera.

The author's data assembled between 1948 and 1960 are summarized in Table 30.1.

Cold-agglutinin titres using normal erythrocytes varied from 2048 to 16 000 at the height of the patients' illness and, in the cases in which it

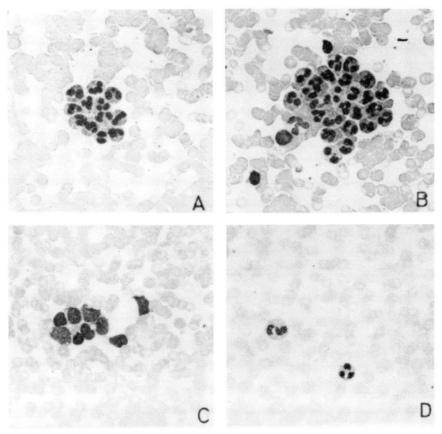

Fig. 30.1 **Photomicrographs of blood films of a patient who had formed high-titre cold agglutinins following *M. pneumoniae* infection.**
(A) shows neutrophil auto-agglutination, (B) mixed neutrophil and erythrocyte auto-agglutination, (C) lymphocyte auto-agglutination, and (D) absence of neutrophil agglutination. (A), (B) and (C) were photographs of a film made at room temperature; (D) was made at 37°C. [Reproduced by permission from Feizi et al. (1966).]

was tested for, agglutination was demonstrable to at least 30°C. Auto-agglutination did not, however, occur at 37°C.

The antibodies are potentially lytic and in severely ill patients they typically bring about rapid lysis of normal erythrocytes at 20°C and 30°C, usually, however, only if the serum is suitably acidified (optimum, pH 6.5–7.0). In the first patient studied (Dacie, 1949), lysis occurred so rapidly at 20°C and 30°C that it was not realized at first that the lysin was a cold one and that lysis of normal erythrocytes did not take place at 37°C. Trypsinized erythrocytes are strongly lysed by the antibodies at 20°C and 30°C, and with four out of nine sera there was clear lysis at

37°C. PNH cells were lysed by seven out of eight sera at 37°C.

The DAT was positive in each case at the height of the patients' illness even if the blood was collected directly into saline previously warmed to 37°C: the reaction was of the non-γ-globulin type. The IAT was always strongly positive at 20°C, and the reaction was sometimes but by no means invariably stronger using acidified serum. With five out of eight acidified sera the reaction was positive at 37°C and in two out of seven instances positive using unacidified serum.

These results and the rapid lysis of normal erythrocytes at 30°C, and of trypsinized cells and PNH cells often at 37°C, illustrate the high

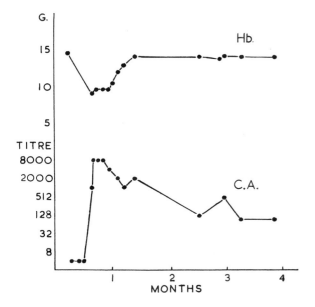

Fig. 30.2 Rise and fall in the cold-agglutinin titre and accompanying changes in haemoglobin in a patient who developed acute haemolytic anaemia following 'virus' pneumonia, M. A. (Case 15 of Dacie, 1954).
    C.A. = cold-agglutinin titre at 2°C.

thermal amplitude and the unusual lytic potency of the antibodies.

In many respects the reactions of the antibodies are similar to those present in patients suffering from CHAD. There are, however, some differences: in the post-mycoplasma pneumonia cases the antibody titres at 2–4°C are usually lower than in CHAD; their thermal amplitude is, however, often higher than in typical CHAD. The differences in the ability of the antibodies in post-mycoplasma pneumonia cases and in CHAD and in PCH (paroxysmal cold haemoglobinuria) to bring about agglutination or lysis *in vitro* are illustrated in Table 28.6 (p. 226).

Other serological findings. Lind and McArthur (1947) reported that the anti-T agglutinin titre was significantly higher in sera from patients suffering from atypical pneumonia than in sera from normal adults; they showed, too, that the anti-T agglutinins and the cold antibodies were distinct entities.

Aaron (1952) reported a temporary rise in serum globulins to 5.6 g/dl in one case. Christenson and Dacie (1957) studied the sera of 10 patients by paper electrophoresis. The protein

pattern was generally that of an infective disease: albumin was low and the α and γ globulins were raised, but no abnormal peaks or cryoglobulins were detected.

Positive Wassermann and Kahn reactions were reported by Florman and Weiss (1945), Kreis (1947) and Aaron (1952). Aaron (1952) reported, too, a transitory rise in serum heterophile antibodies (presumably against sheep erythrocytes) in one case.

Individual differences in the ability of the antibodies to bring about agglutination or lysis *in vitro*

As illustrated in Table 30.1, the reactions of the antibodies *in vitro* vary considerably from patient to patient.

The serum of Case 16 of Dacie (1954) was particularly interesting. Although it undoubtedly contained a high-titre cold agglutinin, normal erythrocytes were apparently sensitized, in the presence of fresh serum only, to agglutination by an antiglobulin serum as intensely at 37°C as at 2°C or 20°C. The serum of Case 15 of Dacie and de Gruchy (1951) (A.S., Table 30.1) was also unusual. At the time of this patient's haemolytic crisis her serum contained a factor which lysed trypsinized normal erythrocytes as actively at 37°C as at 20°C. The 'warm' lytic factor disappeared from the patient's serum during convalescence. The other sera the author investigated between 1948 and 1960, with the exception of that of G.A. (Table 30.1), behaved in exactly the opposite and more orthodox way, i.e., lysis of trypsinized cells took place at 20°C, but not at all or to a markedly lesser degree at 37°C.

As with sera from patients with the CHAD, lysis of normal erythrocytes is usually far better demonstrated at room temperature (15–20°C) or 30°C, preferably using acidified serum, than by the cold–warm (0°C →37°C) Donath–Landsteiner (D–L) procedure using unacidified serum (Table 28.6, p. 226). The orthodox D–L test may thus give negative results. In the case described by Stewart and Friedlander (1957), lysis was, however, apparently best demonstrated in this way.

Specificity

The cold auto-antibodies found in the sera of post-mycoplasma pneumonia patients are typically anti-I. However, the relative ability of the patients' antibodies to react with I and i cells varies considerably, as it does in CHAD. This variability is illustrated in Table 30.2 in which the agglutination titres at 20°C, using I, i (adult) and i (cord) erythrocytes in three post-mycoplasma pneumonia patients are compared with those given by a typical CHAD patient. Whereas serum I.P. contains an antibody that reacts clearly as anti-I, as does the antibody in the CHAD serum (A.D.), the Ii status of the antibodies in sera M.T. and E.F. is less certain (and more interesting).

Further data on the heterogeneity of anti-I cold agglutinins associated with mycoplasma pneumonia were provided by Feizi (1969). She studied the sera of 15 patients, using OI erythrocytes from a single adult donor and Oi (cord) cells from six infants. Higher titres at 4°C were obtained with the OI cells except in four cases in which the titres with the OI and Oi cells overlapped. There were also differences between the agglutinability of the different Oi cells. With eight sera this was marked (particularly so with two sera), with differences in titre up to 128-fold.

A more recent study of König and co-workers (1988) provided further evidence as to complexicity of the specificity of cold auto-antibodies. They had reinvestigated 192 sera known to contain anti-I antibodies for the presence of concomitant antibodies which reacted with sialic-acid-dependent antigens: 35 examples of anti-Fl and three of anti-Gd were detected. It is especially interesting to note that 53% of 32 sera containing anti-I and anti-Fl together had been obtained from patients who had suffered from pneumonia; in 39% of these sera IgM antibodies against *Mycoplasma pneumoniae* were present. König et al. commented: 'since Fl and Gd antigens are identical with the structures identified as receptors for *M. pneumoniae*, the findings support the hypothesis that postinfectious CA [cold agglutinins] are directed against the receptor of the infectious agent' (see also p. 369).

Specificities other than anti-I: anti P

Boccardi and co-workers (1977) described the transitory occurrence of the clinical syndrome of paroxysmal cold haemoglobinuria (PCH) in a 7-year-old boy who had suffered from mycoplasma pneumonia. While other patients had developed haemoglobinuria under similar circumstances (see p. 302), this appears to be the first report implicating anti-P as the causal antibody.

Species specificity

It is interesting to note that both Clough and Richter (1918) and Wheeler, Gallacher and Stuart (1939), in their descriptions of patients who may have suffered from mycoplasma pneumonia, reported that their patients' sera agglutinated animal erythrocytes, as well as human cells, to high titres. Of the species tested, rabbit cells were the most sensitive.

The increased sensitivity of rabbit erythrocytes compared with the cells of other species was confirmed by Turner and Jackson (1943) in a careful study. In order to avoid possible confusion due to agglutination by hetero-antibodies present in normal human sera they tested eluates prepared at 37°C from human erythrocytes derived from blood containing cold agglutinins which had been cooled at 0°C. In seven cases rabbit erythrocytes were found to be as agglutinable as human cells; guinea-pig and pig cells were less agglutinable; sheep and mouse cells were agglutinated by two only of the sera, and horse and ox cells were not agglutinated.

IMMUNOCHEMISTRY OF COLD AGGLUTININS IN *MYCOPLASMA PNEUMONIAE* INFECTION

The antibodies are typically (? invariably) IgM in nature. The light chain pattern is, however, variable: in some patients monotypic kappa chains have alone been demonstrable; in other patients both kappa and lambda chains have been present.

Feizi (1967b) reported on 10 sera obtained from patients with mycoplasma pneumonia. The light chains of the antibodies in four patients who had suffered from transient haemolytic anaemia were kappa in type in three and kappa plus lambda in one; in four patients who did not develop haemolytic anaemia, both kappa and lambda chains were present.

Further studies were described by Feizi and Schumacher (1968). Two sera containing cold agglutinins derived from patients who had suffered from mycoplasma infection, and one serum from a patient who had suffered from an unspecified infection, and three patients suffering from CHAD, were studied. One of the mycoplasma infection cold agglutinins was indistinguishable from the CHAD cold agglutinins: its light chains were monotypic kappa; they had restricted

Table 30.2 Comparative sensitivity of I-positive, I-negative and cord-blood erythrocytes to agglutination by sera from three patients suffering from haemolytic anaemia following 'virus' pneumonia and a serum from a patient suffering from the cold-haemagglutinin disease.

Serum and cells	Temperature (°C)	Serum dilutions					
		1 in 1	1 in 4	1 in 16	1 in 64	1 in 256	Control (saline)
I.P.							
I-positive	20	+++	++	+	±	−	−
I-negative	20	±	Trace	−	−	−	−
Cord	20	±	Trace	−	−	−	−
M.T. (Case 16, Dacie, 1954)							
I-positive	20	+++	++	±	−	−	−
I-negative	20	+++±	+++	+	−	−	−
Cord	20	+	±	−	−	−	−
E.F.							
I-positive	20	+++±	++	++	+	±	−
I-negative	20	+++±	+++	+±	±	−	−
Cord	20	++	++	Trace	−	−	−
A.D. (Case 9, cold-haemagglutinin disease)							
I-positive	20	++++	+++±	+++	++	+	−
I-negative	20	++	+	−	−	−	−

+++ + denotes very intense naked-eye agglutination; +++±, +++, ++, +±, + and ± denote lesser degrees of agglutination; − denotes no agglutination.

mobility on electrophoresis and produced a narrow light-chain zone on starch gel electrophoresis. The other two post-infective cold agglutinins were bitypic with kappa and lambda light chains, but they were relatively homogeneous on immunoelectrophoresis and in starch gell electrophoresis they produced sharper bands than the light-chain zone of normal human IgM.

Further data on the light chains of the IgM cold antibodies of mycoplasma pneumonia haemolytic anaemia were reported by Jacobson, Longstreth and Edgington (1973), Fiala et al. (1974) and Louie et al. (1985).

Jacobson, Longstreth and Edgington reported that in their patient immunoelectrophoresis indicated homogeneity and clonal restriction of the antibody; both kappa and lambda light chains were, however, demonstrable. In the patient of Fiala et al., however, kappa light chains predominated. The patient of Louie et al. was most unusual in that low-grade haemolysis persisted long after the patient had recovered from an acute haemolytic crisis. She had in fact formed a warm IgG kappa auto-antibody in addition to a IgM lambda high-thermal-amplitude high-titre cold auto-agglutinin.

Interaction between *Mycoplasma pneumoniae* and the I antigen

An important question is the reason and mechanism by which infection with *Mycoplasma pneumoniae* so commonly results in a rise in cold auto-agglutinin titre. While it is true that a rise in titre quite commonly follows other types of infection, as has already been emphasized (p. 297), infection with *Mycoplasma pneumoniae* stands out as being an exceptionally potent stimulus, and one which occasionally results in the formation of antibodies of sufficiently high thermal amplitude as to be clinically important.

In attempting to explain the exceptional role of *Mycoplasma pneumoniae* infection, attention has been focused particularly on two possible mechanisms. One is that the organism itself possesses an I-like antigen which stimulates the formation of [cross-reacting] anti-I antibodies in the individual it infects. The second possibility is that the organism acts on and modifies in some way the I antigen on the erythrocyte membrane so that it becomes unusually (auto) antigenic.

There is evidence that both mechanisms appear to play a part in the formation of the cold antibodies.

Schmidt, Barile and McGinniss (1965) added a range of micro-organisms to human I-positive erythrocytes *in vitro* with the aim of seeing whether the agglutinability of the erythrocytes was affected. Eighteen of 25 strains of mycoplasma were found to block or destroy I antigen receptors on the normal erythrocytes tested, as judged by the subsequent agglutinability of the cells by an anti-I antibody present in the serum of an I-negative individual. In contrast, adding mycoplasma strains to sera containing cold antibodies did not affect the potency of the antibodies. Schmidt, Barile and McGinniss concluded, therefore, that the mycoplasma was acting on anti-I receptor sites on the erythrocytes, perhaps by enzyme action. Possible support for this contention was obtained by Smith, McGinniss and Schmidt (1967) who inoculated 27 volunteers with *Mycoplasma pneumoniae* vaccine. The thermal amplitude of anti-I in their serum was increased in 12 of the volunteers and in seven the titre of their antibodies increased fourfold or more. None, however, developed signs of increased haemolysis. The I agglutinogen activity was transitorily reduced in five.

Further indirect evidence in favour of the hypothesis that *Mycoplasma pneumoniae* is capable of modifying the I antigen on erythrocytes so as to render it more antigenic was provided by Feizi and Darrell (1966) and Feizi and Taylor-Robinson (1967). The organism was found to be incapable of absorbing anti-I from human sera and it appeared unlikely, therefore, that the organism carried an I-like antigen. The experiments of Feizi and her co-workers (1969) provided additional evidence. They inoculated a series of rabbits with human OI erythrocytes, with or without viable *Mycoplasma pneumoniae* in addition, and followed any changes in anti-I cold-agglutinin titre in the rabbit sera that might result. As in man affected with *Mycoplasma pneumoniae* a minority of rabbits [nine out of 28 (32%)] inoculated with OI cells and *Mycoplasma pneumoniae* developed fourfold or greater rises in cold-agglutinin titre. In contrast, rabbits inoculated with the organism alone did not produce cold agglutinins in response, nor did rabbits inoculated with human OI cells and an allied organism, *Mycoplasma hominis*.

In 1984, Loomes and co-workers provided additional evidence in favour of the modified antigen hypothesis by their finding that the receptors for *Mycoplasma pneumoniae* on the erythrocyte membrane are sialylated oligosaccharides of Ii antigen type.

However, evidence that *Mycoplasma pneumoniae* does after all bear an I-like antigen was adduced by Costea, Yakulis and Heller (1969, 1972).

Costea, Yakulis and Heller (1969) reported that the injection of suspensions of *Mycoplasma pneumoniae* stimulated the formation of cold agglutinins in rabbits and in a strain of mouse. Cold agglutinins were also formed by rabbits, but not by mice, following inoculation with *Listeria monocytogenes* [see also Costea, Yakulis and Heller (1965)]. They also reported that the cold agglutinins thus formed and isolated from erythrocytes by thermal elution reacted with the micro-organism responsible for their production as well as with the animals' erythrocytes.

Costea, Yakulis and Heller (1972) found that cold antibodies raised in rabbits or mice, as described above, were absorbable by either intact *Mycoplasma pneumoniae* or by mycoplasma lipopolysaccharide and that the same was true of *Listeria monocytogenese*. As reported by Feizi and Taylor-Robinson (1967), Costea, Yakulis and Heller (1972) found that intact *Mycoplasma pneumoniae* were unable to absorb cold agglutinins from the sera of patients who had had mycoplasma pneumonia. When, however, mycoplasma lipopolysaccharide was used as absorbent in place of the intact organism, this caused a sixfold or more reduction in titre. They also reported that neither intact *Mycoplasma pneumoniae* or mycoplasma lipopolysaccharide absorbed cold agglutinins from the sera of CHAD or Waldenström's macroglobulinaemia patients. Costea, Yakulis and Heller concluded that the antigens in *Mycoplasma pneumoniae* with which cold agglutinins react are hidden in the organism's 'limiting membrane' and that the development of cold agglutinins in man and animals as the consequence of infection with a variety of micro-organisms is a consequence of immunization by cross-reacting antigens.

Lind (1973) reported similar findings, i.e. that *M. pneumoniae* and *L. monocytogenes* (and *Streptococcus MG*) stimulate cold-agglutinin production when administered intravenously to rabbits. Absorption experiments suggested that the organisms possess antigens related to the erythrocyte I antigen. The results of the in-vivo experiments were the same irrespective of whether live *M. pneumoniae* had been injected or, alternatively, autologous erythrocytes that had been exposed *in vitro* to the organisms. Lind conceded that an interaction might take place *in vivo* between the organisms and rabbit erythrocytes. However, he pointed out that *L. monocytogenes* and *Strept. MG* do not adsorb to erythrocytes, a finding in favour of the hypothesis that 'CA [cold-agglutinin] triggering I-like antigens are present on these micro-organisms'.

Further evidence was provided by Janney, Lee and Howe (1978) in support of the hypothesis that the development of cold agglutinins following *M. pneumoniae* infection represents a cross-reaction between determinants common to erythrocyte glycoprotein containing I antigen and the membrane of *M. pneumoniae*. Sera from patients convalescing from *M. pneumoniae* infection, rabbit antisera to *M. pneumoniae* and to human erythrocyte glycoprotein were found to contain cold agglutinins that reacted with human erythrocytes.

PROGNOSIS IN MYCOPLASMA PNEUMONIA HAEMOLYTIC ANAEMIA

The prognosis in haemolytic anaemia following mycoplasma pneumonia is generally good, for haemolysis is essentially short-lived. Although some deaths have been recorded, e.g. by Horstmann and Tatlock (1943), Finland et al. (1945b), Parker, Joliffe and Finland (1947), Maisel (1967), Schubothe et al. (1970), most patients recover completely. Sacks, Workman and Jahn (1952) stated that this was so in 33 out of 35 patients.

The onset of anaemia and recovery, and the rise and fall in cold-agglutinin titre of one of the author's patients, is illustrated by Fig. 30.2, and the changes in antibody activity during recovery is shown, in another patient, in Fig. 30.3. The loss of the serum's ability to agglutinate normal cells at 27°C is believed to be particulary significant in relation to recovery, the titre at 2°C at that time having fallen off only by one tube, i.e. only halved.

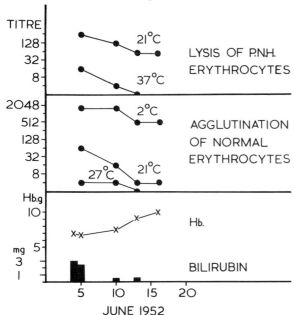

Fig. 30.3   Changes in cold-antibody concentration in the serum of a patient suffering from 'virus' pneumonia (Case 16 of Dacie, 1954).

TREATMENT

The patients should be kept warm in bed. This is particularly important as chilling is likely to cause an increase in haemolysis. This is illustrated by the case report of Colmers and Snaveley (1947) whose patient was sponged with iced alcohol in an attempt to treat her hyperpyrexia. On the following morning she was moribund. Niejadlik and Lozner (1974) described a similar experience. In an attempt to alleviate hyperpyrexia their patient had been nursed on a cooling mattress. This resulted in chills and spiking fever and haemoglobinuria.

Transfusion should be reserved for the most severely anaemic patients, and it is probably advisable to warm the transfused blood to body temperature before administration. (The selection and cross-matching of blood for transfusion in cases of AIHA is considered in Chapter 35, p. 489.)

There seems to be no reason to contemplate splenectomy in post-mycoplasma pneumonia haemolytic anaemia. Most patients, too, recover quickly without the help of corticosteroid drugs. However, if haemolysis is unusually severe or prolonged, or not apparently responding to keeping the patient warm, the drugs should be used (see p. 510). In an early report, Moeschlin and co-workers (1954) considered that ACTH therapy appeared to have been life-saving.

In relation to antibiotic therapy, by the time the patient develops haemolytic anaemia his or her respiratory problem will almost certainly have resolved, either spontaneously or helped by antibiotic therapy. However, if it has persisted, this is an indication for continuing with antibiotics.

REFERENCES

AARON, R. S. (1952). Hemolytic anemia in viral pneumonia with high cold-agglutinin titer. *Arch. intern. Med.*, **89**, 293–296.

ANDREWS, B. E. (1965). Human infections with *Mycoplasma pneumoniae* (Eaton's agent). *Proc. roy. Soc. Med.*, **58**, 80–82.

ANTOPOL, W., APPLEBAUM, I. & GOLDMAN, L. (1939). Two cases of acute hemolytic anemia with auto-agglutination following sulfanilamide therapy. *J. Amer. med. Ass.*, **113**, 488–489.

BATTAGLIA, B. (1947). Hemolytic anemia complicating primary atypical pneumonia with cold isohemagglutinins. *Ann. intern. Med.*, **27**, 469–471.

BELL, C. A., ZWICKER, H. & ROSENBAUM, D. L. (1973). Paroxysmal cold hemoglobinuria (P. C. H.) following mycoplasma infection; anti-I specificity of the biphasic hemolysin. *Transfusion*, **13**, 138–141.

BERLIN, R. (1950). Akut hämolytisk anämi vid viruspneumoni med hög köldagglutinationstiter. *Nord. Med.*, **44**, 1480–1482.

BESTERMAN, E. & BRIGDEN, W. (1949). Haemolytic anaemia complicating virus pneumonia. *Thorax*, **4**, 134–136.

BOCCARDI, V., D'ANNIBALI, S., DI NATALE, G., GIRELLI, G. & SUMMONTI, D. (1977). Mycoplasma pneumoniae infection complicated by paroxysmal cold hemoglobinuria with anti-P specificity of biphasic hemolysin. *Blut*, **34**, 211–214.

BOULET, P., SERRE, H., MIROUZE, J. & FABRE, S. (1956). Association d'une pneumopathie atypique, d'une glomérulo-néphrite aiguë et d'un syndrome hémolytique paroxystique grave. *Montpellier. méd.*, **99**, 123–128.

CAREY, R. M., WILSON, J. L. & TAMERIN, J. A. (1948). Gangrene of feet and hemolytic anemia associated with cold hemagglutinins in atypical pneumonia. *Harlem Hosp. Bull.*, **1**, 25–32.

CHANOCK, R. M., DIENES, L., EATON, M. D. et al. (15 authors). (1963). Mycoplasma pneumoniae: proposed nomenclature for atypical pneumonia organism (Eaton agent). *Science*, **140**, 662.

CHANOCK, R. M., HAYFLICK, L. & BARILE, M. F. (1962). Growth on artificial medium of an agent associated with atypical pneumonia and its identification as a PPLO. *Proc. natn. Acad. Sci. U.S.A.*, **48**, 41–49.

CHRISTENSON, W. N. & DACIE, J. V. (1957). Serum proteins in acquired haemolytic anaemia (auto-antibody type). *Brit. J. Haemat.*, **3**, 153–164.

CLOUGH, M. C. & RICHTER, I. M. (1918). A study of an autoagglutinin occurring in a human serum. *Johns Hopk. Hosp. Bull*, **29**, 86–93.

COLMERS, R. A. & SNAVELEY, J. G. (1947). Acute hemolytic anemia in primary atypical pneumonia produced by exposure and chilling. *New Eng. J. Med.*, **237**, 505–511.

COMMISSION ON ACUTE RESPIRATORY DISEASES (12 authors) (1944). Cold hemagglutinins in primary atypical pneumonia and other respiratory infections. *Amer. J. med. Sci.*, **208**, 742–750.

COPPS, S. C. (1964). Primary atypical pneumonia with hemolytic anemia and erythema multiforme. *Clin. Pediat.*, **3**, 491–495.

CORELLI, F. & RUGGIERI, P. (1951). Demonstration of auto-antibodies (by Coombs's test) in acute haemolytic anemia in the course of virus pneumonia. *Acta haemat. (Basel)*, **5**, 151–157.

COSTEA, N., YAKULIS, V. & HELLER, P. (1965).

Experimental production of cold agglutinins in rabbits. *Blood*, **26**, 323–339.

COSTEA, N., YAKULIS, V. & HELLER, P. (1969). The mechanisms of induction of cold agglutinins by *M. pneumoniae. Blood*, **34**, 829 (Abstract 15).

COSTEA, N., YAKULIS, V. J. & HELLER, P. (1972). Inhibition of cold agglutinins (anti-I) by *M. pneumoniae* antigens. *Proc. Soc. exp. Biol. Med.*, **139**, 476–479.

DACIE, J. V. (1949). Diagnosis and mechanism of hemolysis in chronic hemolytic anemia with nocturnal hemaglobinuria. *Blood*, **4**, 1186–1195.

DACIE, J. V. (1954). *The Haemolytic Anaemias: Congenital and Acquired*, 525 pp. Churchill, London.

DACIE, J. V. & DE GRUCHY, G. C. (1951). Auto-antibodies in acquired haemolytic anaemia. *J. clin. Path.*, **4**, 253–271.

DAMESHEK, W. (1943). Cold hemagglutinins in acute hemolytic reactions in association with sulfonamide medication and infection. *J. Amer. med. Ass.*, **123**, 77–80.

DAUSSET, J. & COLOMBANI, J. (1959). The serology and the prognosis of 128 cases of autoimmune hemolytic anemia. *Blood*, **14**, 1280–1301.

EATON, M. D., MEIKLEJOHN, G., & VAN HERICK, W. (1944). Studies on the etiology of primary atypical pneumonia. A filterable agent transmissible to cotton rats, hamsters and chick embryos. *J. exp. Med.*, **79**, 649–668.

EATON, M. D., MEIKLEJOHN, G., VAN HERICK, W. & COREY, M. (1945). Studies on the etiology of primary atypical pneumonia. II. Properties of the virus isolated and propagated in chick embryos. *J. exp. Med.*, **82**, 317–328.

EVANS, R. S. & WEISER, R. S. (1957). The serology of autoimmune hemolytic disease. Observations on forty-one patients. *Arch. intern. Med.*, **100**, 371–399.

EYQUEM, A. (1950). Les agglutinines froides. Leur signification clinique—Leur importance biologique dans les pneumonias atypiques primitives à virus. *Sem. Hôp. Paris*, **26**, 2523–2531.

FAVOUR, C. B. (1944). Autohemagglutinins—'cold agglutinins'. *J. clin. Invest.*, **23**, 891–897.

FEIZI, T. (1967a). Cold agglutinins, the direct Coombs' test and serum immunoglobulins in *Mycoplasma pneumoniae* infection. *Ann. N. Y. Acad. Sci.*, **143**, 801–812.

FEIZI, T. (1967b). Monotypic cold agglutinins in infection by *Mycoplasma pneumoniae. Nature (Lond.)*, **215**, 540–542.

FEIZI, T. (1969). Antibody heterogenicity of anti-I cold agglutinins as shown by cord cell studies. *Nature (Lond.)*, **222**, 1288–1289.

FEIZI, T. & DARRELL, J. H. (1966). Failure to demonstrate blocking of I antigen by *Mycoplasma pneumoniae in vitro* and *in vivo. Nature (Lond.)*, **211**, 1159–1160.

FEIZI, T., MACLEAN, H., SOMMERVILLE, R. G. &

SELWYN, J. G. (1966). The role of mycoplasmas in human disease. *Proc. roy. Soc. Med.*, **59**, 1109–1112.

FEIZI, T. & SCHUMACHER, M. (1968). Light chain homogeneity of post-infective cold agglutinins. *Clin. exp. Immunol.*, **3**, 923–929.

FEIZI, T. & TAYLOR-ROBINSON, D. (1967). Cold agglutinin anti-I and *Mycoplasma pneumoniae. Immunology*, **13**, 405–409.

FEIZI, T., TAYLOR-ROBINSON, D., SHIELDS, M. D. & CARTER, R. A. (1969). Production of cold agglutinins in rabbits immunized with human erythrocytes treated with *Mycoplasma pneumoniae. Nature (Lond.)*, **222**, 1253–1256.

FIALA, M., MYHRE, B. A., CHINH, L. T., TERRITO, M., EDGINGTON, T. S. & KATTLOVE, H. (1974). Pathogenesis of anemia associated with *Mycoplasma pneumoniae. Acta haemat. (Basel)*, **51**, 297–301.

FINLAND, M. & BARNES, M. W. (1951). Cold agglutinins. VII. Tests for cold isohemagglutinins in pneumonia and other acute respiratory infections over a four-year period. *Amer. J. med. Sci.*, **221**, 152–157.

FINLAND, M. & BARNES, M. W. (1954). Cold agglutinins. VIII. Occurrence of cold isohemagglutinins in patients with primary atypical pneumonia or influenza viral infection. *Arch. intern. Med.*, **101**, 462–466.

FINLAND, M., PETERSON, O. L., ALLEN, H. E., SAMPER, B. A., BARNES, M. W. & STONE, M. B. (1945a). Cold agglutinins. I. Occurrence of cold isohemagglutinins in various conditions. *J. clin. Invest.*, **24**, 451–457.

FINLAND, M., PETERSON, O. L., ALLEN, H. E., SAMPER, B. A. & BARNES, M. W. (1945b). Cold agglutinins. II. Cold isohemagglutinins in primary atypical pneumonia of unknown etiology with a note on the occurrence of hemolytic anemia in these cases. *J. clin. Invest.*, **24**, 458–473.

FLORMAN, A. L. & WEISS, A. B. (1945). Serologic reactions in primary atypical pneumonia. *J. Lab. clin. Med.*, **30**, 902–909.

GINSBERG, H. S. (1946). Acute hemolytic anemia in primary atypical pneumonia associated with high titer of cold agglutinins. *New Engl. J. Med.*, **234**, 826–828.

GIORDANO, A. S. & BLUM, L. L. (1937). Acute hemolytic anemia (Lederer type). *Amer. J. med. Sci.*, **194**, 311–326.

GROBBELAAR, B. G. (1957). Cold haemagglutination in primary atypical pneumonia. *S. Afr. med. J.*, **31**, 1069–1071.

HELWIG, F. C. & FREIS, E. D. (1943). Cold autohemagglutinins following atypical pneumonia producing the clinical picture of acrocyanosis. *J. Amer. med. Ass.*, **123**, 626–628.

HORSTMANN, D. M. & TATLOCK, H. (1943). Cold agglutinins: a diagnostic aid in certain types of primary atypical pneumonia. *J. Amer. med. Ass.*, **122**, 369–370.

JACOBSON, L. B., LONGSTRETH, G. F. & EDGINGTON, T. S. (1973). Clinical and immunologic features of transient cold agglutinin hemolytic anemia. *Amer. J. med.*, **54**, 514–521.

JANNEY, F. A., LEE, L. T. & HOWE, C. (1978). Cold hemagglutinin cross-reactivity with *Mycoplasma pneumoniae*. *Infection and Immunity*, **22**, 29–33.

JANSSON, E. & WAGER, O. (1964). Cold agglutinins in pneumonia. *Acta med. scand.*, **175**, 747–750.

JANSSON, E., WAGER, O., STENSTRÖM, R., KLEMOLA, F. & FORSSELL, P. (1964). Studies on Eaton PPLO pneumonia. *Brit. med. J.*, **i**, 142–145.

KIBUKAMUSOKE, J. W. & SOMERS, K. (1962). Haemolytic anaemia and venous gangrene. *Lancet*, **ii**, 1005–1007.

KÖNIG, A. L., KREFT, H., HENGGE, U., BRAUN, R. W. & ROELCKE, D. (1988). Co-existing anti-I and anti-Fl/Gd cold agglutinins in infections by *Mycoplasma pneumoniae*. *Vox Sang.*, **55**, 176–180.

KREIS, B. (1947). Les manifestations sérologiques de la pneumonie atypique primitive. *Rev. Hémat.*, **2**, 520–534.

KUMAR, S., SINGH, M. M. & BHATIA, B. B. (1958). Symmetrical peripheral gangrene in acquired hemolytic anemia. *Acta haemat. (Basel)*, **19**, 369–377.

LAWSON, D. H., LINDSAY, R. M., SAWERS, J. D., LUKE, R. G., DAVIDSON, J. F., WARDROP, C. J. & LINTON, A. L. (1968). Acute renal failure in the cold-agglutination syndrome. *Lancet*, **iii**, 704–705.

LIND, K. (1973). Production of cold agglutinins in rabbits induced by *Mycoplasma pneumoniae*, *Listeria monocytogenes* or *Streptococcus MG*. *Acta path. microbiol. scand. B*, **81**, 487–496.

LIND, P. E. & MCARTHUR, N. R. (1947). The distribution of 'T' agglutinins in human sera. *Aust. J. exp. Biol. med. Sci.*, **25**, 247–250.

LOOMES, L. M., UEMURA, K.-i., CHILDS, R. A., PAULSON, J. C., ROGERS, G. N., SCUDDER, P. R., MICHALSKI, J.-C., HOUNSELL, E. F., TAYLOR-ROBINSON, D. & FEIZI, T. (1984). Erythrocyte receptors for *Mycoplasma pneumoniae* are sialylated oligosaccharides of Ii antigen type. *Nature (Lond.)*, **307**, 560–563.

LOUIE, E. K., AULT, K. A., SMITH, B. R., HARDMAN, E. L. & QUEENSBERRY, P. J. (1985). IgG mediated haemolysis masquerading as cold agglutinin-induced anaemia complicating severe infection with *Mycoplasma pneumoniae*. *Scand. J. Haemat.*, **35**, 264–269.

MCNEIL, C. (1945). The relationship of cold agglutinins to the course of primary atypical pneumonia. *Amer. J. med. Sci.*, **209**, 48–54.

MAISEL, J. C. (1967). Fatal *Mycoplasma pneumoniae* infection with isolation of organisms from lung. *J. Amer. med. Ass.*, **202**, 287–290.

MEIKLEJOHN, G. (1943). The cold agglutinin test in the diagnosis of primary atypical pneumonia. *Proc. Soc. exp. Biol. Med.*, **54**, 181–184.

MOESCHLIN, S., SIEGENTHALER, W., GASSER, C. & HÄSSIG, A. (1954). Immunopancytopenia associated with incomplete cold hemagglutinins in a case of primary atypical pneumonia. *Blood*, **9**, 214–226.

MUFSON, M. A., MANKO, M. A., KINGSTON, J. R. & CHANOCK, R. M. (1961). Eaton agent pneumonia—clinical features. *J. Amer. med. Ass.*, **178**, 369–374.

NEELY, F. L., BARIA, W. H., SMITH, C. & STONE, C. F. JNR (1951). Primary atypical pneumonia with high titer of cold hemagglutinins, hemolytic anemia, and false positive Donath–Landsteiner test. *J. Lab. clin. Med.*, **37**, 382–387.

NIEJADLIK, D. C. & LOZNER, E. L. (1974). Cooling mattress induced acute hemolytic anemia. *Transfusion*, **14**, 145–147.

PARKER, F., JOLIFFE, L. S. & FINLAND, M. (1947). Primary atypical pneumonia; report of eight cases with autopsies. *Arch. Path.*, **44**, 581–608.

PEPINO, L. (1942). Gangrena acuta simmetrica Raynaud-simile in corso di polmonite crupale. *Minerva med. (Torino)*, **2**, 543–546.

PETERSON, O. L., HAM T. H. & FINLAND, M. (1943). Cold agglutinins (autohemagglutinins) in primary atypical pneumonias. *Science*, **97**, 167.

PISCIOTTA, A. V., DOWNER, E. & HINZ, J. (1955). Cold hemagglutination in acute and chronic hemolytic syndromes. *Blood*, **10**, 295–311.

PLATT, W. R. & WARD, D. S. JNR (1945). Cold isohemagglutinins. Their association with hemolytic anemia and multiple thromboses in primary atypical pneumonia. A brief review of the clinical and laboratory problems involved. *Amer. J. clin. Path.*, **15**, 202–209.

REIMANN, H. A. (1947). The viral pneumonias and pneumonias of probable viral origin. *Medicine (Baltimore)*, **26**, 167–219.

RØNNOR-JESSEN, V. (1950). Et tilfaelde af primaer atypisk pneumoni med haemolytisk anaemi og akrogangraen. *Ugeskr. Laeg.*, **112**, 1548–1551.

SACKS, M. S., WORKMAN, J. B. & JAHN, E. F. (1952). Diagnosis and treatment of acquired hemolytic anemia. *J. Amer. med. Ass.*, **150**, 1556–1559.

SAVONEN, K. (1948). Cold haemagglutination test and its clinical significance. *Ann. Med. exp. Fenn.*, **26** (Suppl. 3), 100 pp.

SCHMIDT, P. J., BARILE, M. F. & MCGINNISS, M. H. (1965). Mycoplasma (pleuropneumonia-like organisms) and blood group I; associations with neoplastic disease. *Nature (Lond.)*, **205**, 371–372.

SCHNEIDER, W. (1967). Zur Klinik und Serologie der Kälteantikörper (ein kasuistischer Beitrag). *Hippokrates (Stuttgart)*, **38**, 362–365.

SCHUBOTHE, H., MERZ, K. P., WEBER, S., DAHM, K., SCHMITZ, W. & ALTMANN, H. W. (1970). Akute autoimmunhämolytische Anämie vom Kälteantikörpertyp nach Mykoplasmapneumonie mit tödlichem Ausgang. *Acta haemat. (Basel)*, **44**, 111–123.

SHONE, S. & PASSMORE, R. (1943). Pneumonitis associated with autohaemagglutination. *Lancet*, **ii**, 445–446.

SIEGENTHALER, W. (1952). Ueber eine immunkörperbedingte hämolytische Anämie nach Viruspneumonie. *Schweiz. med. Wschr.*, **82**, 1100.

SMITH, C. B., McGINNISS, M. H. & SCHMIDT, P. J. (1967). Changes in erythrocyte I agglutinogen and anti-I agglutinins during *Mycoplasma pneumoniae* infection in man. *J. Immunol.*, **99**, 333–339.

SPRINGARN, C. L. & JONES, J. P. (1945). Cold hemagglutination in primary atypical pneumonia and other common infections. *Arch. intern. Med.*, **76**, 75–87.

STATS, D., WASSERMAN, L. R. & ROSENTHAL, N. (1948). Hemolytic anemia with hemoglobinuria. *Amer. J. clin. Path.*, **18**, 757–777.

STEWART, J. W. & FRIEDLANDER, P. H. (1957). Haemoglobinuria and acute haemolytic anaemia associated with primary atypical pneumonia. *Lancet*, **ii**, 774–775.

STREETER, G. A., FARMER, T. W. & HAYES, G. S. (1944). Cold hemagglutination in primary atypical pneumonia. *Bull. Johns Hopk. Hosp.*, **75**, 60–66.

SUSSMAN, S. J., MAGOFFIN, R. L., LENNETTE, E. H. & SCHIEBLE, J. (1966). Cold agglutinins, Eaton agent, and respiratory infections of children. *Pediatrics*, **38**, 571–577.

TURNER, J. C. (1943). Development of cold agglutinins in atypical pneumonia. *Nature (Lond.)*, **151**, 419.

TURNER, J. C. & JACKSON, E. B. (1943). Serological specificity of an auto-antibody in atypical pneumonia. *Brit. J. exp. Path.*, **24**, 121–126.

TURNER, J. C., NISNEWITZ, S., JACKSON, E. B. & BERNEY, R. (1943). Relation of cold agglutinins to atypical pneumonia. *Lancet*, **i**, 765–767.

WALSH, R. J. (1961). The concept of auto-immunisation in haematology. *N. Z. med. J.*, **60**, 253–256.

WHEELER, K. M., GALLAGHER, H. J. & STUART, C. A. (1939). An unusual case of autoagglutination. *J. Lab. clin. Med.*, **24**, 1135–1138.

WIENER, A. S., SAMWICK, A. A., MORRISON, M. & LOEWE, L. (1952). Acquired hemolytic anemia. *Amer. J. clin. Path.*, **22**, 301–312.

YOUNG, I. E. (1946). The clinical significance of cold hemagglutinins. *Amer. J. med. Sci.*, **211**, 23–39.

Auto-immune haemolytic anaemia (AIHA): cold-antibody syndromes IV: haemolytic anaemia following infectious mononucleosis and other viral infections

Early descriptions of haemolytic anaemia following infectious mononucleosis *313*

Recent descriptions *314*

Clinical features: a summary *314*
    Association with hereditary haemolytic anaemias *314*

Haematological findings *315*

Biochemical findings *315*
    Serum proteins *315*
    Serum bilirubin *316*
    Serum haptoglobins *316*

Serological findings *316*
    Antibodies against sheep erythrocytes *316*

Auto-antibodies against human erythrocytes: early observations *316*

Auto-antibodies against human erythrocytes: recent observations and the role of anti-i *318*
    Variation in the ability of sera from patients with haemolytic anaemia complicating infectious mononucleosis to agglutinate I and i erythrocytes *318*

Auto-antibodies with specificities other than anti-i causing haemolytic anaemia complicating infectious mononucleosis *319*
    'Anti-not-I' (anti-Pr) *319*
    Anti-N *319*

Auto-antibodies in infectious mononucleosis bringing about cold–warm (Donath–Landsteiner type) lysis *319*

Immunochemistry of cold auto-antibodies in infectious mononucleosis *320*
    Immunoglobulin class *320*

Auto-antibodies against leucocytes *321*

Treatment *321*

Raised cold-agglutinin titres and cold-antibody haemolytic anaemia associated with viral infections other than infectious mononucleosis *321*
    Adenovirus *322*
    Cytomegalovirus (CMV) *322*
    'Encephalitis' *322*
    Influenza viruses *322*
    Ornithosis *323*
    Rubella *323*
    Varicella *323*
    Cold agglutinins in acquired immune deficiency syndrome (AIDS) *323*

Acute transient AIHA of possibly infective origin apparently brought about by a non-complement-fixing cold antibody *324*

Raised cold-agglutinin titres and cold-antibody haemolytic anaemia associated with bacterial infections *324*
    Legionnaires' disease *325*
    Esch. coli infection *325*

EARLY DESCRIPTIONS OF HAEMOLYTIC ANAEMIA FOLLOWING INFECTIOUS MONONUCLEOSIS

According to Worlledge and Dacie's (1969) review at least 49 patients who had developed haemolytic anaemia as a complication of infectious mononucleosis had been described before it was found that anti-i played an important role in pathogenesis. Some of these early publications are listed below.

Dameshek (1943) had described a possible case (the patient had also received sulphadiazine); other patients who had developed haemolytic anaemia were reported by Riva (1946), Ellis, Wollenman and Stetson (1948), Petrides (1948), Appelman and Morrison (1949), Wilson, Ward and Gray (1949), Sawitsky, Papps and Wiener (1950), Small and Hadley (1950), Berté (1951), Huntington (1951), Mermann (1952), Hall and Archer (1953), Samuels (1953), Appelman and Gordon (1954), Punt and Verloop (1955), Thurm and Bassen (1955), Crosby and Rappaport (1956), Fordham (1956), Bean (1957), Evans and Weiser (1957), Di Piero and Arcangeli (1958) Ess, Gramlich and Mohring (1958), Hortemo (1958), Rossi (1958), Hyman (1959), Perrier and Rousso (1959), Schjøth (1959), Green and Goldenberg (1960) and Houk and McFarland (1961). It is interesting to note that only one such patient had been investigated in the author's laboratory between 1946 and 1960—a reflection of the comparative rarity of the condition.

Acute haemolytic anaemia developing in the course of infectious mononucleosis is now a well-recognized entity. Its incidence is, however, low; but taking into account the frequency of infectious mononucleosis it is of considerable clinical importance, and it has a relatively large literature. Dacie and Worlledge (1969) concluded that less than 1 in 1000 patients developed overt haemolysis, but conceded that minor degrees of increased haemolysis were possibly much more frequent. Hoagland (1967), in a personal study of 500 West Point cadets, had in fact reported an incidence of 3%. From the serological point of view, the finding in 1965 of the association of haemolysis with the formation of anti-i cold auto-antibodies has proved to be of particular interest.

Recent descriptions

Noteworthy accounts of patients who developed haemolytic anaemia associated with infectious mononucleosis include those of Smith, Abell and Cast (1963), Mengel, Wallace and McDaniel (1964), Fekete and Kerpelman (1965), Jenkins et al. (1965), Brafield (1966), Troxel, Innella and Cohen (1966), Casey and Main (1967), Deaton, Skaggs and Levin (1967), Hossaini (1970), Tonkin et al. (1973), Wilkinson, Petz and Garratty (1973), Wishart and Davey (1973), Bowman et al. (1974), Woodruff and McPherson (1976), Burkhart and Hsu (1979), Lee et al. (1980) and Gronemeyer et al. (1981).

CLINICAL FEATURES: A SUMMARY

As with haemolytic anaemia following mycoplasma pneumonia, haemolysis associated with infectious mononucleosis, although it may be severe, is typically transient and recovery may be expected within a few weeks. An exception to this is the history of Thurm and Bassen's (1955) Case 2: in this patient, a male aged 21, who also had moderately severe Mediterranean anaemia

(? thalassaemia intermedia), haemolysis lasted for at least 3 months.

The clinical features seem to be less uniform than in haemolytic anaemia following mycoplasma pneumonia. For one thing, although in most instances the signs of increased haemolysis have developed 1–2 weeks after the onset of the illness, this does not seem always to be so, and in some instances features of infectious mononucleosis and haemolytic anaemia appear to have developed simultaneously. Occasionally, however, haemolytic anaemia has first become obvious as late as 2 months after the initial symptoms.

The clinical symptoms and signs of infectious mononucleosis have been indefinite in many instances, although sore throat and enlargement of lymph nodes and the spleen have usually been found at some stage in the illness. Of the patients whose history had been reviewed by Worlledge and Dacie (1969), 28 out of 38 patients (74%) who developed haemolytic anaemia had a palpable spleen and 23 out of 31 (also 74%) had an enlarged liver.

Most of the patients who developed increased haemolysis were at first acutely ill, with high fever, and then became weak, anaemic and jaundiced. The patients of Ellis, Wollenman and Stetson (1948), Appelman and Morrison (1949), Crosby and Rappaport (1956), Green and Goldenberg (1960), Smith, Abell and Cast (1963), Wishart and Davey (1973) and Woodruff and McPherson (1976) had haemoglobinuria; in most reports the urine has been said to contain urobilin but not bile.

Association with hereditary haemolytic anaemias

Hereditary spherocytosis (HS). Several patients have been described who developed signs of overt haemolysis during an attack of infectious mononucleosis and were subsequently found to have been suffering from previously clinically inapparent or unimportant HS (Young, Izzo and Platzer, 1951, Case 10; Bean, 1957; DeNardo and Ray, 1963; Godal and Skaga, 1969; Gehlbach and Cooper, 1970; Taylor, 1973). Except in the case of DeNardo and Ray's (1963) patient, there was no evidence in the other patients that the increased haemolysis had been caused by an auto-immune mechanism. [Infections, perhaps of any type, are a well-known cause of exacerbation of haemolysis in HS (see Vol. 1 of this book, p. 141).]

Hereditary elliptocytosis. Ho-Yen (1978) described a 12-year-old girl with HE who developed a mild haemolytic anaemia associated with infectious mononucleosis. Blood films showed well-marked elliptocytosis as well as atypical lymphocytes. (The patient's father also had elliptocytic erythrocytes.) The DAT was positive with anti-C sera and the girl's serum contained an antibody which agglutinated i erythrocytes at 4°C to a titre of 128 and to titres of 16 and 4 at 21°C and 37°C, respectively. The patient's own cells were agglutinated at 4°C to a titre of 16 and at 21°C to a titre of 2, but they were not agglutinated at 37°C. The (anti-i) antibody was shown to be an IgM. The patient's heparinized blood, chilled at 4°C and then incubated at 37°C, was examined for evidence of erythrophagocytosis. Many more erythrophages (monocytes and neutrophils) were noted than in control samples (75 compared with two erythrophages per 10 000 cells).

HAEMATOLOGICAL FINDINGS

Anaemia. This is usually moderately severe, but a haemoglobin level as low as 3.2 g/dl was recorded by Tonkin et al. (1973). The reticulocyte count is typically raised commensurate with the haemoglobin level; however, reticulocytopenia may be present at the start of the illness (Crosby and Rappaport, 1956; Bowman et al. 1974; Woodruff and McPherson, 1976).

The 15-year-old youth described by Mengel, Wallace and McDaniel (1964) was unusual in that he appeared to become folate-deficient. His marrow was megaloblastic and the reticulocyte count was low (2.8%), He responded to folic acid.

Spherocytosis. This has quite often been reported, e.g. by Appelman and Morrison (1949), Green and Goldenburg (1960) and Tonkin et al. (1973). Increased osmotic fragility has less often been mentioned; it was, however, reported by Crosby and Rappaport (1956) in their Case 4.

Minor degrees of both spherocytosis and increased autohaemolysis have been reported in infectious mononucleosis uncomplicated by overt increased haemolysis. Kostinas and Cantow (1966) had investigated 41 consecutive patients with infectious mononucleosis. None had suffered from overt increased haemolysis, and the DAT had been negative in each case. Spherocytosis, the MCHC and autohaemolysis were assessed.

Thirty-three patients had a slight degree of spherocytosis (1–5% of cells, designated 1+); 14 had a moderate degree (5–10% of cells, designated 2+). The MCHC had exceeded 35% in 15 patients. The rate of autohaemolysis was above their normal range in 10 out of the 41 patients (24%). Usually (9 out of 12 cases) the increase in lysis was 'corrected' in the presence of glucose. The increase in autohaemolysis was found to correlate well with the presence of spherocytosis and with a raised MCHC, and Kostinas and Cantow concluded that occult haemolysis was a common event in infectious mononucleosis.

Auto-agglutination. This has only occasionally been mentioned, e.g. by Hall and Archer (1953) and Crosby and Rappaport (1956); it may, however, cause spurious macrocytosis in automated counts (Gleeson and McSherry, 1983). Erythrophagocytosis was described and illustrated by Bowman et al. (1974).

Leucocyte count. This varies but is usually above normal. A count as high as $42.6 \times 10^9/1$ was recorded by Green and Goldenberg (1960). A variable but often large proportion of the cells present are abnormal lymphocytes typical of infectious mononucleosis. Leucopenia (2.7×10^9 cells per litre) was reported by Smith, Abell and Cast (1963) in a patient in whom leucoagglutinins at low titre were detected in her serum.

Platelet count. This is often normal, but in some patients thrombocytopenia has accompanied increased haemolysis (Thurm and Bassen, 1955; Smith, Abell and Cast, 1963; Casey and Main, 1967). In Smith, Abell and Cast's patient antibodies against platelets were demonstrated by means of an antiglobulin consumption test.

BIOCHEMICAL FINDINGS

Serum proteins

Belfrage (1963), who had studied 107 cases of infectious mononucleosis, reported that the γ-globulin concentration was increased initially, i.e. at diagnosis, in about 80% of cases and reached a maximum at about 2–3 weeks after the onset, at a time when the heterophile-antibody titre was also at its highest. The increase in γ globulin was found to persist for 3 months in about 50% of cases; it was described as being electrophoretically heterogeneous, i.e. polyclonal.

Wollheim and Williams (1966) reported data

for IgG, IgM and IgA separately, based on studies carried out on 36 students at the University of Minnesota: the mean concentration of IgG was approximately 50% above the normal mean; that of IgM was approximately 100% above, and IgA was not increased. Wollheim and Williams showed by measuring the IgM levels in sera before and after absorption with i and sheep erythrocytes that the two corresponding antibodies accounted for only 1–5% of the increase in IgM.

Further data were reported by Wollheim (1968), this time based on 45 patients studied at Malmö, Sweden. γM was shown to reach its highest levels (mean 286% of the normal mean) 1–20 days after the clinical onset of the disease and γG to reach its peak (mean 163% of the normal mean) somewhat later (10–30 days after the onset). γA was found to increase also and to reach its peak (158% of the normal mean) at about the same time as γG, but to fall more rapidly to normal levels. There was no apparent correlation between γM levels and anti-i titres, and none of the patients studied had had overtly increased haemolysis.

In patients who have developed haemolytic anaemia as a complication the serum Ig levels seem seldom to have been measured. However, Houk and McFarland (1961) reported a γ-globulin concentration of 2.25 g/dl, and Deaton, Skaggs and Levin (1967) an IgM level as high as 960 mg/dl—eight times the control value, with normal IgG and IgA levels. The heterophile antibody titre (229 376!) was extremely high in this case and the anti-i titre at 5°C 1024. Woodruff and McPherson (1976) recorded an IgM level of 510 mg/dl.

Serum bilirubin. As in other haemolytic anaemias, the serum bilirubin concentration is raised in patients with infectious mononucleosis who have developed overt haemolysis. The rises probably reflect both haemolysis and impaired liver function. According to Finch (1969), the serum bilirubin is slightly raised in 30–50% of cases even in the absence of overt haemolysis; however, the total bilirubin level is usually less than 3 mg/dl.

Serum haptoglobins. According to Nyman (1959), low serum haptoglobulin levels and even ahaptoglobulinaemia are commonly found in infectious mononucleosis. Thus out of 246 ahaptoglobulinaemic sera, 11 were from patients with infectious mononucleosis. It was not clear, however, whether the absence was attributable to increased haemolysis or hepato-cellular damage or both mechanisms.

SEROLOGICAL FINDINGS

Antibodies against sheep erythrocytes

Heterophile agglutinins at high or very high titres have been present in the sera of all the patients at some time in their illness, and their titre has often been shown to fall as the patient recovered. When tested, the antibodies have been shown *not* to be absorbed by guinea-pig kidney but to be absorbed by ox cells—findings characteristic of infectious monocleosis.

Auto-antibodies against human erythrocytes: early observations

The results of tests for auto-antibodies have been far less uniform than those for heterophile antibodies. The reports of early investigators were described by the author (Dacie, 1962, p. 536) as divergent and confusing, with no single pattern standing out. They were, however, of considerable interest; and a summary of some of these findings is reproduced below.

Dameshek (1943) reported that an auto-agglutinin was present in the serum of his patient which was most active at room and ice-box temperature. Appelman and Morrison (1949), on the other hand, stated that tests for cold agglutinins and the Donath–Landsteiner test were negative. Sawitsky, Papps and Wiener (1950) reported that both the direct and indirect antiglobulin tests were positive, and Huntington (1951) stated that the direct test was positive. Mermann (1952), on the other hand, observed a rise in the cold-agglutinin titre of his patient's serum from 128 to 2084. Hall and Archer (1953) reported the presence of auto-agglutination and mentioned that the DAT was positive.

Additional reports in which the DAT was stated to be positive include those of Samuels (1953), Crosby and Rappaport (1956), Fordham (1956),

Ess, Gramlich and Mohring (1958), Hortemo (1958), Perrier and Rousso (1959) and Green and Goldenberg (1960), while reports in which the reaction was stated to have been negative include those of Punt and Verloop (1955), Thurm and Bassen (1955), Evans and Weiser (1957), Bean (1957) and Di Piero and Arcangeli (1958).

Cold agglutinins at a moderate titre (128 at 15°C), which disappeared on recovery, were reported by Punt and Verloop (1955), and auto-agglutination which prevented blood grouping and a cold-agglutin titre of 64 were mentioned by Crosby and Rappaport (1956). A rise in agglutinin titre against trypsinized erythrocytes, followed by a fall, was observed by Di Piero and Arcangeli (1958) and a cold-agglutinin titre of 256 at 3°C by Green and Goldenberg (1960).

The observations of Ellis, Wollenman and Stetson (1948), Evans and Weiser (1957), Ess, Gramlich and Mohring (1958) and Rossi (1958) were extensive and important.

The history of Ellis, Wollenman and Stetson's patient suggested mycoplasma pneumonia, but the blood picture was in favour of a diagnosis of infectious mononucleosis; the antibody appeared to resemble the Donath–Landsteiner antibody.

Their patient was a man aged 21 years who was admitted into hospital with a history of having passed 'bloody' urine for the previous 8 days, and of having become weak and breathless upon exertion. Two weeks previously he had had an upper respiratory tract infection, associated with headache and anorexia, for which he had had no treatment.

On examination he was found to be pale and slightly icteric. The liver and spleen were just palpable and were tender. An enlarged lymph node was palpable in the left auricular region, but elsewhere his lymph nodes did not seem to be enlarged. His temperature was 99.4°F.

The day following admission an acute haemolytic episode developed; haemoglobinuria was intense and the patient's haemoglobin fell from 12.1 g/dl to 5.9 g/dl in 5 hours. The total leucocyte count rose to $24.3 \times 10^9/l$, 64% of the cells being lymphocytes similar to those seen in infectious mononucleosis. Agglutinins against sheep erythrocytes were present to a titre of 1024. Cold agglutinins against adult human group-O cells were also present, their titre at 4°C being 256. Agglutination also took place at room temperature and this did not completely disperse at 37°C. Normal

human erythrocytes suspended in fresh patient's serum and chilled at 4°C underwent lysis when subsequently incubated at 37°C (a positive Donath–Landsteiner test). This test was still positive 7 weeks later at a time when the patient had practically recovered; it was negative when repeated 2 years later. The Wassermann and Kahn tests were negative. The patient was critically ill for 2 week during which time he was transfused with 7 litres of blood. Eventually he made a complete recovery.

Evans and Weiser's (1957) observations on two patients were largely negative but are of great interest nevertheless. The erythrocytes of the first patient gave at the most a trace of agglutination in antiglobulin serum, which disappeared later, and trypsinized normal cells were also weakly, but transitorily, agglutinated at 37°C in the patient's undiluted serum. The tests were entirely negative with the cells and serum of the second patient. Evans and Weiser concluded that the haemolysis was unlikely to be due to the direct effect of a virus. They concluded that an auto-antibody of unusual type, not readily demonstrable by the currently available tests, was more likely to be responsible.

Rossi (1958) reported on some detailed studies carried out in the author's laboratory on the patient whose history was reported by Hyman (1959). This patient, a boy aged 16, was admitted into hospital with a fortnight's history of pyrexia, enlarged lymph nodes and jaundice. On admission, his haemoglobin was 6.5 g/dl, the reticulocyte count was 39%, and total leucocytes $7 \times 10^9/l$, including atypical lymphocytes. The Paul–Bunnell test was positive to a titre of 5120.

Rossi found that the DAT was negative with the standard sera used but was weakly positive, using glycerol-preserved cells, when carried out subsequently using an antiglobulin serum prepared against the patient's own whole serum. No abnormal anti-human erythrocyte antibodies could be demonstrated using albumin, the IAT or trypsinized cells. Rossi, however, found that the patient's erythrocytes were insensitive, compared with normal cells, to sensitization by incomplete anti-D or by the warm auto-antibodies in the sera of certain AIHA patients or by warm-antibody-containing eluates derived from their cells.

Rossi's results, unless explained by the high proportion of possibly insensitive reticulocytes present in the original specimen of patient's blood tested, suggested that the patient's erythrocytes may have been 'coated' by an unusual type of 'blocking' auto-antibody.

Ess, Gramlich and Mohring (1958) and Ess and Friederici (1958) described a dramatic rise in cold-agglutinin titre in a 31-year-old man diagnosed as suffering from a lymphotropic virus infection (? infectious mononucleosis). The antibody titre at its maximum was recorded as >128 000 at 4°C, 512 at 22°C, 8 at 34°C and 4 at 37°C. It was shown to cause lysis of normal erythrocytes in acidified serum (pH 6.5) at 22°C. The specificity of the antibody was not determined. It persisted in the patient's serum for at least 11 months; its presence was accompanied by an increase in serum γ_1 globulin.

AUTO-ANTIBODIES AGAINST HUMAN ERYTHROCYTES: RECENT OBSERVATIONS AND THE ROLE OF ANTI-i

The finding that the sera of patients with infectious mononucleosis quite frequently contained a cold antibody that agglutinated cord-blood erythrocytes more strongly than adult cells, i.e. was anti-i in specificity, provided a new approach to the investigation of patients with infectious mononucleosis complicated by haemolytic anaemia.

The association of anti-i antibodies with infectious mononucleosis was described independently in 1965 in the U.K. and in the U.S.A.

Jenkins and his co-workers (1965) reported that the serum of an 18-year-old girl with infectious mononucleosis complicated by a severe haemolytic anaemia contained a cold antibody which agglutinated at 12°C cord-blood erythrocytes more strongly than adult cells. The titres were: OI cells 8; O cord cells 128; Ai cells 64 and AI cells 8. Cynamolgus monkey cells were agglutinated to a titre of 512. The DAT was strongly positive: it was of the non-γ type. Absorption experiments showed that the heterophile antibody that was present (titre 33 000) and the cold autoantibody were distinct entities. This observation led Jenkins et al. to test the serum of 85 other patients who had uncomplicated infectious mononucleosis for anti-i. It was present in seven of them (8%). The titre was low in all but one patient in whom there was evidence of hepatocellular damage: in this case the titre was 80. Jenkins et al. suggested that the development of anti-i reflected proliferation of reticulo-endothelial tissues.

Calvo and co-workers (1965) reported in an abstract that they had identified an anti-i agglutinin in the serum of a 16-year-old girl with thalassaemia trait who had developed infectious mononucleosis complicated by haemolytic anaemia. The DAT was positive with anti-C sera. The anti-i antibody in her serum was shown to be IgM and to be distinct from the heterophile antibody also present. The patient's own erythrocytes were agglutinated by both anti-i and anti-I sera. Their reaction with anti-i became stronger during convalescence parallel with the reduction in strength of the positive DAT. Subsequently, similar anti-i agglutinins were found in the sera of 23 out of 38 unselected patients with infectious mononucleosis. Further details of these investigations were reported by Rosenfield et al. (1965).

Costea, Yakulis and Heller (1966) reported that the serum of seven out of 30 patients with infectious mononucleosis agglutinated cord erythrocytes to a titre of 40 or more 'in the cold'.

Deaton, Skaggs and Levin (1967) recorded an anti-i titre of 1024 in a 16-year-old girl. Her haemoglobin dropped to 5 g/dl with up to 13% reticulocytes. The non-gamma DAT was negative. Deaton, Skaggs and Levin reviewed the serological literature then available and suggested that the negative DAT in their case might have been due to depletion of complement during the 7–10 days of haemolysis before the test was carried out.

Worlledge and Dacie (1969) reported that they had tested the sera of 30 patients with infectious mononucleosis and had found that 14 of the sera (47%) agglutinated cord erythrocytes at 4°C to a titre of 32. Hossaini (1970) reported finding anti-i in the serum of 35 out of 52 patients (69%) with infectious mononucleosis. Using cord-blood cells, the agglutinin titres at 4°C were <16 in 28 of them; seven had titres of 32–64, one a titre of 256. Twelve patients were retested 4–6 weeks after the onset of their symptoms: anti-i had disappeared in each case.

Horwitz and co-workers (1977) tested the sera of 157 patients with infectious mononucleosis: 32% of the sera contained anti-i agglutinins compared with 0.3% of 1022 controls (500 healthy adults, 22 hospital employees and 500 patients in whom tests for heterophile antibodies were negative).

Variation in the ability of sera from patients with haemolytic anaemia complicating infectious mononucleosis to agglutinate I and i erythrocytes

Worlledge and Dacie (1969) described their

findings in four patients. Agglutinin titrations were carried out using I-positive adult erythrocytes and i cord cells. The results are shown in Table 31.1. All four antibodies reacted as anti-i but I cells were agglutinated, too, although to lower titres. Patients 1 and 2 had mild easily compensated haemolysis; patients 3 and 4, whose antibodies were more active at 28°C, suffered from active haemolysis and became anaemic.

Wilkinson, Petz and Garratty (1973) also emphasized how variable the antibody pattern might be. They cited three patients. The serological findings in the first patient were considered to be characteristic: his serum agglutinated cord i erythrocytes to a titre of 512 at 4°C and to titres of 64 at 22°C and 4 at 31°C; it also agglutinated adult I cells to a titre of 64 at 4°C and 2 at 22°C. The two other patients had formed anti-i antibodies but they were of low titre at 4°C and did not cause agglutination at 22°C. Both patients had, however, formed also cold-reacting anti-IgG antibodies, but only one reacted at room temperature (27°C).

Woodruff and McPherson (1976) described a patient who had developed severe intravascular haemolysis leading to haemoglobinuria whose antibody pattern was unusual. His serum agglutinated both i cord and I adult cells to titres at 4°C of 128 and 64, respectively; at room temperature the titres were 16 and 32, and at 37°C 0 and 4. On recovery, the reaction with I cells fell more slowly than with i cells.

Table 31.1 Anti-i titres in the sera of four patients with infectious mononucleosis complicated by haemolytic anaemia

Patient	Erythrocytes	Titre of serum giving + agglutination after 2 hours incubation at			
		4°C	20°C	28°C	37°C
1	Adult I	32	4	0	0
	Cord-blood i	512	16	8	0
2	Adult I	64	2	0	0
	Cord-blood i	512	16	8	2
3	Adult I	32	16	4	0
	Cord-blood i	256	128	64	8
4	Adult I	128	8	2	0
	Cord-blood i	512	64	16	0

Patients 1 and 2 developed compensated haemolysis; patients 3 and 4 became anaemic.
[Data from Worlledge and Dacie (1969).]

AUTO-ANTIBODIES WITH SPECIFICITIES OTHER THAN ANTI-i CAUSING HAEMOLYTIC ANAEMIA COMPLICATING INFECTIOUS MONONUCLEOSIS

'Anti-not-I' (anti-Pr)

Brafield (1966), in a letter, described a young man with infectious mononucleosis and haemolytic anaemia whose serological findings were most unusual. He was found to have formed a high-titre high-thermal-amplitude cold auto-antibody the specificity of which, in contrast to the reports listed above, appeared to be neither that of anti-i nor anti-I. The titre at 2°C was 20 480, at room temperature 1280, and at 30°C 10. The antibody reacted similarly with a large range of erythrocytes including cord, adult Oi and Bombay cells. Agglutination was strikingly reduced by prior exposure of the test cells to ficin or papain; it was markedly sensitive, too, to pH: at 12°C and pH 5.0 the titre was 10 240; at pH 7.2 it was 160, and at pH 9.0 30. Jenkins and Marsh (1966), in commenting on the specificity of Brafield's antibody, pointed out that this seemed to be the same as that they had described as 'anti-not-I' (see p. 265).

Anti-N

As already referred to on p. 270, Bowman and co-workers (1974) described finding an auto-anti-N in the serum of a patient who was suffering from haemolytic anaemia following infectious mononucleosis.

Auto-antibodies in infectious mononucleosis bringing about cold–warm (Donath–Landsteiner type) lysis

As referred to earlier (p. 317), Ellis, Wollenman and Stetson (1948) had described a patient who had developed intravascular haemolysis in whom the Donath–Landsteiner (D–L) reaction had been positive for at least 7 weeks, and, as also referred to earlier (p. 314), Wishart and Davey (1973) had described a similar occurrence. Their patient was a 17-year-old male. His serum contained a high-thermal-amplitude cold antibody which agglutinated erythrocytes to a titre of 256 in the cold; it also caused agglutination at room temperature, and the agglutinates did not disperse entirely at 37°C. The antibody did not appear to have any identifiable specificity. The D–L reaction was positive, and it remained so for at least 7 weeks. The Wassermann reaction was also transitorily positive; other tests for syphilis were, however, negative.

Burkhart and Hsu (1979) described a further patient, a 23-year-old man, in whom the D–L reaction was positive. In this case the antibody in his serum was identified as an anti-i and to be an IgM globulin. The titre at 4°C with i (cord) erythrocytes was 16 384 and with I cells 512. At 22°C the titre with the i cells was 64; at 32°C it was zero. The cold–warm (4–37°C) procedure using i cells was positive to a titre of 64. The DAT was positive with anti-C3 and anti-C4 sera: it was negative with anti-IgG sera. The IAT was positive at 4°C and 22°C with anti-IgM and anti-IgA sera but it was negative with anti-IgG sera; in the presence of fresh serum, complement was fixed. A rheumatoid-like factor was present, but its removal did not affect the ability of the serum to agglutinate or lyse i cells.

IMMUNOCHEMISTRY OF COLD AUTO-ANTIBODIES IN INFECTIOUS MONONUCLEOSIS

Immunoglobulin class

Both IgM and IgG antibodies have been described and also cold-reactive IgM rheumatoid-like factors (anti-antibodies) which, reacting with IgG antibodies, act as a complex cold agglutinin.

Mullinax and co-workers (1966) gave a brief account of a young man who developed severe haemolytic anaemia associated with infectious mononucleosis. The DAT was positive with anti-C sera only. At 20°C, however, the IAT was positive with anti-IgG, anti-IgM as well as with anti-C sera. An anti-i antibody caused massive agglutination at 4°C. A cryoprecipitate formed when his serum was chilled: when solubilized at room temperature it was found to contain IgG, IgM and complement (C) components, of sedimentation constants 7, 18.2 and 30.4. Eluates from erythrocytes sensitized by serum at 4°C also contained IgG, IgM and C components. The serum contained a rheumatoid-like factor, and Mullinax et al.

concluded that the auto-agglutination and in-vivo haemolysis may have been brought about by fixation to erythrocytes of a complement-fixing 7S–19S complex.

Goldberg and Barnett (1967) reported that an antibody eluted from the erythrocytes of a patient with haemolytic anaemia complicating infectious mononucleosis consisted of both γM and γG components; they also found that both components were required to be present for agglutination to take place and that normal γM or γG could not be substituted for one of these components. The patient's serum agglutinated Rh-sensitized erythrocytes to a titre of 1024 at 4°C; and Goldberg and Barnett suggested that the γM component was a cold anti-antibody which reacted with the γG component. The patient's whole serum agglutinated normal I-positive erythrocytes strongly at 4°C (titre 128): cord cells were in contrast only weakly agglutinated. The antibody thus (surprisingly) had anti-I specificity. The agglutinin titre (with I-positive cells) was significantly reduced by adding either anti-γG or anti-γM to the serum or eluate. The IAT, using anti-γG serum, was 1024 at 4°C and 2 at 37°C.

Capra and co-workers (1968, 1969) reported findings similar to those described by Goldberg and Barnett (1967), i.e. that cold-reactive γG auto-antibodies might be developed by patients who had contracted infectious mononucleosis. In the patients they themselves had investigated, the specificity of the antibodies was, however, anti-i — not anti-I as in Goldberg and Barnett's patient. Their initial patient was a 20-year-old woman whose serum agglutinated cord erythrocytes at 4°C to a titre of 1000 and adult cells to a titre of 4. After the serum had been fractionated its anti-i activity could only be demonstrated if the 7S and 19S fractions were pooled. Subsequently, the same techniques were applied to 50 more sera from patients suffering from infectious mononucleosis: 19S complete anti-i agglutinins were present in 35%, 7S incomplete anti-i in 90%, 19S cold-reactive anti-γ-globulin in 72%, and mixed 7S anti-i plus 19S anti-γ-globulin (which only cause agglutination when both antibodies are present) in 66%.

Capra et al. concluded that although 19S anti-i may be produced by some patients, in many instances the 19S is a cold-reactive anti-γ-globulin reacting with incomplete (7S) anti-i. The 7S anti-i seemed, too, to be more important clinically than the 19S anti-i. Thus of the five sera with the highest 7S anti-i titres, four had been derived from patients with haemolytic anaemia and the fifth from a patient with thrombocytopenic purpura.

A further patient suffering from infectious mononucleosis and haemolytic anaemia who had formed an incomplete IgG anti-i of low thermal range and a cold IgM rheumatoid-like factor was described by Gronemeyer et al. (1981). The DAT was strongly positive with anti-C sera but doubtful or negative with anti-IgG sera. The cold-agglutinin titre at 4°C with cord i cells was 2560, falling to 128 at 24°C and zero at 37°C; with I cells the titres were 256 at 4°C and zero at 24°C. Fractionation of the patient's serum allowed the IgG fraction and IgM fraction to be tested separately and in combination. The IgG fraction failed to agglutinate i erythrocytes at 4°C and only sensitized them moderately strongly to agglutination by an anti-IgG serum at that temperature. At 24°C there was no agglutination in either procedure. In contrast, the IgM fraction agglutinated i erythrocytes to a titre of 20 at 4°C and the IgG and IgM fractions when present together agglutinated the i cells to a titre of 160. The IgM (rheumatoid) fraction, although most active at a low temperature, was able to react at 37°C.

Auto-antibodies against leucocytes

Lalezari and Murphy (1967) described finding cold antibodies capable of agglutinating at 4°C normal leucocytes in 17 plasma samples from patients with infectious mononucleosis that contained anti-i erythrocyte agglutinins. The reactions were temperature-sensitive; at 22°C only seven out of the 17 plasma samples agglutinated the test leucocytes; at 30°C only one sample. Lalezari and Murphy also stated that weak auto-agglutination of leucocytes was demonstrable at 4°C (but not at 22°C) by their technique in 25% of normal individuals.

TREATMENT

As already mentioned, early spontaneous recovery may be confidently expected in haemolytic anaemia complicating infectious mononucleosis and where haemolysis is of only moderate intensity and adequately compensated for by the patient no treatment seems necessary. In more serious cases corticosteroids should be given exactly as in idiopathic AIHA (see p. 496). Transfusion should be reserved for the most seriously ill patients, but as the transfused blood may be expected to have a very short survival [e.g. $^{51}Cr\ T_{50}$ 4 days and 6 days, respectively, in Evans and Weiser's (1957) two patients], benefit will be transitory.

Splenectomy need not normally be contemplated — spontaneous recovery should make consideration of this unnecessary. This has, however, been carried out at least twice, by Wilson, Ward and Gray (1949) and in Case 2 of Thurm and Bassen (1955). The latter patient was, however, exceptional for he was known to have Mediterranean anaemia (thalassaemia minor) and the complicating infectious mononucleosis appeared to initiate a hypersplenic syndrome. Splenectomy was undertaken with some benefit after the illness had lasted 3 months, during which time the patient had received six transfusions.

RAISED COLD-AGGLUTININ TITRES AND COLD-ANTIBODY HAEMOLYTIC ANAEMIA ASSOCIATED WITH VIRAL INFECTIONS OTHER THAN INFECTIOUS MONONUCLEOSIS

As already referred to on p. 31, there is much circumstantial evidence for the occasional development of transient, usually acute, haemolytic anaemia following a variety of viral infections. Although in most cases warm auto-antibodies have appeared to be responsible,[*] in a minority high-titre cold auto-antibodies have been identified (see below).

In addition to the small number of patients who form cold antibodies transiently and do in fact suffer from increased haemolysis, there are other patients — the great majority — in whom the formation of cold antibodies following an infection is not overtly harmful. The reason for this is not wholly understood, but the nature and concentration of the antibodies and their thermal range, and their complement-

---

[*]Patients who have developed AIHA of the warm-antibody variety, apparently closely following a viral infection, are referred to on p. 336 in Chapter 33 when the role of viruses in the aetiology of AIHA is discussed.

fixing ability, are all important factors (see p. 429).

Adenovirus

As already mentioned (p. 301), Lawson and co-workers (1968) described two patients with acute cold-antibody haemolytic anaemia who developed acute renal failure. The first patient had had mycoplasma pneumonia, the second patient, a woman aged 64, had also had a lung infection. Her haemoglobin was 4.0 g/dl, leucocyte count $51 \times 10^9/l$ and blood urea 570 mg/dl. Her blood underwent intense auto-agglutination at room temperature and the DAT was positive. Viral studies showed that she had had a recent adenovirus infection, with a rise in antibody titre from < 8 to 64; there was no rise in titre against *Mycoplasma pneumoniae*. The patient was kept warm, dialysed and transfused with blood warmed to 37°C and eventually made a complete recovery.

Cytomegalovirus (CMV)

Infection with CMV is now recognized as a possible cause of haemolytic anaemia, and in some at least of the cases that have been reported a raised titre of cold agglutinins has been recorded.

Kantor and co-workers (1970) recorded the clinical and immunological findings in 10 patients who had developed post-perfusion CMV infection; three of them developed transient haemolytic anaemia. The DAT was positive in two out of seven patients tested, and the cold-agglutinin titre was raised in two patients (512 and 2048). Cryoglobulins were present in two patients and rheumatoid factors in three patients.

Reller (1973) described a patient who developed granulomatous hepatitis in association with CMV infection. This was associated with mild haemolysis: the packed-cell volume fell to 30% and the reticulocyte count rose to 6%. The cold-agglutinin titre rose from 16 to 512 during the course of the illness; the antibody was identified as anti-I.

Berlin, Chandler and Green (1977) described a patient suffering from spontaneously developing acute CMV infection who developed mild haemolysis. Her haemoglobin fell to 8.3 g/dl and the reticulocyte count rose to 5.6%. The DAT was negative. However, an anti-i agglutinin had developed: the IAT (at an unspecified temperature) rose to a titre of 128 with cord-blood (i) erythrocytes and remained steady at a titre of 8 with adult group-O cells.

Horwitz and co-workers (1984) described two patients with spontaneously developing CMV infection in whom increased haemolysis was an important feature of their illness. The haemoglobin of the first patient, a young woman aged 18, fell to 5.2 g/dl; numerous microcytes, spherocytes and normoblasts were present in blood films, and also atypical lymphocytes. The reticulocyte count, which was at first low (0.4–2.3%), eventually rose to 13.6%. A high-thermal-amplitude cold agglutinin was present: its titre at 4°C was 112 (with both cord-blood and adult cells); at 25°C, the titres were 56 and at 37°C, 7 with cord cells and 14 with adult cells. The plasma haemoglobin was raised, and the ^{51}Cr T_{50} with the most compatible donor blood was as short as 5.5 days. The DAT was positive with an anti-IgG serum but not with an anti-C3 serum. The second patient of Horwitz et al. was not so severely affected. His minimum haemoglobin was 8.8 g/dl and maximum reticulocyte count 11.3%. Occasional spherocytes and many abnormal lymphocytes were noted in blood films. The DAT was negative and cold agglutinins were not present at a raised titre.

Horwitz et al. also reviewed 20 additional patients with CMV-mononucleosis who had been studied in their laboratory during an 11-year period. They concluded that there had been evidence for subclinical increased haemolysis in at least 50%. DATs had been carried out on 10 patients and the test had been positive in three of them (in two with anti-IgG and anti-C sera and in one with an anti-C serum alone). Ten of the 20 patients had had cold-agglutinin titres exceeding 56, the highest titre being 1792; seven of the cold agglutinins were anti-I, one was anti-I plus anti-Pr and two were 'not Ii'. The lowest haemoglobin recorded was 10.6 g/dl, and eleven of the patients had had reticulocyte counts exceeding 2.5%, the maximum being 11.1%.

'Encephalitis'

Unger, Wiener and Dolan (1952) reported the occurrence of haemolytic anaemia in an infant born with signs of encephalitis. Cold agglutinins were present in the child's serum to titres exceeding 1000 units. No abnormal antibodies were found in the mother's serum.

Influenza viruses

Laroche and co-workers (1951) described a patient who developed an acute haemolytic episode in the course of influenzal pneumonia.

Serological tests indicated influenza type-A infection. The onset of the patient's anaemia was associated with the formation of high-titre cold antibodies. Ventura and Aresu (1957) reported a similar case. Their patient was acutely ill and developed haemoglobinuria and was found to have formed high-titre high-thermal-amplitude lytic cold auto-antibodies. Influenza was not proved serologically, but the illness occurred during an outbreak of 'Asiatic' influenza from which the patient's brother had suffered a few days previously.

According to Eyquem and co-workers (1953), infection with influenza viruses is a common cause of raised cold-agglutinin titres. Of 54 patients resident in or near Paris who had suffered from pulmonary infections in 1950 and 1951 and whose sera contained cold agglutinins at abnormally high titres, 21 gave positive Hirst reactions for influenza viruses.

Ornithosis

Vanherweghem, DeJonghe and van Geel (1977) described the occurrence of fever, pulmonary infection and transient acute haemolysis in a woman aged 37 who had apparently contracted ornithosis from a budgerigar which had died 15 days previously. Her haematocrit fell from 30% to 15% in 2 days and the reticulocyte count reached 17%. There was temporary renal impairment. The cold-agglutinin titre was 1000 and lysis *in vitro* was demonstrated up to 32°C. A rise and subsequent fall in antibody titre against ornithosis virus was demonstrated; tests for Coxsackie virus, mycoplasma, and Q fever and VDRL and Paul–Bunnell tests were negative.

Rubella

Geisen and co-workers (1975) reported the formation of high-titre cold agglutinins in a 19-year-old patient following an attack of rubella. There appeared to be mild compensated increased haemolysis: the haemoglobin was 15.3 g/dl, reticulocyte count 3.7% and serum bilirubin 0.9 mg/dl. The cold-agglutinin titre reached 8000 following the subsidence of the skin eruption; it fell to normal within the next 20 weeks. The antibody was an IgM, and was shown to be capable of bringing about lysis *in vitro* at pH 6.5. It appeared to be a monoclonal protein with only kappa light chains demonstable. Its specificity was anti-Pr.

Varicella

Northoff, Martin and Roelcke (1987) described the occurrence of a transient attack of acute haemolysis affecting a 43-year-old woman who was suffering from a pustulous skin infection diagnosed clinically and serologically as varicella. Her haemoglobin fell from 14.4 to 11.1 g/dl, and in her serum a cold antibody was present which had anti-Pr_{1h} specificity; it was IgG in type, had kappa light chains and appeared to be monotypic. The DAT was positive with anti-C sera but negative with anti-IgG, -IgA and -IgM sera. The patient's serum agglutinated all erythrocytes tested at 22°C, but not at 37°C; the antibody titre at 0°C was 256. In confirmation of the diagnosis of varicella, the patient's 15-year-old daughter developed all the signs of varicella a few days after her mother had been admitted to hospital.

Cold agglutinins in acquired immune deficiency syndrome (AIDS)

Several reports have indicated that raised cold-agglutinin titres are a frequent feature of AIDS. To what extent the increased titres are due to infection with HIV directly or to opportunistic infection with CMV, EB virus or other agents seems to be uncertain.

McGinniss and co-workers (1986) described their findings in 28 hospitalized AIDS patients of whom 25 had Kaposi sarcoma and 14 had *Pneumocystis carinii* pneumonia or were infected with *Mycobacterium avium intracellulare* or other opportunistic organism. Tests for CMV were positive in 25 patients, and 16 out of 16 were infected with EB virus. Eighteen out of 25 patients had formed anti-i and in three patients the anti-i was active at 37°C; their haemoglobin ranged between 7.2 and 9.2 g/dl. Nine of the 28 patients had formed an auto-anti-U antibody, demonstrable by the use of enzyme-treated erythrocytes. One patient's serum contained a strongly-reacting anti-U as well as a weak panagglutinin, and in this patient the DAT was strongly positive with an anti-IgG serum. He had the lowest haemoglobin (7.2 g/dl) of the whole series, and anti-U could be eluted from his erythrocytes.

Pruzanski and co-workers (1986) reported on studies carried out on 81 patients positive for HTLV-III antibody: 19 had AIDS, 20 chronic lymphadenopathy syndrome (CLS), 10 AIDS-related complex (ARC) and 32 were free of symptoms. Cold agglutinins at raised titres (>64) were present in four of the AIDS patients, in four of the CLS patients, in two of the ARC patients, and in two of the symptom-free patients. The highest titre recorded was 2048 at 4°C (in a CLS patient). Seven of the antibodies were anti-I, four anti-i, and one anti-GD. In 11 out of 12 patients the antibodies persisted at raised titres for 6 months or more. Pruzanski et al. concluded that their experience suggested that the enhanced cold-agglutinin titres were associated with the HTLV-III infection rather than with intercurrent infections.

Lima and co-workers (1986), commenting on the report of Pruzanski et al. (1986) summarized above, referred to their own observations on 40 drug-addicted patients positive for HIV: one had AIDS, five CLS, eight ARC and 26 were symptom-free. Anti-i cold agglutinins were present in five of these patients. Tests showed that none of them was infected with a mycoplasma, CMV or EB virus.

Acute transient AIHA of possibly infective origin apparently brought about by a non-complement-fixing cold antibody

Donovan and co-workers (1983) described what must be a very rare occurrence: namely, acute haemolysis associated with livedo reticularis brought about by a high-thermal-amplitude cold auto-antibody which apparently did not have the capacity to fix complement. Their patient was a 68-year-old man who had suffered from an afebrile episode of malaise, myalgia and chills 8 days before admission to hospital with a diffuse mottling of the skin diagnosed as livedo reticularis. During the next 4 days his haemoglobin fell from 11.7 to 6.9 g/dl, and the reticulocyte count rose to 10.2%. Spherocytes were noted in blood films. Serum haptoglobulins were markedly reduced but serum complement was normal. Serum IgM was raised; IgG and IgA were normal. The DAT was negative using polyspecific and anti-IgG, anti-C3d and anti-IgM sera. A radio-labelled antiglobulin test using ^{125}I anti-IgG was also negative. His serum contained a high-thermal-amplitude cold antibody which agglutinated normal I and i erythrocytes to titres of 512 at room temperature and 64 at 37°C. Agglutination was enhanced by treating the test cells with ficin; it was abolished by dithiothreitol. The patient was treated with 60 mg of prednisone daily and recovered. One year later his haemoglobin was 14.8 g/dl and cold agglutinins were no longer detectable. The DAT was, however, weakly positive using an anti-IgG serum and an eluate was found to contain an agglutinin which reacted with all cells tested.

The exact cause and mechanism of haemolysis in this case remains uncertain: it seems likely that auto-agglutination was taking place at 37°C—the presence of livedo reticularis certainly suggests this. Whether this alone could explain the in-vivo haemolysis is uncertain, as indeed is the reason for, and the role played by, the spherocytosis. [It is possible that small amounts of IgG antibody were in fact playing a part in haemolysis at an early stage of this patient's illness but were not detected.]

RAISED COLD-AGGLUTININ TITRES AND COLD-ANTIBODY HAEMOLYTIC ANAEMIA ASSOCIATED WITH BACTERIAL INFECTIONS

Evidence of cold-agglutinin formation leading to increased haemolysis following bacterial infections is less well documented than in the case of viral infections. However, Pruzanski and Katz (1984), in their review of the occurrence of raised titres of cold agglutinins, listed 17 infections. Aside from viral, spirochaetal and protozoal diseases, they listed listeriosis, Legionnaires' disease, sub-acute bacterial endocarditis, *Esch. coli* pneumonia and 'sepsis' as bacterial infections in which the transient formation of cold agglutinins had been reported. The findings in two patients—one with Legionnaires' disease and one with an *Esch. coli* lung infection—are summarized briefly below.

Legionnaires' disease. King and May (1980) described an 88-year-old man with a 2-week history of cough, fever and increasing confusion. His haematocrit was 31% and there were 6.6% reticulocytes. The DAT was negative, but an IgM anti-I cold agglutinin was present at a titre of 2084; it was active, too, at 20°C. Serological tests for *L. pneumophila* became positive in the course of his illness and infection with influenza A virus, *Mycoplasma pneumoniae* or an adenovirus were excluded.

***Esch. coli* infection**. Poldre and co-workers (1985) described a patient, a woman aged 57, with an *Esch. coli* lung infection. Her haemoglobin was 9.9 g/dl and the reticulocyte count 3–8%. Spherocytes were noted in blood films. The DAT was positive with an anti-C3d serum. A cryoglobulin—an IgM/IgG complex—was present. The cold-agglutinin titre at 4°C was 2048 with I cells and 1024 with i (cord) cells; at 15°C the titre was 128 with both I and i cells. The highest temperature at which agglutination occurred was 22°C. The patient eventually recovered and 6 months after the onset of her illness the cold-agglutinin titre was normal and the DAT negative.

REFERENCES

APPLEMAN, D.H. & MORRISON, M. M. (1949). Concomitant infectious mononucleosis and hemolytic anemia. *Blood*, **4**, 186–188.

APPLEMAN, D. H. & GORDON, G. B. (1954). Acute hemolytic anemia complicating infectious mononucleosis: report of two cases. *Ann. intern. Med.*, **41**, 371–376.

BEAN, R. H. D. (1957). Haemolytic anaemia complicating infectious mononucleosis, with report of a case. *Med. J. Aust.*, **i**, 386–389.

BELFRAGE, S. (1963). Plasma protein patterns in course of acute infectious disease. *Acta med. scand.*, **173** (Suppl. 395), 1–169.

BERLIN, B. S., CHANDLER, R. & GREEN, D. (1977). Anti-'i' antibody and hemolytic anemia associated with spontaneous cytomegalovirus mononucleosis. *Amer. J. clin. Path.*, **67**, 459–461.

BERTÉ, S. J. (1951). Acute hemolytic anemia in infectious mononucleosis. *N. Y. St. J. Med.*, **51**, 781–782.

BOWMAN, H. S., MARSH, W. L., SCHUMACHER, H. R., OYEN, R. & REINHART, J. (1974). Auto anti-N immunohemolytic anemia in infectious mononucleosis. *Amer. J. clin. Path.*, **61**, 465–472.

BRAFIELD, A. J. (1966). Glandular fever and cold agglutinins. *Lancet*, **ii**, 982 (Letter).

BURKHART, P. T. & HSU, T. C. S. (1979). IgM cold-warm hemolysins in infectious mononucleosis. *Transfusion*, **19**, 535–538.

CALVO, R., STEIN, W., KOCHWA, S. & ROSENFIELD, R. E. (1965). Acute hemolytic anemia due to anti-i; frequent cold agglutinins in infectious mononucleosis. *J. clin. Invest*, **44**, 1033 (Abstract).

CAPRA, J. D., DOWLING, P., COOK, S. & KUNKEL, H. G. (1968). Cold reactive antibodies in infectious mononucleosis: delineation of an incomplete γG antibody with i specificity. *Clin. Res.*, **16**, 300 (Abstract).

CAPRA, J. D., DOWLING, P., COOK, S & KUNKEL, H. G. (1969). An incomplete cold-reactive γG antibody with i specificity in infectious mononucleosis. *Vox Sang.*, **16**, 10–17.

CASEY, T. P. & MAIN, B. W. (1967). Thrombocytopenia and haemolytic anaemia in infectious mononucleosis. *N. Z. med. J.*, **66**, 664–667.

COSTEA, N., YAKULIS, V. & HELLER, P. (1966). Light-chain heterogeneity of cold agglutinins. *Science*, **152**, 1520–1521.

CROSBY, W. H. & RAPPAPORT, H. (1956). Reticulocytopenia in autoimmune hemolytic anemia. *Blood*, **11**, 929–936.

DACIE, J. V. (1962). *The Hemolytic Anaemias: Congenital and Acquired. Part II—The Auto-immune Hemolytic Anaemias*, 2nd edn, 377 pp. Churchill, London.

DACIE, J. V. & WORLLEDGE, S. M. (1969). Auto-immune hemolytic anemias. In *Progr. Hemat. VI* (ed. by E. B. Brown and C. V. Moore), pp. 82–120. Grune and Stratton, New York.

DAMESHEK, W. (1943). Cold hemagglutinins in acute hemolytic reactions in association with sulfonamide medication and infection. *J. Amer. med. Ass.*, **123**, 77–80.

DEATON, J. G., SKAGGS, H. JNR & LEVIN, W. C. (1967). Acute hemolytic anemia complicating infectious mononucleosis: the mechanism of hemolysis. *Tex. Rep. Biol. Med.*, **25**, 309–317.

DENARDO, G. L. & RAY, J. P. (1963). Hereditary spherocytosis and infectious mononucleosis, with acquired hemolytic anemia. Report of a case and review of the literature. *Amer. J. clin. Path.*, **39**, 284–288.

DI PIERO, G. & ARCANGELI, A. (1958). Anemia emolitica acquista con auto-anticorpi incomplete a freddo in corso di mononucleosi infettiva. *Haematologica*, **43**, 91–96.

DONOVAN, D. C., COLLIER, V. U., BAUMANN, C. G. & KICKLER, T. S. (1983). Coombs' negative autoimmune hemolytic anemia associated with diffuse livedo reticularis. *Maryland med. J.*, **32**, 846–848.

ELLIS, L. B., WOLLENMAN, O. J. & STETSON, R. P. (1948). Autohemagglutinins and hemolysins with hemoglobinuria and acute hemolytic anaemia, in an illness resembling infectious mononucleosis. *Blood*, **3**, 419–429.

ESS, H. & FRIEDERICI, L. (1958). Klinische und serologische Relationen bei erworbenen hämolytishen Anämien. *Ärzl. Wschr.*, **13**, 457–468.

ESS, H., GRAMLICH, F. & MOHRING, D. (1958). Serologische und physikochemische Eigenshaften eines Kälteagglutinins. *Klin. Wschr.*, **36**, 852–856.

EVANS, R. S. & WEISER, R. S. (1957). The serology of auto-immune hemolytic anemia. Observations in forty-one patients. *Arch. intern. Med.*, **100**, 371–399.

EYQUEM, A., CATEIGNE, G., HANNOUN, CL. & FAUCONNIER, B. (1953). Les problèmes sérologiques et immunologiques concernant les pneumonies atypiques à virus et leurs complications. *Sém. Hôp. Paris*, **29**, 105–109.

FEKETE, A. M. & KERPELMAN, E. J. (1965). Acute hemolytic anemia complicating infectious mononucleosis. *J. Amer. med. Ass.*, **194**, 1326–1327.

FINCH, S. C. (1969). Laboratory findings in infectious mononucleosis. In *Infectious Mononucleosis* (ed. by R. L. Carter and H. C. Penman), pp. 47–62. Blackwell Scientific Publications, Oxford.

FORDHAM, C. C. III (1956). Acute hemolytic anemia complicating infectious mononucleosis. *U. S. Armed Forces med. J.* 7, 98–100.

GEHLBACH, S. H. & COOPER, B. A. (1970). Haemolytic anaemia in infectious mononucleosis due to inapparent congenital spherocytosis. *Scand. J. Haemat.*, 7, 141–144.

GEISEN, H. P., ROELCKE, D., REHN, K. & KONRAD, G. (1975). Hochtitrige Kälteagglutinine der spezifität Anti-Pr nach Rötelninfection. *Klin. Wschr.*, **53**, 767–772.

GLEESON, S. E. & MCSHERRY, J. A. (1983). Spurious macrocytosis in infectious mononucleosis. *Canad. med. Ass. J.*, **129**, 1260–1261 (Letter).

GODAL, H. C. & SKAGA, E. (1969). Aggravation of congenital spherocytosis during infectious mononucleosis. *Scand. J. Haemat.*, **6**, 33–35.

GOLDBERG, L. S. & BARNETT, E. V. (1967). Mixed γG-γM cold agglutinin. *J. Immunol.*, **99**, 803–809.

GREEN, N. & GOLDENBERG, H. (1960). Acute hemolytic anemia and hemoglobinuria complicating infectious mononucleosis. *Arch. intern. Med.*, **105**, 108–111.

GRONEMEYER, P., CHAPLIN, H., GHAZARIAN, V., TUSCANY, F. & WILNER, G. D. (1981). Hemolytic anemia complicating infectious mononucleosis due to the interaction of an IgG cold anti-i and an IgM cold rheumatoid factor. *Transfusion*, **21**, 715–718.

HALL, B. D. & ARCHER, F. C. (1953). Acute hemolytic anemia associated with infectious mononucleosis. *New Eng. J. Med.*, **249**, 973–976.

HARRIS, A. I., MEYER, R. J. & BRODY, E. A. (1975). Cytomegalovirus-induced thrombocytopenia and hemolysis in an adult. *Ann. intern. Med.*, **83**, 670–671.

HO-YEN, D. O. (1978). Auto-immune haemolytic anaemia complicating infectious mononucleosis in a patient with hereditary elliptocytosis. *Acta haemat. (Basel)*, **59**, 45–51.

HOAGLAND, R. J. (1967). *Infectious Mononucleosis*, 132 pp. Grune and Stratton, New York and London.

HORTEMO, T. (1958). Hemolytisk anemi ved mononucleosis infectiosa. *Nord. Med.*, **59**, 468–469.

HORWITZ, C. A., MOULDS, J., HENLE, W., HENLE, G., POLESKY, H., BALFOUR, H. H. JNR, SCHWARTZ, B. & HOFF, T. (1977). Cold agglutinins in infectious mononucleosis and heterophil-antibody-negative mononucleosis-like syndromes. *Blood*, **50**, 195–200.

HORWITZ, C. A., SKRADSKI, K., REECE, E., LEWIS, F. B., SCHWARTZ, B., KELTY, R. & POLESKY, H. (1984). Haemolytic anaemia in previously healthy adult patients with CMV infections: report of two cases and an evaluation of subclinical haemolysis in CMV mononucleosis. *Scand. J. Haemat.*, **33**, 35–42.

HOSSAINI, A. A. (1970). Anti-i infectious mononucleosis. *Amer. J. clin. Path.*, **53**, 198–203.

HOUK, V. N. & MCFARLAND, W. (1961). Acute autoimmune hemolytic anemia complicating infectious mononucleosis. *J. Amer. med. Ass.*, **177**, 210–212.

HUNTINGTON, P. W. JNR (1951). Hemolytic anemia in infectious mononucleosis. A case report. *Delaware med. J.*, **23**, 165–167.

HYMAN, R. A. (1959). Acute hemolytic anaemia complicating infectious mononucleosis. *Practitioner*, **182**, 615–617.

JENKINS, W. J., KOSTER, H. G., MARSH, W. L. & CARTER, R. L. (1965). Infectious mononucleosis: an unsuspected source of anti-i. *Brit. J. Haemat.*, **11**, 480–483.

JENKINS, W. J. & MARSH, W. L. (1966). Glandular fever and cold agglutinins. *Lancet*, **i**, 1158 (Letter).

KANTOR, C. L., GOLDBERG, L. S., JOHNSON, B. L., DERECHIN, M. M. & BARNETT, E. V. (1970). Immunologic abnormalities induced by postperfusion cytomegalovirus infection. *Ann. intern. Med.*, **73**, 553–558.

KING, J. W. & MAY, J. S. (1980). Cold agglutinin disease in a patient with Legionnaires' disease. *Arch. intern. Med.*, **140**, 1537–1539.

KOSTINAS, J. E. & CANTOW, E. F. (1966). Studies on infectious mononucleosis. II. Autohemolysis. *Amer. J. med. Sci.*, **252**, 296–300.

LALEZARI, P. & MURPHY, G. B. (1967). Cold reacting

leukocyte agglutinins and their significance. In *Histocompatibility Testing* (ed. by S. E. Curtoni, P. L. Mattius and R. M. Tosi), pp. 421–427. Williams and Wilkins, Baltimore.

LAROCHE, C., MILLIEZ, P., DREYFUS, B., DAUSSET, J. & LAPRAT, J. (1951). Ictère hémolytique aigu post-grippal. *Bull. Soc. méd. Hôp. Paris*, **67**, 779–784.

LAWSON, D. H., LINDSAY, R. M., SAWERS, J. D., LUKE, R. G., DAVIDSON, J. F., WARDROP, C. J. & LINTON, A. L. (1968). Acute renal failure in the cold-agglutination syndrome. *Lancet*, **iii**, 704–705.

LEE, C. H., HAGEN, M. A., CHONG, B. H., GRACE, C. S. & ROZENBERG, M. C. (1980). Lewis system and secretor status in autoimmune hemolytic anemia complicating infectious mononucleosis. *Transfusion*, **20**, 585–588.

LIMA, J., RIBERA, A., GARCIA-BRAGADO, F., MONTEAGUDO, M. & MARTIN, C. (1986). Cold agglutinins in parenteral drug-addicts positive for HIV antibody. *Acta haemat. (Basel)*, **76**, 235 (Letter).

McGINNISS, M. H., MACHER, A. M., ROOK, A. H. & ALTER, H. J. (1986). Red cell autoantibodies in patients with acquired immune deficiency syndrome. *Transfusion*, **26**, 405–409.

MENGEL, C. E., WALLACE, A. G. & McDANIEL, H. G. (1964). Infectious mononucleosis, hemolysis, and megaloblastic arrest. *Arch. intern. Med.*, **114**, 333–335.

MERMANN, A. C. (1952). Acute hemolytic anemia with infectious mononucleosis. *U. S. Armed Forces med. J.*, **3**, 1551–1553.

MULLINAX, F., JAMES, G. W. III, MULLINAX, G. L. & HIMROD, B. (1966). Hemolytic anemia, cold agglutination and cryoprecipitation in infectious mononucleosis. *Arth. Rheum.*, **9**, 526 (Abstract).

NORTHOFF, H., MARTIN, A. & ROELCKE, D. (1987). An IgG K-monotypic anti-Pr$_{1h}$ associated with a fresh varicella infection. *Europ. J. Haemat.*, **38**, 85–88.

NYMAN, M. (1959). Serum haptoglobin: methodological and clinical studies. *Scand. J. clin. lab. Invest.*, **11** (Suppl. 39), 150.

PERRIER, C. V. & ROUSSO, C. (1959). Un cas de mononucleose infectieuse avec anémie hémolytique et test de Coombs positif. *Schweiz. med. Wschr.*, **89**, 766–769.

PETRIDES, A. S. (1948). Akute hämolytische Anämie (Typ Lederer-Brill) bei Pfeifferschem Drüsenfieber. *Mschr. Kinderheilk.*, **97**, 56–59.

POLDRE, P., PRUZANSKI, W., CHIU, H. M. & DOTTEN, D. A. (1985). Fulminant gangrene in transient cold agglutinemia associated with *Escherischia coli* infection. *Canad. med. Assoc. J.*, **132**, 261–263.

PRUZANSKI, W. & KATZ, A. (1984). Cold agglutinins— antibodies with biological diversity. *Clin. Immunol. Rev.*, **3**, 131–168.

PRUZANSKI, W., ROELCKE, D., DONNELLY, E. & LUI,

L.-C. (1986). Persistent cold agglutinins in AIDS and related disorders. *Acta haemat. (Basel)*, **75**, 171–173.

PUNT, K. & VERLOOP, M. C. (1955). Een geval van acute haemolytische anaemie bij mononucleosis infectiosa. *Ned. T. Geneesk.*, **99**, 3128–3130.

RELLER, L. B. (1973). Granulomatous hepatitis associated with acute cytomegalovirus infection. *Lancet*, **i**, 20–22.

RIVA, C. (1946). Zur Frage der Autoagglutination der roten Blutkörperchen: erworbener hämolytischer ikterus bei Drüsenfieber. *Helvet. med. Acta*, **13**, 446–450.

ROSENFIELD, R. E., SCHMIDT, P. J., CALVO, R. C. & McGINNISS, M. H. (1965). Anti-i, a frequent cold agglutinin in infectious mononucleosis. *Vox Sang.*, **10**, 631–634.

ROSSI, V. (1958). Anemia emolitica in corso di mononucleosi infettiva: osservazioni sieroimmunologiche. *Boll. Soc. ital. Ematol.*, **6**, 12–17.

SAMUELS, M. L. (1953). Hemolytic anemia complicating infectious mononucleosis. Report of three cases. *U. S. Armed Forces med. J.*, **4**, 1778–1782.

SAWITSKY, A., PAPPS, J. P. & WIENER, L. M. (1950). The demonstration of antibody in acute hemolytic anemia complicating infectious mononucleosis. *Amer. J. Med.*, **8**, 260–262.

SCHJØTH, A. (1959). Infeksiøs mononucleose med hemolytisk anemi. *T. norske Laegeforen.*, **79**, 401–403.

SMALL, C. S. & HADLEY, G. G. (1950). Acute hemolytic anemia complicating infectious mononucleosis; report of a case. *Amer. J. clin. Path.*, **20**, 1056.

SMITH, D. S., ABELL, J. D. & CAST. I. P. (1963). Auto-immune haemolytic anaemia and thrombocytopenia complicating infectious mononucleosis. *Brit. med. J.*, **ii**, 1210–1211.

TAYLOR, J. J. (1973). Haemolysis in infectious mononucleosis: inapparent congenital spherocytosis. *Brit. med. J.*, **iv**, 525–526.

THURM, R. H. & BASSEN, F. (1955). Infectious mononucleosis and acute hemolytic anemia; report of two cases and review of the literature. *Blood*, **10**, 841–851.

TONKIN, A. M., MOND, H. G., ALFORD, F. P. & HURLEY, T. H. (1973). Severe acute haemolytic anaemia complicating infectious mononucleosis. *Med. J. Aust.*, **ii**, 1048–1050.

TROXEL, D. B., INNELLA, F. & COHEN, R. J. (1966). Infectious mononucleosis complicated by hemolytic anemia due to anti-i. *Amer. J. clin. Path.*, **46**, 625–631.

UNGER, L. J., WIENER, A. S. & DOLAN, D. (1952). Anémie auto-hémolytique chez un nouveau-né. *Rev. Hémat.*, **7**, 495–504.

VANHERWEGHEM, J. -L., DEJONGHE, M. & VAN GEEL,

P. (1977). Syndrome hémolytique aigu par agglutinines froids: manifestation inhabituelle d'une ornithose. *Nouv. Pr. méd.*, **6**, 851–852 (Letter).

VENTURA, S. & ARESU, G. (1957). Grave anemia immuno-emolitica in decorso di influenza cosidetta 'asiatica'. *Rass. med. Sarda*, **59**, 609–617.

WILKINSON, L. S., PETZ, L. D. & GARRATTY, G. (1973). Reappraisal of the role of anti-i in haemolytic anaemia in infectious mononucleosis. *Brit. J. Haemat.*, **25**, 715–722.

WILSON, S. J., WARD, C. E. & GRAY, L. W. (1949). Infectious lymphadenosis (mononucleosis) and hemolytic anemia in a negro; recovery following splenectomy. *Blood*, **4**, 189–192.

WISHART, M. M. & DAVEY, M. G. (1973). Infectious mononucleosis complicated by acute haemolytic anaemia with a positive Donath–Landsteiner reaction. *J. clin. Path.*, **26**, 332–334.

WOLLHEIM, F. A. (1968). Immunoglobulin changes in the course of infectious mononucleosis. *Scand. J. Haemat.*, **5**, 97–106.

WOLLHEIM, F. A. & WILLIAMS, R. C. JNR (1966). Studies on the macroglobulins of human serum. I. Polyclonal immunoglobulin M (IgM) increase in infectious mononucleosis. *New Engl. J. Med.*, **274**, 61–66.

WOODRUFF, R. K. & McPHERSON, A. J. (1976). Severe haemolytic anaemia complicating infectious mononucleosis. *Aust. N. Z. J. Med.*, **6**, 569–570.

WORLLEDGE, S. M. & DACIE, J. V. (1969). Haemolytic and other anaemias in infectious mononucleosis. In *Infectious Mononucleosis* (ed. by R. L. Carter and H. G. Penman), pp. 82–98. Blackwell Scientific Publications, Oxford.

YOUNG, L. E., IZZO, M. J. & PLATZER, R. F. (1951). Hereditary spherocytosis. 1. Clinical hematologic and genetic features in 28 cases, with particular reference to the osmotic and mechanical fragility of incubated erythrocytes. *Blood*, **6**, 1073–1098.

Auto-immune haemolytic anaemia (AIHA): cold-antibody syndromes V: paroxysmal cold haemoglobinuria (PCH)

History   *329*
Donath and Landsteiner's and Eason's discovery   *330*
Early reviews and incidence   *331*
More recent incidence   *332*
Relationship of PCH to syphilis   *332*
PCH: a classification   *333*
Recent reviews   *334*
Clinical features of syphilitic PCH   *334*
   Haemoglobinuria: the paroxysm   *334*
   Course of the disease   *335*
Clinical features of non-syphilitic PCH   *336*
Acute transient PCH   *336*
   Early reports   *336*
   More recent reports   *338*
Chronic non-syphilitic PCH   *339*
Blood picture   *341*
   Chronic syphilitic PCH   *341*
   Acute transient PCH   *342*
Serological findings   *345*
   Early studies   *345*
   Role of complement in the cold phase   *346*
   Role of complement in the warm phase   *347*
Recent studies on the D–L reaction   *347*
   Thermolability of D–L antibodies   *348*

Effect of pH on lysis by D–L antibodies   *348*
Time required for sensitization in the cold phase   *349*
Degree of chilling required for sensitization in the cold phase   *349*
Optimum temperature for lysis in the warm phase   *350*
Lysis by D–L antibodies of enzyme-treated and PNH erythrocytes   *350*
D–L antibodies as a cause of agglutination   *351*
D–L antibodies as a cause of sensitization to agglutination by antiglobulin sera   *352*
Specificity of D–L antibodies   *353*
   Demonstration of anti-P specificity   *354*
   Chemical nature of the P antigen   *354*
Immunochemistry of D–L antibodies   *354*
Relationship between D–L antibodies and the material in the serum of syphilitics reacting positively with the WR and Kahn test antigens etc.   *355*
   'False positive' tests for syphilis in acute transient PCH   *355*
Serum complement in PCH   *355*
Correlation of D–L antibody titre and thermal range and the severity of haemolysis *in vivo*   *355*
Treatment of patients with PCH   *356*
   Chronic PCH   *356*
   Acute transient PCH   *357*

The repeated passage of urine containing haemoglobin and/or methaemoglobin in solution (haemoglobinuria) as the result of exposure to cold is *the* clinical feature of paroxysmal cold haemoglobinuria (PCH). Haemoglobinuria occurs of course from time to time in other types of acquired haemolytic anaemia and is often a significant feature in patients suffering from a variety of types of cold-haemagglutinin syndrome. PCH is, however, unusual in several ways: in the nature of its antibody, which acts as a powerful lysin rather than as an agglutinin; in the specificity of the antibody, which is anti-P, rather than anti-I or i or Pr, and in its strong past association with syphilis. The qualification 'past' is necessary because with the effective treatment of syphilis and the virtual elimination of the congenital form, 'classical' syphilitic PCH is now an extremely rare disorder. Thus, virtually all cases of PCH now met with are of the one-time less familiar non-syphilitic variety, which clinically presents as a rule in children as a transient episode of acute anaemia with haemoglobinuria following a virus infection rather than as recurrent haemoglobinuria brought about by exposure to cold.

HISTORY

Of all the haemolytic anaemias, PCH was the first

to be recognized, and there are in fact excellent clinical accounts of the disease in the 19th century medical literature. At first sight this seems remarkable, but when it is remembered how striking a symptom and sign is haemoglobinuria, compared with pallor or jaundice, the relatively easy recognition of PCH (and a little later of march haemoglobinuria and paroxysmal nocturnal haemoglobinuria) becomes understandable. Dressler (1854) is generally credited with the differentiation from haematuria of a case of intermittent 'chromaturia'. His 10-year-old patient may have been a congenital syphilitic. In England the disease had been imperfectly described earlier by Elliotson (1832), whose patient had heart disease and cold 'fits' and passed bloody urine 'whenever the east wind blew.' It was remarkably accurately described by Harley (1865), Dickinson (1865) and Hassall (1865). All three physicians realized that exposure to cold precipitated their patients' attacks and that the urine contained blood pigment but no blood corpuscles. Dickinson considered that the disorder was due to an alteration in the blood and likened the urine to that in arsine poisoning! They, nevertheless, described the condition as (intermittent or winter) haematuria. The term haemoglobinuria was, according to Nabarro (1954), first used by Secchi (1872), but it is by no means certain that his patient was in fact suffering from PCH. The first observation indicating that the blood pigment in the urine might be derived from haemoglobin liberated into the plasma and that it was not of renal origin seems to have been made by Kuessner (1879) who found that serum obtained by cupping was tinged red if obtained during an attack of haemoglobinuria. It was at about this time that Rosenbach (1879, 1880) published his account of the production of attacks of haemoglobinuria by immersion of the patient's feet in ice-containing water — Rosenbach's test. This work was extended by Ehrlich (1881a, b, 1891) who showed that if an elastic ligature was placed around a finger which was then chilled in ice-water, serum subsequently obtained from the finger would be stained with haemoglobin — a positive 'Ehrlich's test.'

Götze (1884) and Murri (1885) seem to have been the first to have called attention to the aetio-logical relationship between syphilis and paroxysmal haemoglobinuria.

The disease was the subject of a monograph by Chvostek in 1894, and by the end of the 19th century its clinical features were fairly well known. Nothing was, however, known of its pathogenesis although Ehrlich and Morgenroth in 1899 had suggested that paroxysmal haemoglobinuria might be due to amboceptor-alexin lysis. This prophecy does not in fact amount to much. Referring to the lytic properties of normal serum, they had written: 'It is very probable that certain forms of haemoglobinuria originate through analogous haemolysins' [Bolduan's translation]. However, they diluted the prophecy by going on to write that: 'Many years ago Ehrlich showed that the haemoglobinuria ex frigore was caused, not by any particular sensitiveness of the erythrocytes to cold, but by certain poisons produced, especially by the vessels, as a result of cold.'

DONATH AND LANDSTEINER'S AND EASON'S DISCOVERY

In 1904, Donath and Landsteiner published their classical paper. They had studied three patients and showed that the haemolysis was in all probability due to an autolysin which united with the patient's erythrocytes at low temperatures, and that labile serum factors (alexin or complement) caused lysis of the sensitized cells if the temperature was subsequently raised. This work represents the greatest single step forward that has been made in the understanding of PCH. Further confirmatory studies by Donath and Landsteiner were published in 1906 and 1908. Similar and apparently independent observations were described by Eason (1906a, b).

Eason's two papers, published in 1906, were based on his M.D. thesis* (1905). His experiments, which had been carried out in 1903, had been the subject of a communication read at a meeting of the Galenian Society, Edinburgh, in January 1904. He stated that '10 months after the results had been communicated by me the most important of them were confirmed by Donath and Landsteiner whose research on these lines had been conceived independently of mine'. He added that these collaborators furthermore proved that it is in the 'process of anchoring of the intermediary body to the red corpuscles which required the low temperature.'

Eason's 1906 papers contain an interesting review of contemporary thought as to the mechanism of paroxysmal haemoglobinuria and a detailed description of his own experiments which had been based on observations made on two patients under his care at Leith Hospital. In discussing the role of intermediary body (I.B.) and complement, he concluded that the intermediary body anchors to the erythrocyte when exposed together *in vitro* at a temperature lower than that of the body, that union may take place at room temperature or at 0°C, and that washed cells from patients with paroxysmal haemoglobinuria do not become destroyed at 0°C. In his own words: 'The further combination of complement with R.B.C. + I.B. does not occur at 0°C, but does so freely at blood temperature and haemolysis then results'. 'Similarly *in vivo* atmospheric cold and stasis in the peripheral circulation probably cause a reduction of the temperature of the limbs sufficient to permit the union of the intermediary body and red corpuscle. The further union of complement probably occurs most rapidly when the blood returns to the central organs'.

Eason also appreciated that normal erythrocytes exposed to his patients' serum might undergo adhesion to leucocytes in in-vitro preparations — in accordance with observations that had been described earlier by certain continental experimental immunologists, e.g., he quoted the work of Levaditi, Savtchenko, Gruber and Ruziczka. Eason's illustration (Fig. 1 of his 1906a paper) is particularly revealing: it shows as a result of adding his own blood cells to the serum of one of his patients, contracted, densely staining erythrocytes adhering to neutrophils. In his own words: 'In many

cases the red cells appear to be partly nibbled away'. 'The significance which I attach to those changes which I have observed in the red and white cells is that they have probably to do with the activities of an intermediary body in the serum of individuals affected with paroxysmal haemoglobinuria.' Further details of leucocyte–erythrocyte interaction were given by Eason (1907). In this paper he stressed that both polymorphs and mononuclears participated in the phagocytic action and also that the phagocytosis is 'as much dependent on the previous chilling of the blood as is the extra-cellular lysis, another indication that the amboceptor is the cause of both processes'.

Donath and Landsteiner's and Eason's observations were soon confirmed in their essentials by workers in many parts of the world, and the diagnostic cold–warm procedure for the demonstration of the lysin is still widely referred to as the Donath–Landsteiner test. The antibody is conveniently called the D–L antibody.

EARLY REVIEWS AND INCIDENCE

Paroxysmal cold haemoglobinuria has a large literature. Reviews (in English) include those of Macalister (1908–1909), Mackenzie (1929a), Becker (1948), Dacie (1954, p. 272), Nabarro (1954) and Dacie (1962, p. 545). Nevertheless, the disease is a rare one. Howard, Mills and Townsend (1938), for instance, reported that only two patients out of 209 879 admissions to the Montreal General Hospital within a 38-year period had been diagnosed as suffering from PCH. One was known to have suffered from syphilis. Becker (1948) stated that only one patient had been recognized as suffering from PCH out of a total of 130 000 patients admitted to the University of Chicago Clinic in 20 years. It had been considered, too, to be a rare disease in the 1920s, for Thurmon and Blain (1931) could find only three cases out of 74 186 consecutive admissions to the Peter Bent Brigham Hospital in Boston. In Britain the disease was undoubtedly also rare: Nabarro (1954) reported seeing only 13 cases of typical PCH and five atypical ones during his very extensive experience at the Great Ormond Street Hospital for

---

* Dr John Eason was awarded a gold medal by Edinburgh University for his thesis and also the Milner–Fothergill medal in therapeutics. He was born in 1874 and graduated M.B. with first-class honours in 1896. His work on paroxysmal haemoglobinuria was thus carried out while he was a relatively young man. His later career was that of a distinguished general physician; he developed, however, a particular interest in endocrinology. He was elected a Fellow of the Royal College of Physicians of Edinburgh in 1902 at the early age of 28 and died in 1964, aged 90, the College's Senior Fellow.

Children in London between the years 1912 and 1939.

More recent incidence

PCH remains a rare disease, but, nevertheless, many cases have been described since the author (1962) wrote his review for the 2nd edition of this book. Some idea of the frequency of the disorder may be judged from the proportion of cases of PCH relative to other types of AIHA as listed in reviews.

van Loghem and his co-workers (1958) reported that they had studied 17 patients with PCH out of a total of 168 patients with various types of AIHA, a percentage of approximately 10%: eleven of the cases were attributed to syphilis, six were judged to be idiopathic or secondary.

Dacie (1962, p. 342) reported that eight out of 175 patients with AIHA that he had investigated between 1947 and 1961 had been suffering from PCH, an incidence of 4.6%; later, Dacie and Worlledge (1969) gave an incidence of 5.1%, i.e., 15 out of 295 patients had had PCH, of which eight appeared to be idiopathic and seven secondary cases.

Pirofsky (1969, p. 272), in referring to PCH as a rare disease, stated that he had only encountered two cases during 15 years he had spent in New York and Oregon. Petz and Garratty (1980, p. 54) reported a somewhat similar small incidence—six patients only with PCH out of a total of 347 AIHA patients.

The differences in incidence between the above-quoted series depend probably on several factors: a known interest, for instance, of the investigator in PCH; whether he or she sees many children, who are particularly prone to PCH, or whether among a particular series of patients with AIHA is a disproportionate number who have an underlying haematological malignancy, in which type of case the development of PCH is extremely unlikely. A further potential cause of difference is the definition of PCH—whether this is based on clinical criteria supported by a positive D–L test or, more specifically, by a positive D–L test brought about by an antibody of anti-P specificity.

Relationship of PCH to syphilis

As already referred to, PCH was at one time regarded more often than not as a complication of syphilis (see below). In contrast, most, at least, of the cases that are diagnosed at the present time are attributed, usually with good reason, to viral infections of various sorts rather than to syphilis. This suggests the strong possibility that some of the patients diagnosed in the past as having had PCH as a complication of syphilis had in reality developed the disease instead as a response to a viral infection.

Early reports. In the late 19th century syphilis was certainly suspected of being an important aetiological factor (Götze, 1884; Murri, 1885). Murri, for instance, reviewed 36 cases and thought that there was evidence of syphilis in fifteen of them. The frequency of the disease in congenital syphilitic children and the occasional presence of lesions of acquired syphilis in adult patients all seemed to bear this out. The improvement in diagnosis resulting from the introduction of the Wassermann reaction (WR) likewise appeared to furnish further support for this contention. It is interesting, however, to note that Donath and Landsteiner as early as 1908 suggested that the disease might be caused by infections other than syphilis.

The WR was positive in five out of the six patients of Browning and Watson (1912–1913); five were children with congenital syphilis and it is interesting to note that in two of them there was no other manifestation of syphilis, aside from the positive serological tests (see below). Donath and Landsteiner (1925), in a review of 99 patients, considered that there was evidence of syphilis in 95; in 81 patients the WR was positive, and in 24 there was clinical evidence of syphilis. It seems possible that in the past the sera of an appreciable proportion of patients with late syphilis contained the D–L lysin, even if the patients did not themselves suffer from clinical PCH. Donath and Landsteiner (1908) had reported one such instance out of 28 patients suffering from general paralysis. Kumagai and Namba (1927), too, found the D–L antibody in the sera of seven out of 35 patients with late syphilis and that Ehrlich's finger test was also positive. Mackenzie (1929a) concluded (1) that PCH was 'usually and perhaps always a manifestation of syphilis' and (2) 'that a small percentage of patients with late syphilis have the latent form of paroxysmal hemoglobinuria.' He also stressed that PCH appeared only in the quiescent stage of late syphilis. Thurmon and Blain (1931) made the point that PCH could be the only sign of syphilis. They cited in support of this contention the finding of the D–L antibody in the serum of a boy, without clinical or serological evidence of syphilis, whose half-brother was a proved congenital syphilitic and who also suffered from PCH.

Becker (1948) also concluded that syphilis was the cause of PCH. He reviewed 37 reports in the literature published since 1930 and added a case of his own. Ten of the patients were children; the parents of eight of the children were investigated and clinical or serological evidence of syphilis established in each case. In none of the 37 patients was there clinical evidence of active syphilis at the time of the development of the haemoglobinuria, although some gave a history of infection years previously. On the other hand, in eleven of the patients cited, positive serological reactions were the only signs of the syphilis, their personal histories and clinical examination being negative. In eight of the patients anti-syphilitic therapy was associated with amelioration or disappearance of the haemoglobinuria.

Nabarro's (1954) conclusions were very similar to those of Becker. He stressed in particular that when PCH occurs in congenital syphilis the underlying disease is practically always latent. Nabarro had studied 13 cases of PCH, all in children believed on other grounds to have congenital syphilis, as well as three possible examples, and two others not thought to be associated with syphilis. Of the fathers of these children, five were old soldiers, two had positive WR's and three negative; the others were not tested. Of the mothers, four were themselves probably congenital syphilitics and six had positive WR's; in one who was dead there was a history of syphilis and two were not tested. Nabarro made the point that in most instances the parental infection had occurred many years before the affected child was born.

Not much is known as to the latent period for the development of PCH in acquired syphilis. It may be many years but is sometimes comparatively short. The shortest recorded period from primary infection to PCH is probably the 1 year recorded by Mumme (1940). Perhaps the longest is the 55-year gap between infection and clinical evidence of haemoglobinuria in the patient recorded by Hill (1951).

Burmeister's (1921) conclusion as to the role of syphilis in PCH had differed from those of Mackenzie (1929a), Becker (1948) and Nabarro (1954). Of 207 case reports in the literature he considered that there were indications of syphilis in only 79 (38%), although the WR was positive in 95% of the cases in which it had been carried

out. Contrary to other observers (see p. 355), Burmeister found that when the lysin was absorbed with erythrocytes in the cold, the Wassermann-reacting substance was also absorbed and that when the lysin was dissociated from the sensitized corpuscles by warming, the eluate gave a positive WR. Burmeister concluded that some cases of PCH occurred in the absence of syphilis, even though the WR was positive.

Burmeister's (1921) conclusion, although against most contemporary opinion, that PCH quite commonly occurred in the absence of syphilis, even though the WR might be positive, is now generally accepted to be correct. As already described (p. 81), there is now abundant evidence that the WR, and other non-specific tests for syphilis, are not infrequently positive in AIHA and in other types of auto-immune disease, too. The occurrence of these so-called 'biologically false-positive' tests in auto-immune disorders makes it difficult to assess the contention (in the older literature, see above) that PCH, coupled with a positive WR, may be the *only* manifestations of latent syphilis. Clearly at the present time, if the question of the existence of syphilis in a patient with PCH arises, a more specific test for the disease, e.g. a TPI (treponema immobilization) test needs to be undertaken.

It may be asked, in view of the possibility of biologically false-positive tests for syphilis in PCH, whether cases of PCH genuinely associated with syphilis ever really occurred. The answer to this question must surely be that they did, the strongest evidence in favour being not a positive WR but clinical evidence of congenital or acquired syphilis in the patient in question, as described repeatedly in the early literature on the subject (see above).

PCH: A CLASSIFICATION

It seems justifiable to consider PCH as a syndrome of variable aetiology of which three main types exist: a chronic syphilitic type—now very rare, and both acute transient and chronic non-syphilitic types (Table 32.1). The clinical and haematological features of the three types differ and will be discussed separately. The three types

Table 32.1   A classification of paroxysmal cold haemoglobinuria (PCH).

Type	Frequency	Aetiology
1. Chronic syphilitic	Very rare, at one time relatively common	A complication of both congenital and acquired syphilis
2. Acute transient non-syphilitic	Relatively common	Usually a complication of viral infections, but occasionally idiopathic
3. Chronic non-syphilitic	Rare	Usually idiopathic, rarely secondary

have in common the nature of the causal antibody, which in each type appears to represent an immune response to infection.

RECENT REVIEWS

Reviews published in recent years include those of Pirofsky (1969), Bird (1977), Djaldetti (1978), Petz and Garratty (1980), Sokol, Hewitt and Stamps (1982), Heddle (1989), Göttsche, Salama and Mueller-Eckhardt (1990) and Rosse (1990).

CLINICAL FEATURES OF SYPHILITIC PCH

Race, age and sex. Little is known of any racial predisposition to PCH. Most of the case reports have dealt with patients of Northern European, North American (white or black) or Japanese origin. By its nature the disease is unlikely to make itself manifest or be diagnosed in tropical or subtropical countries. There are, however, reports of its existence in South African Bantu (Watson and Laurie, 1956) and in Brazil (Landmann, 1958).

The disease affected all ages, but as many of the cases had occurred in congenital syphilitics it had been more common in childhood. The youngest of Nabarro's patients was $1\frac{1}{2}$ years of age at the onset of the disease. The youngest recorded seems to be that of Wiltshire (1867); this patient was an infant aged 7 months who passed bloody urine (free from red cells in the sediment) when

the 'weather was particularly inclement.' It is even possible that haemolytic disease in the newborn has been caused by the presence of the D–L antibody in the maternal serum. Hoppe and Witte (1960) recorded a possible example of this, but actual neonatal haemoglobinuria was not noticed.

Both sexes are affected and there is no evidence that one sex is affected more frequently than the other.

Familial incidence. There are several reports of more than one member of a family suffering from syphilitic PCH. Matsuo (1912) described two such families; in one the propositus, his sister and two cousins, and in the other a father and his daughter, were affected. Thurmon and Blain (1931) referred to two half-brothers, one of whom, however, had serological but not clinical evidence of the disease.

Haemoglobinuria: the paroxysm

A typical attack consists of constitutional symptoms as well as of the passage of haemoglobin in the urine. However, each feature can occur without the other. The necessary degree of chilling varies from patient to patient; sometimes a brief exposure to a minor degree of cold is all that is necessary. Usually there is a pause of a few minutes up to several hours before the patient experiences symptoms. First, pains in the back and legs develop or there may be abdominal cramps or headache. The patient may then experience a rigor during which his temperature may rise as high as 104°F. The pyrexia may last up to several hours. Usually the first specimen of urine passed after the start of the rigor contains haemoglobin and perhaps methaemoglobin also; it may be dark red in colour or almost black. As a rule the haemoglobinuria disappears within a few hours; exceptionally, it may persist for a day or more. If paroxysms occur frequently, significant amounts of haemosiderin are present in the urine even in the absence of overt haemoglobinuria.

During the attack and for a short time afterwards the patient's spleen may be palpable, and on the following day he or she may be slightly jaundiced.

Abortive attacks. Haemoglobinuria may occur in some patients without other symptoms;

in other patients the constitutional symptoms may occur in the absence of overt haemoglobinuria. Kaznelson (1921) described such attacks as paroxysmal 'Kälteikterus'. Probably, however, if plasma haemoglobin concentrations were estimated in such patients, haemoglobinaemia would always be demonstrable, as was found by Mackenzie (1929a) when he attempted to induce attacks by immersing his patients' hands and feet in ice-water. Transitory albuminuria is also usually found in association with abortive attacks.

As Nelson and Nicholl (1960) pointed out, the constitutional symptoms associated with attacks of haemoglobinuria in PCH are generally more severe than when patients suffering from CHAD develop haemoglobinuria in cold weather. Presumably this is the consequence of the sudden intensity of haemolysis in PCH, which is perhaps paralleled by the remarkable lytic potency of the antibody *in vitro*.

Vasomotor phenomena. Many authors have reported the association of vasomotor phenomena with attacks of haemoglobinuria, and it seems clear that these disturbances may develop in typical PCH as well as in CHAD. Tingling of the hands and feet, urticarial weals, 'cold-urticaria', 'goose-skin', cyanosis, Raynaud's phenomena of the extremities and gangrene have all been described. Rohrer's (1901) well-illustrated case of gangrene of the ear, associated with haemoglobinuria, is an early example of a severe vasomotor disturbance in a probable case of PCH.

Bywater (1930) described how in a child, whose father had syphilis, exposure to cold would initiate cyanosis of the fingers, toes and ears and subsequent haemoglobinuria, while Hunt (1936), in a review of the causes of Raynaud's phenomena, made the point that involvement of the nose or ears in a child, or the occurrence of haemoglobinuria with Raynaud's phenomena, suggested congenital syphilis as the diagnosis. Harris, Lewis and Vaughan (1929) suggested that 'cold urticaria' might be due to an antibody, a dermolysin, which injured the cells of the skin on exposure to cold. They found that the serum of one particular patient, when injected intradermally into a non-sensitive subject, caused the formation of a pruritic erythematous weal when the site was chilled and then warmed. Becker (1948) made similar observations in one case. One of the two patients studied by Jordan, Pillemer and Dingle (1951a) described that after having been exposed to cold 'he had a shaking chill; his skin

"prickled", "tingled" and was sensitive to touch, and he voided dark urine'.

The vasomotor phenomena, referred to above, which were also well known to 19th century physicians, e.g. Wiltshire (1867) and Lichtheim (1876), do not, however, necessarily occur. They were not observed, for instance, by Nabarro (1954) in his series of 18 patients.

Course of the disease

Syphilitic PCH was a long-continued comparatively benign disease and rarely by itself caused death and seldom was a cause of severe chronic anaemia. The severity and frequency of the attacks of haemoglobinuria varied greatly: in some patients they occurred only occasionally and then only in exceptionally cold weather; other patients suffered almost daily attacks as a result of moderate cold. The attacks might be spread over many years without altering much in their frequency or in the circumstances which brought them about.

Glushien (1949), Peterson and Walford (1952) and Nelson and Nicholl (1960) described, for instance, patients who gave a history of suffering from the disease for 41, 14 and 27 years, respectively. Glushien's and Nelson and Nicholl's patients probably had congenital syphilis.

Banov (1960), too, reported an interesting case. The patient, a man aged 51, suffered from attacks of haemoglobinuria each winter between 1945 and 1955. Splenectomy was then performed for a lacerated spleen. Thereafter he kept free from haemoglobinuria. When examined in 1959 the Donath–Landsteiner test was strongly positive.

Other patients with long-standing disease who had or probably had had syphilis include those described by Parish and Mitchell (1960) and Weintraub et al. (1962).

Renal function. This is seldom impaired despite the long-drawn-out course of the disease. Sussman and Kayden (1948) did, however, record a patient who died of renal failure thought to be due to past haemoglobinuria.

Mohler, Farris and Pearre (1963) described a patient who went into acute renal failure associated with an episode of acute haemolysis with haemoglobinuria for which she had been massively transfused. She recovered after 17 days of oliguria. The D–L was positive and the WR strongly positive. She had been treated for syphilis 29 years previously.

Rosse (1990) described a further variant of the association of PCH and renal disease. The patient, a man aged 28, was diagnosed as having secondary syphilis and nephrotic syndrome. D–L antibodies were demonstrated both in his serum and in urine.

CLINICAL FEATURES OF NON-SYPHILITIC PCH

In the great majority of non-syphilitic cases the onset is acute and haemolysis is severe but of short duration. Almost all the recorded cases have been in children. Chronic cases of non-syphilitic PCH are rare: in the majority there has been no obvious cause; in a very few cases only a possible associated disorder had been present or developed subsequently.

ACUTE TRANSIENT PCH

The typical history is of a child who during the preceding 1–2 weeks had suffered from what appeared to be an undefined or 'flu'-like viral illness or an exanthem such as varicella or measles. Usually the onset of haemolysis is signalled by a recurrence of pyrexia or perhaps even a rigor and then the passage of red-brown urine, i.e. haemoglobinuria. Anaemia and jaundice then become noticeable and the spleen may be palpable. Further haemoglobinuria may follow exposure to cold, but the first episode quite often occurs in the absence of any obvious chilling. Haemolysis typically lasts for a few days only and recovery thereafter is usually uninterrupted. Treatment should be directed primarily to keeping the child warm. Corticosteroid therapy should be reserved for children whose haemoglobin falls below 8 g/dl. Blood transfusion is seldom necessary (see p. 510).

Acute transient PCH has been the subject of several recent comprehensive reviews, e.g. by Sokol, Hewitt and Stamps (1982), Heddle (1989) and Göttsche, Salama and Mueller-Eckhardt (1990). It is interesting (but puzzling) to note that the disorder is apparently more common in boys than girls. Adding together the information on sex given in the reviews quoted above gives a boy-to-girl ratio of 2.1:1 — 52 boys to 25 girls (see also p. 31).

Acute transient PCH is a rare disorder in adults, but if there has been a well-defined prodromal infection, spontaneous recovery may be confidently expected.

Early reports

Kaiser and Bradford's (1929) patient was a boy aged $2\frac{1}{2}$ years who sustained a severe haemolytic crisis (haemoglobin 15%; leucocyte count 61×10^9/l) in the prodromal stage of chicken-pox (varicella). The D–L test was positive during the attack and became negative subsequently. The same was true of the WR and Kahn tests. Five days after admission chicken-pox eruptions appeared—he had been exposed to the infection 17 days previously.

Ellis, Wollenman and Stetson's (1948) patient, a young man apparently suffering from infectious mononucleosis has already been referred to.

Gasser (1951, p. 140, Case 46) described and beautifully illustrated the clinical, haematological and serological findings in a $2\frac{3}{4}$-year-old boy who, without any obvious prodromal illness, developed haemoglobinuria acutely following exposure to cold in the street for about 1 hour on a cold winter's afternoon. Both the D–L test and the WR were transitorily positive. He recovered spontaneously within 10 days (Fig. 32.1).

Sweetnam, Murphy and Woodcock's (1952) patient was a boy aged $3\frac{1}{2}$ years who complained of headache and abdominal pain and suffered from a rigor. Haemoglobinuria was present but persisted for 12–18 hours only. The D–L test was positive but the WR and Kahn test were negative. Haemoglobinuria was provoked by placing the child's arm in cold water (5–10°C) for 10 minutes.

Dacie's (1954, p. 288) Case 18 was a girl aged 3 years who developed haemoglobinuria 9 days after the onset of measles. The D–L test, DAT and WR were

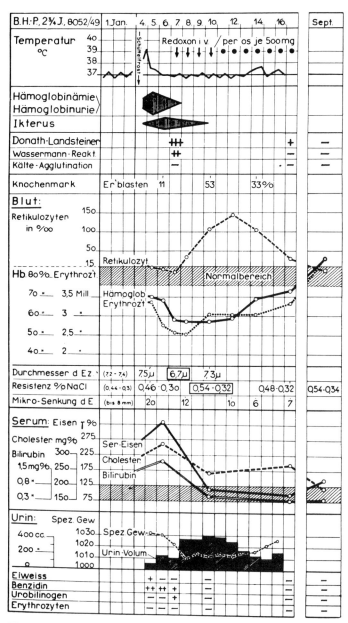

Fig. 32.1 Chart illustrating the clinical and laboratory findings in the case of a small boy who had developed acute transient PCH.

[Reproduced by permission from Gasser (1951).]

transitorily positive (see Fig. 32.2) She recovered spontaneously.

Nabarro (1954) referred to two children who had suffered from transient haemoglobinuria. In one of them the attack had followed a cold and sore throat. Both had positive WRs which became negative subsequently.

van Loghem, van der Hart and Dorfmeier (1958) referred to six non-syphilitic patients whose sera they had investigated, but except for giving the ages of the patients, 5 months to 18 years, five being 3 years or younger, no clinical details were appended. One child, however, subsequently developed a chronic haemolytic anaemia associated with the presence of a warm auto-

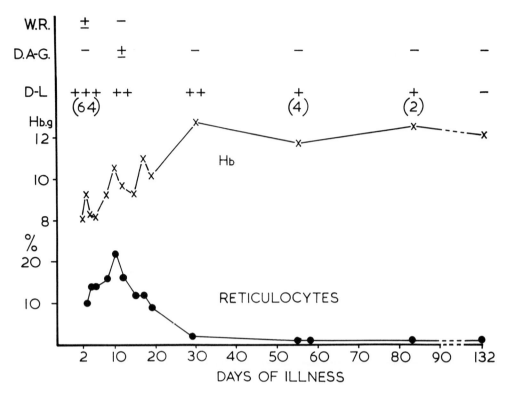

Fig. 32.2   Chart illustrating the haematological and serological findings in the case of a small girl who had developed acute transient PCH following measles.
W.R. = Wassermann reaction; DAT= direct antiglobulin test; D–L = Donath–Landsteiner test—the figures in parentheses are lysis titres.
[From Dacie (1954).]

antibody after having formed a biphasic lysin at the start of the illness.

Marstrander and Halvorsen's (1959) patient was a 4-year-old girl who suffered from a transient haemoglobinuria. The D–L reaction and DAT were positive; both tests became negative on her recovery.

Nelson and Marshall's (1960) patient was a 61-year-old man who had developed haemoglobinuria after a 'flu'-like illness and later on exposure to cold. Tests for syphilis, including a TPI test, were negative. The D–L test was transitorily positive. He recovered spontaneously.

More recent reports

Clinical and serological descriptions published between 1961 and 1991 include those of Schubothe and Haenle (1961), Colley (1964), Weiner, Gordon and Rowe (1964), O'Neill and Marshall (1967), Gelfand et al. (1971), Bunch, Schwartz and Bird (1972), Vogel, Hellman and Moloshok (1972), Niederhoff et al. (1974),

Rausen et al. (1975), Bird et al. (1976), Boccardi et al. (1977), Johnsen, Brostrøm and Madsen (1978), Miyagawa et al. (1978), Wolach et al. (1981), Sokol, Hewitt and Stamps (1982), Sokol et al. (1984), Hernandez and Steane (1984), Nordhagen et al. (1984), Lindgren et al. (1985), Heddle (1989), Göttsche, Salama and Mueller-Eckhardt (1990) and Nordhagen (1991).

In almost all the above-described cases the onset of haemolysis was acute and had followed by a few days to several weeks a well-defined infection, usually of the upper respiratory tract. More often than not the exact nature of the infection had not been determined, although thought to have been of viral origin. In the following cases identification had, however, been possible.

Colley's patient had had mumps, O'Neill and Marshall's patient measles, Bunch, Schwartz and Bird's patient had received measles vaccine, and the patient described by Boccardi et al. had had mycoplasma pneumonia. Sokol, Hewitt and Stamps listed influenza virus A, adenovirus and chicken pox virus as being isolated from three out of 13 patients. Wolach and co-workers, who had described five children, reported that cytomegalovirus had been cultured from one and *H. influenzae* from two others. They stressed that the onset of haemoglobinuria had not in their cases been clearly related to cold and suggested that the disorder be referred to as 'Donath–Landsteiner haemolytic anaemia' rather than PCH. [The difficulty about this title is that Donath and Landsteiner (1904) definitely associated in their original report the paroxysms of haemoglobinuria as occurring under the influence of cold.]

It is interesting to note that in recent years acute non-syphilitic PCH has become recognized as being a relatively frequent cause of acute transient AIHA in childhood. At one time it was looked upon as a rarity. Thus the D–L antibody was recognized as the causal antibody in only four out of 34 children with acute AIHA reviewed by Habibi et al. (1974) and in only one out of 17 children with acute transient AIHA reviewed by Buchanan, Boxer and Nathan (1976). In contrast to the data in these series studied in North America, Niederhoff and co-workers (1974) reported that seven out of 13 children with acute AIHA had had PCH and Nordhagen and co-workers (1984) suggested that PCH was perhaps the most common acute AIHA affecting children. Data from the U.K. and from Germany support its relative frequency. Sokol and co-workers (1984) stated that 17 out of 42 (40%) of patients less than 16 years of age with AIHA had formed D–L antibodies and Göttsche, Salama and Mueller-Eckhardt (1990) reported only a slightly lower percentage, i.e. 32% (22 out of 68 children). Heddle (1989), who reviewed 42 reported cases of acute transient PCH, had concluded that PCH was indeed one of the most common causes of acute AIHA in young children.

The reason why acute transient PCH appears now to be a more common type of childhood AIHA than it was several decades ago is obscure. Improvements in laboratory technique (see p. 351) and the realization that D–L antibodies are worth testing for in every case and are sometimes only transitorily present may have contributed to

this. The possibility that the causal pathogen or pathogens are more widespread than they used to be is a possible hypothesis but evidence for this is lacking.

CHRONIC NON-SYPHILITIC PCH

This is a rare disorder. The symptoms complained of have been variable but haemoglobinuria has always been an important feature. In some cases exposure to cold has clearly been a precipitating factor; in other cases this has not been obviously so. The following case summaries illustrate the wide difference in presentation and severity from case to case.

Dacie (1954, p. 287) described a young man aged 18 who had experienced a single episode of haemoglobinuria in December 1949 following exposure to severe cold. This did not recur, and he did not become significantly anaemic. The D–L test was found to be positive soon after the initial episode and remained so until 1957, although the titre of the antibody fell from 16 to 2. There was no clinical or serological evidence of syphilis: the WR and Kahn test on his blood and CSF were negative and blood WR and Kahn tests were negative, too, when carried out on both parents and a sister.

Leonardi and Andolfatto-Zaglia (1960) reported on a more seriously affected chronic case. The patient was a woman aged 37 and all tests for syphilis were negative. The D–L antibody present had a relatively high thermal range (up to 20°C) and was shown to act *in vitro* also as a cold leuco-agglutinin. The cold-agglutinin titre, using the patient's or normal erythrocytes, was 64.

Schmidt and Clifford (1960) described briefly the serological findings in Case II of Hinz, Picken and Lepow (1961a). This patient was a 32-year-old woman with no clinical or serological stigmata of syphilis, suffering from chronic PCH. The antibody was described as acting as a 'monothermic hemolysin' due to the overlapping activity of amboceptor and complement.

Kissmeyer-Nielson and Schleisner (1963) described a woman aged 65 who had had a series of attacks of haemoglobinuria within an 11-month period. Her haemoglobin had ranged between 7.7 and 12.2 g/dl. The D–L test was positive and sensitization took place at temperatures up to 20°C. The cold-agglutinin titre was normal. The WR and TPI reactions were negative.

Sirchia, Ferrone and Mercuriali (1965) described a most unusual case—unusual both with respect to the patient's history and to the serological findings. Their patient was a 35-year-old woman who had complained in the winter of 1963 of the passage of dark urine (haemoglobinuria) following exposure to severe cold. Her past history had been uneventful except that when aged 23 she had had several attacks of haemoglobinuria similarly brought on by exposure to cold. In 1963 the haemoglobin was found to be 12.5 g/dl with only 1.2% reticulocytes. Tests for syphilis were negative, including the TPI test; Rosenbach's test was positive, i.e. it provoked an episode of haemoglobinuria. The DAT was positive and was of the non-γ type. Her serum lysed normal erythrocytes, but a 2-stage procedure (cold stage optimum 2–10°C, range 0–30°C; warm stage optimum 30°C, range 10–37°C). The antibody was a 7S globulin. Its specificity could not be determined: it did not appear to be anti-I, anti-i, anti-H or anti-Tj[a].

Fisher (1969) also reported a most unusual case. A 19-year-old girl had presented with a long-standing moderately severe haemolytic anaemia of obscure origin. Six years previously she had had a 1500 g spleen removed with apparent benefit. Slight to moderate anaemia had, however, recurred and this had been, for the last 3 years, worse in winter-time. The D–L test was positive and the responsible antibody was found to be an IgG globulin with lambda light chains. The relationship between this finding and the preceding haemolytic anaemia and splenomegaly is uncertain.

Ries and co-workers (1971) described another unusual case. Their patient was a 60-year-old who had a chronic moderately severe haemolytic anaemia. Haemoglobinuria occurred from time to time and this did not seem to be connected with exposure to cold. However, the D–L test was found to be positive, and, in vitro, lysis took place in a 2-stage reaction with the temperature of the first stage ranging from 0°C to the exceptionally high temperature of 32°C. Lysis also took place readily in monophasic tests at temperatures from 10 to 32°C; the optimum was 15–20°C (Fig. 32.3). Lysis was not enhanced by acidification to pH 6.5. The specificity of the antibody was shown to be typical of that of D–L antibodies, namely anti-P. The antibody caused agglutination as well as lysis; at 20°C the IAT was 1+ with an anti-IgG serum and 4+ with an anti-C serum.

Another most unusual patient was described by Djaldetti and co-workers (1975). A 25-year-old woman gave a history of chronic haemolytic anaemia extending back to infancy, for which splenectomy had been carried out when she was aged 9 years. When aged 25, the haemoglobin was 7.6 g/dl and there were 14.5% reticulocytes. The DAT was negative but the D–L reaction was positive, and marked erythrophagocytosis developed if her blood was allowed to stand in vitro at 15°C. The WR and VDRL tests for syphilis were negative.

A further unusual case was described by Lau et al.

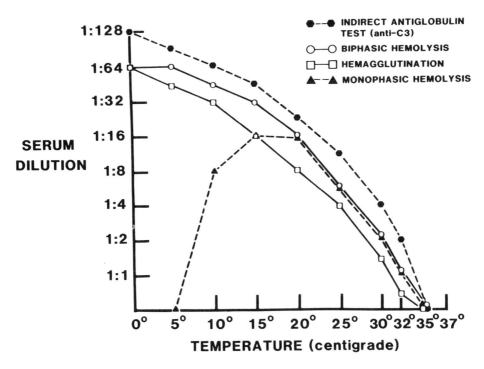

Fig. 32.3 Chart illustrating the temperature requirements for lysis, agglutination and the IAT given by a D–L antibody of exceptionally high thermal activity.
[Reproduced by permission from Ries et al. (1971).]

(1983). A man aged 60 who had been operated on for an aortic aneurism developed a series of post-operative complications including acute renal failure and klebsiella pneumonia. A total of 12 units of packed erythrocytes had been transfused. Later, erythrophagocytosis was noted in the peripheral blood and he became anaemic and had haemoglobinuria. The D–L test and DAT were positive; a VDRL test for syphilis was negative. The antibody was shown to have anti-P specificity and to have a high thermal amplitude: it was active against normal erythrocytes up to 22°C and lysed ficinized cells at 37°C. Lau and his co-workers considered that the appearance of the D–L antibody during a fulminating klebsiella infection was strongly suggestive of a causal relationship.

Rosse (1990) referred to two adults who had formed D–L antibodies. Their clinical histories were very different. The first, a 23-year-old student, presented with a severe haemolytic anaemia. The DAT was positive with an anti-C serum and the D–L test was positive, too. In the patient's serum was a polyclonal paraprotein. He subsequently developed a refractory hypoproliferative anaemia and a mediastinal mass which was found to consist of a proliferation of normal plasma cells. Ten years after the finding of the positive D–L test he developed symptoms similar to those of multiple sclerosis. Rosse's second patient was a slightly anaemic 67-year-old man; his haemoglobin was 12 g/dl and there were 2.6% reticulocytes. He gave a history of passing almost black urine several times following exposure to cold. When tested for several months after his last episode of haemoglobinuria, a D–L antibody was found in his serum, which at that time lysed PNH but not normal erythrocytes.

BLOOD PICTURE

Chronic syphilitic PCH

Erythrocytes. Patients suffering from chronic PCH may become anaemic during cold weather if they have frequent attacks, and in seriously affected patients steep falls in haemoglobin and erythrocyte count can occur following a paroxysm. Donath and Landsteiner (1925), for instance, reported that in one patient the haemoglobin fell from 85% to 55% as the result of a single paroxysm. Other early data were quoted by Mackenzie (1929a).

On recovery from a haemolytic episode the usual signs of blood regeneration, such as a raised reticulocyte count and polychromasia, are found. Between attacks the haemoglobin is often within the normal range.

Erythrophagocytosis. This has repeatedly been remarked on as an unusual feature in peripheral blood films. Ehrlich (1891) seems to be the first to have noticed it. This was in films made from a patient's finger which had been chilled while the circulation through it was obstructed (Ehrlich's test.)

Subsequent early reports include those of Eason (1907), Meyer and Emmerich (1909) and Uchida (1921). Eason reported that neutrophils as well as monocytes acted as erythrophages and that *in vitro* erythrophagocytosis might take place even if the serum had been inactivated. More recently, however, Jordan and his colleagues (1952) and Bonnin and Schwartz (1954) concluded that complement had to be present for phagocytosis by neutrophils and monocytes of erythrocytes sensitized by D–L antibodies.

Leucocytes. Interesting leucocyte changes occur during a paroxysm of haemolysis, leucopenia being followed by a neutrophil leucocytosis. This was recognized by Widal, Abrami and Brissaud as early as 1913(b). Uchida (1921) found that the lowest counts were reached 5–20 minutes after exposure to cold, the percentage fall being as much as 72% in his most severe case; the leucopenic phase lasted from 10 minutes to 2 hours. The greatest fall in leucocyte count observed by Bjørn-Hansen (1936) was from 10 000 to 2100 cells per μl 20 minutes after the commencement of cooling. Bjørn-Hansen (1936), Tötterman (1946) and Jordan and co-workers (1952) found that the total monocyte and eosinophil counts also fall, as does the lymphocyte count to a lesser extent.

The mechanism of the leucopenia has been the subject of much debate. Jordan and his co-workers reviewed the earlier literature and concluded that anaphylaxis, the pyrogenic reaction and the 'alarm' reaction all probably contribute to the leucopenia, with erythrophagocytosis playing an important part in bringing about the trapping of leucocytes in the capillaries of internal organs. The work of Jandl and Tomlinson (1958) suggested that the changes seen in PCH are no different, except perhaps in degree, from those that occur in many other erythrocyte antigen–antibody reactions, and that the adhesion of leucocytes to agglutinated erythrocytes as demonstrated by Swisher (1956) may be one way by which the leucopenia is brought about. Whether the ability of the D–L antibody, or an additional antibody, to cause direct leuco-agglutination, as observed in a non-syphilitic case reported by Leonardi and Andolfatto-Zaglia (1960), is a common additional mechanism is uncertain.

Platelets. Possible changes in the platelet count during or following the paroxysm of haemolysis deserve study. Marx (1954) reported agglutination and lysis of platelets and Bjørn-Hansen (1936) mentioned a decrease in coagulation time. Tötterman (1946) referred to hypercoagulability. Some effect on the blood-coagulation system seems certain to follow the sudden intravascular liberation of thromboplastic material derived from the lysed erythrocytes.

Acute transient PCH

The blood picture is similar in most respects to that found in children suffering from acute AIHA caused by warm auto-antibodies (p. 25). Anaemia is often severe.

Haemoglobin. Levels as low as 5 g/dl, or even lower, have been quite commonly recorded, e.g. by Kaiser and Bradford (1929) 15%, Schubothe and Haenle (1961) 4 g/dl, O'Neill and Marshall (1967) 4.8 g/dl, Bunch, Schwartz and Bird (1972) 3.3 g/dl, Wolach et al. (1981) 2.5 g/dl, Sokol, Hewitt and Stamps (1982) 3.9 g/dl and Lindgren et al. (1985) 3.2 g/dl.

Sokol, Hewitt and Stamps (1982) reported that the minimum haemoglobin level had been less than 5 g/dl in seven out of 13 personally investigated cases, and Heddle (1989), in her review of 42 published cases, gave a haemoglobin range on admission to hospital of 2.5–12.5 g/dl. Göttsche, Salama and Mueller-Eckhardt (1990) reported haemoglobin levels less than 5 g/dl in six out of 22 cases, the minimum being 4.4 g/dl.

Reticulocytes. Reticulocytopenia quite commonly occurs during the first few days of illness, as it does in warm-antibody AIHA in children (p. 69). In acute PCH it was observed, for instance, by Gasser (1951) (Fig. 32.1), O'Neill and Marshall (1967) and by Wolach et al. (1981)

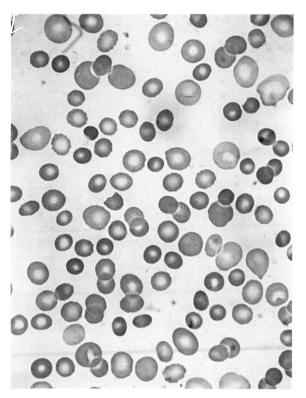

Fig. 32.4   Photomicrograph of the blood film of a small girl who had developed acute transient PCH following measles (Case 18 of Dacie, 1954).
There is a marked degree of anisocytosis and definite spherocytosis. × 700.

in four out of five cases. A reticulocytosis is, however, typically present in the recovery phase (Fig. 32.2).

Spherocytosis and osmotic fragility. Spherocytes are commonly visible transitorily in the peripheral blood of severely affected patients (Fig. 32.4). Their presence, for instance, was noted by Gasser (1951), Dacie (1954, p. 289), O'Neill and Marshall (1967), Bird et al. (1976), Johnsen, Brostrøm and Madsen (1978), and by Wolach et al. (1981) in four patients assessed on the basis of the appearance of their erythrocytes fixed in glutaraldehyde, and by Sokol, Hewitt and Stamps (1982). Osmotic fragility is increased commensurate with the spherocytosis present (Dacie, 1954, p. 289), but has seldom been recorded.

Auto-agglutination. This has not generally been considered to be a characteristic or common feature in acute PCH. However, it has been recorded, e.g. by Rausen et al. (1975), Wolach et al. (1981) and Sokol, Hewitt and Stamps (1982) in three out of 13 cases. As described by Wolach et al., 'Microspherocytosis, erythrocyte autoagglutination and adherence of red cells to leucocytes and platelets were prominent and consistent abnormalities detected on examination of peripheral blood smears from all five patients'.

Erythrophagocytosis. As in chronic syphilitic PCH after a paroxysm, erythrophagocytosis visible in peripheral blood or buffy-coat films is sometimes a conspicious feature in acute transient PCH. It was recorded, for instance, by O'Neill and Marshall (1967), Gelfand et al. (1971), Sokol, Hewitt and Stamps (1982) and Hernandez

and Steane (1984) (Fig. 32.5). In the case of the 5-year-old boy studied by Gelfand et al. (1971), phase-contrast microscopy of buffy-coat preparations revealed erythrophagocytosis and also erythrocytes bound to monocytes in a rosette pattern (Fig. 32.6).

Leucocytes. A predominantly polymorphonuclear leucocytosis is commonly found. In the 12 patients investigated by Sokol, Hewitt and Stamps (1982) total leucocyte counts of between 8.9 and 70.0 × 10^9/l were recorded, three being greater than 20 × 10^9/l. Göttsche, Salama and Mueller-Eckhardt (1990) reported counts of between 10.5 and 38.6 × 10^9/l in their series of 21 patients; nine counts exceeded 30 × 10^9/l. Initial leucopenia, as in chronic paroxysmal PCH, was not noted in either of the two series quoted above.

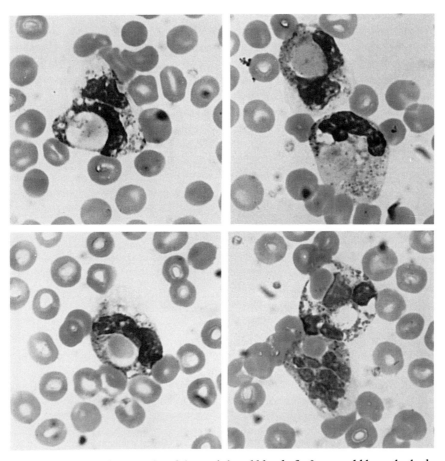

Fig. 32.5 Photomicrographs of the peripheral blood of a 2-year-old boy who had developed acute transient PCH, showing erythrophagocytosis by neutrophils.
[Reproduced by permission from Hernandez and Steane (1984).]

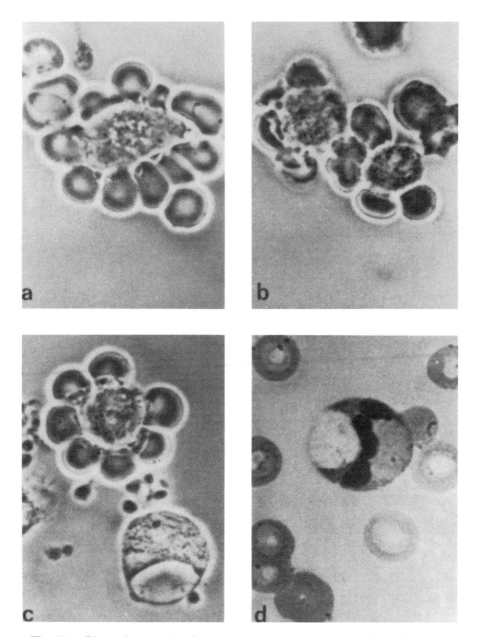

Fig. 32.6 Photomicrographs of the phase-contrast appearances of a buffy-coat preparation of the blood of a 5-year-old boy who had developed acute transient PCH, showing rosette formation around monocytes and erythrophagocytosis by a neutrophil.

[Reproduced by permission from Gelfand et al. (1971).]

Platelets. Platelet counts seem seldom to have been carried out in cases of acute PCH. Göttsche, Salama and Mueller-Eckhardt (1990) do, however, record the counts of 20 patients at the time of their admission to hospital. In only one patient was there slight thrombocytopenia — 139×10^9/l; in the remaining 19 patients the counts ranged between 210 and 559×10^9/l.

SEROLOGICAL FINDINGS

Although the clinical histories and blood pictures of patients suffering from chronic or acute transient PCH differ markedly, there seems to be no reason to suppose that the causal anti-erythrocyte antibodies differ except in detail. For that reason the antibodies present in both categories of patient will be discussed together in the subsequent sections. The marked clinical differences between patients in the two categories—a chronic episodic illness or a severe acute transient one—can be readily explained by the persistence or otherwise of the antibody, the amount formed—its titre, and its thermal range and ability to fix complement.

Before discussing the nature of the causal antibody and its behaviour *in vitro*, it is necessary to clarify what has been meant by a biphasic* or a monophasic* lysin. These terms have been extensively used in the past to describe an antibody producing lysis *in vitro* by a 2-stage (cold to warm) procedure or one producing lysis (say at 18 –25°C) without the necessity of any preliminary cooling (van Loghem et al., 1952; Schubothe, 1956, 1958, 1959; Dausset, Colombani and Evelin, 1957; Hennemann, 1957). In the author's view it is unnecessary and unwarranted to divide lytic cold antibodies into two categories in this way.

Whether an antibody is able to bring about lysis biphasically or monophasically depends primarily on its thermal range: if a cold antibody can attach itself to its target erythrocyte firmly at temperatures up to 15–20°C (or even at a higher temperature)—temperatures at which complement will bring about lysis—preliminary cooling is unnecessary. On the other hand, if the upper limit of antibody attachment is 15°C or below, preliminary cooling is essential. Thus the D–L antibody, the 'classic' biphasic antibody, will produce lysis monophasically, if its thermal amplitude is sufficiently high (Fig. 32.3) (see also Table 32.3, p. 350).

---

* Alternative terms are 'bithermic' and 'monothermic' (see also p. 275).

Looking at the problem from another angle, the author thinks that it is unwarranted to refer to antibodies which differ from the 'classical' antibody of PCH in their nature or specificity as being Donath–Landsteiner (D–L) antibodies or as bringing about D–L haemolysis, simply because they readily cause haemolysis *in vitro* biphasically. In the author's view they are cold antibodies that are highly complement-fixing but have a relatively low thermal range. Several examples of antibodies of this type have been referred to in Chapter 9.

In the following section the author defines the 'classical' antibody of Donath and Landsteiner as an IgG antibody of anti-P specificity that is highly complement-fixing and is thus potentially a powerful lysin.

EARLY STUDIES

The seminal observations of Donath and Landsteiner (1904) and of Eason (1906a, b) have already been referred to. Donath and Landsteiner showed that lysis took place when the erythrocytes of the patient, or those from a normal subject, were chilled at 5°C in the serum of the patient and then subsequently warmed at 37°C. They also showed that previous heat-inactivation of the patient's serum prevented the onset of lysis. The lytic reaction thus appeared to be of the ambiceptor–complement type, and two phases, a cold sensitizing first phase and a second warm lytic phase, were clearly differentiated. Subsequent work has fully confirmed this basic concept. There have, however, been some differences of opinion in matters of detail.

Controversy has centred in particular on (1) the role played by complement in the cold phase of the reaction, (2) the thermolability of the antibody, (3) the effect of exposure to CO_2 or acidification of the serum on lysis and (4) on the highest temperature at which the antibody could be bound. Early work on these and other matters of detail were reviewed by Mackenzie (1929a) and also by the author in early editions of this book

(Dacie, 1954, p. 276; Dacie, 1962, p. 552) and by Schubothe (1958) and Hinz, Picken and Lepow (1961a, b).

Role of complement in the cold phase

Hoover and Stone (1908) reported observations which suggested that the union of lysin and erythrocytes took place in the cold only if complement was present. This view was supported by the experiments of Moss (1911), Cooke (1912) and of Dennie and Robertson (1915) and by the work of others. This conclusion was, however, disputed by Mackenzie (1929a) who, nevertheless, admitted that more lysis occurred if complement was present during both phases of the reaction.

More recently the problem has been re-investigated. Siebens, Zinkham and Wagley (1948) concluded that at least one component of complement was necessary in the cold phase for fixation of the antibody, and Jordan, Pillemer and Dingle (1951a) claimed that it was the C4 component of complement which was required for fixation of antibody in the cold. van Loghem and his co-workers (1952) in their Case 1 found that, although lysis was maximal if fresh human complement was present in the cold phase, a certain amount of lysis followed sensitization in heat-inactivated serum. Schubothe (1958) came to the same conclusion in an elegant experiment in which lysis was measured quantitatively. Approaching the problem in a different way, Baxter and Jordan (1954) concluded that Mg^{2+} ions were not essential for antibody fixation in the cold phase of the D–L reaction. Thus when Mg^{2+} ions were removed from the serum by means of an ion-exchange column subsequent lysis was only slightly reduced.

The author (Dacie, 1962, p. 553) considered that complement was not necessarily essential for the fixation of antibody in the cold phase although more was bound in its presence; he concluded that in some cases at least a variable amount was bound even if the heat-labile fractions of complement had been destroyed and that the discrepancies in the literature seemed likely to be due to qualitative differences in the antibodies of different patients and to variations in the potency

Table 32.2   Experiment demonstrating that the Donath–Landsteiner antibody is adsorbed at 0°C in the absence of thermolabile components of complement.

Stage of experiment	Procedure	Lysis
I	Sensitization at 0°C	–
II	Incubation at 37°C (elution of antibody)	–
III	Sensitization of fresh erythrocytes in eluate at 0°C	–
IV	Incubation at 37°C	+

For explanation, see text.

(titre) of the antibodies as well as to differences in technique.

He had studied the role of complement in the cold phase using serum from two patients. In both Cases 17 and 18 of Dacie (1954, p. 287) no lysis developed unless fresh serum was present in the cold phase. However, it was possible to demonstrate with one of the sera that lytic antibody *was* adsorbed in the cold phase in the absence of thermolabile constituents of complement even though no lysis occurred subsequently (Table 32.2).

The patient's serum was inactivated and normal erythrocytes were sensitized in it for 30 minutes at 0–2°C (Stage I). The cells were washed twice in a large volume of ice-cold saline. The button of cells was then placed in a water-bath at 37°C and fresh normal serum added. No lysis developed after 30 minutes' incubation (Stage II). The suspension of cells was then rapidly centrifuged, the serum was separated, and fresh normal erythrocytes added to the serum. The suspension of fresh cells was then chilled at 0°C for 30 minutes (Stage III) and finally rewarmed (Stage IV). Lysis rapidly developed. This experiment indicated that antibody is, or can be, adsorbed in the cold phase in the absence of thermolabile constituents of complement. Under these circumstances, however, the antibody was thought to be so rapidly eluted at 37°C as to prevent lysis occurring.

Hinz, Picken and Lepow (1961a) confirmed and elaborated the above-mentioned studies in some elegant experiments. They used two D–L sera of different potencies, human serum as a source of complement and normal and PNH erythrocytes. With normal cells, none of the antibody preparations caused more than a trace of lysis (on the addition of complement) in the warm phase when complement was omitted from the cold phase. PNH cells, however, were lysed to some extent by both sera under these conditions, and other experiments suggested that they were 4–8 times as sensitive as normal cells. Hinz, Picken and Lepow concluded that the requirement for complement in the cold phase is a quantitative one, depending on the potency of the antibody and the sensitivity of the erythrocytes.

In further studies, Hinz , Picken and Lepow (1961b), using human serum or guinea-pig serum as a source of complement, showed that contrary to the observations of Jordan, Pillemer and Dingle (1951a), it is the complement fraction C1 and Ca^{2+} ions which are essential in the cold phase (not C4—which fitted in with the observation that no lysis generally results if heat-inactivated serum is used in the cold phase), that C4 reacts in both the warm and cold phases, but is not essential in the cold phase, and that C2 (and Mg^{2+} ions) and C3 are essential in the warm phase.

It is interesting to recall that the conclusions of Hinz, Picken and Lepow (1961a) using PNH cells were similar to those arrived at by Dacie (1952) [quoted by Dacie (1954, p. 257)], who used PNH cells in an attempt to define the role of complement fractions in lysis by high-titre cold antibodies. It was then concluded that C1 was essential in the cold phase but not in the warm phase and that C2 and C4 (+ C3) were essential in the warm phase but not in the cold phase. It was found, too, that PNH cells, if sensitized in the cold in the presence of fresh serum, underwent lysis if subsequently warmed in saline alone, which suggested that these cells were capable of adsorbing in the cold phase all the complement fractions required for lysis. It was also observed that PNH cells could adsorb a certain amount of antibody in the cold in the complete absence of complement fractions and that lysis would then take place provided that whole fresh serum was available in the warm phase.

Role of complement in the warm phase

All authors agree that lysis takes place in the warm phase of the D–L reaction through the agency of complement. It had been claimed, however, that sometimes sufficient complement can be adsorbed in the cold phase to bring about lysis when the corpuscles are subsequently warmed (Widal, Abrami and Brissaud, 1913a; Émile-Weil and Stieffel, 1927). Most workers, e.g. Siebens, Zinkham and Wagley (1948), have not substantiated this claim. Jordan, Pillemer and Dingle (1951a), however, stated that there is a reciprocal relationship between the amounts of complement

required in the two phases. As already mentioned, the author found, using the very sensitive PNH erythrocytes and high-titre anti-I cold antibodies, that sufficient complement might be fixed or adsorbed to the cells in the cold phase to produce lysis on subsequent warming.

Recent studies on the role of complement in the D-L reaction

Further studies on the role of complement in the D–L reaction include those of Hinz (1963), Weiner, Gordon and Rowe (1964), Hinz and Mollner (1964) and Rosse, Adams and Logue (1977).

Hinz (1963) had studied six sera: all produced much more lysis in the warm phase when complement was present in the cold phase and some of the sera were inactive in the absence of complement in the cold phase. Hinz and Mollner (1964) described experiments that demonstrated the importance of the 11S component of complement (C1q) in initiating the first stage of the D–L reaction.

Rosse, Adams and Logue (1977) described the time and temperature requirements for the lysis by two D–L antibodies of both normal and PNH erythrocytes, using sophisticated techniques designed to measure the amount of antibody, and of the C4, C3 and C5 components of complement, bound to the erythrocyte membranes. In summary, they showed that C1 and C4 (but not C3) are fixed to erythrocytes in the presence of the D–L antibody at temperatures below 15°C. During warming at 37°C both antibody and C1 elute. C3 is fixed during warming but its fixation ceases once the temperature reaches 37°C. Similarly, the fixation of C4 ceases once the temperature reaches 37°C, and the amount of active C3 diminishes rapidly as incubation at 37°C continues. C5 is rapidly fixed during warming and for a short while after the temperature reaches 37°C, but it is unstable. Rosse (1990), in his review, stressed how important for the occurrence of lysis is the establishment of the amplification complex C4b2a before the antibody and C1 are eluted during warming. [Rosse, Adams and Logue (1977) did not determine whether C2 is also fixed at a low temperature; but as, however, C2 is bound to C4 by the action of C1, this step must take place before C1 is eluted during warming.]

Thermolability of D–L antibodies

Yorke and Macfie (1921), Mackenzie (1929a) and Siebens, Zinkham and Wagley (1948) reported that heating at 56°C to inactivate complement appeared in some cases to destroy the lysin also. Yorke and Macfie (1921) stated that the thermolability of one serum appeared to fluctuate from time to time and Mackenzie (1929a) reported that heating at 45°C for 30 minutes destroyed the lysin in the serum of one of his patients and that in another the lysin was destroyed at a temperature of 47.5°C. Siebens, Zinkham and Wagley (1948) found that whilst one serum they studied was more sensitive than complement to inactivation by heating, another serum was less sensitive. Jordan, Pillemer and Dingle (1951a) investigated two sera from this point of view. They found that some lytic activity was still demonstrable after the sera had been heated at 62°C for 30 minutes if sufficient complement was subsequently added. The lytic activity of two sera studied by the author (Dacie, 1954, p. 278) was not affected by heating at 56°C for 30 minutes.

Schubothe (1958) studied one serum. He found that heating for 10 minutes at 60°C made little difference to the serum's lytic ability but that almost all activity was destroyed by exposure for 10 minutes at 70°C. Hinz, Picken and Lepow (1961a) likewise concluded that the D–L antibody was thermostable. They attributed moderate and inconstant inhibition of lysis to the anticomplementary effect of heat-inactivation rather than destruction of antibody.

These observations lead to the conclusion that, although the lysins in the sera of patients with PCH may well vary in their thermolability, most antibodies are probably unaffected by a temperature as high as 56°C for 30 minutes. Of the thermolabile ones, it is probably true that some lytic activity can usually be demonstrated after exposure to quite high temperatures, if large amounts of complement are added subsequently.

Effect of pH on lysis by D–L antibodies

The possibility that lysis by D–L antibodies might be affected by pH was first raised as far back as 1909 by Hijmans van den Bergh who reported that if the whole blood of a patient described as suffering from paroxysmal haemoglobinuria, or the erythrocytes of the patient suspended in serum, were exposed to CO_2, they underwent lysis at 16°C. On the other hand, no lysis devel-

oped at 16°C without CO_2 or at 37°C, with or without CO_2. In this account there is no mention of the possible occurrence of auto-agglutination. However, in retrospect it seems from the results reported that the patient was more likely to have been suffering from a form of CHAD rather than from PCH caused by a D–L antibody. Moreover, according to Mackenzie (1929a), subsequent investigators studying presumed cases of PCH mostly failed to confirm Hijmans van der Bergh's observations. Hannema and Rytma (1922), however, stated that they obtained increased lysis in the presence of CO_2, and Wagley, Zinkham and Siebens (1947) and Siebens, Zinkham and Wagley (1948) reported that in one of two cases lysis at 27°C occurred only in the presence of carbon dioxide.

Carbon dioxide probably affects lysis by decreasing pH. The author (Dacie, 1954, p. 279) described pH–lysis curves based on observations made on three sera, using HCl as acidifying agent (Fig. 32.7). In each case lysis was almost maximal

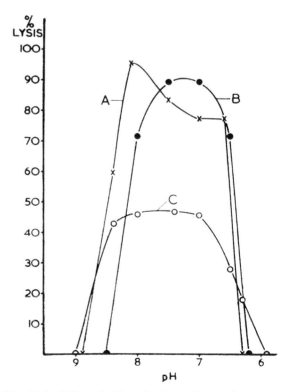

Fig. 32.7   Effect of pH on the lysis of normal erythrocytes by three D–L antibodies (A, B and C).

in unacidified serum (pH 8.0), only slightly more lysis developing at the optimum pH of approximately 7.0–7.5. Adsorption of the antibody was inhibited at a pH above 8.7 and below 6.2. Almost identical pH–lysis curves were illustrated by Schubothe (1958), and Hinz, Picken and Lepow (1961a) recorded similar data, i.e. inhibition at pH less than 5.2 and greater than 9.7, the optimum range in both phases with normal cells being pH 7.5–8.5. With PNH cells the optima were wider, i.e. pH 6.0–8.0 in the cold phase and pH 6.5–8.5 in the warm phase.

Schubothe and Haenle (1961) compared the pH requirement for lysis by two D–L antibodies, one from a non-syphilitic acute transient case and one from a syphilitic case: the pH–lysis curves were identical, the optimum for antibody-binding being pH 7.7. Kissmeyer-Nielsen and Schleisner (1963), who had studied a chronic non-syphilitic case, investigated the effect of pH on the cold and warm phases of the D–L reaction separately. For the cold phase the optimum pH was approximately 7.5, with a comparatively wide range of just below pH 6.0 to just above pH 9; for the warm phase the optimum appeared to be the same, approximately 7.5, but the range, just above 6.0 to about 8.5, was a little more restricted.

Time required for sensitization in the cold phase

Yorke and Macfie (1921) reported that sensitization was maximal, as judged by subsequent lysis, if erythrocytes were suspended in serum for relatively short periods: they found, for instance, that more lysis followed chilling for 5–7 minutes than for 30 minutes. The author, and van Loghem and co-workers (1952), failed to confirm these observations: thus with the serum from Case 17 of Dacie (1954), maximum lysis did not occur unless the cold phase was prolonged for at least 20 minutes (Fig. 32.8). However, antibody is without doubt rapidly bound. Schubothe (1958), for instance, found that approximately half-maximal binding took place after only 1 minute at 0°C; binding was, nevertheless, increased to a small extent if the exposure time was increased from 30 to 60 minutes. Hinz, Picken and Lepow (1961a) made similar observations. Almost maximal lysis followed 10 to 15 minutes' exposure in the cold phase, with a more gradual increase up to 30 minutes.

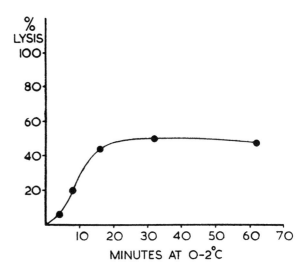

Fig. 32.8 Effect of duration of sensitization at 0–2°C on lysis produced by a D–L antibody (Case 17 of Dacie, 1954).

Degree of chilling required for sensitization in the cold phase

The highest temperature at which sensitization takes place varies from patient to patient and it is likely that the height of the sensitizing temperature is correlated with the severity and frequency of clinical attacks. In the early literature the maximum temperature at which antibody attaches itself to erythrocytes was recorded generally as 10–15°C. Thus Mackenzie (1929a) observed this to be 10–12°C in the three cases he studied, Grafe's (1911) report of 20°C being exceptional. Schubothe (1958) concluded that 20°C was the highest temperature likely to be observed with sera derived from proved syphilitic cases.

In acute transient non-syphilitic cases considerably higher maximum cold-phase temperatures have quite often been reported: 25°C, 25°C, 24°C, 25°C, 18°C, 25°C, 16°C and between 20° and 30°C were the maximum temperatures recorded, respectively, by Dacie (1954), Schubothe and Haenle (1961), Colley (1964), Bunch, Schwartz and Bird (1972), Vogel, Hellman and Moloshok (1972), Bird et al. (1976), Boccardi et al. (1977) and Lindgren et al. (1985) in the patients (all children) they had studied, while 20°C, 30°C and 32°C were the maximum temperatures recorded by Kissmeyer-Nielson and Schleisner (1963), Sirchia, Ferrone and Mercuriali (1965) and Ries et al. (1971) in three adult patients with chronic non-syphilitic PCH.

In vitro, irrespective of the highest sensitizing temperature, maximum lysis is obtained by immersing the cell–serum suspensions in water containing crushed ice.

Optimum temperature for lysis in the warm phase

It has generally been assumed that 37°C is the optimum temperature for lysis in the warm phase. There seems to be in fact little information on the point. Schubothe (1958) showed curves indicating more lysis occurring at 40°C than 30°C, while Hinz, Picken and Lepow (1961a) found that 32°C was the optimum, that some lysis occurred even at 10°C and that it might be almost maximal at 20°C.

As already referred to, Sirchia, Ferrone and Mercuriali (1965) found in their unusual case that 30°C appeared to be optimal for the warm phase with a range of 10°C to 37°C.

Lysis by D–L antibodies of enzyme-treated and PNH erythrocytes

Enzyme-treated and PNH erythrocytes are more sensitive than are normal cells to lysis by D–L antibodies, and in view of this it is recommended that in testing sera for the presence of D–L antibodies these cells should always be used before reporting that the D–L reaction is negative.

Dacie (1954, p. 283) described his findings in two patients. The serum of Case 17 lysed trypsinized normal (TN) erythrocytes slightly more readily than fresh normal untreated cells (lytic titre × 2), and PNH erythrocytes rather more actively (lytic titre × 2–4). The results with the serum of Case 18 were similar; TN and PNH cells were each about twice as sensitive as normal cells. Some data obtained with the serum of a third patient, a girl aged 9 years suffering from syphilitic PCH, were illustrated by Dacie (1955). This serum (Ca) lysed normal cells at 18°C to a titre of 2 and PNH cells to a titre of 16 at that temperature. With the cold–warm (2° → 37°C)

Table 32.3 Differences in the lytic ability of sera containing cold auto-antibodies.

	Temperature, °C	Serum A.D.* (Case 9)	Serum E.F.†	Serum B.C. (D–L antibody)
Agglutinin titre	30	0	2	0
Normal cells	18	4000	1000	4
	2	64 000	4000	16
Lysin titre	30	1	2	0
Normal cells	18	16	64	1
pH 7.0	0→37	1	4	16
Lysin titre	30	32	256	1
PNH cells	18	4000	4000	8
pH 8.0	0→37	8000	8000	32

* Cold-haemagglutinin disease.
† Post-'virus' pneumonia haemolytic anaemia.

procedure the titres were 32 with normal cells and 64 with PNH cells.

In Table 32.3 are shown for comparison the reactions under different experimental conditions of normal and PNH cells when exposed to three sera containing cold antibodies. Two of the sera contained high-titre anti-I antibodies: one (A.D.) had been derived from a patient with CHAD and one (E.F.) derived from a patient with post-'virus' pneumonia haemolytic anaemia. The third serum (B.C.) contained a D–L antibody. The titration figures emphasize the relatively great lytic activity of the D–L antibody against normal cells, for the differences in sensitivity to lysis between normal and PNH cells are markedly less in the case of the D–L antibody than those observed with the strongly agglutinating high-titre cold antibodies.

Hinz, Picken and Lepow (1961a) re-affirmed the unusual sensitivity of PNH erythrocytes to lysis by D–L antibodies. They recorded with the two sera they investigated that 10°C was the maximum temperature at which detectable lysin was bound to normal cells; with PNH cells, on the other hand, binding occurred up to at least 17°C. In a later paper, Hinz (1963) reported on the use of PNH cells in six cases: the D–L antibody titres with these cells ranged from 6 to 128.

Ries and co-workers (1971) compared the sensitivity of normal and papainized erythrocytes to agglutination and lysis by a D–L antibody of exceptionally high thermal range. Testing the serum monophasically at 20°C, agglutination and lysis were considerably stronger with the papainized cells than with the normal unmodified cells, i.e. they were scored as 4+ or 3+ compared to 3+ or 2+.

Wolach and co-workers (1981) reported that they had studied the sera of five children with transient 'Donath–Landsteiner haemolytic anaemia'. The indirect D–L reaction was positive in all five: however, with two of the sera it was positive only if papainized cells rather than unmodified cells had been used.

Göttsche, Salama and Mueller-Eckhardt (1990) had tested the sera of 22 children with acute AIHA attributable to D–L antibodies. They recorded the remarkable finding that while indirect D–L tests carried out in a standard way were clearly positive in all 22 cases using bromeline-treated erythrocytes, the tests were positive in only 12 cases when unmodified cells had been used. Göttsche, Salama and Mueller-Eckhardt emphasized that in their experience D–L antibodies in acute AIHA in childhood were always weak and only transitorily present in the patients' serum. Their data, and the earlier report of Wolach et al. (1981), underline the desirability of always using enzyme-treated, or PNH cells, in testing sera for the presence of D–L antibodies.

D–L antibodies as a cause of agglutination

D–L antibodies often cause agglutination at low temperatures: they act, however, usually far less strongly as agglutinins then they do as lysins. This facet of their activity has, however, received relatively little attention. One reason has been the assumption that agglutination brought about at a low temperature by a serum known to contain a D–L antibody may have been due to the concomitant presence of an anti-I antibody; another reason has been that when sera containing D–L antibodies have been titrated in saline and agglutinin titres measured the titres have seldom exceeded the normal range for cold auto-agglutinins (Stats and Wasserman, 1943; Becker, 1948). There are, nevertheless, some reports of definitely raised titres in otherwise acceptable cases. Siebens, Zinkham and Wagley (1948), for instance, reported titres of 160 and 320 in two cases, Hill (1951) a titre of 320, Hennemann and Seifert (1957) a titre of 128 and Marstrander and Halvorsen (1959) a titre of 1024.

The cold-agglutinin titres of the patients described as Cases 17 and 18 by Dacie (1954) were 16 and 32, respectively. However, significantly, the ability of the serum of Case 18 to agglutinate normal erythrocytes at 18°C, and to cause their lysis at this temperature, diminished in

Table 32.4   Serial serological observations carried out with the serum of Case 18 of Dacie (1954): acute transient paroxysmal cold haemoglobinuria.

Day of illness	Temperature of sensitization (°C)	Lysis (30 min. at 37 °C)	Agglutination (at temperature of sensitization)	Antiglobulin reaction*
+3	2	+++	++	++++
	18	++	+	++++
	25	+	±	+++
	30	–	trace	+
	37	–	–	–
+55	2	++	+	++++
	18	–	–	–
	37	–	–	–
+83	2	+±	++	++++
	18	–	–	–
	37	–	–	–
+132	2	–	–	+
	18	–	–	–
	37	–	–	–

*The antiglobulin reactions were carried out on any cells remaining unlysed, after washing them in several changes of saline warmed to 37°C.

+ + + +, + + +, + +, + ±, + and ± denote intensities of agglutination or lysis; – denotes no agglutination or lysis.

a parallel manner as the patient recovered (Table 32.4). The author (Dacie, 1962, p. 560) concluded that it seemed likely 'that the D–L antibody regularly causes agglutination as well as lysis; it would perhaps be surprising if it did not'.

More recent reports in which auto-agglutination has been mentioned or cold-agglutinin titrations carried out include those of Hinz (1963), Knapp (1964), Ries et al. (1971), Rausen et al. (1975), Wolach et al. (1982), Sokol, Hewitt and Stamps (1982) and Lindgren et al. (1985).

Hinz (1963) recorded cold-agglutinin titres of 4–32 in six cases: all except one (titre 32) were lower than the D–L lysin titres (using PNH cells.)

Knapp (1964) gave details of titration scores at 4°C, using P_1, P_2 and pp erythrocytes, obtained with the sera of three PCH patients. Significantly, the P_1 and P_2 cells were strongly and about equally agglutinated while three samples of pp cells were not agglutinated at all— a finding indicating that the agglutination was being brought about by D–L antibodies and not by anti-I. Knapp reported that treatment of two of the sera with 2-ME destroyed their ability to cause agglutination completely, and partially destroyed the activity of the third serum—which had been the most active of the three (titre 128 at 4°C and 8 at 20°C) (see p. 355).

Ries and co-workers (1971) also reported some most significant observations. The serum they had studied, which was exceptional in its high thermal activity, acted strongly as both agglutinin and lysin at 20°C when tested with erythrocytes of a wide range of phenotypes, including i cells. While P_1 and P_2 cells were strongly agglutinated and lysed, pp cells and P^k cells were not agglutinated. They concluded: 'Thus, the specificity of the cold antibody was shown to be directed against P, with both agglutination and hemolysis mediated by the same antibody.'

Lindgren et al. (1985) reported that agglutination and lysis paralleled each other in the case of another high-thermal-amplitude D–L antibody; in fact, weak agglutination was discernable at 30°C while lysis did not take place at this temperature (although it was possible to demonstrate binding on of complement by means of the IAT).

D–L antibodies as a cause of sensitization to agglutination by antiglobulin sera

Fisher (1950), Jordan, Pillemer and Dingle (1951a), Peterson and Walford (1952), van Loghem et al. (1952), Dacie (1954, p. 289) and Parish and Mitchell (1960) reported that erythrocytes sensitized with the D–L antibody *in vitro* became agglutinable by antiglobulin sera.

Jordan, Pillemer and Dingle (1951a) also described how the erythrocytes of their patients gave strongly positive DATs at the time of haemolytic attacks produced by chilling. The reactions, however, became negative shortly after the attacks. Both Jordan, Pillemer and Dingle (1951a) and van Loghem et al. (1952) reported that the antiglobulin reactions were not inhibited in high concentrations of antiglobulin serum, i.e. a prozone was not observed.

The IAT was studied in some detail by Jordan, Pillemer and Dingle (1951b). In two patients the antibody titres as measured by lysis, and by agglutination using a constant amount of antiglobulin serum, were identical or agglutination was higher by a factor of 2. Jordan and his co-workers concluded that the lytic antibody and the sensitizing antibody were probably the same substance.

Dacie (1954, p. 290), in serial studies on the child who developed a potent D–L antibody following measles, showed that the DAT, which was positive at the onset of the haemolysis, became negative as the child recovered, but well before the D–L antibody disappeared from her serum. He also showed that the IAT, which

seemed to be a more sensitive way of demonstrating antibody activity than looking for lysis, diminished in strength parallel to the disappearance of the antibody (Table 32.4).

It has subsequently become clear that positive DATs and IATs in patients with PCH (of all types) are mainly brought about by a reaction between anticomplement antibodies in antiglobulin sera and complement components fixed to the erythrocytes through the agency of the D–L antibody, as they are with other types of complement-fixing cold antibodies (Dacie, Crookston and Christenson, 1957). In the case of PCH the DAT is thus likely to be positive in patients recently exposed to cold sufficient to cause adsorption of antibody *in vivo* and to be negative in patients who are symptom-free in warm weather or when the thermal range of the antibody is low. IATs are often exceedingly strongly positive if carried out on the residue of cells which are not lysed in a positive D–L test. Maximal agglutination takes place in high concentrations of potent antiglobulin serum and agglutination persists even if relatively large amounts of human γ globulin (IgG) are added to the antiglobulin serum ('non-γ' reaction). However, strongly sensitized cells may be agglutinated, albeit weakly, by specific anti-IgG sera, as well as being very strongly agglutinated by anti-'non-γ' sera (Table 32.5). Whether the reaction with an anti-IgG serum is positive or negative will depend on the completeness with which the antibody is eluted in the washing process; and this will depend on the thermal range of the antibody and also on the temperature of the saline used in washing. The author suspects that the IAT using an anti-IgG serum would always be positive if the serum tested contained an appreciable amount of a D–L antibody, with the proviso that the sensitized cells had been washed in saline at 0–4°C. However, the test needs to be carefully controlled, for many sera give positive results under these circumstances if a broad-spectrum antiglobulin serum is used, due to the presence in the human sera of the normal incomplete cold antibody (p. 276). It is important therefore to be sure that the anti-IgG serum used is completely free from antibodies reacting with complement components.

Table 32.5 Agglutination by antiglobulin sera of erythrocytes sensitized at 0°C in serial dilutions of a Donath–Landsteiner (D–L) antibody.

Type of antiglobulin serum	Dilutions of D–L antibody					
	1 in 2	1 in 4	1 in 8	1 in 16	1 in 32	Control (saline)
Anti-γ	+	±	–	–	–	–
Anti-non-γ	+ + + +	+ + +	+	±	–	–

+ + + + denotes very intense agglutination by antiglobulin serum; + + +, + and ± denote lesser degrees of agglutination; – denotes no agglutination.

Two recent reports of PCH have emphasized the value of the IAT in demonstrating the presence of D–L antibodies acting at body temperature.

Lindgren and co-workers (1985) described the occurrence of acute transient intravascular haemolysis in a 14-year-old boy following an acute febrile illness of probable viral origin. His haemoglobin fell to 3.2 g/dl; in his serum was an anti-P high-thermal-amplitude D–L antibody. Lysis was demonstrable by a two-stage 20°C–37°C procedure but not at 30°C. The IAT was strongly positive at all temperatures up to 37°C.

Nordhagen (1991) briefly described the occurrence of transient acute anaemia accompanied by haemoglobinuria in two small children following acute upper respiratory tract infections. The DAT was positive with an anti-C3 serum and in one of the children also with an anti-IgG serum. The IAT was positive, at 37°C in both cases, using an anti-IgG serum and erythrocytes suspended in a low-ionic-strength medium.

Monocyte monolayer assays in PCH

Lindgren and co-workers (1985) carried out a direct monocyte monolayer assay, using normal donor monocytes, in the case referred to above and obtained a strongly positive result. Garratty and co-workers (1989) reported on assays carried out on four PCH patients using the patients' own monocytes (a homologous assay) and compared the results with similar tests carried out with the serum and cells of four CHAD patients. The results of the tests with the CHAD monocytes and erythrocytes were negative whereas they were clearly positive in three out of the four PCH patients, suggesting that the erythrocytes of the PCH patients were carrying small amounts of IgG

despite the DAT, carried out in a routine way, being negative.

SPECIFICITY OF D–L ANTIBODIES

For many years, that is up to 1963, it had been assumed that D–L antibodies were 'non-specific' in the sense that they appeared to react with human erythrocytes irrespective of their known blood groups or types. In 1963, however, Levine, Celano and Falkowski showed that this concept was incorrect, for they had found in four cases that the sera failed to react with the very rare *pp* cells (see below).

Early observations

van Loghem and his co-workers (1952) reported that the serum of an adult with syphilitic PCH gave a weak to moderately strong D–L reaction when the patient's own erythrocytes were used in the test: the results with 20 other different samples of group-O erythrocytes were in contrast negative. There do not seem to be any other reports of this unexpected finding.

Schubothe (1958) reported some interesting findings. Using a panel of ten samples of human blood of known and various genotypes, he found that although all were lysed, lysis measured quantitatively varied from as much as 14% to 62%. Schubothe, too, tested various animal erythrocytes against an eluted D–L antibody. Human and pig cells were approximately equally sensitive to lysis; ox, horse and sheep cells were but weakly lysed. Guinea-pig, rat, mouse and dog cells were not lysed, and of two rabbit-blood samples only one was weakly lysed. Schubothe's result with rabbit cells thus indicated a major difference in specificity between D–L and anti-I antibodies, which regularly react with rabbit cells at least as strongly as with human erythrocytes.

The author (Dacie, 1962, p. 564) tested four sera containing D–L antibodies for their ability to lyse adult I, cord i and adult i erythrocytes. All three types of cells were lysed, but it was interesting to note that with three of the four sera the cord i cells appeared to be the most sensitive.

Demonstration of anti-P specificity

Levine, Celano and Falkowski (1963, 1965) reported that they had tested the sera of six patients with PCH, two at least being non-syphilitic cases, and found that the D–L antibodies in the sera appeared to have the specificity anti-P + P_1 (anti-Tj^a). They had been able to demonstrate this specificity by looking for lysis in the classical cold–warm procedure and also by carrying out IATs on the residue of unlysed erythrocytes. In one case, too, the specificity was evident in agglutination tests carried out at 5°C. Levine, Celano and Falkowski also reported that one blood sample of P^k specificity failed to react when tested with three of the sera.

Levine, Celano and Falkowski's discovery was soon confirmed, and it is now generally accepted that the D–L antibody has in fact anti-P specificity. Indeed, in the author's view, its anti-P specificity is an essential criterion for labelling an auto-antibody as a D–L antibody.

As noted above, Levine, Celano and Falkowski had found that three of the D–L sera they had tested had failed to react with P^k erythrocytes as well as failing to react with *pp* cells. Worlledge and Rousso (1965) studied 10 sera from PCH patients, two of whom were known to have had syphilis and were able to show that none of the sera reacted with P^k cells; all had failed, too, to react with *pp* cells. P_1 and P_2 cells were, however, lysed by, and appeared to be equally sensitive to, the antibodies; their sensitivity was not enhanced by treating the cells with papain. PNH cells were used to test one serum and were found to be somewhat more sensitive (lysin titre × 2). Worlledge and Rousso pointed out that the behaviour of the antibodies resembled closely that of the anti-P antibody that had occurred as a natural iso-antibody in subjects with the very rare P^k phenotype. In support of this view they instanced the failure of the antibody to react more strongly with enzyme-treated cells, as would be expected of an anti-P_1 antibody, and the finding that the antibody was not inhibited by pig hydatid cyst fluid, which usually inhibits anti-P_1. Worlledge and Rousso also used the D–L sera to sensitize Bombay and i_2 cells, in addition

to P_1, P_2, p and P^k cells, in IATs. The tests were positive only with cells bearing the P antigen, irrespective of their content of the H or I antigen. In other tests positive results were obtained with certain rare erythrocytes devoid of public antigens, e.g. D-negative, S^uS^u, Cellano-negative, Kp^b-negative, Lu (a− b−) and Vel-negative cells.

Chemical nature of the P antigen

Chemical studies have shown that the P antigen is a glycosphingolipid globoside (Naiki and Marcus, 1974, 1975) and it has subsequently been shown that the auto-anti-P (D–L) antibody in the serum of patients with PCH can be inhibited by this globoside and also by the chemically quite similar Forssman glycolipids which are present in various types of micro-organisms (Schwarting, Kundu and Marcus, 1979).

Schwarting, Kundu and Marcus (1979) studied four D–L antibodies: two were inhibited more effectively by globoside than by Forssman glycolipid and two more effectively by Forssman glycolipid than by globoside, indicating heterogeneity. They suggested that some human anti-P antibodies are formed as immune responses to Forssman antigens that are widespread in animal tissues and micro-organisms.

Globoside is known to be present as a soluble glyco-lipid in the serum of P-positive individuals, and this raises the possibility that adding fresh normal human serum as a source of complement in D–L tests could result in inhibition of the antibody and hence a false-negative result (Heddle, 1989). In relation to this possibility, Wolach and co-workers (1981) had noted partial inhibition as the result of adding fresh normal serum to one of the PCH sera they were investigating.

Immunochemistry of D–L antibodies

It is now generally accepted that the D–L antibody is a 7S (IgG) globulin.

Early data established that the antibody was a γ globulin but whether of the 7S or 19S variety was at first uncertain.

Jordan, Pillemer and Dingle (1951b) found that antibody activity was concentrated in the water-soluble (pseudoglobulin) fraction of serum. Gouttas and his co-workers (1958) made eluates of a patient's serum submitted to paper electrophoresis and found the highest D–L antibody activity in the γ-globulin fraction. Leonardi and Andolfatto-Zaglia (1960) stated that an eluted D–L antibody (from a non-syphilitic case) migrated on paper electrophoresis as a γ_1 globulin.

Subsequent studies showed clearly that the D–L antibody molecules that bring about complement fixation and lysis are 7S (IgG) globulins (Hinz, 1963; Kissmeyer-Nielsen and Schleisner, 1963; van der Hart et al. 1964; Weiner, Gordon and Rowe, 1964; Ries et al., 1971, etc.).

The antibodies seem likely to be polyclonal, but conclusive proof of this seems to be lacking. Gelfand and co-workers (1971) tested the erythrocytes of one child, with acute PCH, with antisera against IgG subtypes. A weak 1+ reaction was obtained with anti-IgG_3; in contrast, the anti-IgG_1, -IgG_2 and -IgG_4 sera failed to bring about agglutination.

It seems likely that the D–L antibodies that can bring about agglutination are not always or necessarily IgG molecules. Knapp (1964) reported that she had tested the ability of three anti-P + P_1 sera obtained from patients with PCH with P_1 erythrocytes before and after treating the sera with 2-mercapto-ethanol. The ability of two of the sera to cause agglutination was inhibited completely; with the third serum the agglutinin score was reduced from 45 to 8. Her findings suggest that the agglutination had been wholly or largely brought about by IgM molecules.

Possibility of an erythrocyte abnormality in PCH

Jordan and Schlesinger (1955) reported that in one case (of syphilitic origin) the patient's own erythrocytes were more sensitive to lysis *in vitro* than normal cells; it also appeared as if there were two populations of cells present, one more sensitive than the other. Jordan and Schlesinger also reported that the Crosby test — the lysis of the patient's cells in acidified normal serum to which thrombin had been added — was positive, and that the test became negative after anti-syphilitic treatment.

Relationship between D–L antibodies and the material in the serum of syphilitics reacting positively with the WR and Kahn test antigens, etc

The evidence indicates that the D–L antibody and the material in serum giving positive reactions for syphilis are separate entities. Thus early workers absorbed out the D–L antibody and showed that the positive tests for syphilis persisted (Moro and Noda, 1909; Matsuo, 1912; Mackenzie, 1929b; Thurmon and Blain, 1931; Jordan, 1952, etc). Subsequently, the separability of the D–L antibodies and the material giving positive reactions for syphilis has been confirmed by means of sophisticated methods of serum separation, e.g. by Hinz, Picken and Lepow (1961a) and Hinz (1963).

'False -positive' tests for syphilis in acute transient PCH

As already mentioned (p. 336), the WR and Kahn test for syphilis have occasionally been found to be positive in transient PCH during the acute phase of the illness and to become negative during the patient's recovery, e.g. as described by Kaiser and Bradford (1929), Gasser (1951) and Dacie (1954) (Fig. 32.2). In this respect acute PCH resembles other types of AIHA and auto-immune disease in which false-positive tests for syphilis are not uncommon and well authenticated (see p. 81). The nature of the reacting material and the exact reason for its formation in PCH remains obscure, as indeed it does in other types of AIHA.

Serum complement in PCH

It has been known for a long time that the serum-complement concentration may be abnormally low in PCH, particularly following repeated attacks of haemolysis (Meyer and Emmerich, 1909). The serum may even be anti-complementary (Mackenzie, 1929a). More recently, Jordan (1958) reported low complement levels in three out of four patients and van Loghem, van der Hart and Dorfmeier (1958) low levels in all of 17 patients, 11 syphilitic and six non-syphilitic.

Vogel, Hellman and Moloshok (1972) reported low complement levels in two children with acute transient PCH. Wolach and co-workers (1981) estimated serum C3 and C4 separately in three children, also suffering from acute PCH: the C3 level was normal in all three children but the C4 level was markedly subnormal in two of them. Clearly, the possibility of a low complement level has to be taken into account in interpreting the result of direct D–L tests carried out at the time of a haemolytic attack.

CORRELATION OF D–L ANTIBODY TITRE AND THERMAL RANGE WITH THE SEVERITY OF HAEMOLYSIS *IN VIVO*

Antibody titre and especially thermal range are closely correlated with the severity and frequency of haemolysis *in vivo*. This has been appreciated for many years. According to Kumagai and Namba (1927), for instance, a lysin titre greater than 8 was associated with spontaneous attacks of haemoglobinuria; at a titre of 4, haemoglobinuria could be induced by artificial chilling; at a titre of 2–4, albuminuria could be induced by chilling, but with antibodies weaker than this no changes of any kind could be produced. Mackenzie (1929a), too, stated that he had observed an inverse relationship between the titre of the lysin and susceptibility to haemolysis in two patients, and also that improvement following therapy in one patient seemed to be paralleled by a diminution in the titre of the D–L antibody.

The child described as Case 18 by Dacie (1954) was followed in some detail. In this (non-syphilitic) case spontaneous cure was closely correlated with diminution in the antibody concentration and in the temperature at which it would produce sensitization (Fig. 32.2; Table 32.4).

It is no coincidence, too, that in acute transient PCH the maximum temperature at which sensitization takes place *in vitro* in the cold phase of a D–L test has often exceeded 20°C (see p. 349). Temperatures exceeding 32°C have, however, not been recorded; and it is legitimate to ask why haemolysis in such cases should be so severe, and often not obviously provoked by exposure to cold, when the maximum sensitizing temperature *in vitro* has not exceeded 20–25°C. Perhaps the explanation is that the antibody population of molecules is heterogeneous with respect to temperature requirements for sensitization, with some molecules reacting with the patient's erythrocytes at temperatures up to, or almost up to, 37°C. These high-thermal-amplitude molecules would inevitably attach themselves to erythrocytes *in vivo* and be no longer detectable in serum in in-vitro tests.

TREATMENT OF PATIENTS WITH PCH

Chronic PCH

It seems logical to treat patients in whom there is definite evidence of syphilis with anti-syphilitic treatment and to combine this with avoidance of exposure to cold as far as this is practicable. In the early literature there are in fact many reports of clinical improvement following anti-syphilitic treatment, with the attacks of haemoglobinuria diminishing in frequency or disappearing altogether.

Kumagai and Namba (1927), in a comprehensive early report on the effect of anti-syphilitic therapy, stated that ten out of 14 patients were clinically cured. Mackenzie (1929a), in reviewing earlier reports of failure of therapy or equivocal results, pointed out that this could generally be attributed to treatment being insufficiently intensive and prolonged. Mackenzie added that in three personal cases the clinical manifestations ceased, the WR became negative and the lysin disappeared from serum in the order named. Nabarro's (1954) series of 13 congenital syphilitics with PCH were treated intensively with arsenicals and/or mercury. The attacks of haemoglobinuria eventually ceased in every case and the serological reaction became negative in at least nine instances.

Penicillin has been used, too, with success: for example, by Nichols and Williams (1949) and Cattan, Frumusan and Dausset (1955) and, combined with arsenicals and bismuth, by Nelson and Nicholl (1960). In contrast Milić (1957) reported no benefit from two courses of 15 000 000 units of penicillin.

Schweitzer (1957), too, reported that treatment with penicillin had no apparent effect on haemolysis, although alleviating other signs of syphilis.

Nelson and Nicholl (1960), in a review of the effect of treatment of syphilitic cases, stated that of 36 patients who had been treated with arsenic or heavy metals 23 had been reported as either cured or improved, while of 10 treated with penicillin, six had been cured or improved.

Other treatments

Corticosteroid or ACTH therapy seems to have no place normally in the treatment of chronic PCH, and the same applies to blood transfusion and splenectomy. Some early reports on the use of steroids (and antihistamines) are summarized below.

Becker (1948) stated that antihistamines would control to some extent urticarial lesions but had no effect on the haemoglobinuria. Carey and co-workers (1950) similarly reported that a short (5-day) course of ACTH (450 mg) controlled itching and urticaria but did not effect the ease with which haemoglobinuria could be provoked by chilling a foot. Milić (1957), in another early report on the use of steroids, reported that a course of cortisone (2.5 g in total) did not affect the ease with which haemolysis could be provoked by local chilling.

Protection from cold

As in the management of patients with CHAD, protection from cold, as far as is practicable, is a simple and in theory an effective way of controlling the severity of chronic PCH. Its likely effectiveness clearly depends upon the thermal range of the antibody. That the environmental temperature can have a significant effect on a patient's haemoglobin is admirably illustrated in Fig. 17 of Djaldetti's (1978) review: in this case (described by Djaldetti et al., 1975) the patient's haemoglobin was at its lowest in three successive midwinters and paralleled the external temperature. The swing in haemoglobin with the seasons is reminiscent of that of one of the author's own patients suffering from CHAD.

Acute transient PCH

Many patients get better quickly and spontaneously without any therapy except rest in bed in a warm room. However, blood transfusion should not be withheld if the haemoglobin appears to be falling to a dangerously low level. Whether corticosteroids should be used is more problematical; the difficulty has been to assess their value in a disease normally of short duration. They have, however, been quite widely given. Sokol, Hewitt and Stamps (1982) in their review, reported that they had been administered to eight out of 13 children: of these, one child died within 12 hours of admission. Probably the right course of action is to administer effective doses of corticosteroids, even intravenously, if the child's condition is a cause of anxiety, particularly if he or she does not seem to be responding to blood transfusion and haemoglobinuria persists.

In relation to blood transfusion, it would theoretically be best undoubtedly to tranfuse P-negative (*pp*) blood. However P-negative blood is so rare as to not be normally available. P-positive blood has, therefore, per force usually to be transfused; in fact this does not seem to have done harm, even if the rise in haemoglobin following transfusion is short-lived. In any case, the blood should be given slowly and if possible warmed up to body temperature. Ideally, too, in a patient likely to have a low complement level, plasma-depleted blood (e.g. packed or washed cells) should be administered rather than whole blood.

The following authors described children with acute PCH who derived benefit from blood transfusion, despite, almost certainly, receiving P-positive blood: Kaiser and Bradford (1929), O'Neill and Marshall (1967), Bird et al. (1976), Johnsen, Brostrøm and Madsen (1978), Wolach et al. (1981), Sokol, Hewitt and Stamps (1982), Nordhagen et al. (1984) and Lindgren et al. (1985).

The report of Rausen et al. (1975) is particularly interesting in that both of their patients received Tj(a−) (*pp*) erythrocytes. In the second patient these cells had been given after two transfusions with Tj(a+) (P+) cells had resulted in only temporary rises in haematocrit; following the transfusion of the Tj(a−) cells this became stabilized.

Sokol, Hewitt and Stamps (1982), in their review, reported that seven out of 13 children had been transfused; no details of their response is given but all recovered.

Nordhagen and co-workers (1984) transfused four children, two with erythrocyte concentrates and two with washed cells. The fourth child needed three transfusions; the last was of P-negative (*pp*) cells, following which his condition stabilized.

REFERENCES

BANOV, C. H. (1960). Paroxysmal cold hemoglobinuria: apparent remission after splenectomy. *J. Amer. med. Ass.*, **174**, 1974–1975.

BAXTER, J. A. & JORDAN, W. S. JNR (1954). Role of magnesium ions in Donath–Landsteiner hemolytic reaction of paroxysmal cold hemoglobinuria. *Proc. Soc. exp. Biol. Med. (N. Y.)*, **85**, 648–651.

BECKER, R. M. (1948). Paroxysmal cold hemoglobinuria. *Arch. intern. Med.*, **81**, 630–648.

BIRD, G. W. G. (1977). Paroxysmal cold haemoglobinuria. *Brit. J. Haemat.*, **37**, 167–171 (Annotation).

BIRD, G. W. G., WINGHAM, J., MARTIN, A. J., RICHARDSON, S. G. N., COLE, A. P., PAYNE, R. W. & SAVAGE, B. F. (1976). Idiopathic non-syphilitic paroxysmal cold haemoglobinuria in children. *J. clin. Path.*, **29**, 215–218.

BJØRN-HANSEN, H. (1936). Über die paroxysmale Kältehämoglobinurie. Mit besonderm Hinblick auf die leukoztären Blutveränderungen, die hämolyse und den Blutdruck in Anschluss an experimentelle Abkühlungversuche. *Acta med. Scand.*, **88**, 129–179.

BOCCARDI, V., D'ANNIBALI, S., DI NATALE, G., GIRELLI, G. & SUMMONTI, D. (1977). Mycoplasma pneumoniae infection complicated by paroxysmal cold hemoglobinuria with anti-P specificity of biphasic hemolysin. *Blut*, **34**, 211–214.

BONNIN, J. A. & SCHWARTZ, I. (1954). The combined study of agglutination, hemolysis and erythrophagocytosis. With special reference to acquired hemolytic anemia. *Blood*, **9**, 773–788.

BROWNING, C. H. & WATSON, H. F. (1912–13). Paroxysmal haemoglobinuria: (1) its relation to syphilis as shown by the Wassermann reaction; (2) the action of the serum-haemolysin. *J. Path. Bact.*, **17**, 117–118.

BUCHANAN, G. R., BOXER, L. A. & NATHAN, D. G. (1976). The acute and transient nature of idiopathic immune hemolytic anemia in childhood. *J. Pediat.*, **88**, 780–783.

BUNCH, C., SCHWARTZ, F. C. M. & BIRD, G. W. G. (1972). Paroxysmal cold haemoglobinuria following measles immunization. *Arch. Dis. Childh.*, **47**, 299–300.

BURMEISTER. J. (1921). Über paroxysmale Hämoglobinurie und Syphilis; zugleich ein Beitrag zum Problem der Erkältungskrankheiten. *Z. klin. Med.*, **92**, 19–40.

BYWATER, H. G. (1930). Haemoglobinuria with Raynaud's disease. *Lancet*, **ii**, 632.

CAREY, R. A., HARVEY, A. MC., HOWARD, J. E. &

WAGLEY, P. F. (1950). The effect of adrenocorticotropic hormone (ACTH) and cortisone on drug hypersensitivity reactions. *Bull. Johns Hopk. Hosp.*, **87**, 354–386.

CATTAN, R., FRUMUSAN, P. & DAUSSET, J. (1955). Hémoglobinurie paroxystique à frigore chez un syphilitique guéri par la pénicilline. *Sang*, **26**, 714–719.

CHVOSTEK, F. (1894). *Ueber das Wesen der paroxysmalen Hämoglobinurie.* 105 pp. Deuticke, Leipzig and Wien.

COLLEY, E. W. (1964). Paroxysmal cold haemoglobinuria after mumps. *Brit. med. J.*, **i**, 1552–1553.

COOKE, R. A. (1912). Paroxysmal hemoglobinuria. *Amer. J. med. Sci.*, **144**, 203–219.

DACIE, J. V. (1952). Auto-antibodies in acquired haemolytic anaemia. Thesis for degree of Doctor of Medicine (University of London).

DACIE, J. V. (1954). *The Haemolytic Anaemias: Congenital and Acquired*, 525 pp. Churchill, London.

DACIE, J. V. (1955). The haemolytic activity of cold antibodies. *Proc. roy. Soc. Med.*, **48**, 211–215.

DACIE, J. V. (1962). *The Haemolytic Anaemias: Congenital and Acquired. Part II—The Auto-immune Haemolytic Anaemias*, 377 pp. Churchill, London.

DACIE, J. V., CROOKSTON, J. H. & CHRISTENSON, W. N. (1957). 'Incomplete' cold antibodies: role of complement in sensitization to antiglobulin serum by potentially haemolytic antibodies. *Brit. J. Haemat.*, **3**, 77–87.

DACIE, J. V. & WORLLEDGE, S. M. (1969). Auto-immune hemolytic anemias. In *Progress in Hematology, VI* (ed. by E. B. Brown and C. V. Moore), pp. 82–120. Grune and Stratton, New York.

DAUSSET, J., COLOMBANI, J. & EVELIN, J. (1957). Technique de recherche des auto-hémolysines immunologiques. *Rev. franç. Ét. clin. biol.*, **11**, 735–745.

DENNIE, C. C. & ROBERTSON, O. H. (1915). Study of a case of paroxysmal hemoglobinuria: serum reactions: urobilin and hemoglobin excretion. *Arch. intern. Med.*, **16**, 205–212.

DICKINSON, W. H. (1865). Notes on four cases of intermittent haematuria. *Lancet*, **i**, 568–569.

DJALDETTI, M. (1978). Paroxysmal cold hemoglobinuria. *CRC Crit. Rev. clin. lab. Sci.*, **9**, 49–83.

DJALDETTI, M., ELION, D., BESSLER, H. & FISHMAN, P. (1975). Paroxysmal cold hemoglobinuria. Transmission and scanning electron microscopy features of erythrocytes. *Amer. J. clin. Path.*, **63**, 804–810.

DONATH, J. & LANDSTEINER, K. (1904). Ueber paroxysmale Hämoglobinurie. *Münch. med. Wschr.*, **51**, 1590–1593.

DONATH, J. & LANDSTEINER, K. (1906). Ueber paroxysmale Hämoglobinurie. *Z. klin. Med.*, **58**, 173–189.

DONATH, J. & LANDSTEINER, K. (1908). Weitere Beobactungen über paroxysmale Hämoglobinurie. *Zbl. Bakt. I Abt. Orig.*, **45**, 205–213.

DONATH, J. & LANDSTEINER, K. (1925). Über Kältehämoglobinurie. *Ergebn. Hyg. Bakt.*, **7**, 184–228.

DRESSLER, DR. (1954). Ein Fall von intermittirender Albuminurie und Chromaturie. *Virchow's Arch. Path. Anat.*, **6**, 264–266.

EASON, J. (1906a). The pathology of paroxysmal haemoglobinuria (preliminary communication). *Edin. med. J.*, **19**, 43–52.

EASON, J. (1906b). The pathology of paroxysmal haemoglobinuria. *J. Path. Bact.*, **11**, 167–202.

EASON, J. (1907). Phagocytosis of erythrocytes and the question of opsonin in paroxysmal haemoglobinuria. *Edinb. med. J.*, **21**, 440–442.

EHRLICH, P. (1881a). Über paroxysmale Hämoglobinurie. *Z. klin. Med.*, **3**, 383–385.

EHRLICH, P. (1881b). Über paroxymale Hämoglobinurie. *Dtsch. med. Wschr.*, 7, 224–225.

EHRLICH, P. (1891) Ueber paroxysmale Haemoglobinurie. In *Farbeanalytische Untersuchungen zur Histologie und Klinik des Blutes*, pp. 110–113. August Hirschwald, Berlin.

EHRLICH, P. & MORGENROTH, J. (1899). Ueber Haemolysine. Zwiete Mittheilung. *Berl. klin. Wschr.*, **36**, 481–486.

ELLIOTSON, J. (1832). Diseases of the heart united with ague. *Lancet*, **i**, 500–501.

ELLIS, L. B., WOLLENMAN, O. J. & STETSON, R. P. (1948). Autohemagglutinins and hemolysins with hemoglobinuria and acute hemolytic anaemia, in an illness resembling infectious mononucleosis. *Blood*, **3**, 419–429.

ÉMILE-WEIL, P. & STIEFFEL, R. (1927). Étude analytique et critique de la réaction de Donath et Landsteiner. *Sang*, **1**, 123–133.

FISHER, B. (1950). Positive Coombs' test in cold hemoglobinuria. *J. Urol. (Baltimore)*, **64**, 816–817.

FISHER, S. (1969). Paroxysmal cold hemoglobinuria. Case report with characterization of the Donath-Landsteiner hemolysin. *Amer. J. Med.*, **46**, 475–479.

GARRATTY, G., NANCE, S., ARNDT, P. & POSTAWAY, N. (1989). Positive direct monocyte monolayer assays associated with positive Donath Landsteiner tests. *Transfusion*, **29**, Suppl. 49 S (Abstract S 175).

GASSER, C. (1951). *Die hämolytische syndrome im Kindesalter*, 332 pp. Georg Thieme, Stuttgart.

GELFAND, E. W., ABRAMSON, N., SEGEL, G. B. &

NATHAN, D. G. (1971). Buffy-coat observations and red cell antibodies in acquired hemolytic anemia. *New Engl. J. Med.*, **284**, 1250–1252.

GLUSHEIN, A. S. (1949). Syphilitic paroxysmal cold hemoglobinuria of forty-one years' duration associated with syphilitic heart disease. *Amer. J. Syph.*, **33**, 444–449.

GÖTTSCHE, B., SALAMA, A. & MUELLER-ECKHARDT, C. (1990). Donath–Landsteiner autoimmune hemolytic anemia in children. A study of 22 cases. *Vox Sang.*, **58**, 581–586.

GÖTZE, L. (1884). Beitrag zur Lehre von der paroxysmalen Haemoglobinurie. *Berl. klin. Wschr.*, **21**, 716–718.

GOUTTAS, A., TSEVRENIS, H., POUGGOURAS, P., RENIÉRI, N. & PAPATHANASSION, S. (1958). Hémoglobinurie paroxystique à frigoré avec coexistence d'un anticorps froid incomplet à grande marge thermique. *Sang*, **29**, 53–56.

GRAFE, E. (1911). Zur Kenntnis der paroxysmalen Hämoglobinurie. *Dtsch. med. Wschr.*, **37**, 2035–2036.

HABIBI, B., HOMBERG, J. -C., SCHAISON, G. & SALMON, C. (1974). Autoimmune hemolytic anemia in children. A review of 80 cases. *Amer. J. Med.*, **56**, 61–69.

HANNEMA, L. S. & RYTMA, J. R. (1922). Some investigations into a case of paroxysmal haemoglobinuria. *Lancet*, **ii**, 1217–1220.

HARLEY, G. (1865). Notes of two cases of intermittent haematuria: with remarks upon their pathology and treatment. *Lancet*, **i**, 568.

HARRIS, K. E., LEWIS, T. & VAUGHAN, J. M. (1929). Haemoglobinuria and urticaria from cold occurring singly or in combination; observations referring especially to the mechanism of urticaria with some remarks on Raynaud's disease. *Heart*, **14**, 305–336.

HASSALL, A. H. (1865). On intermittent, or winter haematuria. *Lancet*, **ii**, 368–369.

HEDDLE, N. M. (1989). Acute paroxysmal cold hemoglobinuria. *Transf. Med. Rev.*, **3**, 219–229.

HENNEMANN, H. H. (1957). *Erworbene hämolytische Anämien. Klinik und Serologie*, 198 pp. George Theime, Leipzig.

HENNEMANN, H. H. & SEIFERT, J. (1957). Immunohämatologische untersuchungen bei einer syphilitischen paroxysmalen Kältehämoglobinurie. *Folia haemat. (Lpz)*, **75**, 52–68.

HERNANDEZ, J. A. & STEANE, S. M. (1984). Erythrophagocytosis by segmented neutrophils in paroxysmal cold hemoglobinuria. *Amer. J. clin. Path.*, **81**, 787–789.

HIJMANS VAN DEN BERGH, A. A. (1909a). Untersuchungen über die Hämolyse bei der paroxysmalen Hämoglobinurie. *Berl. klin. Wschr.*, **46**, 1251–1253.

HIJMANS VAN DEN BERGH, A. A. (1909b). Ueber die Hämolyse bei der paroxysmalen Hämoglobinurie. *Berl. klin. Wschr.*, **46**, 1609–1610.

HILL, N. P. (1951). Syphilitic paroxysmal cold hemoglobinuria causing a transfusion reaction: response to penicillin. *Amer. J. Syph.*, **35**, 329–333.

HINZ, C. F. JNR (1963). Serologic and physicochemical characterization of Donath–Landsteiner antibodies from six patients. *Blood*, **22**, 600–605.

HINZ, C. F. JNR & MOLLNER, A. M. (1964). Studies on immune human hemolysis. III. Role of 11 S component in initiating the Donath–Landsteiner reaction. *J. Immunol.*, **91**, 512–517.

HINZ, C. F. JNR, PICKEN, M. E. & LEPOW, I. H. (1961a). Studies on immune human hemolysis. I. The kinetics of the Donath–Landsteiner reaction and the requirement for complement in the reaction. *J. exp. Med.*, **113**, 177–192.

HINZ, C. F. JNR, PICKEN, M. E. & LEPOW, I. H. (1961b). Studies on immune human hemolysis. II. The Donath–Landsteiner reaction as a model system for studying the mechanism of action of complement and the role of C'1 and C'1 esterase. *J. exp. Med.*, **113**, 193–218.

HOOVER, C. F. & STONE, G. W. (1908). Paroxysmal hemoglobinuria. Account of two cases. *Arch. intern. Med.*, **2**, 392–404.

HOPPE, H. H. & WITTE, A. (1960). Hämolytische Erkrankung eines Neugeborenen bei paroxysmaler Kältehämoglobinurie der Mutter. *Vox Sang.*, **5**, 425–433.

HOWARD, C. P., MILLS, E. S. & TOWNSEND, S. R. (1938). Paroxysmal hemoglobinuria. With report of a case. *Amer. J. med. Sci.*, **196**, 792–796.

HUNT, J. H. (1936). The Raynaud phenomena: a critical review. *Quart. J. Med.*, **5**, 399–444.

JANDL, J. H. & TOMLINSON, A. S. (1958). The destruction of red cells by antibodies in man. II. Pyrogenic, leukocytic and dermal responses to immune hemolysis. *J. clin. Invest.*, **37**, 1202–1228.

JOHNSEN, H. E., BROSTRØM, K. & MADSEN, M. (1978). Paroxysmal cold haemoglobinuria in children: 3 cases encountered within a period of 7 months. *Scand. J. Haemat.*, **20**, 413–416.

JORDAN, F. L. J. (1958). The role of complement in immunohemolytic disease. *Proc. 6th int. Congr. int. Soc. Hemat.*, *Boston, 1956*, pp. 825–832. Grune and Stratton, New York.

JORDAN, F. L. J. & SCHLESINGER, F. G. (1955). Studies on the destruction of red blood cells in paroxysmal cold haemoglobinuria of the Donath–Landsteiner (syphilitic) type. *Acta med. scand.*, **151**, 107–116.

JORDAN, W. S. JNR (1952). Separate identities of the Donath–Landsteiner hemolysin (PCH antibody) and Treponemal immobilizing antibody. *Proc. Soc. exp. Biol. Med. (N. Y.)*, **80**, 357–359.

JORDAN, W. S. JNR, PILLEMER, L. & DINGLE, J. H. (1951a). The mechanism of hemolysis in paroxysmal cold hemoglobinuria. I. The role of complement and its components in the Donath–Landsteiner reaction. *J. clin. Invest.*, **30**, 11–21.

JORDAN, W. S. JNR, PILLEMER, L. & DINGLE, J. H. (1951b). The mechanism of hemolysis in paroxysmal cold hemoglobinuria. II. Observations on the behavior and nature of the antibody. *J. clin. Invest.*, **30**, 22–30.

JORDAN, W. S. JNR, PROUTY, R. L., HEINLE, R. W. & DINGLE, J. G. (1952). The mechanism of hemolysis in paroxysmal cold hemoglobinuria. III. Erythrophagocytosis and leukopenia. *Blood*, **7**, 387–403.

KAISER, A. D. & BRADFORD, W. L. (1929). Severe haemoglobinuria in a child, occurring in the prodromal stage of chickenpox. *Arch. Pediat.*, **46**, 571–577.

KAZNELSON, P. (1921). Beobactungen über paroxysmale Kälthämoglobinurie und Kälteikterus. *Dtsch. Arch. klin. Med.*, **138**, 46–57.

KISSMEYER-NIELSON, E. & SCHLEISNER, P. (1963). Paroxysmal cold haemoglobinuria of non-syphilitic type. Report of a case with haemolytic anaemia and a normal cold haemagglutinin titre. *Dan. med. Bull.*, **10**, 52–58.

KNAPP, T. (1964). The laboratory investigation of three cases of paroxysmal cold haemoglobinuria. *Canad. J. med. Technol.*, **26**, 172–187.

KUESSNER, B. (1879). Paroxymale Hämoglobinurie. *Dtsch. med. Wschr.*, **5**, 475–478.

KUMAGAI, T. & NAMBA, M. (1927). Weitere Beitrage zur Kenntnis der paroxysmalen Hämoglobinurie. *Dtsch. Arch. klin. Med.*, **156**, 257–271.

LANDMANN, J. (1958). Estudo sobre a hemoglobinuria paroxistica a frio (segundo caso observado no Brazil). *Gaz. méd. port.*, **11**, 77–111.

LAU, P., SERERAT, S., MOORE, V., MCLEISH, K. & ALOUSI, M. (1983). Paroxysmal cold hemoglobinuria in a patient with Klebsiella pneumonia. *Vox Sang.*, **44**, 167–172.

LEONARDI, P. & ANDOLFATTO-ZAGLIA, G. (1960). Emoglobinuria parossistica a frigore non luetica da anticorpo bifasico tipo Donath e Landsteiner. *Minerva med. (Torino)*, **51**, 453–459.

LEVINE, P., CELANO, M. J. & FALKOWSKI, F. (1963). The specificity of the antibody in paroxysmal cold hemoglobinuria. *Transfusion*, **3**, 278–280.

LEVINE, P., CELANO, M. J. & FALKOWSKI, F. (1966). The specificity of the antibody in paroxysmal cold hemoglobinuria (P. C. H.). *Ann. N. Y. Acad. Sci.*, **124**, 456–461.

LICHTHEIM, L. (1876). Ueber periodische Hämoglobinurie. *Sammlung klin. Vörtrage* (ed. by R. Volkmann), **134**, 1147–1168.

LINDGREN, S., ZIMMERMAN, S., GIBBS, F. & GARRATTY, G. (1985). An unusual Donath–Landsteiner antibody detectable at 37°C by the antiglobulin test. *Transfusion*, **25**, 142–144.

MACALISTER, G. H. K. (1908–1909). The pathology of paroxysmal haemoglobinuria. A critical review. *Quart. J. Med.*, **2**, 368–395.

MACKENZIE, G. M. (1929a). Paroxysmal

hemoglobinuria. A review. *Medicine (Baltimore)*, **8**, 159–191.

MACKENZIE, G. M. (1929b). Observations on paroxysmal hemoglobinuria. *J. clin. Invest.*, 7, 27–43.

MARSTRANDER, J. & HALVORSEN, K. (1959). Paroxysmal kuldehemoglobinuri. *Nord. Med.*, **61**, 276–277.

MARX, R. (1954). Zur Therapie idiopathischer Hämoglobinurien. *Med. Mschr.*, **8**, 807–812.

MATSUO, J. (1912). Über die klinischen und serologischen Untersuchungen der paroxysmalen Hämoglobinurie, zugleich ein Beitrag zur Kenntnis der Isolysine. *Dtsch. Arch. klin. Med.*, **107**, 335–356.

MEYER, E. & EMMERICH, E. (1909). Über paroxysmale Hämoglobinurie. *Dtsch. Arch. klin. Med.*, **96**, 287–327.

MILÍC, N. (1957). Paroxysmal cold hemoglobinuria with positive treponema immobilization test. Report of a case. *Blood*, **12**, 907–912.

MIYAGAWA, Y., YAMADA, S., KOMIYAMA, A. & AKABANE, T. (1978). Measurement of Donath–Landsteiner antibody-producing cells in idiopathic nonsyphilitic paroxysmal cold hemoglobinuria (PCH) in children. *Blood*, **52**, 97–101.

MOHLER, D. H., FARRIS, B. L. & PEARRE, A. A. (1963). Paroxysmal cold hemoglobinuria with acute renal failure. *Arch. intern. Med.*, **112**, 36–40.

MORO, E. & NODA, S. (1909). Paroxysmale Hämoglobinurie und Hämolyse in vitro. *Münch. med. Wschr.*, **56**, 545–549.

MOSS, W. L. (1911). Paroxysmal hemoglobinuria: blood studies in three cases. *Johns Hopk. Hosp. Bull.*, **22**, 238–247.

MUMME, C. (1940). Über paroxysmale Kältehämoglobinurie und über einen besonderen Fall von Hämoglobinurie bei Glomerulonephritis. *Z. klin. Med.*, **138**, 334–354.

MURRI, A. (1885). Emoglobinuria e sifilide. *Riv. clin. Bologna*, Serie **3**, 241–259, 321–342.

NABARRO, D. (1954). *Congenital Syphilis*, pp. 247–261. Arnold, London.

NAIKI, M. & MARCUS, D. M. (1974). Human erythrocyte P and P^k blood group antigens: identification as glycosphingolipids. *Biochem. biophys. Res. Commun.*, **60**, 1105–1111.

NAIKI, M. & MARCUS, D. M. (1975). An immunochemical study of the human blood group P_1, P and P^k glycosphingolipid antigens. *Biochemistry*, **14**, 4837–4841.

NELSON, M. G. & NICHOLL, B. (1960). Paroxysmal cold haemoglobinuria. *Irish J. med. Sci.*, Sixth Series, No. 410, 49–57.

NICHOLS, F. T. JNR & WILLIAMS C. J. (1949). Paroxysmal cold haemoglobinuria associated with dementia paralytica. Report of treatment with penicillin. *J. Amer. med. Ass.*, **140**, 1322–1324.

NIEDERHOFF, H., SCHUBOTHE, H. & WEBER, S. (1974). Akute autoimmunhämolytische Anämien vom Donath–Landsteiner-Typ. *Mschr. Kinderheik.*, **122**, 651–652.

NORDHAGEN, R. (1991). Two cases of paroxysmal cold hemoglobinuria with a Donath–Landsteiner antibody reactive by the indirect antiglobulin test using anti-IgG. *Transfusion*, **31**, 190–191 (Letter).

NORDHAGEN, R., STENSVOLD, K., WINSNES, A., SKYBERG, D. & STOREN, A. (1984). Paroxysmal cold haemoglobinuria. The most frequent acute autoimmune haemolytic anaemia in children. *Acta paediat. scand.*, **73**, 258–262.

O'NEILL, B. J. & MARSHALL, W. C. (1967). Paroxysmal cold haemoglobinuria and measles. *Arch. Dis. Childh.*, **42**, 183–186.

PARISH, D. J. & MITCHELL., J. R. A. (1960). Syphilitic paroxysmal cold haemoglobinuria. Case report and study of the Coombs test. *J. clin. Path.*, **13**, 237–240.

PETERSON, E. T. & WALFORD, R. L. (1952). Serologic properties of a cold hemolysin and an acid hemolysin occurring in a case of syphilitic paroxysmal cold hemoglobinuria. *Blood*, 7, 1109–1116.

PETZ, L. D. & GARRATTY, G. (1980). *Acquired Immune Hemolytic Anemias*, 458 pp. Churchill Livingstone, New York.

PIROFSKY, B. (1969). *Autoimmunization and the Autoimmune Hemolytic Anemias*, 537 pp. Williams and Wilkins, Baltimore.

RAUSEN, A. R., LEVINE, R. HSU, T. C. S. & ROSENFIELD, R. E. (1975). Compatible transfusion therapy for paroxysmal cold hemoglobinuria. *Pediatrics*, **55**, 275–278.

RIES, C. A., GARRATTY, G., PETZ, L. D. & FUDENBERG, H. H. (1971). Paroxysmal cold hemoglobinuria: report of a case with an exceptionally high thermal range Donath–Landsteiner antibody. *Blood*, **38**, 491–499.

ROHRER, F. (1901). Ueber ein Symptom der Hämoglobinurie: Cyanose und Gangrän am äusseren Ohr. *Z. Ohrenheilk*, **39**, 165–167.

ROSENBACH, O. (1879). Zur Lehre von der periodischen Hämoglobinurie. *Dtsch. med. Wschr.*, **5**, 613.

ROSENBACH, O. (1880). Beitrag zur Lehre von der periodischen Hämoglobinurie. *Berl. klin. Wschr.*, **17**, 132–134, 151–153.

ROSSE, W. F. (1990). Autoimmune hemolytic anemia due to cold-reacting antibodies: paroxysmal cold hemoglobinuria. In *Clinical Immunohematology: Basic Concepts and Clinical Applications*, pp. 583–589. Blackwell Scientific Publications, Boston.

ROSSE, W. F., ADAMS, J. & LOGUE, G. (1977). Hemolysis by complement and cold-reacting antibodies: time and temperature requirements. *Amer. J. Hemat.*, **2**, 259–270.

SCHMIDT, J. & CLIFFORD, G. O. (1960). Studies of the antibody in paroxysmal cold hemoglobinuria. *Clin. Res.*, **8**, 217 (Abstract).

SCHUBOTHE, H. (1956). Die Serologie der

Kältehämolysine. *5th Kongr. Europ. Ges. Hämat.*, *Freiburg I. Br.*, Sept. 1955, p. 781. Springer-Verlag, Berlin.

SCHUBOTHE, H. (1958). *Serologie und klinische Bedeutung der Autohämantikörper*, 284 pp. Karger, Basel.

SCHUBOTHE, H. (1959). Serologie und Klinik der Autoimmunhämolytischen Erkrankungen. *Ergebn. inn. Med. Kinderheilk.*, **11**, 466–624.

SCHUBOTHE, H. & HAENLE, M. (1961). Serologische Studien über die nichtsyphilitische Varainte des Donath-Landsteinerschen Hämolysins. *Vox Sang.*, **6**, 455–468.

SCHWARTING, G. A., KUNDU, S. K. & MARCUS, D. M. (1979). Reaction of antibodies that cause paroxysmal cold hemoglobinuria (PCH) with globoside and Forssman glycosphingolipids. *Blood*, **53**, 186–192.

SCHWEITZER, I. L. (1957). Syphilitic paroxysmal cold hemoglobinuria. *Ann. intern. Med.*, **46**, 590–594.

SECCHI (1872). Ein Fall von Hämoglobinurie aus der Klinik des Geh. Rath Prof. Dr. Lebert. *Berl. klin. Wschr.*, **9**, 237–239.

SIEBENS, A. A., ZINKHAM, W. H. & WAGLEY, P. F. (1948). Observations on the mechanism of hemolysis in paroxysmal (cold) hemoglobinuria. *Blood*, **3**, 1367–1380.

SIRCHIA, G., FERRONE, S. & MERCURIALI, F. (1965). A case of paroxysmal cold haemoglobinuria with unusual serological findings. *Haematologica latina*, **8**, 103–112.

SOKOL, R. J., HEWITT, S. & STAMPS, B. K. (1982). Autoimmune haemolysis associated with Donath–Landsteiner antibodies. *Acta haemat. (Basel)*, **68**, 268–277.

SOKOL, R. J., HEWITT, S., STAMPS, B. K. & HITCHEN, P. A. (1984). Autoimmune haemolysis in childhood and adolescence. *Acta haemat. (Basel)*, **72**, 245–257.

STATS, D. & WASSERMAN, L. R. (1943). Cold hemagglutination—an interpretive review. *Medicine (Baltimore)*, **22**, 363–424.

SUSSMAN, R. M. & KAYDEN, H. J. (1948). Renal insufficiency due to paroxysmal cold hemoglobinuria. *Arch. intern. Med.*, **82**, 598–610.

SWEETNAM, W. P., MURPHY, E. F. & WOODCOCK, R. C. (1952). Acute idiopathic paroxysmal cold haemoglobinuria of non-syphilitic type in a child. *Brit. med. J.*, **i**, 465–466.

SWISHER, S. N. (1956). Nonspecific adherence of platelets and leukocytes to antibody-sensitized red cells: a mechanism producing thrombocytopenia and leukopenia during incompatible transfusion. *J. clin. Invest.*, **35**, 738 (Abstract).

THURMON, F. & BLAIN, D. (1931). Paroxysmal hemoglobinuria; observations based upon the study of three cases. *Amer. J. Syph.*, **15**, 350–367.

TÖTTERMAN, L. E. (1946). A contribution to the knowledge of paroxysmal cold hemoglobinuria. *Acta med. scand.*, **124**, 446–465.

UCHIDA, H. (1921). Uber die Erythrophagocytose der Leukozyten, besonders bei der paroxysmalen Hämoglobinurie. *Mitt. med. Fak. Tokyo*, **26**, 503–586.

VAN DER HART, M., VAN DER GIESSEN, M., VAN DER VEER, M., PEETOM, F. & VAN LOGHEM, J. J. (1964). Immunochemical and serological properties of biphasic haemolysins. *Vox Sang.*, **9**, 36–39.

VAN LOGHEM J. J. JNR, MENDES DE LEON, D. E., FRENKEL-TIETZ, H. & VAN DER HART, M. (1952). Two different serologic mechanisms of paroxysmal cold hemoglobinuria, illustrated by three cases. *Blood*, 7, 1196–1209.

VAN LOGHEM, J. J. JNR, VAN DER HART, M. & DORFMEIER, H. (1958). Serologic studies in acquired hemolytic anemia. *Proc. 6th int. Congr. int. Soc. Hemat., Boston, 1956*, pp. 858–868. Grune and Stratton, New York.

VOGEL, J. M., HELLMAN, M. & MOLOSHOK, R. E. (1972). Paroxysmal cold hemoglobinuria of nonsyphilitic etiology in two children. *J. Pediat.*, **81**, 974–977.

WAGLEY, P. F., ZINKHAM, W. H. & SIEBENS, A. A. (1947). A note on studies of hemolysis in paroxysmal (cold) hemoglobinuria. *Amer. J. Med.*, **2**, 342–346.

WATSON, K. C. & LAURIE, W. (1956). Syphilitic cold haemoglobinuria, *S. Afr. med. J.*, **30**, 1001–1002.

WEINER, W., GORDON, E. G. & ROWE, D. (1964). A Donath–Landsteiner antibody (non-syphilitic type). *Vox Sang.*, **9**, 684–697.

WEINTRAUB, A. M., PIERCE, L. E., DONOVAN, W. T. & RATH, C. E. (1962). Paroxysmal cold hemoglobinuria. Two cases of interest, one with red blood cell lipid studies. *Arch. intern. Med.*, **109**, 589–594.

WIDAL, F., ABRAMI, P. & BRISSAUD, E. (1913a). Recherches sur l'hémoglobinurie paroxystique 'à frigore'. *Sem. méd. (Paris)*, **33**, 585.

WIDAL, F., ABRAMI, P. & BRISSAUD, E. (1913b). L'auto anaphylaxie. Son rôle dans l'hémoglobinurie paroxystique. Traitement anti-anaphylactique de l'hémoglobinurie. Conception physique de l'anaphylaxie. *Sem. méd. (Paris)*, **33**, 613–619.

WILTSHIRE, A. (1867). Urine from a case of intermittent haematuria. *Trans. path. Soc. Lond.*, **18**, 180.

WOLACH, B., HEDDLE, N., BARR, R. D., ZIPURSKY, A., PAI, K. R. M. & BLAJCHMAN, M. A. (1981). Transient Donath–Landsteiner haemolytic anaemia. *Brit. J. Haemat.*, **48**, 425–434.

WORLLEDGE, S. M. & ROUSSO, C. (1965). Studies on the serology of paroxysmal cold haemoglobinuria (P. C. H.), with special reference to its relationship with the P blood group system. *Vox Sang.*, **10**, 293–298.

YORKE, W. & MACFIE, J. W. S. (1921). The mechanism of autolysis in paroxysmal haemoglobinuria. *Brit. J. exp. Path.*, **2**, 115–130.

33

Auto-immune haemolytic anaemia (AIHA): aetiology

The classic studies of Ehrlich and Morgenroth   364
Definition of an auto-antibody   364
Acquired haemolytic anaemia: often an auto-immune disease? Early views   365
Recent reviews   365
Aetiology of acute transient AIHA   366
Modes of action of viruses or bacteria, or viral or bacterial products, in bringing about haemolysis   367
  Direct damage to the erythrocyte surface by micro-organisms   367
  Newcastle disease virus (NDV)   368
  Altered erythrocyte antigenicity   368
  Exposure of antigens that are normally present but not normally available   369
  Development of cross-reacting antibodies   369
  The critical role of the individual   369
Aetiology of chronic AIHA   369
Clinical clues to the aetiology of chronic AIHA   370
  Possible role of prophylactic immunization   370
  Genetic factors   371
  Occurrences of AIHA and another auto-immune disease in the same patient   371
  Development of AIHA in patients with a malignant disease   371
  Development of AIHA in association with deficiencies in immunoglobulins   372
Serological clues to the aetiology of chronic AIHA   372

Unusual propensity to form antibodies   372
Allo-immunization to blood-group antigens as a factor in the production of auto-antibodies   372
Specificity of the auto-antibodies   372
Disturbed T-cell function   374
Damage to erythrocytes by mechanisms not involving micro-organisms   375
Role of viruses in chronic AIHA   376
Milgrom's anti-antibody hypothesis   376
In-vitro studies of auto-antibody formation   377
Aetiology of chronic cold-haemagglutinin disease (CHAD)   377
Experimental studies in animals that relate to the aetiology of AIHA   378
  Attempts to produce AIHA in normal animals   378
  Production of auto-antibodies by immunization with the erythrocytes of an allied species   378
  Occurrence of anti-erythrocyte auto-antibodies in grafted animals   379
Naturally-occurring AIHA in species other than man   380
  Canine AIHA   380
  Canine SLE   381
AIHA in New Zealand (NZB/BL) mice   381
  Occurrence of lymphomas and C-type oncogenic viruses in NZB/BL mice   382
Summary   384

The Oxford English Dictionary defines *Aetiology* in relation to medicine as 'that branch of medical science which investigates the causes and origin of diseases'. In this chapter an attempt will be made to discuss the aetiology of AIHA, a difficult and complicated assignment, which is made all the more difficult by the fact that the term AIHA embraces several groups of diseases which, although united by the fact that they all depend upon the formation of anti-erythrocyte auto-antibodies, differ markedly with respect to the type of antibody formed, their clinical expression and the age of patient affected. No attempt, therefore, will be made in this chapter to discuss the aetiology of AIHA under a single entity. Instead the problem will be discussed under three main headings: (1) the aetiology of acute transient AIHA; (2) the aetiology of chronic warm-antibody AIHA and (3) the aetiology of chronic cold-antibody AIHA (CHAD). First, however, reference will be made to the history of the subject, which dates back to the beginning of the century, and then to the remarkable resurgence in interest in AIHA (and in other types of auto-immune disease) that occurred in the late 1940s and 1950s and which provided the basis on which current ideas have been formulated.

THE CLASSIC STUDIES OF EHRLICH AND MORGENROTH

It is now over 90 years since the classic studies of Ehrlich and Morgenroth on haemolysins were published. Ehrlich and Morgenroth (1900), in their third publication, described how they had injected goats intraperitoneally with the laked blood of other goats and looked for the development of lysins in the blood of the recipient goats. These lysins were regularly found, and blood samples of all the goats tested, except that of the recipients, were found to be sensitive to lysis. This led Ehrlich and Morgenroth to distinguish clearly between an 'isolysin'—capable of lysing the cells of animals of the same species, and an 'autolysin', capable of lysing the cells of the experimental animal itself. The potential importance of an autolysin was immediately apparent to them. They wrote (English translation by Bolduan of Ehrlich's (1906) *Collected Studies on Immunity*, p. 25):

'It is therefore of the highest pathological importance to determine whether the absorption of its *own* body material can excite reactive changes in the organism, and what the nature of the change is. The simplest conditions and those most accessible to experimental study are those which arise on the absorption of blood-cells. But here we face a curious dilemma. If an animal organism, when injected with blood-cells of a foreign species, always produces a specific haemolysin for each of these species, it must surely be following a natural law; and it is improbable that the law which applies in any particular number of cases should be suspended in the case of blood-cells of the same individual.'

A little later they wrote: 'It cannot be doubted that the organism seeks a way out of this difficulty by means of certain regulating contrivances, whose determination will be of the highest interest.' Later, they refer to their experimental work as an example of the general law that autolysins are not capable of existence in an organism and they speculated that 'anti-autolysins' might play a part in neutralizing autolysins, if they should be formed, and also that the receptors might disappear. The celebrated phrase 'horror autotoxicus' is not mentioned as such. This came later (Ehrlich and Morgenroth, 1901). In Bolduan's (1906, p. 82) English translation of Ehrlich's (1904) *Collected Studies on Immunity*: 'In the third communication, on isolysins, we pointed out that the organism possesses certain contrivances by means of which the immunity reaction, so easily produced by all kinds of cells, is prevented from acting against the organism's own elements and so give[s] rise to autotoxins. Further investigations made by us have confirmed this view, so that one might be justified in speaking of a 'horror autotoxicus' of the organism. These contrivances are naturally of the highest importance for the existence of the individual.' Earlier, Ehrlich and Morgenroth (1900), in referring to the possibilities of auto-intoxication occurring in man, made the point that: 'Only when the internal regulating contrivances are no longer intact can great dangers arise' (Bolduan, 1906, p. 35).

Ehrlich and Morgenroth's concept as given above can hardly be faulted even today. The 'law' of 'horror autotoxicus', so often quoted still stands and even if the 'internal regulating contrivances' may not be those that they conceived, their suggestion that their breakdown could lead to great dangers seems exactly right.

Definition of an auto-antibody

It is important to clarify what is meant by an auto-antibody. In its most narrow sense, in relation to erythrocytes, it could be defined (Dacie, 1958) as an antibody formed by normal antibody-forming cells against the subject's own normal erythrocytes, acting as antigen, in apparent direct contradiction of the law of 'horror autotoxicus'; in a broader sense, it could be held merely to mean an antibody capable of being adsorbed by autologous cells at 37°C, or even below this temperature, and causing agglutination, lysis or sensitization to agglutination by antiglobulin serum, without specifying either that the erythrocytes themselves or the antibody-forming mechanism was necessarily normal. If the later viewpoint is accepted, and this to the author seems the right way to look at the problem, the concept of 'horror autotoxicus' can still be accepted as valid under normal conditions, for there is no reason whatever to suppose that auto-immune haemolytic anaemia ever develops on the basis of strictly normal erythrocytes or a strictly normal antibody-forming tissue.

ACQUIRED HAEMOLYTIC ANAEMIA: OFTEN AN AUTO-IMMUNE DISEASE? EARLY VIEWS

The discovery in the late 1940s and 1950s that many cases of acquired haemolytic anaemia were apparently bought about by the development of anti-erythrocyte antibodies led to much discussion as to whether such cases should be looked upon as valid examples of auto-immune disease. They also led to renewed interest into the important problem of the how and why of auto-antibody formation.

Of seminal importance at that time were the theoretical discussions of Burnet (Burnet and Fenner, 1949; Burnet, 1956, 1957, 1959a,b,c, 1961) and the pioneer experimental studies of transplantation immunity of Medawar and his colleagues (see Billingham, Brent and Medawar, 1953; Medawar, 1961).

Witebsky (1959), a pioneer in research into thyroid auto-immunity and a strong supporter of the concept of 'horror autotoxicus', accepted the D–L antibody of PCH as a genuine auto-antibody but argued against the uncritical acceptance of the warm antibody of acquired haemolytic anaemia as an auto-antibody on several grounds, including the fact that the erythrocyte antigen was at the time uncertain or unknown. Other contemporary reviews dealing with the genesis and mechanism of auto-immune disease, with reference to acquired haemolytic anaemia, include the following: Eyquem (1956), Moeschlin (1957), Dixon (1958), Dausset (1958), Grabar (1959), Burnet (1959b,c) and Dameshek and Schwartz (1959).

The author's own view was summarized in the 2nd edition of this book (Dacie, 1962, p. 583). He then wrote as follows: 'The concept of "horror autotoxicus" needs no defence. It is unassailable as an integral part of health. The "internal regulating contrivances" of Ehrlich and Morgenroth comprise, as we now know, the foetal "actively acquired tolerance" of Billingham, Brent and Medawar (1953) and possibly also other at present less tangible homeostatic mechanisms (Burnet, 1959a). Auto-immune haemolytic anaemia develops in consequence of a breakdown of "horror autotoxicus"; it is a question of the exception proving the rule.' With 30 year's hindsight this still seems a tenable view.

Since the above paragraph was written, the auto-immune diseases, of which AIHA (in particular PCH) can claim to be the prototype, have continued to be a focus of great interest for immunologists and clinicians throughout the world. However, despite remarkable advances in knowledge of cellular and molecular immunology, a complete solution to the problem of the exact sequence of events that lead to the development of auto-immune diseases, and the reason why some individuals, but not others, suffer from them, remains elusive.

Four main hypotheses for the development of the 'auto-antibodies' of AIHA have been advanced. These are: (1) an alteration in the patient's erythrocyte antigens so that they appear 'foreign' or 'not-self' to his or her normal antibody-forming apparatus which in consequence forms antibodies against them; (2) the formation by the patient of antibodies primarily directed against an invading micro-organism, which nevertheless cross-react with an antigen or antigens normally present on the erythrocyte surface; (3) the formation of anti-erythrocyte antibodies not due to any alteration in erythrocyte antigens but due to an intrinsic abnormality of the immune system leading to a breakdown in immune tolerance, and (4) the formation of antibodies in large amounts as the result of the monoclonal proliferation of antibody-forming cells already dedicated to the formation of an auto-antibody, as in the case of the anti-I of CHAD.

RECENT REVIEWS

The published literature on the aetiology of the auto-immune diseases is now extensive. The following authors have provided wide-ranging reviews that illustrate how understanding has evolved during the last three decades: Burnet (1962, 1966*, 1967, 1972a,b), Milgrom and Witebsky (1962), Dameshek (1964*, 1965a*,b*), Good et al. (1965), Haurowitz (1965), Milgrom (1965, 1969), van Loghem (1965*), Fudenberg (1966), Schwartz and Costea (1966), Zuelzer et al. (1966*, 1970*), Holborow (1967), Mitchison (1967), Asherson (1968), Pirofsky (1968*, 1969*), Weigle (1968), Weir (1969), Glynn (1970), Dmochowski (1971), Hong and Ammann (1972), Allison (1974), Levy (1974), Weens and Schwartz (1974), Playfair (1975), Barnes and Wills (1976), Talal (1976), Waldmann et al. (1978), Teale and MacKay (1979), Cox and Howles (1981*), Lippman et al. (1982), Nossal (1983), Plotz (1983), Smith and Steinberg (1983), Bias et al. (1986), Rosse (1990*) and Viard and Bach (1991). The articles marked with an asterisk (*) deal primarily with the aetiology of AIHA. There seems, however, no reason to suppose that the aetiology of AIHA differs in any substantial way from that of other auto-immune diseases.

AETIOLOGY OF ACUTE TRANSIENT AIHA

As has been repeatedly stressed in previous chapters of this book, there is a great deal of circumstantial evidence that acute transient warm-antibody AIHA may closely follow an acute infection, particularly if this is of viral origin. This is especially true of AIHA affecting children. Most commonly this has followed an upper respiratory tract infection of indeterminate causation, but occasionally it has been associated with measles or varicella, or with influenza virus-A or Coxsackie virus-A or cytomegalovirus (CMV) infection (see below). Reference, too, has been made in Chapters 30–32 to acute transient cold-antibody AIHAs developing as sequelae to mycoplasma pneumonia, infectious mononucleosis and other viral infections.

Amongst the case reports of acute transient warm-antibody AIHAs which developed as rare complications of identified viral infections are those described in the 1950s and 1960s by Betke et al. (1953) (Coxsackie-virus-A), Todd and O'Donohoe (1958) (herpes simplex), Beickert and Sprössig (1959) (Asiatic influenza), d'Oelsnitz, Vincent and Lippman (1959) (influenza virus-A) and Goudemand, Voisin and Marchandise (1962) (virus pneumonia, ? ornithosis).

More recently, a number of patients have been described suffering from generally transient haemolytic anaemia in whom there has been evidence of cytomegalovirus (CMV) infection; but whether the CMV has been the primary initiator of the haemolysis or a secondary invader associated with immune deficiency is unclear.

Toghill and co-workers (1967) described two such patients (in whom the DAT was negative) and Harris, Meyer and Brody (1975) a patient whose DAT was negative, too, who also became severely thrombocytopenic.

Coombs's (1968) patient, a man aged 45, suffered from severe haemolysis and was also reticulocytopenic and thrombocytopenic. The DAT was positive, and a panagglutinin active at 37°C was present in his serum. At necropsy there was evidence of widespread CMV infection and Candida infection of the lungs.

Other patients with DAT-positive AIHA and CMV infection were described by Houston et al. (1980) and Dietz (1981).

An important point that needs to be made in connection with AIHA apparently occurring as a sequal to an acute viral infection is that the great majority of children (or indeed adults) who contract such infections do not suffer from acute haemolysis subsequently. There are, therefore, two important questions that require answers: one is concerned with the mechanisms(s) by which the infective agent brings about the haemolysis, the other with the reason why only certain individuals — a very small minority—are affected.

MODES OF ACTION OF VIRUSES OR BACTERIA, OR VIRAL OR BACTERIAL PRODUCTS, IN BRINGING ABOUT HAEMOLYSIS

There seem to be several possible ways by which micro-organisms, or products, e.g enzymes derived from them, could bring about haemolysis: (1) by a direct damaging effect on the erythrocyte surface; (2) by altering the cell surface in some way, e.g. by modifying a surface antigen (or antigens) so that the cell becomes antigenic; (3) by affecting the cell surface so that antigens that are not normally available (cryptic antigens) become exposed and react with antibodies that are normally present and harmless, and (4) by causing the production of antibodies directed against the invading micro-organism that react, too, with erythrocyte antigens that are normally present (cross-reacting antibodies).

Direct damage to the erythrocyte surface by micro-organisms

Viruses have for long been known to exert profound effects on erythrocytes *in vitro* (e.g., see Briody, 1952), and lysis may be produced *in vitro* by the mumps virus (Morgan, Enders and Wagley, 1948; Moberley et al. (1958) and by the Newcastle disease (NDV) virus (Kilham, 1949). There is no doubt, therefore, but that viruses can produce lysis as well as agglutination by a direct effect on erythrocytes. *In vivo*, too, erythrocytes modified by influenza virus (Stewart, Petenyi and Rose, 1955), or NDV (Wright and Gardner, 1960) have been shown to have a reduced survival time.

There is, however, little or no positive evidence of direct damage being a pathogenetic mechanism in man. For instance, in haemolytic anaemia following mycoplasma pneumonia it is characteristic that the anaemia develops during convalescence when the titre of cold agglutinins, a manifestation of the immune response to the infection, is at its maximum and when the concentration of mycoplasma in the body would be minimal.

A possible variation of the direct-action hypothesis is one in which the virus (or viral or bacterial product) is adsorbed to the erythrocytes with the result that the cell surface may become later the site of interaction between virus, acting as antigen, and a corresponding anti-virus antibody. This mechanism appeared to be at least part explanation for the haemolysis observed in dogs when transfused with influenza-virus-modified erythrocytes (Stewart, Petenyi and Rose, 1955). Ceppellini and de Gregorio (1953), too, carried out some interesting experiments with bacterial antigens. In rabbits immunized against the Vi antigen of *Salm. ballerup*, they found that autologous erythrocytes exposed *in vitro* to the Vi antigen were rapidly destroyed when reinjected into the immunized animal. They failed, however, to demonstrate this by injecting the Vi antigen, even in large amounts, directly into the animal. Presumably, under these circumstances, the antigen combined with free antibody in the rabbit serum and was unable to attach itself to the erythrocytes.

Suzuki and co-workers (1964) described the results of further experiments on the lines of those of Ceppellini and de Gregorio (1953), referred to above. Rabbits were immunized with an antigen common to many Enterobacteriaceae and then injected with autologous erythrocytes that had been exposed to the antigen. Intravascular haemolysis resulted. Suzuki et al. pointed out that antibodies to the antigen have been identified in the serum of healthy human individuals and that rises in titre have been detected in children with enterobacterial infections. Whether the above mechanism is a cause of haemolysis in human enterobacterial infections is unclear; it seems likely to be important in *Esch. coli* septicaemia.

The sequence of events in man in cases where anti-viral antibodies have been demonstrated does not seem, however, to favour a virus–antibody interaction at the erythrocyte surface. For instance, in the child carefully studied by Betke et al. (1953), in whom haemolysis appeared to be associated with, or at least coincidental with, Coxsackie virus-A infection, the DAT, which was positive at the height of the child's illness, could not be explained by the binding on by virus of anti-viral antibodies to the erythrocyte surface as the antibodies did not appear in the child's serum until convalescence when the haemolytic episode had subsided.

More recently, Mulhearn, Rothschild and Freeman (1975) described some findings in an unvaccinated 9-month-old boy, who had suffered from a recurrent and eventually fatal warm-antibody AIHA, which appeared possibly to reflect direct virus or virus–antibody interaction at the erythrocyte surface.

Polio III virus had been recovered from the stools on two separate hospital admissions, although no anti-polio antibodies had been identified in his serum. When, however, his erythrocytes were incubated *in vitro* in his serum in the presence of guinea-pig complement and type III polio virus, the increase in osmotic fragility was substantially greater than in control preparations in which normal erythrocytes and normal serum were substituted for the patient's cells and serum.

Newcastle disease virus (NDV)

In the 1950s attention was focussed on NDV as a possible aetiological factor in human AIHA, e.g. by Moolten and Clark (1952a,b) and Moolten et al. (1953). This possibility does not seem, however, to have been substantiated by later work.

Auto-agglutination was a marked feature in Moolten and Clark's (1952a) first case and was attributed by them to adsorption of virus on to erythrocyte surfaces, and not to the presence of abnormal auto-agglutinins. Subsequently, not only NDV but the virus of herpes simplex, and other unidentified viruses, were isolated from other patients suffering from various types of haemolytic anaemia (Moolten and Clark, 1952b; Moolten et al. (1953).

Other attempts at the time to isolate viruses were, however, less successful. Thus Morgan (1952) searched for viruses in the blood of six patients and in the spleens of three patients with acquired haemolytic anaemia but was unable to isolate any. Eyquem and Dausset (1952) studied the sera of 120 patients suffering from various types of anaemia. Seven sera inhibited the agglutination of erythrocytes by NDV: three of them contained a powerful inhibitor but only one of these was from a patient with acquired haemolytic anaemia; the other two were from patients suffering from HS and PNH, respectively. Morgan (1955) reported on further negative studies carried out on eight patients.

Further experiments with Newcastle disease virus were described by Wright and Gardner (1960). They reported that both chicken and human erythrocytes exposed to the virus were more readily phagocytosed by cultured rabbit spleen cells than were unmodified cells; also that human erythocytes, exposed to the virus and then used to immunize rabbits, led to antibodies being formed which could not be completely absorbed by normal human cells. This led them to suggest that exposure to the virus had resulted in antigenic modification.

Gardner, Wright and Williams (1961) demonstrated that rabbit erythrocytes exposed to NDV or influenza virus *in vitro* had an impaired survival when injected back into the donor animals. Cells that had been exposed to influenza virus survived longer in splenectomized rabbits.

Altered erythrocyte antigenicity

It has for many years been considered to be a conceivable and reasonable hypothesis that erythrocytes might be altered and rendered auto-antigenic by the adsorption to their surfaces of viruses or viral or bacterial enzymes, or products of their metabolism, and that antibodies might be produced in response to the presence of the damaged cells. Similarly, it was considered reasonable to suppose that a chemical or drug might, after adsorption to the surface of an erythrocyte, so alter the surface of the cell that it became antigenic, or that a combination of the drug and a component of the cell surface might together function as antigen in the same sort of way that many chemicals are known to combine with proteins and to impart to them greater or lesser degrees of 'foreignness' and antigenicity (see Wright, 1953). The question is whether these types of mechanism actually produce AIHA in man.

In the case of certain drug-dependent immune haemolytic anaemias they certainly seem to do so, and stemming from the stimulus of the pioneer studies of Harris (1954, 1956) with the anti-bilharzial drug stibophen (Fuadin), a great deal of work has been undertaken in recent years with the aim of elucidating the details and consequences of drug–erythrocyte interactions. The subject is a large one and will be considered in Volume 4 of this book.

Exposure of antigens that are normally present but not normally available

The phenomenon of polyagglutinability, i.e. the acquired property of erythrocytes to be agglutinated by adult human sera irrespective of blood group—the so-called Hübener–Thomsen–Friedenreich phenomenon—has been discussed already in Chapter 27 (p. 201). The basis of the phenomenon is the unmasking of an antigen—the T antigen—that is normally present, as the result of the action of enzymes of bacterial origin. Anti-T antibodies exist normally apparently in the serum of adults; they are absent, however, in the serum of newborns. As discussed on p. 203, there is some evidence that

T–anti-T interaction is a rare cause of haemolytic anaemia.

Development of cross-reacting antibodies

It is an attractive hypothesis that infection with a micro-organism, which carried an antigen similar to an antigen present on normal human erythrocytes, might cause the development of antibodies that would react not only with the invading micro-organism but also with the host's erythrocytes. This is the mechanism probably responsible for the normally occurring anti-A and anti-B antibodies and for the development of the anti-I cold antibodies found in most normal human sera; it is probably, too, at least partly responsible for the development of the high-titre anti-I antibodies following infection with *Mycoplasma pneumoniae*, as described on p. 298. This concept, too, had been considered in the 1950s and found favour with some virologists, e.g. Vivell (1954), at that time. This is, too, probably the mechanism responsible for the development of cold antibodies in listeria infections (p. 307) and also in the rare cases of transient acute cold-antibody haemolytic anaemias of uncertain origin. On the other hand, there seems to be no evidence that cross-reacting antibodies formed in response to microbial infection are ever responsible for warm-antibody acute AIHA.

Whether the anti-i antibodies that are sometimes developed in infectious mononucleosis (p. 318) are cross-reacting antibodies is uncertain. Their occurrence in infectious mononucleosis as well as occasionally in association with poorly differentiated malignant lymphomas (p. 251), points to some relationship with the proliferation of primitive lymphoid cells, but the exact nature of this relationship remains obscure.

The critical role of the individual

A point that has to be made in relation to the role of micro-organisms in the genesis of AIHA is that, irrespective of the exact mechanism by which infection with the organism leads to the production of erythrocyte auto-antibodies, it is the individuality of the affected person that determines whether or not he or she develops the antibodies and, if so, whether the antibodies, by virtue of the quantity formed and their nature—whether IgG or IgM, have the ability to lead to clinically important haemolysis. Thus, while many patients who develop mycoplasma pneumonia develop high-titre cold antibodies, only a few suffer from overt haemolytic anaemia; and of the very many young people who develop infectious mononucleosis only a very small number suffer from haemolytic anaemia; and of the thousands of children who suffer from measles or varicella only a tiny fraction develops PCH. In a nutshell, the infection provides the trigger, the patient's own immune system determines the outcome.

AETIOLOGY OF CHRONIC AIHA

In chronic AIHA, whether idiopathic or associated with an underlying disease, the available evidence points strongly to a breakdown in the mechanisms that normally prevent an individual from forming antibodies against his or her own normal tissues. As already referred to (p. 364), the concept that a breakdown in immune tolerance can lead to 'great dangers' stems from the beginning of this century (Ehrlich and Morgenroth, 1900).

A detailed consideration of how normal immunological tolerance is attained and maintained by an antibody-forming system which responds readily to non-self antigens is beyond the scope of this book. That tolerance is a process which starts *in utero* and involves probably the elimination of self-reacting clones of immunocytes, and that thymus-derived (T) lymphocytes play an important role in this, seems to be well established. The process is, however, without doubt complicated. In his 1983 review Nossal summarized the situation as follows: 'The complex process of self-tolerance is probably an amalgam of repertoire purging, suppression, sequestration of self antigens, and blockade of receptors by monovalent, non-immunogenic self molecules and other regulating loops, possibly including anti-idiotype networks'.

The basic problem in AIHA, and in other auto-immune diseases, is how this normal process of tolerance is abrogated. As mentioned earlier in this chapter, Burnet's (1959c) somatic-mutation hypothesis implied the formation of 'forbidden clones' of antibody-forming cells that reacted with normal erythrocyte antigens. The cause of the hypothetical somatic mutation was a matter for speculation. Burnet considered that it might be induced by virus infections. The frequent association of auto-antibody formation in malignant lymphoproliferative diseases (see below) was an important point in favour of Burnet's hypothesis. Burnet's (1972a) later interpretation of auto-immune disease included the following summary:

'Autoimmune disease represents a breakdown of normal intrinsic tolerance associated with the proliferation of clones of immunocytes derived from 'initiator cells' of abnormal character. These are cells which would normally be inactivated by early contact with the antigenic determinant normal to the body with which their immune receptors can unite specifically. The abnormality responsible for their resistance to this process is probably often in part genetic, in the form of a generally increased resistance to tolerigenic stimuli, but will generally include somatic mutational change as well.'

'In addition to the appearance of potential initiator cells of appropriate (somatic) genetic quality there must also be an appropriate source of accessible autoantigen and the necessary micro-environmental conditions to allow the proliferative stimulation by autoantigen which will provoke the development of a pathogenic forbidden clone.'

'Many factors, including various types of infection and certain drugs, can modify one or other aspect of the autoimmune process to significant degrees.'

CLINICAL CLUES TO THE AETIOLOGY OF CHRONIC AIHA

There are several clinical associations which if and when fully understood should provide important clues to the aetiology of chronic AIHA. One such clue is the occurrence of more than one case of AIHA within a family or the occurrence of AIHA in one member of a family and another type of auto-immune disease in another closely related member. These associations point strongly to genetic factors playing an important part in aetiology. Another association indicating an individual proneness to auto-immune diseases is the occurrence of AIHA and another auto-immune disease in the same patient. Other important clues to aetiology are the development of AIHA in patients suffering from malignant lymphoproliferative diseases and in patients who have congenital or acquired deficiencies of immunoglobulin.

Possible role of prophylactic immunization

In other patients the onset of chronic AIHA has seemed to have been precipitated by some event involving stimulation of the immune system by, for instance, vaccination. Thus vaccination against smallpox (Kölbl, 1955) or poliomyelitis (Dameshek and Schwartz, 1959) has appeared to be responsible in rare instances and, in a somewhat different category, relapse following bee-stings (Christen and Jaccottet, 1958). It has also for long been recognized that in patients with established haemolytic anaemia major or minor exacerbations of haemolysis were likely to follow intercurrent upper respiratory tract or other infections (Kissmeyer-Nielsen, 1957; Pisciotta, Downer and Hinz, 1959; Wright and Gardner, 1960).

Gedikoğlu and Cantez (1967) described in a brief report how a 6-year-old boy, who had developed warm-antibody AIHA and had responded well to prednisolone, had relapsed 1 year later 7 days after receiving a D.T.T. (diphtheria–tetanus–typhoid) injection. He responded once more to prednisolone only to relapse again after developing typical pertussis.

Genetic factors

The occurrence of AIHA in identical twins or in more than one closely related member of a family has been discussed and documented in Chapter 22 (p. 12 and Table 22.2). The possibility of the association of AIHA with a particular ABO or Rh blood group or with an HLA antigen or haplotype is also discussed in Chapter 22 on p. 14. The early work quoted indicated the absence of any simple association. More recent work, reviewed for instance by Bias et al. (1986), has pointed to an interplay of several intrinsic factors, including sex and age as well as environmental factors. Bias and co-workers had subjected to genetic analysis 18 kindreds in which auto-immune disorders had occurred. Consideration of the data provided by these families, combined with other published reports, led them to suggest that there is a primary human auto-immune gene inherited as an autosomal dominant which is carried by approximately 20% of the population. In addition, secondary interacting or modifying genes, including MHC (major histocompatibility complex) genes, notably HLA-DR3, are required to confer specificity to the auto-antibody and for clinical expression. Bias et al. also concluded that an early-onset auto-immune state requires the presence of the primary gene plus at least two secondary auto-immune genes and that, although environmental challenges cannot overcome the need for the primary gene, an environmental trigger may be necessary for clinical expression.

Occurrences of AIHA and another auto-immune disease in the same patient

It has been widely recognized since the early 1950s that warm-antibody AIHA may occasionally complicate other diseases thought to be of auto-immune origin, with the result that both disorders occur in the same patient simultaneously or successively. The associations will be dealt with in detail in Volume 4 of this book: the accompanying diseases include systemic lupus erythematosus (SLE), polyarteritis nodosa, scleroderma — so-called collagen diseases — as well as rheumatoid arthritis, pernicious anaemia, thyrotoxicosis and ulcerative colitis. These occurrences point strongly to an unusual proneness by the patient to develop auto-antibodies. As postulated by Bias et al. (1986), and referred to above, secondary auto-immune genes seem likely to be responsible for the specificity of the tissues affected by the auto-immune process.

Development of AIHA in patients with a malignant disease

The association of AIHA with malignant lymphoproliferative diseases is well known and has been recognized since the 1930s, if not earlier. Both warm-antibody and cold-antibody AIHA have been recorded. These associations will be described and documented in Volume 4 of this book, as will the less frequent occurrences of AIHA in association with types of leukaemia other than chronic lymphocytic leukaemia and in patients suffering from various types of carcinoma or other tumours. The nature of these associations is obscure; but a breakdown in immune surveillance, manifesting itself in a failure to eliminate damaging clones forming auto-antibodies, as well as overtly malignant clones, is a possibility.

This important topic was reviewed by Schwartz (1972): he pointed out that not only was there a relationship between malignant lymphomas and auto-immune disease but that lymphomas also developed with unusual frequency in patients who had received allografts, as in renal transplantation. Schwartz raised the question of the activation of latent oncogenic viruses in such cases. [The possibly analogous situation in NZB/BL mice in which AIHA is also associated with lymphomas in some of the older animals is referred to on p. 382.]

The possibility that X-irradiation or treatment with an alkylating agent may act as a 'trigger' and break immunological tolerance in some patients was suggested by Lewis, Schwartz and Dameshek (1966). They had observed that of 100 patients suffering from a malignant lymphoproliferative disease, seven had developed an auto-immune complication (in six AIHA) soon after commencing such treatment.

Development of AIHA in association with deficiencies in immunoglobulins

The occurrence of AIHA in patients suffering from immune deficiency syndromes has been described and documented in Chapter 22 (p. 39) of this book. The association has been noted in children suffering from congenital or familial immunoglobulin deficiencies as well as in adults with hypogammaglobulinaemia of apparently acquired origin. As also referred to in Chapter 22 (p. 43), there is evidence, too, that many patients with apparently idiopathic AIHA have unsuspected deficiencies of, or less commonly form excessive amounts of, serum immunoglobulins. The data of Blajchman et al. (1969), for instance, indicated that in only 14 out of 48 patients with idiopathic AIHA were the results normal. IgA was the immunoglobulin that was most commonly present in abnormally low concentration.

The significance of these observations is not fully understood. They certainly point to immune dysfunction; but the link between the failure to synthesize normal immunoglobulins in normal amounts and the synthesis, nevertheless, of unwanted immunoglobulins acting as auto-antibodies remains obscure.

SEROLOGICAL CLUES TO THE AETIOLOGY OF CHRONIC AIHA

Unusual propensity to form antibodies

The critical role of the individual in determining whether microbial infection is followed by auto-antibody formation has already been stressed in relation to the aetiology of acute transient AIHA (p. 369). There is evidence, too, that in health individuals vary widely in their response to similar immunological stimuli, as, for instance, in responding to prophylactic immunization. It has also been known for a long time that some patients form allo-antibodies with remarkable ease following blood transfusions (Callender and Race, 1946; Malone and Cowan, 1950; Collins et al., 1950; Waller and Race, 1951; Cleghorn, 1959). It can hardly be a coincidence that some of the patients referred to in the publications cited above had suffered from SLE or AIHA; they

certainly appear to have had a 'highly-reactive' antibody-forming system. Other things being equal, such patients would seem to be much more likely to form auto-antibodies than patients who fail to form allo-antibodies readily after transfusion. It seems possible, therefore, that the principle that the patient who develops AIHA is an unusually 'good' antibody producer applies irrespective of whether the stimulus for the formation of the antibody is exogenous, as in the case of *Mycoplasma pneumoniae* infection, or more subtle as in idiopathic AIHA. As long ago as 1955, Gear, in referring to auto-immune diseases including AIHA, emphasized the importance with respect to aetiology of a hyperreactive antibody-forming system.

Allo-immunization to blood-group antigens as a factor in the production of auto-antibodies

Dameshek and Levine (1943) suggested that the formation of iso-(allo-) antibodies following repeated transfusions might in some way lead to auto-immunization and the perpetuation of haemolysis. There is some evidence that, exceptionally, this may happen. Hennemann (1955) reported, for instance, that a rise in titre of the anti-Rh antibodies anti-C + anti-D from 1000 to 65 000 occurred concurrently with the development of auto-antibodies and clinically severe AIHA. It is tempting to conclude that the exceptional vigour of the response to the allo-antigens in this case had been a manifestation of a hyper-reactability, another facet of which was a breaking of tolerance to self-antigens.

Further evidence of the breaking of tolerance was provided by the experiments of Mohn et al. (1963, 1965), who infused into a R_2R_2 (*cDE/cE*) recipient an exceptionally powerful anti-CD antibody. On the 70th post-infusion day anti-E antibodies were detected in an eluate of the recipient's erythrocytes, and antibody of this specificity was still detectable on the 229th post-infusion day. Mohn and his co-workers suggested that 'the E receptors [at the Rh sites on the erythrocyte membrane] were sufficiently close to the D receptors to be altered by the reactions of the transfused anti-CD antibodies on the D receptors and, thus, became involved in the autoimmunization process.'

Another interesting example of the apparent breaking of tolerance as shown by the widening of the specificity of an antibody was recorded by Isbister, Ting and Seeto (1977). A patient who had formed anti-Rh(D) allo-antibodies as the result of immunization during pregnancy was treated by repeated phasmaphereses. Eventually her DAT became positive and eluates from her erythrocytes were found to react with erythrocytes of all Rh genotypes tested except Rh null cells. A second patient similarly treated but less closely investigated appeared to show the same phenomenon. Isbister, Ting and Seeto suggested that the repeated plasmaphereses in the presence of persisting strong antigenic stimulation had allowed a widening of the specificity of the antibody by removing feedback inhibition — in their own words the patients had been 'pushed from alloantibody production to autoantibody production'.

Sosler and co-workers (1989) referred in a brief report to two more instances of blood transfusions apparently breaking tolerance. Two patients with sickle-cell disease had formed several allo-antibodies as the result of past transfusions. Their DAT, too, was weakly (1+) positive. Transfusion with apparently compatible blood was followed in each case by a severe haemolytic crisis in which both donor and recipients' erythrocytes were destroyed; in the first patient the DAT and IAT were recorded as becoming strongly (4+) positive.

Specificity of the auto-antibodies

One of the as yet unsolved mysteries of chronic AIHA is the curious specificity of the antibodies formed by the patient. The predilection for Rh antigens, in cases in which specificity could be demonstrated, and the absence of auto-antibody formation directed against the A and B allo-antigens, led the present author (Dacie, 1958) to suggest that auto-antibodies to Rh antigens might develop in post-natal life in consequence of a failure (complete or partial) to acquire the normal tolerance to these antigens in utero. It was consid-

ered that such an occurrence would be most unlikely to occur with the soluble A, B, H and Lewis antigens but could perhaps happen in the case of the Rh antigens because of their insolubility. It was thought that this type of mechanism might be the explanation for the instances of AIHA developing in infants of a few months of age onwards, at a time when their maturing antibody-forming system would be expected to react against the antigens to which tolerance had not been achieved in utero. This hypothesis remains unproved. The concentration and effectiveness of the antigen was thought to be important in relation to the forbidden clone hypothesis. Burnet (1959c) had emphasized that for the production of forbidden clones an essential requirement is an accessible source of antigen in amounts adequate to act as a stimulant but not in high enough concentration to inhibit. This requirement provides perhaps the answer to the question as to why auto-antibodies against the A and B antigens are very rarely formed while auto-antibodies against Rh antigens are relatively common. Heni and Blessing (1954) had suggested that specificity depended upon the 'strength' of the antigens to which antibodies are formed: thus those formed against strong antigens were likely to be but slightly specific (panagglutinins), while those formed against weaker antigens were more specific, and those formed against the weakest antigens would react only with the patient's own erythrocytes.

Swisher (1959) put forward some interesting ideas. He conceived that two events were necessary to initiate auto-immunization: (1) a permanent or temporary alteration in erythrocyte antigens, and (2) the occurrence of this alteration at a time when the body is capable of recognizing the antigenic stimulus and is capable of responding to it. He suggested that there might normally be antigens which are so structurally located that they are normally functionally inaccessible, and that antigens of this type, even with blood-group specificity, might develop late enough in fetal life for them to be regarded immunologically as 'not-self'. Swisher went on to suggest that the post-natal unmasking of antigens of this type might be the first step in auto-immunization.

Disturbed T-cell function

Allison, Denman and Barnes (1971), under the title Hypothesis, postulated that T-lymphocytes play a key role in antibody responses and that they achieve this by two mechanisms — cooperation with B cells in the formation of antibodies and a feedback control limiting antibody formation. In health, these two mechanisms, which are now referred to as 'helper' and 'suppressor' functions, were considered to be opposed and balanced; relaxation of this control was suggested as an important contributory factor in the development of auto-immunity.

Subsequent studies have indicated that a series of suppressor cell systems regulate immunological processes, and there is evidence, too, that a reduction in the number of suppressor T-cells plays a part in the genesis of many auto-immune disorders, including AIHA (see Waldmann et al, 1978). Some studies that have indicated abnormalities in T-cell function are summarized below.

Fagiolo and Laghi (1970) studied the response of peripheral-blood lymphocytes to phythaemagglutinin (PHA) in 15 patients with AIHA, 12 of whom suffered from the idiopathic disease. The blastogenic response was markedly deficient in 13 of the patients.

Krüger and co-workers (1976) reported data on 15 patients with chronic warm-antibody AIHA. Lymphocytopenia ($<1 \times 10^9$/cells per litre) was present in 11 of the patients and the spontaneous binding of sheep cells to lymphocytes (rosette formation) was deficient in 36 out of 41 tests. There was, however, no correlation between the reduction in rosette formation and lymphoblastogenesis induced by PHA. Lymphocytoxic antibodies were present in eight patients and were correlated, with one exception, with reduced rosette formation.

Parker, Stuart and Dewar (1977) tested the peripheral-blood mononuclear cells of 14 patients with active warm-antibody AIHA for their ability to cause rosetting with homologous and autologous erythrocytes. In 12 of the patients the percentage of rosettes was abnormally high, and in 10 patients, followed for periods of up to 2 years, the number of rosettes formed appeared to be directly related to the activity of haemolysis. The cells giving rise to the rosettes were identified as T-lymphocytes.

The results of a more detailed study of 10 warm-antibody AIHA patients were reported by Krüger and Desaga (1978). The tendency to lymphocytopenia was confirmed: the absolute number of T and B cells was less than the normal mean in all 10 patients and in three of them the counts were less than −2 S.D. of the normal mean. In-vitro cellular activity was evaluated with PHA, concanavalin A (ConA) and pokeweed mitogen (PwM). The results showed 'a blend of general or selective depression and sometimes a normal or increased activity with no definite correlation with both the number of circulating T cells and the extent of the hemolytic activity of the disease.' In eight of nine patients tested, sheep-cell rosette formation was, however, strikingly subnormal. One difficulty in interpreting the above results is that seven out of the 10 patients were receiving low doses of corticosteroids. Krüger and Desaga pointed out, however, that there appeared to be no major differences in the results in the treated and untreated patients; also, that blood samples were always withdrawn 24 (or 48) hours after an oral dose of prednisone.

A remarkable example of severe AIHA in a child suffering from a rare genetically determined condition — purine nucleoside phosphorylase deficiency — which was associated with T-cell dysfunction, was described by Rich et al. (1979). There was severe lymphopenia, and the T-cell response to mitogens was markedly subnormal, as were the responses in skin tests to Candida antigens, etc.

The availability of monoclonal antibodies specifically directed against sub-populations of T-lymphocytes has allowed more detailed investigations into the number and types of circulating T cells in patients with AIHA. In a substantial proportion of patients, but not in all of them, a significant imbalance in T-cell helper to suppressor ratio has been identified.

Phan-Dinh-Tuy and co-workers (1983) reported on a comprehensive study of 30 patients with warm-antibody AIHA, of whom 24 had idiopathic AIHA. Three monoclonal antibodies were employed: OKT3 which reacts with all peripheral-blood T cells, OKT4 which recognizes only T cells with helper-inducer function, and OKT8 which recognizes T cells with suppressor and cytotoxic activity. The OKT4-to-OKT8 (helper-to-suppressor) ratio was found to be abnormally low in seven patients and abnormally high in seven other patients. The high values were found chiefly in untreated patients; treatment with corticosteroids or immunosuppressive agents tended to decrease the ratio. The existence of two groups of patients, with contrasting T-cell helper-to-suppressor ratios, did not correspond to clinical differences. Phan-Dinh-Tuy et al. emphasized that the results of their studies underlined the heterogeneity of AIHA. The finding of T-cell imbalance, particularly the suppressor T-cell deficit in some cases, could explain in their view why AIHA patients often present with other signs of auto-immunity in addition to forming anti-erythrocyte antibodies.

Molaro and co-workers (1983) investigated 13 patients with warm-antibody AIHA of which 10 had suffered from the idiopathic disease. In eight of the patients the T-cell helper-to-suppressor ratio was abnormal: in seven of them this was, however, the result of an increase in the number of T-helper cells rather than a deficit of T-suppressor cells.

Further evidence of T-cell abnormality was provided by Conte, Tazzari and Finelli (1985), who had studied 10 patients with idiopathic AIHA. All responded subnormally in autologous mixed lymphocyte reactions (MLRs), despite normal responsiveness in allogeneic MLRs. There was, too, a marked decrease in lymphocyte responsiveness to PHA and evidence of imbalance in T-cell subsets due to reduction in OKT4 reactivity.

Conte and his co-workers (1989) reported on the state of the natural killer (NK) cell population in warm-antibody type AIHA. Nine patients, all of whom had been off treatment for at least 3 months, had been studied. Despite being present in normal numbers, the NK-cell function was found to be markedly decreased in all the patients compared with that of age- and sex-matched controls.

Damage to erythrocytes by mechanisms not involving micro-organisms

Interest in the possibility that damage to erythrocytes other than by micro-organisms might render the cells antigenic stems from the early 1950s. Extraversation of blood outside blood vessels, leading presumably to possible enzyme action, and very severe trauma to erythrocytes have been suggested as possible mechanisms.

Liu and Evans (1952) reported that the DAT had become transiently positive in a patient who had suffered from an intraperitoneal haemorrhage as the result of an ectopic pregnancy. This observation led them to attempt to reproduce the phenomenon experimentally. Twelve rabbits were given intraperitoneal injections of their own blood once a week for 4 weeks. Four developed transiently positive DATs; none, however, became anaemic. Dameshek and Schwartz (1959) referred to possible examples of the same sequence of events described in earlier publications.

Dodd and co-workers (1953) reported observations which could be taken as indicating that the erythrocytes from patients with acquired haemolytic anaemia have abnormal surfaces. Rabbits were immunized with normal human erythrocytes or trypsinized human erythrocytes, respectively. It was then found that both types of rabbit sera, absorbed with normal human erythrocytes, still reacted with the trypsinized cells, suggesting that as the result of trypsinization some previously hidden antigens had been revealed. Especially interesting was the finding that the erythrocytes of 15 out of 19 patients with acquired haemolytic anaemia were also agglutinated by the rabbit sera previously absorbed with normal cells. Whether this meant that the cells which reacted positively had modified surface antigens or whether agglutination was merely a sign of damage to the cells' surfaces which might have been caused by the adsorption of auto-antibodies was not clear; it is interesting to note that positive results were also obtained in three out of 13 patients with HS.

Theoretical discussions on the question of modified antigenicity of erythrocytes as a factor in auto-antibody formation are to be found in many early reviews. Amongst those published in the 1950s are those of Stats and Wasserman (1952), Dubert (1957), Campbell (1957) and Burnet (1959c).

Stats and Wasserman (1952) discussed the concept in the light of the evidence available to them at that time, and concluded that the hypothesis was unproved. As already mentioned, they considered that there was no theoretical reason why antibodies developed against partially damaged erythrocytes should not cross-react with normal cells. Dubert (1957) came to a similar conclusion. He conceived that the structure of normal body constituents could be slightly altered as the result of infection or metabolic abnormality so as to render them antigenic, and that antibodies formed in consequence might react not only against the modified constituent but against the normal constituent itself. It was also suggested that under these circumstances the constituent might remain antigenic in its normal state and antibody formation would persist. Some experimental evidence in support of this hypothesis was cited.

Campbell's (1957) paper was concerned with the role of antigenic fragments in immune mechanisms. He made the point that autologous proteins could become antigenic if they contained faulty or abnormal configurations; he also suggested that erythrocytes could become antigenic not only by 'faulty' protein synthesis but also by adsorption to their surfaces of abnormal antigenic fragments, which might be an infectious agent or derived from one, or even denatured autologous protein.

Burnet (1959c), however, considered that the evidence was against the hypothesis of alteration of antigenicity and emphasized that this concept was difficult to reconcile with the fact that the antibodies were known to react on occasions with Rh antigens. He concluded, too, that modification of antigenicity by virus was most unlikely in human disease.

The idea that extraversation of blood might render erythrocytes immunogenic was resuscitated by Jerne, Sørvin and Hansen (1973) who had observed that of 69 patients, suffering from a variety of disorders, in whom the DAT was positive, 17 had bled into the upper gastro-intestinal tract. This association was, in their view, unlikely to be fortuitous and indicated that 'some processing (i.e., physical, chemical, or microbial) of the erythrocyte surface antigens must take place for the antigens to become immunogenic, and that this processing occurs, at least in part, in the digestive tract above the duodenum.'

The question as to whether very severe trauma to erythrocytes could render the cells auto-antigenic was raised by Pirofsky et al. (1965) and Pirofsky (1965). They had studied seven patients, submitted to aortic-valve surgery, who had developed signs of AIHA subsequently. The DAT had been transitorily positive in six of the patients and eluted antibody was shown to react as a panagglutinin. Four of the patients had benefited from treatment with corticosteroids. In addition to the patients who had been operated on, two additional patients had been found to give a positive DAT or bromelin test before operation. Pirofsky et al. suggested two possible explanations for the auto-antibody development. One was that it was part of a graft-*versus*-host phenomenon resulting from the infusion of many viable donor lymphocytes during blood transfusion in the course of the operation—four of the patients had shown evidence of the febrile lymphocyte–splenomegaly syndrome; the other was that it was the very severe trauma to erythrocytes associated with the aortic-valve disease and surgical procedure that had caused changes in the cells' surface membrane rendering them antigenic. Proof of either mechanism was lacking, but the latter hypothesis seemed in their view to be the more likely.

Role of viruses in chronic AIHA

This is a very large subject, and no attempt will be made to deal with it in detail. As mentioned earlier in this chapter (p. 370), Burnet (1959c) considered that somatic mutation leading to the formation of forbidden clones might be engendered by virus infection, and the discovery that C-type RNA viruses chronically infect the NZB/BL

mice that develop AIHA and renal lesions resembling human lupus nephritis, and malignant lymphomas (see p. 383), provided further support for this hypothesis. Then there is the undoubted association of transient AIHA with acute virus infections (see p. 366). However, it has been difficult to prove without doubt that virus infection plays a role in the aetiology of chronic human AIHA, and in other chronic auto-immune disorders, despite the possibility receiving a great deal of attention. Nevertheless, it seems possible, even probable, that virus infection, by one means or another, could be an important factor in a chain of events leading to the breaking of self-tolerance. As Dmochowski (1971) wrote, after listing some of the immune-deficiency, malignant and auto-immune diseases in which viruses have been thought to play a part, a great deal remains to be explored. This seems still to be true.

Milgrom's anti-antibody hypothesis

Milgrom, Dubiski and Woźniczko (1956) observed that human sera occasionally had the property of agglutinating erythrocytes which had previously adsorbed incomplete anti-D. This was interpreted as due to the presence in the sera of a factor (an 'anti-antibody') which agglutinated denatured immune globulin. This observation led to a concept of auto-antibody formation in which the body forms antibodies against immune globulin developed originally against (say) a foreign protein, which in the case of haemolytic anaemia was envisaged as being adsorbed to erythrocytes. The essence of the hypothesis (Milgrom and Dubiski, 1957; Milgrom, 1959) was that the immune globulin itself is altered in the course of the serological reaction in the sense that it becomes denatured; receptors are thought perhaps to be exposed or produced as the result of antigen–antibody interaction, and are capable of stimulating further antibody formation. A chain reaction was thus postulated. Some experimental evidence in support of this concept was given in the papers referred to above.

This hypothesis aroused a good deal of interest, and Milgrom and Dubiski (1957), in meeting the objection that, if true, the antibodies against denatured immunoglobulin should be frequently demonstrable in patients suffering from a microbial infection, conceded that only 'good' antibody producers would respond in this way—which implied a peculiarity of the antibody-forming mechanism. In fact, it seems that anti-antibodies have not been demonstrated in serum* in human AIHA except in the perhaps special case of AIHA following infectious mononucleosis. In this condition, as described on p. 320, cold anti-antibodies appear to be uniquely formed. Milgrom and Dubiski (1957) also pointed out that [warm-acting] anti-antibodies might be difficult to detect in serum, because they would be continuously adsorbed to erythrocytes at body temperature *in vivo*.

IN-VITRO STUDIES OF AUTO-ANTIBODY FORMATION

Attempts have been made to demonstrate the synthesis of anti-erythrocyte antibodies by immunocytes in culture *in vitro*.

Hernandez-Jodra and co-workers (1990) described the results of cultivating peripheral-blood mononuclear cells in the presence or absence of activators, such as pokeweed mitogens. At the end of 2-week's cultivation the concentration of IgG and IgM was estimated by means of a radiolabelled binding assay using ^{125}I-staphylococcal protein A. Anti-erythrocyte auto-antibodies were detected in the cultures obtained from the peripheral blood of four out of eight AIHA patients, in the absence of additives. In two AIHA patients antibody formation was augmented in the presence of pokeweed mitogen and in two other patients it was only detected in the presence of the mitogen. However, there was evidence, too, of auto-antibody formation, and its augmentation in the presence of mitogen, in three out of four cultures derived from the blood of normal individuals. Auto-antibodies were also demonstrated in the supernatants of cultures of EB-virus-transformed lymphocytes derived from either AIHA patients or normal individuals. The amount of antibody formed was, however, greater in the case of the AIHA patients. Hernandez-Jodra et al. interpreted their data as indicating that the lymphocytes of some people are primed for auto-antibody formation and are sensitive to polyclonal activation; they concluded that both polyclonal B-cell activation and antigen-driven responses play a part in the genesis of auto-immune diseases.

AETIOLOGY OF CHRONIC COLD-HAEMAGGLUTININ DISEASE (CHAD)

As described in Chapters 28 and 29, CHAD is typically a very chronic disease of predominantly elderly subjects that is brought about by the formation of very large amounts of a monoclonal IgM cold auto-antibody, almost always of anti-I specificity. There are close similarities between CHAD and Waldenström's macroglobulinaemia, except for one important difference—that is that the monoclonal paraprotein in CHAD acts as a cold antibody. The fact that some CHAD patients, after perhaps many years of a relatively benign illness, develop a lymphoma suggests a link between CHAD and malignant lymphoproliferative disease. The exact sequence of events

that lead to the development of CHAD is unknown—as is the case with Waldenstrom's macroglobulinaemia and the more malignant lymphoproliferative diseases. However, it seems reasonable to regard CHAD as a relatively benign lymphoproliferative disease resulting from a somatic mutation taking place in an antibody-forming cell (a B lymphocyte) already dedicated to the formation of a cold anti-erythrocyte antibody.

Evidence for the participation of lymphocytes in the production of the cold auto-antibodies was elegantly provided by Feizi and her co-workers (1973), who showed that some of the small or medium-sized lymphocytes circulating in the peripheral blood of four CHAD patients formed rosettes with human erythrocytes at 4°C, a phenomenon not demonstrable with the blood of

---

*As decribed on p. 320, anti-antibodies have been demonstrated in eluates made from DAT-positive erythrocytes.

normal subjects or of patients with macro-globulinaemia not associated with abnormal cold-antibody formation. By a number of criteria it was shown that the surface receptors of the reacting lymphocytes were indistinguishable from the CHAD patients' serum antibodies.

EXPERIMENTAL STUDIES IN ANIMALS THAT RELATE TO THE AETIOLOGY OF AIHA

A great deal of work has been undertaken in animals in an attempt to throw light on the mechanisms underlying the development of anti-erythrocyte auto-immunization. These will be considered under three headings: (1) attempts to produce AIHA in normal animals; (2) studies carried out in grafted animals, and (3) studies of naturally-occurring AIHA in animals.

Attempts to produce AIHA in normal animals

Early studies. There is some evidence that manipulation or modification of the erythrocytes of laboratory animals *in vitro* will, exceptionally, produce positive antiglobulin reactions. However, only in the case of the experiments carried out by Suzuki (1960) did overt anaemia develop (see below).

Wagley and Castle (1949) found that one out of four dogs injected with various antigens composed of autologous erythrocytes and streptococcal toxin or staphylo-coccal-culture filtrate, or with Freund's antigen (erythrocytes, lanolin, *Myco. tuberculosis* and pig serum), respectively, developed a transiently positive DAT. The dog did not, however, show any signs of haemolysis.

Liu and Evans (1952) inoculated 12 rabbits intraperitoneally for 4 weeks with their own blood*. Four of the animals developed a positive DAT but none became anaemic. Erythrocyte stroma exposed to a streptococcal filtrate was injected into another series of animals but none of the rabbits showed any signs of auto-sensitization.

---

*The intraperitoneal injection of an animal's blood is a well-tried experimental technique. Lüdke (1918) claimed to have demonstrated the temporary appearance of isolysins and autolysins in two dogs injected intraperitoneally with their own laked blood, while the present author observed marked spherocytosis in one out of six rabbits treated in the same way (unpublished observations).

Motulsky and Crosby (1954) injected guinea-pigs with erythrocytes which had been exposed to Freund's adjuvant mixture or influenza virus. In both series of animals the DAT became positive after six or seven weekly injections. The tests became negative when the injections were stopped and positive again in some animals when they were recommenced. Haemolytic anaemia did not, however, develop. Cajano and co-workers (1955) likewise failed to produce anaemia in guinea-pigs injected with autologous erythrocytes plus Freund's adjuvant. Stadsbaeder (1956) also injected guinea-pigs with erythrocytes treated with Freund's adjuvant, with or without the addition of pyramidon, formalin or a sulphonamide. The animals received the mixtures at 3-week intervals over a period of several months. The results were generally negative; only two animals became severely anaemic and gave positive DATs, and these animals had pneumococcal infections.

Suzuki (1960) gave rabbits a long series of injections of egg albumin. Splenomegaly and portal hypertension resulted. Severe anaemia developed in animals which had received more than 30 injections, with increase in osmotic fragility and positive DATs. Antibodies to albumin were accompanied by 'auto-antibodies' to phospholipid fractions of liver, spleen, erythrocytes and cardiolipin.

Production of auto-antibodies by immunization with the erythrocytes of an allied species

Experimentally, it has been found possible to cause the production of anti-erythrocyte auto-antibodies by immunizing an animal with the erythrocytes of another, but closely allied, species.

Zmijewski (1965) described how young adult chimpanzees immunized with human erythrocytes produced antibodies which reacted not only with human erythrocytes but also with the cells of a proportion of the chimpanzees. The DAT was positive in the animals forming the auto-antibodies and there was evidence that complement was fixed; there were, however, no signs of increased haemolysis.

Playfair and Marshall-Clarke (1973) reported that

mice injected with rat erythrocytes developed a positive DAT. The mice did not, however, become severely anaemic. (Milder evidence of auto-immune disease was not looked for.) Their observation was confirmed by Cox and Keast (1973, 1974), who reported that mice given weekly injections of rat erythrocytes for 6 (or 12) weeks not only developed positive DATs but also signs of increased haemolysis. Splenectomized mice were more severely affected than mice with the spleen *in situ*. Eventually however, if the weekly immunizations were persisted with, the blood pictures of the immunized mice returned to normal, although the DAT remained positive. Eleven mouse strains were tested, and although animals from each strain developed a positive DAT, the strains varied in their susceptibility. Cox and Keast concluded that their experiments showed that immunological tolerance can be broken temporarily by immunization with antigens related to self-antigens and that their results supported the concept that clones of antibody-producing cells potentially reactive against self-antigens exist in the normal mouse.

This work and other work in the same field was extensively reviewed by Cox and Howles (1981) in an important review.

The experimental breaking of self-tolerance in normal animals seems to parallel the human cases in which auto-antibodies have been formed by patients forming allo-antibodies in response to transfusion with allo-antigens (see p. 372).

Occurrence of anti-erythrocyte auto-antibodies in grafted animals

The many experiments that have been undertaken in the field of transplantation immunity have led to the recognition of 'runt' disease. Haemolytic anaemia is one feature of the syndrome, and many interesting parallels can be drawn between it and spontaneously occurring human AIHA.

It has been believed for many years that if animals are joined in parabiosis antibodies against one or other of the partner's erythrocytes are demonstrable in 'parabiosis poisoning' (Mayeda, 1921), and Chute and Sommers (1952) described in detail the haematological and serological features of parabiosis haemolytic disease in rats.

The possibility that grafts of living cells rather than the whole animal might likewise react against the host was subsequently recognized, and graft-*versus* (*v*)-host (GVH) disease is now only too familiar as an important and dangerous complica-

tion of kidney and bone-marrow grafts, etc. in human patients.

In 1953 Simonsen, in carrying out transplantation experiments in dogs, observed a positive DAT in one dog after transplantation of the spleen of another dog. In discussing the cause of this, he concluded that the occurrence was 'consistent with the theory of antibody formation in the transplant against the recipient's individual specific antigens.' At about the same time, Ahrengot (1953), who studied the serum of a patient suffering from haemolytic anaemia associated with an abdominal cyst, postulated as an explanation of the haemolysis a difference in gene content (a gene deficit) in the antibody-producing tissue compared with the rest of the body. He made the point that if the excised tumour was a teratoma, it was reasonable to assume that it might have a haploid chromosome content and be able to produce antibody against the host, but even if it was not a teratoma the gene-deficit theory could still be an acceptable explanation for the antibody formation. Muirhead and Groves (1955), too, observed unexplained positive DATs in dogs in which kidney grafts had been carried out. The tests became positive usually within 5–10 days of the graft at a time when deterioration and resorption of the transplant were beginning to take place.

Simonsen (1957) later showed that adult chicken spleen cells injected into chick embryos generally led to the death of the recipient by producing haemolytic disease in the newborn chick during the first or second week of life. In mice, too, he was able to show that splenomegaly in the newborn resulted only if the adult spleen cells injected into the mouse fetuses were genetically different from the cells of the recipients. These experiments clearly demonstrated that adult antibody-forming cells introduced into embryos or fetuses, and tolerated by them by virtue of their immature antibody-forming tissues, might nevertheless react against the host and cause haemolytic anaemia amongst other complications.

Kaplan and Smithers (1959) drew the analogy between homologous (runt) disease in animals and malignant lymphomas in man. They pointed out that the consequences of malignant lymphomas were similar to those of homologous disease in animals and suggested that the lymphoma cells might be immunologically distinct from the cells of the host, perhaps by 'antigenic deletion', but could still retain the capacity to make antibodies, and that the anaemia of chronic lymphomas could be the result of immunological reactions of the lymphoid cells against the normal haemopoietic cells of the host.

Porter (1960a,b) described detailed studies of secondary (homologous) disease in rabbits injected with homologous spleen cells after X-irradiation, and in fetal rabbits injected with spleen cells. He was able to show by ^{51}Cr studies that the host's erythrocytes were acted upon by antibodies and had a diminished life-span whilst erythrocytes derived from the donors of the spleens survived normally. The DAT became positive in the injected animals and eluted antibodies were shown to be specific for the host's blood group. Similar observations were made in animals, grafted in fetal life, which developed runt disease. In both series the abnormal antibody was incomplete in type.

The results of similar studies were briefly reported by Piomelli and Brooke (1960), using rabbits which were irradiated and then transfused with bone marrow. Some animals survived and in these the DAT became negative — presumably the grafted tissue had died out or possibly had become tolerant of the host.

Oliner, Schwartz and Dameshek (1961) reported detailed studies of the clinical and laboratory features of runt disease in the mouse. Hybrid mice, 6–14 weeks old, were injected with parental mouse spleen-cell emulsions. Haemolytic anaemia, mild to moderate in degree, resulted in many of the animals. The DAT was often positive and eluted antibodies were shown to react with the erythrocytes of the contralateral parent but not with the cells of the donor of the spleen emulsion. It was particularly interesting that some animals recovered and their anaemia disappeared although the DAT remained positive, raising the possibility of at least partial tolerance of the host on the part of the grafted cells. Three such animals relapsed after 6 months.

Somewhat similar studies were described by Harriss and her co-workers (1961), but with the difference that irradiated F_1 hybrid mice were used and injected with parental lymphoid tissue. Wasting disease and anaemia

followed, but ^{51}Cr studies demonstrated relatively rapid loss of both hybrid and parental (donor) cells — which was unexpected if the anaemia was due to haemolysis of hybrid (recipient) cells as the result of graft-v-host reaction.

Oliner, Schwartz and Dameshek (1961) discussed the similarities between the haemolytic anaemia experimentally produced in grafted animals and the spontaneously occurring disease in man. They quoted Billingham's (1959) suggestion that in man lymphoid cells of the mother might be implanted *in utero* into the fetus and later (i.e. after birth) might give rise to trouble by reacting against the host, and also reiterated the possible importance of somatic mutation (of spontaneous origin or due to the effects of virus, chemicals or radiation) as a mechanism leading to gene deletion and to the formation of a strain of cell, tolerated by the individual, yet capable of forming antibodies against normal autologous tissue, including erythrocytic antigens.

Fudenberg and Solomon (1961), in reporting two cases of 'acquired hypogammaglobulinemia' associated with AIHA, discussed various possible aetiological mechanisms and similarly put forward the possibility of a graft-v-host reaction as the basis of the syndrome.

Lindholm, Rydberg and Strannegård (1973) described how they had induced GVH disease in newborn F_1 hybrid mice by injecting them with parental thymus or spleen tissue. Plasma cells were seen to proliferate in lymph nodes of the recipients and the DAT became positive 15–20 days after the induction of the GVH disease. It was established that some at least of the proliferating plasma cells were of host origin and that this was true of the Ig causing the positive DAT. Similar results were obtained by Streilein, Stone and Duncan (1975) who had experimented with hamsters. Anti-erythrocyte auto-antibodies were formed, and it was suggested that the donor T lymphocytes, reacting with host B lymphocytes, had stimulated self-reactive clones.

NATURALLY-OCCURRING AIHA IN SPECIES OTHER THAN MAN

Of considerable interest is AIHA developing spontaneously in animals.

CANINE AIHA

It was in 1955 that Miller and his co-workers described in a dog what appeared to be a close

counterpart of chronic AIHA in man. An incomplete panagglutinin was demonstrable, and when plasma containing the antibody was transfused to normal dogs this was shown to 'block' the recipients' cells and to prevent them from undergoing agglutination (by the panagglutinin) *in vitro*. In *vitro*, the panagglutinin produced a strong antiglobulin reaction but not *in vivo*, although the 'blocked' cells became osmotically fragile and had a shortened life-span. Miller et al. concluded that spherocytosis and cell destruction were brought about by factors other, or in addition to, the amount of antibody on the cells or in plasma. A temporary remission followed the administration of ACTH, but the beneficial effect of ACTH did not seem to be mediated through suppression of antibody formation.

A further description of spontaneous canine AIHA was given by Lewis, Schwartz and Gilmore (1965), based on the study of 19 dogs. Most of the dogs were seriously anaemic, six having a haemoglobin of less than 4 g/dl. The leucocyte count was high, exceeding 30×10^9 cells per litre in eight of the dogs. Fifteen dogs were thrombocytopenic. The DAT was positive in all the dogs and auto-agglutination was noted in some of them. The dogs responded initially favourably to treatment with corticosteroids, but relapses were frequent and 11 of the dogs died.

Canine SLE

Systemic lupus erythmatosis (SLE) also affects dogs, and Lewis, Schwartz and Gilmore (1965) and Lewis, Schwartz and Henry (1965) gave details of seven dogs with an illness the features of which closely paralleled human SLE. All the dogs had a DAT-positive haemolytic anaemia, and also thrombocytopenia, and five out of six were azotaemic. The LE cell factor was demonstrable in six out of seven dogs and rheumatoid factor in two out of six dogs. Four out of six dogs had formed anti-thyroid antibodies, too. In a footnote, hypergammaglobulinaemia was reported to be present in four out of eight dogs.

The aetiology of chronic canine AIHA and canine SLE is obscure, but there is some evidence that canine SLE is caused by a virus and can be transmitted to other animals (see Bull, 1976).

AIHA IN NEW ZEALAND (NZB/BL) MICE

The discovery that AIHA developed apparently spontaneously in a strain of mice by Bielschowsky, Helyer and Howie (1959) proved to be the starting point of a great deal of experimental work, and the subject has now a very large literature. To describe the findings and ramifications of this work in detail is beyond the scope of this book.

In their original paper, Bielschowsky, Helyer and Howie (1959) reported that they had observed the very frequent occurrence of AIHA in an inbred strain of mice, the NZB/BL strain, so much so that by 9 months of age almost every mouse gave a positive DAT. Subsequently, Holmes, Gorrie and Burnet (1961) showed that whereas the DAT did not usually become positive until the mice were 10 weeks of age, positive tests could be regularly obtained much earlier in newborn or young mice inoculated with spleen-cell emulsion derived from DAT-positive isologous donors. These positive transmission experiments were considered to support the hypothesis that the production of the auto-antibody was the result of the emergence of clones of antibody-forming cells intrinsically resistant to control by immunological homeostasis.

Important reviews include those of Burnet (1963), Helyer and Howie (1963), Holmes and Burnet (1963a), Howie and Helyer (1968), Howie and Simpson (1974), De Heer and Edgington (1976) and Talal (1976).

Burnet (1963) referred to the gift of NZB/BL mice [by the Bielschowskys and Sir Charles Hercus] to the Walter and Eliza Hall Institute of Medical Research, Melbourne as 'the finest gift the Institute has ever received'.

Howie and Helyer (1968) had concluded that there was 'as yet no acceptable explanation of how self-recognition fails in these mice and what sort of disturbance results in autoantibody-producing clones being selected and permitted to proliferate.' Howie and Simpson (1974), in their review, listed as many as 218 references, the great majority being directly concerned with NZB/BL mice. Talal (1976) concluded that 'genetic, viral and hormonal influences appear to interact with immunologic regulatory mechanisms to determine the nature and severity of the autoimmune disorder. Androgenic hormones may maintain a more favourable regulatory equilibrium.' All authors have viewed the natural occurrence of the murine disease as being highly relevant to human auto-immune disease. As is summarized below, affected NZB mice not only develop haemolytic anaemia, some also suffer from renal lesions resembling human lupus nephritis; and a proportion of older mice develop malignant lymphomas. They are infected, too, with C-type RNA viruses.

The next advance in knowledge was the report

by Helyer and Howie (1963) that the majority of affected NZB/BL mice developed renal lesions which resembled closely those of human SLE and that some of the animals gave positive LE-cell tests. Cross-breeding resulted in a hybrid strain in which the incidence of haemolytic anaemia was lower but that of florid renal lesions was higher. The incidence of renal failure in these animals was high and at least one-third of them gave positive LE-cell tests. In this paper, too, Helyer and Howie gave further clinical, haematological, serological and morbid-anatomical details. Anaemia in the affected animals was progressive and was accompanied by a reticulocytosis which might even reach 100%, and in the more anaemic animals there was notable microspherocytosis and increased osmotic fragility. Auto-antibodies were readily demonstrable in the serum of affected animals and their presence was in fact the first sign of abnormality; antibodies could, too, be eluted from their erythrocytes. The antibodies were principally incomplete in nature and were best demonstrable with ficinized erythrocytes; in about 50% of animals weak complete antibodies were present also. The antibodies reacted equally at temperatures between 18°C and 37°C; they were less active at 4°C and did not appear to fix complement.

The influence of splenectomy on NZB mice was described by Holmes and Burnet (1963b). Early splenectomy was found to increase the incidence of lethal nephritis in both males and females; and it delayed the onset of a positive DAT in males and diminished other mainfestations of haemolysis. Late splenectomy, i.e. when the DAT had become positive, had little or no effect.

Holmes and Burnet (1964) described the effect on NZB mice of thymectomy carried out in the first few days of life. Removing the thymus did not prevent the onset of auto-immune phenomena; however, the onset of a positive DAT was delayed by 2–3 months.

Further details of the serological findings in NZB mice were reported by Long, Holmes and Burnet (1963). Affected mice gave positive DATs, and of those giving positive tests, 37% gave positive IATs and 96% positive tests for free antibodies in serum using papainized cells. Eluted antibodies were found to react with mouse erythrocytes of all strains tested. They slightly cross-reacted with rat cells; there was, however, no reaction with human cells. Norins and Holmes (1964) reported that the erythrocyte-coating material giving the positive DATs was a γ globulin.

Burnet and Holmes (1965a) reported that they had been able to confirm that NZB/NZW hybrid mice suffered from a high incidence of renal disease which closely resembled that developing in human SLE; there was evidence, too, of polyarteritis affecting not only vessels in the kidney, but also in the spleen, the medulla of the thymus and lymph nodes.

Burnet and Holmes (1965b) reported on the effect of the genetic make-up on the onset of auto-immune phenomena in NZB mice. The time of appearance of a positive DAT was compared in hybrid strains and back crosses with that in the original NZB strain. The median time for conversion to positivity was in female mice 188 days in the NZB strain compared with 310–510 days in seven hybrid and back-cross strains.

Evidence of immunological hyperactivity on the part of 6-week-old NZB and NZB/NZW F_1 mice was provided by Staples and Talal (1969) who demonstrated hyperreactivity to bovine γ globulin and failure to become tolerant to human γ globulin compared with the responses of other strains. They suggested that 'this immunological hyperactivity and lack of experimental tolerance may be related to lack of self-tolerance, autoimmunity, and lymphomas that develop in these mice at a later age.'

Occurrence of lymphomas and C-type oncogenic viruses in NZB/BL mice

East, de Sousa and Parrott (1965) had described in detail the post-mortem macroscopic and microscopic findings in 43 NZB/BL mice that had developed a positive DAT and haemolytic anaemia. The spleen and lymph nodes tended to be markedly enlarged and infiltrated with proliferating plasma cells and reticulum cells, and the serum IgM was markedly elevated. Seven animals, aged between 15 and 32 weeks, had developed thymomas. Cell suspensions from the thymomas caused lethal lymphocytic leukaemia 14–18 days after intraperitoneal injection into 1–28-day-old NZB recipients. It was subsequently realized that lymphomas in fact developed quite commonly in older mice already affected by haemolytic anaemia and renal disease.

Mellors (1966) reported that the lymphomas were of two histological types — reticulum-cell sarcomas and pleomorphic malignant lymphomas. The incidence was high, lymphomas being found in four out of 20 NZB/BL mice selected for necropsy at 9–11 months of age, as compared with a 2–4% incidence of lymphomas in the original NZB stock (Howie and Simpson, 1974). The observation that lymphomas quite commonly developed led to studies being undertaken to see whether viruses could be identified in NZB/BL mice in which the tumours had developed, as was known to be the case in other types of murine leukaemia or lymphomas. Mellors and Huang (1966) were in fact able to separate from transplantable malignant lymphomas of NZB/BL mice a filtrable agent which, when inoculated into pre-weaning NZB/ BL mice, was capable of inducing lymphoid-cell hyperplasia, hypergammaglobulinaemia and renal lesions similar to the changes spontaneously developing in older NZB/BL mice. Electron microscopy showed that particles were present in the affected mice which closely resembled typical 'C'-type murine oncogenic viruses. Subsequently, Mellors and Huang (1967) reported that haemolytic anaemia associated with a positive DAT and renal lesions could be produced in Swiss mice by the intraperitoneal inoculation of cell-free filtrates prepared from the spleens of old NZB/BL mice, and that some of the recipients developed lymphoid- and plasma-cell hyperplasia as well as hypergammaglobulinaemia. Type-'C' murine oncogenic virus-like particles were identified by electron microscopy in the spleen of a recipient Swiss mouse.

Further data on the distribution of virus particles in NZB mice were given by Mellors in his 1971 review. He and his colleagues had demonstrated 'C'-type Gross leukaemia virus-like particles in the thymus, spleen and kidneys of the mice throughout their life-span and in all the malignant lymphomas they had studied. They had attributed the glomerulitis of the affected mice to the formation of antibodies to antigens of the Gross virus system and to deposition of immune complexes within the glomeruli.

East and her associates (East and Prosser, 1967; East et al., 1967a,b; East, 1969) independently provided evidence for the presence of virus-like particles in the tissues of NZB/BL mice. East and Prosser (1967) also reported the successful passage of cell suspensions from the enlarged spleens or lymph nodes of affected mice into newborn NZB mice. The recipients developed enormously enlarged spleens and lymph nodes and died within 2–6 months of the injec-

tions. Repeated passages resulted in a shortening of the time between inoculation and death, and it then became possible to transfer the lymphoid tissue to young adult instead of newborn recipients.

Evidence pointing to the possible presence of virus in the thymus of newborn NZB/BL mice was provided by Masters and Spurling (1967). They implanted into mice of four strains which had been thymectomized soon after birth Millipore diffusion chambers containing thymus tissue from newborn NZB/BL mice. Of 60 surviving animals, 50 developed a positive DAT and other evidence of haemolytic disease.

East and co-workers (1967a) and East and Branca (1969) reported that they had succeeded in rearing NZB/BL mice in a sterile environment. The auto-immune phenomena developed, nevertheless, in much the same way, although less intensely, than in mice reared in a normal environment. Particles resembling the murine leukaemia virus were found in germ-free as well as in the not-germ-free mice. East (1969) reviewed the significance of the finding of virus-like particles in the tissues of NZB/BL mice; she stressed that there was, at the time of writing, no firm experimental proof of a direct or indirect causal relationship between the presence of the 'C'-type virus particles and any of the auto-immune phenomena affecting the mice; she accepted, however, that there were 'considerable precedents for assuming that the virus may be responsible for the malignant proliferation of the reticulum cells, notably its ultrastructural similarity to other murine leukaemia viruses known to cause lymphocytic, erythroid, or myeloid leukaemia.'

Further evidence of an infective aetiology for the auto-immune phenomena of NZB/BL mice was provided by Barnes and Tuffrey (1969) who reported that they had transplanted fertilized ova of CFW (white) mice into female NZB/BL mice: six of the 19 CFW progeny that had been nutured *in utero* developed a (usually) transient positive DAT.

In a later valuable review, East and Harvey (1975) restated the view that the association of murine leukaemia virus and auto-immune haemolysis in NZB mice is highly speculative; also that it was difficult to sustain a link between the auto-immunity and malignancy as a 'wide spectrum of malignancies develops in Coombs negative as well as in Coombs positive NZB hybrids.' They concluded: 'Despite so much work and agonized theorizing we still do not know what triggers the autoimmune reaction, or why the red cells should be targets for this suicidal activity.'

The occurrence of active AIHA in NZB/BL mice has provided the opportunity to compare the effect of immunosuppressive drugs in this convenient model. Several studies in which corticosteroids, cyclophosphamide, 6-mercaptopurine and anti-lymphocyte globulin have been used are referred to in Chapter 35 (p. 471).

SUMMARY

On pp. 602–604 of the 2nd (1962) edition of this book the author attempted to summarize his thoughts on the aetiology of AIHA. Thirty years later this summary makes quite interesting reading. It was pointed out that the term AIHA describes a group of conditions, not a single disease, and that as such AIHA is unlikely to have a single or simple aetiology. A complicated train of events was thought to be necessary for it to occur.

It was also suggested that one necessary circumstance was proneness to develop antibodies and that this could be genetically determined. It was not thought likely, however, that this proneness could by itself lead to auto-antibody formation. It was considered that 'aberrations in the antibody-forming tissues' were more likely to be the cause of the formation of the auto-antibodies than an alteration in erythrocyte antigenicity. Somatic mutation leading to the development of forbidden clones of antibody-forming cells was considered to be perhaps the most probable mechanism by which this could be brought about. It was pointed out, however, that although somatic mutation provided a very acceptable explanation for chronic cold-haemagglutinin disease, it was less satisfactory as a cause of warm-antibody AIHA because of the latter's wide age incidence—from infancy to old age—and its very variable course. It was pointed out, too, that although in some cases auto-antibody formation might continue for years unchanged, in other patients, particularly if they were children, the whole disturbance might be over in a few weeks or months. This meant that forbidden clones, if indeed responsible, could be quickly eliminated. It was concluded that the natural history of

AIHA—its variable course, with auto-antibody formation sometimes ceasing altogether, was more in accord with the concept of an immune response to a stimulus involving a change in erythrocyte antigenicity, which might be temporary, than with the somatic-mutation hypothesis. It was conceded, however, that there was little or no evidence as to the existence, nature or cause of the postulated antigenic alteration (which could involve the unmasking of antigens to which tolerance *in utero* had not been achieved); it was concluded, nevertheless, that it would be premature to discard the concept altogether.

It is interesting to compare current views as to the aetiology of AIHA with the ideas summarized above, which were written 30 years ago in the early 1960s.

That AIHA is a group of disorders is beyond dispute, and in the discussions in this chapter it has seemed justifiable to divide the disorders into three subgroups—acute transient AIHA, chronic warm-antibody AIHA and chronic cold-haemagglutinin disease (CHAD). Each subgroup differs substantially in clinical and laboratory findings and, to some extent at least, probably in aetiology. They are all, however, rare disorders, and this rarity seems to indicate that a complicated series of events is necessary for their development.

To deal with CHAD first. This disorder is best regarded as a clonal lymphoproliferative disease and its aetiology seems likely to be closely similar to that determining the development of other types of malignant lymphoma. Somatic mutation (of unknown causation) affecting an immunocyte already dedicated to producing a cold antibody such as anti-I seems to be a likely explanation.

The aetiology of the two other types of AIHA—the acute transient type and the chronic type—is undoubtedly complicated and multifactorial. Both types share, however, at least one aetiological factor in common: this is an unusual propensity on the part of the patient to develop antibodies. This is well illustrated in the case of the cold agglutinins that are formed after mycoplasma pneumonia. Many patients develop the antibodies at a low titre during convalescence; only a few form enough antibody, of sufficient thermal range, to lead to clinical haemolysis.

Acute transient AIHA, irrespective of whether the causal auto-antibodies are warm or cold in type and of their specificity, seems to depend on polyclonal anti-erythrocyte antibodies developing as a response to the stimulus of microbial infection in a patient who has an unusual propensity to form antibodies. Immunological self-tolerance is broken by one means or another, e.g. by the antibodies engendered by the invading organism cross-reacting with erythrocyte antigens, or by the organism modifying the antigenicity of erythrocyte antigens, or by unmasking antigens that are not normally available. This seems to be true not only of post-mycoplasma pneumonia haemolytic anaemia but also of acute AIHAs following viral infections, including PCH.

The aetiology of chronic AIHA, whether idiopathic or secondary, is clearly complicated. Essentially, its occurrence, too, depends on breaking immunological self-tolerance. Recent studies have concentrated on the mechanisms by which tolerance of self antigens is organized and maintained, with particular reference to the surveillance role of T-lymphocytes. In chronic AIHA self-tolerance is broken. How exactly this happens is the central problem. There is evidence in many cases of chronic AIHA of immunoglobulin abnormalities, particularly perhaps of deficiency of IgA, and also of impaired T-cell function or an abnormal T-suppressor to T-helper ratio. Somatic mutation leading to the formation of forbidden clones seems an unlikely explanation. For one thing the auto-antibodies are usually polyclonal. It has proved difficult to exclude the possibility that viral infection may be a factor in breaking tolerance. That genetic factors play a significant role is certain, in some cases at least; and an unusual propensity to form antibodies, which may, too, be genetically determined, is also probably an important requisite.

REFERENCES

AHRENGOT, V. (1953). De serologiske forhold hos en patient med immunologisk haemolytisk anaemi og en antistofholdig abdominalcyste. *Nord. Med.*, **50**, 1570–1571.

ALLISON, A. C. (1974). Mechanisms underlying tolerance and autoimmunity. *Boll. Ist. sieroterap. milan.*, **53** (Suppl.), 123–130.

ALLISON, A. C., DENMAN, A. M. & BARNES, R. D. (1971). Cooperating and controlling functions of thymus-derived lymphocytes in relation to autoimmunity. *Lancet*, **ii**, 135–140.

ASHERSON, G. L. (1968). Autoimmunity. *Sci. Basis Med. ann. Rev.*, 109–126. Athlone Press, London.

BARNES, R. D. & TUFFREY, M. A. (1969). A transplacental factor in the disease of the autoimmune NZB/BL mouse. *Lancet*, **i**, 1240–1242.

BARNES, R. D. & WILLS, E. J. (1976). 'Normal' elimination of aberrant autoimmune clones. *Lancet*, **ii**, 20–22.

BEIKERT, A. & SPRÖSSIG, M. (1959). Immunohämatologische und virologisch—serologische Beobactungen bei erworbener hämolytischer Anämie im Verlaufe einer 'asiatischen' Grippe. *Klin. Wschr.*, **37**, 146–150.

BETKE, K., RICHARZ, H., SCHUBOTHE, H. & VIVELL, O. (1953). Beobactungen zu Krankheitsbild, Pathogenese und Ätiologie der akuten erworbenen hämolytischen Anämie (Lederer–Anämie). *Klin. Wschr.*, **31**, 373–380.

BIAS, W. B., REVEILLE, J. D., BEATY, T. H., MEYERS, D. A. & ARNETT, F. C. (1986). Evidence that autoimmunity in man is a Mendelian dominant trait. *Amer. J. hum. Genet.*, **39**, 584–602.

BIELSCHOWSKY, M., HELYER, B. J. & HOWIE, J. B. (1959). Spontaneous haemolytic anaemia in mice of the NZB/BL strain. *Proc. Univ. Otago med. Sch.*, **37**, 9–11.

BILLINGHAM, R. E. (1959). Reported at American Society of Hematology meeting, St. Louis, November 22, 1959. (Quoted by Oliner, Schwartz and Dameshek, 1961).

BILLINGHAM, R. E., BRENT, L. & MEDAWAR, P. B. (1953). 'Actively acquired tolerance' of foreign cells. *Nature (Lond.)*, **172**, 603–606.

BLAJCHMAN, M. A., DACIE, J. V., HOBBS, J. R.,

PETTIT, J. E. & WORLLEDGE, S. M. (1969). Immunoglobulins in warm-type autoimmune haemolytic anaemia. *Lancet*, **ii**, 340–344.

BORBOLLA, L. & CHEDIAK, A. B. (1953). Anemia hemolitica de etiologia viral. (Revisión de la literatura). Presentación de un caso en la convalescencia de una varicela con Coombs positivo. *Rev. cubana Lab. clin.*, 7, 124–130.

BRIODY, B. A. (1952). Action of viruses on red blood cells. *Trans. N.Y. Acad. Sci.*, *Series II*, **14**, 231.

BULL, R. W. (1976). Animal models of autoimmune hemolytic disease. *Seminars Hemat.*, **13**, 349–353.

BURNET, F. M. (1956). *Enzyme, Antigen and Virus. A Study of Macromolecular Pattern in Action*, 193 pp. Cambridge University Press.

BURNET, F. M. (1957). A modification of Jerne's theory of antibody production using the concept of clonal selection. *Aust. J. Sci.*, **20**, 67–79.

BURNET, M. (1959a). Auto-immune disease. I. Modern immunological concepts. *Brit. med. J.*, **ii**, 645–650.

BURNET, F. M. (1959b). Auto-immune disease. II. Pathology of the immune response. *Brit. med. J.*, **ii**, 720–725.

BURNET, M. (1959c). *The Clonal Selection Theory of Acquired Immunity*, 209 pp. Cambridge University Press.

BURNET, F. M. (1961). The new approach to immunology. *New Engl. J. Med.*, **264**, 24–34.

BURNET, M. (1962). Autoimmune disease—experimental and clinical. *Proc. roy. Soc. Med.*, **55**, 619–626.

BURNET, F. M. (1963). An experimental model of autoimmune haemolytic anaemia. *Aust. Ann. Med.*, **12**, 3–5.

BURNET, M. (1966). The Harben Lectures 1966. Implication for autoimmune disease in man of studies on NZB mice and their hybrids. 1. Autoimmune haemolytic anaemia. *J. roy. Inst. publ. Hlth*, **29**, 87–94.

BURNET, M. (1967). Concepts of autoimmune disease and their implications for therapy. *Perspect. Biol. Med.*, **10**, 141–151.

BURNET, F. M. (1972a). A reassessment of the forbidden clone hypothesis of autoimmune disease. *Aust. J. exp. Biol. med. Sci.*, **50**, 1–9.

BURNET, M. (1972b). *Auto-immunity and auto-immune disease. A survey for physician or biologist*, 234 pp. Medical and Technical Publishing Co. Ltd., Lancaster.

BURNET, F. M. & FENNER, F. (1949). *The Production of Antibodies*, 2nd Edn, p. 142. Macmillan, Melbourne.

BURNET, F. M. & HOLMES, M. C. (1965a). The natural history of the NZB/BL F$_1$ hybrid mouse: a laboratory model of systemic lupus erythematosus. *Aust. Ann. Med.*, **14**, 185–191.

BURNET, M. & HOLMES, M. C. (1965b). Genetic investigations of autoimmune disease in mice. *Nature (Lond.)*, **207**, 368–371.

CAJANO, A., MILLER, A., FINCH, S. C. & ROSS, J. F. (1955). Auto-immunization to blood cells. *Sang*, **26**, 141–142.

CALLENDER, S. T. & RACE, R. R. (1946). A serological and genetical study of multiple antibodies formed in response to blood transfusion by a patient with lupus erythematosus diffusus. *Ann. Eugen. (Lond.)*, **13**, 102–117.

CAMPBELL, D. H. (1957). Some speculations on the significance of formation and persistence of antigen fragments in tissues of immunized animals. *Blood*, **12**, 589–592.

CEPPELLINI, R. & DE GREGORIO, M. (1953). Crisi embolitica in animali batterio-immuni trasfusi con sangue omologo sensibilizzato in vitro mediante l'antigene batterico specifico. *Boll. Ist. sieroter. milan.*, **32**, 445–453.

CHRISTEN, J., -P., JACCOTTET, M. & WIULLERET, B. (1958). Anémie hémolytique immunologique par auto-anticorps. I^e partie: clinique. *Helv. paediat. Acta*, **13**, 131–149.

CHUTE, R. N. & SOMMERS, S. C. (1952). Hemolytic disease and polycythemia in parabiosis intoxication. *Blood*, 7, 1005–1016.

CLEGHORN, T. E. (1959). A 'new' human blood group antigen, SWa. *Nature (Lond.)*, **184**, 1324–1325.

COLLINS, J. O., SANGER, R., ALLEN, F. H. JNR & RACE, R. R. (1950). Nine blood group antibodies in a single serum after multiple transfusions. *Brit. med. J.*, **i**, 1297–1299.

CONTE, R., DINOTA, A., TAZZARI, P. L., BELETTI, D. & SERMASI, G. (1989). Analysis of natural killer cells in patients with idiopathic autoimmune hemolytic anemia. *Vox Sang.*, **56**, 270–273.

CONTE, R., TAZZARI, P. L. & FINELLI, C. (1985). Deficiency of autologous mixed lymphocyte reaction in patients with idiopathic autoimmune hemolytic anemia. *Vox Sang.*, **49**, 285–291.

COOMBS, R. R. H. (1968). Cytomegalic inclusion-body disease associated with autoimmune haemolytic anaemia. *Brit. med. J.*, **i**, 743–744.

COX, R. O. & HOWLES, A. (1981). Induction and regulation of autoimmune hemolytic anemia in mice. *Immunol. Rev.*, **55**, 31–53.

COX, K. O. & KEAST, D. (1973). Erythrocyte autoantibodies in mice immunized by rat erythrocytes. *Immunology*, **25**, 531–539.

COX, K. O. & KEAST, D. (1974). Autoimmune haemolytic anaemia induced in mice immunized with rat erythrocytes. *Clin. exp. Immunol.*, **17**, 319–327.

DACIE, J. V. (1958). Auto-immune haemolytic anaemias. *Acta haemat. (Basel)*, **20**, 131–136.

DACIE, J. V. (1962). *The Haemolytic Anaemias: Congenital and Acquired. Part II—The Auto-immune Haemolytic Anaemias*, 377 pp. Churchill, London.

DAMESHEK, W. (1964). Recent studies in autoimmunity. *Acta haemat. (Basel)*, **31**, 187–199.

DAMESHEK, W. (1965a). Autoimmunity: theroretical aspects. *Ann. N.Y. Acad. Sci.*, **124**, 6–28.

DAMESHEK, W. (1965b). In *Conceptual Advances in Immunology and Oncology*, pp. 37–65. Hoeber Medical Division, Harper and Row, New York.

DAMESHEK, W. & LEVINE, P. (1943). Isoimmunization with Rh factor in acquired hemolytic anemia. Report of a case. *New Engl. J. Med.*, **228**, 641–644.

DAMESHEK, W. & SCHWARTZ, R. (1959). Hemolytic mechanisms. *Ann. N.Y. Acad. Sci.*, 77, 589–614.

DAUSSET, J. (1958). Le problème des auto-anticorps. *Rev. franç. Étud. clin. biol.*, **3**, 825–828.

DE HEER, D. H. & EDGINGTON, T. S. (1976). Cellular events associated with the immunogenesis of anti-erythrocyte autoantibody responses of NZB mice. *Transplant. Rev.*, **31**, 116–155.

DIETZ, A. J. (1981). Cytomegalovirus infection with carditis, hepatitis and anemia. *Postgrad. Med.*, 70, 203–208.

DIXON, F. J. (1958). Allergy and immunology: autoimmunity in disease. *Ann. Rev. Med.*, **9**, 257–286.

DMOCHOWSKI, L. L. (1971). Review of the clinical implications of the virus–autoimmune response. *Amer. J. clin. Path.*, **56**, 261–264.

DODD, M. C., WRIGHT, C. -S., BAXTER, J. A., BOURONCLE, B. A. & WINN, H. J. (1953). The immunologic specificity of antiserum for trypsin-treated red blood cells and its reactions with normal and hemolytic anemia cells. *Blood*, **8**, 640–647.

D'OELSNITZ, M., VINCENT, L. & LIPPMANN, C. (1959). Ictère hémolytique et hémoglobinurie d'origine grippale. *Arch. franç. Pédiat.*, **16**, 391–394.

DUBERT, J. M. (1957). La tolérance immunitaire. *Rev. franç. Étud. clin. biol.*, **2**, 889–893.

EAST, J. (1969). Viruses and autoimmunity. *Vox Sang.*, **16**, 318–324.

EAST, J. & BRANCA, M. (1969). Autoimmune reactions and malignant changes in germ-free New Zealand black mice. *Clin. exp. Immunol.*, **4**, 621–635.

EAST, J., DE SOUSA, M. A. B. & PARROTT, D. M. V. (1965). Immunopathology of New Zealand black (NZB) mice. *Transplantation*, **3**, 711–729.

EAST, J., DE SOUSA, M. A. B., PROSSER, P. R. & JAQUET, H. (1967a). Malignant changes in New Zealand black mice. *Clin. exp. Immunol.*, **2**, 427–443.

EAST, J. & HARVEY, J. J. (1975). Autoimmune haemolytic anaemia in New Zealand black mice. *Brit. J. Haemat.*, **31** (Suppl.), 37–46.

EAST, J. & PROSSER, P. R. (1967). Autoimmunity and malignancy in New Zealand black mice. *Proc. roy. Soc. Med.*, **60**, 823–825.

EAST, J., PROSSER, P. R., HOLBOROW, E. J. & JAQUET, H. (1967b). Autoimmune reactions and virus-like particles in germ-free NZB mice. *Lancet*, **i**, 755–757.

EHRLICH, P. (1904). *Gesammelte Arbeiten zur Immunitätsforschung.* 776 pp. August Wirschwald, Berlin. [Translated from the German by Dr. Charles Bolduan (1906). John Wiley and Sons, New York.]

EHRLICH, P. & MORGENROTH, J. (1900). Ueber Hämolysine. Dritte Mittheilung. *Berl. klin. Wschr.*, **37**, 453–458.

EHRLICH, P. & MORGENROTH, J. (1901). Ueber Hämolysine. Fünfte Mittheilung. *Berl. klin. Wschr.*, **38**, 251–257.

EYQUEM, A. (1956). La gènese des auto-anticorps. *5th Kongr. Europ. Ges. Hämat., Freiburg I Br., 20–24 Sept. 1955*, p. 861. Springer, Berlin.

EYQUEM, A. & DAUSSET, J. (1952). Recherche des propriétés inhibitrices de l'agglutination par le virus de la maladie de Newcastle dans les sérums de malades atteints d'anémie hémolytique acquise. *Ann. Inst. Pasteur*, **83**, 407–408.

FAGIOLO, E. & LAGHI, V. (1970). Studio dell'immunita cellulare in pazienti affetti da anemia emolitica autoimmune. *Progr. med. (Napoli)*, **26**, 331–334.

FEIZI, T., WERNET, P., KUNKEL, H. G. & DOUGLAS, S. D. (1973). Lymphocytes forming red cell rosettes in the cold in patients with chronic cold agglutinin disease. *Blood*, **42**, 753–762.

FUDENBERG, H. H. (1966). Immunologic deficiency, autoimmune disease, and lymphoma: observations, implications, and speculations. *Arthr. Rheum.*, **9**, 464–472.

FUDENBERG, H. & SOLOMON, A. (1961). 'Acquired agammaglobulinemia' with autoimmune hemolytic disease: graft-versus-host reaction? *Vox Sang.*, **6**, 68–79.

GARDNER, E., WRIGHT, C.-S. & WILLIAMS, B. Z. (1961). The survival of virus-treated erythrocytes in normal and splenectomized rabbits. *J. Lab. clin. Med.*, **58**, 743–750.

GEAR, J. (1955). Autoantibodies and the hyper-reactive state in the pathogenesis of disease. *Acta med. scand.*, **152** (Suppl. 306), 39–55.

GEDIKOĞLU, A. G. & CANTEZ, T. (1967). Haemolytic-anaemia relapses after immunisation and pertussis. *Lancet*, **ii**, 894–895.

GLYNN, L. E. (1970). The breakdown of immunological tolerance. *J. roy. Coll. Phycns*, **4**, 134–139.

GOOD, R. A., PETERSON, R. D. A., MARTINEZ, C., SUTHERLAND, D. E. R., KELLUM, M. J. & FINSTAD, J. (1965). The thymus in immunobiology: with special reference to autoimmune disease. *Ann. N.Y. Acad. Sci.*, **142**, 73–94.

GOUDEMAND, M., VOISIN, C. & MARCHANDISE, C. (1962). Anémie hémolytique aiguë au cours d'une ornithose. *Sem. Hôp. Paris*, **38**, 2235–2236.

GRABAR, P. (1959). Le problème de l'auto-antigénicité. *Immunopathology: 1st International Symposium* (ed. by P. Grabar and P. Miescher), pp. 20–28. Schwabe, Basel.

HARRIS, A. I., MEYER, R. J. & BRODY, E. A. (1975). Cytomegalovirus-induced thrombocytopenia and hemolysis in an adult. *Ann. intern. Med.*, **83**, 670–671.

HARRIS, J.W. (1954). Studies on the mechanism of a drug-induced hemolytic anemia. *J. Lab. clin. Med.*, **44**, 809–810. (Abstract).

HARRIS, J.W. (1956) Studies on the mechanism of a drug-induced hemolytic anemia. *J. Lab. clin. Med.*, **47**, 760–775.

HARRISS, E., CURRIE, C., KRISS, J. P. & KAPLAN, H. S. (1961). Studies on anemia in F_1 hybrid mice injected with parental strain lymphoid cells. *J. exp. Med.*, **113**, 1095–1113.

HAUROWITZ, F. (1965). Immunological unresponsiveness and autoantibody formation. *Ann. N.Y. Acad. Sci.*, **124**, 50–55.

HELYER, B. J. & HOWIE, J. B. (1963). Spontaneous auto-immune disease in NZB/BL mice. *Brit. J. Haemat.*, **9**, 119–131.

HENI, F. & BLESSING, K. (1954). Die Bedeutung der Glutinine für die erworbenen hämolytischen Anämien. *Dtsch. Arch. klin. Med.*, **201**, 113–135.

HENNEMANN, H. H. (1955). La formation d'anticorps multiples au cours d'anémies hémolytiques acquises. *Rev. belg. Path.*, **24**, 479–484.

HERNANDEZ-JODRA, M., HUDNALL, S. D. & PETZ, L. D. (1990). Studies of in vitro red cell autoantibody production in normal donors and in patients with autoimmune hemolytic anemia. *Transfusion*, **30**, 411–416.

HOLBOROW, E. J. (1967). An ABC of modern immunology. VII. Defects and evasions. *Lancet*, **i**, 1208–1210.

HOLMES, M. C. & BURNET, F. M. (1963a). The natural history of autoimmune disease in NZB mice. A comparison with the pattern of human autoimmune manifestations. *Ann. Intern. Med.*, **59**, 265–276.

HOLMES, M. C. & BURNET, F. M. (1963b). The influence of splenectomy in NZB mice. *Aust. J. exp. Biol. med. Sci.*, **41**, 449–456.

HOLMES, M. C. & BURNET, M. (1964). Experimental studies of thymic function in NZB mice and the F1 hybrids with C3H. *Aust. J. exp. Biol. Med. Sci.*, **42**, 589–600.

HOLMES, M. C., GORRIE, J. & BURNET, F. M. (1961). Transmission by splenic cells of autoimmune disease occurring spontaneously in mice. *Lancet*, **ii**, 638–639.

HONG, R. & AMMANN, A. J. (1972). Autoimmune phenomena and autoimmune disease. *Amer. J. Path.*, **69**, 491–496.

HOUSTON, M. C., PORTER, L. L. III, JENKINS, D. E. JNR & FLEXNER, J. M. (1980). Acute immune hemolytic anemia in adults after cytomegalovirus infection. *South. med. J.*, **73**, 1270–1274.

HOWIE, J. B. & HELYER, B. J. (1968). The immunology and pathology of NZB mice. *Adv. Immunol.*, **9**, 215–266.

HOWIE, J. B. & SIMPSON, L. O. (1974). Autoimmune

haemolytic disease in NZB mice. *Series Haemat.*, **7**, 386–426.

ISBISTER, J. P., TING, A. & SEETO, K. M. (1977). Development of Rh-specific maternal autoantibodies following intensive plasmapheresis for Rh immunisation during pregnancy. *Vox Sang.*, **33**, 353–358.

JERNE, D., SØRVIN, B. & HANSEN, J. K. (1973). Can gastrointestinal bleeding provoke erythrocyte autoantibodies? *Lancet*, **i**, 79–81.

KAPLAN, H. S. & SMITHERS, D. W. (1959). Auto-immunity in man and homologous disease in mice in relation to the malignant lymphomas. *Lancet*, **ii**, 1–4.

KILHAM, L. (1949). A Newcastle disease virus (NDV) hemolysin. *Proc. Soc. exp. Bio. Med. (N.Y.)*, **71**, 63–66.

KISSMEYER-NIELSEN, F. (1957). Specific auto-antibodies in immunohemolytic anaemia. With a note on the pathogenesis of auto-immunization. In *P. H. Andresen. Papers in Dedication of his Sixtieth Birthday*, pp. 126–137. Munksgaard, Copenhagen.

KÖLBL, H. (1955). Klinik und Therapie der akuten erworbenen hämolytischen Anämien im Kindersalter. *Ost. Z. Kinderheilk.*, **11**, 27–51.

KRÜGER, J. & DESAGA, F. J. (1978). Functional and surface characteristics of lymphocytes from patients with warm-antibody type autoimmunhemolytic anemia (AIHA). *Blut*, **36**, 315–323.

KRÜGER, J., RAHMAN, A., MOGK, K.-U. & MUELLER-ECKHARDT, C. (1976). T cell deficiency in patients with autoimmune hemolytic anemia ('warm type'). *Vox Sang.*, **31**, 1–12.

LEVY, J. A. (1974). Autoimmunity and neoplasia. The possible role of C-type viruses. *Amer. J. clin. Path.*, **62**, 258–280.

LEWIS, F. B., SCHWARTZ, R. S. & DAMESHEK, W. (1966). X-radiation and alkylating agents as possible 'trigger' mechanisms in the autoimmune complication of malignant lymphoproliferative disease. *Clin. exp. Immunol.*, **1**, 3–11.

LEWIS, R. M., SCHWARTZ, R. S. & GILMORE, C. E. (1965). Autoimmune diseases in domestic animals. *Ann. N. Y. Acad. Sci.*, **124**, 178–200.

LEWIS, R. M., SCHWARTZ, R. S. & HENRY, W. B. (1965). Canine systemic lupus erythematosus. *Blood*, **25**, 143–160.

LINDHOLM, L., RYDBERG, L. & STRANNEGÅRD, O. (1973). Development of host plasma cells during graft-versus-host reactions in mice. *Europ. J. Immunol.*, **3**, 511–515.

LIPPMAN, S. M., ARNETT, F. C., CONLEY, C. L., NESS, P. M., MEYERS, D. A. & BIAS, W. B. (1982). Genetic factors predisposing to autoimmune diseases. Autoimmune hemolytic anemia, chronic thrombocytopenic purpura, and systemic lupus erythematosus. *Amer. J. Med.*, **77**, 827–840.

LIU, C. R. & EVANS, R. S. (1952). Production of positive antiglobulin serum tests in rabbits by intraperitoneal injection of homologous blood. *Proc. Soc. exp. Biol. Med. (N.Y.)*, **79**, 194–195.

LONG, G., HOLMES, M. C. & BURNET, F. M. (1963). Autoantibodies produced against mouse erythrocytes in NZB mice. *Aust. J. exp. Biol. med. Sci.*, **41**, 315–321.

LÜDKE, H. (1918). Klinische und experimentelle Untersuchungen über den hämolytischen Ikterus. *Münch. med. Wschr.*, **65**, 1098–1102.

MALONE, R. H. & COWAN, J. (1950). Multiple antibody response to repeated transfusions. *Brit. med. J.*, **i**, 1299–1300.

MASTERS, J. M. & SPURLING, C. L. (1967). Induction of autoimmune hemolytic disease by diffusible substances from the thymus of NZB/BL mice. *Blood*, **30**, 569–575.

MAYEDA, T. (1921). Untersuchungen über Parabiose mit besonderer Berücksichtigung der Transplantation und Hypernephrektomie. *Dtsch. Z. Chir.*, **167**, 295–347.

MEDAWAR, P. B. (1961). Immunological tolerance. *Nature (Lond.)*, **189**, 14–17.

MELLORS, R. C. (1966). Autoimmune disease in NZB/BL mice. II. Autoimmunity and malignant lymphomas. *Blood*, **27**, 435–448.

MELLORS, R. C. (1971). Wild-type Gross leukemia virus and heritable autoimmune disease of New Zealand mice. *Amer. J. clin. Path.*, **56**, 270–279.

MELLORS, R. C. & HUANG, C. Y. (1966). Immunopathology of NZB/BL mice. V. Viruslike (filtrable) agent separable from lymphoma cells and identifiable by electron microscopy. *J. exp. Med.*, **124**, 1031–1038.

MELLORS, R. C. & HUANG, C. Y. (1967). Immunopathology of NZB/BL mice. VI. Virus separable from spleen and pathogenic for Swiss mice. *J. exp. Med.*, **126**, 53–62.

MILGROM, F. (1959). Antigenicity of antibodies. *Proc. 7th Congr. int. Soc. Blood Transfusion, Rome, Sept. 3–6, 1958*, pp. 512–515. Karger, Basel.

MILGROM, F. (1965). When does self-recognition fail? *Series Haemat.*, **9**, 17–25.

MILGROM, F. (1969). Autoimmunity. *Vox Sang.*, **16**, 286–298.

MILGROM, F. & DUBISKI, S. (1957). Méchanisme de l'auto-immunisation au cours des anémies hémolytiques. *Sang.*, **28**, 11–23.

MILGROM, F., DUBISKI, S. & WOŹNICZKO, G. (1956). Human sera with 'anti-antibody'. *Vox Sang.*, **1**, 172–183.

MILGROM, F. & WITEBSKY, E. (1962). Autoantibodies and autoimmune diseases. *J. Amer. med. Ass.*, **181**, 706–716.

MILLER, G., FURTH, F. W., SWISHER, S. N. & YOUNG, L. E. (1955). Studies on destruction of red cells by canine autoantibodies in normal dogs and in a dog with naturally occurring auto-immune hemolytic disease. *J. clin. Invest.*, **34**, 953 (Abstract).

MITCHISON, N. A. (1967). The concept of auto-immunity. *Practitioner*, **199**, 143–149.

MOBERLY, M. L., MARINETTI, G. V., WITTER, R. F. & MORGAN, H. R. (1958). Studies of hemolysis of red blood cells by mumps virus. III. Alterations in lipoproteins of red blood cell wall. *J. exp. Med.*, **107**, 87–94.

MOESCHLIN, S. (1957). Die Auto-immunerkrankungen (Autoaggressionskrankheiten). *Acta haemat. (Basel)*, **18**, 13–27.

MOHN, J. F., LAMBERT, R. M., BOWMAN, H. S. & BRASON, F. W. (1963). Production of specific anti-E autoantibodies in experimental iso-immune haemolytic anaemia in man. *Nature (Lond.)*, **199**, 705–706.

MOHN, J. F., LAMBERT, R. M., BOWMAN, H. S. & BRASON, F. W. (1965). Experimental production in man of autoantibodies with Rh specificity. *Ann. N.Y. Acad. Sci.*, **124**, 477–483.

MOLARO, G., SANTINI. G., DE PAOLI, P. & DA PONTE, C. (1983). T lymphocyte subsets and autoimmune hemolytic diseases. *Haematologica*, **68**, 167–178.

MOOLTEN, S. E. & CLARK, E. (1952a). Viremia in acute hemolytic anemia and in autohemagglutination; report of case and review of literature, with special reference to virus of Newcastle disease. *Arch. intern. Med.*, **89**, 270–292.

MOOLTON, S. E. & CLARK, E. (1952b). The red blood cell as a vehicle of virus transport. II. Role of blood-borne viruses in autohemagglutination and in hemolytic anemia. *Trans. N.Y. Acad. Sci., Series II*, **14**, 235–238.

MOOLTON, S. E., CLARK, E., GLASSER, M. F., KATZ, E. & MILLER, B. S. (1953). Blood stream invasion by Newcastle disease virus associated with hemolytic anemia and encephalopathy. Report of three cases. *Amer. J. Med.*, **14**, 294–306.

MORGAN, H. R. (1952). Acquired hemolytic anemia and viremia. *J. Lab. clin. Med.*, **40**, 924 (Abstract).

MORGAN, H. R. (1955). Acquired hemolytic anemia and viremia. *J. Lab. clin. Med.*, **46**, 580–582.

MORGAN, H. R., ENDERS, J. R. & WAGLEY, P. F. (1948). A hemolysin associated with the mumps virus. *J. exp. Med.*, **88**, 503–514.

MOTULSKY, A. G. & CROSBY, W. H. (1954). Experimental production of red cell autoimmunization. *Amer. J. Med.*, **17**, 102 (Abstract).

MUIRHEAD, E. E. & GROVES, M. (1955). Homologous renal transplantation in dogs; associated positive Coombs test and anemia. *Arch. Path. (Chicago)*, **59**, 223–231.

MULHEARN, T., ROTHSCHILD, H. & FREEMAN, J. (1975). An in vitro method to study the participation of various components in autoimmune hemolytic anemia. *Acta haemat. (Basel)*, **53**, 309–314.

NORINS, L. C. & HOLMES, M. C. (1964). Globulins on NZB mouse erythrocytes. *J. Immunol.*, **93**, 897–901.

NOSSAL, G. J. V. (1983). Cellular mechanism of immunologic tolerance. *Ann. Rev. Immunol.*, **1**, 33–62.

OLINER, H., SCHWARTZ, R. & DAMESHEK, W. (1961). Studies in experimental autoimmune disorders. I. Clinical and laboratory features of autoimmunization (runt disease) in the mouse. *Blood*, **17**, 20–44.

PARKER, A. C., STUART, A. E. & DEWAR, A. E. (1977). Activated T-cells in autoimmune haemolytic anaemia. *Brit. J. Haemat.*, **36**, 337–345.

PHAN-DINK-TUY, F., HABIBI, R., BACH, M. A., CHATENOUD, L., SALMON, C. & BACH, J. F. (1983). T cell subpopulations defined by monoclonal antibodies in autoimmune hemolytic anemia. *Biomed. Pharmacother.*, **37**, 75–80.

PIOMELLI, S. & BROOKE, M. S. (1960). Studies on 'secondary disease' in X-irradiated rabbits transfused with homologous bone marrow. *Blood*, **15**, 424 (Abstract).

PIROFSKY, B. (1965). Aortic valve surgery and autoimmune hemolytic anemia. *Amer. Heart J.*, **70**, 426–428 (Annotation).

PIROFSKY, B. (1968). Autoimmune hemolytic anemia and neoplasia of the reticuloendothelium. With a hypothesis concerning etiologic relationships. *Ann. intern. Med.*, **68**, 109–121.

PIROFSKY, B. (1969). *Autoimmunization and the Autoimmune Hemolytic Anemias*, pp. 313–337. Williams and Wilkins, Baltimore.

PIROFSKY, B., SUTHERLAND D. W., STARR, A. & GRISWOLD, H. E. (1965). Hemolytic anemia complicating aortic-valve surgery. An autoimmune syndrome. *New Engl. J. Med.*, **272**, 235–239.

PISCIOTTA, A. V., DOWNER, E. M. & HINZ, J. E. (1959). Clinical and laboratory correlation in severe autoimmune hemolytic anemia. *Arch. intern. Med.*, **104**, 264–276.

PLAYFAIR, J. H. L. (1975). The cellular basis of autoimmunity. *Brit. J. Haemat.*, **31** (Suppl.), 29–35.

PLAYFAIR, J. H. L. & MARSHALL-CLARKE, S. (1973). Induction of red cell autoantibodies in normal mice. *Nature New Biology*, **243**, 213–214.

PLOTZ, P. H. (1983). Autoantibodies are anti-idiotype antibodies to antiviral antibodies. *Lancet*, **ii**, 824–826.

PORTER, K. A. (1960a). Immune haemolysis in rabbit radiation-chimaeras. *Brit. J. exp. Path.*, **41**, 72–80.

PORTER, K. A. (1960b). Immune hemolysis: a feature of secondary disease and runt disease in the rabbit. *Ann. N.Y. Acad Sci.*, **87**, 391–402.

RICH, K. C., ARNOLD, W. J., PALELLA, T. & FOX, I. H. (1979). Cellular immune deficiency with autoimmune hemolytic anemia in purine nucleoside phosphorylase deficiency. *Amer. J. Med.*, **67**, 172–176.

ROSSE, W. F. (1990). *Clinical Immunology: Basic Concepts and Clinical Applications*, pp. 427–435. Blackwell Scientific Publications, Boston.

SCHWARTZ, R. S. (1972). Immunoregulation, oncogenic viruses and malignant lymphomas. *Lancet*, **i**, 1266–1269.

SCHWARTZ, R. S. & COSTEA, N. (1966). Autoimmune hemolytic anemia: clinical correlations and biological implications. *Seminars Hemat.*, **3**, 2–26.

SIMONSEN, M. (1953). Biological incompatibility in kidney transplantation in dogs. II. Serological investigations. *Acta path. microbiol. scand.*, **32**, 36–84.

SIMONSEN, M. (1957). The impact on the developing embryo and newborn animal of adult homologous cells. *Acta path. microbiol. scand.*, **40**, 480–500.

SMITH, H. R. & STEINBERG, A. D. (1983). Autoimmunity—a perspective. *Ann. Rev. Immunol.*, **1**, 175–210.

SOSLER, S. D., PERKINS, J. T., SAPORITO, C., UNGER, P. & KOSHY, M. (1989). Severe autoimmune hemolytic anemia induced by transfusion in two alloimmunized patients with sickle cell disease. *Transfusion*, **29**, Suppl. 49 S (Abtract).

STADSBAEDER, S. (1956). Différences des auto-anticorps au cours des anémies hémolytiques. *Acta clin. belg.*, **11**, 78–80.

STAPLES, P. J. & TALAL, N. (1969). Relative inability to induce tolerance in adult NZB and NZB/NZW F_1 mice. *J. exp. Med.*, **129**, 123–139.

STATS, D. & WASSERMAN, L. R. (1952). A critique on our knowledge of the etiology of hemolytic anemia. *Trans. N.Y. Acad Sci.*, Series II, **14**, 238–241.

STEWART, W. B., PETENYI, C. W. & ROSE, H. M. (1955). The survival time of canine erythrocytes modified by influenza virus. *Blood*. **10**, 228–234.

STREILEIN, J. W., STONE, M. J. & DUNCAN, W. R. (1975). Studies on the specificity of autoantibodies produced in systemic graft-vs-host disease. *J. Immunol.*, **114**, 255–260.

SUZUKI, T. (1960). Morbus Banti and autoimmune hemolitic anemia. *Programme VII Congr. Soc. int. Hemat. Roma, 7–13 Sept. 1958*, pp. 46–47 (Abstract). 'Il Pensiero Scientifico', Roma.

SUZUKI, T., GORZYNSKI, E. A., WHANG, H. Y. & NETER, E. (1964). Hemolysis in immune rabbits of autologous erythrocytes modified with common enterobacterial antigen. *Experientia*, **20**, 75–76.

SWISHER, S. N. (1959). Autoimmune hemolytic disease: some experiences and some unsolved problems. In *Mechanisma of Hypersensivity, a Henry Ford Hospital International Symposium* (ed. by J. H. Shaffer, G. A. LoGrippo and M. W. Chase), pp. 349–360. Churchill, London.

TALAL, N. (1976). Disordered immunologic regulation and autoimmunity. *Transplant. Rev.*, **31**, 240–263.

TEALE, J. M. & MACKAY, I. R. (1979). Autoimmune disease and the theory of clonal abortion. *Lancet*, **ii**, 284–287.

TODD, R. M. & O'DONOHOE, N. V. (1958). Acute

acquired haemolytic anaemia associated with herpes simplex infection. *Arch. Dis. Childh.*, **33**, 524–526.

TOGHILL, P. J., BAILEY, M. E., WILLIAMS, R., ZEEGEN, R. & BROWN, R. (1967). Cytomegalovirus hepatitis in the adult. *Lancet*, **i**, 1351–1354.

VAN LOGHEM, J. J. (1965). Concepts on the origin of autoimmune diseases. The possible role of viral infection in the aetiology of idiopathic autoimmune diseases. *Series Haemat.*, **9**, 1–16.

VIARD, J.-P & BACH, J.-F. (1991). Clonality in autoimmune diseases. *Seminars Hemat.*, **28**, 57–65.

VIVELL, O. (1954). Ergebnisse virologischer Studien bei Fällen von akuter hämolytischer Anämie (Lederer–Brill). *Mschr. Kinderheilk.*, **102**, 113–115.

WAGLEY, P. F. & CASTLE, W. B. (1949). Destruction of red blood cells. VII. Apparent autosensitization to dog red blood cells. *Proc. Soc. exp. Biol. Med. (N.Y.)*, **72**, 411–413.

WALDMANN, T. A., BLAESE, R. M., BRODER, S. & KRAKAUER, R. S. (1978). Disorders of suppressor immunoregulatory cells in the pathogenesis of immunodeficiency and autoimmunity (N.I.H. Conference). *Ann. intern. Med.*, **88**, 226–238.

WALLER, R. K. & RACE, R. R. (1951). Six blood-group antibodies in the serum of a transfused patient. *Brit. med. J.*, **i**, 225–226.

WEENS, J. H. & SCHWARTZ, R. S. (1974). Etiologic factors in autoimmune hemolytic anemia. *Series Haemat.*, **7**, 303–327.

WEIGLE, W. O. (1968). Immunologic unresponsiveness. In *Textbook of Immunopathology* (ed. by P. Meischer and H. Müller-Eberhard), pp. 60–75. Publication 170, Scripps Clinic and Research Foundation, La Jolla.

WEIR, D. M. (1969). Altered antigens and autoimmunity. *Vox Sang.*, **16**, 304–313.

WITEBSKY, E. (1959). Historical roots of present concepts of immunopathology. *Immunopathology: 1st International Symposium* (ed. by P. Grabar and P. Miescher), pp. 1–13. Schwabe, Basel.

WRIGHT, C.-S. & GARDNER, E. JNR (1960). A study of the role of acute infections in precipitating crises in chronic hemolytic states. *Ann. intern. Med.*, **52**, 530–537.

WRIGHT, G. PAYLING (1953). Hypersensitivity reactions. In *Recent Advances in Pathology* (ed. by G. Hadfield), 6th edn, pp 23–58. Churchill, London.

ZMIJEWSKI, C. M. (1965). The production of erythrocyte autoantibodies in chimpanzees. *J. exp. Med.*, **121**, 657–670.

ZUELZER, W. W., MASTRANGELO, R., STULBERG, C. S., POULIK, M. D., PAGE, R. H. & THOMPSON, R. I. (1970). Autoimmune hemolytic anemia. Natural history and viral–immunologic interactions in childhood. *Amer. J. med.*, **49**, 80–93.

ZUELZER, W. W., STULBERG, C. S., PAGE, R. H., TERUYA, J. & BROUGH, A. J. (1966). Etiology and pathogenesis of acquired hemolytic anemia (The Emily Cooley Lecture). *Transfusion*, **6**, 438–461.

34

Auto-immune haemolytic anaemia (AIHA): pathogenesis

Clinical evidence as to pathogenesis   393
 Splenomegaly   393
Blood picture: evidence as to pathogenesis   393
 Auto-agglutination   393
 Erythrophagocytosis   394
 Spherocytosis   394
Warm auto-antibodies: role in haemolysis *in vivo*   394
 Auto-agglutination: early studies   394
 Auto-agglutination brought about by 'incomplete' antibodies   395
 Auto-agglutination brought about by 'complete' antibodies   395
 Relevance of experiments with allo-antibodies to haemolysis in AIHA   396
 Antiglobulins (rheumatoid factors): possible role in haemolysis *in vivo*   398
 Intravascular haemolysis in severe AIHA possibly mediated by non-complement-binding IgG auto-antibodies   398
Role of the spleen and liver in haemolysis in AIHA   399
 Erythrophagocytosis (EP)   400
 Role of erythrostasis in the spleen   401
 Possible role of tissue lysins   401
 Mechanism of sequestration of antibody-coated erythrocytes   401
Possibility of metabolic damage to erythrocytes from the attachment of antibodies to the cell membrane   402
Spherocytosis   402
 Early views as to causation   402
 A more up-to-date view as to causation   403
Correlation between amount of auto-antibody formed by an AIHA patient and severity of haemolysis *in vivo*   404
 Flow cytofluorometry   405
Distribution of antibody-binding sites on the erythrocyte membrane: a possible determinant of the severity of haemolysis   406
Role of complement in haemolysis *in vivo*   406
Complement : its nature and activation   407
 Alternative pathway of complement activation   408
Nature of complement components detectable on the erythrocytes of AIHA patients   409
Interaction between IgG-coated or complement-coated erythrocytes and phagocytic cells   410

Receptors for the Fc portion of IgG and for complement components   417
 Receptors for IgGFc   417
 Receptors for complement components   418
Antibody-dependent cell-mediated cytotoxicity (ADCC) : possible role in haemolysis in AIHA   418
In-vitro monocyte/macrophage erythrocyte assays and haemolysis *in vivo*   418
Hyperactivity of the patient's monocyte/macrophage system in AIHA: a factor possibly influencing severity   420
Erythrocyte rosetting around mononuclear cells in AIHA   421
Erythrocyte rosetting around neutrophils in acquired haemolytic anaemia   421
AIHA associated with IgA auto-antibodies: mechanism of haemolysis   422
Effect of antibodies on erythropoiesis   422
Cold-antibody AIHA : mechanisms of haemolysis *in vivo*   423
 Early observations   423
 Sites of haemolysis *in vivo* in cold-antibody AIHA   426
 Possible protective mechanisms   426
 More recent observations   427
DAT-negative cold-antibody AIHA   429
Pathogenesis of leucopenia and thrombocytopenia in AIHA   430
Morbid-anatomical and histological findings in AIHA   431
 Findings in cold-antibody AIHA   432
Mechanism of reticulo-endothelial (RE) cell hyperplasia in AIHA   433
Experimental immune haemolytic anaemia in animals   433
 The pioneer experiments   433
 More recent studies   436
 Resistance to hetero-immune sera   437
 Antiglobulin reactions in experimental haemolytic anaemia   437
Experimental haemolytic anaemia produced by allo-antibodies   439
 Experimental allo-immune haemolytic anaemia in man   439
The pathogenesis of AIHA : a brief summary of the growth of knowledge in the 20th century   440

In the Oxford English Dictionary, *pathogenesis* is defined as the 'production or development of disease' and as 'the process or manner of origination of a disease or bodily affection'. In relation to the AIHAs, the central problem is how exactly erythrocyte life-span is curtailed as the result of the action on the erythrocyte membrane of the various types of auto-antibody that are formed. Subsidiary problems include the role of complement; the role of organs such as the spleen and liver which are rich in phagocytic cells; the mechanism of phagocytosis; the significance of spherocytosis, and the effect of auto-antibodies on the erythrocyte precursor cells. In the following pages all the problems listed above will be considered and, in addition, some experimental studies carried out on animals that have a bearing on the spontaneous disease in man. First, however, certain clinical features that are significant in relation to pathogenesis will be briefly discussed.

CLINICAL EVIDENCE AS TO PATHOGENESIS

As discussed in Volume 1 of this book (pp. 39–50), effete or damaged erythrocytes can be disposed of in one of two ways: by undergoing lysis while circulating in the blood stream and liberating their haemoglobin into the plasma (intravascular haemolysis), or by being ingested by phagocytes in organs rich in reticulo-endothelial cells and being destroyed within the phagocytes' cytoplasm (extravascular haemolysis). In health, extravascular haemolysis predominates and intravascular haemolysis is minimal, with the result that the plasma haemoglobin concentration is normally very low. In AIHA, the plasma haemoglobin is likely to be raised: often the rise is quite small, but sufficient to reduce the plasma haptoglobin concentration significantly; in some patients, however, the rise is sufficient to lead to haemoglobinuria, which, if present, suggests that the antibody present is strongly complement-fixing.

The fact that two types of increased haemolysis could be recognized clinically, an intravascular type and an extravascular type, was appreciated early in this century. This distinction has often been made use of in classifications of the haemolytic anaemias, so much so that the 'haemoglobinurias' have sometimes been referred to and discussed as a distinct group of diseases,

e.g. by Witts (1936). The presence of haemoglobinuria is certainly characteristic of some types of haemolytic anaemia (Stats, Wasserman and Rosenthal, 1948; Ham, 1955), whilst its absence is characteristic of others, e.g. HS. The careful studies made by Crosby and Dameshek (1951) on plasma haemoglobin levels in a variety of types of haemolytic anaemia supported this concept. However, their data also suggested that whether haemolysis appeared to be predominantly intravascular or extravascular could depend on quantitative differences in the rate of haemolysis and was not necessarily a characteristic of any particular disease. This was borne out by their observations in AIHA of various types. Raised plasma haemoglobin levels were found at one time or another in 15 out of 17 patients, with the level being generally higher in patients in whom haemolysis was active than in those in clinical remission.

Splenomegaly

The spleen is typically enlarged in AIHA and is often palpable (p. 18). Its enlargement, and the clinical improvement that often follows splenectomy (p. 471), are good evidence that it plays a significant role in the increased haemolysis. This applies, although to a variable extent, irrespective of the type of auto-antibody that is being formed.

BLOOD PICTURE: EVIDENCE AS TO PATHOGENESIS

Auto-agglutination. In haemolytic anaemia, the presence of auto-agglutination is important evidence that the anaemia is likely to be of auto-antibody origin. In cold-antibody AIHA massive agglutination is often visible to the naked eye in blood that has been allowed to cool down towards room temperature after withdrawal and is characteristically extremely obvious in blood films made at room temperature (Fig. 28.8, p. 220). In warm-antibody cases agglutination is seldom visible to the naked eye; in blood films, however, minor degrees of the phenomenon are not infrequent. The film illustrated in Fig. 23.5 (p. 58) is unusual with respect to the intensity of the agglutination, but the accompanying presence of spherocytosis is a typical finding.

Erythrophagocytosis. This phenomenon was described and illustrated in Volume 1 of this book (p. 80) and has also been referred to earlier in this volume, in relation particularly to acute AIHA in children (p. 59), in CHAD, and in PCH (p. 343). Its obvious presence in peripheral-blood or buffy-coat preparations is strongly indicative of an AIHA. Monocytes predominate as erythrophages but in some cases, usually when haemolysis is particularly severe, neutrophils act similarly. Small numbers of erythrophages may be seen occasionally in conditions other than AIHA, e.g. in chemical poisonings, septicaemia, protozoal infections and in haemolytic disease of the newborn.

Spherocytosis. As discussed and illustrated, too, in Volume 1 of this book (p. 65), spherocytosis is an important sign of damage to the erythrocyte and is a common phenomenon in many types of haemolytic anaemia. In AIHA it is often, but not always, conspicuous in warm-antibody AIHA (Fig. 23.5, p. 58); it may be seen, too, in PCH (Fig. 32.4, p. 342) but is usually not obvious in other types of cold-antibody AIHA. The significance and mode of production of spherocytosis in AIHA is considered on p. 402.

WARM AUTO-ANTIBODIES: ROLE IN HAEMOLYSIS *IN VIVO*

It will be convenient to discuss haemolysis due to warm antibodies separately from that brought about by cold antibodies. As already described in Chapter 25, warm antibodies react most frequently *in vitro* as incomplete antibodies: they act much less commonly as auto-agglutinins and only rarely as agglutinins and lysins.

Auto-agglutination: early studies

The possible importance of auto-agglutination *in vivo* as a haemolytic mechanism in acquired haemolytic anaemia was emphasized by Ham and Castle (1940a,b), who conceived the idea that agglutination could, by causing erythrostasis, initiate changes leading to haemolysis, particularly in the presence of spherocytosis and increased osmotic fragility. In a later paper (Castle, Ham and Shen, 1950), the thesis of the importance of agglutination as a haemolytic mechanism was developed further and tissue injury secondary to erythrostasis was invoked as an important mechanism in the chain of events leading to haemolysis. Castle, Ham and Shen remarked on the discrepancy between the results of tests for antibody activity *in vitro* and the observable effects of the antibodies *in vivo*—as had many previous authors in connection with experimental work carried out on animals (see p. 434). They suggested that the discrepancy might be resolved if the antibody which *in vitro* appeared to be incapable of bringing about lysis initiated the following sequence of events *in vivo*:

'(1) Red cell agglutination in the peripheral blood; (2) red cell sequestration and separation from plasma in tissue capillaries; (3) ischemic injury of tissue cells with release of substances that increase the osmotic and mechanical fragilities of red cells *locally*; (4) local osmotic lysis of red cells or subsequent escape of mechanically fragile red cells into the blood stream where the traumatic motion of the circulation causes their destruction.'

Wasastjerna (1951) similarly concluded on the basis of experimental work in animals that intravasal agglutination was an important mechanism by which the destructive effect of an immune antibody was potentiated, and this concept was further elaborated in relation to human cases of acquired haemolytic anaemia by Wasastjerna (1953) and Wasastjerna, Dameshek and Komninos (1954). It was pointed out, however, that 'auto-agglutination' in the circulating blood in AIHA might not be more conspicuous than in other seriously ill patients, not suffering from excessive haemolysis, in whom a similar degree of clumping might be due to excessive rouleaux formation. [This observation had in fact no great bearing on Castle, Ham and Shen's (1950) hypothesis which stressed the importance of agglutination in bringing about the arrest of the circulation in organ capillaries and initiating a complicated series of events, rather than the presence of agglutination in circulating blood being of any particular importance in pathogenesis.]

Auto-agglutination brought about by 'incomplete' antibodies

Wiener (1945) seems to have been the first to demonstrate that erythrocytes sensitized by an incomplete type of auto-antibody might undergo agglutination in a medium of high protein content. In a paper largely devoted to the conglutination test for Rh sensitization he mentioned that 'in a case of acquired hemolytic anemia, by using the conglutination technique, I succeeded in demonstrating auto-agglutination in vitro at body temperature as well as in the refrigerator.' Subsequently, Wagley and co-workers (1948) reported that the erythrocytes from three patients with acquired haemolytic jaundice underwent spontaneous auto-agglutination in normal serum but not in saline. Later, Jandl (1955) and Jandl and Castle (1956) published detailed studies on the phenomenon of the agglutination in colloidal media of erythrocytes coated with incomplete antibodies.

As has already been referred to (p. 58), some degree of auto-agglutination is quite commonly found in patients with warm-antibody AIHA who are suffering from a serious degree of haemolysis. Jandl and Castle's (1956) work went a long way in providing an explanation for the phenomenon. Working with erythrocytes sensitized *in vitro* with anti-Rh(D) as well as with cells sensitized *in vivo* obtained from cases of AIHA, they found that concentrating whole plasma or serum to the extent of 10–20% was sufficient to agglutinate the antibody-coated cells, as were increases in fibrinogen or globulin to levels only slightly in excess of the normal. Fibrinogen was most active in this respect and γ globulin, other globulins and albumin were less active in this order (concentration for concentration), the order being that of diminishing molecular weight and axial ratio.

Auto-agglutination brought about by 'complete' antibodies

As referred to on p. 95, occasionally, auto-antibodies are developed which cause strong auto-agglutination of the patient's blood at 37°C as well as agglutinating normal erythrocytes in saline suspension. Such patients are invariably seriously ill, for haemolysis occurs at a very rapid rate. These clinical observations had their parallel in the experimental studies carried out by Jandl and Mollison and their colleagues in the late 1950s.

It was repeatedly shown that agglutinating or agglutinating and lytic antibodies bring about more rapid haemolysis than do incomplete antibodies. Moreover, this occurs widely throughout the body in organs rich in reticuloendothelial cells of which the liver, by virtue of its size, is the most important. It is thus easy to understand why patients forming agglutinating antibodies may be so severely affected and also why splenectomy often fails in AIHA patients who are seriously ill.

There is an interesting parallel in this experimental work with the occurrence of auto-agglutination of erythrocytes heavily coated with incomplete antibodies. Jandl and Kaplan (1960) showed for instance, with an allo-antibody such as anti-D, and also with heterophile antibodies injected into rats, that increasing the degree of sensitization, or dose of antibody injected, quickens sequestration in the spleen and eventually leads to sequestration in the liver as well. Again, in the disease in man, it is the patients whose cells are very heavily coated with incomplete antibodies, and who are most seriously ill, who show accumulation of radioactivity in the liver as well as in the spleen, when their own erythrocytes are tagged with ^{51}Cr and surface counting is carried out (see p. 478).

Jandl (1960a) and Jandl and Kaplan (1960) assessed the role of the spleen and liver from the quantitative standpoint. They concluded that sequestration depends on, amongst other factors, the strength and size of the agglutinates, the 'pore' size of the splenic and hepatic filters, and pressure gradients. With relatively large agglutinates, the liver is predominantly important and the spleen unimportant because of its much smaller blood flow. The smaller and weaker agglutinates (and unagglutinated cells sensitized with incomplete antibodies) appear to pass through the liver sinuses without harm, only to get caught up by the more sensitive filtering mechanism of the spleen.

Relevance of experiments with allo-antibodies to haemolysis in AIHA

While it is legitimate to stress the analogies and similarities between the presumed course of events in AIHA in man and the experimental work with allo-antibodies, it must not be forgotten that the time scale is vastly different.

The half-time of disappearance of D-positive or K-positive cells injected into subjects with anti-D or anti-K in their circulation was shown by Mollison and Cutbush (1955) to be within the range of 20–30 minutes, and it was suggested that if 3% of the circulating blood passes through the spleen each minute, and if the blood in passage was cleared completely of incompatible cells, it would take approximately 25 minutes to remove half the cells from the circulation. Hughes Jones, Mollison and Veall (1957), Cutbush and Mollison (1958), Mollison and Hughes Jones (1958) and Mollison (1959b) published more extensive and confirmatory data. Hepatic removal of strongly agglutinating antibodies or complement-fixing antibodies was found to occur within half-times of 2–6 minutes. Weak agglutinating antibodies which did not fix complement were associated with half-times of 20 minutes or more. Predominantly splenic destruction brought about by incomplete antibodies was found to be associated with half-times of 15–22 minutes.

Similar results were obtained by Jandl and his colleagues. The half-time of disappearance of D-positive cells injected into subjects with anti-D in their circulation was shown by Jandl, Richardson Jones and Castle (1957) to range from 8 to 24 minutes (mean, 14 minutes), while cells coated with anti-D *in vitro* gave a half-time of disappearance which averaged 26 minutes. Jandl and Kaplan (1960) also concluded that the spleen would remove cells coated with incomplete antibodies, when the splenic filter was unsaturated, at the rate of 3±1% per minute. This rate was thought to approach the maximum possible, taking into account the splenic blood flow, and to indicate removal of sensitized cells in a single passage through the spleen. Erythrocytes coated

by agglutinating allo-antibodies were found to be removed by the hepatic mechanism in 4±2 minutes (Jandl, Richardson Jones and Castle, 1957; Jandl, 1960a).

Fortunately for the patient, in contrast to the experimental work carried out with allo-antibodies, in human AIHA half-times of erythrocyte survival are measured in days rather than in minutes, and the erythrocytes, or most of them, must make many passages through the spleen (and liver) before being finally taken out of circulation.

There are several possible explanations for the different time-scale in the experimental work with allo-antibodies and that in patients with naturally-occurring AIHA. Amongst them are: (1) differences in the relative proportion of erythrocyte antigen to available antibody; (2) qualitative differences between the auto-antibodies and allo-antibodies; (3) differences in 'saturation' of the splenic (or hepatic) filter; (4) a varying sensitivity of erythrocytes to the action of antibodies, and (5) the relative insensitivity of reticulocytes.

1. Most important factors are the volume (mass) of antigen, the titre of the antibody and the ratio of antigen to antibody.

In the experiments with allo-antibodies small volumes of incompatible cells were usually injected, 1–5 ml as a rule, and these cells would be exposed to a large volume of circulating antibody. Even so, under these circumstances, which are so favourable for haemolysis, a definite relationship between the titre of antibody and the rate of haemolysis can be demonstrated. Mollison and Cutbush (1955) and Mollison (1959b), for instance, showed when D-positive cells were injected into recipients who had anti-D in their circulation that a titre of 64 or more was associated with a half-time of removal of approximately 20 minutes, a titre of 16 with a half-time of 60–70 minutes and a titre of 4 with a half-time of several days. In human cases of AIHA not only are high titres of free antibody in the serum rarely met with but the amount of antigen with which the antibody has to react is relatively very great. Very rapid rates of destruction can hardly be expected under these circumstances.

2. It is possible that auto-antibodies in AIHA are, in some instances at least, less effective in causing damage to erythrocytes than are the specific allo-antibodies (e.g. anti-Rh(D)) with which they have usually been compared.

As already described, the auto-antibodies often lack easily definable specificity and not infrequently they react preferentially or occasionally react only with enzyme-treated erythrocytes. The relative effectiveness of the 'non-specific' auto-antibodies and the Rh-specific auto-antibodies is uncertain, but there is no reason to suppose that titre for titre as measured *in vitro* they are necessarily equally harmful *in vivo*. It is certainly true in AIHA that the patient may be in clinical remission and yet his or her erythrocytes still give a clearly positive and often a quite strongly positive DAT. However, it is also true that cells, or a high proportion of them, sensitized with low concentrations of anti-Rh may similarly survive normally (Mollison and Paterson, 1949; Mollison, 1959b). This type of evidence is thus inconclusive with respect to the relative potency *in vivo* of the two types of antibody.

Culp and Chaplin (1960) reported on some interesting experiments. They prepared an eluate from the erythrocytes of a patient with AIHA and succeeded in sensitizing normal cells with the eluate so that they gave a '4+' antiglobulin reaction. These cells were then reinjected to the patient; there was no immediate splenic sequestration, and they were only slowly eliminated. The ^{51}Cr T_{50} was 7 days. When, however, normal cells were sensitized with anti-D to a degree judged by the antiglobulin test to be comparable with that of the cells sensitized by the auto-antibody, and then injected into a normal recipient, there was splenic uptake of radioactivity; the ^{51}Cr T_{50} was 1.3 hours, and all the cells had disappeared in 24 hours. Culp and Chaplin concluded: 'that in vitro behavior in the antiglobulin test gives limited insight into the physiologic alterations brought about on the red cell surface by different antibodies.' They did not mention whether they had been able to demonstrate that the auto-antibody had any specificity; presumably it had not.

3. It seems probable that one factor which retards the rate of haemolysis in the spleen is the degree to which the organ is saturated or choked with erythrocytes. The histological evidence is that although congestion with blood is a variable feature, occasionally this may be very great indeed.

That this is relevant was demonstrated by Jandl, Richardson Jones and Castle (1957), who compared the survival of ^{51}Cr-labelled erythrocytes, derived from a patient with acquired haemolytic anaemia, in the patient himself, in a normal subject and in a patient with hyperglobulinaemia due to multiple myeloma. Destruction was most rapid in the patient with multiple myeloma and far slower in the patient with acquired haemolytic anaemia. Jandl and his co-workers pointed out that in the normal subject and, to a greater extent in the patient with multiple myeloma, the initial splenic sequestration resembled the pattern seen in normal subjects injected with erythrocytes previously sensitized with anti-D. They concluded that the relatively slow rate of sequestration of the labelled cells in the patient himself probably reflected 'the competition of the patient's circulating unlabelled cells for the splenic sequestering site.'

4. Variation within a population of erythrocytes in their sensitivity towards antibody action seems likely to be an additional mechanism by which the patient can protect himself or herself from the worst effects of the auto-antibodies. The wide range of sensitivity of individual cells to agglutination and lysis in conventional tests *in vitro* needs no emphasis. It is usually impossible to achieve 100% agglutination or lysis, and, at the other end of the scale, the extreme sensitivity of some cells makes it difficult to define titre end-points accurately.

In vivo, the same phenomenon was demonstrated repeatedly by Cutbush and Mollison (1958) and Mollison (1959b) in their experiments with allo-antibodies. With some antibodies, depending on their titre, and depending, too, on the genotype of the erythrocytes, it seemed that a proportion of the cells might be so little affected by the antibody that their survival was unimpaired.

It seems probable, therefore, that the circulating population of erythrocytes in a patient with AIHA will contain a higher than normal proportion of relatively resistant cells because of the continuing and relatively rapid elimination of the most sensitive cells. This could explain, at least in part, the often poorer initial survival of transfused normal erythrocytes compared with that of the patient's own cells, as measured by labelling a random sample of his peripheral blood (see Mollison, 1959a).

5. Another possible protective mechanism is the increased resistance to antibody-complement action of young as compared with old erythrocytes. Cruz and Junquiera (1952), London (1960), Rice and Mathies (1960), Gower and Davidson (1963) and Dudok de Wit and van Gastel (1969), in experimental systems using dog, sheep, guinea-pig and human erythrocytes, all obtained evidence that young cells are more resistant than old cells.

More recent studies using ^{125}I IgG have shown that anti-D binds to reticulocytes less well than to mature erythrocytes. Gray, Kleeman and Masouredis (1983) reported, too, that testing density-fractionated blood from four out of five patients with AIHA revealed less IgG bound to reticulocytes than to mature erythrocytes. However, this reduction in antibody binding can only have relative value, for in certain patients reticulocytopenia is found and it is generally thought that auto-antibodies not infrequently damage erythrocyte precursor cells in the bone marrow. Moreover, there is evidence that reticulocytes, because of their surface properties, tend to be sequestered (normally only temporarily) in the spleen (Berendes, 1959; Jandl, 1960b) and this would be expected to nullify any benefit from the cells' inherent insensitivity to antibody action.

To summarize, the apparent relatively long survival of auto-antibody-sensitized erythrocytes in AIHA compared with the much shorter survivals observed when normal incompatible cells are exposed to allo-antibodies, is probably due to a combination of factors. These include the large mass of erythrocytes at risk in AIHA, the possible relative impotency (in some instances at least) of the auto-antibodies, the limited capacity of the splenic filtering mechanism and resistance to the action of antibodies of a proportion of the erythrocytes formed by the patient.

Antiglobulins (rheumatoid factors) : possible role in haemolysis *in vivo*

As referred to on p. 320, cold-acting rheumatoid-like antiglobulins have been described in the sera of some patients who have developed haemolytic anaemia following infectious mononucleosis, and it is possible that they have played a part in bringing about haemolysis in some of these cases. It is possible, too, that similar antibodies have been a rare cause of increased haemolysis in warm-antibody cases (see below).

They were the subject of an experimental study reported by Kaplan and Jandl (1963, 1964). In the rat they showed that the interaction between anti-rabbit antiglobulins and rat erythrocytes sensitized with rabbit antisera brought about agglutination *in vitro* and accelerated destruction of the sensitized cells *in vivo*. In man, however, naturally-occurring rheumatoid antiglobulins (macroglobulins), although causing the agglutination *in vitro* of erythrocytes coated with anti-Rh antibodies, did not accelerate their destruction *in vivo*.

Goldberg and Fudenberg's (1968) patient, who had previously been described by Fialkow, Fudenberg and Epstein in 1964, had had moderately severe AIHA associated with the formation of a warm IgG(7S) auto-antibody. His serum had contained in 1961 an anti-γ globulin (rheumatoid factor) at a high titre (28 000 in a latex test). When he was reinvestigated in 1968, in complete clinical remission, the DAT was still strongly positive; the anti-γ globulin had, however, almost disappeared (titre 20). Goldberg and Fudenberg suggested that the anti-γ globulin had been of importance in relation to the severe haemolysis from which the patient had earlier suffered.

The idea that anti-Ig antibodies might play a role in mitigating the effect of the coating of erythrocytes with IgG (Masouredis, Branks and Victoria, 1987) and that their presence might help to explain why some individuals giving positive DATs show no signs of in-vivo haemolysis (see p. 195) has received further support from the work of Victoria et al. (1990). They labelled the auto-antibodies of two AIHA patients with ^{125}I and used the labelled antibodies to identify epitope-bearing erythrocyte membrane polypeptides. These were found within band 3, the major membrane protein resolved by SDE PAG electrophoresis. The auto-antibodies bound with affinities comparable to those of blood-group allo-antibodies to all the human erythrocytes they tested including rare Rh types. Victoria et al. were not, however, able to identify any non-erythrocyte-adsorbable (anti-idiotype) IgG, and they suggested that an absence of a significant anti-idiotypic IgG population in auto-antibodies associated with AIHA may be an important factor in promoting haemolysis.

Intravascular haemolysis in severe AIHA possibly mediated by non-complement-binding IgG auto-antibodies

As has been referred to earlier (e.g. p. 32), haemoglobinuria, the consequence of severe intravascular haemolysis, is a frequent sign in some types of AIHA—in PCH it is in fact often the patient's initial complaint. In such cases it is generally possible to demonstrate *in vitro* that the haemolysis is being mediated by complement, by showing that the patient's serum contains a complement-fixing antibody and/or by finding that the patient's erythrocytes are coated with complement components. It is often possible, too, to demonstrate a reduction in complement activity in the patient's serum.

The question arises as to whether auto-antibodies which totally lack complement-fixing ability, if present in high enough concentration, can lead to intravascular haemolysis of sufficient intensity to produce haemoglobinuria. Luthringer, Jenkins and Wallis (1969) reported a probable instance of this and mentioned a small number of other possibly similar cases that had been described in the literature. Their patient was an 84-year-old woman who had developed a haemolytic anaemia described as fulminating. Her haemoglobin on admission was 4.5 g/dl and there were 34% reticulocytes. Her plasma was dark brown and she had haemoglobinuria. The peripheral blood film was described as showing macrocytosis and polychromasia; spherocytosis and auto-agglutination were not mentioned. The DAT and IAT were strongly positive with anti-γ sera but negative with an anti-non-γ serum. The antibody was identified as being IgG—it was not inhibited by 2-ME.

All attempts to demonstrate that the antibody in her serum had lytic potentiality, including the use of PNH erythrocytes, failed. However, two early measurements of serum complement activity gave subnormal results. Luthringer, Jenkins and Wallis suggested two possible explanations for their patient's intravascular haemolysis; either that a 'hemolysin' had been present in the early stages of her illness or that the antibody was not complement-fixing but had produced haemolysis extravascularly at such an intensity that the patient was unable to metabolize all the liberated haemoglobin. Of these two possibilities the second was thought more likely to be correct. They cited in support of this contention experimental work that had been carried out earlier with anti-D allo-antibodies.

ROLE OF THE SPLEEN AND LIVER IN HAEMOLYSIS IN AIHA

The important role played by organs rich in potentially phagocytic reticulo-endothelial cells in the disposal of effete erythrocytes has been known for many years and has been referred to many times already in this book. The advent of radioactive chromium (^{51}Cr) in the early 1950s and its ready availability as a research tool provided, however, a powerful means of studying the relationship between the type of antibody and the site in vivo of erythrocyte destruction. In the case of incomplete antibodies the spleen was soon shown to be the organ where most destruction took place. Of particular importance were the early reports of Jandl (1955, 1956, 1958), Mollison and Cutbush (1955), Jandl, Richardson Jones and Castle (1957), Cutbush and Mollison (1958), Mollison and Hughes Jones (1958), Mollison (1959a), Jandl and Kaplan (1960) and Crome and Mollison (1964) who had studied

patients with AIHA and also, to a larger extent, normal volunteers who had been injected with small volumes of incompatible blood or with erythrocytes previously sensitized in vitro with allo-antibodies, e.g. with incomplete anti-Rh(D). Both experimental approaches gave comparable results. In particular, it was shown that whereas strongly agglutinated erythrocytes or cells exposed to complement-fixing potentially lytic antibodies are removed from the circulation rapidly, predominantly by the liver, cells coated by incomplete antibodies are removed almost quantitatively by the spleen.

The time taken for haemolysis to occur once antibody-coated cells have become irreversibly trapped in the spleen was studied by Jandl (1956) and Jandl, Richardson Jones and Castle (1957). Human reticulocytes were labelled in vitro with ^{59}Fe and then sensitized with the allo-antibody anti-D. They were injected into a normal recipient and also into a patient with AIHA. Radioactive iron was detected in the peripheral blood of the recipient, i.e. in erythrocytes newly delivered from the bone marrow, in 34–36 hours in the normal recipient and within 8 hours in the patient with AIHA. Jandl and his co-workers calculated that the sensitized cells probably underwent lysis within a few minutes and that their haemoglobin was transformed to bilirubin in 1–2 hours, and that the liberated iron was available for erythropoiesis in 6–8 hours.

In addition to the experimental studies referred to above, many other studies have been carried out on patients with AIHA, a primary reason being to assess the spleen's role in haemolysis and the likely response of the patients to splenectomy (see p. 477).

How and why the spleen is so effective in sequestering cells coated by incomplete antibodies was, and still is, an interesting question. One obvious reason is the large number of phagocytic cells present with which the antibody-coated cells can come into intimate contact and the unique splenic circulation which ensures that many of the cells passing through the organ take a long time to do so (see Vol. 1, p. 36). There are, however, other possible reasons why the spleen is so effective is sequestering cells coated by incomplete antibodies. One possible reason is a higher concentration of plasma protein in spleen blood than in mixed arterial blood. Jandl (1955) reported that in dogs there might be as much as a 1.5 times increase in concentration, and he suggested, too, that haemoconcentration in the spleen pulp might in itself favour sequestration. The spleen also is in all probability a source of auto-antibody and cells circulating through it will of necessity be exposed to high concentrations of antibody possibly over relatively prolonged periods. In favour of this concept were the observations of Wagley et al. (1948) who showed in three patients with AIHA that erythrocytes derived from their spleen were more strongly agglutinated by an antiglobulin serum than were cells obtained from peripheral venous blood, and the finding of Wright et al. (1951), who demonstrated that the titre of antibody in spleen-pulp blood was higher than in peripheral blood in a series of patients with AIHA. Jandl, Richardson Jones and Castle (1957), too, reported that auto-agglutination might be an obvious feature of splenic blood although none was visible in peripheral blood.

Another factor which must be of importance is spherocytosis. A greater or lesser degree is almost the rule in warm-type AIHA, and it seems highly likely that the spherocytosis predisposes to splenic sequestration.

In the following sections the actual way in which antibody-affected erythrocytes are destroyed within the spleen, or sustain damage by their passage through the organ, will be discussed. There seem to be three possible mechanisms: contact with phagocytic cells; erythrostasis leading to metabolic damage, and exposure to tissue 'lysins' and enzymes.

Erythrophagocytosis (EP)

For many years phagocytosis by fixed tissue macrophages and by macrophages in the peripheral blood has been known to be a striking phenomenon in experimental haemolytic anaemia in animals. In man, too, as has been described earlier, EP is occasionally visible in the peripheral blood in severely affected patients with warm-antibody AIHA (p. 61) or CHAD (p. 221) or paroxysmal cold haemoglobinuria (PCH) (p. 343), and it can be regularly seen in PCH in blood withdrawn from a chilled finger around

which a ligature had been placed (Ehrlich's test) (as described in Vol. 1, p. 80). In histological sections of spleens removed at operation, and in the liver, lymph nodes and bone marrow of fatal cases of AIHA, evidence of EP can be usually seen without much difficulty.

The occurrence of EP in AIHA has attracted a great deal of attention, especially since the early 1950s. Particular attention has been focused on the part played by the class and subclass of immunoglobulin coating the erythrocyte, and the role of complement, in causing the sensitized erythrocytes to adhere to phagocytes prior to phagocytosis. In Volume 1 of this book on pp. 80–84 a selected series of papers dealing with EP which had been published between 1954 and 1978 were summarized. The following account is based on these summaries and brought further up-to-date.

Bonnin and Schwartz (1954) studied the auto-antibodies of some of the author's AIHA patients and compared the ability of the antibodies to cause EP with that of allo-antibodies such as anti-A. In general, antibodies which did not fix complement *in vitro* failed to produce EP, while those which fixed complement and lysed normal or enzyme-treated erythrocytes did so. The results paralleled the presence of EP in peripheral-blood or buffy-coat preparations. Monocytes were found to be more active as erythrophages than neutrophils, for the latter appeared to be only capable of phagocytosing erythrocytes sensitized with high concentrations of antibody.

Bessis (1954) used phase-contrast microscopy in the study of phagocytosis by living cells *in vitro*. Human erythrocytes sensitized by a rabbit antiserum were noted first to adhere to monocytes or granulocytes and then to undergo complete or partial phagocytosis. Bessis noted, too, that sometimes a sensitized cell might be lysed a moment after being attached to a phagocyte, i.e. without being phagocytosed.

Schubothe and Müller (1955) applied Ehrlich's test to a variety of haemolytic disorders and exposed the finger to a range of temperatures. In PCH, 10 minutes at 5°C, followed by 10 minutes at 40°C, gave rise to marked lysis and EP; in CHAD, 10–30 minutes at 20°C led to marked lysis and a little phagocytosis; in warm-antibody

AIHA, 10–30 minutes at 40°C gave rise to a moderate amount of phagocytosis but no lysis. In paroxysmal nocturnal haemoglobinuria 10–30 minutes at 40°C led to marked lysis but doubtful EP. These results paralleled closely what had been observed experimentally *in vitro*.

Further details of the process of EP as viewed by microcinematography and by transmission and scanning electron microscopy were described by Bessis and de Boisfleury (1970) and illustrated by excellent photographs. They used as a model the phagocytosis by human peripheral blood leucocytes of homologous erythrocytes sensitized by sublytic amounts of a rabbit anti-human erythrocyte serum. Several stages in phagocytosis were identified: (1) initial attachment of a small part of the erythrocyte surface; (2) the transformation of the biconcave discocyte to a spherocyte; (3) the surrounding of the erythrocyte by a hyaloplasmic veil which 'by moving forward transforms the spherocyte into a characteristic pear shape'; (4) the enclosure of the entire cell within the phagocyte. They reported, too, that frequently 'the hyaloplasmic veil, in surrounding the erythrocyte, compresses it at its median and actually cuts the cell in two, liberating a spherocyte schizocyte to the medium.'

Role of erythrostasis in the spleen

In addition to the damaging effect of the macrophage–erythrocyte interaction (see p. 410), it seems likely that sequestration *per se* of antibody-coated and spherocytic erythrocytes within the spleen plays a significant role in their destruction.

Ham and Castle (1940a,b,c) had argued that erythrostasis was probably an important mechanism leading to haemolysis and that erythrocytes with increased osmotic fragility would be unusually sensitive to its effects. In AIHA both sequestration of erythrocytes and increased osmotic fragility are found, and it seemed reasonable to suppose that relatively slow haemolysis could be brought about by these means alone, as in hereditary spherocytosis (HS). The erythrostasis would also permit a relatively long exposure to locally formed auto-antibodies and this, too, would be a factor in accelerating haemolysis.

Possible role of tissue lysins

The fact that tissue extracts could cause the lysis of erythrocytes has been known for many years (see Ponder, 1951, 1952). The lytic substances in tissues appear to exist in life as lysin–inhibitor complexes, from which lysins can be extracted by chemical solvents (Laser, 1950) or by saline if the tissues have undergone autolysis (Brückmann and Wertheimer, 1945). As Ponder (1951) pointed out, they are thus laboratory creations, whose importance in pathological processes is uncertain. Nevertheless, such substances have been thought of from time to time as being possibly of significance in physiological haemolysis in the spleen (Fåhraeus, 1939) and in haemolytic states in man (Maegraith, Martin and Findlay, 1943; Castle, Ham and Shen, 1950).

The possibility that tissue enzymes may increase the sensitivity of erythrocytes to agglutination by auto-antibodies has also been considered. Leroy and Spurrier (1954, 1955), for instance, stressed that β-glucuronidase, of which the spleen is a rich source, could act in this way. *In vitro*, cells exposed to the enzyme were more strongly agglutinated by specific allo-antibodies, and cold auto-antibodies acted to a higher temperature than on untreated cells—there are analogies here with the effect of trypsinization. *In vitro*, the agglutination-enhancing effect of β-glucuronidase was inhibited by cortisone acetate, and other known inhibitors of the enzyme.

Magalini, Blumenthal and Stefanini (1956) studied extracts of normal and pathological spleens. Lytic fractions containing long-chain fatty acids were found to produce sphering of the erythrocytes and then lysis. Other extracts inhibited lysis. They speculated that this 'balanced hemolytic system' might operate in physiological haemolysis, and in pathological states imbalance might be an additional mechanism promoting haemolysis within the spleen. Torp (1956) stated that the spleen contains acetylcholine and suggested that the fall in pH resulting from the action of erythrocyte acetylcholinesterase on the acetylcholine might be important in haemolysis. Fall in pH resulting from erythrostasis *per se* or from any other mechanism might certainly accelerate haemolysis in the spleen pulp, if the trapped cells were spherocytes.

Mechanism of sequestration of antibody-coated erythrocytes

One mechanism, is auto-agglutination occurring in the spleen pulp; a second mechanism is spherocytosis which probably impedes the passage of the cells from the splenic pulp into the splenic sinuses (see Vol. 1, p. 36); a third possible mechanism is loss of plasticity of erythrocytes coated with incomplete anti-bodies.

Experimentally, there is some evidence that coating with incomplete antibodies may impair plasticity. Nicolau, Teitel and Fotino (1959) tested the ease with which erythrocytes coated with increasing amounts of anti-D passed through the pores of filter paper. A straight-line relation-ship on semilog paper was established between the speed of filtration and the concentration of antibody. They suggested that the increasing difficulty in filtration was due not to auto-aggluti-nation but to loss of plasticity resulting from the antibody coating and that this could explain the selective trapping of sensitized cells within the spleen.

Possibility of metabolic damage to erythrocytes from the attachment of antibodies to the cell membrane

In addition to the antibodies bringing about erythrostasis (by promoting auto-agglutination or spherocytosis or both) there is some evidence that the presence of adsorbed antibody damages the metabolic efficiency of the erythrocytes—which itself could lead to spherocytosis. A pointer to metabolic damage is the behaviour of the erythro-cytes when AIHA blood is incubated *in vitro*. Not only may the rate of autohaemolysis be acceler-ated but the addition of glucose to the suspension may fail to diminish the rate of lysis as it does normally (Dacie, 1954, p. 174). More detailed studies have provided further evidence in favour of metabolic damage.

Swisher (1954) found in dogs transfused with a powerful dog 'anti-A' antibody that the in-vitro uptake of ^{32}P-labelled phosphate by the recipient's erythro-cytes was markedly deranged subsequently, and further disturbances of carbohydrate metabolism of antibody-affected cells were mentioned by Young (1958) and Altman, Tabechian and Young (1958).

Storti, Vaccari and Baldini (1956) described how D-positive erythrocytes exposed to the antibody anti-D *in vitro* suffered an approximately 25–30% reduction in the rate of glycolysis. Agglutination *per se* appeared to

have nothing to do with the effect and it could not be reproduced with the allo-antibody anti-A. Nicolau and Teitel (1959) took the experiments of Storti and his co-workers as a starting point. They suggested that adsorp-tion of antibodies might render a cell 'diabetic' by the antibody protein adsorbed to the surface of the cell acting as a mechanical barrier to the passage of glucose molecules. Nicolau and Teitel then described how the addition of insulin to incubating cells retarded the onset of change in osmotic fragility, and they suggested that insulin, by enhancing glucose metabolism, might accel-erate the rate of entry of glucose molecules through uncovered areas of the cell surfaces.

That antibody coating of erythrocytes impairs their metabolism is thus a possibility. If metabolic damage in fact occurs, it could not but fail to be a factor in acceler-ating erythrocyte destruction within the spleen and possibly elsewhere, too, in the body. Abnormalities in erythrocyte carbohydrate metabolism have also been demonstrated in experimental animals given anti-erythrocyte immune sera. Pipitone, Russo and Dailly (1959) and Pipitone and co-workers (1959), for instance, reported that the ATP-ase activity of rabbit erythrocytes and the rate of glycolysis, respectively, are substantially reduced.

SPHEROCYTOSIS

The phenomenon of erythrocyte spherocytosis has been mentioned frequently in the preceding pages as being more or less conspicuous in most patients with AIHA of the warm-antibody type; it is also a striking feature of the blood picture in experimentally produced immune haemolytic anaemia in animals (see p. 434). It can be looked upon as a sign that the erythrocyte has been damaged by antibody action and, as has already been explained, the shape change itself probably leads to sequestration within the spleen. As Crosby (1952) pointed out, in acquired haemolytic anaemias the degree of spherocytosis may be more extreme than in HS (e.g. Fig. 23.5).

Early views as to causation

It has been realized for many years that although the injection of an anti-erythrocyte serum into an animal would produce spherocytosis with great regularity, the phenomenon could not be repro-duced *in vitro* by the addition of antiserum to erythrocytes (Banti, 1913: Wasastjerna, 1948; Castle, Ham and Shen, 1950). Dameshek and

Schwartz's (1938) original view that spherocytosis was the result of a direct effect of 'hemolysin' on the erythrocyte surface thus had to be discarded.

Evans (1946) made the significant observation that after normal blood was transfused to a persistently anaemic patient, who had earlier undergone colectomy for ulcerative colitis and splenectomy for acquired haemolytic anaemia, the transfused normal erythrocytes rapidly—within a day or so—became spherocytic and osmotically fragile. On the other hand, there was no difference in the rate at which normal erythrocytes became osmotically fragile when incubated *in vitro* in the patient's serum or normal serum, respectively. In discussing the nature of the (unknown) lytic substance which was clearly able to act on the transfused normal erythrocytes as well as on the patient's own erythrocytes, Evans commented: 'Since it is not easily demonstrable in the peripheral blood there is less difficulty in supposing it to be an immune body type of hemolysin than a simple lytic substance'. How the 'hemolysin' could cause spherocytosis and increased osmotic fragility *in vivo* but not *in vitro* was, however, unknown at the time. Evans suggested that 'the primary effect of the lytic substance was damage to the cell which caused or permitted the absorption of fluid'.

As already described (p. 401), Castle, Ham and Shen (1950) concluded that spherocytosis might develop when agglutinated erythrocytes became exposed to injurious substances derived locally from tissues made ischaemic due to the auto-agglutination blocking small blood vessels. This mechanism still seems a plausible part explanation. The same is true of the metabolic damage hypothesis also referred to earlier (p. 402).

Jandl (1960a), in referring to the occurrence of spherocytosis in AIHA in man, considered that the spherocytosis and concomitant increase in osmotic fragility were a comparatively slow and indirect metabolic effect of antibody-coating. He felt that the tissues were in some way involved.

A more up-to-date view as to causation

An interesting observation that was at one time (e.g. in the 1950s) as intriguing as it was puzzling was that in haemolytic anaemias induced by auto-antibodies the intensity of spherocytosis and increased osmotic fragility varied markedly from case to case. While it was true that in warm-antibody AIHA the changes were more marked in the more severely affected patients, this did not seem always to be so. In contrast, in CHAD due to anti-I antibodies, despite a great deal of auto-agglutination, spherocytosis was inconspicuous. In PCH on the other hand, it was often a marked feature. It was also appreciated that spherocytosis was typically well marked in haemolytic disease of the newborn caused by ABO incompatibility, but not in cases in which the cause was Rh incompatibility. With the present knowledge of the role of IgG antibody and of complement in bringing about adhesion of sensitized erythrocytes to macrophages and spherocytosis developing in consequence of this (see p. 410), these differences are more easily understood. They depend upon whether the causal antibody is IgG rather than IgM (for which the macrophages lack receptors) and the degree to which the antibody brings about the fixation of complement.

How exactly adhesion of antibody- or complement-coated erythrocytes to macrophages damages the cells and causes them to become spherocytic is an interesting question. According to Fleer et al. (1978a), it is the release of lysosomal enzymes at the point of contact between the erythrocyte membrane and the macrophage that causes the damage. In experiments *in vitro* with human anti-D allo-antibodies, the damage responsible for the spherocytosis, as reflected by increase in osmotic fragility, appeared to be complete within 1 hour, although for the full expression of the damage a much longer period of contact was necessary.

To summarize, the major cause of the presence of spherocytes in the peripheral blood in AIHA is the recirculation of erythrocytes, coated with IgG auto-antibody and/or with complement, that have been damaged earlier by contact with phagocytic cells. The effects of sequestration within the spleen and (possibly) of metabolic damage secondary to the presence of antibodies on the erythrocyte membrane seem likely to contribute to the changes. An important point to note is that although a spleen *in situ* probably always contributes to the development of spherocytosis, this usually persists, sometimes to a marked degree, in patients in whom increased haemolysis has continued after splenectomy. Case 12 of Dacie (1954, p. 202) provided a striking example of this persistence.

CORRELATION BETWEEN AMOUNT OF AUTO-ANTIBODY FORMED BY AN AIHA PATIENT AND SEVERITY OF HAEMOLYSIS *IN VIVO*

Common sense suggests strongly that the clinical severity of an AIHA patient's illness should be closely correlated with the amount of auto-antibody he or she is forming. In fact, a great deal depends, too, on the nature, i.e. the quality, of the antibody—in particular whether it is an IgG, IgM or IgA globulin and if an IgG, its subclass. Its nature determines aspects of its activity which are critically important *in vivo*, and which can be readily demonstrated *in vitro*: as shown for instance, by its ability to cause direct agglutination of the patient's erythrocytes, as opposed to sensitizing them to agglutination by antiglobulin sera; by its ability to fix complement; by the temperature range at which these reactions can take place and its ability to promote macrophage/monocyte adhesion. Then there is the efficiency of the patient's macrophage/ monocyte phagocytic system, and finally his or her ability to compensate for developing anaemia by accelerating erythropoiesis.

In each and all of the aspects of antibody activity which have been mentioned above, there are patient-to-patient differences. It is these differences which lead to the wide variation in clinical severity of the auto-immune haemolytic anaemias. As in aetiology, so in pathology and pathogenesis it is the individual who determines the course and outcome of his or her illness— whether haemolysis is short-lived or long-continued, whether the patient's illness is clinically mild or devastatingly severe and perhaps fatal.

In later sections of this Chapter, the role of complement activation and of the macrophage/ monocyte system, and the effect of auto-antibodies on erythropoiesis, will be discussed. Before this is attempted, however, reference is made to some important early and more recent studies that have been carried out on the relationship between erythrocyte sensitization and in-vivo haemolysis.

Early evidence of a close relationship between the amount of antibody bound to erythrocytes and in-vivo haemolysis was provided by Evans and his colleagues (1961, 1963) and Constantoulakis et al. (1963).

Evans, Bingham and Boehni (1961) studied the rate of transference of auto-antibody from the erythrocytes of AIHA patients to normal erythrocytes *in vitro*. They concluded that the rate of transference reflected the amount of bound antibody and was correlated with the rate of haemolysis. There were, however, patient-to-patient differences. Evans, Bingham and Turner (1965) reported on three closely studied patients with warm-antibody AIHA. In two of the patients who had responded well to prednisone the antibody transference test indicated a marked diminution in the amount of auto-antibody; in the third patient who had responded only partially to dexamethasone the diminution in antibody transference was less impressive.

Constantoulakis and co-workers (1963) studied the quantitative relationship between erythrocyte sensitization with incomplete antibodies and in-vivo survival as assessed by ^{51}Cr labelling and a radioactive antiglobulin test. They worked with allo-antibodies, e.g. anti-Rh(D) and anti-K, and also with auto-antibodies eluted from the erythrocytes of AIHA patients. Antibodies of the same specificity, obtained from different sources and used to coat erythrocytes in similar amounts, were found to cause different degrees of impairment of in-vivo survival. This was the case with both the allo-antibodies and the auto-antibodies they had experimented with. The term 'hemolytic effectiveness' was used to describe the antibodies' biological activity.

Rosse (1971) set out to determine the relationship between erythrocyte-bound antibody and in-vivo haemolysis by means of a complement (C1) fixation and transfer test, i.e. by estimating the number of molecules of C1 fixed by the reaction of a rabbit anti-human IgG antibody with bound human IgG, a reaction which can provide a quantitative assessment of the number of IgG molecules coating erythrocytes. Thirty patients with various types of AIHA were studied in this way and the data obtained were related to the severity of haemolysis in the individual patients as assessed by their haemoglobin concentration and reticulocyte count and as measured by the production of endogenous CO. In general, the rate of haemolysis was closely correlated with the concentration of cell-bound antibody, and it was interesting to note that in splenectomized patients the rate of haemolysis was very much reduced in relation to the amount of erythrocyte-bound antibody. The effect of prednisone on haemolysis and cell-bound antibody was also studied with most interesting results. These data are described on p. 463.

Rosse (1975), in a review, also dealt with the correlation of in-vivo and in-vitro measurements of immune haemolysis; he expanded his discussion to include, too, the role of complement in both warm and cold-antibody AIHA.

Flow cytofluorometry

In recent years flow cytofluorometry has been used to measure quantitatively the degree to which cells have been coated with antibodies. Leucocytes as well as erythrocytes have been the targets. Garratty (1990b) outlined the general principles of the technique and its many applications. In relation to AIHA, the key questions have been the degree to which antibody coating, as revealed by cytofluorometry, reflects in-vivo haemolysis and whether the results of cytofluorometry are more reliable in this respect than assessment by the positivity of the DAT, as indicated by the strength of the reaction or its titre.

van der Meulen and co-workers (1980) studied 29 patients whose erythrocytes gave a positive DAT due to coating with IgG1: 17 had suffered from haemolytic anaemia; 12 appeared to be free from increased haemolysis. Twelve of the 29 patients had been treated with α-methyldopa: seven had haemolytic anaemia, five showed no signs of increased haemolysis. With only one exception, the two groups of patients—those with and those without signs of overt haemolysis — were separable on the basis of erythrocyte fluorescence and antibody cytotoxicity towards monocytes. Using allo-anti-D an excellent linear correlation was found between dilution of anti-D and the resultant fluorescence, but the correlation between the fluorescence score and the titre (end-point) of the corresponding antiglobulin reaction was poor.

Nance and Garratty (1984) reported on the use of cytofluorometry in the study of 50 individuals whose erythrocytes had given a positive DAT. They comprised patients with idiopathic AIHA, patients receiving α-methyldopa, newborn infants whose mothers had developed allo-antibodies, and normal blood donors. Although the fluorescence score was higher in the presence of overt haemolysis, there were considerable overlaps between the various groups.

Further and more complete data were described by Garratty and Nance (1990). Seventy-three individuals had by then been studied, all giving positive DATs: some were suffering from overt haemolysis; in others there was no evidence of this. Their conclusions were the same as in their earlier report: namely, that there was considerable overlap in fluorescence in patients with or without overt haemolysis in each group and that it was not possible to define a fluorescence threshold which would define clearly individuals suffering from increased haemolysis. Garratty and Nance concluded that although flow cytofluorometry provided more accurate and reproducible data than antiglobulin scores, neither of the two approaches provided a precise measurement of in-vivo haemolysis. [This is not surprising as neither measurement takes into account the uniqueness of the individual in his or her ability to dispose of the antibody-affected erythrocytes.]

Chaplin's (1990) recent review dealt with the same question that the earlier workers cited above had attempted to answer—namely, the correlation between erythrocyte-bound IgG and the severity of in-vivo haemolysis and the value of measuring bound IgG as a predictor of severity. In commenting on Garratty and Nance's paper on the value of flow cytometry (quoted above), Chaplin stated that he agreed with their conclusion, namely, that the amount of bound IgG cannot serve as the sole predictor of haemolysis in many cases of AIHA. In Chaplin's words 'The pathogenesis is too complex ... for an expectation that measurement of a single factor will be predictive of the combined effects of all the factors'.

DISTRIBUTION OF ANTIBODY-BINDING SITES ON THE ERYTHROCYTE MEMBRANE: A POSSIBLE DETERMINANT OF THE SEVERITY OF HAEMOLYSIS

Another aspect of the uniqueness of the individual which could be a factor in determining the severity of haemolysis is the distribution of antibody-binding sites on the patient's erythrocytes. Davis and co-workers (1968) applied immuno-electron microscopy, using ferritin-labelled antiglobulin sera, to determine the fine structural characteristics of the binding of IgG and C3 to the erythrocytes membrane. Erythrocytes sensitized with high-titre anti-Rh (D or CD) antibodies and cells from DAT-positive patients with idiopathic AIHA were studied. Both qualitative and quantitative differences in the periodicity and intensity of labelling were observed with the cells of different AIHA patients, and the periodicity of labelling with penicillin- and α-methyldopa-induced antibodies differed from each other and from the antibodies of the idiopathic AIHA patients.

ROLE OF COMPLEMENT IN HAEMOLYSIS *IN VIVO*

As referred to on p. 136, in cases in which lysis depending on the presence of complement can be demonstrated *in vitro* at 37°C, the patient is usually seriously ill and may well be suffering from haemoglobinuria. Intravascular haemolysis dominates the picture, although there is every reason to believe that erythrocytes which have been agglutinated by the antibody and/or which have been coated by sublytic amounts of complement are also removed from circulation, predominantly by the liver. The early experimental studies of Jandl, Richardson Jones and Castle (1957), Cutbush and Mollison (1958) and Jandl and Kaplan (1960) with lytic or potentially lytic allo-antibodies, e.g. anti-A, anti-B, anti-Le^a, showed that the rate of haemolysis and the proportion of cells lysed in the blood stream or filtered from the circulation by the liver can be correlated with the lytic potency of the antibody *in vitro*.

In man, most of the restraints to the rate of haemolysis already referred to above probably operate in the case of lytic antibodies as they do with incomplete and non-complement-fixing agglutinating antibodies. However, it seems doubtful whether 'saturation' of the liver is as important a restraint as is 'saturation' of the spleen, and no physical restraint can operate in the circulating blood stream. Here, however, lack or even apparent absence of complement is often found in the presence of severe intravascular haemolysis, and this is likely to be important in retarding haemolysis, as was so well demonstrated in dogs by Young, Ervin and Yuile (1949) and Christian et al. (1951).

That complement plays a dual role in the destruction of erythrocytes in AIHA was indirectly first demonstrated in the late 1950s as the result of investigations into the nature and meaning of the 'non-γ' positive antiglobulin reactions. These studies showed that the non-γ reaction was in fact brought about by interaction between anti-complement antibodies in the antiglobulin serum and complement components attached to erythrocytes that had been exposed to a complement-fixing antibody that was insufficiently potent to cause actual lysis (see p. 406).

Summarized simply, the two mechanisms referred to above by which complement can bring about erythrocyte destruction in AIHA are as follows:

(1) if the complement sequence is completed after attachment to the erythrocyte surface as the result of antibody action, the affected cells undergo lysis in the blood stream (intravascular haemolysis);

(2) if, on the other hand, complement is attached but the sequence is not completed, residual complement components on the erythrocyte surface may cause erythrocytes to become

attached to the surface of phagocytic cells (which have receptors for complement components) and to sustain damage with loss of surface and consequent spherocytosis and possibly to undergo phagocytosis (extravascular haemolysis).

It is possible, too, that coating with complement components may affect the deformability of the erythrocyte and in this way lead to its potentially harmful sequestration in the microvasculature (Durocher, Gockerman and Conrad, 1975).

Mechanisms (1) and (2), summarized above, are discussed in more detail below, following a brief description of the nature of complement and its activation by antibody–erythrocyte interaction.

COMPLEMENT: ITS NATURE AND ACTIVATION

To attempt to describe the complement system and its activation in any detail would be beyond the scope of this book. The subject has a very large literature, and its nature and complexity, and its activation and significance in relation to human disease, have been dealt with in many publications.

Valuable reviews on complement and on the role it plays in the pathogenesis of blood diseases, which have been published in the last three decades, include those of Stratton (1965), Müller-Eberhard et al. (1966), Yachnin (1966), Garratty (1968, 1984), Müller-Eberhard (1969, 1975), Rosse (1979, 1990) and Lachmann and Peters (1982). The following account is a summary of the main facts.

That serum contains a heat-labile constituent which acts as a necessary co-factor in the lysis of erythrocytes by antibodies has been known since the end of the 19th century. Referred to as 'complement' according to Müller-Eberhard since the days of Ehrlich and Bordet, it is now known to comprise a whole series of plasma proteins, distinguishable by their molecular weight, electrophoretic mobility and concentration, which act in concert when complement is activated. These proteins, referred to as complement (C) components, are now designated by the symbols C1, C1q, C1r, C1s, and C2, C3, C4, C5,

C6, C7, C8 and C9. C3 is present in serum in the greatest concentration, c 1500 µg/ml; C4 is present in the next greatest concentration, c 500 µg/ml; the other components are present in small or minute amounts, c 25–180 µg/ml. In addition, there are several inhibitors and inactivators and at least three other components which operate within the alternative activation pathway (see p. 408).

Complement can be activated in one of two ways: by the classical or by the alternative pathway. In relation to its role in AIHA, it is the classical activation pathway that is involved.

Activation by the classical pathway by antibody–erythrocyte interaction can be conveniently broken down into five stages; functionally, it is an enzymatic cascade culminating in a 'membrane attack unit'.

1. The attachment of antibody (A) to erythrocyte (E) leads to activation of C1, a macromolecular complex of C1q, C1r and C1s held together by Ca^{2+} ions. C1q has binding sites for IgG and for IgM. When C1 makes contact with an antigen–antibody complex (EA), it becomes attached to the Fc fragment of the antibody molecule. For this to happen at the surface membrane of an erythrocyte the antibody has to be an IgM molecule or two IgG molecules have to be closely adjacent on the membrane (Borsos and Rapp, 1965). The attachment of C1q to the antibody results in the activation of C1r and subsequently of C1s which acts as an enzyme, $C\overline{1s}$;* the attachment of $C\overline{1s}$ to the membrane is a relatively loose one and it can move from site to site.

2. The next stage in activation is the generation of the enzyme C3 convertase by the action of activated $C1(C\overline{1s})$ on two further complement components, C4, the primary substate, and C2. $C\overline{1s}$ splits C4 into two fragments, a minor fragment, C4a, and a major fragment, C4b. A large number of C4b fragments may be produced by a single $C\overline{1s}$ molecule, so that although only a small proportion of the fragments attach themselves to the membrane each EAC1 site may

---

*A bar over the component, e.g. $C\overline{1s}$, identifies the component as an enzyme.

be surrounded by a cluster of C4b molecules. Activated C1($\overline{\text{C1s}}$), as well as acting on C4, also splits C2 into two fragments, C2a and C2b. The larger fragment, C2a, combines, if Mg^{2+} ions are available, with C4b on the cell membrane to form the active enzyme $\overline{\text{C4b2a}}$; this is C3 convertase.

3. C3 convertase next acts on C3, the major protein of the complement system, and splits it into two parts, C3a and C3b. C3b, the larger component, attaches itself to the membrane which has, as it has for C4b, binding sites for it. As C3 convertase is an enzyme it is capable of producing a large number of C3b molecules. A small proportion of these bind in the vicinity of the EAC1 site.

4. The next stage in activation is the generation of 'the heat-stable intermediate complex' or C5 convertase by the combination of $\overline{\text{C4b2a}}$ with C3b. C5 convertase splits C5 into C5a and C5b. C5b then binds to C6 and C7 to form the enzyme $\overline{\text{C567}}$, some molecules of which attach themselves to the cell membrane.

5. The last stage in activation involves the attachment of C8 to $\overline{\text{C567}}$ and of C9 to C8. This final complex, the 'membrane attack unit' acts on the cells' lipid membrane so as to produce 'holes', visible in electron micrographs, at the site of interaction between erythrocyte membrane antigen, the corresponding antibody and complement (Borsos, Dourmashkin and Humphrey, 1964, Dourmashkin and Rosse (1966) (Fig. 34.1). These holes are the morphological micro-equivalent of lysis. How exactly they are caused is uncertain, as is how exactly their presence leads to lysis. The holes seem to be too small in diameter for haemoglobin molecules to escape, and lysis may result from the unrestricted entry of sodium and water through the holes into the cell interior, which could lead to membrane rupture by osmotic forces (see Sears, Weed and Swisher, 1963, 1964).

Rosse's (1990) recent account of complement and complement-dependent mechanisms in immune destruction is particularly comprehensive: it includes, in addition to some historical notes, a list of 458 relevant references.

Rosse (1990) summarized in a table the biochemical details of as many as 21 components of complement, all proteins of molecular weight between 18–560 kD. Of these 21 components, seven are designated inhibitors or regulators: these are C1 inh, which inhibits C1r and C1s; Factor H, which binds C3b and regulates the alternative pathway; C4 BP(binding protein) which binds C4b and regulates the classical pathway; DAF (decay accelerating factor), which disrupts convertases; vitronectin (S protein), which inhibits C5b–7 in serum; C8 BP, which inhibits C9 polymerization; and MIRL (membrane inhibitor of reactive lysis), which inhibits C5b–7 binding.

Vitronectin, by binding to the C5b–7 complex, prevents its insertion into the lipid bilayer, so that for lysis to occur a very large number of activated components have to be formed. In any case the membrane normally binds the C5b–7 complex poorly, the protein MIRL contributing to this. DAF and C8 BP also help to frustrate the development of the final sequence. The net result of the action of these inhibitors and regulators, and of the instability of some of the complexes, e.g. the antibody–antigen and C1q–antibody interactions, the C1q–C1r, C1s interaction, and convertase activity, is that the normal human erythrocyte is relatively resistant to lysis by homologous complement, as opposed to the remarkable PNH cell in which some of the above-mentioned regulators are absent or deficient.

Alternative pathway of complement activation

Pillemer and his co-workers reported in 1954 that a hitherto undescribed substance in normal plasma would react with certain polysaccharides and lipopolysaccharides so as to activate complement in the absence of antibody. They called this substance properdin. Subsequently, several other distinct factors normally present in plasma were found to be necessary for activation to proceed. This 'alternative-pathway' mechanism activates C3 and leads to the formation of C5 convertase which with C6, C7, C8 and C9 is capable of bringing about the same cell damage as is achieved by C3 activated via the classical pathway involving C1, C4 and C2. As already referred to, the alternative pathway appears to play no part in complement activity in AIHA, and for this reason

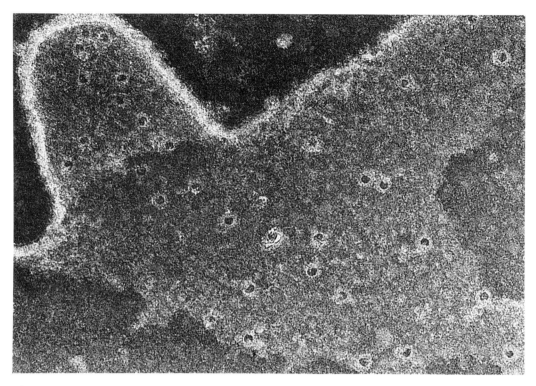

Fig. 34.1   Electron micrograph of part of the membrane of a PNH erythrocyte after lysis by complement in acidified serum.
    The 'holes' in the membrane are similar to those produced by anti-I antibody and complement.
[Reproduced by permission from Rosse, Dourmashkin and Humphrey (1966).]

will not be discussed further at this point. Alternative-pathway activation is, however, important in the pathogenesis of paroxysmal nocturnal haemoglobinuria (PNH), and it will be dealt with in more detail when PNH is described in Volume 4 of this book.

Rosse (1990) gives a short but interesting account of the controversy and eventual vindication of Pillemer's concept of an alternative pathway of complement activation that followed the identification of properdin. Rosse suggests that the (alternative) pathway that does not require antibody for activation is probably more important for immune protection than the (classical) pathway that does. In support of this contention, he cites the occurrence of congenital deficiences of C1, C4, and C2 without appreciable immune deficiency. He summarizes the situation as follows: 'In reality, what we call the alternative pathway is, in fact, the real pathway, and the "classical pathway" is the alternative that is used if antibody happens to be present'!

NATURE OF THE COMPLEMENT COMPONENTS DETECTABLE ON THE ERYTHROCYTES OF AIHA PATIENTS

This interesting problem has been considered at some length in Chapter 29 (p. 280). To recapitulate, the use of monoclonal antibodies that react with specific complement components has resulted in more precise information being available. Thus it has been shown that a hitherto unrecognized compound C3d,g (α-2D globulin) is detectable on the erythrocytes of CHAD patients. C3d,g is formed as the result of the splitting of iC3b, which is itself derived from the rapid breakdown of cell-bound C3b by the combined action of C3b inhibitor (factor I) and a further factor named H. iC3b is relatively slowly broken down on the cell surface into two components, C3c, which is released into the circulation, and C3d,g which is retained on the cell surface. In in-vitro systems, C3d,g can be split into C3d and C3g. *In vivo*, C3d,g seems to be the final product of C3 breakdown (Lachmann, Pangburn and Oldroyd, 1982; Lachmann et al., 1983).

INTERACTION BETWEEN IgG-COATED OR COMPLEMENT-COATED ERYTHROCYTES AND PHAGOCYTIC CELLS

A great deal is now known as to how and why erythrocytes coated with antibodies and/or complement adhere to, and are phagocytosed by, peripheral-blood leucocytes and fixed tissue macrophages. Briefly, the phagocytic cells have specific receptors for the Fc portion of IgG molecules, particularly those of IgG3 and IgG1; and they also have receptors for the C3b component of complement. These antibody–receptor interactions are responsible not only for erythrocyte adhesion and phagocytosis but also for the spherocytosis which is so prominent a feature in some patients with AIHA and in animals injected experimentally with hetero-immune anti-erythrocyte sera. However, not all erythrocytes that adhere to phagocytes undergo phagocytosis. Some cells are released before this can take place, as the result of the intervention of fluid-phase IgG or the inactivator of C3b. During the period of contact, however, adherent cells lose surface so that if and when they break free they circulate as spherocytosis.

How this remarkable story has been built up in recent years is outlined in the following pages.

In 1958 Jandl and Tomlinson described how leucocytes adhered to agglutinated erythrocytes when human group-A cells were suspended in incompatible (group-O) plasma in the presence of leucocytes, and they also observed that the erythrocytes in contact with the leucocytes underwent sphering and that some might be phagocytosed. When the experiment was repeated with plasma containing incomplete anti-D and D-positive cells, there was no agglutination, but some of the erythrocytes formed rosettes around individual leucocytes and tended also to become spherocytic. Some years were to pass before these key observations were re-investigated and extended. In the meanwhile, in animal systems the concepts of 'cytophilic antibody', i.e. a type of antibody binding sensitized cells to macrophages, had been elaborated (Boyden, 1964; Berken and Benacerraf, 1966). Archer (1965) extended Jandl and Tomlinson's observations: he centrifuged D-positive erythrocytes, anti-D antibody and leucocytes and showed that human monocytes ingested the sensitized cells [erythrophagocytosis (EP)] and that the phenomenon was independent of the presence of serum factors other than the antibody. When sensitized cells were suspended in saline containing leucocytes in suspension, EP did not occur; instead, clusters of erythrocytes formed around monocytes.

LoBuglio and Jandl (1967) and LoBuglio, Cotran and Jandl (1967) reported important new information. Human monocytes, macrophages and certain lymphocytes were found to be capable of binding on erythrocytes coated with IgG whether or not the IgG was acting as antibody. The binding to monocytes was found to be specific for the Fc-fragment of IgG and was not necessarily a prelude to phagocytosis; the binding, nevertheless, injured the bound cells, as was shown by spherocytosis, increased osmotic fragility and deformation and fragmentation. The binding was inhibited by serum. Cells coated with IgM antibodies were not bound and it was concluded that mononuclear cells have specific receptors for IgG and that this provides a mechanism by which cells coated with antibody can be 'apprehended' and destroyed. LoBuglio and co-workers suggested that the inhibition of the reaction by serum, which was thought to be due to competition by normal IgG for the receptors, might be ineffective in the pulp of the spleen where many macrophages would be present and the haematocrit would be high, and they concluded that the IgG-coated erythrocyte–macrophage interaction provided a mechanism for the sphering and destruction *in vivo* of erythrocytes coated with allo- or auto-IgG antibodies.

Cline and Lehrer (1968) similarly reported that

the ingestion of anti-D-sensitized cells by human peripheral-blood monocytes is inhibited by whole serum or IgG; it was in contrast not inhibited by IgM or albumin. They also stressed that *in vitro* adherence to a surface appeared to be critical for the phagocytosis of erythrocytes, but not for the ingestion of bacteria.

Huber, Douglas and Fudenberg (1969), using erythrocytes sensitized with an anti-Rh antibody, concluded that the receptor could be looked upon as an immunological marker for mononuclear cells, and they showed that it was present on human peripheral-blood monocytes, and on hepatic and splenic macrophages.

The next step in this unfolding story was the demonstration that the binding of erythrocytes to phagocytes was influenced by the subtype of the sensitizing immunoglobulin. Ig of subtypes IgG_1 and IgG_3 were found to bind readily, IgG_2 and IgG_4 much less readily or not at all (Huber and Fudenberg, 1968; Huber et al., 1971; Abramson et al., 1970 a,b; Abramson and Schur, 1972; Hay, Torrigiani and Roitt, 1972).

Huber and Fudenberg (1968) reported that erythrocytes sensitized by IgG antibodies, but not by IgM, were readily phagocytosed by human peripheral-blood monocytes. They also showed that phagocytosis was dependent on the Fc fragment and that IgG in the incubation medium inhibited the phagocytosis of IgG-sensitized erythrocytes. Their experiments also indicated that IgG of subclasses IgG_1 and IgG_3 were many times more effective in binding to the monocytes than IgG_2 or IgG_4.

Abramson and co-workers (1970b,c) studied the interaction between anti-D erythrocytes and human peripheral-blood mononuclear cells. Rosette formation was inhibited by free IgG globulin and by IgG_1 and IgG_3; IgG_4 was less inhibiting and IgG_2 caused little inhibition. Erythrocytes coated with IgG_1 and IgG_3 bound readily to the phagocytes; cells coated with IgG_4 or IgG_2 bound poorly. Rosette formation of D–L-antibody- or penicillin-antibody-sensitized erythrocytes was similarly inhibited by free IgG_1 or IgG_3. Rosettes were also inhibited by the Fc fragment of IgG and partly inhibited by the $F(ab)_2$ fragment. Abramson and co-workers concluded that the receptor site for IgG on human mononuclear cells is specific for IgG_1 and IgG_3 and that it may react with the IgG molecule near the disulphide hinge of the Fc fragment.

Abramson and co-workers (1970c) reproduced excellent transmission electron micrographs showing the distortion and damage to the erythrocyte membrane at the point of adhesion to a monocyte and how the membranes of the two cells might interdigitate; they pointed out that the deformation of a large number of erythrocytes by a single mononuclear cell, leading to spherocytosis or fragmentation, was likely to be a more efficient mechanism of cell destruction than the phagocytosis of a small number of cells.

In addition to the monocyte/macrophage receptor for IgG referred to above, it is now known that the same cells bear receptors for the C3b component of complement.

Lay and Nussenzweig (1968) showed that whereas sheep cells coated with 7S Forssman antibodies would bind to mouse macrophages this did not happen with 19S Forssman antibody unless complement was present. Then, rosettes were formed with the macrophages as well as with polymorphs, some monocytes and with 10–25% of lymph-node lymphocytes (but not with thymic lymphocytes). It seemed that only the early components of complement were involved as C5-deficient mouse serum and C6-deficient rabbit serum were both active. Lay and Nussenzweig's (1968) electron micrographs showed that the damage to the adherent erythrocyte at the point of contact with a macrophage was very similar to, if not identical with, that resulting from IgG (Fc)-macrophage interaction: 'finger-like processes [surround] the red cell, which appears deformed and fragmented.' Mantovani, Rabinovitch and Nussenzweig (1972), working with the same system, concluded that the complement factor involved (C3) brought about attachment rather than phagocytosis and stressed that the C3 and IgG receptor sites played different roles.

Huber and co-workers (1968) showed that with human complement the receptor was specific for C3; also that it was distinct from, and functioned independently of, the receptor for IgG, although it could cooperate with it. They found that for the phagocytosis of C3-coated cells many more molecules of C3 were required than for adhesion and rosette formation.

Huber and Douglas (1970) gave further details of the interaction between human monocytes and erythrocytes coated with complement by exposure to a high-titre anti-I antibody. The effect of temperature on erythrocyte–monocyte rosette formation and lysis was found to be comparable. Less antibody was, however, required for rosette formation than for lysis. The complement-coated cells were found to bind to monocytes irrespective of whether the cold antibody had been eluted. Binding took place, too, when the cells had been coated with complement in the absence of antibody, by using, for instance, low ionic strength isotonic sucrose as a suspending medium.

Michlmayr and Huber (1970) comfirmed that receptor sites for complement are present on some lymphocytes, as had been reported earlier by Lay and Nussenzweig (1968). In the case of human peripheral blood, the receptors could be demonstrated on small lymphocytes, but were absent on 95% of those of medium or large size.

Brown, Lachmann and Dacie (1970) showed that EC43(5) rabbit erythrocytes would attach to macrophages, irrespective of whether the sensitizing (IgM) antibody was present or not. They had carried out two series of experiments on normal, C6-deficient, and C3-depleted rabbits. In the first series they injected intravenously a potent human IgM anti-I cold antibody. In the normal rabbits the injection was followed by significant falls in haemoglobin and rises in plasma haemoglobin as well as severe transient thrombo-

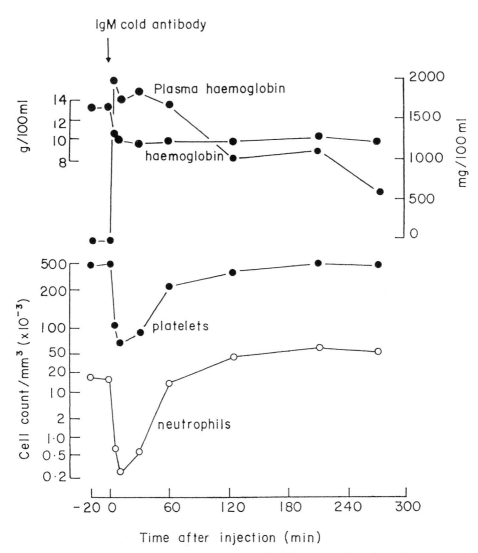

Fig. 34.2a   Haematological changes in a normal rabbit (34.2a), in a C6-deficient rabbit (34.2b) and in a C3-depleted rabbit (34.2c) following the intravenous injection of a human IgM anti-I cold antibody.

[Reproduced by permission from Brown, Lachmann and Dacie (1970)].

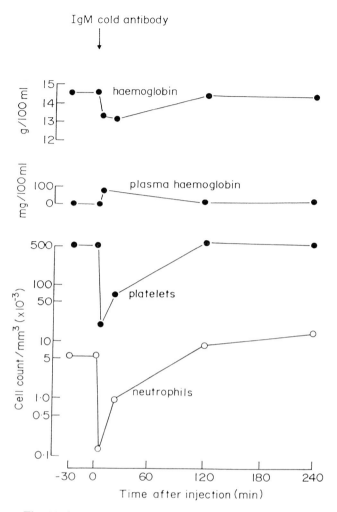

Fig. 34.2b

cytopenia and neutropenia (Fig. 34.2a). In the C6-deficient rabbits the changes were similar except that the falls in haemoglobin and rises in plasma haemoglobin were less marked (Fig. 34.2b). In both cases there was a sharp fall in plasma C3 and the erythrocytes became coated with C3(C3b). In the C3-depleted rabbits injection of the same IgG cold antibody had no significant effects (Fig. 34.2c). In the second series of experiments rabbit erythrocytes were sensitized *in vitro* with the cold antibody so as to be in the form EC43(5) or EC4. They were then injected intravenously into the donor rabbits and their fate followed. The EC4 cells survived normally, whereas the EC43(5) cells rapidly left the circulation (T_{50} 1.5–4 min) at sites in the RE-

cell system. The liver was the main source of sequestration and EC43(5) cells could be seen attached to Kupffer cells; some were phagocytosed (Fig. 34.3). In time, unphagocytosed cells returned to the circulation at a slow exponential rate (T_{50} 25–100 min), apparently as spherocytes.

The adhesion of C3b-coated erythrocytes to the C3 receptor of macrophages is not inhibited by the C3 in plasma. The reason for this is that the receptor is directed against C3b and not against native C3. Another most interesting feature of C3b–macrophage interaction, as demonstrated in the experiments of Brown, Lachmann and Dacie (1970) outlined above, is that it is transient. This is due to cell-bound C3b being broken down rapidly by the combined action of two additional

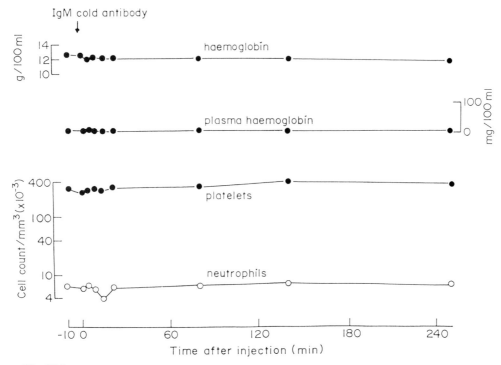

Fig. 34.2c

plasma factors—C3b inhibitor (factor I or KAF) and factor H (p. 408). It is the breakdown of C3b that explains the reappearance in the peripheral blood of C3b(C3b,g)-coated erythrocytes after transient sequestration in organs, such as the liver, that are rich in phagocytic cells.

Evidence that the adhesion of C3b-coated erythrocytes to phagocytic cells could be transient had been obtained earlier in man.

Jandl, Richardson Jones and Castle (1957), in a study of a healthy donor injected with his own group-B erythrocytes which had been exposed to anti-B *in vitro*, found that many of the sensitized cells appeared to be held temporarily in the liver for an hour or so, with only a fraction of the retained cells ultimately undergoing haemolysis.

Lewis, Dacie and Szur (1960) described the same phenomenon in a CHAD patient whose ^{51}Cr-labelled erythrocytes were reinjected into her circulation after being exposed *in vitro* under conditions allowing, respectively, auto-agglutination only or a minor or major amount of complement adsorption. Auto-agglutination by itself did not seem to produce any irreversible

damage to the erythrocytes as judged by their subsequent survival in the patient; agglutination plus a minor amount of complement adsorption resulted in the reinjected cells undergoing temporary retention in the liver without impairment of their survival; auto-agglutination plus a major amount of complement adsorption was followed by the relatively rapid haemolysis of about 30% of the reinjected cells.

Brown and Nelson (1971, 1973) reported on an electron-microscopic study of the interaction between C3(C3b)-coated rabbit erythrocytes and the Kupffer cells in the liver of rabbits. Within 2 minutes of the intravenous injection of the cells protrusions of erythrocyte membrane were surrounded by macrophage cytoplasm, while at 5–25 minutes apparently separated round fragments of erythrocyte could be seen to have been engulfed by the macrophage (Fig. 34.4). The loss of these fragments, or 'microspheres', without lysis appeared to be contributing to the spherocytic appearance of the adherent erythrocytes, as the result, it was thought, of a proportionately greater loss of cell surface than of

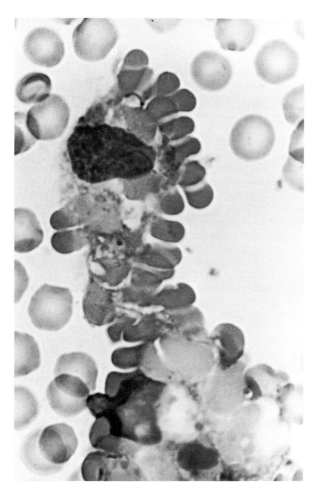

Fig. 34.3 Photomicrograph of a smear prepared from the liver of a C6-deficient rabbit which had been injected intravenously with C3-coated rabbit erythrocytes.
Two Kupffer cells are present: they are surrounded by spherocytic erythrocytes some of which have been phagocytosed. [Reproduced by courtesy of Dr. D. L. Brown.]

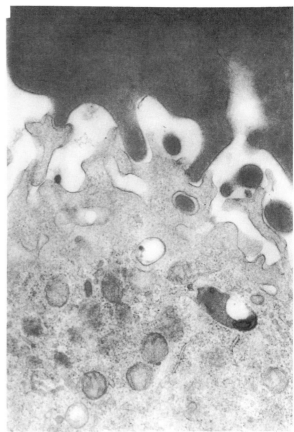

Fig. 34.4 Electron micrograph of the point of contact of a C-3 coated rabbit erythrocyte (top) and a Kupffer cell (bottom).
Same material as in Fig. 34.3. [Reproduced by courtesy of Dr. D. L. Brown and Professor D. Nelson.]

volume. The time-course of the sphering of the adherent erythrocytes was consistent with the appearance of spherocytes in the peripheral blood.

Further details of immune clearance of antibody-sensitized cells in an experimental system were given by Schreiber and Frank (1971, 1972a,b). Guinea-pig erythrocytes were sensitized with rabbit IgG or IgM antisera and transfused back into the donor guinea-pigs. At least 60 C1-fixing sites per cell were required for the accelerated clearance of IgM-sensitized cells, Most of the cells were sequestered in the liver within 5 minutes, then returned to the circulation where they

survived normally. In C4-deficient guinea-pigs similarly sensitized cells were not cleared at an accelerated rate. In contrast to the findings with IgM-sensitized cells, only 1.4 (on average) C1-fixing sites per cell were required for the accelerated clearance of erythrocytes sensitized with IgG antibodies. However, as many as about 2000 IgG molecules were required to yield a single C1-fixing site. The accelerated clearance of the IgG-sensitized cells was achieved by their progressive trapping and destruction within the spleen. Schreiber and Frank concluded that their data indicated that IgG and IgM antibody molecules interact with erythrocytes and complement *in vivo* by mechanisms that are qualitatively and quantitatively different and produce different effects.

In further experiments with guinea-pigs, Atkinson and Frank (1974a) compared the in-vivo clearance of antibody-sensitized erythrocytes in normal animals and in animals that had been inoculated with BCG Mycobacterium vaccine. The BCG-infected animals were more efficient in clearing both IgM- and IgG-sensitized cells. Also, in contrast to normal animals, cells sensitized with moderate amounts of IgM antibodies and sequestered in the liver were not released—a pattern of behaviour only seen in normal animals receiving unusually highly sensitized cells. In the case of cells sensitized with IgG antibodies the pattern of clearance (mostly in the spleen), although accelerated, was not altered. Atkinson and Frank concluded that their data suggested that increased macrophage activation in the BCG-infected animals had played a critical role in determining the consequence of the cells' sensitization.

Atkinson and Frank (1974b) reported on the immune clearance and destruction of human erythrocytes sensitized by IgM anti-A or anti-B antibodies and complement. Cells sensitized with as few as 20 C1-fixing sites were cleared from the circulation, and with 40 sites 45–62% of the cells were cleared; with 80 C1-fixing sites 75% of the cells were cleared within 10 minutes. In each case cells were rapidly sequestered in the liver. This was followed by some of the cells gradually returning into the circulation and subsequently surviving apparently normally.

Excellent summaries of the early (1958–1974) work on the interaction of erythrocytes coated with IgG(EIgG) or complement (EC3b) and the corresponding receptors at the surface of phagocytes are to be found in the reviews of Huber and Fudenberg (1969, 1970), Rosse (1973) and Brown (1973, 1974).

Many additional significant papers have since been written on EIgG and EC3b interaction and on the nature of the receptors on the surface of the macrophages.

Rosse, de Boisfleury and Bessis (1975) and Rosse and de Boisfleury (1975) described the sequence of adherence, deformation, scission and ingestion, as seen under the scanning electron microscope, and concluded that there were many differences in the way antibody-coated and complement-coated cells, respectively, were dealt with.

Griffin, Bianco and Silverstein (1975) demonstrated differences in the character of the receptors for IgG and C3b in respect of the requirement for Mg^{2+} ions and resistance to trypsin. They stressed that the C3 receptors mediated binding and not ingestion, except under special circumstances, and concluded that the two receptors were chemically and physically separate entities.

von dem Borne, Beckers and Engelfriet (1977) described experiments which underlined the importance of the Fc antibody fragment in respect of monocyte adhesion. They showed that if IgG anti-D was degraded so that it was almost entirely converted to $F(ab)_2$, the fragment, although it bound to erythrocytes, was not capable of causing the cells to adhere to monocytes *in vitro* or of causing elimination of the cells *in vivo*.

Fleer and co-workers (1978b) studied the interaction between anti-D-sensitized erythrocytes and monocytes with particular reference to the intensity of antibody sensitization and the ratio between the number of sensitized erythrocytes and the number of available monocytes. It was found that the greater the number of sensitizing antibody molecules per erythrocyte the less the interaction was inhibited by free IgG; also that when the number of sensitized erythrocytes per monocyte was increased the inhibition caused by a standard amount of IgG decreased significantly. These findings were thought to be relevant to conditions within the spleen where haemoconcentration would be expected to diminish the ability of the plasma IgG to inhibit macrophage–erythrocyte interaction.

Schreiber and McDermott (1978) experimented with monocyte monolayers and human erythrocytes sensitized with rabbit anti-human IgM and coated with human complement (C). With large amounts of C, the ability of serum inactivating factors to effect the removal of the C-coated cells from the surface of the monocytes was diminished, with the result that persistently bound cells were eventually phagocytosed.

Kurlander, Rosse and Logue (1978), working with IgG anti-D and anti-A and -B, related the number of IgG molecules on erythrocytes with the lysis of the cells which results from contact with, or phagocytosis by, monocytes *in vitro*, measuring lysis by ^{51}Cr release. Lysis was found to increase linearly with increase in the number of IgG antibody molecules, but the addition of unbound IgG could abolish this even at maximum levels of sensitization with anti-D. *In vivo*, cells were lysed by densities of antibodies less than could be demonstrated to produce any lysis *in vitro*, and Kurlander, Rosse and Logue suggested that this was brought about by repeated and intimate contacts (they calculated at least 40 a day) between weakly sensitized cells and macrophages within the spleen, resulting in cumulative damage, a type of exposure which could not be mimicked in in-vitro experiments.

Kurlander and Rosse (1979b) also investigated quantitative aspects of the inhibition by IgG of the monocyte-mediated destruction of anti-D-coated erythrocytes. Undiluted human serum or purified IgG1, at a concentration 1000 μg/ml, was used. Both sources of IgG were effective in inhibiting phagocytosis. However, neither medium inhibited phagocytosis completely; moreover, this was found to be augmented parallel with increase in erythrocyte concentration up to 20%, and also to be augmented by increasing the degree to which the cells were sensitized. Phagocytosis was, too, markedly increased by concurrent coating of the erythrocytes with complement—which in the absence of antibody caused very little ingestion. ^{51}Cr

release occurred in parallel with phagocytosis in the presence of serum. Kurlander and Rosse concluded that their experiments *in vitro* demonstrated that the destruction by monocytes of antibody-sensitized erythrocytes could occur under in-vivo conditions.

Kurlander and Batker (1982) reported on the relative binding of ^{125}I-labelled preparations of IgG1 to human peripheral-blood monocytes and polymorphonuclears (PMN). They found that although the PMN bound many more molecules of IgG1 at saturation point than did monocytes, the mean association constant for the PMN was 100–1000 times lower than for the binding of the same preparation to monocytes. They also found that the binding of the labelled IgGI to monocytes was 10–100-fold more easily inhibited by unlabelled IgG1 than was the binding to PMN.

Rosse (1982) included in his Philip Levine Award Lecture a thoughtful discussion of key issues relevant to the haemolytic potentiality of Rh antibodies. He pointed out that fluid phase IgG1 and IgG3 are more effective against monomers than dimers or oligomers in preventing IgGFc–macrophage interaction and that the limited number of Rh antigen sites had, too, an inhibiting effect. He stressed the importance for successful interaction of a high concentration of sensitized erythrocytes, as would be found locally in the spleen, and the relevance of this to the successful outcome of splenectomy in AIHA patients forming auto-antibodies of Rh specificities. He also referred to the finding that whereas pure IgG inhibits lysis by lymphocytes, whole serum does not, apparently because serum contains a small-molecular-weight substance which enhances the interaction between antibody and the lymphocytes' IgGFc receptor. He suggested that lymphocytes might, therefore, play a significant role in the destruction of Rh-antibody-coated erythrocytes.

Further data on the effect of unbound IgG on the interaction between bound IgGFc and macrophages were provided by Kelton et al. (1985), who related the rate of clearance *in vivo* of radio-labelled autologous erythrocytes coated with anti-D IgG and the concentration of IgG free in the plasma. A close relationship was demonstrable: clearance was slowest in hypergammaglobulinaemia and fastest in hypogammaglobulinaemia. They also confirmed that the rate of clearance was positively correlated with the number of molecules attached to the test cells. An equilibrium was postulated between plasma IgG, IgG bound to circulating cells and IgG interacting with receptors on monocytes and macrophages.

More recently, studies on the binding of human IgG1 and IgG3 antibodies to monocytes has been facilitated and refined by the availability of monoclonal antibodies against the two IgG subclasses, and experiments carried out with monoclonal antibodies of anti-D specificity have confirmed the relative superiority of IgG3 antibodies in achieving the binding of erythrocytes to monocytes. Thus Wiener and co-workers (1987) reported that whereas IgG3 antibodies opsonized erythrocytes at a density of approximately 100 molecules per erythrocyte, IgG1 antibodies needed as many as 10 000 molecules to achieve the same effect.

Receptors for the Fc portion of IgG and for complement components

Advances in technology and the availability of monoclonal antibodies have allowed during the last decade or so the identification and characterization of receptors for both the Fc portion of IgG and for complement (C) components. This topic has been dealt with, along with other aspects of the immune destruction of erythrocytes, in a number of recent reviews. Those of Unkeless, Scigliano and Freedman (1988) and Anderson and Kelton (1989) are particularly informative. The following is a brief summary. As already mentioned, there are separate receptors for erythrocytes coated with immunoglobulin or with complement.

Receptors for IgGFc

Receptors are present on macrophages, neutrophils, platelets, natural killer (NK) cells and B lymphocytes. At least three different receptors exist, identifiable by monoclonal antibodies; each has a different function.

HuFcγRI (human Fcγ receptor I) is present on monocytes and macrophages. It is involved in the rosetting of IgG-sensitized erythrocytes but may not be important in phagocytosis. Its interaction with IgG-sensitized cells can, however, lead to ADCC (antibody-dependent cell-mediated cytotoxicity).

HuFcγRII is also found on many types of blood cell. It is implicated both in phagocytosis and in ADCC and will weakly rosette IgG-sensitized cells.

HuFcγRIII is present in high concentration on the macrophages of the liver and spleen, as well as on monocytes, neutrophils and NK cells; it is probably the most important, at least in relation to AIHA, of the three receptors.

Neutrophils bear both the RII and RIII receptors. Their activity is increased by the lymphokinine γ interferon; this increases, too, the expression of the RI receptors on monocytes and macrophages.

According to Zupańska and her co-workers (1985) almost all peripheral-blood mononuclear cells carry receptors for the Fc portion of both IgG1 and IgG3 anti-Rh antibodies. However, the percentage of cells that are able to bind IgG3 molecules is higher; also, lymphocytes bind only or mainly IgG1. Subsequently, Zupańska, Thomson and Merry (1986) reported that the minimum number of IgG3 molecules required for erythrocyte adherence (as demonstrable in a rosette test) is 180–460 for monocytes and 520–1300 for lymphocytes, compared with 1180–4300 for monocytes and 3400–14200 for lymphocytes in the case of IgG1 molecules. Comparable quantitative data were reported by Zupańska et al. (1987a) for the numbers of IgG1 and IgG3 molecules required for erythrophagocytosis by monocytes.

Receptors for complement components

There are at least four different receptors.

CR1 (complement receptor 1) is present on neutrophils, monocytes, macrophages and lymphocytes, and also on erythrocytes, which carry large numbers of the receptors. CR1 binds C3b and C4b and (weakly) C3bi. The receptors on neutrophils and monocytes are implicated in both adherence and phagocytosis.

CR2 is present on B lymphocytes; it binds C3dg.

CR3 is present on neutrophils, monocytes, macrophages and large granular lymphocytes. It binds primarily C3Bi and possibly also C3dg, and seems to be the most important receptor for the phagocytosis of C-coated erythrocytes.

CR4 is present on neutrophils and binds C3dg.

ANTIBODY-DEPENDENT CELL-MEDIATED CYTOTOXICITY (ADCC): POSSIBLE ROLE IN HAEMOLYSIS IN AIHA

That antibody-sensitized erythrocytes might undergo lysis in the absence of complement, apparently as the result of direct contact between erythrocyte and effector cell was apparently first described about 20 years ago (Holm, 1972; MacLennan, 1972; Perlmann, Perlmann and Wigzell, 1972; Holm and Hammerstrom, 1973).

A lymphocyte of null type (i.e. neither B nor T) later termed a K (killer) or NK (natural killer) cell, appears to be particularly implicated; but monocytes and neutrophils, too, seem able to bring about lysis similarly. A considerable literature is now available concerning K-cell activity, based on experiments with allo-antibodies; and it has been shown that K-cells have specific receptors for IgGFc, but not for IgM or IgA. The question arises, but remains unsettled, as to the role, if any, of K-cell lysis in erythrocyte destruction in AIHA.

More recent papers giving further information about K-cell lysis (ADCC) and technical information include those of Urbaniak (1976, 1979a,b), Handwerger, Kay and Douglas (1978), Shaw, Levy and LoBuglio (1978), Kurlander and Rosse (1979a) and Bakács et al. (1984).

Shaw, Levy and LoBuglio (1978) reported that ADCC was dependent on the amount and distribution of the antibody fixed to the erythrocyte as well as on the effector cell: target cell ratio. They concluded that the Fc receptors on lymphocytes have more stringent criteria than have the receptors on monocytes for the recognition of, and interaction with, antibodies attached to the erythrocyte surface.

Urbaniak (1979a) showed that treatment with papain increased erythrocyte lysis, and Urbaniak (1979b) reported that the K-cell receptor reacted with IgG1 and IgG3, reacted slightly with IgG2 but failed to react with IgG4, IgA and IgM. Hydrocortisone was found to inhibit lysis, and Urbaniak speculated that this in-vitro inhibition might be relevant to the beneficial effect of corticosteroid therapy in AIHA.

Kurlander and Rosse (1979a) reported that although lymphocyte-mediated lysis was markedly inhibited by pure monoclonal IgG1 (at a concentration of 1000 μg/ml) added to the culture medium, lysis persisted or was even enhanced by the addition of undiluted human serum. In contrast, monocyte-mediated lysis was inhibited by the serum. Kurlander and Rosse suggested that lymphocytes played a more important role *in vivo* in the immune destruction of erythrocytes than had hitherto been appreciated.

IN VITRO MONOCYTE/MACROPHAGE ERYTHROCYTE ASSAYS AND HAEMOLYSIS *IN VIVO*

In recent years attempts have been made to use in-vitro indices of monocyte/macrophage activity as indicators of in-vivo haemolysis. Most of the work has been undertaken in relation to allo-antibodies, but some studies relevant to AIHA are available. Garratty (1990a) has recently reviewed the history and technical aspects of cellular assays. Amongst the variables that have to be considered and standardized in monocyte/macrophage monolayer assays are the source of the monocytes or macrophages — human or otherwise, autologous or homologous, the freshness of the cells, how long they should be cultured before the addition of the sensitized cells, how long the suspensions should be incubated, whether the tests should be carried out in the presence of complement, the optimum pH of the incubation mixture, whether the number of cells adhering or erythrophagocytosis is assessed, and how the results are expressed.

In an early study, Wright and co-workers (1953) assessed the ability of a 3–5-day-old culture of rabbit macrophages to phagocytose human erythrocytes. The percentage of macrophages so doing was taken as a phagocytic index. In 59 normal individuals the index was up to 12%, median 3%: in 16 patients with acquired haemolytic anaemia the index ranged from 9 to 74%, median 35.5%. However, high values were also obtained with the erythrocytes of patients with hereditary spherocytosis, and in various types of leukaemia, Hodgkin's 'syndrome' and carcinoma, and tuberculosis and other infections.

The results of more detailed and sophisticated studies were reported in the 1970s and 1980s.

Mason (1976) used human peripheral-blood monocytes and recorded the number of erythrocytes ingested per 100 normal monocytes. Eleven patients with warm-antibody AIHA were studied, all but one of them actively haemolysing, as well as three infants with haemolytic disease of the newborn and six patients receiving α-methyldopa and three apparently healthy blood donors, in all of whom the DAT was positive. Unexpectedly perhaps, Mason found that the erythrocytes of the non-haemolysing individuals were as avidly ingested by the normal monocytes as were the cells of the haemolysing patients.

In contrast to Mason's experience, which is summarized above, most subsequent reports have indicated a definite parallelism between monocyte activity *in vitro* and haemolysis *in vivo*.

Kay and Douglas (1977) studied 17 patients with AIHA: eleven had idiopathic AIHA, six secondary AIHA. They used human peripheral-blood monocytes and compared the results obtained with their patients' erythrocytes with those given by normal control erythrocytes in two ways: by a 'morphologic' ratio, which reflected combined rosette formation and phago-cytosis, and by a radioactive ratio based on ^{51}Cr release. Twelve of the 17 patients gave elevated ratios in the morphologic assay and in 15 the radioactive ratio was abnormally high. Kay and Douglas also reported that in the majority of cases higher ratios were obtained with autologous compared with homologous monocytes.

van der Meulen and co-workers (1978) used homologous peripheral-blood monocytes and assessed rosette formation. Twenty-two patients who had formed IgG non-complement-binding auto-antibodies were suffering from increased haemolysis: adherence was recorded as present in all of them. In contrast, in 26 patients forming similar antibodies but not suffering from increased haemolysis adherence was recorded as absent.

Brojer, Zupańska and Michalewska (1982) studied 23 patients with warm-antibody AIHA of varying severity with the aim of comparing the degree of sensitization of their erythrocytes, as estimated in an AutoAnalyser, with erythrocyte adhesion to monocytes, as measured by the percentage formation of rosettes. Whereas a close correlation was demonstrated between the degree of sensitization *in vitro* of normal erythrocytes by anti-Rh (D or CD) sera and rosette formation, no such close relationship was demonstrable in the case of AIHA patients' erythrocytes sensitized *in vivo*. Thus the erythrocytes of some of the patients failed to adhere to the monocytes although apparently strongly sensitized and, on the other hand, the cells of some patients adhered although their apparent sensitization was weaker than that of control erythrocytes sensitized with an amount of anti-CD serum which did not cause adhesion. Nevertheless, Brojer, Zupańska and Michalewska concluded that adherence was probably correlated with the rate of haemolysis *in vivo* and with the treatment the patients had received. Thus they had found that the erythrocytes of most patients who were actively haemolysing, and who had not been treated or were receiving only small doses of prednisone, formed rosettes, while the cells of most patients in remission failed to form significant numbers of rosettes. The source of the monocytes—whether from the patients or from normal donors—did not seem to affect the results.

Hunt and co-workers (1982) studied eight patients, all giving a positive DAT. Four had AIHA (one had SLE) and four were receiving α-methyldopa. With the erythrocytes of the α-methyldopa patients there was insignificant phagocytosis in a peripheral-blood monocyte assay; in contrast, with the erythrocytes of the AIHA patients, phagocytosis was significantly increased above the normal in all four cases using autologous monocytes and increased in two out of the four using homologous normal monocytes. Hunt et al. concluded that both the amount of antibody on the erythrocytes and the source of the monocytes affect the results of in-vitro assays of monocyte activity, and that patients' monocytes rather than normal monocytes should be used in assays designed to predict the fate of erythrocytes transfused to patients forming erythrocyte auto-antibodies.

Nance and Garratty (1982) described the results of subjecting the erythrocytes of a large number of normal donors and patients to a monocyte-monolayer assay in which both erythrocyte adhesion and phagocytosis were measured. The normal mean total (monocyte) reactivity (MTR) was 0.3%. Forty-four patients who gave a positive DAT had been studied: 19 were suffering from increased haemolysis and in these the MTR was 11.4%; in contrast, in 25 other patients in whom the DAT was positive but in whom there was no evidence of increased haemolysis the MTR was 3.8%.

Gallacher and co-workers (1983) related in-vitro monocyte/macrophage–erythrocyte interaction with in-vivo haemolysis in 22 patients with DAT-positive AIHA and in 11 patients with DAT-negative acquired haemolytic anaemia. In sixteen of the DAT-positive patients there was evidence of increased haemolysis: all of them had raised association (adherence) and phago-cytosis indices. In contrast, the phagocytosis index was normal in six patients whose DAT was positive but in whom there was no evidence of increased haemolysis, and the association index was but slightly raised in two of them. The results with the 11 DAT-negative patients were especially interesting, for in seven of them both indices were above normal.

Herron and co-workers (1986) have provided more data. A phagocyte association test was found to give abnormally high results in 22 out of 24 patients suffering from warm-antibody AIHA, and the results were above normal, too, in four out of 14 patients with a positive DAT but in whom there was no evidence of increased haemolysis. In three patients suspected of suffering from DAT-negative AIHA the results were normal.

Zupańska and co-workers (1987a) reported studies carried out on 48 DAT-positive AIHA patients and also on three DAT-positive but otherwise normal blood donors. Monocyte–erythrocyte interaction was assessed by phagocytosis and rosette assays. Phagocytosis was found to be increased in 16 out of 23 patients in whom haemolysis was classified as acute and not increased in 25 out of 29 patients in remission. Zupańska et al. stressed that although there was in general a good correlation between increased phagocytosis and haemolysis, there were exceptions in both directions. Their data did not indicate that the patients' cells adhered better to autologous than to normal homolo-gous monocytes.

The data quoted in the foregoing paragraphs show that carefully executed monocyte/macrophage monolayer assays provide results which, with but few (interesting) exceptions, parallel the severity of haemolysis in DAT-positive

warm-antibody AIHA. The fact that some DAT-negative acquired haemolytic anaemia patients have given positive results supports the concept of an auto-immune origin for the illness in these particular patients, and it indicates, too, that in certain circumstances a mononuclear/macrophage assay can be more sensitive than a DAT in indicating that a patient's erythrocytes are coated with IgG auto-antibodies.

As already referred to (p. 411), it is the Fc portion of IgG1 and IgG3 molecules bound to erythrocytes that make contact with the corre-sponding receptors on the phagocytes, and it has been shown that IgG3 molecules are more successful than IgG1 molecules in achieving this. Some quantitative data are available as to how many molecules are required for visible interac-tion. Zupańska and co-workers (1987b) reported that phagocytosis was detectable with more than 2000 IgG1 molecules per erythrocyte; with IgG3 antibodies, this would take place, however, with as little as 230 molecules per cell. A simular ratio was demonstrable in the case of rosette assays. Adhesion takes place, too, faster with IgG3 molecules than with IgG1. Brojer, Merry and Zupańska (1989) reported that maximum adhesion or phagocytosis took place within 30 minutes with IgG3 antibodies compared with up to 2 hours with IgG1 antibodies.

Hyperactivity of the patient's monocyte/macrophage system in AIHA: a factor possibly influencing severity

MacKenzie (1975) had reported in an abstract that 10–50% of normal peripheral blood mono-cytes acted as erythrophages, when tested with a standard suspension of anti-D-sensitized erythro-cytes. In AIHA the percentage of reacting cells was greater, varying between 40 and 80%. Similarly high values were obtained, however, with the monocytes of patients suffering from other types of haemolytic anaemia.

Fries, Brickman and Frank (1983) estimated the number of Fcγ receptors on the surface of monocytes isolated from the peripheral blood of normal adults and from 23 patients suffering from a variety of types of haemolytic anaemia. In health, more receptors were present on the monocytes of females than in males: in AIHA, in both sexes, significantly more receptors were present, while in the cases of non-immune haemolytic anaemia the numbers were intermediate. A significant reduction in receptor numbers was recorded in two AIHA patients and in five volunteers after the administration of prednisone, and Fries, Brickman and Frank concluded that this may be one way by which treatment with corticosteroids influences the course of AIHA. They pointed out, however, that their data were obtained with peripheral-blood monocytes, not with tissue macrophages.

Munn and Chaplin (1977) investigated the problem using ^{51}Cr-labelled erythrocytes coated with IgG anti-D and peripheral-blood monocyte–monolayer preparations. Rosette formation was estimated indirectly from the residual radioactivity after eluting the preparation with saline. The results with 10 different donors varied considerably, and the same was true when the monocytes of the same donor were tested sequentially. Striking increases in activity were found in four donors who contracted viral infections. High values were obtained, too, in AIHA, but also in cases of leukaemia and myelofibrosis. In AIHA, although the highest value was obtained with the monocytes of the patient suffering from the most active haemolysis, the correlation between monocyte activity and clinical haemolysis was not close. Nor was there an absolute correlation between the number of IgG molecules per erythrocyte and monocyte activity. In thirteen out of 17 experiments, monocyte activity was enhanced if the test erythrocytes had also been coated with complement components.

Erythrocyte rosetting around mononuclear cells in AIHA

The occurrence in the peripheral blood of unusual numbers of mononuclear cells around which autologous erythrocytes would rosette was described by Gluckman (1970). Compared with negative results in 33 controls, tests with the autologous erythrocytes of five AIHA patients were positive (4–22 rosettes per 1000 mononuclears).

Hamlin and Verrier Jones (1970) reported, in contrast, that they had failed to detect rosetting in seven cases of warm-antibody AIHA, although they had been successful in doing so in two cases of CHAD. They had, however, used homologous rather than autologous erythrocytes in their tests.

Dewar and co-workers (1974), on the other hand, reported positive tests using normal (homologous) erythrocytes. Fourteen AIHA patients were studied, six being under treatment: 0.4–17% of rosettes were noted, compared with 0.1–4.6% in controls; of the six patients under treatment, three gave normal results, three outside the normal range. The cells to which the erythrocytes were adhering were judged to be predominantly lymphocytes.

Parker and Stuart (1978) also used normal erythrocytes and the mononuclear cells of 10 AIHA patients. Of 172 rosette-forming cells studied by transmission electron microscopy, 144 were lymphocytes: 44% of these were identified as T cells. Contact between erythrocyte and lymphocyte was point-like and the erythrocytes were not deformed; with monocytes the contact point was also narrow but the erythrocytes were deformed. As the target erythrocytes (being normal) were thought not to be carrying any IgGFc, it was suggested that the cell rosetting was being brought about by the mononuclear cells (in AIHA) being unusually activated.

Erythrocyte rosetting around neutrophils in acquired haemolytic anaemia

Rarely, erythrocytes may be seen in stained blood films adhering to a neutrophil so as to form a rosette around it. One such rosette was illustrated by Dacie and Lewis (1975, p. 115), who had noticed the phenomenon in the films of an adult male suffering from a DAT-negative acquired haemolytic anaemia of obscure origin.

A similar occurrence was described and illustrated by Pettit, Scott and Hussein (1976). Their patient was a 28-year-old man also suffering from chronic acquired haemolytic anaemia. In this case, however, the DAT was positive with anti-C sera and the patient's serum contained a weak cold agglutinin which agglutinated cord-blood and adult erythrocytes up to 20°C and sensitized them to agglutination by anti-C sera up to 30°C. The erythrocyte rosetting was consistently noted in films made over a 2-year period. Up to 75% of the neutrophils were surrounded with from five to 40 erythrocytes. The rosetting occurred irrespective of whether the blood sample had been kept at 15°C or 37°C before films were made. A remarkable feature was that the phenomenon only occurred with blood anticoagulated with EDTA. It was not seen in films made from native (uncoagulated) blood or in films made from blood to which heparin or sodium citrate had been added, and it was not seen in films made from a mixture of patient's plasma and ABO-compatible normal blood. The nature of this type of rosetting is obscure. However, it presumably represents some type of immune adherence.

AIHA ASSOCIATED WITH IgA AUTO-ANTIBODIES: MECHANISM OF HAEMOLYSIS

As described earlier (p. 111), AIHA apparently brought about by IgA auto-antibodies is a rarity. Little is known of the haemolytic mechanism, but there is evidence that this may not be uniform. That subpopulations of human peripheral-blood granulocytes and monocytes, and lymphocytes, express receptors for IgA was demonstrated by Fanger et al. (1980), using ox cells sensitized with rabbit IgG, IgA and IgM. Purified human IgA blocked the IgA receptors. The findings in three human AIHA cases in which IgA antibodies appeared to be responsible for the haemolysis are given below.

In the patient described by Suzuki et al. (1981) the antibody fixed complement. Erythrocyte–macrophage interaction was demonstrated and it was concluded that this was mediated mainly via C3 receptors. A cooperative effect of receptors for FcIgA and C3 could, however, not be excluded. In the case described by Clark et al. (1984), the IgA antibody involved failed to fix complement. However, antibody eluted from the patient's erythrocytes caused normal erythrocytes to be lysed by human monocytes in a system designed to demonstrate antibody-dependent cell-mediated cytotoxicity (ADCC). That the antibody involved was IgA was shown by the fact that lysis could be inhibited by small amounts of normal serum IgA. The eluted antibody was shown also to be capable of sensitizing normal erythrocytes to phagocytosis by monocytes. This interaction, too, was inhibited by IgA, but not by IgG at the same concentration.

More recently, Salama, Bhakdi and Mueller-Eckhardt (1987) described the occurrence of acute haemolytic anaemia with haemoglobinuria in a boy aged 6 who was forming predominantly IgA auto-antibodies. Intravascular haemolysis was attributed to 'reactive lysis', i.e., C5b6 complexes generated in plasma lysing bystander erythrocytes by an antibody- and C3-independent mechanism. The DAT was weakly positive with anti-IgG and strongly positive with anti-IgA sera, and IgA auto-antibodies were present in serum to a titre of 512 and demonstrable, too, along with weak anti-IgG antibodies, in eluates. The DAT with anti-C3 and anti-IgM sera was negative. The antibody had no definable specificity.

EFFECT OF ANTIBODIES ON ERYTHROPOIESIS

The occurrence and serious nature of reticulocytopenia in the course of AIHA in man has already been referred to (p. 69). Experimental observations support the concept that this may be due, at least in part, to a direct effect of the antibodies on erythrocyte precursor cells.

Linke (1952), for instance, who administered rabbit anti-rat-erythrocyte serum to rats found evidence in 18 out of 45 rats of marrow aplasia and reticulocytopenia which developed within a few hours of giving the serum. Previous splenectomy did not prevent it. Wagner (1956), who also worked with rats, demonstrated inhibition of the reticulocyte response when he increased the dose of serum he administered. Najean, Ruvidic and Bernard (1959) compared the erythropoietic response of rats to comparable degrees of anaemia produced by haemorrhage and by the administration of immune serum, respectively. They found the reticulocyte response to be more vigorous and the incorporation of ^{59}Fe more complete in the rats whose anaemia was due to bleeding. Porter (1960a,b), who studied runt disease in newborn rabbits injected as fetuses with adult spleen cells, reported that their marrow became hypoplastic or aplastic after birth.

In vitro, too, erythrocyte precursor cells can be shown to be affected by antibodies. Steffen (1955) reported that he had found the bone-marrow erythroblasts in two patients with acquired haemolytic anaemia to be coated with the same globulins as were peripheral erythrocytes; both types of cell gave strongly positive DATs. Pisciotta and Hinz (1956) showed that normoblasts derived from a patient with AIHA were agglutinable by allo-antibodies such as anti-A and anti-D as well as by sera containing warm or cold auto-agglutinins; and Rossi, Diena and Sacchetti (1957) and Sacchetti, Diena and Rossi (1957), who also carried out experiments *in vitro*, were able to demonstrate agglutination of erythroblasts by auto-antibodies of both the warm and cold varieties.

In rabbits, Borsook, Ratner and Tattrie (1969) showed that the sensitivity to lysis of erythroblasts by goat anti-rabbit-erythrocyte sera depended upon the cells' maturity, less mature basophilic erythroblasts being less sensitive than mature acidophilic cells.

All the experiments quoted above point to marrow damage as being of considerable importance in the genesis of anaemia brought about by immune sera. In man, aside from reticulocytopenia and the occasional overt megaloblastic change which may occur (see p. 68), nuclear fragmentation and excessive intracytoplasmic iron granulation may be seen in films made from the blood or marrow of severely affected patients (Fig. 23.16, p. 68). How these unusual appearances are produced and whether they are related directly to antibody activity is uncertain.

COLD-ANTIBODY AIHA: MECHANISMS OF HAEMOLYSIS *IN VIVO*

As described in Chapters 28 and 29, the concentration of cold antibodies in the sera of patients suffering from AIHA may be very high indeed, whilst the temperature at which the antibodies are active *in vitro* may extend almost, if not quite, up to 37°C.

As described on p. 273, anti-I antibodies are capable of causing both agglutination and lysis of normal erythrocytes *in vitro* as well as sensitization to antiglobulin sera. Normal erythrocytes are, however, much less sensitive to lysis than to agglutination, even if the pH for lysis is adjusted to the optimum (usually pH 6.5–7.0). Nevertheless, in some cases lysis may be observed to take place *in vitro* at a relatively high temperature (e.g. at 30°C) and at the physiological pH of blood.

It is interesting to note that the highest temperature at which auto-agglutination can usually be demonstrated in a test-tube in the laboratory in patients suffering from CHAD (29–32°C) corresponds closely to the subcutaneous temperature of the unclothed limb exposed to normal environmental temperatures in Britain. Barcroft and Edholm (1946) found that the temperature of the skin, subcutaneous tissue and deep muscle immediately after baring the human forearm was 33°C, 33.6°C and 36.2°C, respectively. However, after the limb had been exposed for 2 hours to rather cool room temperature (18.5°C) the temperatures were: skin, 27.9°C, subcutaneous tissue, 28.5°C and muscle, 30.7°C. The occurrence of auto-agglutination *in vivo* in the presence of high-thermal-amplitude auto-antibodies and the consequent development of acrocyanosis are thus hardly surprising.

The episodes of haemoglobinuria which may be brought about by cold weather and the more constant presence in chronic cases of haemosiderin in the urinary deposit (Fig. 28.5, p. 217) indicate that part at least of the haemolysis takes place in some cases in the blood stream. A point of considerable interest is the relative importance of auto-agglutination and of complement lysis in bringing about the haemolysis.

Early observations

The importance of auto-agglutination as an important mechanism of haemolysis was stressed by Stats (1945) who in an elegant series of experiments clearly showed that *in vitro* mechanical trauma applied to agglutinated erythrocytes in strong suspension would bring about their lysis (see also p. 274). Whittle, Lyell and Gatman (1947) reported, too, that when agglutinated erythrocytes in suspension were placed between a slide and cover-glass, tapping the cover-glass would cause some of the cells to fragment.

In vivo, however, it proved difficult to establish without any doubt that the sensitivity of agglutinated cells to mechanical trauma is important in relation to haemolysis. (Agglutination, on the other hand, was held to be undoubtedly responsible for the acrocyanosis).

That complement action was likely to be responsible not only for overt intravascular haemolysis but also for the less dramatic continuing haemolysis was strongly suggested by the surviving circulating erythrocytes of patients in whom there was clinical evidence of haemolysis being agglutinable by anticomplement sera.

As far back as 1948, Ham and his co-workers concluded that mechanical trauma causes lysis *in vivo* only when the erythrocytes are already sensitized by incomplete antibodies. [In fact, the patients' cells were agglutinated by antiglobulin sera probably by virtue of their coating with complement components.]

They had studied two patients whose sera contained cold agglutinins at the same concentration (titre, 5000). One patient was anaemic; her erythrocytes gave a positive DAT. The other patient, convalescing from 'virus' pneumonia, was not anaemic and her erythrocytes were not agglutinated by an antiglobulin serum. Chilling the patients' arms for 20 minutes resulted in haemoglobinaemia in the first patient but not in the second.

Observations made by the author in the 1950s on patients with CHAD or with post-*Mycoplasma pneumoniae* haemolytic anaemia, summarized by Dacie (1962), strongly supported the concept that it is the ability of the antibodies to react with erythrocytes at a relatively high temperature (e.g. up to 28–32°C) and to fix complement and to bring about lysis at the physiological pH of blood which determine the occurrence and severity of haemolysis. The actual height of the agglutination titre at a low temperature, i.e. 2–4°C, seemed to be of little importance, except as an indicator as to how much antibody was being formed.

Table 34.1   Comparisons between the agglutinin and lysin titres of the sera of five patients who probably suffered from mycoplasma pneumonia.

Patient	Agglutination of normal erythrocytes (titre, 17°C)	Lysis of PNH erythrocytes (titre, 17°C)
W.R.	256	64
W.B.	512	32
I.P.	512	256
E.M.	512	256
A.S.	512	256

Patients I.P., E.M. and A.S. developed acute haemolytic anaemia; patients W.R. and W.B. did not become anaemic.

Evidence indicating a correlation between clinical haemolysis and the lytic power of the patients' sera *in vitro* is summarized in Table 34.1. In this Table are compared the agglutinating and lytic activities of five sera obtained from patients who probably had suffered from mycoplasma pneumonia, titrated with normal and paroxysmal nocturnal haemoglobinuria (PNH) erythrocytes, respectively. The agglutinin titres were about the same in each instance. The lysis titres, using the PNH cells, varied: in Cases I.P., E. M. and A. S. they were close to the agglutinin titres — the patients all suffered from haemolytic anaemia; in Cases W. R. and W. B. the lysin titres were significantly less — neither patient suffered from haemolytic anaemia.

A patient probably suffering from haemolytic anaemia following mycoplasma pneumonia (Dacie, 1954, Case 16) provided an opportunity for studying the reactions of his antibody *in vitro* in relation to the progress of his clinical recovery (Fig. 30.3, p. 308). Four samples of serum were compared for their ability to lyse PNH erythrocytes at 37°C—a measure of antibody action at the upper limit of its thermal range—and for their ability to agglutinate normal erythrocytes at 2°C. Clinical recovery was associated with loss of activity at 37°C but only a small change in the agglutinin titre at 2°C.

Pannacciulli, Rossi and Tizianello (1958a,b) tagged with ^{51}Cr the erythrocytes of a man, aged 61, who had formed high-titre cold agglutinins and studied the consequences of immersing all four limbs in water at 4°C for 20 minutes. There was a fall in the haematocrit in the general circulation which was attributed largely to pooling of blood in his limbs and probably in the liver also. Temporary rises in radioactivity were detected by in-vivo counting over the liver and spleen but the effect on erythrocyte survival was insignificant, although transitory haemoglobinaemia associated with an increased excretion of ^{51}Cr in the urine occurred.

Lewis, Dacie and Szur (1960) investigated the relative importance of agglutination and the fixation of complement in leading to haemolysis in CHAD by studying the effect on the survival of erythrocytes when reinjected into a patient's circulation after exposing the cells *in vitro* to different environmental conditions.

Serum and erythrocytes were freshly obtained from an elderly patient suffering from typical CHAD. The erythrocytes were labelled with ^{51}Cr and then resuspended as an approximately 15% suspension in the patient's serum which had been heat-inactivated at 56°C for 30 minutes (Expt. 1). The cells were then allowed to undergo massive auto-agglutination by chilling the suspension to 4°C for 15 minutes. The suspension was then warmed at 37°C and when the cells were no longer agglutinated the supernatant serum was pipetted off, replaced by saline and the suspension was reinjected into the patient. The survival of the formerly agglutinated cells was found to be unimpaired (Fig. 34.5). The experiment was repeated on two further occasions using fresh serum which had not been heat-inactivated (Expt. 2) and using fresh serum the pH of which had been adjusted to approximately 7.0 by the addition of a one-tenth volume of 0.2 N-hydrochloric acid (Expt. 3). In Experiment 3 the suspension was not cooled below 20°C. No in-vitro lysis was noted in Experiment 2 but definite lysis occurred in Experiment 3.

In Experiment 2, there were evidence from surface counting of the temporary sequestration of erythrocytes in the liver but no substantial degree of cell destruction occurred; in Experiment 3 there was a major degree of hepatic sequestration and some accumulation of ^{51}Cr in the spleen, too, and this was followed by considerable cell destruction (Fig. 34.6).

The experiments described above demonstrated that agglutination *per se* may not

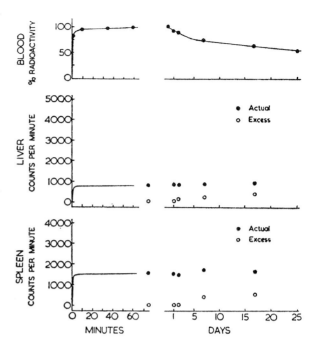

Fig. 34.5 **Radioactivity over the liver and spleen and in the blood after labelling a CHAD patient's erythrocytes with ^{51}Cr and reinjecting them after exposure at 4°C to heat-inactivated autologous serum.**
[Reproduced by permission from Lewis, Dacie and Szur (1960).]

harm erythrocytes and that agglutinated cells, once agglutination has been reversed, are not sequestered in the liver. The experiments did show, however, that if the antibodies are able to fix complement on the cell surfaces in sublytic amounts whilst undergoing agglutination, then, despite reversal of agglutination, sequestration in the liver will take place and, if the coating with complement is sufficient, this will lead to erythrocyte destruction, presumably mainly by phagocytosis.

While the above experiments seemed to dispose of the idea that agglutination by itself is harmful, it was thought possible that it could produce haemolysis indirectly by the lysis locally of agglutinated erythrocytes in small blood vessels in which auto-agglutination had brought the circulation to a standstill. It was also thought possible that if auto-agglutination took place at or near body temperature mechanical forces could lead to lysis of some of the cells in circulating agglutinates.

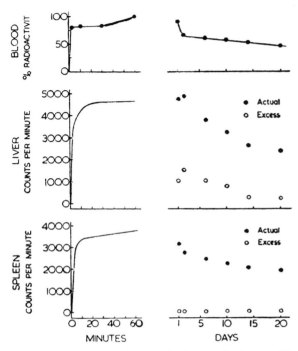

Fig. 34.6 Radioactivity over the liver and spleen and in the blood after labelling a CHAD patient's erythrocytes with ^{51}Cr after exposure at 20°C to acidified fresh autologous serum.

[Reproduced by permission from Lewis, Dacie and Szur (1960).]

Sites of haemolysis in vivo in cold-antibody AIHA

In the few patients suffering from CHAD in whom surface counting had been carried out after labelling the patients' erythrocytes with ^{51}Cr, excess of radioactivity had been demonstrated in the liver as well as in the spleen (Miescher et al. 1962) (Fig. 34.7).

Possible protective mechanisms

At least two mechanisms were thought likely to protect the patient against the worst effects of his or her auto-antibodies in cold-antibody AIHA. One was complement depletion; the other was the presence in the patient's erythrocyte population of a significant number of relatively insensitive cells.

As already referred to (p. 282), there had been reports of low complement levels in the serum of patients forming high-titre cold auto-antibodies;

sometimes the serum had even appeared to be devoid of complement activity. By analogy with the observations of Christian et al. (1951) in dogs this seemed likely to put a brake on haemolysis.

The second possibly protective mechanism is illustrated in Table 28.4. The results with the serum of E.W. were most illuminating. This particular patient's cold antibody agglutinated normal erythrocytes at 37°C, but, fortunately, did not agglutinate her own cells at temperatures exceeding 32°C. Clinically, she was not very severely affected. In other cases studied by the author autologous erythrocytes similarly appeared to be significantly less sensitive than normal adult control cells. It was felt that this was most likely to have been the result of selective cell destruction *in vivo*, the more sensitive cells, i.e. those acted on at the highest temperature, being eliminated whilst the less sensitive ones survived.

The studies carried out in the 1940s, 1950s and early 1960s that have been outlined above established that the severity of in-vivo haemolysis brought about by cold auto-antibodies depended on two factors: the temperature up to which the antibody could act, i.e. its thermal range, and its ability to fix complement. It was realized that individual antibodies varied considerably with respect to both these properties, and that a combination of a high-thermal-amplitude and a strongly complement-fixing antibody led inevitably to clinically important haemolysis and to intravascular haemolysis and haemoglobinuria in the worst cases. The titre of the antibody, as estimated at a low temperature, while providing a measure of the amount of antibody produced, was by itself known to be of little clinical importance, but if auto-agglutination occurred at a relatively high temperature this, it was realized, could lead to serious acrocyanosis and even local gangrene. Auto-agglutination in the absence of concurrent complement fixation did not seem to be an important cause of haemolysis, unless perhaps it occurred at a temperature approaching 37°C. The role of complement, while thought to be of great importance, was, however, not wholly understood. While complement lysis was known to be clearly responsible for the episodes of overtly intravascular haemolysis, the part it played in

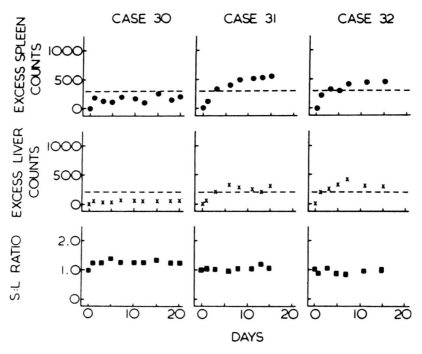

Fig. 34.7   Radioactivity over the liver and spleen after labelling three CHAD patients' erythrocytes with ^{51}Cr.
[Reproduced by permission from Lewis, Szur and Dacie (1960).]

bringing about less dramatic chronic haemolysis and its role in the adhesion of cold-antibody-affected erythrocytes to macrophages and in the cells' subsequent phagocytosis was at the time unknown. The important role that the liver played in the sequestration and destruction of complement-coated cold-antibody-affected erythrocytes was, however, appreciated.

More recent observations

Work subsequent to that summarized in the preceding paragraph has provided new insights into the pathogenesis of cold-antibody AIHA.

Evans, Turner and Bingham (1964, 1965) labelled the cold agglutinins of 10 patients with ^{131}I. This procedure enabled them to conduct some elegant experiments. They confirmed that equilibrium between cold agglutinins and erythrocytes was dependent on pH as well as on temperature. In five experiments (four with anti-I, one with anti-i), they showed that the adsorption of the antibody at 25°C increased steadily as the pH was reduced from 7.4 to 6.6. They also showed

that the fixation of complement as the result of exposing erythrocytes to cold antibodies did not effect the dissociation of the antibody caused by warming. In three patients complement depletion appeared to be a limiting factor in in-vivo haemolysis. The erythrocytes of normal individuals were found to differ considerably in the amount of ^{131}I-labelled cold antibody adsorbed at 25°C as well as in their susceptibility to lysis by complement.

In a subsequent important paper, Evans, Turner and Bingham (1967) described the results of further experiments carried out with ^{131}I-labelled cold antibodies. They showed that the erythrocytes of two CHAD patients forming anti-I, which were coated with complement components, were abnormally resistant to lysis by anti-I and complement, and also that normal erythrocytes exposed to anti-I and complement *in vitro* became similarly resistant. Evans, Turner and Bingham postulated that this could be due to steric hindrance to the adsorption of antibody by the accumulation on the erythrocyte membrane of complement complexes. They concluded that this was the most important factor in causing the abnormal resistance of CHAD erythrocytes to complement lysis, and that heterogeneity within the erythrocyte population was of only minor significance.

Some further interesting experiments were described

by Evans et al. (1968). The sera of four CHAD patients forming anti-I antibodies were shown to coat normal erythrocytes with complement components at 37°C *in vitro*; and that this was occurring *in vivo* at or near body temperature was suggested by the abrupt fall in the serum complement level of two patients after they had been transfused with large volumes of normal erythrocytes. Auto-survival studies of ^{51}Cr-labelled erythrocytes revealed T_{50} values of 7–19 days. Normal erythrocytes were removed in part by sequestration in the liver during the first few hours after transfusion; subsequently, they survived more normally, parallel with the accumulation of complement complexes on their surface. Normal erythrocytes coated with complement *in vitro* were shown to survive significantly better after transfusion to the patients than the same cells that had not been coated with complement. The levels of serum complement were subnormal in all four patients.

The experiments carried out by Brown, Lachmann and Dacie (1970) on rabbits injected with rabbit erythrocytes exposed *in vitro* to human IgM anti-I antibodies and rabbit complement have already been referred to (p. 412). Briefly, the reinjected cells left the circulation rapidly, being sequestered particularly in the liver where some cells were immediately phagocytosed by Kupffer cells. With time, some of the cells re-entered the circulation at a slow exponential rate ($T_{\frac{1}{2}}$ 25–100 min). The return of these cells to the circulation from sites of attachment to fixed macrophages was attributed to the inactivation of fixed C3. It was concluded that the presence of fixed active C3 is essential for the non-lytic sequestration of erythrocytes that have been exposed to IgM cold antibodies.

Logue, Gockerman and Rosse (1971) and Logue, Rosse and Gockerman (1973) studied three patients suffering from CHAD with the aim of determining the role that C3 bound to erythrocytes played in haemolysis. Bound C3 was measured quantitatively and the effect of plasmapheresis assessed: the cold-agglutinin titre was reduced by 70% and the rate of haemolysis, as determined by endogenous CO production, was decreased, but the amount of bound C3 did not alter appreciably. When normal erythrocytes were transfused, C3 accumulated on the transfused cells and reached the levels on the patient's cells within 48 hours. When the patients were subjected to acute cold stress, by immersing an arm in an 8°C water-bath for 2–5 minutes or by the patient being placed in a cold room at 10°C for 25 minutes, there was evidence of acute intravascular haemolysis and an abrupt increase in C3 fixation to erythrocytes. The conclusion was reached that the *rate* of attachment of C3 is important, because of the activity of C3 inactivator, and that, in the absence of cold stress, membrane-bound C3 is continually inactivated with the result that the amount of C3

present is insufficient for the complement sequence to proceed to completion.

Engelfriet and his co-workers (1972) reported that they, too, had been able to demonstrate that the erythrocytes of CHAD patients were remarkably resistant to the lytic activity of anti-I antibodies. Experimenting with several antibodies specifically directed against complement components, namely, an anti-β_1E(C4) serum and three antibodies against determinants of C3, namely, anti-β_1A, anti-α_2D and anti-β_1C sera, they were only able to detect α_2D as a residual C3 component on the erythrocyte membrane. They doubted whether this could cause much steric hindrance, and proposed instead that resistance was due to sites on the cell membrane (that once had reacted with complement components β_1E and β_1A and from which these components had subsequently been eluted) no longer being able to react with new β_1E and β_1A molecules, thus effectively blocking complement action.

Further observations on the role of C3b on the clearance from the circulation of cold-antibody-sensitized erythrocytes were described by Jaffe, Atkinson and Frank (1976). Human volunteers were injected with their own ^{51}Cr-labelled erythrocytes after they had been exposed *in vitro* to a purified IgM anti-I cold antibody and fresh human serum as a source of complement. The cells, as reinjected, were coated with C3b but free from cold antibody. They were initially sequestered in the liver; subsequently, a proportion of the cells was released into the general circulation in which they survived normally. Both phenomena—the sequestration and the release—were shown to be dose-dependent, and the sequence of events closely followed the results that Atkinson and Frank (1974b) had obtained with anti-A and anti-B IgM allo-antibodies. Functionally, intact C3b was required for hepatic sequestration; cells coated with C3d were not cleared from the circulation. Jaffe, Atkinson and Frank also showed that in two patients who were severely complement-deficient hepatic sequestration failed to take place.

Rosse and Adams (1980) described experiments carried out with purified anti-I antibodies derived from six patients with CHAD of very variable severity: three of the patients suffered from marked haemolysis and needed transfusion; two suffered from moderate haemolysis and had not been transfused; one patient had minimal haemolysis but suffered from severe acrocyanosis and had even experienced pain in the oesophagus on eating ice cream. The aim of Rosse and Adams's experiments was to define the factors that were responsible for the interpatient differences in clinical severity.

PNH erythrocytes were used in in-vitro tests to indicate the antibodies lytic potential. Five of the antibodies caused the lysis of 80–100% of the test cells under optimum conditions, one antibody only 30%.

There was a close relationship between the amount of purified anti-I in the reaction mixture and consequent lysis, and in a bithermic ($0° \rightarrow 37°C$) test, the optimum temperature for the first stage was found to be $10-20°C$; with five out of six of the antibodies there was some inhibition of subsequent lysis if the first stage had been conducted at $0°C$. The amount of C1 fixed was shown to be directly proportional to the amount of antibody fixed: with four antibodies the relationship between the amount of C1 fixed per μg antibody was similar; with one serum it was considerably less. The amount of C3 fixed after warming to $37°C$—it was only fixed during the warm phrase—varied considerably from antibody to antibody; ultimate lysis was directly related to the amount of C3 fixed. Rosse and Adams confirmed that the presence of C3 on the erythrocyte membrane inhibited the attachment of antibody. However, the extent to which this happened varied from antibody to antibody.

Rosse and Adams concluded that while differences in agglutinin titres at $0°C$ (3200–102 400) did not explain the variation in the clinical severity, this could be correlated with the ability of the antibodies to initiate complement activation—an ability dependent upon the concentration of antibody, its thermal amplitude, the degree to which C3 on the erythrocyte membrane modified antibody fixation and the degree to which antibody once attached was able to fix components of complement.

Rosse (1990), in an account of the mechanism of haemolysis in cold-antibody AIHA, reiterated the importance of the amount of antibody formed and its thermal amplitude and the temperature to which the blood is exposed. But he also stressed the individual patient-to-patient differences in antibody–antigen interaction that influence the amount of C3 fixed and consequent haemolysis, as illustrated by the experiments of Rosse and Adams (1980) referred to above. In an interesting comment on the possible importance of mechanical trauma in bringing about haemolysis, he pointed out that the force required to rupture the erythrocyte membrane is only to be found in the arterial side of the circulation where the blood, coming from the central regions of the body, is warm and auto-agglutination unlikely; in contrast, on the venous side of the circulation in the periphery, where auto-agglutination caused by a high-thermal-amplitude antibody could take place, the force of the circulation would be insufficient to cause the erythrocyte membrane to disrupt.

DAT-NEGATIVE COLD-ANTIBODY AIHA

In relation to the relative importance of agglutination and lysis in the pathogenesis of cold-antibody AIHA the point was made earlier in this Chapter (p. 424) that the ability of the antibody to fix complement and to react with antigen at or near body temperature is of critical importance. In fact, it is most unusual for cold auto-antibodies not to fix complement. For this reason the history of the patient described by Donovan et al. (1983) is of particular interest. This patient, a man aged 68, developed, following a short febrile illness, a moderately severe haemolytic anaemia: his haemoglobin fell from 11.7 to 6.9 g/dl over a 4-day period and the reticulocyte count rose to 10.2%. Spherocytes were noticed a blood films; auto-agglutination was not mentioned. The DAT was repeatedly negative with anti-IgG, anti-C3d and anti-IgM sera. His serum, nevertheless, contained a high-thermal-amplitude cold antibody which agglutinated normal erythrocytes to a titre of 64 at $37°C$ and 512 at room temperature. Serum IgM was elevated (745 mg/dl); serum complement activity was normal. The antibody was inactivated by DTT, i.e. it was an IgM. I and i cells were equally sensitive to agglutination, which was enhanced if the cells were pretreated with ficin. The patient received high doses of prednisone and steadily improved: transfusions were not required.

An interesting feature of the case was the development of well-marked diffuse livedo reticularis, presumably the result of the intracapillary stagnation of agglutinated erythrocytes. The possible occurrence of acrocyanosis and haemoglobinuria, as found characteristically in CHAD, was not mentioned.

One year after the onset of his illness, the patient was well and his haemoglobin 14.8 g/dl. The cold antibody had disappeared; on the other hand, the DAT was now weakly positive with an anti-IgG serum and eluates were shown to contain an agglutinin which reacted with all cells tested.

PATHOGENESIS OF LEUCOPENIA AND THROMBOCYTOPENIA IN AIHA

There seem to be three possible causes:

1. The formation of auto-antibodies directed against leucocyte, e.g. neutrophil, or platelet antigens. Evidence for this has been summarized on p. 36 under the heading 'Immunopancytopenia'.

2. The interaction between cold antibodies and Ii antigens on leucocytes.

As described on p. 303, agglutinates composed of neutrophils or of a mixture of erythrocytes and neutrophils, or of lymphocytes, may occasionally be seen in blood films that have been prepared at room temperature from the blood of patients forming high-thermal-amplitude cold auto-antibodies. Pruzanski and co-workers have shown, too, that anti-I and anti-i antibodies are cytotoxic *in vitro* to both B and T lymphocytes (Pruzanski et al., 1975b) and to neutrophils and monocytes (Pruzanski et al., 1975a; Pruzanski and Delmage, 1977). The toxic effects are temperature-dependent and best demonstrated bithermically ($4°C \rightarrow 25°C$). In experiments with monocytes, however, a substantial kill was noticeable at $37°C$.

3. The immune adherence of neutrophils and

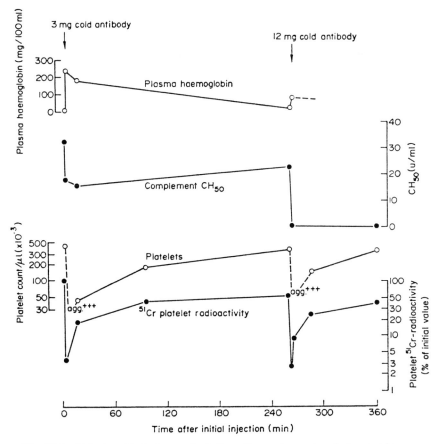

Fig. 34.8 Relationship between depletion of complement and changes in plasma haemoglobin, platelet count and platelet radioactivity after injecting a rabbit with a human IgM anti-I cold antibody.
[Reproduced by permission from Brown (1970).]

platelets, which possess C3 receptors, to C3 fixed to erythrocyte membranes as the result of antibody action. Brown (1970) demonstrated this mechanism in some elegant experiments carried out on rabbits. A direct relationship was shown to exist between complement consumption, as reflected in a fall in CH_{50} (a measure of complement lytic activity) and plasma C3 concentration, and the occurrence of temporary severe leucopenia and thrombocytopenia during acute intravascular haemolysis brought about by the intravenous injection of human IgM anti-I antibody (Figs. 34.2 and 34.8).

MORBID-ANATOMICAL AND HISTOLOGICAL FINDINGS IN AIHA

Typical findings are splenomegaly with varying degrees of vascular engorgement, a lesser degree of hepatomegaly, hyperplasia of the bone-marrow, widespread hyperplasia of reticulo-endothelial cells with evidence of erythrophagocytosis, and haemosiderosis. Oettinger's (1908) account of the necropsy findings in a case of 'ictère hémolytique non congénitale' is perhaps the earliest available.

Spleen. This has usually been described as being twice to five times the normal size. Kremer and Mason (1936) and Israëls and Wilkinson (1938) described the histological findings in the surgically removed spleens of several adult patients suffering from haemolytic jaundice of apparently acquired origin. Dameshek and Schwartz, in their 1940 review of the literature on acute haemolytic anaemia, described the microscopic picture of the spleen as being not as uniform as in patients with hereditary spherocytosis (HS). However, there is usually considerable congestion with blood, and sometimes this approaches in degree that seen in HS. Dameshek and Schwartz mentioned the presence in one of their cases of numerous thromboses of veins and capillaries which had resulted in multiple venous infarctions. Sometimes macroscopic infarcts occur.

Irrespective of the degree of congestion, there is hyperplasia of the reticulum cells of the spleen pulp; in most instances, too, erythrophagocytosis is easily seen. Some of the erythrophages are distended with up to six, or even more, ingested erythrocytes; in other cells abundant brownish iron-containing pigment (haemosiderin) is evidence of past phagocytic activity. In these respects — reticulum-cell hyperplasia and erythrophagocytosis — the histological appearances of the spleen differ from those of HS in which neither reticulum-cell hyperplasia nor evidence of phagocytosis is well marked. Another commonly observed feature is the presence of small islands of myeloid (mostly erythroid) metaplasia. Again, this change is not so commonly seen in HS.

Rappaport and Crosby's (1957) account contained a wealth of detail. Their report included a histological study of 30 spleens (mostly surgical specimens) obtained from patients suffering from AIHA not associated with malignancy. The spleens weighed on an average 650g; five weighed more than 1000 g. In 18 patients the degree of pulp congestion approached in intensity that found in HS; in 11 patients the sinuses were congested and the pulp cords narrow and relatively bloodless. Hyperplasia of the reticulum cells of the splenic cords associated with infiltration by lymphocytes and macrophages were conspicuous in 12 spleens; plasma cells were conspicuous in seven and macrophages in nine. The endothelial cells lining the splenic sinuses were often hyperplastic and invariably contained material reacting positively for ionized iron, and iron-containing macrophages were sometimes to be seen free in the lumina. Erythrophagocytosis was detected in 80% of the spleens; the erythrophages were more easily detected in the sinuses than in the pulp. Extramedullary haemopoiesis was seen in 10 spleens removed at operation and in five post-mortem specimens: erythropoiesis predominated, but in a few instances megakaryocytes were also present.

More recently, Jensen and Kristensen (1986) have again contrasted the histological appearances of the spleen in HS and in AIHA. Surgically removed spleens were perfused with glutaraldehyde and cacodylate fixative, then post-fixed with formaldehyde. Sections were viewed by light and electron microscopy. In both HS and AIHA the red pulp of the spleen was relatively and absolutely increased in volume; the changes were, however, relatively greater in HS than in AIHA. In both disorders the abnormally dense, more regular and almost circular profiles of the erythrocytes (i.e. of the spherocytes) could be easily recognized in electron-micrographs.

Liver. In fatal cases the liver has usually been described as enlarged. The enlargement is mostly due to congestion with blood. There may in addition be areas of focal necrosis, as well as hyperplasia of Kupffer cells with evidence of erythrophagocytosis (Schubothe and Altmann, 1950). Sometimes small islands of erythropoiesis can be detected. Siderosis is often a striking feature, the iron-containing granules being present both in Kupffer cells and in liver-parenchyma cells. The intensity of siderosis depends to some extent on the number of times the patient has been transfused during life.

Occasionally an acute haemolytic process is accompanied by signs of serious liver damage (Farrar, Burnett and Steigman, 1940); the patient may then become quite deeply jaundiced and have bile in the urine. In these patients a serious degree of liver-cell necrosis probably occurs. The sequence of events leading to necrosis is not fully understood. One possible factor is auto-agglutination leading to circulatory stasis and consequent anoxia.

Kidneys. In fatal cases there may be a variable degree of tubular damage. Usually there is a moderate amount of siderosis: this may be a very striking feature in patients in whom the plasma haemoglobin concentration is constantly raised, even in the absence of overt haemoglobinuria. According to Leonardi and Ruol (1960), most of the haemosiderin is in the cells of the proximal convoluted tubules but where large amounts are present the second convoluted tubules, loops of Henle and collecting tubules may be stuffed with granules also. In patients who have died with haemoglobinuria, haemoglobin-containing casts may be conspicuous in the collecting tubules.

Lymph nodes. These are not usually significantly enlarged, and their basic histological structure is normal. However, slight to moderate enlargement may occur and there may be an unusual intensity of erythrophagocytosis by free phagocytic cells in the lymph sinuses. This phenomenon was noted by Oettinger as far back as 1908. [It should be added, however, that some degree of erythrophagocytosis in lymph nodes is a common phenomenon in many diseases, not necessarily involving the haemopoietic system, and it also probably occurs in health (see Smith, 1958).] Extramedullary haemopoiesis may occur in lymph nodes but this is unusual. Rappaport and Crosby (1957) mentioned two instances, and in a patient investigated by the present author extramedullary haemopoiesis appeared to be the pathological change responsible for lymph-node enlargement simulating reticulosarcoma.

Bone marrow. The bone marrow is typically hyperplastic due to normoblastic hyperplasia. Megaloblastic change has, however, occasionally been described (see p. 68). Increased erythrophagocytosis is a typical finding (see below).

Stainable iron is variable in amount depending on the intensity of erythropoiesis and on the extent to which the patient has been transfused. Cases have been described, e.g. by Engel, Schein and Conley (1982), in which bone-marrow biopsy has revealed an absence or almost complete absence of iron, despite there being a large amount of haemosiderin in macrophages in the spleen (as revealed by splenectomy). Crosby (1982), in describing a similar case, made the point that the cordal macrophages of the spleen cannot easily recycle the iron that they load themselves with as the result of their role as phagocytic cells. He cited pulmonary haemosiderosis and the spleen in sickle-cell anaemia as analogous conditions in which there is a great deal of iron locally in the lungs and spleen, respectively, which is not available for erythropoiesis.

According to Schubothe, Raju and Wendt (1966), an increase in 'lymphoid reticular cells' is a common finding in the bone marrow in idiopathic AIHA. In 17 cases the number of such cells per 100 myeloid cells varied from 2.8 to 50.2 compared with 2.0 to 10.2 in six HS patients whose marrows had also undergone erythroblastic hyperplasia. Plasma cells were present in the AIHA marrows in normal numbers, and the same was true of lymphocytes except in one case in which there were 20.6%.

Matsumato and Hiroshige (1986) provided some quantitative data on erythrophagocytosis (EP) by bone-marrow macrophages in haemolytic anaemia. They assessed EP from Wright-stained smears of aspirated marrow cells and also by observing in suspension marrow cells fixed in glutaraldehyde and viewed with a differential interference contrast microscope. EP was found to be increased in AIHA, but also in HS, and to a lesser extent in PNH. In AIHA about 32% of the cells judged to be macrophages had ingested 1 or 2 erythrocytes and a further 10% had ingested 3 or more erythrocytes.

Other organs. The usual effects of anaemia will be present, in addition to a variable degree of siderosis, the latter depending to a great extent on the history of the patient with respect to blood transfusion.

Post-operative thrombosis of veins, particularly of the portal system, may be encountered in patients dying after splenectomy. One of the author's patients [Case 13, Dacie (1954)] died 9 years after splenectomy of pulmonary hypertension consequent on multiple embolization of pulmonary veins [see British Medical Journal (1960)].

Massive fat embolization was described by van Phan and David (1959) in a fatal case. The relationship (if any) between this rare event and haemolysis remains obscure.

Findings in cold-antibody AIHA

The findings summarized in the above paragraphs have referred primarily to patients with warm-antibody AIHA. The findings in cold-antibody cases, e.g. in CHAD, are very similar. Siderosis of the kidneys is, however, likely to be a striking feature, as it is in any patient who has suffered from chronic haemoglobinuria or from a chronically raised plasma haemoglobin even in the absence of haemoglobinuria.

Schubothe, Baumgartner and Yoshimura (1961) reported an increase in the lymphocyte content of the bone marrow in six out of 12 patients diagnosed as suffering from chronic CHAD.

Schubothe and Altmann (1950) described in detail the findings in a fatal case of CHAD: EP in Kupffer cells in the liver was a striking feature. The findings in a further typical case of CHAD were described in 1951 by Ferriman et al. (Case 2). Fig. 28.6 (p. 219) is a photomicrograph of a section of one of this patient's kidneys; there is heavy siderosis.

Mechanism of reticulo-endothelial (RE) cell hyperplasia in AIHA

The enlargement of the spleen and liver and proliferation of RE cells throughout the body, which are characteristic morbid-anatomical and histological features in AIHA, prompted Jandl and his co-workers (1965) to consider how the hyperplasia was brought about. To this end they administered the haemolytic chemical phenylhydrazine to rats and assessed the consequent cellularity and proliferative activity of the spleen and liver by measuring the organs' DNA content and ^{3}H-thymidine incorporation. Their detailed studies indicated that acute erythrocyte sequestration stimulates RE-cell proliferation. In the spleen this was most marked in the marginal zone, which is the initial site of sequestration, and involves several division steps. There was also a generalized stimulation of macrophages and littoral cells involving one or two divisions. Chronic compensated haemolytic anaemia in rats resulted in overactivity of the RE system, with increased sequestering function and hypergammaglobulinaemia. Jandl et al. suggested that the cytoproliferative aspects of immune responses is geared to total 'work load' and depends on 'non-specific', usually particulate, stimuli. After prolonged stimulation, hyperplasia of the RE system was thought likely to become partly irreversible.

EXPERIMENTAL IMMUNE HAEMOLYTIC ANAEMIA IN ANIMALS

Much light has been thrown on the spherocytosis problem and indeed on most aspects of AIHA in man by the numerous observations made on animals to which anti-erythrocyte sera have been administered. The experiments occupy an important place in the history of immunopathology and for this reason they deserve a short account in their own right. They had, too, a considerable effect on the development of thought in relation to human haemolytic anaemia, for little experimental work in man had been possible before the advent of radioactive chromium.

The pioneer experiments

Belfanti and Carbone (1898) were apparently the first to record that the serum of animals injected with the blood cells of a different species acquired a high degree of toxicity for the donor species. Bordet (1898) furnished the explanation: he found that if guinea-pigs were injected with defibrinated rabbit blood the guinea-pig serum would then dissolve and/or agglutinate rabbit cells. He also showed that on heating the serum the lytic power was lost although agglutination persisted, and, in addition, that the serum of injected guinea-pigs was quite unable to lyse guinea-pig cells. These fundamental observations were soon confirmed and elaborated in France and Germany and many of the salient findings associated with the administration of heteroimmune sera accurately described. Cantacuzène (1900) demonstrated how anaemia was produced. Lesné and Ravaut (1901) compared in dogs the effects of haemolytic immune serum with other haemolytic agents such as distilled water and toluylenediamine; they found that while small doses of the serum produced urobilinuria, large doses caused urobilinuria and choluria and the largest doses haemoglobinuria. Kraus and

Sternberg (1902) recorded the occurrence of auto-agglutination in association with haemoglobinaemia, jaundice and bile retention. Levaditi (1902) described the presence of marked erythrophagocytosis, particularly in the spleen.

Pearce (1904) prepared antisera against other tissues as well as against blood cells. Areas of necrosis in the liver were readily produced in dogs when the immune sera were injected intravenously; he considered that the lesions were probably the consequence of venous or capillary thromboses, secondary to the plugging of the vessels with masses of agglutinated erythrocytes. In Britain, Dudgeon, Panton and Ross (1909), too, reported on the pathological changes. They prepared antisera against spleen extracts as well as against erythrocytes and observed similar changes with both types of antisera. Widespread necrosis of the liver and kidney occurred and the spleen was found to be distended with erythrocytes. There was abundant erythrophagocytosis within the spleen and in lymph nodes, which took on the appearance of haemolymph glands.

Christophers and Bentley (1909), in India, injected dogs with antisera prepared in goats, in an attempt to obtain insight into haemolytic mechanisms in man, particularly that of blackwater fever. As already mentioned in Volume 1 (p. 66), they coined the term 'spherocyte'. Christophers and Bentley's remarkable contribution deserves a more detailed description.

At a post-mortem examination carried out on one of their dogs they noted that the blood was auto-agglutinated, that the spleen was markedly congested and that there was abundant erythrophagocytosis. In another animal they carried out serial osmotic fragility studies, and observed that lysis commenced in near-isotonic saline.

Christophers and Bentley recognized that the haemoglobinaemia resulted from intravascular haemolysis, 'lysaemia', in contradistinction to erythrocyte destruction outside the blood stream which they referred to as 'erythrocatalysis' and attributed to erythrophagocytosis without solution of the haemoglobin. The phenomenon of rapid lysis *in vitro* was also recognized and referred to as 'extravascular lysaemia'. Spherocytes were reported in the peripheral blood of some of the dogs receiving the immune serum. Although they were found to be inconspicuous in the initial stages of lysis, they were noted to be present in blood from viscera. When haemoglobin-aemia was present, shoals of ghosts or shadows were seen in blood taken from the renal or hepatic veins. Referring to hepatic-vein blood, they stated: 'The groups of agglutinated cells are all spherocytes' and noted they they were often arranged around one or two leucocytes.

In addition to making these remarkable and prescient observations, Christophers and Bentley went on to discuss the possible causes for the lack of correlation they had observed between the action of haemolytic agents *in vitro* and *in vivo* and cited specific immune sera and cobra venom in illustration.

Christophers and Bentley's work was followed by the extensive and important observations of Muir and McNee (1912) and of Banti (1913).

Muir and McNee worked with rabbits given haemolytic immune sera derived from goats and they described in detail the consequent blood changes. Their paper contains some good photomicrographs (Fig. 34.9), and although they did not actually use the term 'spherocyte', they certainly illustrated them and commented on their presence. The following is part of what they wrote: 'As the anaemia progressed many of the old erythrocytes seem to diminish in size, so that many corpuscles of 3–5 μ in diameter, which stain deeply with eosin, are present. At the same time, the larger newly formed corpuscles gradually lose their basophil reaction, and it would appear that some of them undergo contraction and diminution in size'. Later on in their paper they reported that the microcytes disappeared quickly as the animals recovered and they concluded that this was probably the result of them being destroyed.

Muir and McNee went on to discuss the mechanism of anaemia and to compare the degree to which overt erythrocyte destruction could be produced by experiments *in vivo*, and *in vitro*, as the result of the interaction between erythrocytes, antibody and complement. They made the point that the amount of haemolysis produced *in vivo* by a particular dose of immune serum was always far greater than that which would be expected on the basis of experiments *in vitro* and they reached the important conclusion that the course of events in the experimental animal could not be explained by the principles which governed the development of lysis in the laboratory.

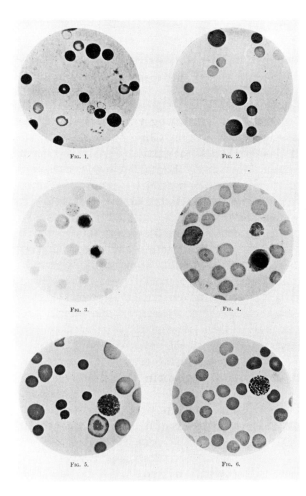

Fig. 34.9 Photomicrographs of the blood cells of rabbits to which haemolytic immune sera had been administered.

[Reproduced by permission from Muir and McNee (1912).]

Banti (1913) used dogs as well as rabbits, and although he did not study erythrocyte morphology closely he measured osmotic fragility and also considered the role of the spleen in haemolysis. Like Christophers and Bentley and Muir and McNee, he was struck by the much greater activity *in vivo* of haemolytic immune sera compared with their ability to cause lysis *in vitro*. He noted, too, that the erythrocytes of the experimental animal became more fragile to osmotic lysis in hypotonic saline and discussed possible causes of this. He rejected the hypothesis, which he attributed to Widal, that the increased fragility was due to adsorbed antibody and considered that the change more probably resulted from a peculiar 'fragilizing activity' which the animal possesses or develops, and that the severe anaemia which a haemolytic serum

might produce after injection was in large part due to the haemolytic potentiality of the animal itself.

Banti then considered where this hypothetical haemolytic potentiality was likely to be located, and concluded that the spleen was the most important organ in this respect. First, he noted that when haemolytic immune sera were given to splenectomized animals the resultant effects were less intense; there was less anaemia, and this occurred more slowly; osmotic fragility changes were less marked and there was less haemoglobinaemia. Secondly, he referred to the well-known fact that the spleen enlarges after the administration of serum and becomes greatly congested. He described how the erythrocytes filled the sinuses and infiltrated the pulp cords in large numbers. He pointed out that the endothelial cells became swollen and acted as erythrophages, and that within the pulp were masses of agglutinated cells, some lacking haemoglobin but others being well-filled small cells. Banti added, significantly, that with large doses of serum the liver showed rather similar changes; the capillaries were dilated and packed with agglutinated cells and Kupffer cells acted as erythrophages. Banti was a most acute observer; almost everything he reported has, in retrospect, been shown to be correct.

Pearce and his colleagues carried out a long series of experimental studies in America, working with dogs and rabbits. Their cumulative experience was set out in a monograph, *The Spleen and Anaemia*, published in 1918 by Pearce, Krumbhaar and Frazier.

Much of their work was concerned with the effect of splenectomy on blood formation and osmotic fragility and on the response of splenectomized animals to haemolytic agents. They concluded, as had Banti in relation to immune sera, that there was a lessened tendency for haemolytic agents to cause severe anaemia, haemoglobinuria and jaundice after splenectomy, but they also noted in the splenectomized dog given immune serum that, although the anaemia might be slow to develop, recovery was also slower so that eventually the anaemia might be more severe and prolonged than in normal dogs. Pearce and Austin (1912) in an early paper described how after splenectomy in dogs many more phagocytes were to be seen in lymph nodes and also in the livers of dogs given immune serum. This they attributed to a compensatory taking over of the spleen's function.

The early experimental work carried out in the first two decades of the century outlined in the preceding paragraphs established clearly the main features of the haemolytic anaemia produced in animals injected with immune sera. The course of events was clarified and the changes in morphology of the blood cells were accurately described. Spherocytes were named and recognized and their significance in relation to the frequency of osmotic fragility changes was appreciated. The occurrence of lysis in the blood stream was well recognized and its relationship to haemoglobinaemia established; auto-agglutination *in vivo* had been noticed, as well as congestion of the spleen and liver, and the part played by phagocytosis in disposing of damaged erythrocytes was described. The effect of splenectomy in alleviating to some extent the worst effects of the immune serum had been established and the discrepancy between the potency of an antibody *in vitro* and its apparently more severe effect *in vivo* was recognized.

More recent studies

The above summary broadly describes the position when Dameshek and Schwartz in 1938 reawakened interest in the experimental approach to haemolytic anaemia. They pointed out the many analogies which could be drawn between the experimental disease in animals and the spontaneous disease, acute (acquired) haemolytic anaemia, in man. No major discoveries had been made in the intervening years, although some experimental work had been carried out, e.g. by Bennati and Pla (1932), who studied leucocyte changes and recorded hyperleucocytosis in dogs, and Filo (1936).

Dameshek and Schwartz's (1938) main contribution, other than causing a general reawakening of interest, was the demonstration of the relationship between the amount of antibody injected into guinea-pigs and the severity of the haemolytic process it produced, and the correlation between the severity of haemolysis and the changes in erythrocyte morphology and osmotic fragility (Fig. 34.10). They pointed out, too, as had Banti (1913), that the effects of the injection of immune serum were not maximal shortly after the time of the injection but developed progressively.

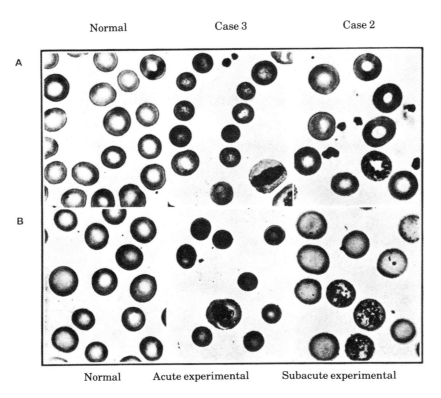

Fig. 34.10 Photomicrographs of blood films illustrating similarities in erythrocyte morphology in acute acquired haemolytic anaemia in man (A) and in guinea-pigs (B) to which haemolytic immune sera had been administered.
[Reproduced by permission from Dameshek and Schwartz (1938).]

The time-sequence of events was also studied in detail in dogs by Tigertt, Duncan and Hight (1940); a diminution in erythrocyte diameter was demonstrable in 12 hours and became marked in 48 hours. Anaemia was maximal in 3–6 days. Signs of regeneration, with the appearance of normal-sized cells or macrocytes, were obvious in 3–4 days, and 2–3 days later a double population of erythrocytes could be seen. Spherocytes gradually decreased in numbers but might be demonstrable up to 1 month following the injection of the immune serum; they were usually devoid of reticulofilamentous material.

Bessis and Freixa (1947), working with rats, made a notable contribution from several points of view. The morphological changes were described in detail, in particular the tendency 3–4 hours after the injection of serum for the erythrocytes of the injected animal to adhere one to another in the form of chains and if subject to tension to assume a fusiform shape and to be joined end to end by a thread (chaîne de fuseaux)—this phenomenon can also be seen in auto-agglutination in man (see Dacie, 1962, p. 355). Later, chains of spherocytes were formed which looked very much like greatly enlarged streptococci; and with larger doses of serum clumps of spherocytes resembling bunches of grapes were formed.

Wasastjerna (1948, 1951, 1953) reported the results of extensive studies. He used guinea-pigs and compared the ability of immune serum, saponin, streptolysin and a bean extract in bringing about haemolysis. Wasastjerna confirmed much of the earlier work. He, too, noted the discrepancy between the in-vitro and in-vivo effects of immune serum but concluded that conditions *in vivo* do not activate the antibody directly; he raised the question as to whether an excess of complement was significant in this respect. He noted that the enhancement of haemolytic activity *in vivo* applied only to the immune serum, not to saponin and streptolysin which if anything were less active *in vivo* than might be expected, and that the haemolysis they produced was not progressive.

Wasastjerna, too, found that the effect of an immune serum was usually less in a splenectomized animal, as also was the spherocytosis. He concluded that the latter change was not the direct effect of the antibody but was produced by the action of the living animal on the 'sensitized' cells. He concluded that intravascular auto-agglutination was an important mechanism by which the effect of the antibody was potentiated.

de Boisfleury and Mohandas (1977) used scanning electron microscopy to study the histology of the spleen of rats responding to the injection of rabbit anti-rat-erythrocyte immune serum. Before the injection of the serum it was possible to demonstrate clearly the passage of erythrocytes from spleen cord to sinus through narrow slits between adjacent endothelial cells. Twenty-four hours after the injection of the immune serum the sinuses were almost empty of erythrocytes; in contrast, the pulp cords were crowded with cells, as the cells, being undeformable, were then unable to pass through the slits. Six days after the injection, the picture was different: many cells were passing through the slits—these were flexible reticulocytes.

Resistance to hetero-immune sera

Bessis and Freixa (1947) failed in their attempts to produce a chronic haemolytic anaemia in rats by the administration of repeated doses of immune serum. Samaille et al. (1952–1953), working with dogs, reported similarly. Arbouys and Eyquem (1954) found, however, that when rats became resistant to one heterospecific serum they would still respond to injections of an immune serum prepared in another animal. However, after about 40 days a general and unexplained resistance developed. Davidsohn, Hermoni and Hanawalt (1957) also showed that guinea-pigs became resistant to immune rabbit serum if they were first immunized against normal rabbit serum. They pointed out that resistance to repeated doses of immune sera had been recorded by Muir and McNee many years earlier, in 1912!

Antiglobulin reactions in experimental haemolytic anaemia

The role of incomplete antibodies and auto-antibodies has been considered by a number of workers. Samaille and co-workers (1952–1953) and Samaille, Ropartz and Eyquem (1953) described some interesting observations using antiglobulin sera directed against rabbit globulin and dog globulin, respectively. They showed in dogs injected with immune sera prepared in rabbits that the dogs' erythrocytes became coated with dog serum protein as well as with rabbit immune protein. The autologous protein remained coating the erythrocytes longer than did the heterologous protein and was particularly noticeable in animals previously immunized against the heterologous (rabbit) protein. Samaille and co-workers discussed whether the autologous coating protein could be complement or anti-antibody directed against the heterologous rabbit protein and considered that the latter was more likely. Analogous observations made in guinea-pigs injected with rabbit immune antibody were reported by Samaille and Richardson Jones (1953).

Muratore, Cervellera and Gardaci (1953), working on parallel lines, made similar observations, also in guinea-pigs. They interpreted their results as indicating that the delayed haemolytic anaemia in the animals they were investigating was brought about by the combined effects of hetero-antibody and incomplete auto-antibody. Similar experimental observations were reported by Lille-Szyszkowicz and Chojnacka (1955). They also concluded that erythrocyte destruction was not wholly due to the introduction of the hetero-immune serum but was supplemented by auto-antibodies formed against the recipient's erythrocytes which had been damaged by adsorbed antibody. Their interpretation was in line with the anti-antibody hypothesis of Milgrom (see p. 376).

Davidsohn, Hermoni and Hanawalt (1957), in acute experiments in which rabbits were injected with anti-rabbit-erythrocyte sera prepared in guinea-pigs, regularly obtained positive DATs as early as 4 hours after the injection of the immune serum. They noted that spherocytosis persisted long after the antiglobulin test had become negative.

It is difficult to assess what part, if any, incomplete antibodies in hetero-immune sera play in erythrocyte destruction in the experimental animal. Certainly, the more severe phases of haemolysis appear to be due to the action of antibodies acting as both agglutinin and haemolysin. Kuroyanagi and Kurisu (1959), however, reported that they had destroyed the agglutinating and haemolytic activity of an immune dog serum by heating it at 65°C for 60 minutes and subsequently obtained a haemolytic syndrome in rabbits by the administration of the heated serum in which incomplete antibody was still present. Significantly perhaps, previous splenectomy protected the animals against the effects of the injected serum.

Morris (1958) described some interesting experiments on young mice injected with rabbit anti-mouse-erythrocyte serum. Massive auto-agglutination took place in the liver, spleen, lungs and bone marrow, and the animals seemed to die from the removal of erythrocytes from circulation rather than from haemolysis. If they survived, haemoglobinaemia occurred 13–34 hours after the injection of the serum, and this was interpreted as due to the lysis of sequestered blood. Liver-cell necrosis was also a noticeable feature. Young mice have little or no demonstrable complement in their serum, and the delay in haemolysis was thought to be due to this. In older animals, whose serum contains complement, haemoglobinaemia was found to be an early feature if sufficient antiserum was given.

Jandl and Kaplan (1960), who had been studying the sites of haemolysis in man brought about by anti-B and anti-D allo-antibodies, turned their attention to the in-vivo survival of rat erythrocytes sensitized in vitro with rabbit anti-rat-erythrocyte sera. With small amounts of antibody the cells underwent relatively slow and incomplete sequestration in the spleen, whereas with large amounts there was rapid, largely hepatic, sequestration. Still larger amounts of antibody led to overt intravascular haemolysis. The results were closely similar to those they had observed in man with erythrocytes sensitized in vitro with anti-B.

Takita (1966) reported on the haemolytic anaemia resulting from injecting rabbits with an anti-rabbit-erythrocyte serum prepared in guinea-pigs. Within 60 minutes of a single injection of the immune serum both guinea-pig γ globulin and rabbit non-γ globulin, thought possibly to be complement, were demonstrable on the recipient rabbit's erythrocytes. In rabbits previously immunized against normal guinea-pig serum, the recipient's erythrocytes became coated with rabbit γ globulin presumably reacting on the erythrocyte surface with the guinea-pig anti-erythrocyte antibody.

Vitale and co-workers (1967) fractionated the sera of rabbits immunized with rat erythrocytes by DEAE and CM cellulose chromatography and succeeded in partially separating the sera into lytic, agglutinating and coating fractions. Rat erythrocytes were labelled with ^{51}Cr and sensitized with the different fractions before injection into isologous rats. The survival of the erythrocytes and their sequestration in the liver depended upon the amount of lytic antibody with which the cells had been sensitized. In contrast, cells sensitized with agglutinating or coating (but non-lytic) fractions survived normally. Lysis in vitro and shortened survival and hepatic sequestration in vivo were abolished or markedly reduced when complement-fixing (lytic) fractions were digested with pepsin or alkylated. These results emphasize the importance and role of complement fixation, and lack of importance of agglutinin, in this type of experimental system.

The experimental studies of Cooper and Brown (1971), who had injected rabbits with purified human anti-I antibodies, have already been referred to in relation to leucopenia and thrombocytopenia accompanying acute haemolysis. Rabbit erythrocytes react strongly with human anti-I, even at 37°C, and the injection of anti-I resulted in intravascular haemolysis. With large doses of antibody the haemolysis was sufficiently severe to lead to complement depletion, so that a second dose of antibody, administered $2\frac{1}{2}$ hours after the first, had little or no effect. Heparin, if given in sufficient dosage, prevented haemolysis, presumably by its anti-complement action. Antibody administered daily became less effective; however, one rabbit given four daily injections of antibody developed sustained haemolysis with well-marked spherocytosis and eventually a reticulocytosis.

R. A. Cooper's (1972) studies were concerned with what happens to the chemical constituents of the erythrocyte membrane when it becomes spherocytic in the course of antibody-induced haemolytic anaemia. Rats given rabbit anti-erythrocyte sera rapidly became anaemic, the PCV falling, for instance, from 40.6% to 27.6%. There was, however, no change in MCV, MCH, K^+ or ATP. On the other hand, accompanying marked spherocytosis, as revealed by a substantial increase in osmotic fragility, there was a striking and progressive loss in membrane constituents and surface area, e.g. major losses of cholesterol (-23.5%) and phospholipids (-26.3%). These changes occurred irrespective of whether the animals had been first splenectomized. Cooper concluded that his findings could not be explained by erythrostasis, which would lead to loss of ATP; they were, on the other hand, consistent with membrane damage resulting from interaction between IgG-coated cells and macrophages.

EXPERIMENTAL HAEMOLYTIC ANAEMIA PRODUCED BY ALLO-ANTIBODIES

Compared with the many reports of the use of hetero-immune sera there are but few descriptions of the effect of allo-antibodies in causing anaemia in animals, other than haemolytic disease of the newborn. The work of Young and his colleagues in dogs (see below) was, however, a notable exception. Almost all possible facets of the effects of allo-antibodies were explored. The consequence of transfusing incompatible erythrocytes was closely studied, and by the transfusion of antibody-containing plasma it was possible to reproduce almost exactly the sequence of events following the transfusion in man of human high-titre potent anti-A antibodies to group-A recipients. Interesting data were accumulated on the relationship between the in-vitro characteristics of an antibody and its effects *in vivo*, and the role of complement deficiency as a possible limiting factor in intravascular lysis was clearly shown.

An account of the early observations of Young and his associates was given by Young, Ervin and Yuile

(1949) and Young et al. (1951a). More detailed observations on the in-vitro activities of the five different dog allo-antibodies studied, anti-A, -B, -C, -D and -E were reported by Christian, Ervin and Young (1951) and Young et al. (1951b). Anti-A, an antibody which is powerfully lytic *in vitro*, caused rapid intravascular haemolysis, with haemoglobinaemia and haemoglobinuria, *in vivo*. When serum containing anti-A was transfused to A-positive dogs, haemolysis of the recipients' erythrocytes took place over a period of a few days, with positive DATs, spherocytosis and increased osmotic fragility persisting for considerably longer. Anti-B, -C and -D act as agglutinins *in vitro* and are insensitive to changes in temperature; they are not lytic *in vitro*, and *in vivo* they seemed to cause little or no lysis of incompatible cells. Anti-C and anti-D may cause sensitization to antiglobulin serum *in vitro* and this is regularly accomplished by anti-E, which is an agglutinin potentiated by cold. Christian, Stewart and their co-workers (1951) demonstrated that if successive transfusions of incompatible A cells were given to a dog whose plasma contained a powerful anti-A, depletion of complement might act as a brake to the rate of disappearance of the transfused cells.

Further details of experiments with six different allo-antibodies were briefly reported by Swisher, O'Brien and Young (1953), who again stressed the discrepancies between the in-vitro and in-vivo activity of an antibody: anti-C, for instance, had no effect *in vivo*, although causing agglutination at 37°C *in vitro*. Swisher (1954), summarizing the group's work on dog allo-antibodies, discussed mechanisms of erythrocyte destruction, as illustrated by their experience in dogs, in relation to the hypotheses which were then current. Later, Swisher (1956), working with canine A cells and anti-A, pointed out that platelets adhere to agglutinated erythrocytes both *in vivo* and *in vitro* and suggested that this might be a mechanism producing thrombocytopenia following incompatible transfusion.

EXPERIMENTAL ALLO-IMMUNE HAEMOLYTIC ANAEMIA IN MAN

The use of ^{51}Cr in following the fate of small volumes of incompatible erythrocytes injected into human subjects has already been discussed (Vol. 1, p. 110). Interesting information has also been obtained from the accidental, or deliberate, intravenous injection of homologous plasma containing antibodies at high titres capable of reacting on the recipient's erythrocytes. Ervin and Young (1950), who also gave details of the earlier literature on 'dangerous universal donors', described a detailed haematological study of a group-A patient who accidentally received 500 ml of group-O blood containing high-titre anti-A, and Ervin, Christian and Young (1950) described further details of three additional cases.

In the first patient haemoglobinaemia persisted for 30 hours and hyperbilirubinaemia, spherocytosis and increased osmotic and mechanical fragility lasted for at least 9 days. The patient's haemoglobin fell from 10.5 to 4.7 g/dl despite further transfusions with group-A blood. The changes noted in the other three subjects were essentially the same: in particular, spherocytosis and increased osmotic fragility; in one case, too, the DAT was found to be transitorily positive.

Mohn and co-workers (1961) and Bowman and co-workers (1961) described extensive comparative studies on the effects of the intravenous administration of high-titre anti-Rh, -K and -M to volunteers. In the first series

of experiments (Mohn et al., 1961), although the recipients' erythrocytes were found to give positive DATs, no significant degree of haemolysis was discernible. In the second paper (Bowman et al., 1961), plasma containing anti-CD antibodies of exceptional potency was transfused, with remarkable results. Anaemia resulted, the PCV falling to 21% by the 7th post-transfusion day, and hyperbilirubinaemia and haemoglobinaemia lasted at least 7 days. Marked spherocytosis developed with accompanying increase in osmotic fragility. A positive DAT persisted for 133 days. Extensive studies for free antibodies in the serum were also carried out and it was extremely interesting to note a resurgence of antibody activity between the 98th and 140th post-transfusion days. Bowman and his colleagues discussed various explanations for these findings, including the possibility of auto-immunization against erythrocyte antigens previously 'altered' as the result of saturation with Rh allo-antibodies.

THE PATHOGENESIS OF AIHA: A BRIEF SUMMARY OF THE GROWTH OF KNOWLEDGE IN THE 20TH CENTURY

In this chapter an attempt has been made to describe how auto-antibodies that react with human erythrocytes damage them so as to shorten their life-span and lead to haemolytic anaemia. During the first few years of this century, experiments with animals injected with hetero-immune sera had provided important information as to the role of the spleen and liver and phagocytic cells in the disposal *in vivo* of antibody-damaged erythrocytes; while *in vitro* the role of a labile serum factor (alexin or complement) had been clearly demonstrated. Spherocytosis was a known accompaniment of immune haemolysis, but why it developed was not understood.

It was not until the late 1930s that Dameshek and Schwartz (1938) in Boston reawakened interest in the causation of acquired haemolytic anaemia by their observations on acute cases in man and by their experiments with guinea-pigs. They concluded that the mechanism of haemolysis in their human cases was likely to be similar to that in experimental animals injected with immune sera and that 'hemolysins' were not only an important cause of acute acquired haemolytic

anaemia in man but also the cause of the notable spherocytosis that was present.

The next seminal step in this exciting story was the observation by Boorman, Dodd and Loutit (1946) that the antiglobulin test of Coombs, Mourant and Race (1945) was positive in many cases of human acquired haemolytic anaemia. This finding clearly established auto-antibody-induced (auto-immune) acquired haemolytic anaemia (AIHA) as a definite and important entity. Then came the realization in the late 1940s and 1950s that AIHA could be caused by more than one type of auto-antibody. From that time on a primary aim of investigators has been to determine the exact way in which the auto-antibodies lead to increased haemolysis. The developments in knowledge in this field have been the subject of this Chapter.

It is now known that of outstanding importance is the phagocytic cell system — the fixed macrophages and the blood monocytes—and the activity of complement.

Phagocytic cells have receptors for the Fc fragment of IgG antibodies, particularly for IgG3 and to a lesser extent IgG1 antibodies, so that erythrocytes coated with these antibodies tend to adhere to macrophages, especially in the spleen, and get damaged as the result of their adhesion. Some of the adherent cells are phagocytosed; others manage to break free from the phagocytes and recirculate for a limited period as spherocytes.

Phagocytic cells have receptors for complement, too. Erythrocytes, if coated with sufficient C3b, adhere to macrophages and undergo damage similar to that sustained by erythrocytes coated with IgG. Some of the cells are phagocytosed; others are able to break free from the phagocytes as the result of the action of the C3b inactivators. This reaction between complement-coated erythrocytes and phagocytes is an important mechanism of in-vivo erythrocyte destruction and takes place particularly in the liver. Only if really large amounts of complement are deposited on the erythrocyte surface can the complement sequence be completed and its membrane breached with the result that lysis (intravascular haemolysis) takes place. In relation to haemolysis caused by complement-fixing cold antibodies, e.g. anti-I and the anti-P D–L antibody of PCH, the thermal amplitude of the antibody, i.e. how close to body temperature the antibody reacts, is all-important. Cold antibodies present in high concentrations, i.e. antibodies that yield high titres *in vitro* at 0–4°C, although they may cause acrocyanosis, only produce important haemolysis if they have a high thermal amplitude, too.

Reviews published since 1960 which reflect the state of knowledge of the mechanisms of erythrocyte destruction in AIHA at the time they were published include those of Dacie (1962), Swisher (1964), Jandl (1965), Leddy (1966), Engelfriet et al. (1974, 1981), Frank et al. (1977), Lalezari (1983), Kelton (1987), Anderson and Kelton (1989), Garratty (1989) and Rosse (1990).

REFERENCES

ABRAMSON, N., GELFAND, E. W., JANDL, J. H. & ROSEN F. S. (1970a). The interaction between human monocytes and red cells: specificity for IgG subclasses and IgG. *J. exp. Med.*, **132**, 1207–1215.

ABRAMSON, N., GELFAND, E. W., ROSEN, F. S. & JANDL, J. H. (1970b). Specificity of monocyte receptor in man and monkey. *Clin. Res.*, **18**, 397 (Abstract).

ABRAMSON, N., LoBUGLIO, A. F., JANDL, J. H. & COTRAN, R. S. (1970c). The interaction between human monocytes and red cells: binding characteristics. *J. exp. Med.*, **132**, 1191–1206.

ABRAMSON, N. & SCHUR, P. H. (1972). The IgG subclasses of red cell antibodies and relationship to monocyte binding. *Blood*, **40**, 500–508.

ALTMAN, K. I., TABECHIAN, H. & YOUNG, L. E. (1958). Some aspects of the metabolism of red blood cells from patients with hemolytic anemias. *Ann. N. Y. Acad. Sci.*, **73**, 142–147.

ANDERSON, D. R. & KELTON, J. G. (1989). Mechanisms of intravascular and extravascular cell destruction. In *Immune Destruction of Red Blood Cells* (ed. by S. J. Nance), pp. 1–52. American Association of Blood Banks, Arlington, VA.

ARBOUYS, A. & EYQUEM, A. (1954). Anémie expérimentale avec crises hémolytiques itératives par injections repétiées d'immun-sérums d'origine polyspecifique. *V. int. Congr. Hémat., Paris.* Programme, p. 230, Abstract 207.

ARCHER, G. T. (1965). Phagocytosis by human monocytes of red cells coated with Rh antibodies. *Vox Sang.*, **10**, 590–598.

ATKINSON, J. P. & FRANK, M. M. (1974a). The effect of bacillus Calmette–Guerin-induced macrophage activation on the in vivo clearance of sensitized erythrocytes. *J. clin. Invest.*, **53**, 1742–1749.

ATKINSON, J. P. & FRANK, M. M. (1974b). Studies on the in vivo effect of antibody. Interaction of IgM antibody and complement in the immune clearance and destruction of erythrocytes in man. *J. clin. Invest.*, **54**, 339–348.

ATKINSON, J. P. & FRANK, M. M. (1977). Role of complement in the pathophysiology of hematologic diseases. *Progr. Hemat.*, **10**, 211–245.

BAKÁCS, T., KIMBER, I., RINGWALD, G. & MOORE, M. (1984). K cell mediated haemolysis: influence of large numbers of unsensitized cells on the antibody-dependent lysis of anti-D-sensitized erythrocytes by human lymphocytes. *Brit. J. Haemat.*, **57**, 447–455.

BANTI, G. (1913). Splenomégalie hémolytique anhémopoiétique: le rôle de la rate dans l'hémolyse. *Sem. méd. (Paris)*, **33**, 313–323.

BARCROFT, H. & EDHOLM, O. G. (1946). Temperature and blood flow in the human forearm. *J. Physiol. (Lond.)*, **104**, 366–376.

BAUMGARTNER, W. (1954). Die erworbenen hämolytischen Anämien und der hämolytische Transfusionzwischenfall. Pathogenese und Klinik unter dem Gesichtpunkt der serologischen

Hämatologie. *Helv. med. Acta*, **21** (Suppl. 35), 192 pp.

BELFANTI, S. & CARBONE, T. (1898). Produzione di sostanze tossiche nel siero di animali inoculati con sangue eterogeneo. *G. Accad. Med. Torino*, **61**, Serie IV, 4, 321–324.

BENNATI, D. & PLA, J. C. (1932). Contribution à l'étude des leucocytoses expérimentales. Action de certains sérums hémolytiques. *C. R. Soc. Biol. (Paris)*, **109**, 150–152.

BERENDES, M. (1959). The proportion of reticulocytes in the erythrocytes of the spleen as compared with those of circulating blood, with special reference to hemolytic states. *Blood*, **14**, 558–563.

BERKEN, H. & BENACERRAF, B. (1966). Properties of antibodies cytophilic for macrophages. *J. exp. Med.*, **123**, 119–144.

BESSIS, M. (1954). Phagocytosis and other phenomena in sensitized red cells, white cells and platelets. Study by phase-contrast microscopy. *Vox Sang. (Amst.)*, **4**, 177–180.

BESSIS, M. & DE BOISFLEURY, S. (1970). Étude des différentes étapes de l'érythro-phagocytose par microcinematographie et microscopie électronique à balayage. *Nouv. Rev. franç. Hémat.*, **10**, 223–242.

BESSIS, M. & FREIXA, P. (1947). Études sur l'ictère hémolytique expérimental par injection et ingestion d'antisérum. *Rev. Hémat.*, **2**, 114–146.

BONNIN, J. A. & SCHWARTZ, L. (1954). The combined study of agglutination, hemolysis and erythrophagocytosis. With special reference to acquired hemolytic anemia. *Blood*, **9**, 773–778.

BOORMAN, K. E., DODD, B. E. & LOUTIT, J. F. (1946). Haemolytic icterus (acholuric jaundice) congenital and acquired. *Lancet*, **i**. 812–814.

BORDET, J. (1898). Sur l'agglutination et la dissolution des globules rouge par le sérum d'animaux injectés de sang défibriné. *Ann. Inst. Pasteur*, **12**, 688–695.

BORSOOK, H., RATNER, K. & TATTRIE, B. (1969). Differential immune lysis of erythroblasts. *Nature (Lond.)* **221**, 1261–1262.

BORSOS, T., DOURMASHKIN, R. R. & HUMPHREY, J. H. (1964). Lesions in erythrocyte membranes caused by immune haemolysis. *Nature (Lond.)*, **202**, 251–252.

BORSOS, T. & RAPP, H. T. (1965). Complement fixation on cell surfaces by 19S and 7S antibodies. *Science*, **150**, 505–506.

BOWMAN, H. S., BRASON, F. W., MOHN, J. F. & LAMBERT, R. M. (1961). Experimental transfusion of donor plasma containing blood-group antibodies into incompatible normal human recipients. II. Induction of iso-immune haemolytic anaemia by a transfusion of plasma containing exceptional anti-CD antibodies. *Brit. J. Haemat.*, 7, 130–145.

BOYDEN, S. V. (1964). Cytophilic antibody in guinea-pigs with delayed-type hypersensitivity. *Immunology*, 7, 474–483.

BRITISH MEDICAL JOURNAL (1960). An obscure case demonstrated at the Postgraduate Medical School of London. *Brit. med. J.*, **ii**, 926–934.

BROJER, E., MERRY, A. H. & ZUPANSKA, B. (1989). Rate of interaction of IgG1 and IgG3 sensitized red cells with monocytes in the phagocytosis assay. *Vox Sang.*, **56**, 101–103.

BROJER, E., ZUPAŃSKA, B. & MICHALEWSKA, B. (1982). Adherence to human monocytes of red cells from autoimmune haemolytic anaemia and red cells sensitized with alloantibodies. *Haematologia*, **15**, 135–145.

BROWN, D. L (1970). Acute complement-mediated haemolysis in the rabbit: relationship between the thrombocytopenia and neutropenia and complement consumption. *Brit. J. Haemat.*, **19**, 499–513.

BROWN, D. L. (1973). The immune interaction between red cells and leucocytes and the pathogenesis of spherocytes. *Brit. J. Haemat.*, **25**, 691–694 (Annotation).

BROWN, D. L. (1974). The behaviour of phagocytic cell receptors in relation to allergic red cell destruction. *Series haemat.*, **7**, 348–357.

BROWN, D. L., LACHMANN, P. J. & DACIE, J. V. (1970). The in vivo behaviour of complement-coated red cells: studies in C6-deficient, C3-depleted and normal rabbits. *Clin. exp. Immunol.*, **7**, 401–422.

BROWN, D. L. & NELSON, D. A. (1971). Surface microfragmentation of erythrocytes as a mechanism of complement-mediated immune spherocytosis. *Blood*, **38**, 811 (Abstract 73).

BROWN, D. L. & NELSON, D. A. (1973). Surface microfragmentation of red cells as a mechanism for complement-mediated immune spherocytosis. *Brit. J. Haemat.*, **24**, 301–305.

BRÜCKMANN, G. & WERTHEIMER, E. (1945). Lysis of red blood cells by tissue slices. *Brit. J. exp. Path.*, **26**, 217–224.

CANTACUZÈNE, J. (1900). Sur les variations quantitatives et qualitatives des globules rouges provoquées chez le lapin par les injections de sérum hémolytique. *Ann. Inst. Pasteur*, **14**, 378–389.

CASTLE, W. B., HAM, T. H. & SHEN, S. C. (1950). Observations on the mechanism of hemolytic transfusion reactions occurring without demonstrable hemolysin. *Trans. Ass. Amer. Phycns*, **63**, 161–171.

CHAPLIN, H. JNR (1990). Red cell-bound immunoglobulin as a predictor of severity of hemolysis in patients with autoimmune hemolytic anemia. *Transfusion*, **30**, 576–577.

CHRISTIAN, R. M., ERVIN, D. M. & YOUNG, L. E. (1951). Observations on the in-vitro behavior of dog isoantibodies. *J. Immunol.*, **66**, 37–50.

CHRISTIAN, R. M., STEWART, W. B., YUILE, C. L., ERVIN, D. M. & YOUNG, L. E. (1951). Limitation of hemolysis in experimental transfusion reactions related to depletion of complement and isoantibody in the recipient. Observations on dogs given successive transfusions of incompatible red cells tagged with radioactive iron. *Blood*, **6**, 142–150.

CHRISTOPHERS, S. R. & BENTLEY, C. A. (1909). *Blackwater Fever. Scientific Memoirs by Officers of the Medical and Sanitary Depts. of the Government of India*. New Series, No. 35. Government Printing, Calcutta.

CLARK, D. A., DESSYPRIS, E. N., JENKINS, D. E. JNR & KRANTZ, S. B. (1984). Acquired immune hemolytic anemia associated with IgA erythrocyte coating: investigation of the hemolytic mechanisms. *Blood*, **64**, 1000–1005.

CLINE, M. J. & LEHRER, R. I. (1968). Phagocytosis by human monocytes. *Blood*, **32**, 423–435.

CONSTANTOULAKIS, M., COSTEA, N., SCHWARTZ, R. S. & DAMESHEK, W. (1963). Quantitative studies of the effect of red-blood-cell sensitization on in vivo hemolysis. *J. clin. Invest.*, **42**, 1790–1801.

COOMBS, R. R. A., MOURANT, A. E. & RACE, R. R. (1945). A new test for the detection of weak and 'incomplete' Rh agglutinins. *Brit. J. exp. Path.*, **26**, 255–266.

COOPER, A. G. & BROWN, D. L. (1971). Haemolytic anaemia in the rabbit following the injection of human anti-I cold agglutinins. *Clin. exp. Immunol.*, **9**, 97–110.

COOPER, R. A. (1972). Loss of membrane components in the pathogenesis of antibody-induced spherocytosis. *J. clin. Invest.*, **51**, 16–21.

CROME, P. & MOLLISON, P. L. (1964). Splenic destruction of Rh-sensitized, and of heated red cells. *Brit. J. Haemat.*, **10**, 137–154.

CROSBY, W. H. (1952). The pathogenesis of spherocytes and leptocytes (target cells). *Blood*, **7**, 261–274.

CROSBY, W. H. (1982). Iron and the macrophage. The monocyte is a metabolic idiot. *Arch. intern. Med.*, **142**, 233–235.

CROSBY, W. H. & DAMESHEK, W. (1951). The significance of hemoglobinemia and associated hemosiderinuria, with particular reference to various types of hemolytic anemia. *J. Lab. clin. Med.*, **38**, 829–841.

CRUZ, W. O. & JUNQUIERA, P. C. (1952). Resistance of reticulocytes and young erythrocytes to the action of specific hemolytic serum. *Blood*, **7**, 602–606.

CULP, N. W. & CHAPLIN, H. JNR (1960). The effects of concentrated eluted anti-red cell antibodies on the in vivo survival of normal red blood cells. *Blood*, **15**, 525–533.

CUTBUSH, M. & MOLLISON, P. L. (1958). Relation between characteristics of blood-group antibodies in vitro and associated pattern of red-cell destruction in vivo. *Brit. J. Haemat.*, **4**, 115–137.

DACIE, J. V. (1954). *The Haemolytic Anaemias. Congenital and Acquired*, 525 pp. Churchill, London.

DACIE, J. V. (1962). The *Haemolytic Anaemias: Congenital and Acquired. Part II— The Auto-immune Haemolytic Anaemias*, 377 pp. Churchill, London.

DACIE, J. V. & LEWIS, S. M. (1975). *Practical Haematology*, 5th edn, 629 pp. Churchill Livingstone, Edinburgh.

DAMESHEK, W. & SCHWARTZ, S. O. (1938). Hemolysins as the cause of clinical and experimental hemolytic anemias. With particular reference to the nature of spherocytosis and increased fragility. *Amer. J. med. Sci.*, **196**, 769–792.

DAMESHEK, W. & SCHWARTZ, S. O. (1940). Acute hemolytic anemia (acquired hemolytic icterus, acute type). *Medicine* (Baltimore), **19**, 231–327.

DAVIDSOHN, I., HERMONI, D. & HANAWALT, E. G. (1957). Experimental hemolytic anemia in rabbits. Protective role of sensitization to the species-specific protein of the heteroimmune hemolytic serum. *Blood*, **12**, 710–725.

DAVIS, W. C., DOUGLAS, S. D., PETZ, L. D. & FUDENBERG, H. H. (1968). Ferritin-antibody localization of erythrocyte antigenic sites in immunohemolytic anemias. *J. Immunol.*, **101**, 621–627.

DE BOISFLEURY, A. & MOHANDAS, N. (1977). Antibody-induced spherocytic anemia. II. Splenic passage and sequestration of red cells. *Blood Cells*, **3**, 197–208.

DEWAR, A. E., STUART, A. E., PARKER, A. C. & WILSON, C. (1974). Rosetting cells in autoimmune haemolytic anaemia. *Lancet*, **ii**, 519–520 (Letter).

DONOVAN, D. C., COLLIER, V. U., BAUMANN, C. G. & KICKLER, P. S. (1983). Coombs negative autoimmune hemolytic anemia associated with diffuse livedo reticularis. *Maryland med. J.*, **32**, 846–848.

DOURMASHKIN, R. R. & ROSSE, W. F. (1966). Morphologic changes in the membranes of red blood cells undergoing hemolysis. *Amer. J. Med.*, **41**, 699–710.

DUDGEON, L. S., PANTON, P. N. & ROSS, E. A. (1909). The action of splenotoxic and haemolytic sera on the blood and tissues. *Proc. roy. Soc. Med.*, **2**, 64–87.

DUDOK DE WIT, C. & VAN GASTEL, C. (1969). Red cell age and susceptibility to immune haemolysis. *Scand. J. Haemat.*, **6**, 373–376.

DUROCHER, J. R., GOCKERMAN, J. P. & CONRAD, M. E. (1975). Alteration of human erythrocyte membrane properties by complement fixation. *J. clin. Invest.*, **55**, 675–680.

ENGEL, P., SCHEIN, O. D. & CONLEY, C. L. (1982). Bone marrow hemosiderin does not always reflect body iron stores. *Arch. intern. Med.*, **142**, 287–288.

ENGELFRIET, C. P., VON DEM BORNE, A. E. G. KR., BECKERS, D., REYNIERSE, E. & VAN LOGHEM, J. J. (1972). Autoimmune haemolytic anaemias. V. Studies on the resistance against complement haemolysis of the red cells of patients with chronic cold agglutinin disease. *Clin. exp. Immunol.*, **11**, 255–264.

ENGELFRIET, C. P., VON DEM BORNE, A. E. G. KR.,

BECKERS, D., VAN DER MEULEN, F. W., FLEER, A., ROOS, D. & OUWEHAND, W. H. (1981). Immune destruction of red cells. *In A Seminar on Immune-Mediated Cell Destruction*, pp. 93–130. American Association of Blood Banks.

ENGELFRIET, C. P., VON DEM BORNE, A. E. G. KR., BECKERS, D. & VAN LOGHEM, J. J. (1974). Autoimmune haemolytic anaemia: serological and immunochemical characteristics of the autoantibodies; mechanisms of cell destruction. *Series haemat.*, 7, 328–347.

ERVIN, D. M., CHRISTIAN, R. M. & YOUNG, L. E. (1950). Dangerous universal donors. II. Further observations on in vivo and in vitro behavior of isoantibodies of immune type present in group O blood. *Blood*, 5, 553–567.

ERVIN, D. M. & YOUNG, L. E. (1950). Dangerous universal donors. I. Observations on destruction of recipient's A cells after transfusion of group O blood containing high titre of A antibodies of immune type not easily neutralizable by soluble A substance. *Blood*, 5, 61–73.

EVANS, R. S. (1946). Chronic hemolytic anemia. Observations on the effect of fat content of the diet and multiple red cell transfusions. *Arch. intern. Med.*, 77, 544–563.

EVANS, R. S., BINGHAM, M. & BOEHNI, P. (1961). Autoimmune hemolytic disease. Antibody dissociation and activity. *Arch. intern. Med.*, 108, 338–352.

EVANS, R. S., BINGHAM, M. & TURNER, E. (1965). Autoimmune hemolytic disease: observations of serological reactions and disease activity. *Ann. N. Y. Acad. Sci.*, 124, 422–440.

EVANS, R. S., TURNER, E. & BINGHAM, M. (1964). Studies with I^{131} tagged cold agglutinins. *Proc. 9th Congr. int. Soc. Blood Transf., Mexico 1962*, pp. 347–351. Karger, Basel.

EVANS, R. S., TURNER, E. & BINGHAM, M. (1965). Studies with radioiodinated cold agglutinins of ten patients. *Amer. J. Med.*, 38, 378–395.

EVANS, R. S., TURNER, E. & BINGHAM, M. (1967). Chronic hemolytic anemia due to cold agglutinins; the mechanism of resistance of red cells to C' hemolysis by cold agglutinins. *J. clin. Invest.*, 46, 1461–1474.

EVANS, R. S., TURNER, E., BINGHAM, M. & WOODS, R. (1968). Chronic hemolytic anemia due to cold agglutinins. II. The role of C' in red cell destruction. *J. clin. Invest.*, 47, 691–701.

FÅHRAEUS, R. (1939). The erythrocytes–plasma interface and the consequences of its diminution. *Lancet*, ii, 630–634.

FANGER, M. W., SHEN, L., PUGH, J. & BERNIER, G. M. (1980). Subpopulations of human peripheral granulocytes and monocytes express receptors for IgA. *Proc. nat. Acad. Sci. U.S.A.*, 77, 3640–3644.

FARRAR, G. E. JNR, BURNETT, W. E. & STEIGMAN, A. J. (1940). Hemolysinic anemia and hepatic degeneration cured by splenectomy. *Amer. J. med. Sci.*, 200, 164–172.

FERRIMAN, D. G., DACIE, J. V., KEELE, K. D. & FULLERTON, J. M. (1951). The association of Raynaud's phenomena, chronic haemolytic anaemia, and the formation of cold antibodies. *Quart. J. Med.*, 20, 275–292.

FIALKOW, P. J., FUDENBERG, H. & EPSTEIN, W. V. (1964). 'Acquired' antibody hemolytic anemia and familial aberrations in gamma globulins. *Amer. J. Med.*, 36, 188–199.

FILO, E. (1936). Anémies hémolytiques provoquées par le sérum érythrolytique. *Sang*, 10, 178–191.

FLEER, A., KOOPMAN, M. G., VON DEM BORNE, A. E. G. KR & ENGELFRIET, C. P. (1978a). Monocyte-induced increase in osmotic fragility of human red cells sensitized with anti-D alloantibodies. *Brit. J. Haemat.*, 40, 439–446.

FLEER, A., VAN DER MEULEN, F. W., LINTHOUT, E., VON DEM BORNE, A. E. G. KR. & ENGELFRIET, C. P. (1978b). Destruction of IgG-sensitized erythrocytes by human blood monocytes; modulation of inhibition by IgG. *Brit. J. Haemat.*, 39, 425–436.

FRANK, M. M., SCHREIBER, A. D., ATKINSON, J. P. & JAFFE, C. J. (1977). Pathophysiology of immune hemolytic anemia. *Ann. intern. Med.*, 87, 210–222.

FRIES, L. F., BRICKMAN, C. M. & FRANK, M. M. (1983). Monocyte receptors for the Fc portion of IgG increase in number in autoimmune hemolytic anemia and other hemolytic states and are decreased by glucocorticoid therapy. *J. Immunol.*, 131, 1240–1245.

GALLACHER, M. T., BRANCH, D. R., MISON, A. & PETZ, L. D. (1983). Evaluation of reticuloendothelial function in autoimmune hemolytic anemia using an in vitro assay of monocyte-macrophage interaction with erythrocytes. *Exp. Hemat.*, 11, 82–89.

GARRATTY, G. (1968). Complement. *J. med. Lab. Technol.*, 25, 313–328.

GARRATTY, G. (1984). The significance of complement in immunohematology. *CRC Crit. Rev. clin. lab. Sci.*, 20, 25–56.

GARRATTY, G. (1989). Factors affecting the pathogenicity of red cell auto- and alloantibodies (The Emily Cooley Memorial Lecture). In *Immune Destruction of Red Blood Cells* (ed. by S. J. Nance), pp. 109–169. American Association of Blood Banks, Arlington, VA.

GARRATTY, G. (1990a). Predicting the clinical significance of red cell antibodies with in vitro cellular assays. *Transf. Med. Rev.*, 4, 297–312.

GARRATTY, G. (1990b). Flow cytometry; its application to immunohaematology. *Baillières' Clinical Haematology*, 3, 267–287.

GARRATTY, G. & NANCE, S. J. (1990). Correlation between in vivo hemolysis and the amount of red cell-bound IgG measured by flow cytometry. *Transfusion*, 30, 617–621.

GLUCKMAN, E. (1970). Rosette tests in autoimmune haemolytic anaemias. *Lancet*, **ii**, 101 (Letter).

GOLDBERG, L. S. & FUDENBERG. H. H. (1968). Warm antibody hemolytic anemia; prolonged remission despite persistent positive Coombs test. *Vox Sang.*, **15**, 443–445.

GOWER, D. B. & DAVIDSON, W. M. (1963). The mechanism of immune haemolysis. I. The relationship of the rate of destruction of red cells to their age, following the administration to rabbits of an immune haemolysin. *Brit. J. Haemat.*, **9**, 132–140.

GRAY, L. S., KLEEMAN, J. E. & MASOUREDIS, S. P. (1983). Differential binding of IgG anti-D and IgG autoantibodies to reticulocytes and red blood cells. *Brit. J. Haemat.*, **55**, 335–345.

GRIFFIN, F. M. Jnr, BIANCO, C. & SILVERSTEIN, S. C. (1975). Characterization of the macrophage receptor for complement and demonstration of its functional independence from the receptor for the Fc portion of immunoglobulin G. *J. exp. Med.*, **141**, 1269–1277.

HAM, T. H. (1955). Hemoglobinuria. *Amer. J. Med.*, **18**, 990–1006.

HAM, T. H. & CASTLE, W. B. (1940a). Relation of increased hypotonic fragility and of erythrostasis to the mechanism of hemolysis in certain anemias. *Trans. Assoc. Amer. Phycns*, **55**, 127–132.

HAM, T. H. & CASTLE, W. B. (1940b). Studies on destruction of red blood cells. Relation of increased hypotonic fragility and of erythrostasis to the mechanism of hemolysis in certain anemias. *Proc. Amer. phil. Soc.*, **82**, 411–419.

HAM, T. H. & CASTLE, W. B. (1940c). Mechanism of hemolysis in certain anemias; significance of increased hypotonic fragility and of erythrostasis. *J. clin. Invest.*, **19**, 788 (Abstract).

HAM, T. H., GARDNER, F. H., WAGLEY, P. F. & SHEN, S. C. (1948). Studies on the mechanism of hemolytic anemia and hemoglobinuria occurring in patients with high concentrations of serum cold agglutinins. *J. clin. Invest.*, **27**, 538–539 (Abstract).

HAMLIN, T. J. & VERRIER JONES, J. (1970). Rosette tests in autoimmune haemolytic anaemias. *Lancet*, **ii**, 314 (Letter).

HANDWERGER, B. S., KAY, N. E. & DOUGLAS, S. D. (1978). Lymphocyte-mediated antibody-dependent cytolysis; role in immune hemolysis. *Vox Sang.*, **34**, 276–280.

HAY, F. C., TORRIGIANI, G. & ROITT, I. M. (1972). The binding of human IgG subclasses to monocytes. *Europ. J. Immunol.*, **2**, 257–261.

HERRON, R., CLARK, M., YOUNG, D. & SMITH, D. S. (1986). Correlation of mononuclear phagocyte assay results and in vivo haemolytic rate in subjects with a positive antiglobulin test. *Clin. lab. Haemat.*, **8**, 199–207.

HOLM, G. (1972). Lysis of antibody-treated human erythrocytes by human leukocytes and macrophages. *Int. Arch. Allergy appl. Immunol.*, **43**, 671–682.

HOLM, G. & HAMMASTRÖM, S. (1973). Haemolytic activity of human blood monocytes. Lysis of human erythrocytes treated with anti-A serum. *Clin. exp. Immunol.*, **13**, 29–43.

HUBER, H. & DOUGLAS, S. D. (1970). Receptor sites on human monocytes for complement; binding of red cells sensitized by cold autoantibodies. *Brit. J. Haemat.*, **19**, 19–26.

HUBER, H., DOUGLAS, S. D. & FUDENBERG, H. H. (1969). The IgG receptor; an immunological marker for the characterization of mononuclear cells. *Immunology*, **17**, 7–21.

HUBER, H., DOUGLAS, S. D., NUSBACHER, J., KOCHWA, S. & ROSENFIELD, R. S. (1971). IgG subclass specificity of human monocyte receptor sites. *Nature (Lond.)*, **229**, 419–420.

HUBER, H. & FUDENBERG, H. H. (1968). Receptor sites of human monocytes for IgG. *Int. Arch. Allergy Appl. Immunol.*, **34**, 18–31.

HUBER, H. & FUDENBERG, H. H. (1969). Die Phagozytose von Erythrozyten–Antikörper-Komplexen in vitro. *Blut*, **19**, 357–364.

HUBER, H. & FUDENBERG, H. H. (1970). The interaction of monocytes and macrophages with immunoglobulins and complement. *Series haemat.*, **3**, 160–175.

HUBER, H., POLLEY, M. J., LINSCOTT, W. D., FUDENBERG, H. H. & MÜLLER-EBERHARD, H. J. (1968). Human monocytes; distinct receptor sites for the third component of complement and for immunoglobulin G. *Science*, **162**, 1281–1283.

HUGHES JONES, N. C., MOLLISON, P. L. & VEALL, N. (1957). Removal of incompatible red cells by the spleen. *Brit. J. Haemat.*, **3**, 125–133.

HUNT, J. S., BECK, M. L., TEGTMEIER, G. E. & BAYER, L. (1982). Factors influencing monocyte recognition of human erythrocyte auto-antibodies in vitro. *Transfusion*, **22**, 355–358.

ISRAËLS, M. C. G. & WILKINSON, J. F. (1938). Haemolytic (spherocytic) jaundice in the adult. *Quart. J. Med.*, 7, 137–150.

JAFFE, C. J., ATKINSON, J. P. & FRANK, M. M. (1976). The role of complement in the clearance of cold agglutinin-sensitized erythrocytes in man. *J. clin. Invest.*, **58**, 942–946.

JANDL, J. H. (1955). Sequestration by the spleen of red cells sensitized with incomplete antibody and with metallo-protein complexes. *J. clin. Invest.*, **34**, 912 (Abstract).

JANDL, J. H. (1956). The rapid destruction of sequestered red cells as determined with Fe^{59}-labelled human reticulocytes. *Clin. Res. Proc.*, **4**, 81 (Abstract).

JANDL, J. H. (1958). Observations on the pathway of destruction of red cells sensitized with incomplete antibodies. *Proc. 6th int. Congr. int. Soc. Hemat., Boston, 1956*, pp. 875–881. Grune and Stratton, New York.

JANDL, J. H. (1960a). Modern views of

immunohematology. *Programme VII Congr. Soc. int. Hemat., Roma, 7–13 Sept. 1958*, pp. 3–5. II Pensiero Scientifico, Roma.

JANDL, J. H. (1960b). The agglutination and sequestration of immature red cells. *J. Lab. clin. Med.*, **55**, 663–681.

JANDL, J. H. (1965). Mechanisms of antibody-induced red cell destruction. *Series haemat.*, **9**, 35–66.

JANDL, J. H. & CASTLE, W. B. (1956). Agglutination of sensitized red cells by large anisometric molecules. *J. Lab. clin. Med.*, **47**, 669–685.

JANDL, J. H., FILES, N. M., BARNETT, S. B. & MacDONALD, R. A. (1965). Proliferative response of the spleen and liver to hemolysis. *J. exp. Med.*, **122**, 299–324.

JANDL, J. H. & KAPLAN, M. E. (1960). The destruction of red cells by antibodies in man. III. Quantitative factors influencing the patterns of hemolysis *in vivo*. J. clin. Invest., **39**, 1145–1156.

JANDL, J. H., RICHARDSON JONES, A. & CASTLE, W. B. (1957). The destruction of red cells by antibodies in man. I. Observations on the sequestration and lysis of red cells altered by immune mechanisms. *J. clin. Invest.*, **36**, 1428–1459.

JANDL, J. H. & TOMLINSON, A. S. (1958). The destruction of red cells by antibodies in man. II. Pyrogenic, leukocytic and dermal responses to immune hemolysis. *J. clin. Invest.*, **37**, 1202–1228.

JENSEN, O. M. & KRISTENSEN, J. (1986). Red pulp of the spleen in autoimmune haemolytic anaemia and hereditary spherocytosis; morphometric light and electron microscopy studies. *Scand. J. Haemat.*, **36**, 263–266.

KAPLAN, M. E. & JANDL, J. H. (1963). The effect of rheumatoid factors and of antiglobulins on immune hemolysis in vivo. *J. exp. Med.*, **117**, 105–125.

KAPLAN, M. E. & JANDL, J. H. (1964). Immune hemolysis in man: the effects of antiglobulins and rheumatoid factors. *Proc. 8th Congr. int. Soc. Blood Transf., Mexico 1962*, pp. 375–380. Karger, Basel.

KAY, N. E. & DOUGLAS, S. D. (1977). Monocyte–erythrocyte interaction in vitro in immune hemolytic anemias. *Blood*, **50**, 889–897.

KELTON, J. G. (1987). Platelet and red cell clearance is determined by the interaction of the IgG and complement on the cells and the activity of the reticuloendothelial system. *Transf. Med. Rev.*, **1**, 75–84.

KELTON, J. G., SINGER, J., RODGER, C., GAULDIE, J., HORSEWOOD, P. & DENT, P. (1985). The concentration of IgG in the serum is a major determinant of Fc-dependent reticuloendothelial function. *Blood*, **66**, 490–495.

KRAUS, R. & STERNBERG, C. (1902). Ueber Wirkungen der Hämolysine im Organismus. *Zbl. Bakt.*, **32**, 903–911.

KREMER, M. & MASON, W. H. (1936). Acholuric jaundice in the adult. *Lancet*, **ii**, 849–852.

KURLANDER, R. J. & BATKER, J. (1982). The binding of human immunoglobulin G1 monomer and small covalently cross-linked polymers of immunoglobulin G1 to human peripheral blood monocytes and polymorphonuclear leucocytes. *J. clin. Invest.*, **69**, 1–8.

KURLANDER, R. J. & ROSSE W. F. (1979a). Lymphocyte-mediated lysis of antibody coated human red cells in the presence of serum. *Blood*, **53**, 1197–1202.

KURLANDER, R. J. & ROSSE, W. F. (1979b). Monocyte-mediated destruction in the presence of serum of red cells coated with antibody. *Blood*, **54**, 1131–1139.

KURLANDER, R. J., ROSSE, W. F. & LOGUE, G. L. (1978). Quantitative influence of antibody and complement coating of red cells on monocyte-mediated cell lysis. *J. clin. Invest.*, **61**, 1309–1319.

KUROYANAGI, T. & KURISU, A. (1959). Evidence for action of incomplete antibodies in experimental immunohemolytic anemia. *Tohoku J. exp. Med.*, **70**, 235–246.

LACHMANN, P. J., PANGBURN, M. K. & OLDROYD, R. G. (1982). Breakdown of C3 after complement activation. Identification of a new fragment, C3g, using monoclonal antibodies. *J. exp. Med.*, **156**, 205–216.

LACHMANN, P. J. & PETERS, D. K. (1982). Complement. In *Clinical Aspects of Immunology*, 4th edn (ed. by P. J. Lachmann and D. K. Peters), pp. 18–49. Blackwell Scientific Publications, Oxford.

LACHMANN, P. J., VOAK, D., OLDROYD, R. G., DOWNIE, D. M. & BEVAN, P. C. (1983). Use of monoclonal anti-C3 antibodies to characterise the fragments of C3 that are found on erythrocytes. *Vox Sang.*, **45**, 367–372.

LALEZARI, P. (1983). Autoimmune hemolytic disease. In *Recent Advances in Clinical Immunology* (ed. by R. A. Thompson and N. R. Rose), pp. 69–90. Churchill Livingstone, Edinburgh.

LASER, H. (1950). The isolation of a haemolytic substance from animal tissues and its biological properties. *J. Physiol. (Lond.)*, **110**, 338–355.

LAY, W. H. & NUSSENZWEIG, V. (1968). Receptors for complement on leukocytes. *J. exp. Med.*, **128**, 991–1007.

LEDDY, J. P. (1966). Immunological aspects of red cell injury in man. *Seminars Hemat.*, **3**, 48–73.

LEONARDI, P. & RUOL, A. (1960). Renal hemosiderosis in the hemolytic anemias: diagnosis by means of needle biopsy. *Blood*, **16**, 1029–1038.

LEROY, E. P. & SPURRIER, W. (1954). Effect of some carbohydrases on hemagglutination—their possible role in some immunohematologic disorders. *J. Lab. clin. Med.*, **44**, 826 (Abstract).

LEROY, E. P. & SPURRIER, W. (1955). Hemolytic property of some carbohydrases; their possible role in red cell destruction. *Blood*, **10**, 912–925.

LESNÉ, & RAVAUT, P. (1901). Des rapports que présentent entre elles hémoglobinurie, la cholurie et l'urobilinurie à l'hématolyse expérimentale. *C. R. Soc. Biol. (Paris)*, **53**, 1106–1107.

LEVADITI, C. (1902). Contribution à l'étude de l'anémie expérimentale. État de la cytase hémolytique dans le plasma des animaux normaux. *Ann. Inst. Pasteur*, **16**, 233–256.

LEWIS, S. M., DACIE, J. V. & SZUR, L. (1960). Mechanism of haemolysis in the cold-haemagglutinin syndrome. *Brit. J. Haemat.*, **6**, 154–159.

LEWIS, S. M., SZUR, L. & DACIE, J. V. (1960). The pattern of erythrocyte destruction in haemolytic anaemia, as studied with radioactive chromium. *Brit. J. Haemat.*, **6**, 122–139.

LILLE-SZYSZLKOWICZ, I. & CHOJNACKA, J. (1955). Anémie hémolytique expérimentale. Étude sérologique. *Sang*, **26**, 13–23.

LINKE, A. (1952). Klinische und experimentelle Beobactungen über aplastische Krisen der Erythropoese bei haemolytischen Anämien. *Verh. dtsch. Ges. inn. Med.*, **58**, 724–727.

LOBUGLIO, A. F., COTRAN, R. S. & JANDL, J. H. (1967). Red cells coated with immunoglobulin G: binding and sphering by mononuclear cells in man. *Science*, **158**, 1582–1585.

LOBUGLIO, A. F. & JANDL, J. H. (1967). Specific binding and sphering of γG-globulin-coated red cells by human monocytes and splenic macrophages. *J. clin. Invest.*, **46**, 1087 (Abstract).

LOGUE, G., GOCKERMAN, J. & ROSSE, W. (1971). Measurement of in vivo attachment of third component of complement (C3) to human red cells by cold agglutinin antibody. *Blood*, **38**, 810 (Abstract 71).

LOGUE, G. L., ROSSE, W. F. & GOCKERMAN, J. P. (1973). Measurement of the third component of complement bound to red blood cells in patients with the cold agglutinin syndrome. *J. clin. Invest.*, **52**, 493–501.

LONDON, I. M. (1960). Metabolism of the mammalian erythrocyte. *Bull. N. Y. Acad. Med.*, **36**, 79–96.

LUTHRINGER, D. G., JENKINS, D. E. JNR & WALLIS, L. A. (1969). Autoimmune hemolytic anemia with hemoglobinemia and hemoglobinuria in the absence of a demonstrable hemolysin or complement-binding antibody. *Vox Sang.*, **16**, 18–31.

MACKENZIE, M. R. (1975). Monocytic sensitization in autoimmune hemolytic anemia. *Clin. Res.*, **23**, 132a (Abstract).

MACLENNAN, I. C. M. (1972). Antibody in the induction and inhibition of cytotoxicity. *Transplantation Rev.*, **13**, 67–90.

MAEGRAITH, B. G., MARTIN, N. H. & FINDLAY, G. M. (1943). The mechanism of red blood cell destruction. *Brit. J. exp. Path.*, **24**, 58–65.

MAGALINI, S. I., BLUMENTHAL, W. & STEFANINI, M. (1956). A splenic hemolytic system of lipidic nature in man. *Clin. Res. Proc.*, **4**, 81–82 (Abstract).

MANTOVANI, B., RABINOVITCH, M. & NUSSENZWEIG, V. (1972). Phagocytosis of immune complexes by macrophages. Different roles of the macrophage receptor sites for complement (C3) and for immunoglobulin (IgG). *J. exp. Med.*, **135**, 780–792.

MASON, D. Y. (1976). Monocyte ingestion of IgG-coated erythrocytes from haemolysing and non-haemolysing subjects. *Acta haemat. (Basel)*, **55**, 1–9.

MASOUREDIS, S. P., BRANKS, M. J. & VICTORIA, E. J. (1987). Antiidiotypic IgG cross-reactive with Rh alloantibodies in red cell autoimmunity. *Blood*, **70**, 710–715.

MATSUMATO, N. & HIROSHIGE, Y. (1986). Erythrophagocytosis by bone marrow macrophages in hemolytic anemias. *Acta haemat. jap.*, **49**, 823–828.

MICHLMAYR, G. & HUBER, H. (1970). Receptor sites for complement on certain human peripheral blood lymphocytes. *J. Immunol.*, **105**, 670–676.

MIESCHER, P. A., BARKER, L., GEVIRTZ, N. R., JENKINS, D., MELTZER, M. & KOEPPEN, M. (1962). Étude du méchanisme de l'érythroclasie dans un cas d'anémie hémolytique provoquée par des autoanticorps froids. *C. R. Soc. Biol. (Paris)*, **156**, 1017–1021.

MOHN, J. F., LAMBERT, R. M., BOWMAN, H. S. & BRASON, F. W. (1961). Experimental transfusion of donor plasma containing blood-group antibodies into compatible normal human recipients. I. Absence of destruction of red cell mass with anti-Rh, anti-Kell and anti-M. *Brit. J. Haemat.*, **7**, 112–129.

MOLLISON, P. L. (1959a). Measurement of survival and destruction of red cells in haemolytic syndromes. *Brit. med. Bull.*, **15**, 59–67.

MOLLISON, P. L. (1959b). Blood-group antibodies and red-cell destruction. *Brit. med. J.*, **ii**, 1035–1041, 1123–1130.

MOLLISON, P. L. & CUTBUSH, M. (1955). Use of isotope-labelled red cells to demonstrate incompatibility in vivo. *Lancet*, **i**, 1290–1295.

MOLLISON, P. L. & HUGHES JONES, N. C. (1958). Sites of removal of incompatible red cells from the circulation. *Vox Sang.*, **3**, 243–251.

MOLLISON, P. L. & PATERSON, J. C. S. (1949). Survival after transfusion of Rh-positive erythrocytes previously incubated with Rh antibody. *J. clin. Path.*, **2**, 109–113.

MORRIS, I. G. (1958). Experimentally induced haemolytic disease in young mice. *J. Path. Bact.*, **75**, 201–210.

MUIR, P. & MCNEE, J. W. (1912). The anaemia produced by a haemolytic serum. *J. Path. Bact.*, **16**, 410–438.

MÜLLER-EBERHARD, H. J. (1969). Complement. *Ann. Rev. Biochem.*, **38**, 389–414.

MÜLLER-EBERHARD, H. J. (1975). Complement. *Ann. Rev. Biochem.*, **44**, 697–724.

MÜLLER-EBERHARD, H. J., NILSSON, U. R., DALMASSO, A. P., POLLEY, M. J. & CALCOTT, M. A.

(1966). A molecular concept of immune cytolysis. *Arch. Path.*, **82**, 205–217.

MUNN, L. R. & CHAPLIN, H. JNR (1977). Rosette formation by sensitized human red cells—effects of source of peripheral leukocyte monolayers. *Vox Sang.*, **33**, 129–142.

MURATORE, F., CERVELLERA, G. & GARDACI, G. (1953). Role of incomplete autoantibodies in production of experimental haemolytic anaemia induced by small doses of haemolytic serum. *Acta haemat. (Basel)*, **10**, 233–238.

NAJEAN, Y., RUVIDIC, R. & BERNARD, J. (1959). Étude de la réaction médullaire à une anémie hémolytique immune. *Rev. franç. Ét. clin. biol.*, **4**, 464–466.

NANCE, S. & GARRATTY, G. (1982). Correlations between an in vitro monocyte monolayer assay and autoimmune hemolytic anemia (AIHA). *Transfusion*, **22**, 410 (Abstract).

NANCE, S. & GARRATTY, G. (1984). Correlates between in vivo hemolysis and the amount of RBC-bound IgG measured by flow cytofluorometry. *Blood*, **64** (Suppl. 1), 88a (Abstract).

NICOLAU, C. T. & TEITEL, P. (1959). Über eine Verbesserung der osmotischen Resistenz von antikörperbeladenen Erythrozyten durch Stoffweckseleffekte des Insulins. *Z. ges. inn. Med.*, **14**, 40–42.

NICOLAU, C. T., TIETEL, P. & FOTINO, M. (1959). Loss of plasticity of erythrocytes coated with incomplete antibodies. *Nature (Lond.)*, **184**, 1808–1809.

OETTINGER, (1908). Ictère hémolytique non congénitale. Autopsie. *Presse méd.*, **16**, 679–680.

PANNACCIULLI, I., ROSSI, V. & TIZIANELLO, A. (1958a). Effet de la réfrigération dans l'anémie hémolytique acquise avec agglutinines froides: étude de l'hémolyse par le ^{51}Cr et étude immunologique. *Sang*, **29**, 695–700.

PANNACCIULLI, I., ROSSI, V. & TIZIANELLO, A. (1958b). Anemia emolitica acquista con crioagglutinine ad alto titolo: osservazioni sul quadro serologico e sul meccanismo di eritrodistruzione. *Haematologica*, **43**, 669–688.

PARKER, A. C. & STUART, A. E. (1978). Ultrastructural studies of leucocytes which form rosettes with homologous erythrocytes in human auto immune haemolytic anaemias. *Scand. J. Haemat.*, **20**, 129–140.

PEARCE, R. M. (1904). The experimental production of liver necroses by the intravenous injection of hemagglutinins. *J. med. Res.*, 12, 329–339.

PEARCE, R. M. & AUSTIN, J. H. (1912). The relation of the spleen to blood destruction and regeneration and to hemolytic jaundice. V. Changes in the endothelial cells of the lymph nodes and liver in splenectomized animals receiving hemolytic serum. *J. exp. Med.*, **16**, 780–788.

PEARCE, R. M., KRUMBHAAR, E. B. & FRAZIER, C. H.

(1918). *The Spleen and Anaemia. Experimental and Clinical Studies.* 418 pp. Lippincott, Philadelphia.

PERLMANN, P., PERLMANN, H. & WIGZELL, H. (1972). Lymphocyte mediated cytotoxicity in vitro. Induction and inhibition of humoral antibody and nature of effector cells. *Transplantation Rev.*, **13**, 91–114.

PETTIT, J. E., SCOTT, J. & HUSSEIN, S. (1976). EDTA dependent red cell neutrophil rosetting in autoimmune haemolytic anaemia. *J. clin. Path.*, **29**, 345–346.

PILLEMER, J., BLUM, L., LEPOW, I. H., ROSS, O. A., TODD, E. A. & WARDLOW, A. C. (1954). The properdin system and immunity: 1. Demonstration and isolation of a new serum protein, properdin, and its role in immune phenomena. *Science*, **120**, 279–285.

PIPITONE, V., RUSSO, R., CRISPO, A. & DAILLY, L. (1959). Anemia emolitica sperimentale da eteroantisieri. (II) Comportamento della glicolisi eritrocitaria. *Boll. Soc. ital. Biol. sper.*, **35**, 1268–1270.

PIPITONE, V., RUSSO, R. & DAILLY, L. (1959). Anemia emolitica sperimentale da eteroantisieri. (I) Comportamento della attivitá adenosintrifosfatasica degli eritrociti. *Boll. Soc. ital. Biol. sper.*, **35**, 1266–1268.

PISCIOTTA, A. V. & HINZ, J. E. (1956). Occurrence of agglutinogens in normoblasts. *Proc. Soc. exp. Biol. Med.*, **91**, 356–358.

PONDER, E. (1951). Certain hemolytic mechanisms in hemolytic anemia. *Blood*, **6**, 559–574.

PONDER, E. (1952). Les hémolysines des tissus et des tumeurs. *Rev. Hémat.*, 7, 436–443.

PORTER, K. A. (1960a). Immune haemolysis in rabbit radiation-chimaeras. *Brit. J. exp. Path.*, **41**, 72–80.

PORTER, K. A. (1960b). Immune hemolysis: a feature of secondary disease and runt disease in the rabbit. *Ann. N. Y. Acad. Sci.*, **87**, 391–402.

PRUZANSKI, W. & DELMAGE, K. J. (1977). Cytotoxic and cytolytic activity of homogeneous cold agglutinins on peripheral blood monocytes. *Clin. Immunol. Immunopath.*, 7, 130–138.

PRUZANSKI, W., FARID, N., KEYSTONE, E. & ARMSTRONG, M. (1975a). The influence of homogeneous cold agglutinins on polymorphonuclear and mononuclear phagocytes. *Clin. Immunol. Immunopath.*, **4**, 277–285.

PRUZANSKI, W., FARID, N., KEYSTONE, E., ARMSTRONG, M. & GREAVES, M. F. (1975b). The influence of homogeneous cold agglutinins on human B and T lymphocytes. *Clin. Immunol. Immunopath.*, **4**, 248–257.

RAPPAPORT, H. & CROSBY, W. H. (1957). Auto-immune hemolytic anemia. II. Morphologic observations and clinicopathologic correlations. *Amer. J. Path.*, **33**, 429–449.

RICE, J. D. JNR & MATHIES, L. A. (1960). Comparison of resistance of reticulocytes and mature erythrocytes to immune hemolysis. Studies in the guinea-pig, rabbit, dog, and man. *Arch. Path.*, **70**, 435–440.

ROSSE, W. F. (1971). Quantitative immunology of immune hemolytic anemia. II. The relationship of cell-bound antibody to hemolysis and the effects of treatment. *J. clin. Invest.*, **50**, 734–742.

ROSSE, W. F. (1973). Correlation of in vivo and in vitro measurements of hemolysis in hemolytic anemia due to immune reactions. *Progr. Hemat.*, **8**, 51–75.

ROSSE, W. F. (1979). Interactions of complement with the red-cell membrane. *Seminars Hemat.*, **16**, 128–139.

ROSSE, W. F. (1982). The lysis of erythrocytes by incomplete antibodies (Philip Levine Award Lecture). *Amer. J. clin. Path.*, **77**, 1–6.

ROSSE, W. F. (1990). *Clinical Immunohematology: Basic Concepts and Clinical Applications*, pp. 43–105. Blackwell Scientific Publications, Boston.

ROSSE, W. F. & ADAMS, J. P. (1980). The variability of hemolysis in the cold agglutinin syndrome. *Blood*, **56**, 409–416.

ROSSE, W. F. & DE BOISFLEURY, A. (1975). The interaction of phagocytic cells and red cells following alteration of their form or deformability. *Blood Cells*, **1**, 359–367.

ROSSE, W. F., DE BOISFLEURY, A. & BESSIS, M. (1975). The interaction of phagocytic cells and red cells modified by immune reactions. Comparison of antibody and complement coated red cells. *Blood Cells*, **1**, 345–358.

ROSSE, W. F., DOURMASHKIN, R. & HUMPHREY, J. H. (1966). Immune lysis of normal human and paroxysmal nocturnal haemoglobinuria (PNH) red blood cells. III. The membrane defects caused by complement lysis. *J. exp. Med.*, **123**, 969–984.

ROSSI, V., DIENA, F. & SACCHETTI, C. (1957). Demonstration of specific and non-specific agglutinogens in normal bone marrow erythroblasts. *Experientia*, **13**, 440–441.

SACCHETTI, C., DIENA, F. & ROSSI, V. (1957). Comportamento degli eritroblasti nella anemia emolitica acquisita. *Haematologica*, **42**, 895–909.

SALAMA, A., BHAKDI, S. & MUELLER-ECKHARDT, C. (1987). Evidence suggesting the occurrence of C3-independent intravascular immune hemolysis. Reactive hemolysis in vivo. *Transfusion*, **27**, 49–53.

SAMAILLE, J. & RICHARDSON [JONES] (1953). Protective mechanisms in experimental haemolytic anaemia induced by hetero-immune sera. *4th Congr. Europ. Soc. Haemat., Amsterdam, 8–12th Sept., 1953.* Abstract of paper 8.

SAMAILLE, J., ROPARTZ, C. & EYQUEM, A. (1953). Anémie hémolytique expérimentale par hétéroimmune sérums chez le chien. Mise en évidence, à l'aide de la reaction de Coombs, de la fixation des protéins de l'animal sur ses propres globules rouges. *Ann. Inst. Pasteur*, **85**, 48–55.

SAMAILLE, J., ROPARTZ, C., EYQUEM, A. &

GOUDEMAND, M. (1952–1953). Anémies hémolytiques expérimentales du chien par hétéroimmunsérums. Étude hémolytique et immunologique. Action de l'exsanguino-transfusion. *Ann. Inst. Pasteur Lille*, **5**, 139–173.

SCHREIBER, A. D. & FRANK, M. M. (1971). Role of antibody and of complement in the immune clearance and destruction of erythrocytes. *Blood*, **38**, 810 (Abstract 72).

SCHREIBER, A. D. & FRANK, M. M. (1972a). Role of antibody and complement in the immune clearance and destruction of erythrocytes. I. In vivo effects of IgG and IgM complement-fixing sites. *J. clin. Invest.*, **51**, 575–582.

SCHREIBER, A. D. & FRANK, M. M. (1972b). Role of antibody and complement in the immune clearance and destruction of erythrocytes. II. Molecular nature of IgG and IgM complement-fixing sites and effects of their interaction with serum. *J. clin. Invest.*, **51**, 583–589.

SCHREIBER, A. D. & McDERMOTT, P. B. (1978). Effect of C3b inactivator on monocyte-bound C3-coated human erythrocytes. *Blood*, **52**, 896–904.

SCHUBOTHE, H. & ALTMANN, H. W. (1950). Kältehämagglutinine als Ursache chronischer hämolytischer Anämien. *Z. klin. Med.*, **146**, 428–479.

SCHUBOTHE, H., BAUMGARTNER, W. & YOSHIMURA, H. (1961). Makroglobulinvermehrung und lymphoide Zellproliferation bei chronischen Kälteagglutininkrankheit. *Schweiz. med. Wschr.*, **91**, 1154–1156.

SCHUBOTHE, H. & MÜLLER, W. (1955). Über die Anwendbarkeit des Ehrlichsen Fingerversuches als Nachweismethode intravitaler Hämolyse und Erythrophagocytose bei hämolytischen Erkrankungen. *Klin. Wschr.*, **33**, 272–276.

SCHUBOTHE, H. RAJU, S. & WENDT, F. (1966). Hyperplasie lymphoider Reticulumzellen im Knockenmark bei idiopathischen autoimmunhämolytischen Anämien vom Wärmeantikörpertyp. *Klin. Wschr.*, **44**, 1319–1320.

SEARS, D. A., WEED, R. I. & SWISHER, S. N. (1963). Characterization of the mechanism of hemolysis of human erythrocytes by antibody and complement. *J. clin. Invest.*, **42**, 977 (Abstract).

SEARS, D. A., WEED, R. I. & SWISHER, S. N. (1964). Differences in the mechanism of in vitro immune hemolysis related to antibody specificity. *J. clin. Invest.*, **43**, 975–985.

SHAW, G. M., LEVY, P. C. & LoBUGLIO, A. F. (1978). Human lymphocyte antibody-dependent cell-mediated cytotoxicity (ADCC) toward human red blood cells. *Blood*, **52**, 696–705.

SMITH, F. (1958). Erythrophagocytosis in human lymph-glands. *J. Path. Bact.*, **76**, 383–392.

STATS, D. (1945). Cold hemagglutination and cold hemolysis. The hemolysis produced by shaking cold agglutinated erythrocytes. *J. clin. Invest.*, **24**, 33–42.

STATS, D., WASSERMAN, L. R. & ROSENTHAL, N. (1948). Hemolytic anemia with hemoglobinuria. *Amer. J. clin. Path.*, **18**, 757–777.

STEFFEN, C. (1955). Untersuchungen über den Nachweis sessiler Antikörper an Knockenmarkzellan bei erworbener hämolytischer Anämie. *Wien. klin. Wschr.*, **67**, 224–228.

STORTI, E., VACCARI, F. & BALDINI, E. (1956). Changes in red cell metabolism in presence of incomplete antibodies. *Experientia*, **12**, 108–109.

STRATTON, F. (1965). Complement in immunohematology. *Transfusion*, **5**, 211–215.

SUZUKI, S., AMANO, T., MITSUNAGA, M., YAGYU, F. & OFUJI, T. (1981). Autoimmune hemolytic anemia associated with IgA autoantibody. *Clin. Immunol. Immunopath.*, **21**, 247–256.

SWISHER, S. N. (1954). Studies of the mechanisms of erythrocyte destruction initiated by antibodies. *Trans. Ass. Amer. Phycns*, **67**, 124–132.

SWISHER, S. N. (1956). Nonspecific adherence of platelets and leukocytes to antibody-sensitized red cells. A mechanism producing thrombocytopenia and leukopenia during incompatible transfusions. *J. clin. Invest.*, **35**, 738 (Abstract).

SWISHER, S. N. (1964). Immune hemolysis. *Ann. Rev. Med.*, **15**, 1–22.

SWISHER, S. N. JNR, O'BRIEN, W. A. JNR & YOUNG, L. E. (1953). Studies of the mechanisms of destruction of transfused incompatible erythrocytes by isoantibodies. *J. clin. Invest.*, **32**, 607 (Abstract).

TAKITA, A. (1966). Studies on experimental hemolytic anemia induced by heteroimmune hemolytic serum. *J. Kyushu hemat. Soc.*, **16**, 74–93.

TIGERTT, W. D., DUNCAN, C. N. & HIGHT, A. J. (1940). Erythrocyte morphology in experimental hemolytic anemia as induced by specific hemolysin. *Amer. J. med. Sci.*, **200**, 173–182.

TORP, H. E. (1956). Has the enzyme system acetycholine–cholinesterase any significance for physiological hemolysis in the spleen? *Scand. J. clin. Lab. Invest.*, **8**, 84–85.

UNKELESS, J. C., SCIGLIANO, E. & FREEDMAN, V. H. (1988). Structure and function of human and murine receptors for IgG. *Ann. Rev. Immunol.*, **6**, 251–281.

URBANIAK, S. J. (1976). Lymphoid cell dependent (K-cell) lysis of human erythrocytes sensitized with Rhesus alloantibodies. *Brit. J. Haemat.*, **33**, 409–413.

URBANIAK, S. J. (1979a). ADCC (K-cell) lysis of human erythrocytes sensitized with rhesus alloantibodies. I. Investigation of *in vitro* culture variables. *Brit. J. Haemat.*, **42**, 303–314.

URBANIAK, S. J. (1979b). ADCC (K-cell) lysis of human erythrocytes sensitized with rhesus alloantibodies. II. Investigation into the mechanism of lysis. *Brit. J. Haemat.*, **42**, 315–328.

VAN DER MEULEN, F. W., DE BRUIN, H. G.,

GOOSEN, P. C. M., BRUYNES, E. C. E., JOUSTRA-MAAS, C. J., TELKAMP, H. G., VON DEM BORNE, A. E. G. KR. & ENGELFRIET, C. P. (1980). Quantitative aspects of the destruction of red cells sensitized with IgG1 autoantibodies: an application of flow cytofluorometry. *Brit. J. Haemat.*, **46**, 47–56.

VAN DER MEULEN, F. W., VAN DER HART, M., FLEER, A., VON DEM BORNE, A. E. G. KR., ENGELFRIET, C. P. & VAN LOGHEM, J. J. (1978). The role of adherence to human mononuclear phagocytes in the destruction of red cells sensitized with non-complement binding IgG antibodies. *Brit. J. Haemat,*. **38**, 541–549.

VAN PHAN, N. & DAVID, N. (1959). Fettembolie bei erworbener hämolytischer Anämie. *Z. ges. inn. Med.*, **14**, 507–508.

VICTORIA, E. J., PIERCE, S. W., BRANKS, M. J. & MASOUREDIS, S. P. (1990). IgG red blood cell autoantibodies in autoimmune hemolytic anemia bind to epitopes on red blood cell membrane band 3 glycoprotein. *J. Lab. clin. Med.*, **115**, 74–87.

VITALE, B., KAPLAN, M. E., ROSENFIELD, R. E. & KOCHWA, S. (1967). Immune mechanisms for destruction of erythrocytes *in vivo*. I. The effect of IgG rabbit antibodies on rat erythrocytes. *Transfusion*, **7**, 249–260.

VON DEM BORNE, A. E. G. KR., BECKERS, D. & ENGELFRIET, C. P. (1977). Mechanisms of red cell destruction mediated by non-complement binding IgG antibodies: the essential role *in vivo* of the Fc part of IgG. *Brit. J. Haemat.*, **36**, 484–493.

WAGLEY, P. J., SHEN, S. C., GARDNER, F. H. & CASTLE, W. B. (1948). Studies on the destruction of red blood cells. VI. The spleen as a source of a substance causing agglutination of the red blood cells of certain patients with acquired hemolytic jaundice by an antihuman serum rabbit serum (Coombs' serum). *J. Lab. clin. Med.*, **33**, 1197–1203.

WAGNER, K. (1956). Die Bedeutung experimenteller serologisch bedingter hämolytischer Anämien für Klinik und Forschung erworbener hämolytischer Anämien. *Wien. Z. inn. Med.*, **37**, 389–408.

WASASTJERNA, C. (1948). On the influence of immune hemolysin on red blood corpuscles in vivo and vitro. *Acta med. scand.*, **132**, 132–149.

WASASTJERNA, C. (1951). The destruction of red blood corpuscles in experimental hemolytic anemia. *Acta med. scand.*, **140**, Suppl. 258. 88 pp.

WASASTJERNA, C. (1953). Immunohemolytic mechanisms in vivo. The mode of destruction of sensitized red cells in the living organism. *Blood*, **8**, 1042–1051.

WASASTJERNA, C., DAMESHEK, W. & KOMNINOS, Z. D. (1954). Direct observations of intravascular agglutination of red cells in acquired autoimmune hemolytic anemia. *J. Lab. clin. Med.*, **43**, 98–106.

WHITTLE, C. H., LYELL, A. & GATMAN, M. (1947). Raynaud's phenomenon, with paroxysmal haemoglobinuria, caused by cold haemagglutination. *Proc. roy. Soc. Med.*, **40**, 500–501.

WIENER, A. S. (1945). Conglutination test for Rh sensitization. *J. Lab. clin. Med.*, **30**, 662–667.

WIENER, E., ATWAL, A., THOMPSON, K. M., MELAMED, M. D., GORICK, B. & HUGHES-JONES, N. C. (1987). Differences between the activities of human monoclonal IgG1 and IgG3 subclasses of anti-D (Rh) antibody in their ability to mediate red cell-binding to macrophages. *Immunology*, **62**, 401–404.

WITTS, L. J. (1936). The paroxysmal haemoglobinurias. *Lancet*, **ii**, 115–120.

WRIGHT, C.-S., DODD, M. C., BOURONCLE, B. A., DOAN, C. A. & ZOLLINGER, R. M. (1951). Studies of hemagglutinins in hereditary spherocytosis, and in acquired hemolytic anemia: their relationship to the hypersplenic mechanism. *J. Lab. clin. Med.*, **37**, 165–181.

WRIGHT, C.-S., DODD, M. C., BRANDT, N. G. & ELLIOTT, S. M. (1953). Erythrophagocytosis: standardization of a quantitative tissue culture test and its application to hemolytic, malignant, and infectious diseases. *J. Lab. clin. Med.*, **41**, 169–178.

YACHNIN, S. (1966). Functions and mechanism of action of complement. *New Engl. J. Med.*, **274**, 140–145.

YOUNG, L. E. (1958). Hemolytic disorders: some highlights of 20 years of progress. *Ann. intern. Med.*, 49, 1073–1089.

YOUNG, L. E., CHRISTIAN, R. M., ERVIN, D. M., SWISHER, S. N., O'BRIEN, W. A., STEWART, W. B. &

YUILE, C. L. (1951a). Erythrocyte–isoantibody reactions in dogs. *Proc. 3rd int. Congr. int. Soc. Hemat., Cambridge, England, Aug. 21–25, 1950*, pp. 226 – 233. Heinemann, London.

YOUNG, L. E., ERVIN, D. M. & YUILE, C. L. (1949). Hemolytic reactions produced in dogs by transfusion of incompatible dog blood and plasma. I. Serologic and hematologic aspects. *Blood*, **4**, 1218–1231.

YOUNG, L. E., O'BRIEN, W. A., MILLER, G., SWISHER, S. N., ERVIN, D. M., CHRISTIAN, R. M. & YUILE, C. L. (1951b). Erythrocyte–isoantibody reactions in dogs. *Trans. N. Y. Acad. Sci.*, **13**, 209–213.

ZUPAŃSKA, B., BROJER, E., MAŚLANKA, K. & HALLBERG, T. (1985). A comparison between Fc receptors for IgG1 and IgG3 on human monocytes and lymphocytes using anti-Rh antibodies. *Vox Sang.*, **49**, 67–76.

ZUPAŃSKA, B., BROJER, E., THOMPSON, E. E., MERRY, A. H. & SEYFRIED, H. (1987a). Monocyte–erythrocyte interaction in autoimmune haemolytic anaemia in relation to the number of erythrocyte-bound IgG molecules and subclass specificity of autoantibodies. *Vox Sang.*, **52**, 212–218.

ZUPAŃSKA, B., THOMPSON, E., BROJER, E. & MERRY, A. H. (1987b). Phagocytosis of erythrocytes sensitized with known amounts of IgG1 and IgG3 anti-Rh antibodies. *Vox Sang.*, **53**, 96–101.

ZUPAŃSKA, B., THOMPSON, E. E. & MERRY, A. H. (1986). Fc receptors for IgG_1 and IgG_3 on human mononuclear cells—an evaluation with known levels of erythrocyte-bound IgG. *Vox Sang.*, **50**, 97–103.

Auto-immune haemolytic anaemia (AIHA): treatment

ACTH and corticosteroids as treatment for warm-antibody AIHA   *453*

Early reports   *453*
  Relative effectiveness of ACTH and cortisone   *455*

Prednisone and the newer synthetic corticosteroids   *455*
  Early personal observations   *456*
  More recent recommendations   *458*

Effect of ACTH or corticosteroids on haematological and serological findings   *461*

Mode of action of ACTH and corticosteroids   *462*
  Inhibition of antibody formation   *462*
  Alteration in affinity of antibody for antigen   *463*
  Interference with erythrocyte–macrophage interaction   *464*
  Possibility of bone-marrow stimulation   *465*

Immunosuppressive alkylating and anti-metabolite drugs as treatment for warm-antibody AIHA   *465*
  Nitrogen mustard   *465*
  6-Mercaptopurine (6MP), 6-thioguanine (6TG) and azathioprine (Imuran)   *466*
  Immunosuppressive drugs as treatment for AIHA in NZB mice   *471*

Splenectomy as treatment for warm-antibody AIHA   *471*
  Early results   *471*
  Some unusual case reports   *472*
  More recent data   *472*
  Complications of splenectomy   *476*
  Assessment of sites of erythrocyte destruction using ^{51}Cr-labelled erythrocytes as a guide to the value of splenectomy   *477*

Treatment of warm-antibody AIHA patients who fail to respond to corticosteroids, splenectomy and immunosuppressive drugs   *479*
  Thorotrast and X-irradiation   *480*
  Radioactive gold   *480*
  Heparin   *480*
  Salicylates and 5-iodosalicylic acid   *482*
  Anti-snake-venom serum   *482*

Thymectomy as treatment for AIHA in infancy and childhood   *483*
Chloroquin   *485*
L-Asparaginase   *485*
Vinca alkaloids   *486*
Danazol   *488*

Blood transfusion in warm-antibody AIHA   *488*
  Early experiences   *488*
  Exsanguination (exchange) transfusion   *489*
  Recent reviews: the problem of incompatibility and selection of blood   *489*
  Auto-antibody specificity and blood transfusion   *490*

Plasmapheresis and plasma exchange as treatment for warm-antibody AIHA   *491*
  Specific immunoadsorption of IgG   *492*

Intravenous γ globulin (IgG) as treatment for warm-antibody AIHA   *494*

Practical management of patients with warm-antibody AIHA   *496*
  Choice of treatment   *496*
  Value of ascertaining sites of haemolysis with ^{51}Cr   *496*

Prognosis in warm-antibody AIHA   *497*

Mortality in idiopathic warm-antibody AIHA   *498*
  More recent data on mortality   *500*

Recovery ('cure') from idiopathic warm-antibody AIHA   *501*

Treatment and prognosis of cold-antibody AIHA   *502*

Chronic cold-haemagglutinin disease (CHAD)   *502*
  Corticosteroids   *503*
  Alkylating and anti-metabolite drugs   *503*
  Mercaptanes   *505*
  α-Interferon   *505*
  Blood transfusion   *505*
  Survival of i erythrocytes in patients forming high-titre anti-I antibodies   *507*
  Plasma exchange   *507*
  Splenectomy   *508*

Treatment and prognosis of acute cold-antibody AIHA   *508*
  Steroid-responsive idiopathic CHAD   *510*

Despite the availability of the corticosteroid drugs and various immunosuppressive agents, and the option of splenectomy, the onset of auto-immune haemolysis is a potentially serious matter. The outcome in any particular patient at the start of his or her illness is uncertain: some patients recover quickly spontaneously; others respond rapidly to treatment and do not relapse; still others respond to treatment but relapse and need continuous supervision for perhaps years thereafter; a small minority develop fulminating haemolysis and, failing to respond to all available treatment, die of their disease. In addition, there is the ever-present possibility of the presence at the time or in the future of an associated or underlying disease — a lymphoma or another autoimmune disease perhaps—which may or may not be easy to treat, and which will affect the outcome of the patient's illness.

These wide variations in clinical expression reflect the fact that the aetiology of AIHA is complicated: a variety of factors, acting alone or in combination, lead to the breakdown of self-tolerance. In addition, there are major differences between patients in their responses to this breakdown, some forming one type of antibody, others an antibody of a quite different nature. Because the type of auto-antibody formed has an important influence on the patient's illness, and on his or her likely response to treatment, in this Chapter the management of warm-antibody and cold-antibody AIHA will be considered separately.

ACTH AND CORTICOSTEROIDS AS TREATMENT FOR WARM-ANTIBODY AIHA

Early reports

The first published reports of favourable responses to treatment with ACTH or cortisone date from the early 1950s.

Dameshek (1950) reported 'startling' improvement as the result of treating with ACTH two patients who were suffering from AIHA associated with generalized lymphosarcoma; the serum bilirubin concentration and the auto-antibody content in their sera diminished, their erythrocyte counts improved and the lymphosarcoma regressed. Dameshek also reported that two other patients with idiopathic AIHA, who had not responded to splenectomy, improved when injected with ACTH. Gardner (1950), too, described improvement in three patients: in one, a girl aged 5 years, the erythrocyte osmotic and mechanical fragilities returned to normal and there was a fall in the 'Coombs titer'.

Details of five patients were given by Dameshek, Rosenthal and Schwartz (1951). In each case the DAT was positive and all had free auto-antibodies in their sera. Three of the patients were suffering from symptomatic haemolytic anaemia associated with lymphosarcoma or lymphocytic leukaemia, whilst in two patients the disease was idiopathic. All received intensive ACTH therapy; the dosage varied from 30 mg to 80 mg given intramuscularly at 6- or 8-hour intervals. Four of the five patients underwent almost complete remission and their antibody titres were markedly diminished. Two of the patients relapsed following cessation of therapy, but re-administration of ACTH resulted in further remissions. In a footnote the authors referred to three other patients suffering from idiopathic AIHA who had responded dramatically to treatment with ACTH.

Gardner and his colleagues (1951) reported detailed studies in three patients suffering from idiopathic AIHA; two were children, one was an adult. The DAT titre and erythrocyte mechanical fragility declined markedly in each case, and in two patients erythrocyte osmotic fragility became normal. Daily treatment with 100 mg of ACTH resulted in the disappearance from the adult patient's serum of an agglutinin and lysin active against normal erythrocytes at pH 6.4. At the same time the serum γ globulin concentration diminished.

Wintrobe and his co-workers (1951) reported the results of treating three patients with ACTH, the maximum dosage being 100–200 mg daily. In one idiopathic case a striking remission lasting more than 9 months followed the daily administration of 200 mg of ACTH; the DAT titre, however, increased. The other patients, suffering from chronic lymphocytic leukaemia and from SLE, respectively, responded moderately well; in the latter patient the DAT became negative.

Ley and Gardner (1951) reported favourable responses in three patients. In two the DAT became weaker or negative but it was unaltered in the third patient, whose remission was maintained on cortisone acetate. Best, Limarzi and Poncher (1951) likewise reported remission in two further patients treated with ACTH and good responses by single patients were described by Unger (1951), Meyer (1951), Etess et al. (1951) and Crary and Beck (1952) whose patient also received cortisone. Sacks, Workman and Jahn (1952) reported remissions in two patients and partial remissions in six others.

Rosenthal and co-workers (1952) used compound F (hydrocortisone). When given intramuscularly, compound F appeared to be less effective than ACTH or cortisone in four patients; when given orally, it produced a good remission in one patient, but in another it seemed less effective than cortisone.

The early observations on the use of steroids, summarized in the preceding paragraphs, were encouraging, although it is true that relapse had usually followed cessation of treatment. The question of dosage remained to be worked out. It was not, however, long before it was realized that a far higher dosage than had been anticipated might be necessary, and with the increased availability of the drugs this became possible.

Meyers and his colleagues (1952) obtained complete remission in six out of seven patients suffering from the idiopathic AIHA, but to obtain this daily doses of 100–160 mg of ACTH or up to 300 mg of cortisone had to be given. One patient remained in complete remission for 15 months after discontinuing therapy, two relapsed partially and four patients relapsed completely and needed further treatment. Meyers and his colleagues concluded that the best results seemed to be obtainable in patients who responded to moderate amounts of the hormones after relatively short periods of treatment. Dameshek (1952) summarized his by then relatively extensive experience by reporting that haemolysis could almost always be controlled, but that a dosage of up to 300 mg of ACTH or cortisone might be necessary. Fourteen out of his 22 patients had had complete haematological and clinical remissions, although the DAT usually remained positive. Frumin and co-workers (1953) showed that cortisone could be safely given in pregnancy; in one patient, whose acquired haemolytic anaemia probably antedated the pregnancy, daily dosages of 25–200 mg were given throughout.

Evans (1955) reported complete or partial remissions in seven patients whom he had treated with up to 400 mg of cortisone or 160 mg of ACTH daily.

This early work was quickly repeated and confirmed outside America. In Britain, a good response in a single patient was reported by Davidson et al. (1951), and Clearkin (1952) described how haemolysis had been controlled by ACTH in one patient but was ineffective in a second. The results in four patients were reported by Davis et al. (1952); two of the patients responded well but two derived little or no benefit.

The results of the trials sponsored in Britain by the Medical Research Council were only moderately encouraging (M.R.C. Haematology Panel, 1952). The usual minimum course of treatment was 1 g of ACTH or 1.5 g of cortisone given over a period of 10 days. Although eight out of 11 patients showed some sort of favourable response to treatment, in only three was the result really good ; in these three cases the improvement was maintained for more than 6 months after stopping treatment. In some of the patients who responded partially the DAT became weaker; in others who responded the test still remained positive. The later history of some of these patients was reported by the British M.R.C. Haematology Panel (1953). Of the three patients who had responded well, one relapsed and died; the other two remained well. Of the five patients who responded partially, one recovered after splenectomy, but three died; one patient was not traced.

In its second (1953) report the British M.R.C. Haematology Panel also reported on 10 further patients; in seven the haemolytic anaemia was idiopathic; in three it was of the secondary type. In seven patients the DAT was positive. Five patients underwent complete remission and three partial remission. Two patients failed to respond (both had negative DATs) ; their resistance could not be ascribed to underdosage. Throughout the latter series the daily dosage of the drugs ranged from 80 to 200 mg of ACTH and from 100 to 300 mg of cortisone, but in the early stages of the trial the patients received smaller doses than this and were clearly inadequately treated, as stressed by Dameshek (1952) at the time.

Rose and Nabarro (1953) studied three children severely ill with acute haemolytic anaemia. Repeated transfusions did not affect the rate of haemolysis; all three, however, responded to relatively large doses of ACTH or cortisone. One child recovered after 5 weeks of ACTH therapy; the other two relapsed when the drug was withdrawn but remitted when ACTH was re-administered. One child recovered after three courses of ACTH and cortisone; haemolysis in the other persisted longer, but was still being controlled by a daily dose of 75 mg of cortisone 30 weeks after the start of his illness. The sera of all three children contained autoantibodies. Aber, Chandler and Hartfall (1954) reported that the last patient was still being maintained in good health on 75 mg of cortisone a day 60 weeks after the start of treatment.

In 1955, the third report of the British M.R.C. Haematology Panel was published. This contained the results of treating 28 further patients: five did not respond, 15 were judged to respond partially and eight completely. They had received from 100 to 300 mg of cortisone daily. The point was made that the response rate might have been 'slightly better' if all the patients had received large doses. It was stressed, however, that two of the patients who had failed to respond had received 300 and 400 mg, respectively, of cortisone daily for 11 and 12 days, and that of the 15 patients who had only responded partially five had received as much as 300 mg for 11 to 30 days.

In Europe ACTH and cortisone were also soon widely used and generally favourable ,results reported, e.g., by Mallarmé et al. (1951), Mallarmé (1952), Heilmeyer (1952), Hansen (1952a), Christol, Eyquem and Colvey (1952), Letman (1953, 1957), Gros (1955) and Verloop (1955). In Australia and New Zealand, improvement or good responses were reported by Saint and Gardner (1952), Gunz and Aiken (1952) and by de Gruchy (1954).

Relative effectiveness of ACTH and cortisone

The question of the relative effectiveness of the two drugs exercised physicians in the early 1950s. ACTH was the first preparation available and, as had been described, very favourable results followed its use, but it had the serious disadvantage that it had to be injected, whereas cortisone could be given by mouth.

In some early reports ACTH had, however, appeared to be the more useful. Also, in theory at least, it seemed likely that the variety of hormones secreted by a stimulated adrenal might well be more effective than a single synthetic (adrenal-suppressing) hormone, even if the latter were given in very large doses.

de Gruchy (1954) referred to four patients who responded to ACTH but not to cortisone, and Meyer and Ritz (1954) mentioned a patient who responded to a daily dose of 80 mg of ACTH after having apparently failed to respond to 150 mg of cortisone given daily for 17 days. Meyer and Ritz also referred to a patient who failed to respond to oral cortisone but who nevertheless responded to the same drug when given by injection. Stein (1957) reported that a patient suffering from severe AIHA failed on two occasions to respond to 200–250 mg of cortisone given daily by injection over a period of 5 days, only to respond immediately when ACTH was substituted. Later, prednisolone was given by mouth in 50 mg daily doses for 5 days without effect; once more, there was a good response to ACTH. Dausset and Colombani (1959) also mentioned that in certain cases ACTH given intravenously might give spectacular benefit when orally administered corticosteroids were ineffective.

One of the difficulties in assessing the validity of these observations was the question of the relative dosages and potencies of the preparations used.

This was emphasized by Aitchison (1953) who described a patient in whom ACTH appeared to be ineffective while cortisone induced a dramatic improvement. Another factor which made comparison difficult was the possibly impaired ability of very sick patients to absorb steroids given by mouth. There was, however, enough in these early descriptions to warrant the use of ACTH in any severely ill patient when orally administered steroids appeared to be ineffective.

Prednisone and the newer synthetic corticosteroids

The next step in this unfolding story was the synthesis of prednisone (δ-cortisone). Reports on its use in AIHA date from 1956.

Sussman and Dordick (1956) described favourable responses to Metacortin in three patients and stressed its relative freedom from side-effects. Dameshek and Komninos (1956) in a larger series of patients also reported favourably but stressed that prednisone and cortisone did not seem to be exactly interchangeable in equivalent dosages (i.e. 40 mg of prednisone might or might not seem to be equivalent to 200 mg of cortisone). Some patients, for instance, appeared to respond better to prednisone. This report was comprehensive and dealt with the responses of 21 idiopathic and 22 secondary cases of AIHA. Doses of 150–300 units of ACTH, 200–400 mg of cortisone, 150–200 mg of hydrocortisone or 40–80 mg of prednisone were used as initial therapy. Three patients did not respond, 12 responded to a limited extent but 28 achieved full haematological and clinical remissions. However, 15 out of the 23 patients who had done well relapsed when their treatment was discontinued.

Other favourable reports on the use of prednisone included those of Marmont and Fusco (1956), Remy (1957) and Martelli, Martinez and Caronia (1959).

Dausset and Colombani (1959) considered that prednisone was the best drug to use in routine treatment: its side-effects, in large doses, were felt to be less severe than those of cortisone and its ability to control haemolysis seemed to be at least as good. Prednisolone appeared to have no advantage over prednisone.

In relation to the relative effectiveness of other newly introduced corticosteroids, Yunis and Harrington (1958) considered that methylprednisolone was as effective as prednisone. Melani and Prenna (1959) reported the successful treatment of a severely affected patient with a very large dose (40 mg daily) of triamcinolone.

In a review, Horster (1961) referred to the results of corticosteroid therapy in 167 cases of idiopathic AIHA: 6.8% of the patients were 'cured', 31.7% were still in remission 1 year after stopping treatment, 51% were in remission only during treatment and 17% were not benefited.

Early personal observations

The present author's experience in the use of corticosteroids in the 1950s was similar to that of most other workers; virtually all the patients so treated were benefited to a greater or lesser degree at one time or another, although in some this did not prevent the patient dying of his or her disease. Often relative failure to respond was converted into successful treatment by increasing the dosage —sometimes though at the expense of unpleasant side-effects. ACTH and cortisone and prednisone were used, the latter almost exclusively in later years, and in at least one patient ACTH appeared to be the more effective drug in the initial stage of treatment. Some typical responses are illustrated in Figs. 35.1–35.4. As described later (p. 498),

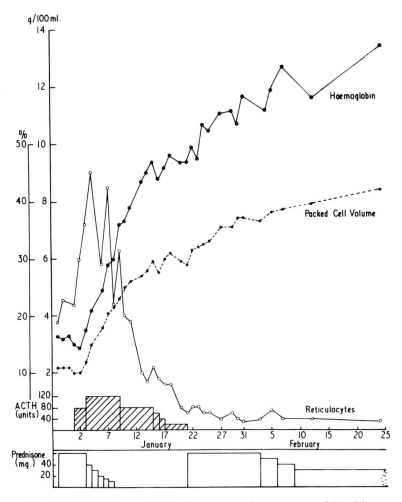

Fig. 35.1 Initial haematological response of a woman aged 26 with a warm-antibody AIHA to treatment with prednisone and ACTH.
    As she did not at first appear to be responding to oral prednisone at a daily dosage of 60 mg, this was supplemented by daily intramuscular injections of ACTH. [Reproduced by permission from Dacie (1959).]

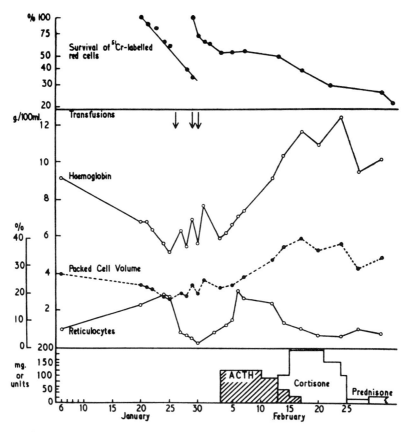

Fig. 35.2   Initial haematological response of a 70-year-old woman with warm-antibody AIHA to treatment with ACTH, cortisone, and finally prednisone.

[Reproduced by permission from Dacie (1959).]

the mortality in patients investigated by the author and treated with corticosteroids (with or without transfusions) was disturbingly high—nine deaths out of 23 patients (39%). Three of the 23 patients were clinically cured, and 14 managed to compensate for continuing haemolysis; in six, however, this did not prove to be possible (Table 35.1).

The author's recommendations based on his experience on the use of corticosteroids in the 1950s, as set out in the 2nd edition of this book (Dacie, 1962, p. 682), are reproduced below verbatim.

'Of the steroids, prednisone is probably the best drug to use—insufficient is known of the newer steroids to recommend any of them for routine use. Large doses may be needed but normally an initial dose of 40–50 mg per day of prednisone should be tried. If the patient is critically ill, it is wise, probably, to give ACTH as well in doses up to 100 units of the gel daily or the equivalent intravenously, for up to 1 week, and then to change over to prednisone alone. If and when the patient responds, the dose of the drug should be cut down to the minimum which enables the patient to maintain a stable haemoglobin, if possible of at least 10–11 g per 100 ml.'

'There seems no point in continuing to give large doses in the hope of achieving normal or near normal haemoglobin levels, for the hormones are in no sense a cure for the disease. The best that can be hoped for is to control the severity of the haemolysis until spontaneous recovery takes place. This may, unfortunately, necessitate continuous hormone treatment over many months or even years.'

'If the patient fails to respond to 40–50 mg of prednisone, particularly if ACTH has also been given, then larger doses should be given, and up to 100 mg of prednisone, given for 10–14 days, should next be tried. Whether still larger doses are ever required or achieve success seems doubtful, but in desperate situations

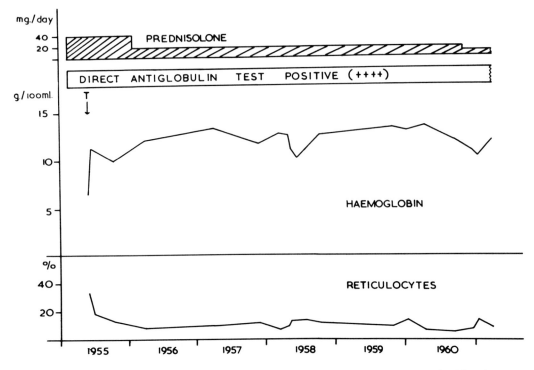

Fig. 35.3   Haematological response of a 59-year-old woman with warm-antibody AIHA to long-term treatment with prednisone.
  A daily dosage of 20 mg allowed her to keep in fair health over a 6-year-period. Haemolysis was compensated but remission was incomplete, and the DAT was strongly positive throughout.

there seems no reason for not increasing the dose to 250 mg daily for 7–10 days. However, it might well prove to be better to try an antimetabolite such as 6-mercaptopurine or 6-thioguanine before proceeding to use doses in excess of 100 mg of prednisone.'

'When a stable and adequate haemoglobin level has been reached, then the dose of steroids should be gradually reduced, the aim being to take the patient off the drugs completely over the next 6–8 week period. A significant proportion of patients will continue with little or no signs of haemolysis without further treatment. If they relapse, then hormone therapy, at the lowest possible level will have to be restarted. After another 2 months, a further attempt to withdraw the drugs should be made. In patients who have to be maintained on steroid hormones for many months, it is at least theoretically advisable to supplement the steroid therapy with a week's course of ACTH, say every 3 months, but this may be difficult to organize in practice.'

More recent recommendations

Before discussing how corticosteroids are currently used, i.e. in the early 1990s, some earlier

recommendations, based on the results being achieved in the 1960s, 1970s and 1980s will be briefly reviewed.

Jandl (1963) stated that three-quarters of the patients treated should experience a full or partial remission as the result of corticosteroid therapy, and that to achieve this a daily dose of 40–50 mg of prednisone (or prednisolone or methylprednisolone), or 200–300 mg of cortisone, was usually sufficient. He also stated that many observers had recommended that up to 100 units of ACTH should be given daily initially. In very ill patients up to 200 mg of prednisone could be given for brief periods. Jandl concluded that approximately one-third of patients should achieve sustained remissions on withdrawal of the corticosteroids; one-third would need long-term treatment and one-third might require other forms of treatment.

Allgood and Chaplin (1967), who reviewed the responses of 44 patients with idiopathic AIHA who had been treated with corticosteroids between 1955 and 1965, recommended an initial dosage of 60–100 mg of prednisone per day maintained for 1–3 weeks. After maximum benefit the dose was to be tapered down to 10 mg per day. If the patient did not respond, or if he or

Table 35.1 Effect of treatment in idiopathic warm-antibody AIHA.

Treatment	No. of patients	Effect of treatment				Direct antiglobulin test in patients clinically cured	
		Clinical cure	Compensated haemolysis	Uncompensated haemolysis*	Deaths	Still positive	Negative
None or transfusion only	1	0	0	1	1 (100%)	...	...
Steroids ± transfusion	23	3	14	6	9 (39%)	1	2
Splenectomy ± transfusion	13	7	1	5	6 (46%)	2	5
Splenectomy + steroids ± transfusion	13	0	7	6	7† (54%)	...	...
Total no. of patients	50	10	22	18	23 (46%)	3	7

The figures refer to the number of patients in each catergory; . . . denotes no observation.
*Includes patients who died with uncompensated haemolysis.
†Includes three patients who died post-operatively.

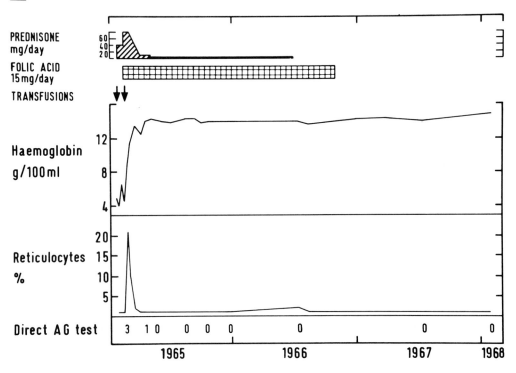

Fig. 35.4   Haematological response of a 15-year-old woman with warm-antibody AIHA to treatment with prednisone, supplemented with folic acid.

Her case is unusual in that all abnormal serological signs had disappeared within 5 months. She subsequently remained in complete remission for at least $2\frac{1}{2}$ years. [Reproduced by permission from Dacie and Worlledge (1969).]

she relapsed while the dosage was being reduced, splenectomy was considered. Eighty-four per cent of their patients had responded partially or completely to this regime, but only 16% remained in remission when no longer on steroids.

Eyster and Jenkins (1969) summarized the results of treating with corticosteroids 37 patients with idiopathic or secondary warm-antibody AIHA. Twenty-seven of the patients had responded satisfactorily to daily dosages of 40–100 mg of prednisone or its equivalent. There appeared to be no real differences in the initial responses of the patients who had suffered from the idiopathic or secondary type of disease.

Pirofsky and Bardana (1974) reported on their personal experience of 150 adequately treated patients suffering from idiopathic or secondary AIHA. The overall response rate was 53%, but 76% of the patients with idiopathic AIHA had responded. In relation to drug dosages, they suggested that 300 mg of cortisone were equivalent to 240 mg of hydrocortisone, to 60 mg of prednisone, to 48 mg of triamcinolone or to 9 mg of dexamethasone. They thought that there was no advantage to be gained by administering ACTH. They

suggested that 60 mg of prednisone was about the right initial dosage and that there was no advantage in giving higher doses. In their experience the patients responded within 2–28 days of starting treatment: the median was 7 days and in only six patients was their response delayed for more than 14 days. Stabilization of haemoglobin (at normal or subnormal levels) was achieved in 30–90 days as a rule. Long-term therapy with 20 mg or more of prednisone was considered to be unwise.

Petz and Garratty (1980) concluded that prednisone was the corticosteroid drug of choice and that there was no clear advantage in using ACTH. They recommended a daily dose of 60–80 mg of prednisone (for an adult) as initial treatment and that this dosage should normally be maintained for 3 weeks. Eighty per cent of patients should respond; lack of response by 3 weeks was equated with failure. At the end of the initial 3 weeks of treatment, they recommended in patients who had responded that the dose of prednisone should be reduced by 10–15 mg weekly until the daily dose was 30 mg. Then the dose should be reduced by 5 mg each week until 15 mg a day was reached; thereafter the dose should be reduced by 2.5 mg each week. If small doses of prednisone were required to maintain remission, they should not exceed 15 mg a day; if more was required, other forms of treatment should be considered. Petz and Garratty considered that there was possibly some advantage, in maintenance treatment, in giving the drug every alternate day rather than daily.

Zupańska, Sylwestrowicz and Pawelski (1981) reviewed the results of treating 97 patients with AIHA (41 idiopathic, 56 secondary). Eighty of these patients received 60–80 mg of prednisone as initial treatment and 55 of them (68.6%) responded favourably. However, in only 28 of them (35%) was the improvement sustained and long-lasting; the remaining patients needed additional or alternative treatment because of intolerance or complications of corticosteroid therapy or an inadequate response.

Worlledge (1982) recommended that adults suffering from overt haemolysis should receive oral doses of 40–100 mg of prednisone or prednisolone daily and children proportionately lower dosages. Very severely ill patients should be treated initially with intravenous infusions of hydrocortisone, 100 mg being given every 6 hours. According to Worlledge, based on her experience at the Royal Postgraduate Medical School in London, 90% of patients so treated show signs of response within 3 weeks. As haemolysis lessens, and the haemoglobin rises and the reticulocyte count falls, she recommended that the prednisone dosage should be reduced to 10–20 mg daily. This dosage should be continued for a minimum of 3–4 months, even if the haemoglobin and reticulocyte count had returned to normal. Most patients, in her experience, needed treatment for much longer than this, and then a regime of alternate day administration was often useful, particularly in children, in mitigating the harmful effects of the prolonged administration of corticosteroids.

Rosse (1990, p. 441) dealt with AIHA and ITP together when considering corticosteroid therapy. He recommended high doses of prednisone, 1–2 mg/kg per day in adults, at the start of treatment, and that the dose be reduced to 60 mg daily 1 week after a normal count (of erythrocytes or platelets) had been achieved. The dose should then be reduced by 10 mg steps every week until 20 mg a day was being given, a dosage which should be maintained for 1 month. Then the dose should be reduced to 10–15 mg per day or less, preferably given on alternate days. Ultimately, the aim should be to reduce the dose to zero by steps of 2.5–5.0 mg in the dose given on alternate days, maintaining each dose for 1 month before reducing it further. Once a minimum necessary dose had been established, this should be maintained for at least 6 months or, if the DAT was still positive, for longer than this. In a pertinent comment Rosse remarked that 'more patients suffer from the effects of too much glucocorticoid steroids than too little'.

The results of treating patients suffering from warm-antibody AIHA with corticosteroids, which have been summarized in the preceding paragraphs, indicate without any doubt that prednisone and prednisolone are most valuable first-line drugs and that, if given in sufficient dosage, 80–90% of patients achieve worthwhile remissions. They are, however, potentially dangerous drugs, and for that reason the large doses that are often required to achieve initial responses, e.g. up to 100 mg daily orally, should be given for as short a period of time as possible— certainly for not more than 3 weeks. What to do next, if the patient has failed to respond to high doses of the corticosteroids, or has only partially responded and has to be maintained for long periods on dosages of prednisone of 20–30 mg daily, is considered on p. 496 under 'Practical management of patients . . .'.

EFFECT OF ACTH OR CORTICOSTEROIDS ON HAEMATOLOGICAL AND SEROLOGICAL FINDINGS

Clinical and haematological benefit from steroid therapy usually takes place, if it is going to occur, within a week; it may be obvious within 5 days. The first haematological signs are usually a rise in reticulocyte count and in total leucocyte count. A day or so later the erythrocyte count and haemoglobin start to rise and thereafter recovery may be spectacular (Figs. 35.1 and 35.2).

As observed when ACTH was first used as treatment, if a patient derives substantial clinical and haematological benefit from ACTH or corticosteroid therapy, this will be reflected in an improvement in the serological findings. The DAT will become less strong and may even eventually become negative, and free antibody in the serum, if originally present, may disappear altogether. This is the general sequence of events in a successfully treated patient in whom complete or almost complete remission has been produced. In patients, however, who derive minor but perhaps nevertheless clinically important benefit, the serological findings—in particular the DAT—may appear unaltered.

Evans (1955) mentioned the results of treatment in seven patients; in one the DAT became negative; in six it was less strong, and in three patients antibody free in the serum disappeared.

Dameshek and Komninos's (1956) series of patients was larger. Twenty-three patients with idiopathic or secondary AIHA were studied intensively. The DAT titre and strength of agglutination lessened in 16 and in two other patients the test became negative, in one permanently; in five patients the strength of the reaction was apparently unaltered despite clinical and haematological benefit. Nineteen patients had warm auto-antibodies demonstrable at 37°C by the albumin or trypsinized-cell technique; these antibodies disappeared in eight and there was a fall in titre in the remainder.

Pisciotta and Hinz (1957), reporting on 33 patients with idiopathic or secondary AIHA, noted a diminution of the strength of the DAT in most of them but a permanently negative reaction only twice. Letman (1957) reported good accord between the strength of the DAT and the intensity of the haemolytic process in seven out of 11 patients.

The favourable effect on the DAT or a diminution in titre or disappearance of free auto-antibody from the serum of a successfully treated patient occurs relatively slowly and may not be discernible within the first week of treatment; therafter the response, if it occurs at all, is usually relatively rapid and should be well marked by the end of the second week. Kissmeyer-Nielsen's (1957) report of a reversal of the serological findings the day after treatment was started is exceptional and unexplained.

MODE OF ACTION OF ACTH AND CORTICOSTEROIDS

How ACTH and the corticosteroid drugs bring about remission in some patients suffering from AIHA (or other auto-immune diseases) has been the subject of considerable interest and research. In relation to AIHA, they appear to act in more than one way, namely, by diminishing the rate of auto-antibody formation, by interfering with the affinity of antibody for antigen, and by restraining macrophage activity.

Inhibition of antibody formation

Soon after the drugs were introduced it was noticed that in patients who were responding satisfactorily to treatment the strength of the DAT often diminished and the titre of auto-antibody free in the serum usually fell significantly. Thus, as mentioned above, Dameshek and Komninos in their 1956 review reported that the 'Coombs titer' and strength of agglutination diminished in 16 out of 23 patients, while in two additional patients the test became negative.

The results in many subsequent studies have been similar, and it seems clear that inhibition of antibody formation is one of the mechanisms that lead to remission in patients who respond favourably to corticosteroid therapy. How exactly the reduction in antibody formation is brought about is less clear. Rosse (1990) suggested that it is more likely that the effect is on cells controlling the production of antibody-producing cells rather than on the antibody-producing cells themselves.

Additional evidence suggesting inhibition of antibody production was forthcoming from early studies of serum globulin concentration in patients being treated with corticosteroids: a fall in the concentration of γ globulin was quite frequently reported, e.g. by Vaughan, Bayles and Favour (1950), Gardner et al. (1951), Saint and Gardner (1952) and Hansen (1952b).

Many studies were, too, carried out in the 1950s in experimental animals, particularly in rodents, which were injected with a variety of antigens with the aim of seeing whether corticosteroids would inhibit antibody formation or inhibit haemolysis. Most of the studies provided evidence in support of inhibition, e.g. those of de Vries (1950), Bjørneboe, Fischel and Stoerk (1951), Germuth, Oyama and Ottinger (1951), Berglund (1956) and Massei and Marinai (1956). In contrast, the studies of Clearkin (1952), Ecklebe and Sander (1952), Feldman and Rachmilewitz (1954) and Wasastjerna and Désy (1954) provided no evidence for inhibition of antibody formation or alleviation of haemolysis.

Kaliss, Hoecker and Bryant (1956) found that in mice cortisone inhibited the primary iso-agglutinin response to the inoculation of tumours but not the secondary response.

Kaplan and Jandl (1961) reported that cortisone inhibited the hepatic sequestration of antibody-coated, and also of incubated, rat erythrocytes, after a latent period of 2 days. Splenic sequestration was, however, not affected.

It seems likely that species and antigenic differences, and the way in which the experiments were carried out, influenced the outcome of the experiments quoted above.

In the spontaneously occurring AIHA of NZB/BL mice the administration of the corticosteroid betamethasone led to the DAT becoming weaker or negative and a fall in the titre of free antibody in serum (Casey and Howie, 1965).

Alteration in affinity of antibody for antigen

The concept that one of the ways that corticosteroids benefit patients with AIHA might be an effect on the affinity of antibody for antigen seems to stem from the observations of Davidsohn and Spurrier (1954). They gave details of two patients responding to treatment with cortisone in whom the Coombs test became negative before the

disappearance of free antibodies in the serum. They stated that in several other patients the administration of corticotropin or cortisone had had a similar effect on the Coombs test and suggested that 'at least in hemolytic anemia, these hormonal substances influence the union of the antigen with the antibody before the antibody production is affected'.

Rosse (1971), in an elegant and important study, estimated the amount of erythrocyte-bound antibody by measuring the fixation of complement component C1 in a series of patients with AIHA. This enabled him to relate quantitatively the changes in cell-bound and serum antibody resulting from the administration of prednisone. Erythrocyte mean life-span was measured at the same time by the CO excretion method. Fifteen patients were treated with daily doses of 60 mg of prednisone. In 10 of them the

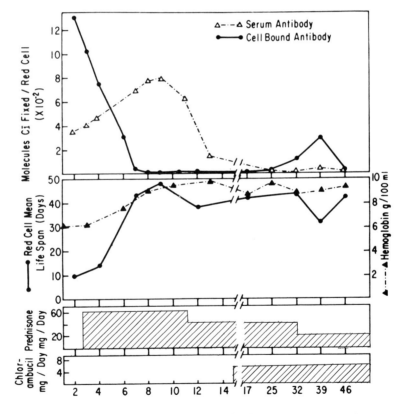

Fig. 35.5   Changes in erythrocyte-bound IgG warm auto-antibody and antibody concentration in serum, haemoglobin concentration and mean erythrocyte life-span, following the administration of prednisone to a 62-year-old man who had AIHA and chronic lymphocytic leukaemia.
[Reproduced by permission from Rosse (1971).]

amount of antibody detectable on their erythrocytes fell rapidly and in eight of them this was accompanied by a rise in the amount of serum antibody (Fig. 35.5). The erythrocyte life-span increased as the amount of antibody in the serum decreased. In one patient the amount of antibody on the cells increased and that in the serum decreased when the dose of prednisone was reduced from 60 mg per day; this relationship was reversed when the dose of prednisone was raised to 60 mg.

How corticosteroids could influence antibody–antigen interaction is unclear. Cregar, Tulley and Hansen (1956) reported that hydrocortisone reversed *in vitro* the accelerated electrophoretic velocity of antibody-coated erythrocytes by, it was suggested, altering the electrical nature of the bond between cell and antibody.

Interference with erythrocyte–macrophage interaction

Evidence is now available which indicates that corticosteroids are able to inhibit the interaction between antibody-sensitized erythrocytes and macrophages.

Packer, Greendyke and Swisher (1960) showed that the ability of normal leucocytes to phagocytose human erythrocytes sensitized by anti-A could be inhibited to a greater or lesser extent by the addition of various corticosteroid compounds to the test suspensions. They were also able to show that the leucocytes recovered from patients receiving steroid drugs were much less active in phagocytosis than cells from normal donors. In one AIHA patient this was demonstrable 24 hours after the administration of 45 mg of prednisone.

Further details of the effects of the administration of ACTH and corticosteroids on the phagocytosis of anti-A-sensitized erythrocytes were given by Greendyke et al. (1965). They confirmed that the oral administration of prednisone or the intravenous infusion of ACTH or cortisol led to significant reductions in the ability of the recipient's leucocytes (neutrophils and monocytes) to phagocytose erythrocytes opsonized by a complement-fixing anti-A antibody. *In vitro*, depression of phagocytic activity could be demonstrated, too, by the addition of glucocorticoids to the test suspensions, but only if the additives were present in grossly unphysiological concentrations. It is interesting to note that Greendyke et al. found consistent significant differences between the leucocytes of individual donors in their ability to act as erythrophages.

Atkinson, Schreiber and Frank (1973) described in an important paper how they had studied the effect of corticosteroids and splenectomy on the in-vivo survival of guinea-pig erythrocytes which had been sensitized with purified rabbit IgG or IgM anti-guinea-pig erythrocyte antibody. The erythrocytes were labelled with ^{51}Cr and the participation of the spleen and liver in their destruction was assessed by surface counting. As expected, IgM-coated cells were rapidly sequestered in the liver and a proportion was then more slowly released into the circulation, while IgG-coated cells were sequestered predominantly in the spleen. It was shown, too, with both classes of antibody that the extent of sequestration was proportional to the degree to which the cells had been coated with the antibodies, as determined by the C1a fixation and transfer test. Giving guinea-pigs daily injections of cortisone acetate increased the survival of cells sensitized by either type of antibody and reduced their sequestration in the liver and spleen, respectively. Five days' treatment with cortisone prior to the administration of the sensitized cells was required for a maximum effect. The cortisone-treated animals appeared to have a lowered sensitivity to erythrocytes coated with antibody and complement, which were in consequence dealt with as if they had been coated with fewer antibody molecules. With heavily sensitized cells the beneficial effect of the standard dose of cortisone was less marked.

Atkinson and Frank (1974) described further significant experiments. The survival of guinea-pig erythrocytes sensitized with rabbit anti-guinea-pig erythrocyte serum was studied in both normal guinea-pig and in animals congenitally deficient in complement component 4 (C4-deficient guinea-pigs). (In the latter animals immune clearance has to be complement-independent.) In the C4-deficient animals at a low level of sensitization cortisone completely prevented the splenic sequestration of IgG-sensitized cells, but as the degree of sensitization was increased more cortisone was required to decrease the rate and magnitude of clearance. Eventually, a degree of sensitization was reached at which cortisone failed to influence clearance. The effect of cortisone was discernible after 3 days treatment but did not become maximal until 5–7 days. Atkinson and Frank concluded that cortisone was not affecting the affinity between antibody and antigen on the erythrocyte membrane. They considered that it was more likely that it affected the interaction between the IgG on the erythrocyte and its receptor on the macrophages of the spleen and liver; they drew attention to the parallelism between their experimental system and warm-antibody AIHA in man in which the most common type of auto-antibody is a non-complement-fixing IgG globulin and inferred that the major mechanism by which corticosteroids benefit human patients is by decreasing complement-independent erythrocyte clearance.

At an NIH conference, Frank (1977), with Schreiber, Atkinson and Jaffe acting as discussants, gave a comprehensive account of current perceptions as to why, how and where antibody and complement-coated erythrocytes are destroyed *in vivo* and the effect that the class of antibody — IgG or IgM — has on the outcome. The results of their work with guinea-pigs (described above), and the conclusions they had reached, were described in detail. In relation to the effect of glucocorticoid therapy they stated that 'Our overall impression from these studies [in guinea-pigs] was that a primary action of glucocorticoid therapy is to decrease erythrocyte clearance'. The glucocorticoids had been most effective in reducing the clearance of IgG-coated cells, moderately effective in the case of IgG plus complement-coated cells and least effective in the case of IgM plus complement-coated cells. In human AIHA, Frank et al. reiterated that the drugs were most effective in warm-antibody cases in which the erythrocytes are coated with IgG and not with C3; they are least effective in CHAD in which the cells are coated with IgM and C3. They suggested, however, that high steroid dosage might be helpful in some CHAD patients.

Possibility of bone-marrow stimulation

The fact that an early sign that a patient with AIHA is responding to AIHA or corticosteroid therapy is a rise in reticulocyte count (Fig. 35.1 p. 456) led to the suggestion that large doses of the hormones act as marrow stimulants (Tischendorf, Ecklebe and Thofern, 1951–1952; Hudson, Herdan and Yoffey, 1952; Heilmeyer, 1952; Thorn et al., 1953). Baikie and Pirrie (1958), working with guinea-pigs in which they had induced hetero-immune haemolytic anaemia, also noted a rise in reticulocyte count when ACTH was administered. However, they considered that this was unlikely to be due to marrow stimulation and suggested premature release from the marrow or a delay in maturation of the reticulocytes as the explanation. They observed, too, that the presence of the spleen appeared to be necessary for the response, as this was not seen in splenectomized animals. To what extent ACTH and corticosteroids act as genuine marrow stimulants remains uncertain; it seems likely that, at the most, marrow stimulation probably plays only a minor part in patients' responses.

IMMUNOSUPPRESSIVE ALKYLATING AND ANTI-METABOLITE DRUGS AS TREATMENT FOR WARM-ANTIBODY AIHA

The anti-mitotic and anti-metabolite drugs which became available in the 1950s provided physicians with a possible effective form of alternative treatment for AIHA patients who had failed to respond satisfactorily to treatment with ACTH or corticosteroids. It seemed possible that the drugs would act as immunosuppressive agents and that their use might be practicable despite the likelihood that they would depress haemopoiesis.

Nitrogen mustard

This was the first immunosuppressive agent used.

Dameshek (1951) reported on the effects of intravenous nitrogen mustard given to four patients in an attempt to reduce, by damaging their lymphoid tissue, the amount of auto-antibody formed. In one patient the treatment was followed by a fall in antibody titre, and although thrombocytopenia and leucopenia caused anxiety, the patient went on to a complete recovery and remained well for at least 2 years subsequently. Dameshek mentioned that urethane and radioactive gold had been tried but found to be ineffective. Meyers and his co-workers (1952) also treated one patient with nitrogen mustard but the only effect was marrow depression. Other patients, suffering from the idiopathic type of disease and treated with nitrogen mustard, were mentioned by Beikert (1957) and Borchers and Eymer (1959).

6-Mercaptopurine (6MP), 6-thioguanine (6TG) and azathioprine (Imuran)

With the synthesis of 6MP, 6TG and later azathioprine, the more dangerous nitrogen mustard was no longer used. Experimentally, 6MP was shown to be a potent inhibitor of antibody formation by Schwartz, Stack and Dameshek (1958) and Schwartz, Eisner and Dameshek (1959). They showed (in rabbits) that the anti-metabolite could block completely the primary response to a purified protein antigen (human serum albumin); it had, however, only a minimal effect on the secondary response. In man, Dameshek and Schwartz (1960) found, however, that both 6MP and 6TG could be of considerable benefit. They described the results of treating six patients: three enjoyed complete remissions (Fig. 35.6), the fourth a partial remission, the fifth improved but there was no follow-up and the sixth died. In three patients remission or improvement lasted at least 3 months after treatment was terminated. In some patients the

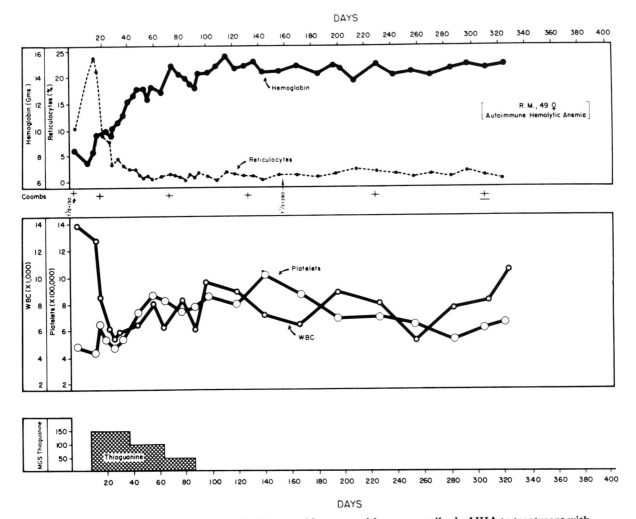

Fig. 35.6 **Haematological response of a 49-year-old woman with warm-antibody AIHA to treatment with thioguanine.**
[Reproduced by permission from Schwartz and Dameshek (1962).]

drugs tended to produce nausea or vomiting and diarrhoea, but these symptoms usually could be controlled by reducing the dosage.

Dameshek and Schwartz also reported success in treating patients with SLE with the same drugs; they stressed that they might be particularly valuable in patients of both groups intolerant of steroids or in whom such large doses of steroids had to be given that side-effects were serious.

Both 6MP and 6TG depress haemopoiesis. Two out of Dameshek and Schwartz's six patients developed leucopenia and a third patient thrombocytopenia, and in two patients megaloblastic change in the bone marrow was noted.

Since this early report, many patients have been treated with anti-metabolites, particularly azathioprine (Imuran), and the drugs have established themselves as valuable second-line agents useful in patients who respond poorly to corticosteroid therapy or experience potentially dangerous side-effects. Their role *vis-à-vis* splenectomy as the next treatment to be tried in such patients is discussed on. p. 496.

Some more recent reports on the use of immunosuppressive agents are summarized below.

Schwartz and Dameshek (1962) reported on the responses of 14 AIHA patients: 10 appeared to have idiopathic AIHA; three had SLE and one chronic lymphocytic leukaemia. Nine of these patients responded to treatment with 6-MP or thioguanine; five failed to respond. Of the responders, three required combined anti-metabolite–corticosteroid treatment or eventually needed to be sustained on small doses of corticosteroids; the other six achieved excellent remissions without the help of corticosteroids. Eight patients experienced unwanted side-effects: five suffered from (mainly mild) nausea or anorexia; three developed leucopenia, one thrombocytopenia and one megaloblastic change in the bone marrow.

Jandl (1963), in a brief review of current concepts of therapy, concluded that many AIHA patients receiving 6-MP or thioguanine would achieve gradual remissions; he stressed, however, that the drugs were potentially toxic to the gastro-intestinal tract and the bone marrow and advised that they should be kept in reserve for patients who did not respond to corticosteroids.

Richmond and his co-workers (1963) described in detail the history of a 28-year-old woman with severe Evans syndrome. She had relapsed with severe thrombocytopenia and auto-immune haemolysis, having almost 6 years before responded successfully to splenectomy for ITP. On her readmission she failed to respond to corticosteroid therapy and needed numerous blood transfusions (42 litres of blood given within 6 weeks). Irradiation to the thymus resulted in temporary improvement, but a second course of irradiation was ineffective. Eventually she responded to treatment with Imuran and actinomycin-C. These dramatic events are illustrated in Fig. 35.7a and b.

Taylor (1963) described a patient, a man aged 67, seriously ill with AIHA who had relapsed after prednisone therapy and had only responded partially to splenectomy. He was then treated successively with triethylenemelamine (TEM), chloramphenicol and cyclophosphamide on and off for the next 6 years, obtaining some benefit after each course of treatment.

Corley, Lessner and Larsen (1966) reviewed the responses of 46 patients suffering from a variety of auto-immune disorders to treatment with azathioprine. Six of these patients had had AIHA: of the four who had received adequate treatment, three had failed to improve, one, who had AIHA and chronic lymphocytic leukaemia, achieved a partial remission on azathioprine and prednisone. Based on their own experience and from a survey of the literature, Corley, Lessner and Larsen concluded that 15 out of 27 AIHA patients who had received anti-metabolite therapy had responded favourably.

Hitzig and Massimo (1966) reported that they had treated three children with azathioprine. They were aged between 3 and 5 years and suffered from chronic AIHA. They had previously responded only partially and temporarily to corticosteroids. Azathioprine was administered at a dosage of between 2 and 5 mg/kg per day: one child responded well and was apparently completely cured; the other two children were significantly improved and could subsequently be maintained on much smaller doses of corticosteroids.

Worlledge and her co-workers (1968) described the results of treating six AIHA patients with azathioprine at a dosage of 100–200 mg per day. One patient had SLE and one thrombocytopenia; all six were treated for a minimum of 6 months. Three patients responded well and this allowed the corticosteroid dosage to be reduced or discontinued; two patients were not benefited by up to 9 and 7 months treatment, respectively, and the anaemia of one patient worsened, perhaps as the result of a reduction in corticosteroid dosage. None of the patients became significantly leucopenic or thrombocytopenic; in two, however, the serum IgM concentration fell and in one that of IgA (Fig. 35.8).

Skinner and Schwartz (1972), in a review of the

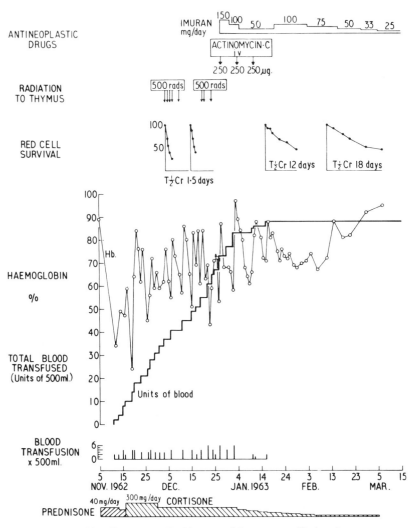

Fig. 35.7a and b   Response of a 34-year-old woman suffering from severe relapsing Evans syndrome to treatment with corticosteroids, irradiation of the thymus, actinomycin C and Imuran.

Splenectomy had been carried out 6 years earlier. [Reproduced by permission from Richmond et al. (1963).]

results of the treatment of AIHA with immunosuppressive drugs, cited 42 AIHA patients described in the literature. Most had been treated with azathioprine and corticosteroids and many had undergone splenectomy before the treatment with azathioprine was started. All had failed to respond adequately to corticosteroids. Twenty of the 42 patients had been reported to have been benefited by the immunosuppressive drugs. Skinner and Schwartz referred to the use of such drugs as a 'rearguard action', implying that they should be used only if treatment with corticosteroids or splenectomy had failed.

Cytotoxic drugs in the treatment of non-malignant diseases were the subject of an NIH conference (Steinberg et al., 1972). The report included a useful general discussion of the drugs then available and their therapeutic uses, side-effects and mechanisms of action. The discussion was not primarily concerned with AIHA.

Habibi and co-workers (1974) reported on the results of treating with azathioprine 13 children suffering from chronic AIHA. Of the seven children who had received regular and sufficient doses for at least 4 months, four had benefited: they had been generally improved and haemolysis had been well compensated on reduced dosages of corticosteroids.

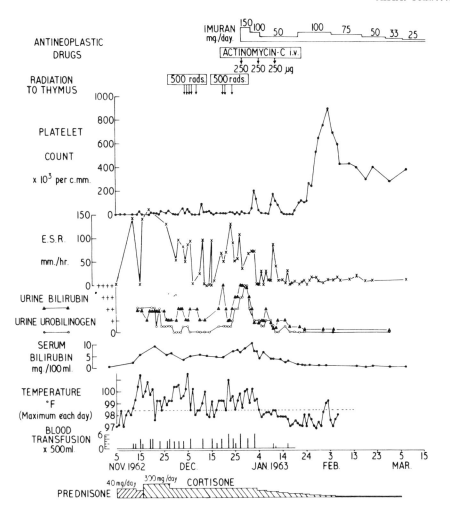

Fig. 35.7b

Pirofsky and Bardana (1974), in a review, referred to nine personally treated AIHA patients who had not responded to corticosteroids. Five of them had experienced remissions on 2.0–2.5 mg of azathioprine per kg after 10 days or more of treatment. Pirofsky and Bardana recommended that if there was no sign of response within 4 weeks of treatment, the daily dose of azathioprine should be increased tentatively by 25 mg every 1–2 weeks until the patient had either responded or there were signs of bone-marrow depression.

Johnson and Abildgaard (1976) reviewed the response of children to anti-metabolite therapy. According to this review, nine out of 17 children had responded favourably.

Murphy and LoBuglio (1976), in a review of the status of immunosuppressive therapy for AIHA, summarized their current recommendations. For the treatment of the 30–40% of the patients who were unable to achieve long-term remissions on corticos-

teroids or were intolerant of the drugs, they recommended splenectomy for those patients considered to be good candidates for the operation, followed by cytotoxic therapy if the splenectomy proved to be a failure. For patients for whom for any reason, such as age, splenectomy appeared to be contraindicated, they recommended cytotoxic therapy as soon as it became clear that corticosteroids were ineffective. Murphy and LoBuglio found it difficult to choose between azathioprine and cyclophosphamide as cytotoxic agents; they pointed out, however, that cyclophosphamide could cause haemorrhagic cystitis, alopecia and sterility. They recommended that either drug should be persisted in for up to 6 months, at the end of which time the alternative drug might be tried if the patient had not responded. They recommended, too, that if the patient relapsed after a good response to a cytotoxic drug, corticosteroids should be tried again before reverting once more to the cytotoxic drug.

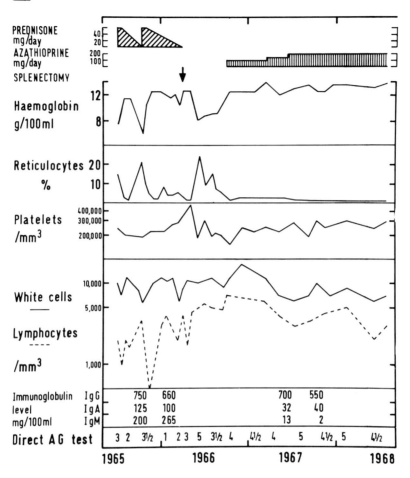

Fig. 35.8   Haematological and serological responses of a 58-year-old man with warm-antibody AIHA to treatment with azathioprine.
He had failed to respond to splenectomy, and prednisone had to be discontinued because of mental depression and a possible peptic ulcer. The azathioprine therapy was followed by a fall in serum IgA and IgM concentration. [Reproduced by permission from Dacie and Worlledge (1969).]

Petz and Garratty (1980) reviewed past experience in the use of immunosuppressive drugs and discussed the pros and cons. They concluded that the drugs had a definite place in therapy, but stressed the not infrequent occurrence of adverse side-effects: they mentioned infection with common or not so common (exotic) organisms—some not normally pathogenic, potential teratogenicity—hence the importance of not using the drugs in pregnancy, the development of malignancies, and sterility.

Zupańska, Sylwestrowicz and Pawelski (1981) reported that of 80 idiopathic and secondary AIHA patients originally treated with prednisone, 43 needed additional treatment with azathioprine or cyclophosphamide: 26 of them (60.5%) responded favourably.

Worlledge (1982), in her last review, summarized her experience of the use of azathioprine as follows: 15 patients had been treated for $3\frac{1}{2}$ months to $2\frac{1}{2}$ years; six patients had responded well, two had responded partially, and six had failed to respond. One patient presented with signs of Hodgkin's disease after $2\frac{1}{2}$ years of treatment; one patient developed leucopenia; none of them became thrombocytopenic.

Heisel and Ortega (1983) reported that seven children with chronic AIHA who were steroid-dependent had been treated with immunosuppressive drugs: only one had achieved a complete remission.

Gibson (1988), in his review, referred to immunosuppressive therapy as an attractive option to splenectomy: in support of this view he listed the patients' variable responses to splenectomy, the relatively advanced ages of many of the patients and the potential complications of the operation. He concluded that cyclophosphamide and azathioprine were likely to be at least partially effective in up to two-thirds of patients who were resistant to splenectomy, but warned of the possibility of unwanted complications.

Immunosuppressive drugs as treatment for AIHA in NZB mice

NZB mice have been used as experimental models in relation to therapy with immunosuppressive drugs and some interesting data relative to human AIHA have been obtained.

Denman, Denman and Holborow (1967) reported that treating the mice from an early age with anti-lymphocyte globulin (ALG) suppressed the development of haemolytic anaemia but it did not, on the other hand, seem capable of influencing the disease once it had become established. They concluded that the results of their experiments argued against ALG being of any benefit to human patients suffering from overt AIHA.

Casey (1968) experimented with 6MP. It was found that when the drug was administered to mice just before AIHA was expected to develop it failed to delay or modify the development of the auto-antibodies or anaemia. Moreover, anaemic mice were found to tolerate the drug poorly: they became more anaemic and the strength of the DAT was unaltered. Casey recommended in consequence that 6MP should be used with caution in human AIHA.

Lemmel, Hurd and Ziff (1971) compared the effects of 6MP and cyclophosphamide when administered to NZB mice. Cyclophosphamide was found to delay the onset of DAT positivity a..u to decrease the strength of the DAT when it became positive. 6MP failed to do this, in confirmation of Casey's (1968) findings. The administration of 6MP resulted in a fall in the peripheral-blood levels of neutrophils, monocytes and large lymphocytes; cyclophosphamide mainly decreased the numbers of small and medium-sized lymphocytes. Cyclophosphamide decreased the intensity of immunofluorescent staining of γ globulin in the mice's kidneys; 6MP failed to do this. Lemmel, Hurd and Ziff concluded that cyclophosphamide was the 'preferable drug where suppression of ongoing cellular and humoral immune reactions is desirable'.

SPLENECTOMY AS TREATMENT FOR WARM-ANTIBODY AIHA

Early results

The beneficial effect of splenectomy in acquired haemolytic anaemia seems to have been reported for the first time by Micheli in 1911. Other favourable accounts soon followed, e.g. those of Antonelli (1913) and Nobel and Steinebach (1914), and by 1940 Dameshek and Schwartz were able to collect together reports of 23 patients suffering from the acute form of the disease (including four patients of their own), 20 of whom had responded favourably to the operation. Later, Dameshek (1943) reported good results in 10 out of 18 personally studied patients.

Subacute and chronic cases were also reported to have benefited greatly from splenectomy. According to Welch and Dameshek (1950), who reviewed 34 cases of idiopathic acquired haemolytic anaemia, splenectomy had been followed by remission in approximately 50% of the patients. Rather similar results based on smaller series of patients were published by

others, e.g. by Stickney and Heck (1948), Robson (1949), Dreyfus, Dausset and Vidal (1951), de Gruchy (1954), Dameshek and Komninos (1956), Stickney and Hanlon (1956), Beikert (1957), Cameron et al. (1957), Krauss, Heilmeyer and Weinreich (1959a,b) and Jamra et al. (1962).

Dausset and Malinvaud (1954) reported on 14 cases: the results were not particularly satisfactory; rapid cure in two patients, clinical cure in four, transient improvement in five and three post-operative deaths.

Dacie and Chertkow (1955) and Chertkow and Dacie (1956) described the effect of splenectomy in 21 patients with idiopathic AIHA. The results were classified as good in four patients, fair in eight, poor in six and doubtful in three. No reliable clinical, haematological or serological data were found which could be used to predict the results of splenectomy beforehand, but it did seem that the chances of success might be worse in the younger patients, in those most severely anaemic, in the presence of thrombocytopenia or in patients who had relatively small spleens.

Crosby and Rappaport (1957), in their review of 57 cases of AIHA, referred to 27 patients with the idiopathic disease who had undergone splenectomy. There had been 10 good responses, seven fair and one poor, and eleven patients had died, two in the immediate post-operative period. Of the 10 patients whose responses had been rated good on the basis of an immediate improvement leading to disappearance of anaemia and reticulocytosis during follow-up, five had suffered from active haemolysis for at least the 9 months preceding splenectomy. Of the patients who had died, this had in some of them been due to causes unrelated to AIHA, but most had died from crises associated with their illness.

Eighteen of Young, Miller and Swisher's (1957) patients were submitted to splenectomy; approximately two-thirds did well.

Dausset and Colombani (1959) reported on 31 patients; eight recovered, twelve died and the disease was stated to be 'in progress' in eleven.

Some unusual case reports

Loeb, Seaman and Moore (1952) described in detail the clinical course of a woman aged 69 with chronic warm-antibody AIHA (Evans syndrome) who had failed to respond satisfactorily to splenectomy and ACTH and cortisone therapy. The presence of an accessary spleen was localized by the use of thorium dioxide (Thorotrast). Laparotomy was carried out and a 2 × 3 cm nodule of splenic tissue was removed from the retroperitoneal region near the pancreas. Her recovery from the operation was uneventful and she remained perfectly well for the next 8 months. Then she suddenly developed the signs of severe thrombocytopenic purpura, the platelet count falling to $15 \times 10^9/l$. Fortunately she responded well to treatment with ACTH and cortisone.

Eisemann and Dameshek (1954) described a 58-year-old woman with chronic severe anaemia and thrombophlebitis, for which she had received many transfusions. There was a profound reticulocytopenia and an almost complete absence of erythroblasts from the bone marrow. The DAT was positive (++). After 10 months of aregenerative anaemia splenectomy was carried out. The spleen weighed 600 g; histologically there was general hyperplasia. Eighteen days after splenectomy reticulocytes appeared in the peripheral blood. No further transfusions were required and the patient eventually recovered. The DAT remained positive but weaker.

Horeau and co-workers (1962) described a 22-year-old woman with severe AIHA who achieved a brief but short-lived remission as the result of corticosteroid therapy. She then suffered intense left-sided abdominal pain, brought about it was thought as the result of massive splenic infarction. She was too ill for laparotomy, but suprisingly improved within a few days markedly spontaneously. Splenectomy was then undertaken and an infarcted spleen removed. Horeau et al. suggested that the in-vivo infarction had, in fact, been responsible for her spontaneous improvement.

The present author's experience (Dacie, 1962, p. 693), based on the results of splenectomy in the late 1940s and throughout the 1950s is incorporated in Table 35.1. Amongst the 50 patients suffering from idiopathic AIHA referred to were some who were extremely ill at a time before corticosteroids were available. Twenty-six of them had undergone splenectomy; thirteen of these had been treated with corticosteroids, thirteen had not. The mortality was high in both series—54% and 46%, respectively. Seven had been clinically cured by splenectomy and eight others had achieved compensation for haemolysis but had not been clinically cured. Splenectomy had been a failure in eleven, and there had been three post-operative deaths (Figs. 35.9–35.14).

More recent data

The results of splenectomy have been referred to in numerous reviews published during the last three decades. Some of the data are summarized below.

Goldberg, Hutchison and MacDonald (1966) reviewed the results taken from the literature of splenectomy in 182 unselected AIHA patients and reported that 95 of them (52%) had been improved. They tabulated data, too, on 21 of their own patients whose ^{51}Cr erythrocyte auto-survival had been measured before and after splenectomy. Eleven out of 13 patients who had idiopathic AIHA had done well; one had died 3 days post-operatively and one patient although improved required continuing treatment with corticosteroids. These 21 patients had raised spleen-to-liver ^{51}Cr surface-counting ratios, in all except two of them the ratio being greater than 2.3—the ratio which Goldberg, Hutchison and MacDonald

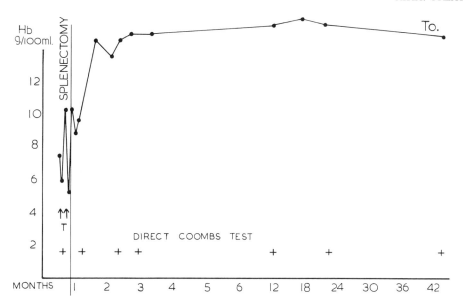

Fig. 35.9 A 'good' response to splenectomy by a patient with warm-antibody AIHA.
The patient remained in good health for more than 3 years after the operation. The DAT, however, remained positive. [Reproduced by permission from Chertkow and Dacie (1956).]

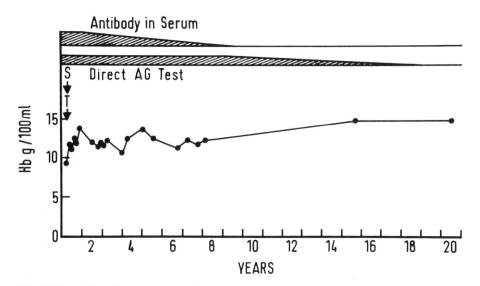

Fig. 35.10 A 'good' response to splenectomy.
The patient, a woman aged 47 when first diagnosed as suffering from warm-antibody AIHA, remained in good health for at least 20 years after splenectomy. The DAT remained positive for 18 years, but eventually became negative; the IAT became negative after 8 years (Case 9 of Dacie, 1954, p. 197).

considered as indicating that splenectomy was likely to be successful.

Allgood and Chaplin (1967), reviewed the clinical course of 44 patients with idiopathic AIHA whom they had treated between 1955 and 1965. Twenty-five of them had undergone

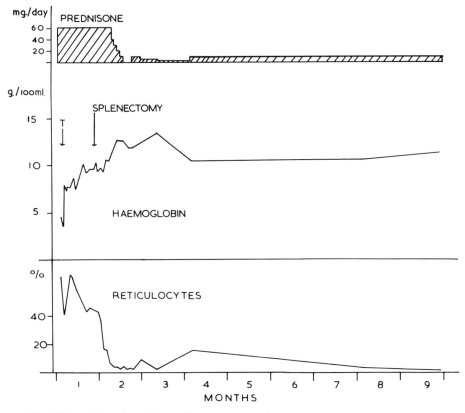

Fig. 35.11 A 'moderately good' response to splenectomy.
The patient was a woman aged 45. Splenectomy allowed her to be kept in remission on a greatly reduced daily dosage of prednisone (Case 12 of Dacie, 1962, p. 684).

splenectomy: 11 (44%) achieved complete remission and this persisted for at least 1 year (although in four of them the DAT remained positive); six (24%) went into remission but subsequently relapsed; one patient achieved a partial remission, and seven (28%) failed to respond. Eight patients died.

Mey and Hesse (1969) reported on the outcome of splenectomy in 38 patients with AIHA. The results were scored as good in 18 (47%), improved in 12 and as a failure in eight. May and Hesse concluded that although therapeutic remissions could not be taken for granted the operative risk of splenectomy was smaller than the danger inherent in the long-term use of immunosuppressive drugs.

Habibi and co-workers (1974) reported on the results of splenectomy in 16 children with chronic corticosteroid-resistant AIHA. Eight were

clinically cured, the DAT remaining positive in three; four were moderately improved, and the results in the remaining four could not be evaluated.

Pirofsky and Bardana (1974) in their review highlighted the then two opposing (rather extreme) views as to the value of splenectomy in AIHA—(1) that it neither cured the disease, nor affected the eventual outcome and (2) that it might induce remission in up to 75% of patients who failed to derive lasting benefit from corticosteroids. They considered that they themselves in the past had been too conservative in recommending splenectomy and not sufficiently appreciative of the deleterious side-effects of prolonged corticosteroid therapy.

Both Bowdler (1976) and Petz and Garratty (1980) discussed the effectiveness of splenectomy and listed in tables remission rates culled from the

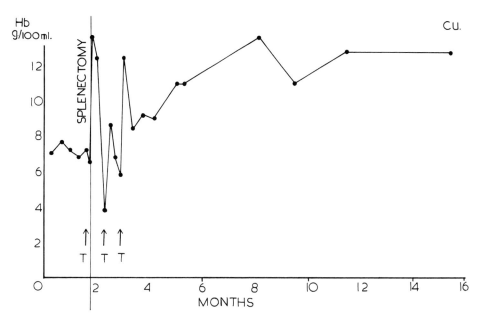

Fig. 35.12   A 'doubtful' response to splenectomy by a patient with warm-antibody AIHA.
The patient enjoyed a remission (? spontaneous) 2 months after the operation. [Reproduced by permission from Chertkow and Dacie (1956).]

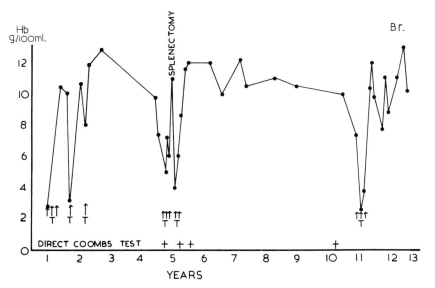

Fig. 35.13   A 'doubtful' response to splenectomy by a patient with warm-antibody AIHA.
The patient had had three haemolytic crises within a 13-year period. Recovery appeared to be spontaneous on possibly all three occasions. [Reproduced by permission from Chertkow and Dacie (1956).]

literature. Petz and Garratty quoted 20 sources reporting in all 316 splenectomies from which an average of 60% of the patients had derived benefit. The data listed by both Bowdler and Petz and Garratty illustrate the different authors' wide divergent experiences as to the effectiveness

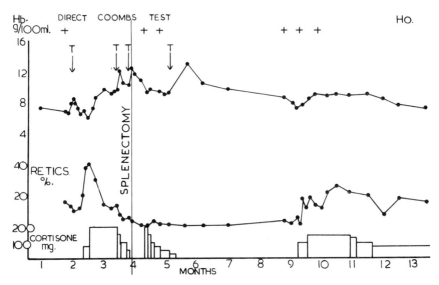

Fig. 35.14   A 'poor' response to splenectomy by a patient with warm-antibody AIHA.

[Reproduced by permission from Chertkow and Dacie (1956).]

of splenectomy—from being virtually ineffective to being successful in a high proportion of patients.

Zupańska, Sylwestrowicz and Pawelski (1981) reported that 21 of their 97 idiopathic and secondary AIHA patients had been splenectomized: excellent to good results followed in 13 (62%). Neither the spleen : liver ^{51}Cr ratio nor the weight of the spleen after its removal seemed to be of much help in predicting the long-term result of splenectomy. One particularly interesting patient was referred to who had enjoyed a 15-year-remission following splenectomy, only for this to be followed by several relapses during the next 13 years. The DAT had been weakly positive during the period of remission.

Gibson (1988), in a review, reported response rates of 30–85%, but added that the responses were often only partial. He added that splenectomy appeared to be in general less successful than in auto-immune thrombocytopenia; also that, in his view, attempts to predict results using ^{51}Cr have generally been unsuccessful.

The place of splenectomy *vis-à-vis* other possible treatments is further discussed on p. 496 under the heading 'Practical management of patients ...'.

Complications of splenectomy

As already referred to (p. 459), three of the author's 26 patients who had undergone splenectomy for AIHA in the late 1940s and 1950s had died of post-operative complications, and the mortality had been similar in other reported series of patients who had been operated on at about the same time. Dameshek and Schwartz (1940), for instance, reported four deaths in 10 cases, Crosby and Rappaport (1957) two deaths in 27 cases and Lorie and Patsiora (1958) five deaths in 21 cases. As after splenectomy for other reasons, evidence of thrombo-embolism is frequent at necropsies (Lorie and Patsiora, 1958; Krauss, Heilmeyer and Weinreich, 1959a,b). Another possible contributing cause of post-operative death is 'adrenal exhaustion' in patients who had been treated with high doses of corticosteroids for long periods of time prior to the operation. To combat this, Moeschlin (1956) recommended the administration of ACTH for 5–6 days prior to the operation and 150–200 mg of hydrocortisone by injection on the day of the operation, reducing the daily dose to 25 mg by the fourth post-operative day.

Occasionally, a patient submitted to splenectomy may subsequently show overt signs of systemic lupus erythematosus (SLE). This was true of two of Dameshek and Komninos's (1956) patients and one of Letman's (1957). SLE is well known sometimes to be accompanied by AIHA, and this may dominate the clinical picture, but whether splenectomy really hastens the progress of SLE or otherwise unmasks it is uncertain.

As described in Volume 1 of this book (p. 116), splenectomy in children seems to lead to an unusual susceptibility to infection subsequently. This has to be borne in mind when considering splenectomy as treatment for AIHA in infants and children. Heisel and Ortega's (1983) experience illustrates the danger: of five children with chronic AIHA submitted to splenectomy, three died of sepsis within 1 year of the operation.

ASSESSMENT OF THE SITES OF ERYTHROCYTE DESTRUCTION USING ^{51}Cr-LABELLED ERYTHROCYTES AS A GUIDE TO THE VALUE OF SPLENECTOMY

The availability of ^{51}Cr, a γ-ray emitter with a half-life of 27.8 days, and its use as a reliable method of labelling erythrocytes, has allowed in-vivo assessment of the relative importance of the spleen and liver as sites of erythrocyte destruction. It had been argued that an excess of radioactivity predominantly in the liver or in the liver as well as in the spleen would make a successful response to splenectomy less likely. The results of early studies in general supported this concept (Korst, Clatanoff and Schilling, 1955; Jandl et al., 1956; Hughes Jones and Szur, 1957; McCurdy and Rath, 1958; Fieschi, Pannacciulli and Tizianello, 1959; Lewis, Szur and Dacie, 1960; Gehrmann and Grobel, 1962; Veeger et al., 1962; Goldberg, Hutchison and MacDonald, 1966; Christensen et al., 1970; Szur, 1970; Habibi and Najean, 1971; Christensen, 1973; von dem Borne et al., 1973).

Jandl and co-workers (1956), in their early and wide-ranging demonstration of the use of ^{51}Cr-labelled erythrocytes in determining the sites of haemolysis in haemolytic anaemias, had included two patients with AIHA in the series of patients they had studied. The first patient had severe acute AIHA associated with auto-agglutination,

intravascular haemolysis and haemoglobinuria. When first investigated it was estimated that approximately 29% of her erythrocytes were being destroyed daily. This was accompanied by a massive uptake of ^{51}Cr by the spleen and also, to only a slightly lesser extent, by the liver. Three weeks later, when auto-agglutination and haemoglobinaemia had disappeared, a repeat study showed that the spleen alone accumulated ^{51}Cr. The second patient had a slightly less severe, but stable chronic haemolytic anaemia. Approximately 20% of the erythrocytes were estimated to be destroyed daily; the ^{51}Cr accumulated markedly in the spleen and only to a small extent in the liver. Jandl et al. concluded that when 'the short survival of labelled red cells in the circulation is accompanied by a progressive increase in radioactivity over the spleen the anemia is relieved by splenectomy'.

Lewis, Szur and Dacie (1960) had carried out surface counting after labelling with ^{51}Cr the erythrocytes of seven warm-antibody AIHA patients. All had a substantial excess of counts over the spleen and four had minor increases of counts over the liver (Fig. 35.15). The spleen: liver ratio was calculated to vary from 0.9 to 2.5. Only one of the patients underwent splenectomy. In her case there had been a substantial accumulation of ^{51}Cr in the spleen; she responded well to the operation. Lewis, Szur and Dacie had also carried out similar studies on patients suffering from cold-antibody AIHA. In two of them there were minor accumulations of radioactivity over both the spleen and the liver; in the third patient no excess counts over either organ were recorded (Fig. 34.7, p. 427).

Goldberg, Hutchison and MacDonald (1966) described the results of surface-counting studies in 13 patients with idiopathic AIHA (two with a negative DAT) who subsequently underwent splenectomy. In each case there was a considerable accumulation of ^{51}Cr in the spleen, and the spleen: liver ratio varied from 2.3 to 4.4. The result of splenectomy was assessed as successful in 11 of the patients; one patient, although improved, still required treatment with corticosteroids and one patient died of a post-operative complication.

Habibi and Najean (1971) reported on studies

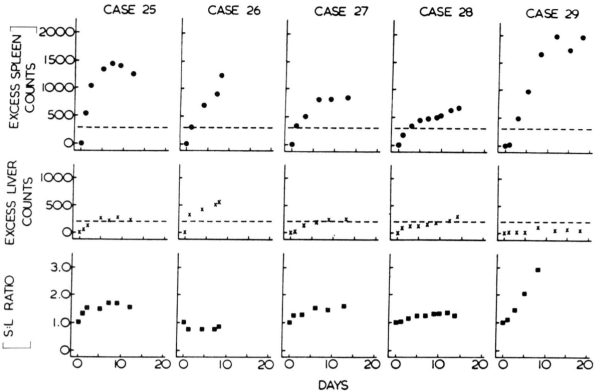

Fig. 35.15 **Surface-counting pattern in five patients with warm-antibody AIHA, after labelling their erythrocytes with ^{51}Cr.**

In each case radioactivity accumulated predominately in the spleen. [Reproduced by permission from Lewis, Szur and Dacie (1960).]

carried out on 37 idiopathic warm-antibody AIHA patients. In 14 of them splenic sequestration was described as 'importante' (with the spleen:liver ratio $\geqslant 2$, and in eight as 'prédominante' (spleen : liver ratio 1.4–1.9). Fourteen of these patients underwent splenectomy; 12 went into remission subsequently. In contrast, in 10 splenic sequestration was 'minime' (with the spleen : liver ratio $\leqslant 1.3$); only three went into complete and long-lasting remission.

Christensen (1973) reported on the pattern of ^{51}Cr accumulation in the spleen and liver in 25 patients, 16 of whom had idiopathic AIHA. Eleven underwent splenectomy. The pattern of accumulation appeared to depend on the intensity of haemolysis and on whether the patient had been treated with corticosteroids. When haemolysis was severe, excess radioactivity was demonstrable over the liver as well as over the spleen, while, after treatment with prednisone, splenic accumulation predominated. Christensen concluded that long-lasting remissions were likely to follow splenectomy carried out on patients in whom splenic accumulation predominated, but that remission was likely to be incomplete in the presence of a 'mixed' (splenic plus liver) accumulation. Of the 11 idiopathic AIHA patients actually subjected to splenectomy, three achieved complete remission—all three gave a splenic pattern of accumulation, seven a partial or temporary remission—two had given a splenic pattern and five a mixed pattern, and one patient, giving a mixed pattern, had failed to respond.

Other observers, while agreeing that ^{51}Cr surface-counting studies were useful in providing an index of the relative importance of the spleen and liver as sites of haemolysis, stressed that the correlation between the radioisotope findings and the actual result of splenectomy was not very close.

Heimpel and Schubothe (1964), who had studied 20 AIHA patients, concluded that while in more than half of them there was evidence of increased ^{51}Cr sequestration in the spleen, the distribution of radioactivity could not be associated with any particular serological or haematological finding. Seven of their patients were splenectomized; five achieved good remissions; in one the operation was a failure and in one the result was in doubt.

Ben-Bassat and co-workers (1967), who had studied 23 patients suffering from various types of haemolytic anaemia, similarly concluded that there was no relationship between ^{51}Cr accumulation in the spleen and any clinical or laboratory finding. They also stressed that surface measurements provided in reality only a very crude index of the accumulation of ^{51}Cr in the spleen: they emphasized the importance in relation to the measurement of radioactivity of the distance of the organ from the surface, its size, scattered radiation from outside the spleen and loss of ^{51}Cr from the spleen by elution. They concluded that patients should not be denied splenectomy simply because the in-vivo counting indices were negative.

Ahuja, Lewis and Szur (1972) reported on the results of splenectomy in 18 patients, including four who had suffered from idiopathic AIHA. All four of them accumulated ^{51}Cr in the spleen and two in the liver also. However, all four responded well or quite well to splenectomy and this was true, also, of 13 out of the 14 remaining patients in their series. Ahuja, Lewis and Szur concluded on the basis of their measurements that it was not possible to predict the *degree* of improvement likely to follow splenectomy on the basis of surface counting.

Parker, Macpherson and Richmond (1977) had carried out surface-counting tests in 12 patients who were subsequently subjected to splenectomy. While it was possible in the case of six patients to discontinue treatment with corticosteroids within 2 months of the operation, they concluded that the radioactivity measurements were not reliable indicators of the likely outcome of the operation. Thus, only three out of the five patients yielding the highest splenic uptakes of radioactivity responded; unexpectedly, however, three out of the five patients yielding the lowest splenic uptakes also responded.

A similar conclusion, namely that presplenectomy surface-counting studies provided only an unreliable indication of the results of splenectomy was reached by Ferrant et al. (1982). Amongst the patients they studied, 11 had suffered from warm-antibody AIHA of whom six had undergone splenectomy. Ferrant and his co-workers estimated the percentage erythrocyte destruction in both liver and spleen and calculated how much was taking place in other sites in the body. In their six AIHA patients who had undergone splenectomy, the spleen had been estimated to have been responsible for 28.4–60.4% of lysis and the liver 7.6–12.4% of lysis. All six patients responded well or partially to splenectomy, but the good and partial responders had not been distinguishable by the presplenectomy ^{51}Cr studies.

TREATMENT OF WARM-ANTIBODY AIHA PATIENTS WHO FAIL TO RESPOND TO CORTICOSTEROIDS, SPLENECTOMY AND IMMUNO-SUPPRESSIVE DRUGS

Severely ill patients suffering from warm-antibody AIHA who continue to haemolyse actively despite intensive therapy with corticosteroids and immunosuppressive drugs and who have undergone splenectomy (or for whom splenectomy has been considered too dangerous) present as serious clinical problems. Under the above circumstances a variety of drugs have been administered or procedures undertaken in a sometimes desperate attempt to keep the patient alive, with the hope that eventually he or she will recover spontaneously. Amongst possible remedies that were tried in the 1940s–1960s, in addition to simple blood transfusion, were exchange transfusion, thorotrast and X-irradiation and radioactive gold, heparin, salicylates and 5-idiosalicylic acid, anti-snake-venom serum and thymectomy. More recently, chloroquin, asparaginase, Vinca alkaloids and danazol have been tried, in addition to plasmapheresis, plasma exchange, the specific immunoadsorption of IgG and the intravenous infusion of high doses of immunoglobulin. Some successes have been claimed for all the above therapies, but there have been failures, too, as the following summaries illustrate.

Thorotrast and X-irradiation

Evans and Duane (1947) described the result of administrating thorotrast to one patient and the effects of irradiation directed to the mediastinum and abdomen in two patients. The patient who received thorotrast had relapsed following splenectomy. She appeared to experience a partial remission, with a transitory slowing in the progress of her anaemia, following the administration of the thorotrast. X-irradiation directed to mediastinal and paraaortic nodes resulted in a fall in total leucocyte and lymphocyte counts and possibly a slight diminution in the rate of haemolysis. In the second patient irradiation seemed to be without effect on the haemolysis.

Heni and Blessing (1954) reported an unfavourable effect of irradiating the spleen — an aggravation of haemolysis, and the same sequence was observed by Sokal (1957) in a patient suffering from 'haemolytic hypersplenism'.

More recently, Markus and Forfar (1986) reported that an elderly man suffering from warm-antibody AIHA and cardiac failure, who had failed to respond to corticosteroids and was considered unfit for splenectomy, had apparently responded well to X-irradiation of the spleen, a midline dose of 2000 cGy being administered in 10 daily treatments. He was, however, receiving 250 mg of azathioprine daily throughout the period he was irradiated, and it is difficult to exclude a delayed response to the drug. The net result of both treatments was that his haemoglobin rose from 6.5 g/dl at the conclusion of the irradiation to 13.7 g/dl 110 days later.

Radioactive gold

Wang, Bowman and Tocantins (1954) and Tocantins and Wang (1956) treated seven patients with ^{198}Au, usually with doses of 10–20 mc given intravenously. Five had idiopathic, two secondary AIHA. The results were moderately encouraging. As with other forms of irradiation, there is a risk of bone-marrow depression.

Heparin

Early studies

Owren (1949) administered heparin to an elderly patient severely ill with AIHA and who required repeated transfusion: 350 mg of heparin given daily for 7 days had no effect on the course of the disease, but 800 mg daily given for 6 days appeared to slow down the rate of erythrocyte destruction. Treatment had to be stopped, however, because of bleeding and a severe haemolytic crisis followed withdrawal of the heparin.

Roth (1954) claimed that heparin added *in vitro* inhibited the auto-agglutination of the erythrocytes of three patients with AIHA. Roth and Frumin (1956) gave details of a patient treated with 50 mg of intramuscular heparin. Within 2 hours the titre of the DAT was reduced by a factor of 4 or 8, the free antibody titre at 37°C was similarly reduced and there was a decrease in serum bilirubin and plasma haemoglobin and improvement in osmotic fragility.

McFarland, Galbraith and Miale (1960) described a patient with severe AIHA, later found to be associated with Hodgkin's disease, in whom daily subcutaneous doses of 150 mg of heparin resulted in stabilization of the haemoglobin and a negative DAT 2 weeks later. Relapse followed cessation of heparin treatment and remission its readministration. It was concluded that heparin interfered in some undefined way with the coating of erythrocytes by immune globulin.

The effect of heparin and other anticoagulants was studied experimentally by Storti and Vaccari (1956) and Storti, Vaccari and Baldini (1956). Storti and Vaccari could not demonstrate any effect of heparin *in vitro* other than its well known anticomplementary effect. Using rabbits injected with immune serum, Storti, Vaccari and Baldini found that anticoagulants, including heparin, postponed the onset of haemolysis, reduced its intensity and shortened its duration. Heparin had a rather inconstant effect and haemorrhages were present in the animals that died. Germanin was more effective; it had high antilytic activity, it was highly anticomplementary, had low anticoagulant activity and little toxicity (to rabbits).

Storti, Vaccari and Baldini also reported on a therapeutic trial of 250 mg of heparin given daily intravenously to a human subject. Treatment was persisted in for 30 days and the erythrocyte count rose from 1.6 to 2.8×10^{12}/l. Relapse followed cessation of treatment.

The studies summarized above suggested that heparin therapy could have a place in the management of severe AIHA. But the high doses required and the risk of haemorrhage were regarded as serious disadvantages.

More recent observations

Some encouraging, but also some discouraging, results of the treatment of AIHA with heparin were described in the 1960s and 1970s.

Hartman (1964) reported that a 29-year-old man with chronic AIHA who had refused splenectomy had responded quickly to 300 mg of heparin given daily subcutaneously. The DAT became quickly negative, there was a fall in plasma haemoglobin and serum bilirubin and the haemoglobin rose from 8.9 to 12.5 g/dl. The DAT became positive again when the heparin therapy was stopped.

Heine, Herrmann and Stobbe (1964) described two patients who appeared to derive moderate benefit from the daily administration of depot heparin for 20 days and $2\frac{1}{2}$ months, respectively.

Ten Pas and Monto (1966) reported that they had treated with remarkable success a 27-year-old man suffering from a disseminated small cell lymphoma complicated by severe AIHA with heparin administered initially in a dose of 100 mg given subcutaneously every 8 hours. Within 2 days the DAT became negative, there was a fall in serum haemoglobin and a rise in serum complement, and the total haemoglobin rose steadily (Fig. 35.16). Ten Pas and Monto observed that if before the heparin had been administered to the patient his erythrocytes were suspended in a heparin–saline solution for 15 minutes before the DAT was carried

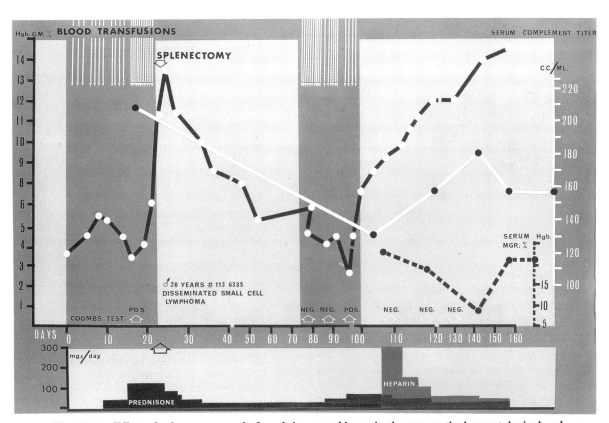

Fig. 35.16 Effect of splenectomy and of prednisone and heparin therapy on the haematological and serological findings in a man aged 20 suffering from AIHA and a lymphoma.
[Reproduced by permission from Ten Pas and Monto (1966).]

out, the result of the DAT, originally positive, became negative. This reversal of the DAT had encouraged Ten Pas and Monto to try the effect of heparin *in vivo*.

In contrast to the favourable responses referred to above, Bardana and co-workers (1970) reported that the seven patients they had treated with subcutaneous injections of heparin in doses up to 300 mg daily had failed to respond favourably. The intensity of haemolysis did not appear to be reduced and the direct and indirect antiglobulin tests and bromelin tests, and the serum complement levels, were unaltered. Six of the patients had formed warm auto-antibodies, one a cold antibody; five had had secondary AIHA, one idiopathic AIHA.

Frimmer and Creger (1970) likewise reported that the two AIHA patients they had treated had appeared to derive no clear benefit: the first patient had received 150 mg of heparin subcutaneously daily for $2\frac{1}{2}$ months; the second patient, who had underlying Hodgkin's disease, had been given 300 mg daily for 3 days.

Honetz and Neumann (1970) described how they had treated six patients (three with idiopathic, three with symptomatic warm-antibody AIHA) with heparin by infusion or depot injections or with the heparinoid SP54 taken orally. Several of these patients improved whilst being so treated, and in one case the ^{51}Cr T$_{50}$ was shown to have increased from 4 to 11 days. The patients were, however, receiving prednisolone at the same time.

It seems clear from the above brief survey of the results of heparin therapy for warm-antibody AIHA that while some patients appear to have responded favourably to doses that can be tolerated, i.e. that do not cause spontaneous haemorrhages, others do not. The cause of these differences must depend upon the way in which heparin acts. It is well known to be anticomplementary and it would be expected, therefore, if present in sufficient concentration, to inhibit haemolysis dependent on complement activity. If that was the only way it affected antibody–antigen interaction, it could hardly be expected to affect favourably haemolysis brought about by the IgGFc–macrophage mechanism. This could be an important reason for its failure in some cases. On the other hand, there have been some reports, e.g. those of Hartman (1964) and Ten Pas and Monto (1966) cited above, indicating a switch from a positive to a negative DAT shortly after commencing heparin therapy, indicating apparently an effect, in some cases, on antibody–antigen interaction.

As already mentioned (p. 480), heparin and Germanin, given to rabbits injected with anti-erythrocyte sera, have been shown to reduce the intensity of haemolysis and shorten its duration (Storti, Vaccari and Baldini, 1956). The subsequent experiments carried out by Rosenfield, Vitale and Kochwa (1967) provided additional data concerning the antihaemolytic action of heparin. They showed that prior heparinization of recipient rats prevented the rapid in-vivo destruction of rat erythrocytes sensitized with rabbit IgG anti-rat-erythrocyte sera. That this appeared to be mediated by an anticomplement mechanism was shown by the fact that rat erythrocytes sensitized *in vitro* by antibody in the presence of complement were lysed rapidly *in vivo* despite the presence of heparin. In that experimental system, heparin appeared to be able neither to block antibody uptake not to increase antibody dissociation from antibody–antigen complexes.

From the practical point of view of treating human patients seriously affected by warm-antibody AIHA, heparin therapy offers a possible means of alleviation, but only as a temporary expedient that is potentially dangerous. Logically it should perhaps be used only if the haemolytic mechanism is clearly complement-dependent, or if heparin can be shown to be capable *in vitro* of rapidly 'reversing' the patient's positive DAT.

Salicylates and 5-iodosalicylic acid

Bateman (1949), who had reported treating with sodium salicylate, without benefit, a patient suffering from CHAD referred to early work on the possible modification of antigen–antibody reactions by salicylates, dating back to 1922. Craddock (1951) described how massive salicylate therapy was given to a patient affected with a serious grade of AIHA. Again, no clear benefit resulted, and there were unpleasant toxic symptoms.

Formijne (1956) reported on the use of the sodium salt of 5-iodosalicylic acid. Four patients were treated: one seemed to be greatly improved, two perhaps obtained partial benefit but the fourth derived no benefit.

On the whole, therefore, salicylates did not seem likely to have been of much value, at any rate in doses which could be tolerated.

Anti-snake-venom serum

Singh and Bird (1960) reported remarkable success as

the result of giving to 27 patients between two and six 20-ml doses of polyvalent anti-snake-venom serum intravenously or intramuscularly. As far as the present author knows these results have not been duplicated.

Thymectomy as treatment for AIHA in infancy and childhood

In 1963 Wilmers and Russell reported that thymectomy had been carried out as a last resort in the case of an infant aged $6\frac{1}{2}$ months who had suffered from extremely severe AIHA for the previous 4 months (see below) and that the excessive haemolysis had ceased approximately 1 month after the operation (Fig. 35.17). In 1964, Karaklis and co-workers reported a similar occurrence. This infant also recovered shortly after thymectomy. The author, too (Dacie and Worlledge, 1969), was personally involved in the management of another infant suffering from severe AIHA who similarly went into remission 2–3 weeks after thymectomy (Figs. 35.18 and 35.19). In all three infants it was impossible to prove that their recovery had been initiated by thymectomy: equally, however, this possibility could not be excluded.

That thymectomy should not be regarded as a 'magic' cure for severe refractory AIHA in infancy was underlined by the experience of Oski and Abelson (1965) and Johnson and Abilgaard (1976) (see later) who reported that the operation had failed to initiate recovery in infants under their care. On the other hand, Hirooka and co-workers (1970) reported that a boy aged 8 years, who had suffered from chronic AIHA since the age of 3 years 6 months, and who had failed to respond satisfactorily to splenectomy and long-term treatment with corticosteroids, seemed to have been benefited by thymectomy. The steroid dosage could be reduced after the operation and transfusions were no longer necessary. Further details of the case histories of the three infants referred to above are summarized below.

Wilmers and Russell's patient was a $2\frac{1}{2}$-month-old female Jamaican infant who appeared moribund when brought into hospital: she was hypothermic and her initial haemoglobin was less than 20% (about 4.8 g/dl). A warm (7S) antibody of no apparent specificity was present in her serum and the DAT was strongly positive. Spherocytes were present in the peripheral blood and erythrophagocytosis was noted in the bone marrow. The infant had been transfused immediately

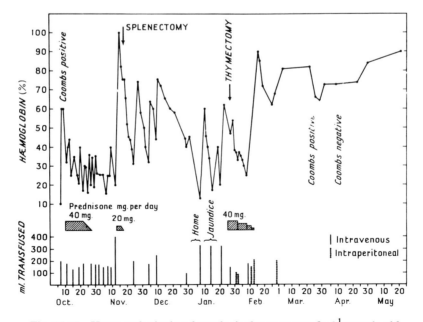

Fig. 35.17 Haematological and serological responses of a $2\frac{1}{2}$ month-old infant with severe warm-antibody AIHA to prednisone therapy, splenectomy and eventually thymectomy.
[Reproduced by permission from Wilmers and Russell (1963).]

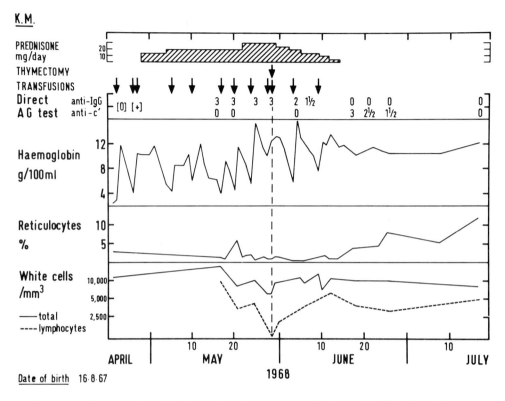

Fig. 35.18 Haematological and serological responses of a 7-month-old infant with severe warm-antibody AIHA to prednisone therapy and eventually to thymectomy.
[Reproduced by permission from Dacie and Worlledge (1959).]

after admission and prednisone administered at the high dose of 40 mg/day without obvious benefit. A succession of transfusions were required to maintain the haemoglobin at about 30% (Fig. 35.17). Splenectomy was carried out 5 weeks after admission. This had little effect and further transfusing was essential. Irradiation of the thymus had been considered but in the end its removal was decided on. The gland weighed only 3 g. Tissue was sent to Sir Macfarlane Burnett who described the organ as 'heavily stressed'. Following thymectomy, several further transfusions were required, the last being given 4 weeks after the operation. Subsequently the infant's recovery was uninterrupted. The DAT was positive 8 weeks after the operation but was negative at 11 weeks. Six months after the operation the haemoglobin was 90% and she appeared to be developing normally.

The male infant described by Karaklis et al. (1964) was 10 months old when admitted to hospital. The haemoglobin was then 6.5 g/dl (after transfusion) and the DAT was positive. Treatment with up to 50 mg of prednisone and 50 units of ACTH daily failed to initiate remission and a series of transfusions were required. Splenectomy was carried out 26 days after admission and for almost 1 month after the operation

the infant did well and did not require transfusion. Then he relapsed; transfusions were ineffective and were followed by haemoglobinuria. Thymectomy was decided on and this was successfully carried out following an exchange transfusion. Sir Macfarlane Burnet reported that sections of the thymus showed that intense immunological activity was taking place and that 'the appearances seemed consistent with the view that the plasmablasts [present] represent a major source of pathogenic antibody'. Haemolysis continued after the operation and two more transfusions were required. The infant then began to improve and the urine became free of haemoglobin. He eventually made a complete recovery.

The infant referred to by Dacie and Worlledge (1969) was aged 7 months. On admission the haemoglobin was less than 4 g/dl and repeated transfusions were required. Prednisone in doses up to 30 mg daily failed to elicit any clear response. The DAT, at first negative, later became strongly positive using an anti-IgG serum. As there seemed to be no immediate prospect of improvement, thymectomy was carried out about 6 weeks after the start of the infant's illness. Two weeks later she went into remission, the DAT became negative and eventually she fully recovered (Fig.

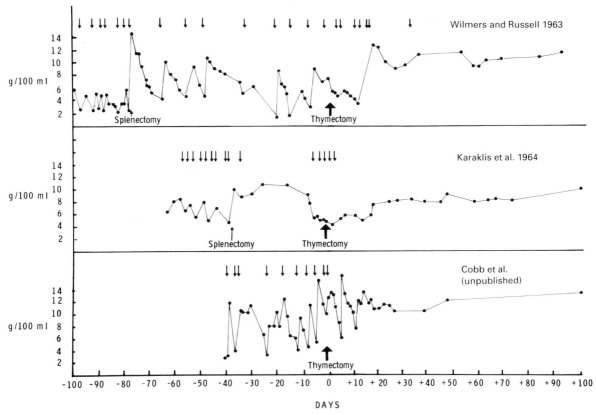

Fig. 35.19   Haematological data from Figs. 35.18 and 35.9 and data from Karaklis et al. (1964), replotted to illustrate the relationship between the infants' remissions and thymectomy.
[Reproduced by permission from Dacie (1970).]

35.18). Ten years later a blood count was reported to be normal.

Johnson and Abilgaard's (1976) patient was an infant boy who was $2\frac{1}{2}$ months of age when he developed severe AIHA. When first admitted to hospital his haemoglobin was as low as 2.2 g/dl. The DAT and IAT were positive; the auto-antibody was 7S, acted at 37°C and lacked apparent specificity. The infant was treated with hydrocortisone, prednisone and cyclophosphamide without benefit, and numerous transfusions were required. When aged 6 months splenectomy was carried out but without benefit. About 1 month later thymectomy was performed, again without benefit (Fig. 35.20). Azathioprine was tried but there was no response, and the infant died aged 7 months of cardiac and hepatic failure.

Chloroquin

Chloroquin had been reported to be of benefit in the treatment of SLE and rheumatoid arthritis. Forrester and Stratton (1970) described how they had administered the drug at a dose of 5 mg twice daily orally to a 10-month-old boy suffering from severe warm-antibody AIHA. The DAT was strongly positive and his serum contained free anti-e auto-antibody. He gradually recovered: by day 180 the DAT had become negative and the treatment with chloroquin was suspended on day 256, by which time the haemoglobin was 11.1 g/dl and reticulocyte count 1.7%. The child's recovery continued and he was found to be well and completely normal $6\frac{1}{2}$ years after the onset of his illness.

L-Asparaginase

Mirecka and co-workers (1972) reported that they had injected two AIHA patients with 500 iu/kg of the enzyme L-asparaginase intravenously and had studied the effects on the strength of the DAT and on the fluorescence of erythrocytes exposed to an anti-human IgG/IgM serum prepared in a sheep. In each patient the DAT was less strongly positive on the 7th day after the injection than before, using both anti-IgG and anti-IgA sera; and erythrocyte fluorescence, too, became

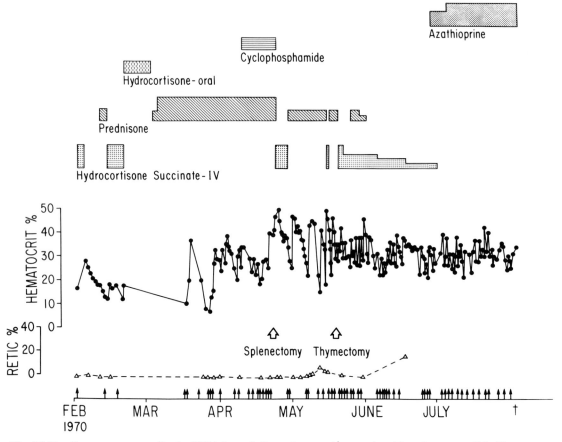

Fig. 35.20   Severe warm-antibody AIHA in an infant who was $2\frac{1}{2}$ months old at the start of his illness.
He failed to respond to a variety of treatments, including splenectomy and thymectomy. [Reproduced by permission from Johnson and Abilgaard (1976).]

temporarily markedly less obvious, particularly on the 3rd day after the injection. No clinical details of the patients were given as to the effect, if any, of the injections. L-asparaginase is, however, well known to be able to affect immunological reactions, e.g. it can inhibit lymphoblastogenesis in culture, and has been shown to be immunosuppressive in experimental systems. In the experiments reported by Mirecka et al., it seemed possible that the enzyme was bringing about the release of immunoglobulin previously attached to erythrocytes.

Vinca alkaloids

Vinblastine and vincristine are known to exert powerful toxic effects on several biological functions, including the activity of the monocyte/macrophage system by inhibiting phagocytosis and interfering with C3 receptors; they also bind to the protein tubulin, which is present in relatively high concentration in

platelets. Their affinity for platelets was exploited in attempts to treat idiopathic thrombocytopenic purpura (ITP) by infusing patients with normal platelets that had been exposed before the infusion to vinblastine (Ahn et al., 1978b). Encouraged by the results of this treatment in ITP, Ahn and co-workers (Ahn et al., 1978a; Ahn and Harrington, 1980) tried the effect of infusing several AIHA patients with Vinca-loaded platelets. In order that the platelets after infusion might make contact with phagocytic cells via their IgGFc receptors, the platelets were exposed before infusion to ABO- and Rh-compatible hepatitis-B surface-antigen-negative plasma from an ITP patient, thought to contain anti-platelet antibodies.

The response of two of them to the Vinca-loaded platelets was scored as excellent and as good in one patient—their remissions extended from 1 to 3 years. The patient who failed to respond had earlier refused splenectomy. The condition of the patients who responded worsened immediately after the injections — perhaps due to the presence of free Vinca alkaloid — before they remitted (Fig. 35.21). Ahn et al. obtained some evidence that vincristine, although more slowly bound to platelets than vinblastine, might be the more effective drug because it dissociated from the platelets more slowly.

Ahn and Harrington (1980) reported that they had administered Vinca-loaded platelets to four patients with warm-antibody AIHA. Three of them appeared to be benefited by the Vinca alkaloid; the fourth patient did not respond. Ahn and Harrington also mentioned that two patients with CHAD had been treated in the same way. The cold-agglutinin titres were reported as being decreased and their intolerance of cold was improved, but no details were given.

Gertz and co-workers (1981) reported using vinblastine-loaded platelets in the case of a 42-year-old female suffering from severe chronic AIHA. She had failed to respond to prednisone, azathioprine, splenectomy and two plasma exchanges. Within 1 week of the infusion of the vinblastine-loaded platelets (and 4 units of erythrocytes) her haemoglobin had risen from 6.1 to 13.9 g/dl. Subsequently haemolysis was controlled satisfactorily by prednisone alone for the next 8 months.

Vinblastine was administered alone, i.e. not bound to platelets, to two patients by Medellin, Patten and Weiss (1982). One patient had Evans syndrome, and had formed an IgG auto-antibody; the other, who had formed an IgM auto-antibody, gave a history of intravenous drug abuse. Both were given vinblastine in 5-mg doses weekly by slow infusions. They appeared to be benefited by the treatment, although the second patient, who was also receiving cyclophosphamide, developed tissue necrosis at the site of the infusion.

Ahn and co-workers (1983a) gave further details of the four patients described briefly by Ahn and Harrington (1980). Three had failed to respond to splenectomy.

Ahn, Harrington and Mylvaganam (1987) reviewed

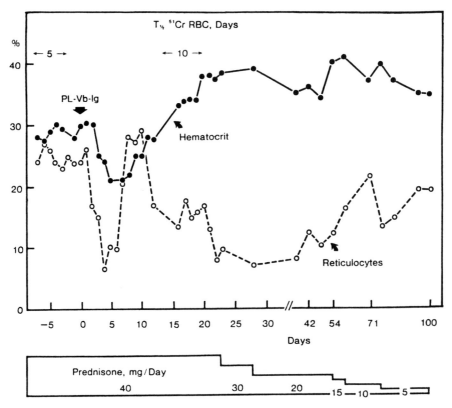

Fig. 35.21 Haematological response of a 72-year-old man suffering from warm-antibody AIHA to treatment with prednisone and an infusion of Vinca-loaded platelets that had been exposed *in vitro* to plasma from a patient with ITP.

[Reproduced by permission from Ahn et al. (1983a).]

the use of Vinca-loaded platelets in ITP, AIHA and in malignant disorders of the mononuclear/macrophage system such as malignant histiocytosis, in which some dramatic, albeit temporary, responses have been reported.

Danazol

Danazol is a modified androgen which has a reduced masculinizing effect. It was used by Ahn et al. (1983b) in the treatment of idiopathic thrombocytopenic purpura (ITP) and the results were sufficiently encouraging for Ahn et al. (1985) to use the drug, at a daily dosage of 600–800 mg, in warm-antibody AIHA in conjunction with high doses of prednisone. Fifteen patients had been treated, and of the twelve with idiopathic AIHA the results were scored as excellent in six, good in three and fair in three; and of the three remaining patients, whose haemolytic anaemia was associated with a malignancy, one responded. In patients who responded the haematocrit started to rise 1–3 weeks after the start of treatment. Erythrocyte-bound IgG and complement (C) had been assayed during the course of treatment: the amount of IgG was not significantly altered but that of C fell. The side-effects of treatment appeared to be less than those produced by corticosteroids, and Ahn et al. suggested that danazol might be used as an alternative to splenectomy in patients not responding well to corticosteroids or in conjunction with lower doses of corticosteroids in patients suffering from the side-effects of high doses of the drugs.

More recently, Ahn (1990) reviewed the use of danazol in a variety of blood disorders, including ITP, AIHA, PNH and myelodysplastic syndrome. Twenty-eight AIHA patients had been treated up to the time of writing. Thirteen of them had had idiopathic AIHA: in ten the responses were scored as excellent or good and in three as fair or poor. (In 15 secondary AIHA patients, mostly with SLE, the responses were not quite so good.) Lasting remissions after all treatment had been discontinued were seen in both AIHA (as well as in ITP) and in most of the patients who were treated with danazol it proved possible to taper off corticosteroids completely. Ahn reported that danazol appeared to affect the erythrocyte membrane, and cited scanning electron micrographs as indicating an increase in surface area as well as increased resistance to osmotic lysis in support of this concept. In a recent abstract, Horstman, Jy and Ahn (1991) reported that treating normal erythrocytes *in vitro* with danazol at very low concentrations (5–20 mg/l) inhibited 'sharply' the binding to the cells of the auto-antibodies of most of the cases of AIHA they had tested.

BLOOD TRANSFUSION IN WARM-ANTIBODY AIHA

Early experiences

Blood transfusion as a means of treating acquired haemolytic anaemia was undoubtedly popularized by the publication of a paper by Lederer (1925) who had described three patients suffering from acute (possibly auto-immune) haemolytic anaemia whose recovery seemed to be initiated by transfusion. In a later report, Lederer (1930) reviewed 12 cases and considered that 11 of the patients had similarly responded to transfusion. In retrospect, it appears doubtful whether transfusion played a decisive part in the recovery of these patients, except in as much as it helped to tide them over anaemic crises; their recovery appears as likely to have been spontaneous as due directly to the transfusions. It is also highly doubtful whether normal plasma or serum ever contains any or sufficient anti-lytic substances to have had a specific inhibitory effect on haemolysis.

The general experience in the 1930s and 1940s failed in fact to confirm Lederer's conclusion as to the value of blood transfusion in initiating remission in acquired haemolytic anaemia. Dameshek and Rosenthal (1951), for instance, reviewing their own experience, stated that in only eight out of 70 cases of mixed pathogenesis were transfusions followed by complete remissions, and in only two of the remitting cases was the disorder of the auto-antibody type.

These early experiences thus indicated clearly that in the great majority of patients with AIHA blood transfusion served only as a palliative measure of short duration and that, while this might indeed be of critical value in transient acute haemolytic anaemia, it was much less often helpful in patients suffering from severe chronic haemolysis. Some of the latter patients actually appeared to be worse after transfusion, for the transfusion of normal erythrocytes, the survival of which was likely to be no better than that of the patient's own cells, perhaps even worse, would increase the formation of bilirubin and lead to a deepening of the patient's jaundice. In patients suffering from intravascular haemolysis, transfusion was likely to lead to increased haemoglobinuria. The author (Dacie, 1954, Case 11, p. 201) described such a patient. He died despite repeated transfusions and was never fit enough for splenectomy to be undertaken.

Exsanguination (exchange) transfusion

The fortunately rare, but nevertheless important, occurrence of critically ill patients at a time when blood transfusion and splenectomy were the only treatments available for severe AIHA led to exsanguination (exchange) transfusion being sometimes undertaken, a heroic undertaking before the advent of automated pheresis equipment. Piney (1950), Ravina et al. (1950), Cattan et al. (1951), Milliez et al. (1951), Bowman (1955) and Wingstrand and Selander (1960) described patients in whom exchange transfusion had been carried out. Unfortunately, the benefit was generally short-lived.

Piney's patient was a woman with AIHA who had not responded to splenectomy. A 30-pint exchange transfusion raised her haemoglobin from 30% to 80%; the DAT, however, remained strongly positive. She gradually relapsed after the exchange but was alive 6 months later and needed simple transfusions every 3 weeks.

Wingstrand and Selander's patient, a woman aged 54, at one time moribund, rallied after a 12-litre exchange and eventually recovered.

In theory exchange transfusion had (and still has) the potential advantage that it not only can raise the patient's haemoglobin substantially (albeit only temporarily) but it also removes some, perhaps much, of the patient's circulating auto-antibody. A modern version of exchange or exsanguination transfusion is plasmapheresis or plasma exchange effected by means of an automated cell separator. Some results of applying this technique in severe AIHA are referred to on p. 491.

RECENT VIEWS: THE PROBLEM OF INCOMPATIBILITY AND SELECTION OF BLOOD

Much has been written in recent years concerning the necessity and practicability of transfusing normal erythrocytes to patients with warm-antibody AIHA and the selection of blood that is likely to have the longest survival *in vivo*. Valuable reviews summarizing the authors' opinions and recommendations include those of Pirofsky (1969), Pirofsky and Bardana (1974), Rosenfield and Jagathambal (1976), Petz and Garratty (1980), Issitt (1981, 1985), Rosenfield and Diamond (1981), Masouredis and Chaplin (1985) and Sokol et al. (1988).

All authors, while agreeing that blood transfusion should be avoided as far as is possible, agree that no patient should be allowed to die of anaemia simply because blood cannot be found that is compatible *in vitro*. All authors also agree that the provision of normal blood that is likely to survive the best is an exacting task and that the chief value of blood transfusion is to gain time for other therapies, particularly the use of corticosteroid drugs in high doses, to work. The major task of the blood-transfusion laboratory is to determine as far as is possible the specificity of the auto-antibody and to identify any allo-antibodies that may be present at the same time in the patient's serum and which may play an important role in shortening the survival of transfused erythrocytes.

Pirofsky (1969) and Pirofsky and Bardana (1974) stated that blood transfusion had been life-saving in several of their patients and that in their experience acute reactions following transfusion had been relatively infrequent despite the transfusion of incompatible blood. Only one of their patients had died (of acute renal failure) as a consequence of a transfusion. They stressed that the decision to transfuse should be based on clinical criteria and they pointed out that severe anaemia in AIHA is generally well tolerated, even by the elderly, if the patients are kept at rest in bed. In their view 'transfusion should not be used to treat either the physician or the hematocrit'!

Rosenfield and Jagathambal (1976) discussed the problem of transfusing AIHA patients from two points of view—that of the blood bank and that of the clinician. They warned against over-transfusing patients and recommended that when transfusion appeared to be essential the volume transfused should always be kept to the minimum that would protect the patient from dying of heart failure brought about by lack of haemoglobin. They suggested 100 ml of packed erythrocytes given twice daily should achieve this purpose. Larger volumes than this were, in their view, unnecessarily dangerous and likened transfusing large volumes 'to "throwing more logs on the fire" of an active red cell destruction process in vivo'.

Petz and Garratty (1980) devoted a whole chapter of their book *Acquired Immune Hemolytic Anemias* to blood transfusion. They discussed in depth the indications (and lack of indications) for transfusion and the unique risks that are inherent in transfusing, i.e. that the presence of auto-antibodies complicates the carrying out of compatibility tests and may make it difficult to detect the concomitant presence of allo-antibodies, and the fact that the auto-antibodies may severely shorten the survival of the transfused normal cells. They emphasized, however, that despite these risks a patient should never be denied a transfusion if threatened by a life-destroying anaemia, even if it meant transfusing the patient with blood that is strongly incompatible *in vitro*. Petz and Garratty described in detail the technical aspects of the selection of donor blood and how it is possible reliably to detect allo-antibodies in sera containing auto-antibodies. A section of their chapter was devoted, too, to the problem of the optimal volume of blood to be transfused. They concluded that transfusion therapy has to be individualized and that it is often necessary to compromise between the impracticability of repeatedly transfusing small volumes of erythrocytes and the dangers inherent in the transfusion of large volumes.

Issitt (1985), writing from the point of view of a serologist, concluded that the decision to transfuse must be made on clinical grounds and not on laboratory values. He emphasized the importance of carrying out exhaustive tests to identify any allo-antibodies present rather than spending time on looking for 'least

incompatible units'. He discussed the interesting question as to whether the transfusion of normal blood, by increasing the antigen load, results in more auto-antibody being formed than might otherwise have been the case and stated that there is anecdotal evidence that transfused patients are more difficult to control by corticosteroid therapy than patients who have not been transfused. Also that premature transfusion may result in the widening of the specificity of the auto-antibody and/or the fixation of complement to the erythrocytes. (These concepts are of course difficult to prove, for it is the worse affected patients who need and receive blood transfusion.) Issitt himself reported, however, that he had seen a series of patients transfused when not severely anaemic, e.g. when their haemoglobin was 9–10 g/dl, who subsequently had stormy courses; he found it difficult to accept that 'their long term problems were not in some way related to the fact that they were transfused too soon'.

Masouredis and Chaplin's (1985) chapter in a volume of the *Methods in Hematology* series was concerned with the detailed technical aspects of what they described as 'one of the most difficult and challenging aspects of transfusion medicine', namely, the provision of compatible erythrocytes for transfusion to patients suffering from AIHA. In discussing the occurrence of post-transfusion haemoglobinuria, they stressed that while the 'knee-jerk' response is to suspect that the haemolysis has been brought about by allo-antibodies, auto-antibody-mediated destruction may be an equally likely cause, as the result of the increase in the total mass of erythrocytes available for destruction.

Sokol and his co-workers (1988) described an 8-year experience in providing blood for 2149 patients who had formed warm or cold auto-antibodies. Allo-antibodies were identified in 294 sera (13.7%), the most frequent being anti-E and anti-K. A total of 7052 units of blood were issued for 1685 patients as 'not compatible but considered suitable'. No haemolytic reactions had been reported.

Auto-antibody specificity and blood transfusion

Soon after it was realized that the auto-antibodies of warm AIHA might possess a well-defined specificity, usually within the Rh system, the possibility was entertained of selecting blood for transfusion lacking the antigens corresponding to the specificity. It was argued that such blood might survive normally and that the patient would correspondingly benefit. That this indeed might be so was demonstrated by Holländer (1954), Crowley and Bouroncle (1956), Wiener, Gordon and Russow (1957), Ley, Mayer and Harris (1958), Mollison (1959) and Högman, Killander and Sjölin (1960).

In Holländer's patient, the auto-antibodies had anti-D specificity; while *cde/cde* blood survived for at least 31 days, *CDe/cde* blood survived for only 3 days. In Crowley and Bouroncle's patient, two auto-antibodies, anti-D and anti-E, were present, and *cde/cde* cells survived normally. In the patient of Wiener, Gordon and Russow the auto-antibody reacted to highest titres with cells containing the **rh'** (C) factor; when transfused with blood lacking this factor, the patient made a complete and lasting recovery. Previously she had been transfused with the blood of randomly selected Rh-positive donors and failed to improve. Ley, Mayer and Harris's patient was group O *cde/cde*. *cDE/cDE* erythrocytes were demonstrated to survive normally (^{51}Cr T$_{50}$ = 25 days), but normal *cde/cde* cells survived even less well than the patient's own cells (^{51}Cr T$_{50}$ 5 days and 13–14 days, respectively).

Mollison's case, studied in collaboration with the present author, was a man of Rh genotype *cde/cde*, whose auto-antibody had the specificity anti-e. Transfused e-negative cells, followed by the Ashby differential agglutination method, survived almost normally while the patient's e-positive cells, labelled with ^{51}Cr and studied simultaneously, were rapidly eliminated.

Högman, Killander and Sjölin's case was a child aged 13 years, of genotype *CDe/CDe*, who had formed auto-anti-e as well as an apparent 'non-specific' component. The latter component did not appear to be of much importance as *cDE/cDE* cells survived normally.

In practice, knowledge of the specificity of the auto-antibodies has proved to be of less value than was at first anticipated. The reason for this is that auto-antibodies of well-defined single specificities, e.g. anti-e or anti-D are rare; almost always, even if antibody molecules of these specificities are present, they are accompanied by other antibodies which have broader specificities within the Rh system (see p. 161).

Another factor which militates against the long-term success of transfusing a patient with blood not containing antigens reacting with a specific auto-antibody is the possibility of immunizing the patient against one or more of the antigens carried by the blood he or she is transfused with. This had been pointed out by Wiener, Gordon and Russow (1957). For instance, if an *rr(cde/cde)* patient forming auto-anti-e is transfused with blood lacking the e antigen, i.e. R_2R_2 (*cDE/cDE*) blood, this means that the patient will very likely form allo-anti-E and perhaps allo-anti-D, the development of which would make any further transfusion an even more difficult problem. This was so in the case of Ley, Mayer and Harris's (1958) patient.

PLASMAPHERESIS AND PLASMA EXCHANGE AS TREATMENT FOR WARM-ANTIBODY AIHA

The development of automated cell separator equipment has made practicable attempts to treat immune disorders by plasmapheresis or plasma exchange, the aim being to remove from the circulation as many harmful immune complexes or auto-antibodies as possible. The technique has been applied in recent years to a number of patients seriously affected by warm-antibody AIHA and some probable or possible successes have been described.

Branda and co-workers (1975) included one patient with AIHA amongst four patients treated by plasma exchange for a variety of immune disorders. The AIHA patient, a 45-year-old man, entered hospital with a Guillian–Barre type polyneuropathy following an acute viral illness. He became anaemic and developed a reticulocytosis during convalescence; the DAT was positive and an anti-e auto-antibody was identified. Because of a history of earlier haemorrhage from a peptic ulcer, corticosteroid therapy was thought to be unwise. A 3-litre plasma exchange was thus carried out, followed by the transfusion of two units of blood. His haemoglobin then stabilized and he eventually recovered.

The technique of, and indications for and scope of, plasma exchange were usefully discussed in a review by Isbister (1979).

Garelli and co-workers (1980) described how they had treated a 43-year-old woman who was suffering from a hyperacute AIHA by means of plasmapheresis and exchange transfusion. Following these procedures her condition stabilized and she eventually recovered. The antibody was an IgG, and this had caused auto-agglutination at 37°C; intravascular haemolysis has resulted.

Herrera and co-workers (1980) described how they had treated a 74-year-old woman suffering from hyperacute warm-antibody AIHA by a 3.5 litre plasma exchange combined with the replacement of her own erythrocytes with 7 units of packed cells—in effect, an exchange transfusion. The patient responded well, and after further transfusions of 5 units of packed cells her haemoglobin rose to 15.1 g/dl.

Patten and Reuter (1980) reported that they had subjected a 48-year-old patient with Evans syndrome to a 9-litre plasma exchange within a period of 12 days. She was desperately ill despite having received blood transfusions, corticosteroids and immunosuppressive drugs and having undergone splenectomy. Following the last exchange, she managed to maintain her haematocrit for approximately 3 weeks. Then, however, she developed pneumonia and experienced a further (and fatal) haemolytic crisis.

Petz and Garratty (1980) described how they had treated two patients by plasma exchange. The first patient was a 13-year-old boy with chronic warm-antibody AIHA. Seven exchanges averaging 2.55 litres of plasma were carried out within a 12-day period. Following this his transfusion requirement diminished and he eventually went into remission. He was, however, being simultaneously treated with 100 mg of prednisone daily. The second patient was a 24-year-old woman who had suffered from AIHA for 7 years, during which time she had experienced a series of acute haemolytic episodes. These continued even after splenectomy. She was treated by an approximate 3-litre plasma exchange every week or so, and on this regime, supplemented by 30 mg of prednisone and 200 mg of azathioprine daily, she experienced no further acute episodes within a 10-month period.

Bernstein, Schneider and Naiman (1981) recounted the history of a 17-year-old patient suffering from very severe AIHA despite being treated by multiple transfusions and high doses of prednisone (2–10 mg/kg/day). Splenectomy was eventually undertaken, preceded by a partial exchange transfusion. This produced, however, only transient benefit. He was next subjected to a plasma exchange: 8.5 litres of blood were processed and 4.24 litres of plasma removed and replaced with 5% albumin–saline. A second exchange was carried out 10 days later, and he was started on azathioprine at a dose-rate of 2 mg/kg/day at about the same time; he continued, too, to receive prednisone. Following the second exchange, his haemoglobin stabilized, and it was eventually found possible to withdraw both the prednisone and azathioprine.

Lundgren and co-workers (1981) reported that they had subjected a 36-year-old woman to six 4-litre plasma exchanges. She had been suffering from end-stage diabetic nephropathy and had developed a fulminating haemolytic anaemia following a renal transplant. The cause of the haemolysis was obscure. The auto-

antibody had anti-A specificity, the patient being group A$_2$. She eventually recovered from the haemolysis and regained renal function; and it seemed likely that the plasma exchange, in addition perhaps to prednisolone and azathioprine, had contributed to her recovery.

Andersen and co-workers (1984) described the progress and treatment of a 5-year-old boy who had developed an extremely severe AIHA. He had failed to respond to prednisone and to splenectomy and had received a total of 93 blood transfusions within a period of 5 months. The intense haemolysis subsided after three plasma exchanges, but azathioprine and cyclophosphamide could have played a part in his recovery, or recovery could have been spontaneous (Fig. 35.22). The DAT had been positive with both anti-IgG and anti-C sera. A weak cold agglutinin had been present, titre 64 at 4°C, which agglutinated I and i erythrocytes equally. At 37°C the antibody was only detectable by the use of enzyme-treated erythrocytes or the IAT. The antibody disappeared on the child's recovery and the DAT became negative. Developing complications associated with iron overload were successfully overcome by the administration of desferrioxamine and vitamin C.

Kutti and co-workers (1984) reported that a 16-year-old patient suffering from severe Evans syndrome had apparently achieved a complete remission following plasmapheresis. She had been severely anaemic and had failed to respond to high doses of corticosteroids and treatment with cyclophosphamide and azathioprine; transfusions had been ineffective, as had five intravenous infusions of 25 g of γ globulin. She was then subjected to three 4-litre plasma exchanges. No further transfusions were required following the last exchange, and there was evidence that haemolysis was gradually subsiding. She eventually recovered apparently completely.

Further patients with severe AIHA who appeared to benefit from plasma exchange have been described by Garelli et al. (1985), von Keyserlingk et al. (1987) and by Govoni et al. (1990).

The patient described by von Keyserlingk et al. (1987) suffered from sickle-cell (AS) trait and had developed a hyperacute immune haemolytic crisis associated with acute renal failure. Immunosuppressive treatment, plasmapheresis and haemodialysis were proceeded with simultaneously. The plasma haemoglobin concentration fell after the third plasma exchange and he was eventually discharged from hospital on maintenance doses of prednisone and azathioprine. His haemoglobin was then stable at about 9 g/dl. The patient described by Govoni et al. (1990) was suffering from a rifampicin-induced drug-immune haemolytic anaemia and acute renal failure.

Specific immunoadsorption of IgG

An alternative to plasmapheresis is specific

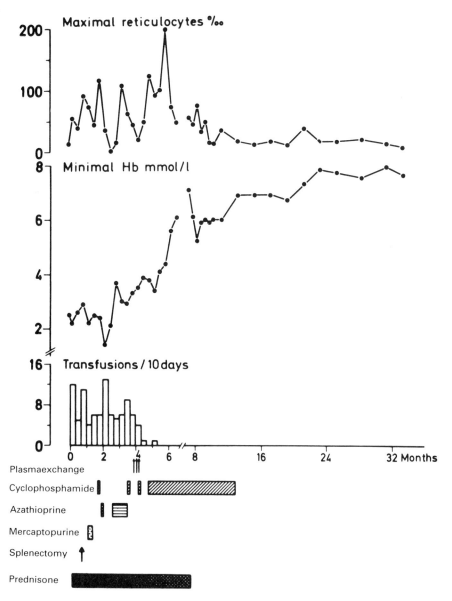

Fig. 35.22   Response of a 5-year-old boy with severe AIHA to treatment by repeated blood transfusion, prednisone, splenectomy, mercaptopurine, azathioprine, three plasma exchanges (totalling 2913 ml) and cyclophosphamide.
[Reproduced by permission from Andersen et al. (1984).]

immunoadsorption of IgG by exploiting the property of 'protein A', a constituent of the cell wall of *Staph. aureus*, to bind to human IgG. Besa and co-workers (1981) employed a continuous-flow cell separator to expose extracorporeally a patient's plasma to a filter containing a formalin-stabilized suspension of *Staph. aureus*. Their

patient was a 65-year-old man with AIHA complicating chronic lymphocytic leukaemia. He was severely anaemic and was suffering, too, from myocardial ischaemia and incipient renal failure. Two immunoadsorption procedures produced some clinical improvement. The first adsorption reduced the plasma IgG by 64% of its original level at the end of 2 hours, the second adsorption by 72% in the first 30 minutes. The IgG concentration returned to 50% of its initial value at the end of 24 hours. As a temporary expedient for critically ill patients immunoadsorption seems to be an effective, if elaborate, procedure. Besa et al. considered it to be more efficient and selective than plasmapheresis.

INTRAVENOUS γ GLOBULIN (IgG) AS TREATMENT FOR WARM-ANTIBODY AIHA

In the early 1980s it was reported that patients suffering from idiopathic thrombocytopenic purpura (ITP) might experience significant rises in platelet count following the intravenous infusion of large amounts of human immunoglobulin (IgG). First described in children (Imbach et al., 1981), this was soon found to be true, too, of adults (Schmidt et al., 1981; Fehr, Hoffmann and Kappeler, 1982; Bussel and Hilgartner, 1984). These results provided the stimulus for testing to see whether similar regimes would bring about remission in patients suffering from AIHA who had failed to respond to more conventional treatment, e.g. the use of corticosteroids or the carrying out of splenectomy.

The results of the use of intravenous IgG in patients with AIHA have been variable. Some patients have responded well, others have failed to respond. At first, dosages similar to those that had been found to be successful in ITP, e.g. courses of 0.4 g/kg/day for 5 days, had been used. Subsequently it was found that higher doses, e.g. up to 1 g/kg/day, might be necessary for a favourable response. Details of some of the published case reports are summarized below.

Bussel and his co-workers (Bussel et al., 1963; Bussel, Cunningham-Rundles and Hilgartner, 1984; Bussel, Cunningham-Rundles and Abraham, 1986; Bussel, 1986) described sustained remissions in two children, a transient response in one adult and failure in one child. They had received up to 1 g/kg/day for 5 successive days.

Salama and co-workers (1984) had treated three patients with, however, no benefit. All three were adults and one of them, who had Evans syndrome and SLE, deteriorated clinically during treatment. They had, however, been given relatively small doses of IgG — namely, 0.4 g/kg/day on 4 or 5 successive days. Further details of these patients, plus one other, were described by Mueller-Eckhardt et al. (1985). ^{51}Cr erythrocyte auto-survival studies, carried out in four of them, showed that the rate of ^{51}Cr elimination had not significantly altered during the period the IgG was being administered. The DAT, too, remained unaltered in each case. Mueller-Eckhardt and his co-workers administered IgG in equivalent doses to five normal volunteers. Their DATs remained negative but the amount of erythrocyte surface IgG increased as determined by radioactive assay. C3 levels were unchanged but those of C4 decreased and the haptoglobin levels fell in two out of the five volunteers. IgG levels rose to 2–3 times baseline levels soon after the infusions were given.

Subsequent reports have included descriptions of possible or probable responses [Macintyre et al., 1985; Oda et al., 1985 (Fig 35.23); Pocecco et al., 1986; Leickly and Buckley, 1987; Majer and Hyde, 1988] and of failure to respond (Richmond, Ray and Korenblitt, 1987; Weinblatt, 1987).

Several mechanisms by which the intravenous infusion of high doses of IgG could induce remission in ITP have been put forward. Salama, Mueller-Eckhardt and Kiefel (1983) and Mueller-Eckhardt et al. (1984) suggested that remission was brought about by competitive inhibition of the reticulo-endothelial system by sequestration of autologous erythrocytes, as the result of the erythrocytes being coated by the infused IgG. Bussel and Hilgartner (1984) discussed four possible mechanisms: reticulo-endothelial Fc receptor blockade (Fehr, Hofmann and Kappeler, 1982); decrease in antibody synthesis; protection of platelets and/or megakaryocytes from platelet antibody, and clearance of persistent viral infection by specific antibody present in the IgG. Evidence reviewed by Bussel and Hilgartner indicated that Fc receptor blockade could result

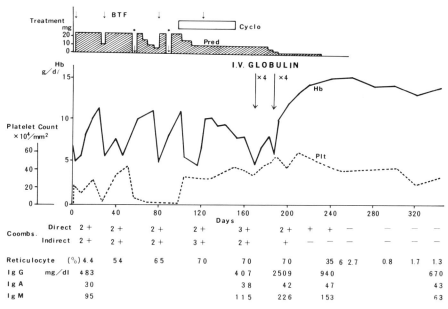

Fig. 35.23   Evans syndrome in a 5-month-old boy.
Response to treatment by blood transfusion (BTF), prednisone, cyclophosphamide and intravenous IgG. [Reproduced by permission from Oda et al. (1985).]

from two mechanisms — decrease in receptor affinity and competition for Fc receptors by the increase in serum IgG; it was unlikely to be responsible for long-term remissions. There appeared to be no hard evidence for the remaining hypotheses.

As it seems likely that the mechanism that is responsible for the occasional remissions that occur in AIHA is very similar if not identical with that that brings about remission in ITP, the question arises as to why the intravenous infusion of IgG is apparently more often successful in ITP than in AIHA and why in AIHA patients who do respond larger amounts of IgG seem to be required than in patients with ITP. A possible reason is that the RE-cell phagocytic system is expanded to a greater extent in AIHA than in ITP and that more Ig would therefore be required to achieve the same degree of Fc receptor blockage (Bussel, Cunningham-Rundles and Abraham, 1986; Majer and Hyde, 1988).

A factor that seems likely to increase rather than inhibit erythrocyte destruction is non-specific coating of erythrocytes with IgG after very high intravenous dosage. As described earlier, Mueller-Eckhardt et al. (1985) had demonstrated this by

means of a radioimmune antiglobulin test; they concluded as the result of their studies of healthy volunteers to whom Ig had been administered that the procedure had led to increased, although clinically inapparent, haemolysis as the result of interaction between IgG-loaded autologous erythrocytes and the volunteers' own mononuclear/macrophage system. Richmond, Ray and Korenblitt (1987) suggested that increased non-specific binding of IgG to erythrocytes may have been responsible for the enhanced haemolysis that supervened after a period of stabilization in the patient whom they had treated with IgG at a dosage of 1 g/kg/day. They also pointed out that IgG preparations contain anti-A and anti-B allo-antibodies at low concentration and that their presence could contribute to in-vivo haemolysis.

Experimental evidence that the intravenous administration of IgG depresses the clearance of IgM-sensitized guinea-pig erythrocytes has been described by Basta et al. (1989b). That the effect is specific for IgG was shown by the failure of another foreign protein, e.g. human serum albumin, to act in the same way. As for the mechanism of the effect, Basta et al. concluded that this was probably due to the IgG retarding the uptake of C3 by the target erythrocytes and modifying the process of complement fragment deposition. Also, it seemed possible that the IgG accelerated the release of erythrocytes adherent to phagocytes. Further evidence that supranormal concentrations of IgG could inhibit, too, the uptake of C3 by IgG-sensitized erythrocytes was obtained by Basta et al. (1989a) as the result of experiments with guinea-pigs injected with anti-Forssman antibody. Intravenous IgG protected the guinea-pigs: no control animal injected with albumin survived.

PRACTICAL MANAGEMENT OF PATIENTS WITH WARM-ANTIBODY AIHA

In this section an attempt will be made to summarize how patients with warm-antibody AIHA should be treated.

Choice of treatment

As already discussed (p. 461), patients who are suffering from overt haemolysis should initially be treated with prednisone or prednisolone at a daily dosage of up to 100 mg for a maximum of 3 weeks. If at the end of this time they show no signs of response, or if it seems clear that doses in excess of 30 mg of prednisone are required to maintain the patient in equilibrium, a change of treatment is imperative. A choice has then to be made between splenectomy and treatment with azathioprine. In favour of splenectomy is that any benefit that results from the operation is likely to be obvious within a matter of days or a week or two at the most, whereas that produced by azathioprine is not likely to show for several weeks or even a month or more. Against splenectomy is the fact that it is a major operation and that post-operative complications, e.g. pulmonary embolism, although not common are a definite hazard, particularly in elderly patients. Against the use of azathioprine is that, as already mentioned, it is slow-acting and that its use, too, may lead to unwelcome complications, e.g. marrow depression. Both splenectomy and azathioprine suffer from a further defect—some patients do not respond to either treatment. And some patients who do respond well relapse later, after perhaps a symptom-free interval of many years (see p. 476 and Fig 35.13).

Value of ascertaining sites of haemolysis with ^{51}Cr

A question of particular interest is the value of ^{51}Cr studies in assessing the role of the spleen and liver as sites of haemolysis. As already referred to, there is a great deal of evidence that indicates that the spleen is a particularly active site of destruction of erythrocytes coated with IgG antibodies as the result of IgGFc–macrophage receptor interaction, whereas the liver plays a predominant role in the destruction of complement-coated erythrocytes (p. 415). The results of pre-splenectomy ^{51}Cr surface-counting studies in AIHA patients have already been referred to (p. 477). A marked uptake of radioactivity by the spleen certainly suggests that splenectomy would be beneficial, and the majority of patients in which this has occurred have in fact responded well. However, in some patients, particularly those in whom haemolysis is most active—and in whom a good response is most eagerly awaited—splenectomy hardly helps, despite the spleen being clearly a site of haemolysis. Whether undertaking splenectomy should be 'vetoed' in a seriously-ill patient by a ^{51}Cr test indicating that the liver is also playing a major role in erythrocyte destruction is more debatable (Fig. 35.24). It depends upon what other options are still available: if no progress is being made with other possible treatments, then splenectomy, in the author's view, should be undertaken; for even if the rate of haemolysis is only slightly to moderately reduced as a result of the operation this may help the patient to achieve a reasonable level of haemoglobin which previously he or she had been unable to sustain or to be

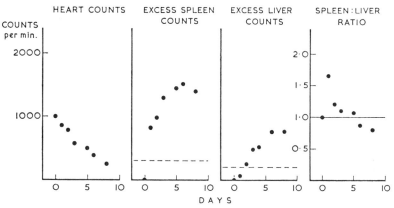

Fig. 35.24   **Surface-counting pattern after labelling the erythrocytes of a patient with warm-antibody AIHA showing accumulation of radioactivity in both the liver and spleen (Case 12 of Dacie, 1962, p. 684).**

in equilibrium on a reduced corticosteroid dosage (Fig. 35.11, p. 474).

The patient who fails to respond adequately to doses of corticosteroids or immunosuppressive drugs that he or she can tolerate, and has also failed to respond significantly to splenectomy, presents the physician with a particularly serious problem. What should be done next? Some possible treatments to which individual patients have responded have been described on pp. 479–488.

Heparin appears to have helped some patients in whom haemolysis has been intravascular and complement-dependent, and plasmapheresis and intravenous γ globulin are obviously worth trying in the case of acutely ill patients. Danazol therapy is simple and although the chance of success is uncertain recent reports are encouraging; treatment with Vinca-loaded platelets is elaborate and difficult to contemplate on a long-term basis. Thymectomy seems to have helped some seriously ill infants, but its curative role is unproved and whether or not to recommend it presents the physician with a difficult decision.

What the physician hopes for, of course, is for the patient to recover spontaneously, as indeed some patients, particularly infants and children, certainly do. The hope is that the various treatments the physician can offer, starting with corticosteroids, will help to sustain the patient (and do at the same time the least possible harm) until recovery takes place; in some patients this may

unfortunately be years ahead, if it ever takes place at all. Blood transfusion is of relatively little value in AIHA, because of the likely short life of the transfused blood, but everybody agrees that to allow a patient to die of anaemia simply because no blood compatible with the recipient's serum can be found is inadmissible. On the other hand, everybody agrees, too, that transfusions of blood should be kept to the minimum; also that it is important to avoid transfusing blood which is incompatible with any allo-antibodies that the patient has formed as the result of earlier transfusions. Techniques in fact are available which facilitate the identification of allo-antibodies in sera also containing free auto-antibodies, so that is a difficulty that can be overcome (see p. 490).

PROGNOSIS IN WARM-ANTIBODY AIHA

In this section the outlook for patients who develop AIHA will be reviewed.

Despite advances in therapy, AIHA must still be regarded as a serious illness even though the resultant mortality is now not so high as it was when the author reviewed the probable outlook for patients 30 years ago (Dacie, 1962, pp. 689–697). However, it is still difficult to provide figures as to the likely mortality or to forecast what will happen to individual patients at the start of his or her illness. For one thing, the auto-immune haemolytic anaemias are a heterogeneous group of disorders which may or may not be secondary to, or associated with, an underlying disease; and the presence of any underlying disease will clearly affect the prognosis. Also, the aetiology of so-called idiopathic AIHA probably varies considerably from case to case, with genetic influences, infection and disturbances of immune regulation of unknown nature all probably playing quantitatively different parts in individual cases. This heterogeneity makes generalizations as to prognosis difficult and forecasting the outlook for any particular patient hazardous.

MORTALITY IN IDIOPATHIC WARM-ANTIBODY AIHA

Early data on the mortality of 'acute hemolytic anemia' were provided by Dameshek and Schwartz in their 1940 review. They cited 106 cases: 18 of these patients were reported to have died, but the ultimate fate of the others is unknown. Twenty-three of the patients were reported as having undergone splenectomy, and 20 to have recovered. In a postscript to this paper Dameshek and Schwartz mentioned 11 patients of their own, five of whom had died. They gave details of four patients who responded to splenectomy, but these patients were only observed for short periods of time, 2 to 8 months, and it is not known whether their remissions were long-continued. Later, Welch and Dameshek (1950) reviewed the result of splenectomy in 34 patients; 50% went into complete remission but the fate of the remainder was not reported.

Dausset and his co-workers in France published extensive data which also indicated that the mortality was high in the 1950s even when the patients had the benefit of treatment with corticosteroids. Dausset and Malinvaud (1954) described the fate of 47 patients, three-quarters having idiopathic AIHA. The mortality, including that of the secondary cases, was stated to have been 37%. Dausset and Colombani (1959) reported on 83 idiopathic cases studied between 1949 and 1958. Twenty-seven were stated to have been cured, 23 were dead (27.7%), and 30 patients still had the disease; three patients had died of causes other than haemolytic anaemia.

Dausset and Colombani added that they thought that the percentage of recovery had risen from 37.5% to 70% as the result of steroid therapy and that allowing for relapse the total recovery rate would be in the region of 50–60%. They found that neither age nor sex nor the intensity of initial haemolysis, nor the clinical signs, had any prognostic value, but they agreed with Chertkow and Dacie (1956) that a low platelet count, and with Crosby and Rappaport (1957) that a low reticulocyte count, were unfavourable prognostic signs. Dausset and Colombani stressed, too, that the presence of free antibody in the serum detectable by the indirect antiglobulin test was a bad sign. Splenectomy, considered as a long-term curative method, seemed not to have had any favourable effect on ultimate prognosis, for 12 patients died out of a total of 31 submitted to the operation and there were four post-operative deaths.

Crosby and Rappaport (1957) reported on the fate of 34 patients treated by various means; 18 had died, a mortality of 53%.

The outlook for infants and children in the 1950s was also serious, although it was realized that haemolysis was more likely to be short-lived than in the case of adults. Negri, Pototschnig and Maiolo (1960) reviewed the case histories of 29 infants and reported that eight (27%) had died.

A major difficulty in attempting to assess prognosis and mortality, which operated in the 1950s and which still is relevant, is that there is almost inevitably an element of selection in the cases a physician sees, because the greater his or

Table 35.2   Mortality in warm- and cold-antibody AIHA. Postgraduate Medical School of London data (1947–1961).

No. of patients	Warm auto-antibodies			Cold auto-antibodies		
	Idio-pathic	Secondary		Idio-pathic	Secondary	
		Infection	Neo-plasm		Infection	Neo-plasm
Total	50	18*	17	16	9	7
Alive†	27	10	2	11	7	0
Dead	23	8	15	5	2	7
Mortality (%)	46	45	88	31	22	100

*Includes six patients with SLE.
†Follow-up of at least 1 year.

Table 35.3 Causes of death in 50 patients suffering from warm-antibody and in 16 patients suffering from cold-antibody idiopathic AIHA.

Type of disease	Treatment			
	None or transfusion only	Steroids ± transfusion	Splenectomy ± transfusion	Splenectomy + steroids ± transfusion
Warm-antibody	Anaemia and pneumonia (1)	Anaemia (4), pneumonia (3), myocardial infarction (2)	Anaemia (5), biliary cirrhosis (1)	Anaemia (2), portal vein thrombosis (1), pneumonia (1), post-operative deaths (splenectomy) (3)
Cold-antibody	Pneumonia (1)	Pulmonary embolism (1), tuberculosis (1)	Anaemia (1)	Carcinoma of breast (1)

her interest or experience the more likely is he or she to be sent patients who are seriously ill or who have already been shown to be refractory to treatment. This was certainly true of the 100 patients the author had investigated between 1947 and 1961. Of the 50 patients in this series who had idiopathic AIHA, 27 were still alive 1 year or more after the onset of their disease and 23 had died (Table 35.2).

In Table 35.1, p. 459 is summarized the effect that the treatment that was then available—corticosteroids and blood transfusion—appeared to have had on the outcome. Ten patients achieved clinical and haematological (but not necessarily serological) cure; seven had undergone splenectomy. Of the other patients, 22 achieved compensation for their haemolysis, i.e., their haemoglobin was maintained at a tolerable level without the necessity for transfusion—most of these patients were receiving maintenance treatment with corticosteroids; 18 further patients remained seriously ill and did not achieve compensation for haemolysis. As mentioned above, 23 of the patients had died. The total mortality rate was thus 46%; it was slightly higher in the patients who had undergone splenectomy than in those receiving steroids only.

The causes of death in these patients are summarized in Table 35.3. Most, perhaps all, of the deaths were connected in one way and another with the patient's haemolytic anemia or the therapeutic attempts to alleviate it.

The high mortality (40–50%) amongst the patients treated by corticosteroids and splenectomy or by corticosteroids or splenectomy alone does not suggest that either of these forms of treatment greatly influenced the final prognosis in this series of patients. It is impossible, however, to believe that they did not help some at least of the patients. However, the dramatic improvement of seriously ill patients as the result of one or other treatment, which was so frequently witnessed in this as in other series of patients, is unfortunately not necessarily well sustained and both the use of corticosteroids and splenectomy have a mortality of their own—infections being exacerbated or masked by the corticosteroids and post-operative deaths occurring not infrequently following splenectomy. Unfortunately, too, neither form of

treatment can be expected to influence fundamentally and permanently auto-antibody formation and both treatments may fail in the worst-affected patients, i.e. in those forming the largest amounts of antibody.

In the present author's series of patients, seen between 1947 and 1961, the majority who died (17 out of 23) did so within 2 years of the onset of their disease (Table 35.4). Data relating prognosis to the presence of free antibody in the serum are given in Table 35.5. Although there was evidence that the intensity of haemolysis, as judged approximately by the haemoglobin level, was correlated with the presence of free auto-antibody in the patient's serum (Dacie, 1959), this did not seem to have affected the ultimate mortality due to the disease. This rather surprising result was contrary to the observations of Dausset and Colombani (1959).

More recent data on mortality

Allgood and Chaplin (1967), in their review of 47 patients with idiopathic AIHA seen between 1955 and 1965, reported that 11 of them (28%) had

Table 35.4 Deaths in idiopathic warm- and cold-antibody AIHA in relation to the duration of the disease.

Type of disease	No. of patients	No. dead within 2 years	No. dead after 2 years	Surviving 2 years or more	Surviving 5 years or more
Warm-antibody	50	17	6	32	19
Cold-antibody	16	2	3	12	10

Table 35.5 Relationship between mortality in warm-antibody AIHA and the presence of free antibody in the patients' serum.

Type of antibody in serum	No. of patients	No. dead	Mortality (%)
Indirect antiglobulin test (+) Agglutination of trypsinized cells (+)	20	9	45
Indirect antiglobulin test (−) Agglutination of trypsinized cells (+)	17	8	47
Both tests (−)	11	5	45

died. They analysed their results from the point of view of the age of the patients and found that 35% of the patients whose disease began when they were 50 years of age or over had died, whereas the mortality of the younger patients was as low as 12.5%—this difference was, however, not statistically significant ($P>0.10$).

Pirofsky (1969) reported that 16 out of his 42 idiopathic AIHA patients had died. Dacie and Worlledge (1975, p. 1152), in their review, mentioned that the mortality rate in the preceding decade—'when corticosteroids were freely available'—had been as low as 10%, but gave no details as to the age of the patients.

Silverstein and co-workers (1972) analysed the mortality rate in respect of 117 patients treated between 1955 and 1965 and calculated that 9% had died within the first year, and 24% within the first 5 years. Thereafter, few had died—73 having survived for 10 years.

Degos, Clauvel and Seligmann (1975) reviewed the survival of 50 warm-antibody AIHA patients whose ages had ranged from less than 10 to over 70. Ten (20%) of these patients had died within the first 4 years but only one had been aged less than 10. In contrast, eight patients who were over 60 had died. The overall mortality at 7 years was approximately 40%.

Petz and Garratty (1980, p. 37) quoted several sets of mortality figures but did not give any personal data and the same is true of Rosse (1990, p. 467). Sokol and co-workers (1984) in their review of AIHA in childhood and adolescence had reported that only two out of 42 children had died; 83% had recovered, usually within 6 months.

Another important factor determining prognosis and mortality is the likelihood of the AIHA patient developing, after having perhaps recovered from increased haemolysis, another auto-immune disorder affecting either the haemopoietic system, e.g. ITP, or other body tissues, leading to SLE, diabetes or ulcerative colitis, etc., or a malignant lymphoma. The chances of this happening are known to be much higher than in the general population, as emphasized particularly by Pirofsky (1969), who also gave figures for the death-rate under these circumstances, Thus, 129 out of the 184 patients

in his series suffering from secondary warm-antibody AIHA had died, an incidence of 70%.

RECOVERY ('CURE') FROM IDIOPATHIC WARM-ANTIBODY AIHA

It is even harder to provide accurate data as to the chances of recovering completely from warm-antibody AIHA, i.e. of achieving a permanent cure, than it is to obtain accurate data on mortality. The problem can be summarized as follows: what are the chances of an AIHA patient who has achieved an apparently complete haematological and serological remission—which had occurred spontaneously or had been aided perhaps by the physician's attempts at treatment—of developing a further similar attack in the near or distant future? Common sense suggests that if the genetic background of the patient had played some part in his or her original illness—which may well have been probable, then he or she would be more likely to develop a similar attack than someone who had never suffered from AIHA.

It seems possible that children who develop AIHA acutely following an overt infection, and who recover rapidly, are no more likely to suffer from a further attack of AIHA than are adults, but more information on this point is required. If it is postulated that an immunological abnormality dictated that an affected child responded to the infection by developing AIHA — whereas hundreds perhaps of apparently similar children exposed to the same environment failed to do this, it is possible that the hypothetical defect might rectify itself as the child matures. If it did not, then the child's vulnerability would persist.

The data in Table 35.1 (p. 459) show that 10 out of the author's 50 warm-antibody AIHA patients (20%) seen in the 1950s were judged to have achieved clinical cure and haematological cure (Dacie, 1962, p. 691). In three of the 10, however, the DAT was still positive when the patients were last investigated; in seven it was negative. Whether any of the patients who had appeared to be cured later relapsed is unknown, as is the number, if any, of those still suffering from increased haemolysis at the time the table was constructed who subsequently achieved cure. Whether improvements in treatment — which certainly seem to have reduced mortality—would result in an increased permanent cure-rate is more doubtful. It seems unlikely, to the author at least, that the temporary use of corticosteroids or immunosuppressive drugs, or splenectomy, or any of the other forms of treatment that have been tried, could influence fundamentally the patient's idiosyncratic tendency to form auto-antibodies once the treatment had been withdrawn. Of course, if the auto-antibody had been derived from the unbridled proliferation of an abnormally functioning monoclone, and if the clone could be totally destroyed by a targeted monoclonal antibody, real cure might be the result. This is a possibility for the future—but hardly likely in any case to be applicable to warm-antibody AIHA where the auto-antibody seems usually (at least) to be polyclonal rather than monoclonal.

Allgood and Chaplin (1967), in their review of 39 warm-antibody AIHA patients, all over the age of 10 years, recorded that 21 of them (54%) had regained normal haemoglobin levels and reticulocyte counts. Three had recovered spontaneously; the remainder had received corticosteroids or had undergone splenectomy. In nine, despite clinical and haematological recovery, the DAT had remained positive.

Pirofsky (1969, p. 31), in discussing the factors that have influenced published survival figures, stressed the importance of the AIHA patient's age, the length of time he or she has been followed up and the possible presence of an underlying disease. Pirofsky went on to write that he considered that the patients in good health whom he had followed up for more than 5 years were 'cases of quiescent hemolytic anemia in "remission"', but that it might be 'equally true to consider the "remission" as complete cure'. He stressed the importance of continual follow-up.

As already mentioned, Silverstein and co-workers (1972), who analysed the records of 117 patients seen between 1955 and 1965 (all except 11 were adults over 20 years of age), concluded that 76% of them were alive 5 years and as many as 73% were alive 10 years after the onset of their illness. How many of these patients were clinically, haematologically and serologically normal when last studied is uncertain.

The more recent data of Heisel and Ortega (1983) and Miyazaki et al. (1983) have confirmed the generally good prognosis of AIHA affecting children. Heisel and Ortega reported that all of nine children aged between 2 and 12 years who had had acute AIHA had recovered within 6 months. Miyazaki et al. had treated 34 children aged between 2 months and 14 years. Sixteen of them had suffered from acute AIHA—in 14 this had followed infections; 18 had had chronic AIHA. Twenty-six (76%) of the children fully recovered, as judged by follow-ups of between 1 and 6 years. Four children (with chronic AIHA) died, all as the result of an underlying disease.

TREATMENT AND PROGNOSIS OF COLD-ANTIBODY AIHA

CHRONIC COLD-HAEMAGGLUTININ DISEASE (CHAD)

These patients present the physician with problems of management which differ considerably from those of patients suffering from warm-antibody AIHA. For one thing almost all the patients are elderly (Fig. 28.1, p. 215), but although this militates against a long survival, some patients manage to live with their disease for 10 years or more (Fig. 28.4, p. 216). Thus 10 out of the 16 patients, details of whom are shown in Table 35.4, survived for at least 5 years. CHAD is in fact essentially a long-continuing and usually only a very slowly progressive disorder which is not necessarily severe. The patients are seldom as anaemic as are warm-antibody AIHA patients but symptoms attributable to in-vivo auto-agglutination, e.g. acrocyanosis, or even gangrene, may be troublesome. Also, it is not rare for a patient who had been considered to be suffering from idiopathic CHAD to develop signs of a lymphoma.

The treatment of CHAD patients is considered below under several headings: general management, use of corticosteroids, use of alkylating and anti-metabolite drugs, use of mercaptanes, blood transfusion, plasma exchange and splenectomy.

General management

It is most important, as is true of course in relation to the care of warm-antibody AIHA patients, that in attempting to help a patient suffering from a very chronic disease such as CHAD, which is as a rule not too incapacitating, to weigh carefully the chances of doing harm against the possible benefits of any particular treatment.

One simple thing that can be done is to counsel the patient to avoid cold as far as is practicable, for example by keeping indoors in wintertime and by maintaining the indoor temperature as high as is practicable, by wearing extra clothing and protecting the hands with mittens and by wearing fur-lined boots and ear-muffs. [The author clearly recollects that a well-known physician stated that he recommended that his patients should spend the winter in a warm tropical or sub-tropical climate—a choice that is not available, unfortunately, to the majority of CHAD patients!]. That warmth by itself can certainly be helpful is illustrated in Fig. 28.3, p. 216, in which the effect of treatment with ACTH and cortisone is compared with that of bed rest in a warm environment.

A novel solution to the paramount importance of avoiding cold was conceived and put into practice by Bartholomew, Bell and Shirey (1987). This was the provision for the patient of an 'environmental suit' within which the patient could be exposed to any temperature between 27°C and 50°C. The idea was that when their (severely affected) patient wished to leave a specially heated room he could don his heated suit. This enabled him to resume a near-normal lifestyle. The patient had suffered from cold-antibody AIHA following mycoplasma pneumonia. The anti-I cold antibody he had formed was active to at least 30°C.

Corticosteroids

That ACTH or corticosteroid therapy was likely to be less successful in CHAD than in warm-antibody AIHA was appreciated soon after the drugs were introduced into medical practice (Hennemann, 1953; Baumgartner, 1955), and, as illustrated in Fig. 28.3, p. 216, it may be difficult to distinguish between the effect of the drugs from that resulting from hospitalization and rest in bed. On the whole, the author feels that, taking into account the likely long-continued course of typical CHAD, it is wise not to start using corticosteroids (see, however, below).

Alkylating and anti-metabolite drugs

As the basis of CHAD is an IgM monoclonal gammopathy, it seems reasonable to expect that CHAD patients would benefit by being treated with drugs that have been used successfully in the treatment of Waldenström's macroglobulinaemia and malignant lymphoproliferative diseases. There is, in fact, evidence that chlorambucil in particular, taken over long periods of time by mouth, has been of help to some, although not to all CHAD patients (Olesen, 1964; Worlledge et al., 1968; Hippe et al., 1970; Evans, Baxter and Gilliland, 1973; Worlledge, 1982).

Worlledge and her co-workers (1968) reported on the use of chlorambucil given orally at a daily dose of 2–10 mg to nine CHAD patients for periods of between 4 and 12 months. Three of the patients responded well, one responded temporarily, two patients were judged to have responded partially and three were not helped. Parallel with a fall in cold-agglutinin titre, in the patients who responded, was a fall in the serum IgM level (Fig. 35.25). Several of the patients experienced unwanted side-effects: in one, pancytopenia developed, in two lymphopenia and in one reticulocytopenia, and one of the patients complained of vertigo. One of the patients who responded temporarily later relapsed and ultimately died of an undifferentiated reticulum-cell sarcoma. Later, Worlledge (1982) reported that of the 11 patients she had by then treated with chlorambucil five had failed to respond. The reason for the varied response is uncertain, nor is it clear whether chlorambucil is best given intermittently in courses or daily continuously. One of Dr Worlledge's patients had been treated with cyclophosphamide at a dose of 100–200 mg daily. This, however, led to neutropenia and was discontinued for this reason. Azathioprine at a

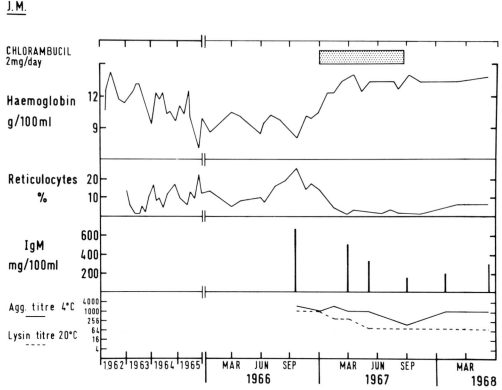

Fig. 35.25   Haematological and serological responses of a 49-year-old man suffering from CHAD to treatment with chlorambucil.
[Reproduced by permission from Dacie and Worlledge (1969).]

dose of 200 mg daily was substituted but while on this regime his haemoglobin fell and the cold-antibody titre and serum IgM level increased.

Hippe and co-workers (1970) reported that four patients had benefited from being treated intermittently or continuously with chlorambucil for from 1 to 7 years. The dose they had received ranged from 20 mg orally per day to 2 mg. None of the patients became thrombocytopenic or leucopenic, but the occurrence of dyspepsia led to the treatment of one of the patients being suspended. The patients' susceptibility to cold improved so that they were able to tolerate the winter (in Denmark) without important acrocyanosis or haemoglobinuria. Their haemoglobin increased and the cold-agglutinin titre decreased by a factor of 3 to 30 times, and the upper thermal limit for antibody activity *in vitro* was calculated to have been reduced by as much as 2.2–7.2°C. The serum IgM levels became almost normal. One of the patients had initially been treated with cyclophosphamide at a dosage of 50 mg three times a day, but the drug had to be discontinued because of dyspepsia and hair loss.

Evans, Baxter and Gilliland (1973) described a detailed study of the results of treating with chlorambucil a 47-year-old man suffering from long-standing CHAD. He responded well first to 6 mg daily and a year later to 4 mg daily. On each occasion the haematocrit rose, the serum IgM content and cold-agglutinin titre fell and the serum complement level, which was too low to measure while haemolysis was active, rose to 50% of the normal level. The ^{51}Cr T_{50} of the patient's erythrocytes increased from 11 days to 15 days after 3 months of therapy. Evans, Baxter and Gilliland mentioned that they had also attempted to treat two other CHAD patients with chlorambucil, but bone-marrow depression rather than any improvement in haemolysis was the result.

An issue of importance to cardiac surgeons is how to avoid damage as the result of auto-agglutination when carrying out open-heart surgery in patients who have formed high-thermal-amplitude cold auto-agglutinins. Various techniques have in fact been employed with success, including plasma exchange and careful control of the systemic perfusion temperature and that of the cardioplegic solution (Klein et al., 1980; Landymore, Isom and Barlam, 1983; Shahian, Wallach and Bern, 1985).

Wertlake, McGinniss and Schmidt (1969) had earlier described the development of intravascular haemolysis as the result of a patient undergoing surgery under hypothermia (29°C) for the insertion of an artificial aortic valve. Unfortunately, the patient, who was group A_1B, had in his plasma an anti-IH cold antibody which agglutinated *in vitro*, and in the presence of complement lysed, group-A_2B erythrocytes up to a temperature of 15°C. Thirteen units of normal group-AB blood were used to cross-circulate with the patient's blood in a chilled heat exchanger. Of these, seven were group A_2B and a further one unit of group A_2B was administered to the patient after the procedure had been completed. Haemoglobinaemia and haemoglobinuria were prominent during the first four post-operative days, and it seemed likely that the patient destroyed all the group A_2B blood he had received during the week following the operation. Fortunately this did not do him any permanent harm. The haemolysis appeared to have occurred in consequence of interaction between group-A_2B cells and the anti-HI antibody taking place *in vivo* at a temperature of 29°C. This was considerably above the highest temperature (15°C) at which interaction was demonstrable *in vitro*.

Mercaptanes

The discovery that mercaptanes can depolymerize macroglobulins (Deutsch and Morton, 1957) led in the early 1960s to their tentative use in patients suffering from CHAD. While their ability to diminish cold-agglutinin activity *in vitro* was readily demonstrated (Fudenberg and Kunkel, 1957; Mehrotra and Charlwood, 1960), their practical value *in vivo* was less clearly established.

Ritzmann and Levin (1961) reported on a comprehensive study of the effect of a variety of SH compounds on cold-agglutinin titres *in vitro*; penicillin G potassium, DL-penicillamine, cyteamine and vitamin B_6-SH (mercaptopyridoxine) were all found to be capable of reducing cold-agglutinin titres substantially. Penicillamine was, too, administered orally in 500 mg doses three times a day for 10 days to a 65-year-old man who had suffered from CHAD for 6 years. This resulted in a substantial decrease in cold-agglutinin titre, e.g. from 131 072 to 32–64 at 25°C, and a reduction, too, in the antibody's lytic activity at 22°C and in

its thermal range. A substantial fall in antibody titre similarly followed the daily intravenous administration of 0.6 g of vitamin B_6-SH. These improvements were, however, only short-lived and the titres had largely returned to their pre-treatment levels a month or so later. A ^{51}Cr erythrocyte auto-survival study had been carried out during the period that the penicillamine and vitamin B_6-SH had been administered, and with each medicament it was clear that the rate of haemolysis was being temporarily slowed.

In subsequent trials, on admittedly only a small number of patients, penicillamine has, however, been found more often than not to be ineffective. Dacie (1962, p. 681) reported that he had treated two patients without success with doses of penicillamine comparable with that used by Ritzmann and Levin (1961) (Fig. 35.26), and Lind, Mansa and Olesen (1963) described how they had similarly treated two patients unsuccessfully. Evans, Bingham and Turner (1965), too, reported that penicillamine had failed to help their patient. On the other hand, Edwards and Gengozian (1965) found that the administration of 500 mg of D-penicillamine four times a day for 7 days resulted in a substantial fall in cold-agglutinin titre and a rise in erythrocyte count in the case of a 71-year-old man who was suffering from AIHA associated with multiple malignancies. In this patient the pre-treatment cold-agglutinin titre was, however, only modestly raised: 128 at 4°C and 32 at 25°C.

α-Interferon

The possibility that α-interferon might be effective in the treatment of chronic CHAD was discussed by Nydegger, Kazatchkine and Miescher (1991) in their review. They quoted in support of this suggestion its apparent value in the treatment of a patient suffering from chronic clonal IgM/polyclonal IgG mixed cryoglobulinaemia who had relapsed after originally responding to cyclophosphamide. A significant reduction in the IgM spike apparent on serum electrophoresis was achieved, and the patient felt well enough to work full-time.

Blood transfusion

Transfusions are seldom necessary in CHAD. This is fortunate because the presence of high-thermal-amplitude cold antibodies makes the selection of donor blood unusually difficult. As in almost all cases the cold antibody will be of anti-I specificity and because I-negative adult blood is extremely rare, in practice it is almost always

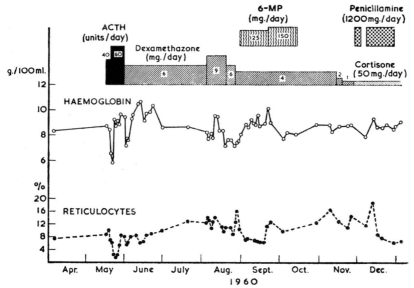

Fig. 35.26 Haematological response of a woman aged 75 with CHAD to treatment with corticosteroids, 6MP and penicillamine (Case 11 of Dacie, 1962, p. 486).

impossible to obtain compatible blood. (See, however, below.) The best that can be done is to screen the patient's serum for the presence of allo-antibodies by means of indirect antiglobulin tests carried out strictly at 37°C and to carry out an in saline cross-match at, say, 32–35°C, using the patient's own erythrocytes as a control. The aim would be to select normal blood samples which are either not agglutinated at that temperature or, if agglutinated, are less strongly agglutinated than are the patient's own cells. Such blood can probably be transfused with safety. It should be run in at a slow drip rate, in which case there is probably no need to attempt to warm it above room temperature.

As referred to already (p. 489), a great deal has been written about the problems of transfusing AIHA patients. In relation to CHAD, Rosenfield and Jagathambal (1976) wrote 'The worst thing that an attending physician can do to a patient who has either severe postviral paroxysmal hemoglobinuria or florid cold agglutinin disease is to administer cold blood', and they went on to refer to some commercially available blood warmers. They stressed that the unmonitored or uncontrolled heating of blood is extremely dangerous and should not be attempted, because of the risk of overheating.

Petz and Garratty (1980) devoted several pages to a detailed discussion of methods of allo-antibody detection in the presence of high-titre cold antibodies, including the inactivation of the IgM cold antibody by 2-mercaptoethanol or dithiothreitol; they also referred to the results of attempts to transfuse CHAD patients with adult I-negative (i) erythrocytes (see below). They stated that in their experience the transfusion of adult I erythrocytes to CHAD patients usually results in an appropriate rise in haemoglobin.

In relation to the question of whether donor blood should be warmed before being administered to CHAD patients, Petz and Garratty stated that their experience had been consistent with the author's view (Dacie, 1962, p. 676), reiterated above — namely, that unwarmed blood can probably be transfused with safety, if given at a slow drip rate. They suggested, however, than an in-line blood warmer should be used in severe PCH or florid CHAD and that it seemed logical to keep the patient warm, even if the value of the manoeuvre had not been proved.

Masouredis and Chaplin (1985), in a review concerned mainly with the technical aspects of transfusing AIHA patients, also described in detail methods for detecting the presence of allo-antibodies in sera containing high-titre cold antibodies, including the adsorption of the cold antibodies by means of rabbit erythrocytes.

Survival of i erythrocytes in patients forming high-titre anti-I antibodies

In relation to the difficulty, referred to above, of obtaining i erythrocytes for the treatment of patients with cold-antibody AIHA who are seriously ill, Woll, Smith and Nusbacher (1974) described a patient to whom two units of warmed previously frozen i erythrocytes were successfully transfused. She was a 51-year-old woman who had probably suffered from mycoplasma pneumonia. Her haematocrit, which had fallen to 9%, was raised to 19% by the transfusion and she was clinically improved and eventually recovered completely. ^{51}Cr labelling of the second unit revealed a ^{51}Cr T_{50} of 24 days.

Earlier, in an elegant experiment, van Loghem and his co-workers (1963) had studied the survival of i erythrocytes in a 57-year-old woman suffering from chronic CHAD: the ^{51}C T_{50} of the i cells was 31 days compared with that of I (donor) cells which was 9 days and I (patient's) cells which was 17 days.

In a comparable experiment carried out on two PCH patients, Silvergleid and co-workers (1978) reported that 53% of a test sample of Tj(a+) erythrocytes were surviving at 48 hours compared with 78% of a test sample of Tj (a−) cells at 96 hours.

Plasma exchange

This has been carried out on a number of occasions in patients suffering from CHAD, and temporary improvement had been recorded. But it seems unlikely that the procedure could be applied on a long-term basis, and the removal from time of time of a substantial mass of cold antibody can hardly be expected to diminish the activity of the monoclone of cells producing the protein. Dealing with plasma containing a high-thermal-amplitude antibody necessitates carrying out the separation at as near body temperature as possible and this renders the whole procedure more experimental than practical.

Published reports of patients suffering from CHAD who have been treated by plasma exchange are referred to below.

Logue, Rosse and Gockerman (1973) reported that following a 3000-ml exchange carried out on two occasions the cold-antibody titre in one patient was reduced by approximately 70% on each occasion and that the rate of haemolysis was reduced in parallel. Unfortunately, however, the titre returned to its original level within 1 week (Fig. 35.27). Rosse (1990, p. 576) pointed out that this was to be expected, bearing in mind the fairly rapid rate of IgM antibody synthesis. However, he also made the point that, although plasmapheresis was a difficult and costly way of treating a CHAD patient, it would be particularly useful if a lowering of antibody titre was urgently needed, as in the case of a patient requiring an immediate surgical operation.

Rosenfield and Jagathambal (1976) reported that they had also found it possible to reduce the concentration of plasma cold agglutinin by plasmapheresis. They

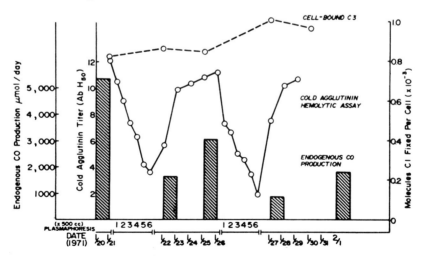

Fig. 35.27   Effect of two 3000-ml plasma exchanges on the cold-agglutinin lytic activity, cell-bound C3 and endogeneous CO production of a man aged 50 with severe CHAD and carcinoma of the lung.
[Reproduced by permission from Logue, Rosse and Gockerman (1973).]

stated that a 'double unit plasmapheresis' performed thrice weekly had reduced the circulating levels of IgM and of mixed cryoglobulins and improved the clinical status of their patients, but they did not give any details. They added, however, that the improvement in patients with K-chain IgM cold-agglutinin disease had not been very great.

Taft, Propp and Sullivan (1977) described their experience of plasma exchange in two CHAD patients. Both had lymphoma. The cold-antibody titres were reduced substantially in each case but neither seemed to derive any substantial clinical benefit. Both patients in fact died of their underlying disease soon after the exchanges.

Isbister, Biggs and Penny (1978) had treated three patients. The first patient had idiopathic CHAD and haemolysis appeared to diminish after a 4-litre exchange. The second patient suffered from immunoblastic lymphadenopathy and had formed a cold antibody active up to 37°C. After two plasmaphereses the cold-agglutinin titre at 4°C had fallen from 128 to 8 and the antibody no longer agglutinated at 37°C. (Both the above patients were being treated with corticosteroids during the period the plasmaphereses were being carried out.) The third patient had also formed a high-thermal-amplitude cold antibody. The antibody titre was reduced, but the patient was not benefited clinically.

Rodenhuis and co-workers (1985) described their experience in treating a transfusion-dependent woman aged 85 suffering from chronic anti-I IgM CHAD. Treatment with chlorambucil had had to be suspended because of marrow depression. Eight weekly plasma exchanges were carried out and significant reductions in cold-agglutinin titre and the thermal amplitude of the antibody resulted. However, the patient's clinical condition did not improve: haemolysis persisted and she continued to require blood transfusions.

Splenectomy

As described on p. 395, agglutinating and/or complement-fixing antibodies lead to the destruction of erythrocytes in many organs of the body, of which the liver because of its size is the most important. Splenectomy, therefore, in theory at least, could hardly be expected to produce much benefit in CHAD, and this has been borne out by clinical experience in patients suffering from typical CHAD (Baumgartner, 1955; McCurdy and Rath, 1960). There are, however, other rare patients forming cold auto-antibodies at moderately high titres, as well as antibodies active at 37°C detectable best by enzyme-treated erythrocytes, who do respond well to splenectomy. Two

such patients were referred to by Dacie and de Gruchy (1951, Cases 5 and 12) and the history of one other similar patient was described in detail by Dacie (1954, p. 205) (Fig. 29.8, p. **000**). These patients had been splenectomized before the advent of ^{51}Cr.

Later studies by Lewis, Szur and Dacie (1960) on three patients suffering from typical CHAD, who had very high-titre cold antibodies in their serum, demonstrated a slight excess of radio-activity in both the liver and spleen in two of them. The data did not, however, suggest that splenectomy would have been of much benefit in these patients, and the operation was in fact not carried out. Similar findings were reported by von dem Borne et al. (1973). Five CHAD patients were investigated: liver sequestration was demonstrated in all five and in three there was also significant sequestration in the spleen. The result of splenectomy, if in fact undertaken, was not recorded.

The possibility that splenectomy may be of value in exceptional CHAD patients in whom there is evidence that the auto-antibody activity extends up to 37°C (as in the three patients of the author mentioned in the preceding paragraph) receives additional support from the detailed description by Evans, Bingham and Turner (1965) of a severely affected man aged 57. He had failed to respond to prednisone, penicillamine and chlorambucil. Splenectomy was carried out and although complicated by a subphrenic abscess and gastric fistula was eventually followed by a sustained remission (Fig. 35.28). An anti-I antibody of high thermal amplitude and high concentration was present in his serum: the agglutinin titre at 5°C was 500 000 and agglutination was detectable up to 31°C. Complement was fixed strongly and normal erythrocytes were lysed: maximal lysis took place at room temperature but some lysis occurred at 37°C; it was most evident at pH 6.6, but took place, too, at pH 7.3. The patient's serum complement level was markedly subnormal.

TREATMENT AND PROGNOSIS OF ACUTE COLD-ANTIBODY AIHA

As described in Chapters 30 and 31, the mortality associated with the transient haemolytic anaemias associated with mycoplasma pneumonia or with infectious mononucleosis, or rarely with other

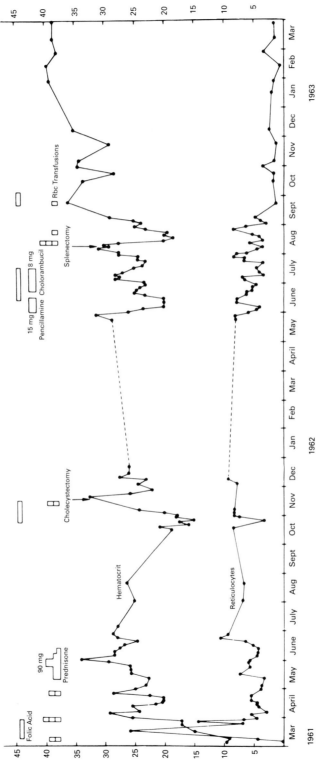

Fig. 35.28 Haematological responses of a man aged 57 with CHAD brought about by a high-thermal-amplitude cold antibody to treatment with prednisone, penicillamine, chlorambucil and eventually splenectomy.
[Reproduced by permission from Evans, Bingham and Turner (1965).]

virus infections, is low; and the chances of a complete recovery occurring within the space of a few weeks is high. Whether the patients should be transfused or receive corticosteroids depends upon the severity of their illness. Neither form of treatment should be withheld if the condition of the patient is judged to be serious. The problems of donor blood incompatibility and the possible advisability of transfusing warm blood to patients who have formed high-thermal-amplitude cold antibodies have been discussed on p. 506.

Rarely, acute cold-antibody AIHA has resulted in the death of the patient. Seldon and co-workers (1980) described such an occurrence.

Their patient, a man aged 21 years, was admitted into hospital giving a 3-day history of progressive lethargy and haemoglobinuria. The haemoglobin was 3 g/dl, and there was marked auto-agglutination. He was jaundiced and livido reticularis was present. His serum contained a low-titre, but high-thermal-amplitude, cold auto-agglutinin without any obvious specificity. The titre was 64 at 4°C and 16 at 37°C. The antibody was shown to be an IgM. Tests for EB and cytomegalovirus and mycoplasma infection were negative, as were the WR and Paul–Bunnell reaction. Treatment with high doses of methylprednisolone (1 g/day), 1.2 g of cyclophosphamide intravenously, blood transfusions and six 5-litre plasma exchanges were unavailing; he developed *Staph. aureus* and *Esch. coli* septicaemia and died 1 week after admission.

As the above case history shows, high-thermal-amplitude cold auto-antibodies, formed for no apparent reason or following no well-defined infection, can pose a serious threat to life, even if the concentration of the antibody, as expressed by its titre at 4°C, is relatively low. Fortunately, such occurrences are rare events. Reference is made below to a small number of published accounts of patients suffering from a similar but less severe syndrome. In each case a cold antibody active at 37°C has been present, and another feature in common has been that the patients responded to treatment with high doses of corticosteroids.

Steroid-responsive idiopathic CHAD

Schreiber, Herskovitz and Goldwein (1977) had described two patients in whom the serological findings were similar to those of the patient of Seldon et al. (1980) described above. Neither was, however, as seriously affected.

The first patient, a woman aged 63, gave a 2-week history of a mild upper-respiratory tract infection. Her haemoglobin on admission was 6.5 g/dl, spherocytes were present in blood films, and the DAT was strongly positive with an anti-C serum but negative with an anti-IgG serum. The cold-agglutinin titre was 256 at 4°C and 32 at 37°C; its specificity was anti-I and it was an IgM. The onset of the second patient's illness, a man aged 35, was more gradual, but the haematological and serological findings were almost identical. Both patients responded to treatment with prednisone, initially at a dose of 100 mg/day. However, the antibody concentration in their plasma persisted unchanged despite clinical improvement and a rise in haemoglobin; and 1 year later, to maintain the haemoglobin at 10 g/dl, the first patient needed a daily dose of at least 20 mg of prednisone and the second patient as much as 40–60 mg.

The sera of both patients were shown *in vitro* to coat human erythrocytes with complement components at 37°C, i.e. with 125 and 160 C1-fixing sites per cell, respectively. Schreiber, Herskovitz and Goldwein showed that the C3-coated erythrocytes, if exposed to monolayers of human mononuclears became spherocytic and had increased osmotic fragility, and that the patients' mononuclear-cell C3 receptor activity was reduced while they were receiving corticosteroids.

A further unusual case was described briefly by Meytes and co-workers (1985). Their patient, a 42-year-old man, suffered from acute haemolysis a few days after a 'flu'-like illness. The DAT was positive and he was shown to have developed a presumably high-thermal-amplitude anti-Pr IgG cold agglutinin: its titre at 4°C was low (4). Despite oral prednisone at a dose of 60 mg daily and blood transfusions the patient's haemoglobin fell to 4.3 g/dl. As a last resort, a single 2.0 g dose of methylprednisolone was administered rapidly intravenously. The acute haemolysis appeared to be arrested and the patient's clinical condition steadily improved: the dosage of oral prednisone was gradually reduced, and 12 months later at follow-up he was found to be well, with no evidence of increased haemolysis, and no demonstrable abnormal antibody.

Another unusual variant of chronic CHAD was

described by Lahav, Rosenberg and Wysenbeek (1989). Their patient, a 69-year-old woman, was admitted to hospital complaining of sudden weakness. There was no history of antecedent infection, and the liver, spleen and lymph nodes were not enlarged. There was evidence of increased haemolysis. The haemoglobin was 8.6 g/dl, with 6.2% reticulocytes; the DAT was strongly positive with anti-C3 sera and weakly positive with anti-IgG sera. Her serum contained a cold antibody active against both I and i erythrocytes; its titre at 4°C was 32; at 20°C, 16; at 37°C, 8. Tests for syphilis, mycoplasma, EB virus and cytomegalovirus were negative. Her haemoglobin fell further to 6 g/dl; she was then transfused with warmed blood and of prednisone at a daily dose of 60 mg administered. Her haemoglobin rose to 11 g/dl. She was followed up for 6 years and it was found that she needed 20 mg of prednisone daily to prevent the recurrence of haemolysis. No signs of a lymphoproliferative or other underlying disease developed during this period.

REFERENCES

ABER, G. M., CHANDLER, G. N. & HARTFALL, S. J. (1954). Cortisone and A.C.T.H. in treatment of non-rheumatic conditions. *Brit. med. J.*, i, 1–8.

AHN, Y. S. (1990). Efficacy of danazol in hematologic disorders. *Acta haemat. (Basel)*, **84**, 122–129.

AHN, Y. S., BYRNES, J. J., BRUNSKILL, D. E., MORITZ, J., HARRINGTON, W. J. & SCHMALE, J. D. (1978a). Selective injury to macrophages: a new treatment for autoimmune hemolytic anemia. *Clin. Res.*, **26**, 340A.

AHN, Y. S., BYRNES, J. J., HARRINGTON, W. J., CAYER, M. L., SMITH, D. S., BRUNSKILL, D. E. & PAUL, L. M. (1978b). The treatment of idiopathic thrombocytopenia with vinblastine-loaded platelets. *New Engl. J. Med.*, **298**, 1101–1107.

AHN, Y. S. & HARRINGTON, W. J. (1980). Clinical use of macrophage inhibitors. *Adv. intern. Med.*, **25**, 453–473.

AHN, Y. S., HARRINGTON, W. J., BYRNES, J. J., PALL, L. & McCRAINIE, J. (1983a). Treatment of autoimmune hemolytic anemia with Vinca-loaded platelets. *J. Amer. med. Ass.*, **249**, 2189–2194.

AHN, Y. S., HARRINGTON, W. J. & MYLVAGANAM, R. (1987). Use of platelets as drug carriers for the treatment of hematologic diseases. In *Methods in Enzymology*, **149**, 312–325. Academic Press, San Diego.

AHN, Y. S., HARRINGTON, W. J., MYLVAGANAM, R., AYUB, J. & PALL, L. M. (1985). Danazol therapy for autoimmune hemolytic anemia. *Ann. intern. Med.*, **102**, 298–301.

AHN, Y. S., HARRINGTON, W. J., SIMON, S. R., MYLVAGANAM, R., PALL, L. M. & SO, A. G. (1983b). Danazol for the treatment of idiopathic thrombocytopenic purpura. *New Engl. J. Med.*, **308**, 1396–1399.

AHUJA, S., LEWIS, S. M. & SZUR, L. (1972). Value of surface counting in predicting response to splenectomy in haemolytic anaemia. *J. clin. Path.*, **25**, 467–472.

AITCHISON, J. D. (1953). Haemolytic anaemia treated by A.C.T.H., cortisone, and splenectomy. *Brit. med. J.*, i, 78–79.

ALLGOOD, J. W. & CHAPLIN, H. (1967). Idiopathic acquired autoimmune hemolytic anemia: a review of forty-seven cases treated from 1955 through 1965. *Amer. J. Med.*, **43**, 254–273.

ANDERSEN, O., TAANING, E., ROSENKVIST, J., MØLLER, N. E. & MOGENSEN, H. H. (1984). Autoimmune haemolytic anaemia treated with multiple transfusions, immunosuppressive therapy, plasma exchange, and desferrioxamine. *Acta paed. scand.*, **73**, 145–148.

ANTONELLI, G. (1913). Intorno agli itteri emolitici. Effetti della splenectomia su di una particulare forma di ittero emolitico acquisato con anemia a tipo pernicioso. *Policlinico, Sez.* med., **20**, 97, 170, 193.

ATKINSON, J. P. & FRANK, M. M. (1974). Complement-independent clearance of IgG-sensitized erythrocytes: inhibition by cortisone. *Blood*, **44**, 629–637.

ATKINSON, J. P., SCHREIBER, A. D. & FRANK, M. M. (1973). Effects of corticosteroids and splenectomy on the immune clearance and destruction of erythrocytes. *J. clin. Invest.*, **52**, 1509–1517.

BAIKIE, A. G. & PIRRIE, R. (1958). The effect of ACTH and cortisone in experimental haemolytic anaemias in guinea-pigs. Studies on anaemias due to heterologous anti-red-cell serum and on the anaemia of chronic lead poisoning. *Scot. med. J.*, **3**, 264–273.

BARDANA, E. J., BAYRAKEI, C., PIROFSKY, B. & HENJYOJ, H. (1970). The use of heparin in autoimmune hemolytic disease. *Blood*, **35**, 377–385.

BARTHOLEMEW, J. R., BELL, W. R., & SHIREY, R. S. (1987). Cold agglutinin hemolytic anemia: management with an environmental suit. *Ann. intern. Med.*, **106**, 243–244.

BASTA, M., KIRSHBOM, P., FRANK, M. M. & FRIES, L. F. (1989a). Mechanism of therapeutic effect of high-dose intravenous immunoglobulin. Attenuation of acute complement-dependent immune damage in a guinea pig model. *J. clin. Invest.*, **84**, 1974–1981.

BASTA, M., LANGLOIS, P. F., MARQUES, M., FRANK, M. M. & FRIES, L. T. (1989b). High-dose intravenous immunoglobulin modifies complement-mediated in vivo clearance. *Blood*, **74**, 326–333.

BATEMAN, J. C. (1949). Symptoms attributable to cold hemagglutination. Report of two cases. *Arch. intern. Med.*, **84**, 523–531.

BAUMGARTNER, W. (1955). Die Kälteagglutinin-krankheit. *Schweiz. med. Wschr.*, **85**, 1157–1162.

BEIKERT, A. (1957). Ergebnisse und Probleme der Behandlung immunologisch bedingter hämolytischer Anämien. *Med. Klin.*, **52**, 1981–1987.

BEN-BASSAT, T., SELIGSOHN, U., LEIBA, H., LEEF, F., CHAITCHIK, S. & RAMOT, B. (1967). Sequestration studies with chromium-51 labeled red cells as criteria for splenectomy. *Israel J. med. Sci.*, **3**, 832–837.

BERNSTEIN, M. L., SCHNEIDER, B. K. & NAIMAN, J. L. (1981). Plasma exchange in refractory acute autoimmune hemolytic anemia. *J. Pediat.*, **98**, 774–775.

BERGLUND, K. (1956). Studies on factors which condition the effect of cortisone on antibody production. 2. The significance of the dose of antigen in primary hemolysin response. *Acta path. microbiol. scand.*, **38**, 329–338.

BESA, E. C., RAY, P. K., SWAIN, V. K., IDICULLA, A., RHOADS, J. E. JNR, BASSETT, J. G., JOSEPH, R. R. & COOPER, D. R. (1981). Specific immunoadsorption of IgG antibody in a patient with chronic lymphocytic leukemia and autoimmune hemolytic anemia. A new form of therapy for the acute critical stage. *Amer. J. Med.*, **71**, 1035–1040.

BEST, W. R., LIMARZI, L. R. & PONCHER, H. G. (1951). Acquired hemolytic anemia treated with corticotropin. *J. Amer. med. Ass.*, **147**, 827–830.

BJØRNEBOE, M., FISCHEL, E. E., & STOERK, H. C. (1951). The effect of cortisone and adrenocorticotrophic hormone on the concentration of circulating antibody. *J. exp. Med.*, **93**, 37–48.

BORCHERS, H. & EYMER, K. P. (1959). Zur Therapie der erworbenen hämolytischen Anämien. *Med. Klin.*, **54**, 498–504.

BOWDLER, A. J. (1976). The role of the spleen and splenectomy in autoimmune hemolytic disease. *Seminars Hemat.*, **13**, 335–348.

BOWMAN, J. M. (1955). Acquired hemolytic anemia; use of replacement transfusion in a crisis. *Amer. J. Dis. Child.*, **89**, 226–232.

BRANDA, R. F., MOLDOW, C. F., McCULLOUGH, J. J. & JACOB, H. S. (1975). Plasma exchange in the treatment of immune disease. *Transfusion*, **15**, 570–576.

BUSSEL, J. B. (1986). Immunoglobulin therapy for autoimmune hemolytic anemia. *J. Pediat.*, **108**, 1043 (Letter).

BUSSEL, J. B., CUNNINGHAM-RUNDLES, C. & ABRAHAM, C. (1986). Intravenous treatment of autoimmune hemolytic anemia with very high dose gammaglobulin. *Vox Sang.*, **51**, 264–269.

BUSSEL, J. B., CUNNINGHAM-RUNDLES, C. & HILGARTNER, M. W. (1984). Intravenous treatment of autoimmune hemolytic anemia with gamma globulin. *Ped. Res.*, **18**, 237A.

BUSSEL, J. B. & HILGARTNER, M. W. (1984). The use and mechanism of action of intravenous immunoglobulin in the treatment of immune haematologic disease. *Brit. J. Haemat.*, **56**, 1–7 (Annotation).

BUSSEL, A., JAISSON, F., JANVIER, M., TRAULLE, C. & SCHENMETZLER, C. (1983). Utilisation des gammaglobulines intraveineuses à fortes doses dans le traitment des anémies hémolytique auto-immunes. *Presse méd.*, **12**, 2628.

CAMERON, D. G., TOWNSEND, S. R., ALBERT, J. R. & HUTCHISON, J. L. (1957). The management of acquired haemolytic anaemia. *Canad. med. Ass. J.*, **76**, 1005–1011.

CASEY, T. P. (1968). 6-Mercaptopurine administration to NZB mice. *Aust. J. exp. Biol. med. Sci.*, **46**, 327–333.

CASEY, T. P. & HOWIE, J. B. (1965). Autoimmune hemolytic anemia in NZB/BL mice treated with the corticosteroid drug betamethasone. *Blood*, **25**, 423–431.

CATTAN, R., FRUMASAN, P., DAUSSET, J. & TRÉLAT, R. (1951). Ictère hémolytique acquis traité notamment par deux exsanguino-transfusions. *Bull. Soc. méd. Hôp. Paris*, **67**, 45–54.

CHERTKOW, G. & DACIE, J. V. (1956). Results of splenectomy in auto-immune acquired haemolytic anaemia. *Brit. J. Haemat.*, **2**, 237–249.

CHRISTENSEN, B. E. (1973). The pattern of erythrocyte sequestration in immunohaemolysis. Effects of prednisone treatment and splenectomy. *Scand. J. Haemat.*, **10**, 120–129.

CHRISTENSEN, B. E., HENSEN, L. K., KRISTENSEN, J. K. & VIDABAEK, A. (1970). Splenectomy in haematology—indications, results, and complications in 41 cases. *Scand. J. Haemat.*, **7**, 247–260.

CHRISTOL, D., EYQUEM, A. & COLVEY, (1952). Action thérapeutique remarquable de l'A.C.T.H. dans un cas d'ictère hémolytique acquis. *Sang*, **23**, 75–80.

CLEARKIN, K. P. (1952). The effect of adrenocorticotropic hormone on clinical and experimental haemolytic anaemia. *Lancet*, **i**, 183–185.

CORLEY, C. C., LESSNER, H. E. & LARSEN, W. E. (1966). Azathioprine therapy of 'autoimmune' disease. *Amer. J. Med.*, **41**, 404–412.

CRADDOCK, C. G. JNR (1951). Acute idiopathic hemolytic anemia; report of a severe fatal case with immunologic observations. *Ann. intern. Med.*, **35**, 912–918.

CRARY, H. I. & BECK, I. A. (1952). Idiopathic acquired hemolytic anemia treated by ACTH and cortisone. *Ann. intern. Med.*, **36**, 1106–1111.

CREGER, W. P., TULLEY, E. H. & HANSEN, D. G. (1956). A note on the effect of hydrocortisone on the microelectrophoretic characteristics of human red cell–antibody unions. *J. Lab. clin. Med.*, **47**, 686–690.

CROSBY, W. H. & RAPPAPORT, H. (1957). Autoimmune hemolytic anemia. I. Analysis of hematologic observations with particular reference to their prognostic value. A survey of 57 cases. *Blood*, **12**, 42–55.

CROWLEY, L. V. & BOURONCLE, B. A. (1956). Studies on the specificity of autoantibodies in acquired hemolytic anemia. *Blood*, **11**, 700–707.

DACIE, J. V. (1954). *The Haemolytic Anaemias: Congenital and Acquired*, 525 pp. Churchill, London.

DACIE, J. V. (1959). Acquired haemolytic anaemia. In *Lectures on the Scientific Basis of Medicine, Volume VII (1957–58)*, pp. 59–79. University of London, Athlone Press, London.

DACIE, J. V. (1962). *The Haemolytic Anaemias: Congenital and Acquired. Part II— The Auto-immune Haemolytic Anaemias*, 2nd edn, 371 pp. Churchill, London.

DACIE, J. V. (1970). Autoimmune haemolytic anaemia (Kettle Memorial Lecture). *Brit. med. J.*, **ii**, 381–386.

DACIE, J. V. & CHERTKOW, G. (1955). Splenectomy in auto-immune haemolytic anaemia. *Trans. Ass. Amer. Phycns*, **68**, 126–130.

DACIE, J. V. & DE GRUCHY, G. C. (1951). Auto-antibodies in acquired haemolytic anaemia. *J. clin. Path.*, **4**, 253–271.

DACIE, J. V. & WORLLEDGE, S. M. (1969). Auto-immune hemolytic anemias. *Progr. Hemat.*, **6**, 82–120.

DACIE, J. V. & WORLLEDGE, S. M. (1975). Autoallergic blood diseases. In *Clinical Aspects of Immunology* (ed. by P. G. H. Gell, R. R. A. Coombs and P. J. Lachmann), 3rd edn, p. 1152. Blackwell Scientific Publications, Oxford.

DAMESHEK, W. (1943). The management of acute hemolytic anemia and the hemolytic crisis. *Clinics*, **2**, 118–165.

DAMESHEK, W. (1950). In discussion on ACTH in leukemia. *Blood*, **5**, 791.

DAMESHEK, W. (1951). Acquired hemolytic anemia: physiopathology with particular reference to autoimmunization and therapy. *Proc. 3rd Congr. int. Soc. Hemat., Cambridge*, 1950, pp. 120–133. Grune and Stratton, New York.

DAMESHEK, W. (1952). Haematological applications of A.C.T.H. and cortisone. *Brit. med. J.*, **ii**, 612 (Letter).

DAMESHEK, W., KOMNINOS, Z. D. & DÉSY L. (1956). The present status of treatment of autoimmune hemolytic anemia with ACTH and cortisone. *Blood*, **11**, 648–664.

DAMESHEK, W. & ROSENTHAL, M. C. (1951). The treatment of acquired hemolytic anemia. With a note on the relationship of periarteritis nodosa to hemolytic anemia. *Med. Clin. N. Amer.*, **35**, 1423–1440.

DAMESHEK, W., ROSENTHAL, M. C. & SCHWARTZ, L. I. (1951). The treatment of acquired hemolytic anemia with adrenocorticotrophic hormone (ACTH). *New Engl. J. Med.*, **244**, 117–127.

DAMESHEK, W. & SCHWARTZ, R. (1960). Treatment of certain autoimmune diseases with antimetabolites; a preliminary report. *Trans. Assoc. Amer. Phycns*, **73**, 113–127

DAMESHEK, W. & SCHWARTZ, S. O. (1940). Acute hemolytic anemia (acquired hemolytic icterus, acute type). *Medicine (Baltimore)*, **19**, 231–327.

DAUSSET, J. & COLOMBANI, J. (1959). The serology and the prognosis of 128 cases of autoimmune hemolytic anemia. *Blood*, **14**, 1280–1301.

DAUSSET, J. & MALINVAUD, G. (1954). Les anémies hémolytiques acquises avec auto-anticorps. Évolution, prognostic et traitment d'après l'étude de 54 cas. *Sem. Hôp Paris*, **30**, 3130–3137.

DAVIDSOHN, I. & SPURRIER, W. (1954). Immunohematological studies in hemolytic anemia. *J. Amer. med. Ass.*, **154**, 818–821.

DAVIDSON, L. S. P., DUTHIE, J. J. R., GIRDWOOD, R. H. & SINCLAIR, R. J. G. (1951). Clinical trials of A.C.T.H. in haemolytic anemia. *Brit. med. J.*, **i**, 657–660.

DAVIS, L. J., KENNEDY, A. C., BAIKIE, A. G. & BROWN, A. (1952). Haemolytic anaemias of various types treated with ACTH and cortisone. Report on ten cases including one acquired type in which erythropoietic arrest had occurred during a crisis. *Glasg. med. J.*, **33**, 263–285.

DE GRUCHY, G. C. (1954). The diagnosis and management of acquired haemolytic anaemia. *Aust. Ann. Med.*, **3**, 106–115.

DE VRIES, J. A. (1950). The effect of adrenocorticotrophic hormone on circulating antibody levels. *J. Immunol.*, **65**, 1–6.

DEGOS, L., CLAUVEL, J. P. & SELIGMANN, M. (1975). Anémies hémolytiques auto-immunes idiopathiques: étude du pronostic des formes chroniques. *Actualités Hématologiques*, *9ᵉ series*, pp. 59–74. Masson, Paris.

DENMAN, A. M., DENMAN, E. J. & HOLBOROW, E. J. (1967). Suppression of Coombs-positive haemolytic anaemia in NZB mice by antilymphocyte globulin. *Lancet*, **i**, 1084–1086.

DEUTSCH, W. H. & MORTON, J. F. (1957). Dissociation of human serum macroglobulins. *Science*, **125**, 600–601.

DREYFUS, B., DAUSSET, J. & VIDAL, G. (1951). Étude clinique et hématologique de douze cas d'anémie hémolytique acquise avec auto-anticorps. *Rev. Hémat.*, **6**, 349–368.

ECKLEBE, G. & SANDER, K. (1952). Der Ablauf der Immunoreaktionen unter ACTH bei experimenteller hämolytischer Anämie. *Z. ges. exp. Med.*, **119**, 338–346.

EDWARDS, C. L. & GENGOZIAN, N. (1965). Autoimmune hemolytic anemia treated with d-penicillamine. Report of a case. *Ann. intern. Med.*, **62**, 576–579.

EISEMANN, G. & DAMESHEK, W. (1954). Splenectomy for "pure red-cell" hypoplastic (aregenerative) anemia associated with autoimmune hemolytic disease. *New Engl. J. Med.*, **251**, 1044–1048.

ETESS, A. D., BASSEN, F., LITWINS, J. & SUSSMAN, L. N. (1951). Acquired hemolytic anemia treated with ACTH prior to splenectomy. *Acta haemat. (Basel)*, **6**, 105–110.

EVANS, R. S. (1955). Autoantibodies in hematologic disorders. *Stamf. med. Bull.*, **13**, 152–166.

EVANS, R. S., BAXTER, E. & GILLILAND, B. C. (1973). Chronic hemolytic anemia due to cold agglutinins: a 20-year history of benign gammopathy with response to chlorambucil. *Blood*, **42**, 463–470.

EVANS, R. S., BINGHAM, M. & TURNER, E. (1965). Autoimmune hemolytic disease: observations of serological reactions and disease activity. *Ann. N. Y. Acad. Sci.*, **124**, 422–440.

EVANS, R. S. & DUANE, R. T. (1947). Observations on the effect of irradiation in chronic acquired hemolytic anemia exhibiting hemolytic activity for transfused erythrocytes. *Blood*, **2**, 72–84.

EYSTER, M. E. & JENKINS, D. E. JNR (1969). Erythrocyte coating substances in patients with positive direct antiglobulin reactions. *Amer. J. Med.*, **46**, 360–371.

FEHR, J., HOFMANN, V. & KAPPELER, U. (1982). Transient reversal of thrombocytopenia in idiopathic thrombocytopenic purpura by high-dose intravenous gamma globulin. *New Engl. J. Med.*, **306**, 1254–1258.

FELDMAN, J. D. & RACHMILEWITZ, M. (1954). The adrenal cortex and hemolysis. II. Immune serum. *Acta haemat. (Basel)*, **11**, 129–133.

FERRANT, A., CAUWE, F., MICHAUX, J. L., BECKERS, C., VERWILGHEN, R. & SOKAL, G. (1982). Assessment of the sites of red cell destruction using quantitative measurements of splenic and hepatic red cell destruction. *Brit. J. Haemat.*, **50**, 591–598.

FIESCHI, A., PANNACCIULLI, I. & TIZIANELLO, A. (1959). L'impiego di emazie marcate con Cr^{51} nello studio della splenomegalia e delle sedi dell'emocateresi. *Minerva nucleare (Torino)*, **3**, 85–94.

FORMIJNE, P. (1956). Clinical applications of 5-iodosalicylic acid in acquired hemolytic anemia and other diseases. *Proc. kon. ned. Akad. Wet., Series C*, **59**, 335–343.

FORRESTER, R. M. & STRATTON, F. (1970). A case of idiopathic autoimmune haemolytic anaemia in an infant treated with chloroquin. *Vox Sang*, **18**, 267–269.

FRANK, M. M., SCHREIBER, A. D., ATKINSON, J. P. & JAFFE, C. J. (1977). Pathophysiology of immune hemolytic anemia. *Ann. intern. Med.*, **87**, 210–222.

FRIMMER, D. & CREGER, W. P. (1970). Heparin and hemolytic anemia. *Amer. J. med. Sci.*, **259**, 412–418.

FRUMIN, A. L., Smith, E. M., TAYLOR, A. G. & DRATMAN, M. B. (1953). Acquired hemolytic anemia in pregnancy treated with ACTH and cortisone. *Amer. J. Obstet. Gynec.*, **65**, 421–423.

FUDENBERG, H. H. & KUNKEL, H. G. (1957). Physical properties of red cell agglutinins in acquired hemolytic anemia. *J. exp. Med.*, **106**, 689–702.

GARDNER, F. (1950). In discussion on "ACTH in leukemia". *Blood*, **5**, 791.

GARDNER, F. H., McELFRESH, A. E., HARRIS, J. W. & DIAMOND, L. K. (1951). The effect of adrenocorticotrophic hormone (ACTH) in idiopathic acquired hemolytic anemia as related to the hemolytic mechanisms. *J. Lab. clin. Med.*, **37**, 444–457.

GARELLI, S., MONTANI, F., NAVASSA, G. & RESTELLI, G. (1985). Exchange transfusion and plasma-exchange in acute autoimmune hemolytic anemia: report of one case. *Haematologica*, **70**, 166–170.

GARELLI, S., MOSIONI, L., VALBONESI, M., SCHIEPPATI, G. & NAVASSA, G. (1980). Plasma exchange for a hemolytic crisis due to autoimmune hemolytic anemia of IgG warm type. *Blut*, **41**, 387–391.

GEHRMANN, G. & GROBEL, P. (1962). The site of red-cell breakdown in haemolytic anaemia. Its significance for predicting the result of splenectomy. *Germ. med. Monthly*, **7**, 5–9.

GERMUTH, J. G. JNR, OYAMA, J. & OTTINGER, B. (1951). The mechanisms of action of 17-hydroxy-11-dehydrocorticosterone (compound E) and of the adrenocorticotropic hormone in experimental hypersensitivity in rabbits. *J. exp. Med.*, **94**, 139–170.

GERTZ, M. A., PETITT, R. M., ALVARO, A., PINEDA, A. A., WICK, M. R. & BURGSTALER, E. A. (1981). Vinblastine-loaded platelets for autoimmune hemolytic anemia. *Ann. intern. Med.*, **95**, 325–326.

GIBSON, J. (1988). Autoimmune hemolytic anemia: current concepts. *Aust. N. Z. J. Med.*, **18**, 625–637.

GOLDBERG, A., HUTCHISON, H. E. & MACDONALD, E. (1966). Radiochromium in the selection of patients with haemolytic anaemia for splenectomy. *Lancet*, **i**, 109–114.

GOVONI, M., MORETTI, M., MENINI, C. & FIOCCHI, F. (1990). Rifampicin-induced immune hemolytic anemia: therapeutic relevance of plasma exchange. *Vox Sang.*, **59**, 246–247.

GREENDYKE, R. M., BRADLEY, E. M., SWISHER, S. N. & TRABOLD, N. C. (1965). Studies of the effects of administration of ACTH and adrenal corticosteroids on erythrophagocytosis. *J. clin. Invest.*, **44**, 746–753.

GROS, H. (1955). Die Loutit-Anämie und ihre Behandlung mit ACTH. *Med. Mschr.*, **9**, 228–232.

GUNZ, F. W. & AIKEN, M. H. (1952). Treatment of acquired haemolytic anaemia by means of ACTH. Report of a case. *N. Z. med. J.*, **51**, 283–290.

HABIBI, B., HOMBERG J.-C., SCHAISON, G. & SALMON, C. (1974). Autoimmune hemolytic anemia in children. *Amer. J. Med.*, **56**, 61–69.

HABIBI, B. & NAJEAN, Y. (1971). Intérêt pratique de l'étude de la cinétique érythrocytaire par marquage au ^{51}Cr in vitro dans les anémies hémolytiques auto-immunes. *Presse méd.*, **79**, 857–862.

HANSEN, K. B. (1952a). Effect of A.C.T.H. on haemolytic anaemia. *Lancet*, **i**, 419 (Letter).

HANSEN, K. B. (1952b). Immuno-haemolytisk anaemi og ACTH. *Nord. Med.*, **47**, 281–283.

HARTMAN, M. M. (1964). Reversal of serologic reactions by heparin. Therapeutic implications. II. Idiopathic acquired hemolytic anemia. *Ann. Allergy*, **22**, 313–320.

HEILMEYER, L. (1952). ACTH und cortisontherapie bei nichtleukämischen Bluterkrankungen. *Acta haemat. (Basel)*, **7**, 206–216.

HEIMPEL, H. & SCHUBOTHE, H. (1964). Die Lokalisation des Erythrozytenabbaus bei autoimmunhämolytischen Anämien. Untersuchungen mit Cr^{51}. *Blut*, **10**, 306–314.

HEINE, K. M., HERRMANN, H. & STOBBE, H. (1964). Die Heparinbehandlung bei erworbener hämolytischer Anämie. *Acta haemat. (Basel)*, **32**, 27–34.

HEISEL, M. A. & ORTEGA, J. A. (1983). Factors influencing prognosis in childhood autoimmune hemolytic anemia. *Amer. J. Pediat. Hemat. Oncol.*, **5**, 147–152.

HENI, F. & BLESSING, K. (1954). Beschreibung zwier schwerer erworbener idiopathischer hämolytischer Anämien. *Klin. Wschr.*, **32**, 481–485.

HENNEMANN, H. H. (1953). Über die Wirkung von ACTH auf unspezifische Kälteagglutinine. *Klin. Wschr.*, **31**, 722.

HERRERA, A., BERNARD, J. F., VROCLANS, M., DHERMY, D., RENOUX, M. & BOIVIN, P. (1980). Les plasmaphérèses et érythrophérèses intensives, thérapeutique d'urgence des anémies auto-immunes suraiguës *Nouv. Presse Méd.*, **9**, 317.

HIPPE, E., JENSEN, K. B., OLSEN, H., LIND, K. & THOMSEN, P. E. B. (1970). Chlorambucil treatment of patients with cold agglutinin syndrome. *Blood*, **35**, 68–72.

HIROOKA, M., YOSHIOKA, K., OHNO, T., KUBOTA, N. & IKEDA, S. (1970). Autoimmune hemolytic anemia in a child treated with thymectomy. *Tohoku J. exp. Med.*, **101**, 227–235.

HITZIG, W. H. & MASSIMO, L. (1966). Treatment of autoimmune hemolytic anemia in children with azathioprine (Imuran). *Blood*, **28**, 840–850.

HÖGMAN, C., KILLANDER, J. & SJÖLIN, S. (1960). A case of idiopathic autoimmune haemolytic anaemia due to anti-e. *Acta paediat. (Uppsala)*, **49**, 270–280.

HOLLÄNDER, L. (1954). Study of the erythrocyte survival time in a case of acquired haemolytic anaemia. *Vox Sang. (Amst.)*, **4**, 164–165.

HONETZ, N. & NEUMANN, E. (1970). Behandlungsergebnisse mit Heparin und SP 54 bei autoimmunhämolytischen Anämien. *Acta haemat. (Basel)*, **43**, 296–308.

HOREAU, J., ROBIN, Cl., GUÉNEL, J., DE FERRON, A. & NICHOLAS, G. (1962). Infarctus splénique au cours d'une anémie hémolytique acquise. Splénectomie. Guerison. *Nouv. Rev. franç. Hémat.*, **2**, 626–629.

HORSTER, J. A. (1961). *Die Korticosteroid-Behandlung hämatologischer und verwandter Erkrankungen*, p. 31. Georg Theime, Stuttgart.

HORSTMAN, L. L., JY, W. & AHN, Y. S. (1991). Danazol inhibits autoantibody binding to erythrocytes in vitro at physiological concentrations. *Clin. Res.*, **39**, 364A (Abstract).

HUDSON, G., HERDAN, G. & YOFFEY, J. M. (1952). Effect of repeated injections of A.C.T.H. upon the bone marrow. *Brit. med. J.*, **i**, 999–1002.

HUGHES JONES N. C. & SZUR, L. (1957). Determination of the sites of red-cell destruction using ^{51}Cr-labelled cells. *Brit. J. Haemat.*, **3**, 320–331.

IMBACH, P., BARANDUN, S., D'APUZZO, U., BAUMGARTNER, C., HIRT, A., MORELL, A., ROSSI, E., SCHÖNI, M., VEST, M. & WAGNER, H. P. (1981). High-dose intravenous gammaglobulin for idiopathic thromboytopenic purpura in childhood. *Lancet*, **i**, 1228–1231.

ISBISTER, J. P. (1979). Plasma exchange: a selective form of blood-letting. *Med. J. Aust.*, **2**, 167–173.

ISBISTER, J. P., BIGGS, J. C. & PENNY, R. (1978). Experience with large volume plasmapheresis in malignant paraproteinemia and immune disorders. *Aust. N. Z. J. Med.*, **8**, 154–164.

ISSITT, P. D. (1981). Red cell transfusions in autoimmunized patients. *Cleveland Clin. Quart.*, **48**, 289–303.

ISSITT, P. (1985). *Applied Blood Group Serology*, 3rd edn, p. 530. Montgomery Scientific Publications, Miami.

JAMRA, M., CILLO, D. M., MAURO, E., BRAGA, F. V. & VASCONCELOS, E. (1962). Esplenectomía en las anemias hemolíticas. Valoración de los resultados. *Sangre (Barcelona)*, **7**, 245–262.

JANDL, J. H. (1963). Current concepts in therapy. Hemolytic anemia. *New Engl. J. Med.*, **268**, 482–486.

JANDL, J. H., GREENBERG, M. S., YONEMOTO, R. H. & CASTLE, W. B. (1956). Clinical determination of the sites of red cell sequestration in hemolytic anemias. *J. clin. Invest.*, **35**, 842–867.

JOHNSON, C. A. & ABILGAARD, C. F. (1976). Treatment of idiopathic autoimmune hemolytic anemia in children. *Acta paediat. scand.*, **65**, 375–379.

KALISS, G., HOECKER, G. & BRYANT, B. F. (1956). The effect of cortisone on isohemagglutinin production in mice. *J. Immunol.*, **76**, 83–88.

KAPLAN, M. E. & JANDL, J. H. (1961). Inhibition of red cell sequestration by cortisone. *J. exp. Med.*, **114**, 921–937.

KARAKLIS, A., VALAES, T., PANTELAKIS, S. N. & DOXIADIS, S. A. (1964). Thymectomy in an infant with autoimmune haemolytic anaemia. *Lancet*, **ii**, 778–780.

KISSMEYER-NIELSEN, F. (1957). A case of autoimmune haemolytic anaemia with a very remarkable course. *Vox Sang.*, **2**, 88–93.

KLEIN, H. G., FALTZ, L. L., McINTOSH, C. L., APPLEBAUM, F. R., DEISSEROTH, A. B. & HOLLAND, P. V. (1980). Surgical hypothermia in a patient with a cold agglutinin. Management by plasma exchange. *Transfusion*, **20**, 354–357.

KORST, D R., CLATANOFF, D. V. & SCHILLING, R. F. (1955). External scintillation counting over the liver and spleen after the transfusion of radioactive erythrocytes. *Clin. Res. Proc.*, **3**, 195–196.

KRAUSS, H., HEILMEYER, L. & WEINREICH, J. (1959a). Ergebnisse und Indikationen der Splenektomie bei verschiedenen Blutkrankheiten. *Folia haemat. (Frankfurt)*, **3**, 243–268

KRAUSS, H., HEILMEYER, L. & WEINREICH, J. (1959b). Splenectomy in blood diseases. Indications and results. *Germ. med. Monthly*, **4**, 300–302.

KUTTI, J., WADENVIK, H., SAFAI-KUTTI, S., BJORKANDER, J., HANSON, L. A., WESTBORG, G., JOHNSEN, S.-A. & LARSSON, B. (1984). Successful treatment of refractory autoimmune haemolytic anaemia by plasmapheresis. *Scand. J. Haemat.*, **32**, 149–152.

LAHAV, M., ROSENBERG, I. & WYSENBEEK, A. J. (1989). Steroid-responsive idiopathic cold agglutinin disease: a case report. *Acta haemat. (Basel)*, **81**, 166–168.

LANDYMORE, R., ISOM, W. & BARLAM, B. (1983). Management of patients with cold agglutinins who require open-heart surgery. *Canad, J. Surg.*, **26**, 79–80.

LEDERER, M. (1925). A form of acute hemolytic anemia probably of infectious origin. *Amer. J med. Sci.*, **170**, 500–510.

LEDERER, M. (1930). Three additional cases of acute hemolytic (infectious) anemia. *Amer. J. med. Sci.*, **179**, 228–236.

LEICKLY, F. E. & BUCKLEY, R. H. (1987). Successful treatment of auto-immune hemolytic anemia in common variable immunodeficiency with high-dose intravenous gamma globulin. *Amer. J. Med.*, **82**, 159–162.

LEMMEL, E., HURD, E. R. & ZIFF, M. (1971). Differential effects of 6-mercaptopurine and cyclophosphamide on autoimmune phenomena in NZB mice. *Clin. exp. Immunol.*, **8**, 355–362.

LETMAN, H. (1953). Behandling af acquisit haemolytisk anaemi med ACTH og cortisone. *Ugeskr. Laeg.*, **115**, 1139–1145.

LETMAN, H. (1957). Auto-immune haemolytic anaemia. *Dan. med. Bull.*, **4**, 143–147.

LEWIS, S. M., SZUR, L. & DACIE, J. V. (1960). The pattern of erythrocyte destruction in haemolytic anaemia, as studied with radioactive chromium. *Brit. J. Haemat.*, **6**, 122–139.

LEY, A. B. & GARDNER, F. H. (1951). The effect of cortisone acetate on idiopathic acquired hemolytic anemia. *J. clin. Invest.*, **30**, 656 (Abstract).

LEY, A. B., MAYER, K. & HARRIS, J. P. (1958). Observations on a 'specific autoantibody'. *Proc. 6th Congr. int. Soc. Blood Transf. Boston, 1956*, pp. 148–153. Karger, Basel.

LIND, K., MANSA, B. & OLESEN, H. (1963). Penicillamine treatment in the cold-haemagglutinin syndrome. *Acta med. scand.*, **173**, 648–660.

LOEB, V. JNR, SEAMAN, W. B. & MOORE, C. V. (1952). The use of thorium dioxide sol (Thorotrast) in the roentgenologic demonstration of accessory spleens. *Blood*, **7**, 904–914.

LOGUE, G. L., ROSSE, W. G. & GOCKERMAN, J. P. (1973). Measurement of the third component of complement bound to red blood cells in patients with the cold agglutinin syndrome. *J. clin. Invest.*, **52**, 493–501.

LORIE, I. I. & PATSIORA, M. D. (1958). The treatment of acquired hemolytic anaemias. *Probl. Hemat. Blood Transf.*, **3**, 1–11.

LUNDGREN, G., ASABA, H., BERGSTRÖM, J., GROTH, C.-G., MAGNUSSON, G., MÖLLER, E., STRINDBERG, J. & WEHLE, G. (1981). Fulminating anti-A autoimmune hemolysis with anuria in a renal transport recipient: a therapeutic role of plasma exchange. *Clin. Nephrol.*, **16**, 211–214.

McCURDY, P. R. & RATH, C. E. (1958). Splenectomy in hemolytic anemia. Results predicted by body scanning after injection of Cr^{51}-tagged red cells. *New Engl. J. Med.*, **259**, 459–463.

McCURDY, P. R. & RATH, C. E. (1960). Selection of patients for splenectomy: evaluation of technic of Cr^{51} spleen localization. *Proc. 7th int. Congr. int. Soc. Hemat., Rome, 7–13th Sept. 1958*, Vol II, pp. 559–563. Il Pensiero Scientifico, Roma.

McFARLAND, W., GALBRAITH, R. G. & MIALE, A. JNR (1960). Heparin therapy in autoimmune hemolytic anemia. *Blood*, **15**, 741–747.

MACINTYRE, E. A., LINCH, D. C., MACEY, M. G. & NEWLAND, A. C. (1985). Successful response to intravenous immunoglobulin in autoimmune haemolytic anaemia. *Brit. J. Haemat.*, **60**, 387–388 (Letter).

MAJER, R. V. & HYDE, R. D. (1988). High-dose intravenous immunoglobulin in the treatment of autoimmune haemolytic anaemia. *Clin. lab. Haemat.*, **10**, 391–395.

MALLARMÉ, J. (1952). L'A.C.T.H. et la cortisone dans le traitment de l'anémie hémolytique acquise et de l'hypersplénisme. *Bull. méd. (Paris)*, **66**, 225–269

MALLARMÉ, J., MARTIN, EYQUEM, & FLEURY, (1951). Le traitement de l'ictère hémolytique acquis par l'A.C.T.H. Son action contre les auto-anticorps. *Sang*, **22**, 580–582.

MARKUS, H. & FORFAR, J. C. (1986). Splenic irradiation in treating warm autoimmune haemolytic anaemia. *Brit. med. J.*, **293**, 839–840.

MARMONT, A. & FUSCO, F. (1956). Nouvi steroidi cortisonici ed anemia emolitiche acquisite. *Minerva med. (Torino)*, **47**, 1679–1695.

MARTELLI, M., MARTINEZ, R. & CARONIA, F. (1959). Il prednisone nelle anemie emolitiche autoimmuni: rilieve clinici e sierologici. *Rif. med.*, **73**, 128–133.

MASOUREDIS, S. P. & CHAPLIN, H. JNR (1985). Transfusion management of autoimmune hemolytic anemia. In *Immune Hemolytic Anemias* (ed. by H. Chaplin), pp. 177–205. Churchill Livingstone, New York.

MASSEI, G. & MARINAI, M. (1956). Effetto del cortisone e dell'ACTH nelle anemie emolitiche sperimentali da siero immune. *Minerva med. (Torino)*, **47**, 593–596.

MEDELLIN, P. L., PATTEN, E. & WEISS, G. B. (1982). Vinblastine for autoimmune hemolytic anemia. *Ann. intern. Med.*, **96**, 123 (Letter).

M.R.C. HAEMATOLOGY PANEL (1952). The treatment of blood disorders with A.C.T.H. and cortisone. A preliminary report to the Medical Research Council by the panel on the haematological applications of A.C.T.H. and cortisone. *Brit. med. J*, **i**, 1261–1263.

M.R.C. HAEMATOLOGY PANEL (1953). Treatment of blood disorders with A.C.T.H. and cortisone. Second report to the Medical Research Council by the panel on haematological applications of A.C.T.H. and cortisone. *Brit. med. J.*, **ii**, 1400–1401.

M.R.C. HAEMATOLOGY PANEL (1955). Treatment of blood disorders with A.C.T.H. and cortisone. Third report to the Medical Research Council by the panel on the haematological applications of A.C.T.H. and cortisone. *Brit. med. J.*, **ii**, 455–457.

MEHROTRA, T. N. & CHARLWOOD, P. A. (1960). Physico-chemical characterization of the cold auto-antibodies of acquired haemolytic anaemia. *Immunology*, **3**, 254–264.

MELANI, F. & PRENNA, G. (1959). Osservazioni cliniche sopre un caso di anemia emolitica auto-immune trattato con triamcinolone. *Riv. Emoterap.*, **3**, 363–375.

MEY, U. & HESSE, P. (1969). Die Splenektomie bei hämatologischem Erkrankungen. *Schweiz. med. Wschr.*, **99**, 1873–1876.

MEYER, J. F. (1951). Idiopathic acquired hemolytic anemia in an infant; successful treatment with corticotropin (ACTH). *Amer. J. Dis. Child.*, **82**, 721–725.

MEYER, L. M. & RITZ, N. D. (1954). Use of corticotropin therapy for idiopathic acquired hemolytic anemia. Report of a case. *J. Amer. med. Ass.*, **155**, 742–743.

MEYERS, M. C., MILLER, S., LINMAN, J. W. & BETHELL, F. H. (1952). The use of ACTH and cortisone in idiopathic thrombocytopenic purpura and idiopathic acquired hemolytic anemia. *Ann. intern. Med.*, **37**, 352–361.

MEYTES, D., ADLER, M., VIRAG, I., FEIGH, D. & LEVENE, C. (1985). High-dose methylprednisolone in acute immune cold hemolysis. *New Engl. J. Med.*, **312**, 318 (Letter).

MICHELI, F. (1911). Unmittelbare Effekte der Splenektomie bei einem Fall von erworbenen hämolytischen splenomegalischen Ikterus, Typus Hayem-Widal. *Wien. klin. Wschr.*, **24**, 1269–1274.

MILLIEZ, P., LAROCHE, C., DUBOST, C., DREYFUS, B., DAUSSET, J. & MOREAU, L. (1951). Maladie neuro-hémolytique apparemment acquise. *Bull. Soc. méd. Hôp. Paris*, **67**, 771–778.

MIRECKA, J., ASTALDI, G., SZMIGIEL, Z., LISIEWICZ, J. & WAZEWSKA-CZYZEWSKA (1972). L-asparaguinase effect on the erythrocyte-immunoglobulin binding in acquired hemolytic anemia. *Acta haemat. (Basel)*, **47**, 71–80.

MIYAZAKI, S., NAKAYAMA, K., AKABANE, T., TAGUCHI, N., AKATSUKA, J., NAGAO, T., TSUJINO, G. & NAKAGAWA, T. (1983). Follow-up study of 34 children with autoimmune hemolytic anemia. *Acta haemat. jap.*, **46**, 6–10.

MOESCHLIN, S. (1956). Indikationen der Splenektomie. *Schweiz. Akad. med. Wiss.*, **12**, 226–241.

MOLLISON, P. L. (1959). Measurement of survival and destruction of red cells in haemolytic syndromes. *Brit. med. Bull.*, **15**, 59–67.

MUELLER-ECKHARDT, C., SALAMA, A., KIEFEL, V., KÜENZLEN, E. & FÖRSTER, C. (1984). A new concept for the effector mechanism of intravenous immunoglobulin in hemocytopenias. *Blut*, **48**, 353–356.

MUELLER-ECKHARDT, C., SALAMA, A., MAHN, I., KIEFEL, V., NEUZNER, J. & GRAUBNER, M. (1985). Lack of efficacy of high-dose intravenous immunoglobulin in autoimmune haemolytic anaemia: a clue to its mechanism. *Scand. J. Haemat.*, **34**, 394–400.

MURPHY, S. & LOBUGLIO, A. F. (1976). Drug therapy of autoimmune hemolytic anemia. *Seminars Hemat.*, **13**, 323–348.

NEGRI, M., POTOTSCHNIG, C. & MAIOLO, A. T. (1960). L'anemia emolitica da autoanticorpi nella prima infanzia. Presentazione di un caso. *Minerva pediat. (Torino)*, **12**, 656–666.

NOBEL, E. & STEINEBACH, R. (1914). Zur Klinik der Splenomegalie im Kindesalter. *Z. Kinderheilk.*, **12**, 75–99.

NYDEGGER, U. E., KAZATCHKINE, M. D. & MIESCHER, P. A. (1991). Immunopathologic and clinical features of hemolytic anemia due to cold agglutinins. *Seminars Hemat.*, **28**, 66–77.

ODA, H., HONDA, A., SUGITA, K., NAKAMURA, A. & MAKAJIMA, H. (1985). High-dose intravenous intact IgG infusion in refractory autoimmune hemolytic anemia (Evans syndrome). *J. Pediat.*, **107**, 744–746.

OLESEN, H. (1964). Chlorambucil treatment of the cold agglutinin syndrome. *Scand. J. Haemat.*, **1**, 116–128.

OSKI, F. A. & ABELSON, N. M. (1965). Autoimmune

hemolytic anemia in an infant. Report of a case treated unsuccessfully with thymectomy. *J. Pediat.*, **67**, 752–758.

OWREN, P. A. (1949). Acquired hemolytic jaundice. *Scand. J. clin. lab. Invest.*, **1**, 41–48.

PACKER, J. T., GREENDYKE, R. M. & SWISHER, S. N. (1960). The inhibition of erythrophagocytosis *in vitro* by corticosteroids. *Trans. Ass. Amer. Physcns*, **73**, 93–102.

PARKER, A. C., MACPHERSON, A.I.S. & RICHMOND, J. (1977). Value of radiochromium investigation in autoimmune haemolytic anaemia. *Brit. med. J.*, **i**, 208–209.

PATTEN, E. & REUTER, F. P. (1980). Evans' syndrome: possible benefit from plasma exchange. *Transfusion*, **20**, 589–593.

PETZ, L. D. & GARRATTY, G. (1980). *Acquired Immune Hemolytic Anemias*, 458 pp. Churchill Livingstone, New York.

PINEY, A. (1950). Acquired haemolytic anaemia. *Sang.* **21**, 229–232.

PIROFSKY, B. (1969). *Autoimmunization and the Autoimmune Hemolytic Anemias*, 537 pp. Williams and Wilkins, Baltimore.

PIROFSKY, B. & BARDANA, E. J. JNR (1974). Autoimmune hemolytic anemia: II. Therapeutic aspects. *Ser. Haemat.*, **7**, 376–385.

PISCIOTTA, A. V. & HINZ, J. E. (1957). Detection and characterization of autoantibodies in acquired auto-immune hemolytic anemia. *Amer. J. clin. Path.*, **27**, 619–634.

POCECCO, M., VENTURA, A., TAMARO, P. & LONGO, F. (1986). High-dose IVIgG in autoimmune hemolytic anemia. *J. Pediat.*, **109**, 726 (Letter).

RAVINA, A., DELARUE, J., MALLARMÉ, J. & EYQUEN, A. (1950). L'anémie hémolytique acquise et les difficultés de son traitement. *Ann. Méd.*, **51**, 655–672.

REMY, D. (1957). Die Prednisonbehandlung erworbener hämolytischer Anämien. *Ärztl. Wschr.*, **12**, 505–509.

RICHMOND, G. W., RAY, I. & KORENBLITT, A. (1987). Initial stabilization preceding enhanced hemolysis in autoimmune hemolytic anemia treated with intravenous gammaglobulin. *J. Pediat.*, **110**, 917–919.

RICHMOND, J., WOODRUFF, M. F. A., CUMMING, R. A. & DONALD, K. W. (1963). A case of idiopathic thrombocytopenia and autoimmune haemolytic anaemia treated by thymic irradiation and by administration of imuran and actinomycin-C. *Lancet*, **ii**, 125–128.

RITZMANN, S. E. & LEVIN, W. C. (1961). Effect of mercaptanes in cold agglutinin disease. *J. Lab. clin. Med.*, **57**, 718–732.

ROBSON, H. N. (1949). Medical aspects of splenectomy. *Edinb. med. J.*, **56**, 381–395.

RODENHUIS, S., MASS, A., HAZENBERG, C. A. M., DAS P. C. & NIEWEG, H. O. (1985). Inefficacy of plasma

exchange in cold agglutinin hemolytic anemia—a case study. *Vox Sang.*, **49**, 20–25.

ROSE, B. S. & NABARRO, S. N. (1953). Four cases of acute acquired haemolytic anaemia in childhood treated with A.C.T.H. *Arch. Dis. Childh.*, **28**, 87–00.

ROSENFIELD, R. E. & DIAMOND, S. H. (1981). Diagnosis and treatment of the immune hemolytic anemias. *Haematologia*, **14**, 247–256.

ROSENFIELD, R. E. & JAGATHAMBAL, (1976). Transfusion therapy for autoimmune hemolytic anemia. *Seminars Hemat.*, **13**, 311–321.

ROSENFIELD, R. E., VITALE, B. & KOCHWA, S. (1967). Immune mechanisms for destruction of erythrocytes in vivo. II. Heparinization for protection of lysin-sensitized erythrocytes. *Transfusion*, 7, 261–264.

ROSENTHAL, M. C., SPAET, T. H., GOLDENBERG, H. & DAMESHEK, W. (1952). Treatment of acquired haemolytic anaemia with compound F acetate. *Lancet*, **i**, 1135–1140.

ROSSE, W. F. (1971). Quantitative immunology of immune hemolytic anemia. II. The relationship of cell-bound antibody to hemolysis and the effect of treatment. *J. clin. Invest.*, **50**, 734–743.

ROSSE, W. F. (1990). *Clinical Immunohematology: Basic Concepts and Clinical Applications*, 677 pp. Blackwell Scientific Publications, Boston.

ROTH, K. L. (1954). Interaction of heparin with auto-agglutinins in idiopathic acquired hemolytic anemia. *Proc. Soc. exp. Biol. Med. (N. Y.)*, **86**, 352–356.

ROTH, K. L. & FRUMIN, A. M. (1956). Effect of intramuscular heparin on antibodies in idiopathic acquired hemolytic anemia. *Amer. J. Med.*, **20**, 968–970.

SACKS, M. S., WORKMAN, J. B. & JAHN, E. F. (1952). Diagnosis and treatment of acquired hemolytic anemia. *J. Amer. med. Ass.*, **150**, 1556–1559.

SAINT, E. G. & GARDNER, H. J. (1952). The successful treatment of severe acquired haemolytic anaemia with adrenocorticotrophic hormone (ACTH). *Med. J. Aust.*, **ii**, 305–307.

SALAMA, A., MAHN, I., NEUZNER, J., GRAUBNER, M. & MUELLER-ECKHARDT, C. (1984). IgG therapy in autoimmune haemolytic anaemia of warm type. *Blut*, **48**, 391–392.

SALAMA, A., MUELLER-ECKHARDT, C. & KIEFEL, V. (1983). Effect of intravenous immunoglobulin in immune thrombocytopenia. Competitive inhibition of reticuloendothelial system function by sequestration of autologous red blood cells. *Lancet*, **ii**, 193–195.

SCHMIDT, R. E., BUDDE, U., SCHÄFER, G. & STROEHMANN, I. (1981). High-dose intravenous gammaglobulin for idiopathic thrombocytopenic purpura. *Lancet*, **ii**, 475–476 (Letter).

SCHREIBER, A. D., HERSKOVITZ, B. S. & GOLDWEIN, M. (1977). Low-titer cold-hemagglutinin disease. Mechanism of hemolysis and response to corticosteroids. *New Engl. J. Med.*, **296**, 1490–1494.

SCHWARTZ, R. & DAMSHEK, W. (1962). The treatment

of autoimmune hemolytic anemia with 6-mercaptupurine and thioguanine. *Blood*, **19**, 483–500.

SCHWARTZ, R., EISNER, A. & DAMESHEK, W. (1959). The effect of 6-mercaptopurine on primary and secondary immune responses. *J. clin. Invest.*, **38**, 1394–1403.

SCHWARTZ, R., STACK, J. & DAMESHEK, W. (1958). Effect of 6-mercaptopurine on antibody production. *Proc. Soc. exp. Biol. Med. (N. Y.)*, **99**, 164–167.

SELDON, W., ISBISTER, J. P., RAIK, E. & BIGGS, J. C. (1980). A fatal case of cold autoimmune hemolytic anemia. *Amer. J. clin. Path.*, **73**, 716–717.

SHAHIAN, D. M., WALLACH, S. R. & BERN, M. M. (1985). Open heart surgery in patients with cold-reactive proteins. *Surg. Clin. N. Amer.*, **65**, 315–322.

SILVERGLEID, A. J., WELLS, R. F., HAFLEIGH E. B., KORN, G., KELLNER, J. J. & GRUMET, F. C. (1978). Compatibility test using ^{51}chromium-labeled red cells in crossmatch positive patients. *Transfusion*, **18**, 8–14.

SILVERSTEIN, M. N., GOMES, M. R., ELVEBACK, L. R., REMINE, W. H. & LINMAN, J. W. (1972). Idiopathic acquired hemolytic anaemia. Survival in 117 cases. *Arch. intern. Med.*, **129**, 85–87.

SINGH, I. & BIRD, G. W. G. (1960). Autoimmune haemolytic anaemia treated with venom antiserum. *Lancet*, **i**, 92.

SKINNER, M. D. & SCHWARTZ, R. S. (1972). Immunosuppressive therapy (First of two parts). *New Engl. J. Med.*, **287**, 211–227.

SOKAL, G. (1957). Hypersplénisme hémolytique. Présence d'un anticorps aux caractères inhabituels. *Rev. belge Path.*, **26**, 95–105.

SOKOL, R. J., HEWITT, S., BOOKER, D. J. & MORRIS, B. M. (1988). Patients with red cell autoantibodies: selection of blood for transfusion. *Clin. lab. Haemat.*, **10**, 257–264.

SOKOL, R. J., HEWITT, S., STAMPS, B. K. & HITCHEN, P. A. (1984). Autoimmune haemolysis in childhood and adolescence. *Acta haemat. (Basel)*, **72**, 245–257.

STEIN, W. (1957). Zur Therapie der durch unvollständige Antikörper bedingten erworbenen hämolytischen Anämien. *Ärztl. Wschr.*, **12**, 450–453.

STEINBERG, A. D., Plotz, P. H., Wolff, S. M., WONG, V. G., AGUS, S. G. & DECKER, J. L. (1972). Cytotoxic drugs in treatment of nonmalignant diseases (NIH Conference). *Ann. intern. Med.*, **76**, 619–642.

STICKNEY, J. M. & HANLON, D. G. (1956). Acquired hemolytic anemia. *Med. Clin. N. Amer.*, **40**, 1015–1024.

STICKNEY, J. M. & HECK, F. J. (1948). Primary nonfamilial hemolytic anemia. *Blood*, **3**, 431–437.

STORTI, E. & VACCARI, F. (1956). Studies on the relationship between anticoagulants and hemolysis. Effect of anticoagulants on hemolysis and on the agglutionation of red blood cells by an anti-erythrocyte serum. *Acta haemat. (Basel)*, **15**, 12–22.

STORTI, E., VACCARI, F. & BALDINI, E. (1956). Studies on the relationship between anticoagulants and hemolysis. Part II. The effect of anticoagulants on the hemolysis caused by antibodies in vivo. *Acta haemat. (Basel)*, **15**, 106–117.

SUSSMAN, L. N. & DORDICK, J. R. (1956). Prednisone (Meticorten) in treatment of acquired hemolytic anemia. *J. Amer. med. Ass.*, **160**, 285–287.

SZUR, L. (1970). Surface counting in the assessment of sites of red cell destruction. *Brit. J. Haemat.*, **18**, 591–595 (Annotation).

TAFT, E. G., PROPP, R. P. & SULLIVAN, S. A. (1977). Plasma exchange for cold agglutinin hemolytic anemia. *Transfusion*, **17**, 173–176.

TAYLOR, L. (1963). Idiopathic autoimmune hemolytic anemia. Response of a patient to repeated courses of alkylating agents. *Amer. J. Med.*, **35**, 130–134.

TEN PAS, A. & MONTO, R. W. (1966). The treatment of autoimmune hemolytic anemia with heparin. *Amer. J. med. Sci.*, **251**, 63–69.

THORN, G. W. and others. (1953). Pharmacologic aspects of adrenocortical steroids and ACTH in man. *New Engl. J. Med.*, **248**, 323–337.

TISCHENDORF, W., ECKLEBE, G. & THOFERN, E. (1951–1952). ACTH und experimentelle hämolytische Anämien. *Z. ges. exp. Med.*, **118**, 203–212.

TOCANTINS, L. M. & WANG, G. C. (1956). Radioactive colloidal gold in the treatment of severe acquired hemolytic anemia refractory to splenectomy. *Progr. Hemat.* **1**, 138–152.

UNGER, L. J. (1951). The effect of ACTH in acquired hemolytic anemia. *Amer. J. clin. Path.*, **21**, 456–459.

VAN LOGHEM, J. J., PEETOM, F., VAN DER HART, M., VAN DER VEER, M., VAN DER GIESSEN, M., PRINS, H. K., ZURCHER, C. & ENGELFRIET, C. P. (1963). Serological and immunochemical studies in hemolytic anemia with high-titre cold agglutinins. *Vox Sang.*, **8**, 33–46.

VAUGHAN, J. H., BAYLES, T. B. & FAVOUR, C. B. (1950). The effect of ACTH on blood complement, gamma globulins and fibrinogen. *J. clin. Invest.*, **29**, 850–851 (Abstract).

VEEGER, W., WORDRING, M. G., VAN ROOD, J. J., EERNISSE, J. G., LEEKSMA, C. H., VERLOOP, M. C. & NIEWEG, H. O. (1962). The value of the determination of the site of red cell sequestration in hemolytic anemia as a prediction test for splenectomy. *Acta med. scand.*, **171**, 507–520.

VERLOOP, M. C. (1955). Ervaringen bij de behandeling van lijders aan verkregen haemolytische anaemie. *Ned. T. Geneesk.*, **99**, 771–783.

VON KEYSERLINGK, H., MEYER-SEBELLEK, W., ARNTZ, R. & HALLER, H. (1987). Plasma exchange treatment in autoimmune hemolytic anemia of the warm antibody type with renal failure. *Vox Sang.*, **52**, 298–300.

VON DEM BORNE, A. E. G. KR., ENGELFRIET, C. P.,

REYNIERSE, E., BECKERS, D. & VAN LOGHEM, J. J. (1973). Autoimmune haemolytic anaemia. VI. [51]Chromium survival studies in patients with different kinds of warm autoantibodies. *Clin. exp. Immunol.*, **13**, 561–571.

WANG, G., BOWMAN, H. S. & TOCANTINS, L. M. (1954). Radioactive colloidal gold for acquired hemolytic anemia refractory to splenectomy. *Trans. Stud. Coll. Phycns Philad.*, **22**, 76.

WASASTJERNA, C. & DÉSY, L. (1954). Corticotropin and cortisone. Influence on experimental immuno-hemolytic anemia in guinea pigs. *Ann. Med. exp. Fenn.*, **32**, 30–41.

WEINBLATT, M. E. (1987). Treatment of immune hemolytic anemia with gammaglobulin. *J. Pediat.*, **110**, 817.

WELCH, C. S. & DAMESHEK, W. (1950). Splenectomy and blood dyscrasias. *New Engl. J. Med.*, **242**, 601–606.

WERTLAKE, P. T., MCGINNISS, M. H. & SCHMIDT, P. J. (1969). Cold antibody and persistent intravascular hemolysis after surgery under hypothermia. *Transfusion*, **9**, 70–73.

WIENER, A. S., GORDON, E. G. & RUSSOW, E. (1957). Observations on the nature of the auto-antibodies in a case of acquired hemolytic anemia. *Ann. intern. Med.*, **47**, 1–9.

WILMERS, M. J. & RUSSELL, A. (1963). Autoimmune haemolytic anaemia in an infant treated by thymectomy. *Lancet*, **ii,**. 915–917.

WINGSTRAND, H. & SELANDER, S. (1960). Exchange transfusion in cases of acquired acute hemolytic anemia. *Acta med. scand.*, **167**, 309–316.

WINTROBE, M. M., CARTWRIGHT, G. E., PALMER, J. G., KUHNS, W. J. & SAMUELS, L. T. (1951). Effect of corticotrophic and cortisone on the blood in various disorders in man. *Arch. intern. Med.*, **88**, 310–336.

WOLL, J. E., SMITH, C. M. & NUSBACHER, J. (1974). Treatment of acute cold agglutinin hemolytic anemia with transfusion of adult i RBCs. *J. Amer. med. Ass.*, **229**, 1779–1780.

WORLLEDGE, S. (1982). Immune haemolytic anaemia (revised by N. C. Hughes Jones and Barbara Bain). In *Blood and its Disorders* (ed. by R. M. Hardisty and D. J. Weatherall), pp. 479–513. Blackwell Scientific Publications, Oxford.

WORLLEDGE, S. M., BRAIN, M. C., COOPER, A. C., HOBBS, J. R. & DACIE, J. V. (1968). Immunosuppressive drugs in the treatment of autoimmune haemolytic anaemia. *Proc. roy. Soc. Med.*, **61**, 1312–1315.

YUNIS, A. A. & HARRINGTON, W. J. (1958). Clinical use of methylprednisolone in certain hematologic disorders. *Metabolism*, 7, 543–568.

YOUNG, L. E., MILLER, G. & SWISHER, S. N. (1957). Treatment of hemolytic disorders. *J. chron. Dis.*, **6**, 307–323.

ZUPAŃSKA, B., SYLWESTROWICZ, T. & PAWELSKI, S. (1981). The results of prolonged treatment of autoimmune haemolytic anaemia. *Haematologia*, **14**, 425–433.

Index

Abnormal serological reactions in auto-immune haemolytic anaemia (AIHA), 81–83
ABO blood groups in AIHA, 14
'Acid-lysins', 138, 274
Acquired haemolytic anaemia as an auto-immune disease, early views, 365
Acrocyanosis, 212, 217, 301
ACTH as treatment for warm-antibody AIHA, 453
  comparison with cortisone, 455
Actinomycin C as treatment for AIHA, 468
AET, effect on Kell antigens, 173
Aetiology of auto-immune diseases, early views, 365
  recent reviews, 366
Aetiology of auto-immune haemolytic anaemia (AIHA), 363–391
  acute transient AIHA, 366–369
    altered erythrocyte antigenicity
    critical role of individual, 369
    cross-reacting antibodies, 369
    damage to erythrocyte surface by micro-organisms, 367
    exposure of antigens not normally available, 368
    Mycoplasma pneumoniae, role, 298
    viruses, role, 366–368
  chronic cold haemagglutinin disease (CHAD), 377
    relationship with malignant lymphoproliferative diseases, 377
  chronic warm-antibody AIHA, 369–377
    allo-immunization to blood-group antigens, 372
    classic studies of Ehrlich and Morgenroth, 374
    clinical clues, 370
    concurrence of another auto-immune disease, 371
    erythrocyte damage not due to micro-organisms, 375
    experimental studies, 378
    genetic factors, 371

Aetiology of auto-immune haemolytic anaemia (*contd*)
  immunoglobulin deficiencies, 39, 372
  in-vitro studies of antibody synthesis, 377
  malignant diseases, association with, 371
  Milgrom's anti-antibody hypothesis, 376
  prophylactic immunization, 370
  serological clues, 373
  T-cell function disturbance, 374
  viruses, 376
  summary, 384
Agglutinability of erythrocytes by cold auto-antibodies, variation in disease, 259–263
  anti-I, 259
  anti-i, 261
    marrow stress, 261
    pernicious anaemia, 262
    thalassaemia, 261
Agglutination as cause of traumatic (mechanical) haemolysis,
  in vitro, 274, 423
  in vivo, 424, 429
AIDS, cold agglutinins in, 323
Albumin, use in enhancing agglutination, 135
'Albumin agglutinins', 148
Allo-antibodies, definition, 1
  as complicating factor in blood transfusion, 490
  in serum of AIHA patients, 135
Anti-antibodies, 320, 376
  hypothetical role in aetiology of AIHA, 376
  in infectious mononucleosis, 320
Anti-C (complement) antiglobulin sera, 106
  anti-C3d sera, 106
Anti-gamma (γ) antiglobulin sera, 104
Anti-IgA antiglobulin serum, 106
Anti-IgG antiglobulin serum, 106
Anti-IgG1–4 antiglobulin sera, 109
Anti-IgM antiglobulin serum, 106
Anti-kappa (k) antiglobulin serum, 106

Anti-lambda (λ) antiglobulin serum, 106
Anti-non-gamma (γ) antiglobulin sera, 104
  nature of non-γ reaction, 105
  role of complement, 105
Anti-snake-venom as treatment for AIHA, 482
Anti-T, 201–204
  as cause of polyagglutination, 201
  detection by use of peanut extract, 201
Anti-Tn, 201
  as cause of polyagglutination, 202
Antibody-binding sites on erythrocyte membrane as determinant of severity of haemolysis, 406
Antibody-dependent cell-mediated cytotoxicity (ADCC), 416
  possible role in haemolysis in AIHA, 418
Antibody elution methods, 142
Antiglobulin (Coombs) Test, 97–114
  discovery and origin, 97
Antiglobulin reactions, 97–105
  early findings in acquired haemolytic anaemia, 97
  in cold-antibody AIHA, 101
  in warm-antibody AIHA, 101
  positive reactions given by healthy people, 189
  positive reactions given by hospital patients, 197
  role of hypergammaglobulinaemia, 198
  prozones, 99
Antiglobulin sera, 99–109
  anti-complement (C), 106
  anti-IgA, 106
  anti-IgG (anti-γ), 104
  anti-IgM, 106
  anti-kappa (k) light chain, 106
  anti-lambda (λ) light chain, 106
  anti-non-γ, 104
  broad-spectrum, 106
  monoclonal, 106, 114
  neutralization by γ globulin, 100
Antiglobulins, possible role in haemolysis *in vivo*, 398

Ashby method of differential
    agglutination,
    results in AIHA, 10, 491
Asparaginase, as treatment for AIHA,
    485
Auto-agglutination, 127, 210, 219,
    393
    'complete' antibodies, role of, 128,
        395
    early observations, 210
    effect of temperature, 143
    in cold-antibody AIHA, 292
    in media of high protein content,
        117
    in warm-antibody AIHA, 128
    'incomplete' antibodies, role of, 127
    of enzyme-treatment erythrocytes,
        119
Auto-agglutinins,
    cold. See Cold auto-agglutinins
    inhibited by ionized calcium, 148
    reactive against stored erythrocytes,
        149
    reactive against washed erythrocytes,
        151
    warm. See Warm auto-agglutinins
Auto-antibodies. See also individual
        antibody specificities
    effect on erythropoiesis, 69, 422
        experimental studies, 422
    in serum in cold-antibody AIHA,
        223–235
    in serum in warm-antibody AIHA,
        129–136
    in-vitro studies of formation, 377
    physiological, 188
    temperature, significance of effect on
        antibody activity, 95
    unitary nature of agglutinins and
        lysins, 96
Auto-antibodies, cold
    anti-A, 268
    anti-AI, 254
    anti-B, 268
    anti-BI, 254
    'anti-cryptic', 257
    anti-D, 272
    anti-Fl, 257
    anti-Gd, 257
    anti-H, 269
        incomplete, with high thermal
            amplitude, 279
    anti-HD, 265
    anti-HI(OI), 254
    anti-I, 250–256
        complement-fixing ability, 273
        cryptic, 257
        effect of enzymes on activity, 224
        experimental production in
            animals, 308
        IgG, 244
        IgM, 241
        immunochemistry, 241–247
        in CHAD, 224
        in mycoplasma pneumonia, 305

Auto-antibodies, cold (contd)
    in normal human sera, 263
    in warm-antibody AIHA, 230
    interaction with isolated antigens,
        253
    lytic potentiality, 224
    thermal amplitude, 224
anti-I^T, 256
    in Hodgkin's disease, 256
    in Melanesian sera, 256, 264
    in Venezuelan sera, 256
anti-i, 250–253
    IgG variant acting as biphasic
        lysin, 245
    in health, 263
    in hospital patients, 264
    in infectious mononucleosis, 318
    in malignant lymphoproliferative
        diseases, 251, 264
    in tropics, 264
anti-Ju, 267
anti-Li, 257
anti-Lud, 257
anti-M, 269
    as cause of CHAD, 269
    cross-reactivity with anti-N, 271
anti-Me, 272
anti-N, 270
    as cause of haemolytic anaemia,
        270
    cross-reactivity with anti-M, 271
    in patients undergoing chronic
        haemodialysis, 270
anti-'Not-I', 265, 319
anti-Om, 272
anti-P, 255, 271, 354
    in paroxysmal cold
        haemoglobinuria (PCH), 354
    rare cause of haemolytic anaemias
        other than PCH, 271
anti-Pr, 266–268
    demonstrable in low-ionic-strength
        saline (LISS), 267
    in routinely tested serum samples,
        267
    subtypes, 266
anti-Sa, 257
anti-Sd^x, 272
anti-Sp_l, 265
anti-Vo, 257
causing lysis. See Cold haemolysins
'incomplete', 244, 276
Auto-antibodies, warm
    anti-dl, 163, 175
    anti-En^a, 169, 175
    anti-Fy(Duffy), 170
    anti-Ge(Gerbich), 170
    anti-Jk(Kidd), 171
    anti-K(Kell), 172
    anti-Lu(Lutheran), 173
    anti-LW(Landsteiner, Wiener),
        173
    anti-nl, 163
    anti-pdl, 163
    anti-protein 4.1, 175

Auto-antibodies, warm (contd)
    anti-Rh, 160, 162–169
        with mimicking specificity, 166
    anti-S, 174
    anti-Sc^3(Scianna), 174
    anti-U, 174
    anti-Vel, 174
    anti-Wr^b, 169
    anti-Xg^a, 175
    causing lysis. See Warm haemolysins
    in serum in AIHA, 129–136
    non-specific, 176
    physiological, 188
    transference from cell to cell, 143
    Type I and Type II, 188
Auto-antibody, definition, 364
Auto-immune haemolytic anaemias
        (AIHAs). See also Warm- and
        Cold-antibody AIHAs
    aetiology, 363–391
    classification, 1
    cold-antibody, 2
    'idiopathic', 1
    in species other than in man,
        380–384
    morbid-anatomical and histological
        findings, 431
    pathogenesis, 392–451
    primary, 1
    secondary, 1
    relative incidence, 2
    treatment, 452–520
    warm-antibody, 2
AIHA in dogs, 380
AIHA in infancy and childhood, 25–34
    age, 30
    course, 31
    duration, 31
    early reports, 25
    prognosis, 31
    role of infection, 25
    serological findings, 26–29
    sex, 31
AIHA in New Zealand [NZB(BL)]
        mice, 381–384
    C-type oncogenic viruses, 382
    lymphomas, 382
    positive DATs, 381
    renal lesions, 382
    splenectomy, 382
    thymectomy, 382
    treatment, 471
AIHA in pregnancy, 19–24
    case reports, 21
    'Coombs-negative' AIHA in
        pregnancy, 22
    effect on infant, 24
        as cause of transient haemolytic
            disease, 24
    prognosis for patient, 24
Auto-immunity,
    Burnet's contributions, 365
    classic studies of Ehrlich and
        Morgenroth, 364
    'Horror autotoxicus', 364

'Auto-specific' antibodies, 159
Azathioprine (Imuran) as treatment for
    AIHA, 466
    in warm-antibody AIHA, 466

Bacterial infections as cause of cold-
    antibody AIHA, 324
Biclonal cold-antibody AIHA, 245
Biological false-positive tests for
    syphilis in AIHA, 81–84, 355
Bithermic (biphasic) cold haemolysins,
    275
Blood transfusion, as treatment for
    AIHA, 488–491
    allo-antibodies, as complicating
        factors, 490
    auto-antibody specificity, 490
    cross-matching, 489
    early experiences, 488
    exchange (exsanguination)
        transfusion, 489
    in cold-antibody AIHA, 505
    incompatibility of blood to be
        transfused, 489
    recent views, 489
    selection of blood to be transfused,
        489
Bone marrow in AIHA, 432
    megaloblastic change, 432
Bovine albumin, use in enhancing
    agglutination, 118
Bromelin, use in enhancing
    agglutination, 11, 119
Bromelin test, 119

Canine AIHA, 380
Canine SLE, 381
Cardiac surgery in CHAD, 504
Chlorambucil as treatment for CHAD,
    503
Chloroquin as treatment for AIHA,
    485
Cold-agglutinin titres, 258
    designation as anti-I or anti-i, 258
    enhancing effect of albumin, 259
    range in health, 263
    source of test erythrocytes, 258
    technical factors affecting, 258
Cold agglutinins. See Cold auto-
    agglutinins
Cold-antibody AIHA,
    associated with more than one Ig
        class of antibody, 244
    associated with lymphoproliferative
        diseases, 234
    associated with neoplasm (excluding
        lymphoproliferative diseases),
        234
    following infectious mononucleosis,
        313–321
    following mycoplasma pneumonia,
        299–309

Cold-antibody AIHA (contd)
    idiopathic in adult. See also Cold-
        haemagglutinin disease
        (CHAD)
    in infants and children, 233
    mechanism of haemolysis in vivo,
        423–429
        auto-agglutination, 423
        complement-mediated lysis, 424,
            427
        DAT-negative cases, 429
        patient-to-patient differences, 429
        protective mechanisms, 426
        sites of haemolysis, 425
        thermal amplitude of antibodies,
            429
        trauma (mechanical) to
            agglutinated erythrocytes, 429
    morbid-anatomical and histological
        findings, 432
    secondary, 2
    splenectomy, 508
    treatment, 502
Cold-antibody AIHA following
    infectious mononucleosis,
        313–321
    anti-i antibodies, 318
    anti-leucocyte antibodies, 321
    anti-N, 319
    anti-not-I(Pr), 319
    association with hereditary
        haemolytic anaemias, 314
    biochemical findings, 316
    blood picture, 315
    clinical features, 314
    cold-agglutinin titres, 316–319
    Donath–Landsteiner reaction, 319
    heterophile (anti-sheep-erythrocyte)
        antibodies, 316
    patient-to-patient differences, 319
    recent descriptions, 314
    serological findings, 316–321
        immunochemistry of antibodies,
            320
    serum proteins, 315
    treatment, 321
Cold-antibody AIHA following
    mycoplasma pneumonia,
        296–312
    blood picture, 302
    clinical features, 299
        acrocyanosis, 301
        gangrene, 299, 301
        phlebothrombosis, 301
        renal involvement, 301
    cold auto-agglutinins, 300
        immunochemistry, 305
        specificity, 305
    early descriptions, 299
    false-positive reactions for syphilis,
        304
    haemoglobinuria, 299
    later case reports of special interest,
        301
    leucocyte auto-agglutination, 303

Cold-antibody AIHA (contd)
    prognosis, 308
    serological findings, 302–308
    treatment, 309
Cold-antibody AIHA following viral
    infections other than infectious
    mononucleosis, 321–324
    adenovirus, 322
    AIDS, 323
    cytomegalovirus (CMV), 322
    'encephalitis', 322
    influenza viruses, 322
    ornithosis, 323
    rubella, 323
    varicella, 323
Cold-antibody AIHA in association
    with bacterial infections,
    Esch. coli, 324
    Legionella pneumophila, 325
Cold-antibody AIHA in infants and
    children, 233. See also
    Paroxysmal cold
    haemoglobinuria
    acute cases, 233
        role of infections, 233
        serological findings, 233
    chronic cases, 234
Cold auto-agglutinins,
    active against 'cryptic' Ii antigens,
        257
    active against stored erythrocytes,
        257
    high titres following acute respiratory
        diseases, 298
    high titres following mycoplasma
        pneumonia, 302
    in AIDS, 323
    in haemolytic anaemia, early reports,
        212
    in health, 263
Cold auto-antibodies. See also Cold
    auto-agglutinins
    as cause of complement-mediated
        lysis, 273, 282
    as cause of sensitization to
        antiglobulin sera, 276
    chemical nature, 241
    IgA type, 245
    IgG type, 244
    IgM lambda (L type), 247
    incomplete. See Incomplete cold
        auto-antibodies
    light chains, 246
    non-complement fixing, 324
    rare variants, 271
    specificity, 247–273. See also
        individual antibody
        specificities
    thermal amplitude, 224
Cold-detectable 'warm' IgG auto-
    antibodies, 245
Cold-haemagglutinin disease (CHAD),
    213–228
    atypical cases, 228
    auto-agglutination, 219

Cold-haemagglutinin disease (contd)
 blood picture, 221
  absolute values, 221
 blood viscosity, 220
 clinical features, 215–218
  acrocyanosis, 217
  age, 215
  chronicity, 216
  nephrotic syndrome, 218
  physical signs, 217
  Raynaud's phenomena, 212, 217
  sex, 215
 early case reports, 213
 erythrocyte mechanical fragility, 223
 erythrophagocytosis, 211
 haemoglobinuria, 218
 haemosiderinuria, 217
 ineffective erythropoiesis, 221
 liver, role, 425
 pathogenesis, 423–429
 prognosis, 502
 serological findings,
  agglutination of enzyme-treated
   erythrocytes, 224
  cold-agglutinin titres, 223
  DAT, 223
  lysis of enzyme-treated
   erythrocytes, 224, 226
  lysis of normal erythocytes, 224,
   228
  lysis of PNH erythrocytes, 224,
   228
  patient-to-patient differences, 228
  resistance of patients' erythrocytes
   to lysis, 226
  temperature, effect on, 224
 serum proteins, 223
 spleen, role, 425
 treatment, 502–508
  alkylating and anti-metabolite
   drugs, 503
  general management, 503
Cold haemolysins (lysins),
 bithermic (biphasic), 275
 Donath–Landsteiner, 330,
  345–351
 effect of pH on lysis, 274
 in cold-antibody AIHA, 225, 273
 monothermic (monophasic), 275
Complement (C), 407–418
 activation, 407
  by alternative pathway, 408
  by classical pathway, 407
 components, 407
 C3-depleted rabbits, 414
 C6-deficient rabbits, 413
 detectable on erythrocyte
  membranes, 195, 409
 receptors for, on phagocytic cells,
  418
 'holes' in erythrocyte membrane
  caused by, 409
 nature, 407
 pH, effect on, 137
 recent studies on fixation, 281

Complement (C) (contd)
 role in haemolysis in vivo, 406–418
 role in non-γ antiglobulin reaction,
  105
 serum complement in AIHA, 282,
  355
 sequence, 407
Complement antiglobulin test, 106
Complement-coated erythrocytes, 406
 interaction with phagocytic cells,
  410–418
Complement components bound to
  erythrocyte membranes
 by anti-Lewis antibodies, 113
 by cold auto-antibodies, 114, 281
 by incomplete cold antibodies, 280
 by warm auto-antibodies, 105
 early studies, 105
 giving rise to positive antiglobulin
  reactions, 106, 113
 in healthy individuals, 195
 in hospital patients, 196
Complement-fixing antibody
  consumption (CFAC) test,
  115
Complete antibodies, 395
Concurrence of warm and cold auto-
  antibodies in AIHA, 230
Conglutination, use in detecting
  erythrocyte sensitization, 117
Coombs-negative (DAT-negative)
  AIHA, 183–187
 case reports, 186
 in pregnancy, 22
 tests for erythrocyte IgG in, 186
Coombs test, 47. See also Antiglobulin
  test
 history of discovery, 97
Corticosteroids as treatment for AIHA,
  453–465
 cold-antibody cases, 503, 510
 mode of action, 462–465
  alteration in affinity of antibody for
   antigen, 463
  bone-marrow stimulation, 465
  inhibition of antibody formation,
   462
  interference with erythrocyte–
   macrophage interaction, 464
 warm-antibody cases, 453–465
  early reports, 453
  effect on haematological findings,
   461
  effect on serological findings, 461
  prednisone and newer synthetic
   corticosteroids, 455
  recent recommendations, 458
Cyclophosphamide as treatment for
  AIHA, 469

Danazol as treatment for AIHA, 488
DAT. See Direct antiglobulin test
DAT-negative cold-antibody AIHA,
 429

DAT-negative warm-antibody AIHA,
 133
 in pregnancy, 22
 with positive indirect enzyme tests,
  133
'Developing test', 99
Direct antiglobulin test (DAT),
 97–109
 'complement', 105
 gamma (γ), 104
 in blood donors, 190
 in cold-antibody AIHA, 223, 302,
  316, 352
 in healthy people, 189
 in hospital patients, 197
  role of hypergammaglobulinaemia,
   198
 in warm-antibody AIHA, 97–109
 modification of MN blood groups as
  cause of positive tests, 193
 number of IgG or complement
  molecules required for positive
  tests, 193
 non-gamma (non-γ), 104
Donath–Landsteiner (D–L) antibodies,
 345–356
 as cause of agglutination, 351
 as cause of lysis, 345
 as cause of positive antiglobulin
  reactions, 352
 immunochemistry, 354
 relationship to WR and Kahn test
  reactants, 355
 specificity (anti-P), 353
 thermal amplitude, 356
 thermolability, 348
 titre, correlation with severity of
  haemolysis in vivo, 355
Donath–Landsteiner (D–L) test, 345
 cold phase, 346, 349
  degree of chilling required, 349
  role of complement, 346
 effect of pH, 348
 lysis of enzyme-treated erythrocytes,
  350
 lysis of PNH erythrocytes, 350
 warm phase, optimum temperature,
  350
  role of complement, 347
Dyke–Young anaemia, 11

Eaton agent, 298
ELACA (enzyme-linked antiglobulin
  consumption assay), 117
ELAT (Enzyme-linked antiglobulin
  test), 116
ELISA (Enzyme-linked
  immunosorbent assay), 116
Eluted antibodies, studies on, 142
Enzyme-treated erythrocytes. See also
  individual enzymes
 factors in normal serum causing
  their agglutination and/or lysis,
  145

Enzyme-treated erythrocytes (*contd*)
  use in demonstrating presence of an antibody, 129–134
Erythrocyte age, effect on binding of antibodies, 187
Erythrocyte antigen depression, 189
  Rh antigens, 187
Erythrocyte–antibody (EA) rosette formation, 119
Erythrocyte antigens, differences in recognition by allo-antibodies and auto-antibodies, 187
Erythrocyte-bound IgG, significance and nature, 194
Erythrocyte membrane protein 4.1, auto-antibody against, 175
Erythrocyte membrane receptors
  for complement components, 418
  for IgGFc, 417
Erythrocyte rosetting
  around mononuclear cells in AIHA, 421
  around neutrophils in acquired haemolytic anaemia, 421
Erythrocytes,
  agglutinability by anti-I, variation in disease, 259
  agglutinability by anti-i, variation in disease, 261
  morphology in cold-antibody AIHA, 220
  morphology in warm-antibody AIHA, 54–63
  senescent, role of physiological auto-antibody in removal from circulation, 188
Erythrophagocytosis (EP), 33, 394, 400
Erythropoiesis, effect of antibodies on, 422
Erythrostasis in spleen, role in haemolysis, 401
Esch. coli infection as cause of haemolytic anaemia, 325
Evans syndrome, 34–36
Experimental allo-immune haemolytic anaemia,
  in dogs, 439
  in man, 439
Experimental immune haemolytic anaemia in animals, 433–439
  antiglobulin reactions, 437
  pioneer experiments, 433
  recent studies, 436
  resistance to hetero-immune sera, 437
Experimental production of AIHA in animals, 378–380
  immunization of an animal with the erythrocytes of another species, 378
  in grafted animals, 378

Ficin, use in enhancing agglutination, 11

Flow cytofluorometry, 193, 405

Gamma globulin (IgG) as treatment for AIHA, 494
Gamma (γ) globulin, effect of adding to antiglobulin sera, 100–103
  γ-globulin neutralization test, 103
Gangrene in AIHA, 218, 299
Gm allotypes in warm-antibody AIHA, 109

Haemoglobinaemia, 84
  in experimental haemolytic anaemia, 412
Haemoglobinuria, 16, 85, 218
Haemolysins (lysins). *See* Cold and Warm haemolysins
Haemosiderinuria, 85, 217
Hayem–Widal anaemia, 11
Hemolysinic icterus, 9
HEMPAS, 262
Heparin as treatment for AIHA, 480
  effect on antibody activity *in vitro*, 144, 480
'Holes' in erythrocyte membranes caused by complement action, 409
Hübener–Thomsen–Friedenreich phenomenon, 201, 368
Hypergammaglobulinaemia, role in causing positive DATs, 198
Hyperleucocytosis in AIHA, 79

i erythrocytes, survival in cold-antibody AIHA, 507
IgA auto-antibodies,
  as cause of cold-antibody AIHA, 246
  as cause of warm-antibody AIHA, 111, 422
  mechanism of haemolysis, 422
IgG auto-antibodies as cause of cold-antibody AIHA, 9, 106–111, 244
IgG1 auto-antibodies as cause of haemolysis in AIHA, 109
IgG2 auto-antibodies as possible cause of haemolysis in AIHA, 110
IgG3 auto-antibodies as cause of haemolysis in AIHA, 109
IgG4 auto-antibodies as possible cause of haemolysis in AIHA, 110
IgM auto-antibodies,
  as cause of haemolysis in cold-antibody AIHA, 95, 243
  as cause of haemolysis in warm-antibody AIHA, 31, 110
  incomplete, 113
IgM lambda cold auto-antibodies, 247
  low molecular weight variant, 247
Ii antigens, 255, 263
  chemical nature, 255

Ii antigens (*contd*)
  cryptic, 257
  I adult (I-positive), 250
  i adult, 250
  i newborn (I-negative), 251
  I^T, 256
  subtypes, 253
  variants, 257
Ii blood-group system, 250, 265
  first description, 250
  recent studies, 253
  relationship with ABH(O) blood groups, 254
  relationship with P blood groups, 255
Immune clearance, 410–418
  experimental studies, 412
  Kupffer cells, role, 415
  liver, role, 415
  of antibody-coated erythrocytes, 410
  of complement-coated erythrocytes, 411
  spleen, role, 415
Immune-deficiency syndromes, association with AIHA, 39–43
Immunoadsorption of IgG as treatment for AIHA, 492
Immunoglobulin (Ig), 95
  classes, 95
  heavy chains, 247
  light chains, kappa(k) and lambda (λ), 246
Immunoglobulin A (IgA or γA), 95
Immunoglobulin G (IgG or γG), 95
  subclasses (IgG1–4), 106–109
Immunoglobulin M (IgM or γM), 95
Immunopancytopenia, 36–39
  serological findings, 39
Immunosuppressive alkylating and antimetabolite drugs as treatment for AIHA, 465–471
  azathioprine (Imuran), 466
  cold-antibody cases, 503
  cyclophosphamide, 469
  in NZ mice, 471
  6-mercaptopurine, 466
  nitrogen mustard, 465
  6-thioguanine, 466
  warm-antibody cases, 465
'Incomplete' cold auto-antibodies, 244, 276
  clinical significance, 279
  do they exist?, 277
  early observations, 276
  in normal sera, 278
  nature, 278
  relationship to cold auto-agglutinins in normal sera, 279
  specificity, 278
  transplacental passage, 279
Incomplete warm (anti-Rh) antibodies, 277, 395
Incomplete IgM warm antibodies, 113
Incomplete warm antibody of Jancović, 147

Indirect antiglobulin test (IAT), 129, 132
  positive tests associated with negative enzyme tests, 134
Ineffective erythropoiesis in CHAD, 221,
Infectious mononucleosis complicated by haemolytic anaemia, 313–321
Interferon, as treatment for CHAD, 505
Intravascular haemolysis, possibly mediated by non-complement-fixing antibodies, 398
Intravenous IgG as treatment for AIHA, 494
Isoelectric focusing, use in demonstrating warm auto-antibody heterogeneity, 109

Kahn test in AIHA, 82
  in PCH, 355
Kälteagglutininkrankheit, 215
Kappa(k) light chains, 246
Kupffer cells, role in haemolysis, 415

Lambda (λ) light chains, 246
Lederer–Brill anaemia, 11
Lederer's anaemia, 11
Leucocytosis in AIHA, 55, 77
Leucopenia in AIHA, 36, 77
  in experimental haemolytic anaemia, 412
  pathogenesis, 430
Leukanemia, 7
LISS (low-ionic-strength saline), 267
Livedo annularis, 18, 267
Livedo reticularis, 18, 266
Liver,
  histological appearances in AIHA, 431
  role in experimental cold-antibody haemolytic anaemia, 415
  role in pathogenesis of AIHA, 399
Loutit anaemia, 11
Lymph nodes, enlargement in AIHA, 432
Lymphoproliferative diseases, association with AIHA, 371
Lysins. See Cold and Warm haemolysins

Megaloblastic erythropoiesis in AIHA, 68, 432
Mercaptanes as treatment for CHAD, 505
6-Mercaptopurine as treatment for AIHA, 466
Metabolic damage to erythrocytes by antibodies, as factor in haemolysis, 402

Micro-organisms, role in aetiology of AIHA, 366–369, 376
  altered erythrocyte antigenicity, 368
  development of cross-reacting antibodies, 369
  direct damage to erythrocyte surface, 367
  exposure of erythrocyte antigens not normally available, 368
'Mixed' warm- and cold-antibody AIHA, 230
  incidence, 232
  severity, 232
Monocyte/macrophage–erythrocyte interaction, 410–421
  hyperactivity of macrophages in patients with AIHA, 420
Monocyte/macrophage monolayer assays, 418
  correlation with haemolysis in vivo, 420
Monocyte/macrophage receptors, 417
  for complement (C3), 418
  for IgG, 417
Monothermic (monophasic) cold haemolysins, 275
Morbid-anatomical and histological findings in AIHA, 431–433
  in cold-antibody cases, 432
Moreschi, Carlo, discoverer of the principle of the antiglobulin reaction, 97
Mortality in warm-antibody AIHA, early data, 498
  recent data, 500
Mycoplasma pneumonia haemolytic anaemia, 299–312
Mycoplasma pneumoniae, 298
  as cause of primary atypical pneumonia, 298
  interaction with I antigen, 307

Naturally-occurring AIHA in species other than man,
  in dogs, 380
  in NZB/BL mice, 381
Newcastle disease virus (NDV), possible role in aetiology of AIHA, 368
Nitrogen mustard as treatment for AIHA, 465
Non-complement-fixing cold auto-antibody as cause of acute transient AIHA, 429
Non-complement-fixing IgG auto-antibodies as cause of intravascular haemolysis, 398
Non-gamma (γ) antiglobulin reaction, nature, 105
'Non-specific' auto-antibodies, 161, 176
Normal serum factors agglutinating and/or lysing erythrocytes treated with enzymes other than trypsin, 147

Normal serum factors causing erythrocytes to be agglutinated by antiglobulin sera, 147
Normal serum factors causing reversible agglutination of trypsinized erythrocytes, 145

P antigen, chemical nature, 354
Papain, use in enhancing agglutination, 11, 131
Paroxysmal cold haemoglobinuria (PCH), 329–362
  abortive attacks, 334
  acute transient PCH, 336–339
    early reports, 336
    recent reports, 338
  age, 334
  blood picture, 341–344
    acute transient PCH, 342
    chronic syphilitic PCH, 341
    erythrophagocytosis, 343
    leucopenia, 341
    spherocytosis, 342
  classification, 333
  clinical features, 334, 336
  complement, serum, 355
  course, 335
  chronic PCH, 335, 339
  Donath–Landsteiner (D–L) antibodies, 348–355
    as cause of agglutination, 351
    as cause of sensitization of antiglobulin sera, 352
    correlation of titre with severity of haemolysis in vivo, 355
    immunochemistry, 354
    specificity, 354
  Donath–Landsteiner (D–L) test, 345–349
    chilling required, 349
    complement, role in cold phase, 346
    complement, role in warm phase, 347
    effect of pH, 348
    lysis of enzyme-treated and PNH erythrocytes, 350
  Donath and Landsteiner's discovery, 330
  early reviews, 331
  Eason's discoveries, 330
  false-positive tests for syphilis, 355
  familial incidence, 334
  haemoglobinuria, 334
  history, 329
  incidence, 332
  monocyte monolayer assays, 353
  non-syphilitic, 336–341
    acute transient, 336
    chronic, 339
  recent reviews and reports, 334, 338
  relation to syphilis, 332
  renal function, 335
  role of viral infections, 336–339

Paroxysmal cold haemoglobinuria (*contd*)
  serological findings. *See also* Donath–Landsteiner antibodies
    early studies, 345
  specificity of auto-antibody (anti-P), 354
  syphilitic, 334
  treatment, 356–358
    acute transient PCH, 357
    chronic PCH, 356
    transfusion of P-negative blood, 357
    warmth, 357
  vasomotor phenomena, 335
Paroxysmal nocturnal haemoglobinuria (PNH) erythrocytes,
  sensitivity to agglutination and lysis by a high-titre cold antibody, 260
  use in detecting lytic antibodies, 137, 139, 224
Pathogenesis of auto-immune haemolytic anaemias, 392–451
  allo-antibodies, relevance of experiments with, 396
  auto-agglutination, role, 394
  clinical evidence, 393
  cold-antibody AIHA, 423–429
  correlation between tests for auto-antibodies *in vitro* and haemolysis *in vivo*, 132, 404
  experimental studies, 433–440
    role of liver and spleen, 399
  summary, 440
  warm-antibody AIHA, 394–406
Peanut extract, value in detecting T antigen, 201
pH, effect on,
  agglutination, 139
  complement, 137
  indirect antiglobulin test (IAT), 143
  lysis, 137, 274
Phagocytosis. *See* Erythrophagocytosis
Plasmapheresis and plasma exchange as treatment for AIHA, 491
  cold-antibody cases, 507
  warm-antibody cases, 491
Polyagglutinability, 201–204, 368
  as cause of haemolytic anaemia in man, 202
  role of bacterial enzymes, 201
  role of T, Tn and Tk antigens, 20
  type 'VA' (Vienna), 204
Polybrene, use in enhancing agglutination, 118
Pr (Sp₁) blood-group system, 265–268
Practical management of patients with warm-antibody, AIHA, 496
Prednisone as treatment for AIHA, 455–465
Primary atypical pneumonia, 296. *See also* Mycoplasma pneumonia
Primary splenic neutropenia, 43
Primary splenic panhaematopenia, 43

Prognosis in AIHA, 497
  acute cold-antibody cases, 508
  chronic CHAD, 502
  chronic warm-antibody cases, 497–502
  in infancy and childhood , 25–34
PVP, use in enhancing agglutination, 118

Radioactive antiglobulin tests, 114
Radioactive chromium (^{51}Cr),
  use as guide to value of splenectomy in AIHA, 477
  use in determining erythrocyte life-span in AIHA, 10, 491
Radioactive gold as treatment for AIHA, 480
Raynaud's phenomena in cold-antibody AIHA, 212
Receptors on erythrocytes for complement components, 418
  Fc portion of IgG, 417
Recovery ('cure') in warm-antibody AIHA, 501
Reticulocyte counts in AIHAs, 55, 67, 69, 221
Reticulocytes,
  ability to bind on antibodies, 188
  resistance to immune haemolysis, 189
Reticulocytopenia in AIHAs, 69–76
Reticulo-endothelial (RE) cell hyperplasia in AIHA, 501
Reversible agglutination of trypsinized erythrocytes, 145
Rheumatoid factors. *See* Antiglobulins
Rh$_{null}$ erythrocytes, 163
Rosetting of erythrocytes around macrophages in AIHA, 421
Rosetting of erythrocytes around neutrophils,
  in AIHA, 421
  in DAT-negative AIHA, 421
Runt disease, 379
  association with AIHA, 380

Salicylates and 5-iodosalicylic acid as treatment for AIHA, 482
Serum-albumin mixtures, use in detecting auto-antibodies, 135
Sequestration of antibody-coated erythrocytes in spleen, 401
Sodium azide as antibody enhancer, 258
Species specificity of human warm auto-antibodies, 176
Specificity of cold auto-antibodies, 247–273
  early studies, 249
  Ii system, 250
  in relation to animal erythrocytes, 247

Specificity of cold auto-antibodies (*contd*)
  in relation to human erythrocytes, 249
  P system, 271, 354
  Pr system, 265
Specificity of warm auto-antibodies, 158–176. *See also* individual specificities
  anti-dl, 163
  anti-nl, 163
  anti-pdl, 163
  anti-Rh, 160, 162–169
  change with time, 166
  early studies, 158
  incidence of specific auto-antibodies, 164
  mimicking specificities, 166–169
  'non-specific' auto-antibodies, 161, 176
  recent studies, 162–169
  reviews, 165
  species specificity, 176
Spherocytosis, 62, 342, 402
  as result of erythrocyte–macrophage interaction, 410–415
  in cold-antibody AIHA, 220
  in experimental immune haemolytic anaemia, 434
  in PCH, 342
  in warm-antibody AIHA, 62
Spleen,
  enlargement in AIHA, 18
  erythrostasis in, 401
  histological findings in AIHA, 431
  role in pathogenesis of AIHA, 399
  value of ^{51}Cr in assessing function, 477
Splenectomy as treatment for AIHA, 471–479
  cold-antibody cases, 508
  complications, 476
  early results, 471
  recent data, 472
  unusual case reports, 472
  use of ^{51}Cr as indicator of outcome, 477
  warm-antibody cases, 471–479
    effect on blood picture, 80
    relapse after, 475
Stercobilin excretion in AIHA, 85
Steroid-responsive chronic CHAD, 510
Stored erythrocytes, agglutination of, 149

Temperature, effect on auto-antibody activity *in vitro*, 144
Thimerosal as antibody enhancer, 258
6-Thioguanine as treatment for AIHA, 466
Thorotrast as treatment for AIHA, 480

Thrombocytopenia, occurrence in
    AIHA, 34–39
  pathogenesis, 430
Thymectomy as treatment for AIHA in
    infancy and childhood, 483
Tissue lysins, possible role in
    haemolysis in AIHA, 401
Trauma (mechanical), as cause of
    haemolysis of agglutinated
    erythrocytes,
  in vitro, 274, 423
  in vivo, 424, 429
Treatment of acute transient cold-
    antibody AIHA, 508
  corticosteroids, 510
  transfusion, 510
Treatment of acute transient warm-
    antibody AIHA, 25–29
Treatment of chronic cold-
    haemagglutinin disease
    (CHAD), 502–508
  alkylating and anti-metabolite drugs,
    503
  blood transfusion, 505
    survival of i erythrocytes, 507
  cardiac surgery in, 504
  chlorambucil, 503
  corticosteroids, 503
  general management, 503
  interferon, 505
  mercaptanes, 505
  penicillamine, 506
  plasma exchange, 507
  splenectomy, 508
  warmth, 503
Treatment of chronic warm-antibody
    AIHA, 453–497
  ACTH and corticosteroids,
    453–465
  immunosuppressive alkylating
    and anti-metabolite drugs,
    465–471
  patients who fail to respond to
    corticosteroids splenectomy and
    immunosuppressive drugs,
    479–488
  practical management of patients,
    496
  splenectomy, 471–479
Trypsin, use in modifying erythrocyte
    agglutinability, 130
Trypsinized erythrocytes, 130
  pH, effect on lysis of, 139
  reversible agglutination of, 145
  use in demonstrating lysis, 139
  use in enhancing agglutination,
    130

Vibrio cholerae filtrate, use in
    detection of antibodies, 130,
    131
Vinca alkaloids as treatment for AIHA,
    486
'Virus' pneumonia, 300
Vitronectin, 408

Warm agglutinins, 128, 395
Warm-antibody auto-immune
    haemolytic anaemia (AIHA),
  abnormal serological reactions,
    81–83
  absolute values, 57
  ABO blood groups, 14
  acute transient, 25–34
  age, 15
  antiglobulin reactions in, 97–109
  'aplastic' crises, 69–76
    role of parvovirus, 76
  association with other diseases, 3
  autohaemolysis, 66
  bilirubin, 85
  biochemical findings, 80
  biological false-positive tests for
    syphilis, 81–83
  blood picture, 54–63
    effect of splenectomy on, 80
    leukaemoid, 34, 77
  bone marrow, 67
    macronormoblasts, 67
    megaloblastic erythropoiesis, 68
  clinical features, 15–19
  complications, unusual, 19
  Coombs test in, 97–109
  course, 16
  early history, 6
  eponyms, 11
  erythroblastaemia, 60
  erythrocyte
    acetylcholinesterase, 86
    membrane lipids, 88
    membrane proteins, 88
    metabolism, 86
    neutrophil rosetting, 78
  erythrocytes,
    absolute values, 57
    auto-agglutination, 57
  erythrophagocytosis, 59
  Evans syndrome, 34
  gangrene, 19
  genetic factors, 12
  haemoglobinaemia, 84
  haemoglobinuria, 16, 25
  haemosiderinuria, 85
  haptoglobins, 84

Warm-antibody auto-immune
    haemolytic anaemia (contd)
  HLA types, 14
  hyperleucocytosis, 77–79
  idiopathic, 2
  immunopancytopenia, 36
  in immune deficiency syndromes,
    39–43
  in infancy and childhood, 25–34
  in pregnancy, 19–24
  incidence in population, 16
  jaundice, 18
  leucocytes, 55, 77–79
  leucopenia, 36–77
  liver, 18
  lymph nodes, 18
  mechanical fragility, 66
  megaloblastic erythropoiesis, 68
  mortality, 498
  occurrence in siblings, 12
  osmotic fragility, 63–66
  physical signs, 17
  platelet count, 55, 78–80
  prognosis, 497
  race, 12
  recovery from, 501
  reticulocytes, 67
  reticulocytopenia, 69
  secondary, 2
  serum proteins, 80
  sex, 15
  siderocytes, 67
  spherocytosis, 58, 62
  spleen, 18
  splenectomy, 471–479
  sterobilin excretion, 85
  symptomatic, 1
  symptoms, 16
  synonyms, 11
  thrombocytopenia, 34–39, 78
  treatment, 452–497
  unusual complications, 19
  urine, 85
Warm haemolysins (lysins), 136, 141
  in warm-antibody AIHA, 136
  inhibition by normal serum, 144
  pH, effect on, 137, 141
  temperature, effect on, 140
Washed erythrocytes, agglutination of,
    151
Wassermann reaction (WR) in AIHA,
    82
  in PCH, 355

X-irradiation as treatment for AIHA,
    469, 480